Li Hongjun

Editor

Radiology of HIV/AIDS

A Practical Approach

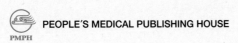 PEOPLE'S MEDICAL PUBLISHING HOUSE

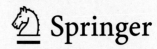 Springer

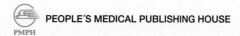

PEOPLE'S MEDICAL PUBLISHING HOUSE

Website: http://www.pmph.com/en

Book Title: Radiology of HIV/AIDS: A Practical Approach

Contact address: No. 19, Pan Jia Yuan Nan Li, Chaoyang District, Beijing 100021, P.R. China, phone/fax: 8610 5978 7352, E-mail: pmph@pmph.com

For text and trade sales, as well as review copy enquiries, please contact PMPH at pmphsales@gmail.com

First published: 2014
ISBN: 978-7-117-18058-0/R · 18059

Cataloguing in Publication Data:
A catalogue record for this book is available from the CIP-Database China.

Printed in The People's Republic of China

ISBN 978-7-117-18058-0

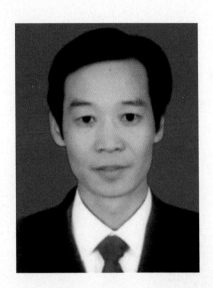

I am reluctant to alienate my wife, my daughter, my friends and my students. But, for the publication of this book, I have to give up enjoying gatherings with my family and friends.

Hereby, this book is dedicated to my wife YING to show my heartfelt thanks for her persistent support, encouragement and trust; as well as to my daughter Zhen. She makes me feel all my contributions are powerful and valuable.

Li Hongjun

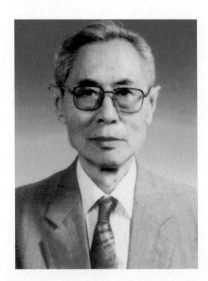

Recently, due to the active measures for prevention and control of AIDS, the number of patients infected with HIV/AIDS has decreased in China. However, the situation is still severe in certain regions and specific populations because of the threats HIV/AIDS has posed. Years of clinical research and practice have proved that the combination of diagnostic imaging with clinical pathology plays an important role in the diagnosis and treatment of HIV/AIDS, especially for concurrent opportunistic infections and neoplasms.

Based on years of clinical practice and applied research, Professor Li Hongjun has already published several relevant monographs. On this basis, he organized an editorial board for another monograph in this field, *Practical Diagnostic Imaging of HIV/AIDS*, which is to be published. The book consists of 3 parts and 26 chapters, with about two million words and more than 2,500 figures. Its contents include a fundamental part about HIV/AIDS as well as the general and systematic clinics on HIV/AIDS. Recent progresses in this field are supplemented into the book, which is clearly structured, comprehensive and detailed.

I sincerely congratulate the publication of the book and expect the book will promote the development of diagnostic imaging on HIV/AIDS in China. Thus, the development of diagnostic imaging on HIV/AIDS will be greatly promoted.

Chinese Engineering Academician
Fuwai Hospital of Chinese Academy of Medical Sciences
Beijing, China
On Oct. 2011

Foreword 2

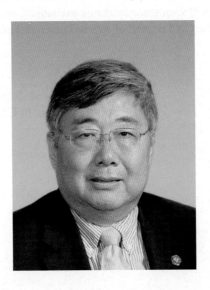

The AIDS epidemic in China has attracted extensive and intensive attention from both the society and government. The epidemic has generally been at a low prevalence, but has a high prevalence in specific populations and some areas. Because the leading cause of death in AIDS patients is the occurrence of AIDS-related diseases, the early diagnosis of AIDS-related diseases constitutes an important measure to improve the patient's quality of life and to prolong their life. AIDS is different from other diseases, in its specificity and complexity, which poses new challenges in its diagnosis and treatment to medical personnel and scientific researchers. Professor Li Hongjun has been studying the diagnostic imaging of HIV/AIDS for up to 13 years, and has already published several monographs, including Clinical and Imaging Diagnosis of HIV/AIDS, Atlas of Differential Imaging Diagnosis of HIV/AIDS, Atlas of Differential Imaging Diagnosis of HIV/AIDS Related Ophthalmopathy, and Comparative Atlas of HIV/AIDS in Anatomy, Diagnostic Imaging and Pathology. In the way of combined theory and practices, the cases data were analyzed in details to guide the related clinical practices. In this book, Professor Li Hongjun further summarizes recent researches and clinical experiences. The finished manuscript, *Practical Diagnostic Imaging of HIV/AIDS* effectively integrates the related resources nationwide, including experts and clinical data. And the book contains more than two million words and more than 2,500 figures, covering 3 parts and 26 chapters. Its content includes the basic sciences of HIV/AIDS, basic clinical sciences and their clinical application. Especially, in the last chapter, functional imaging findings of HIV/AIDS are innovatively demonstrated. Most data in the book is published for the first time.

Professor Li Hongjun and his team have intensively studied the diagnostic imaging data of Chinese with HIV/AIDS. Their achievements include the spectrum of AIDS-related diseases in Chinese, the relationship between the diagnostic imaging and clinical pathology of AIDS-related diseases, the characteristic features of the diagnostic imaging in HIV/AIDS. All his works are valuable for early and accurate diagnosis of AIDS-related diseases, preventing the occurrence of relevant disease and improving the therapeutic efficacy. In addition, it provides scientific theoretical basis and technical support to reduce the morbidity and mortality of AIDS-related diseases. A large number of this valuable first-hand data has laid a solid foundation for the further study of diagnostic imaging of HIV/AIDS in China. The publication of *Practical Diagnostic Imaging of HIV/AIDS* provides valuable reference for clinicians and radiologists internationally. It is a very meaningful work, because it expands a new field of medical imaging in China as a supplement of medical imaging, fills the blank of AIDS imaging.

The authors have devoted several years' time and wisdom in the writing of this book. Its content is rich, comprehensive, systematic, informative, illustrative with clear figures and highly readable to clinicians and radiologists. The book will definitely promote and popularize our understanding of HIV/AIDS, enhance academic exchanges, and promote the progress and development of the prevention and control of AIDS. Therefore I am delighted to write a foreword to this book.

Dai Jianping
American Medical Academician of Sciences
Vice President of Chinese Medical Association
Beijing, China
On Sep. 22nd, 2011

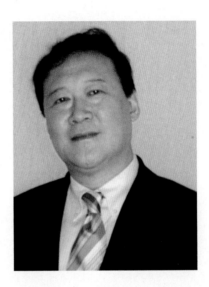

AIDS is globally spreading, constituting a major threat to the health of human being. It is characteristic in term of epidemiology, pathogenesis, and pathology, clinical diagnosis, imaging manifestations, differential diagnosis, treatment and prevention. Based on his 13 years studies, Professor Li Hongjun have published several monographs on the diagnostic imaging of HIV/AIDS. In his works, the national resources in this field have been effectively integrated, including related experts and clinical imaging data. The theoretical research and practical cases studies have been combined. In this way, another monograph, *Practical Diagnostic Imaging of HIV/AIDS* is being published. This book contains more than two million words and more than 2,500 figures, covering 3 parts and 26 chapters. Its content includes the basic sciences of HIV/AIDS, clinical basic sciences of HIV/AIDS and their clinical application. Especially in Chap. 26, the functional imaging studies on HIV/AIDS are firstly introduced into the research field of HIV/AIDS. Most of the data in this book is the frontier research achievements and is published for the first time.

Professor Li Hongjun has done systematic studies on pathological basis of HIV/AIDS imaging during his overseas visiting studies. Based on the previous research, he and his team have intensively studied Chinese with HIV/AIDS. Their achievements include the spectrum of Chinese AIDS-related diseases, diagnostic imaging of HIV/AIDS in Chinese, and the relationship between the diagnostic imaging of HIV/AIDS and their pathological mechanisms, and a large amount of valuable first-hand imaging data. *Practical Diagnostic Imaging of HIV/AIDS* provides valuable first hand data to related clinicians and radiologists. It expands a new field of medical imaging in China and fills the blank in AIDS imaging studies. It further enriches related data for the basic research in HIV/AIDS and for their clinical application. Generally, it is a valuable monograph and important reference book in clinical imaging.

This content-rich, highly readable book integrates efforts and wisdom of the authors. It is promising to promote the progress and development of the prevention and control of HIV/AIDS. I am delighted to write a foreword to this book.

Qi Ji
Former Chair,
Radiology Branch of Chinese Medical Association
Tianjin, China
on Sep. 28th, 2011

Preface

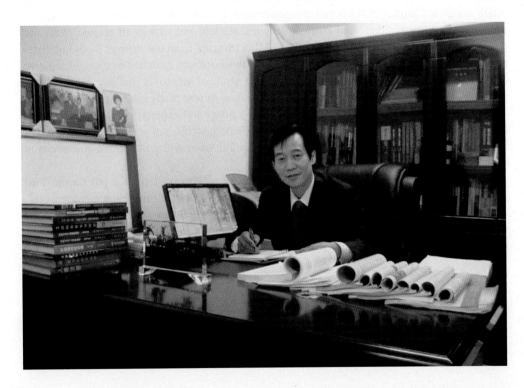

It has been 13 years since I began my research on HIV/AIDS Imaging in 1998. In this period, I and my team members have been collecting substantial first-hand clinical data, retrieving literature, performing comparisons and analysis, assessing these clinical data and integrating the characteristics of Chinese AIDS patients into HIV/AIDS imaging based on the scientific principle of evidence based medicine (EBM). We published six treaties from different perspectives; we finished this treatise based on our research, namely, *Practical HIV/AIDS Imaging*, indicating that the study on HIV/AIDS imaging has grown out of its infancy. In January 2007, we published *Atlas of Imaging Diagnosis in HIV/AIDS*, by People's Medical Publishing House (PMPH), China; and *Clinical AIDS and Diagnostic Imaging*, by Chinese Medical Science Press (CMSP), China. In September 2008, the English version of *Atlas of the Differential Diagnosis in HIV/AIDS* (PMPH) was published by PMPH and was approved by Textbook Office of National Higher Education of China, Textbook office of Health Ministry of China, and Expert Consultation Committee of PMPH, as one of the recommended books of bio-medicine in the project of "International Publication". In June 2008, this book was promoted internationally by Globamid Origination to 160 countries under the bilateral free share agreement. Based on suggestions from PMPH, I cooperated with some ophthalmologists and radiologists to collect substantial amount of clinical imaging data of HIV/AIDS-associated eye diseases. After careful sorting, analyzing and discussing, we published *Atlas of Differential Diagnosis in HIV/AIDS Complicated Eye Diseases*. In August 2008, *Differential Diagnosis in HIV/AIDS: Comparing Imaging with Anatomy and Pathology* was published, which was based on imaging data and combined anatomic and pathologic study for comparative analysis. According to the principles of EBM, HIV/AIDS imaging was scientifically verified for its preciseness and authenticity. It has been more than 7 years since our first treatise on HIV/AIDS imaging was published. At the beginning, the field was still in its infancy, with related treatise having their own focus on one part of the field, while no books on comprehensive analysis of HIV/AIDS imaging. With the advance of the studies in this field, we feel it compulsive to share our findings and experience. On the other hand, during these years, substantial progress has been made on the methodology of HIV/AIDS imaging studies, including new research methods, new techniques, new research design, all of which are reviewed in this book. Another reason of writing this book comes to the establishment of Academic Committee of Medical AIDS Image in China, which has called together more experts and more clinical data to enrich the content of this treatise. And more colleagues, readers and experts of related fields are eagerly expect a more practical book on HIV/AIDS imaging from our team as a guiding blueprint for clinical practice. And lastly, the content of this book was enriched by more summative knowledge, more comprehensive and typical case studies. Moreover, the use of functional imaging in HIV/AIDS diagnosis and differential diagnosis was firstly introduced in this book.

Above all, I would acknowledge the visionary leaders and experts from PMPH for their appreciation of this book, which is systematic, comprehensive and scientific in HIV/AIDS imaging field. The joint effort for its international publication will promote the advancement of this field.

The 24th World AIDS Day (WAD) is coming. We hope this book to be a gift for the 23rd WAD. We expect eradication of AIDS, the new plague of the twenty-first century, in the world.

However, defects in this book are inevitable for our limited understanding of the disease. It will be improved gradually with the general development of scientific discoveries. All comments are welcome to improve our work in the future.

Beijing, China   Li Hongjun

Editors

Chief Editor
Li Hongjun

Honorary Editor
Li Ning

Editors
(in alphabetic order)
Bao Dongwu   Bao Dongying
Chen Dexi   Chen Feng   Chen Longhua   Cheng Jingliang
Feng Shaoyang
Gao Jianbo   Gao Yanqing
He Ning   Huang Shaobiao
Jia Cuiyu   Jin Ronghua
Li Huiqin   Li Hongchen   Li Hongyan   Li Li   Li Ruili   Li Zhen   Li Yunfang
Li Xueqin
Liu Bailu   Liu Baoqin   Liu Chunli   Liu Jinxin   Liu Rongzhi
Lu Puxuan   Lu Zhiyan   Lv Shengxiu   Lv Shuxiu
Mao Lin   Mao Xiaoxi   Mi Haifeng
Niu Guilin
Qi Shi   Qian Nanping
Ren Meiji
Shi Dongli   Shi Dapeng   Shi Daiqiang   Shi Ying   Shi Yuxin
Song Liucun   Song Wenyan   Sun Yan
Wang Lu   Wang Wei   Wang Wen   Wang Xicheng   Wang Yanling   Wang Xing
Xiang Haiping   Xu Fuxia
Yang Xuan   Yang Yiqing   Yang Youyi   Yang Yuxin   Yang Zhou
Yuan Da
Zhang Yanyan   Zhang Lihong   Zhang Aidong   Zhang Na   Zhang Ruichi
Zhang Yuzhong   Zhang Zairen   Zhang Zhiyong
Zhao Dawei   Zhao Jinqi   Zhao Jing   Zhao Qingxia
Zhou Shulin   Zhu Cuiping   Yu Wei   Yao Jinpeng

Proof reader: Li zhen   Xu Jin   Wang Tian   Zhao Mingmeng

Acknowledgement

You'an Hospital, Capital Medical University, Beijing, China

Provincial Hospital for AIDS Patients, Yunnan, China

First Affiliated Hospital, Zhengzhou University, Zhengzhou, Henan, China

Yan'an Hospital, Kunming, Yunnan, China

Provincial Infectious Diseases Hospital, Henan, China (Sixth People's Hospital of Zhengzhou, Henan, China)

Public Health Medical Rescuing Center, Chongqing, China

First Affiliated Hospital, Nanyang Medical Technical College, Nanyang, Henan, China

Infectious Diseases Hospital, Xinjiang Uygur Autonomous Region, China

Traditional Chinese Medicine Hospital, Nanyang, Henan, China

Public Health Medical Rescuing Center, Shanghai, China

Baihe Hospital, Nanyang, Henan, China

Infectious Diseases Hospital, Shenzhen, Guangdong, China

Infectious Diseases Hospital, Chengdu, Sichuan, China

Infectious Diseases Hospital, Hangzhou, Jiangsu, China

Fourth People's Hospital, Nanning, Guangxi Zhuang Autonomous Region, China

Second Affiliated Hospital, Harbin Medical University, Harbin, Heilongjiang, China

Maternal and Child Health Hospital, Lincang, Yunnan, China

First Hospital, Shanxi Medical University, Taiyuan, Shanxi, China

Second People's Hospital, Lincang, Yunnan, China

Provincial People's Hospital, Henan, China

People's Hospital, Shuangjiang, Yunnan, China

University College Cork(UCC) Ireland

Southern of Medical University Guangzhou, China

Peking Union Medical College Hospital, Chinese Academy of Medicine Science, Beijing

Cancer Hospital, Chinese Academy of Medical Sciences &Peking Union Medical College, Beijing, China

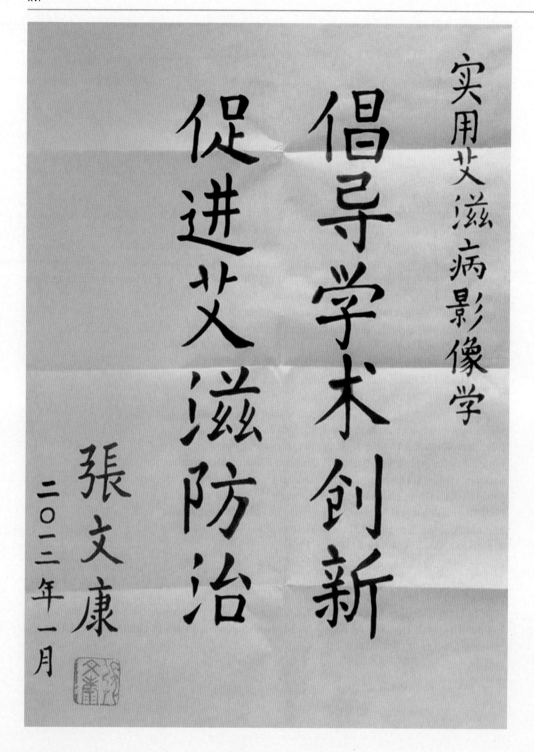

Advocating Academic Innovation and Promoting AIDS Control
By Zhang Wenkang
January 2012

Contents

Definition of AIDS

Acquired immunodeficiency syndrome (AIDS) is a clinical syndrome caused by human immunodeficiency virus (HIV) which leads to compromised human immunity. AIDS can be categorized into two types, namely the type of HIV-1 and the type of HIV-2. HIV can be transmitted via four routes, including sexual transmission, blood-borne transmission, intravenous drug abuse and vertical transmission from mother to child. AIDS has been known as "a plague of twentieth century" as well as "super-cancer" and "killer of the century".

Origination and Development of HIV/AIDS

Origination of HIV/AIDS

Based on research findings, American scholars believe that HIV/AIDS was originated in rural areas of the central African countries. In the early 1970s, a large number of rural population flowed into cities. HIV/AIDS spread rapidly in these cities due to sexual promiscuity and intravenous drug abuse. Of all the 75 sera samples collected in senior areas, 50 contained HIV antibodies, indicating that HIV infection is not accidental and temporary, but a result of long-term extensive prevalence. Such a high detection rate indicated an earlier occurrence of HIV infection in human bodies. Another view holds that AIDS may have occurred in Indians in the Amazon River Basin long time ago without any serious consequences. Some experts pointed out that 4 % of the Indians carrying HIV antibody were asymptomatic. But the study used 3 sera samples from Indians collected in 1968 [1]. However, some others believe that HIV derives from the primates and is a zoonotic disease caused by a mutant strain which is a pathogen of an animal disease before its mutation and can spread into high-risk persons via close contacts with the host animals. In the course of their transmission, some factors cause the viruses to mutate into the highly pathogenic strain. Meanwhile, prostitution, homosexuality and intravenous drug abuse lead to its rapid spread. In Africa, it was found that the Simian T-cell lymphotropic virus (STLV-III) carried by green monkeys is similar to the human T-cell lymphotropic virus (HTLV-III). In the USA, the outbreak of Rhesus AIDS in some American ape centers is similar to human AIDS in terms of epidemiology, virology, and immunology. Some research data implied that HIV is the variants of the primate retrovirus.

Japanese scientists discovered that the way HIV invades human and cat immunocytes is similar, which laid a foundation for the human HIV vaccine development by using cats as the experimental animals. It had been found that cats can also infect AIDS and the pathogen was called feline immunodeficiency virus (FIV). The symptoms of AIDS infected by cats and humans are alike and the targets the viruses attack are both the lymphocytes with immune functions. However, it remains elusive whether the processes of cell infections are also the same. An associate professor, Miyazawa Takayuki [2] from Obihiro University of Agriculture and Veterinary Medicine in Hokkaido, Japan, led a research, which found that the feline immunodeficiency virus firstly binds with protein CD134 on the surface of feline lymphocytes and then invades the lymphocytes with the assistance from a protein called CXCR4. This process shares great similarity to the invasion of HIV into human cells. Some American experts in this field recognized the finding as a breakthrough in understanding AIDS. But the research topics such as where HIV comes from and whether it is characteristically human or is common between human and animals are of great research interests. Gaining some knowledge about the origin of HIV will provide important information for the prevention and control of AIDS.

Retrospective Review of AIDS

From late 1970s to early 1980s, the number of cases with pneumocystis carinii pneumonia (PCP) and Kaposi's sarcoma (KS) suddenly surged among young homosexual men in several big American cities, which were accompanied by immunodeficiency symptoms. The average age of the patients was 36. Rarely did such diseases occur in healthy people in the past and even rarer occurrence in the young. Therefore, the suddenly occurred event caught the attention of Center for Disease Control and Prevention (CDC). By August 1981, CDC had received 111 case reports concerning occurrence of PCP or KS in homosexual men [1]. During the fall in 1981, several PCP cases were reported to be non-homosexual but intravenous drug users in New York.

In Dec. 1981, the *New England Journal of Medicine* (NEJM) reported several cases of cellular immunodeficiency [3]. In January 1982, a 55-year-old man with PCP was reported dead in Miami, America. However, the man was neither homosexual nor drug user and he was not from Haiti but a hemophile who had received the treatment of factor VIII concentrate. Later, another two such cases were reported.

On July 16, 1982, CDC [4] reported and commented such cases on the Morbidity and Mortality Weekly Report (MMWR), concluding that clinical and immunological manifestations of the three hemophile patients were similar to those of the homosexual and non-homosexual drug abusers. It was supposed that the illnesses be caused by the same pathogen and be transmitted through blood and blood products. It was the first time that the illnesses had been caused by the same pathogen and was transmitted through blood. The cases were intensively studied and some features in common were reported as following: serious cellular immunodeficiency, various stimulated opportunistic infections (especially PCP and KS), high death rate. The susceptible populations include homosexuals, intravenous drug user, Haiti immigrants and patients with hemophile (collectively called 4H). The routes of transmission include sexual intercourse and blood. The terms of homosexuality, intravenous drug use, immunodeficiency, PCP and KS are linked together, which was considered as a newly emerging illness unit. Thereafter, a new page was turned to in the history of medicine. A severely infectious disease, acquired immunodeficiency syndrome (AIDS) swept across the world since then. WTO and scientists from each country paid great attention to this disease. In September 1982, CDC of the USA officially nominated the illness as Acquired Immunodeficiency Syndrome (AIDS for short) and its translated version in Chinese as Ai Zi Bing.

In 1983, a prominent scientist, director of Neoplasm Virus Department in French Pasteur Institute, Montagnier, reported his successful isolation of AIDS lymphadenopathy associated virus (LAV) from the lymph node of a male homosexual with lymph node syndrome [5]. In 1984, the researchers [6] from National Cancer Institute of the United States also reported that several strains of retroviruses were isolated from blood samples of AIDS patients. It was nominated as human T-lymphotrophic virus (HTLV-III for short) because the virus invades lymphocytes with immune functions. The two viruses were believed to be the variants of the same antiretrovirus, assured to be the pathogen causing AIDS, which were then named LAV/LTLV-III. On July 25, 1986, WTO announced the decision by the International Committee on the Taxonomy of Viruses [7], that the virus causing AIDS was finally renominated as human immunodeficiency virus (HIV).

HIV refers to the virus that damages human immune system. HIV-infected patients refer to those who carry HIV but with no symptoms of AIDS. AIDS patients refer to those HIV carriers who have symptoms due to compromised immunity after 2–10 years incubation period of HIV. The three terms should be differentially and correctly used.

Nomination and Concept of AIDS Pathogen

Just 3 years after the first AIDS case, scientists successfully isolated and identified the pathogen of AIDS (HTLV-III/LAV). The following four scientific research teams are recognized to be the first ones in isolating and identifying AIDS pathogen.

1. In May 1983 [8], the research team led by Mantagnier from Pasteur Institute in Paris, France, isolated AIDS pathogen from the lymph nodes of a French with lymphadenopathy. The virus was then nominated as lymphadenopathy associated virus (LAV).

2. In April 1984 [9], the research team led by Gallo from US National Cancer Institute isolated the AIDS pathogen from a series of T-cell cultures which was infected by the isolates from 10 AIDS patients. It was then nominated as human T-cell leukemia-virus (HTLV-III).

3. In May 1984 [10], the research team led by Levy from the San Francisco Medical School of the University of California, USA, isolated AIDS pathogen from the blood sample of a local AIDS patient. It was then nominated as AIDS associated retrovirus (ARV).

4. In May 1984 [10], the research team led by Chairman from Pasteur Institute in Paris, France, found AIDS pathogen in the HIV-infected hemophile twins. It was then nominated as immune deficiency associated virus (IDAV). After the scholars decoded its genetic structure, it was found that IDAV and LAV were actually the same virus. HTLV-III can show the genealogy and origin of AIDS, and its discoverer, Galo, is one of the top AIDS researchers, while LAV is the earliest found virus of AIDS. So the Nomenclature Committee held by the International Committee on the Taxonomy of Viruses decided to temporarily name AIDS virus as HTLV-III/LAV. After the earliest isolation and identification of AIDS virus, the Mantagnier team, in early 1985 [11], cloned genes of LAV by genetic engineering techniques and decoded its total 9,193 nucleotides by electronic computer technology. The decoded complicated sequences of nucleotide enable the first gene schematic diagrams of LAV. It was proved by research that the LAV genome is composed of GAG, POL, ENV, Q and S. Gene GAG is responsible for encoding proteins as components of inner nucleus of the virus, which is in charge of ribonucleoproteins for nucleus. Gene POL is responsible for encoding duplicate reverse transcriptase, which is in charge of chromosomes for virus reproduction. Gene ENV is responsible for encoding proteins that comprise HIV envelopes, which is in charge of manufacturing the virus envelopes. Gene Q enables the virus to be in a latent state at disadvantaged conditions, which is in charge of concealing the virus. The functions of gene S are contrary to those of gene Q, which activates the virus. When immune disorders occur, gene S activates the virus, leading to clinical manifestations of AIDS. Meanwhile, the Gallo team decoded the precise genetic sequences of HTLV-III, LAV and ARV successively in early 1985 [12]. They discovered that among nearly 10,000 nucleotide sequences, LAV has only 150 different nucleotides from HTLV-III, but 600 different nucleotides from ARV.

5. In October 1985 [13], the research group led by Martin from the National Institute of Allergy and Infectious Diseases in the USA drew the restriction endonuclease map of HTLV-III, LAV and ARV. It was found that the map of HTLV-III and that of LAV are identical, but ARV's is slightly different from those of HTLV-III and LAV. Current researches have proved that HTLV-III and LAV are of the same virus family. It is still under research as to why slight differences exist in the structure of ARV. That the samples were collected at different time and places may be the reasons why there are slight differences between ARV and HTLV-III/LAV. It is presumed that ARV is actually of the same virus family as HTLV-III/LAV.

6. In 1986 [7], the WTO unified all the nominations of AIDS virus and officially nominated it human immunodeficiency virus (HIV).

HIV, very small biological particles, is only visible under a microscope that magnifies it hundreds of thousands of times. A virion is consisted of a protein layer on the surface and the core component of nucleic acids whose helical structure is the result of two intersecting and entwining long strands. The two long chains can be divided into two single strands which serve as templates for replication to produce new double-stranded nucleic acid molecules. There are two types of nucleic acids, namely DNA and RNA. In general, the transcription of DNA into RNA passes on the genetic information to the next generation. But AIDS virus can transcribe RNA into DNA by a special enzyme called reverse transcriptase. The DNA of this virus can fuse with the chromosomes of the infected people which enables the virus to embed in human cells. When human cells dividing and multiplying in the body, the chromosomes in the nuclei will divide into two to reproduce a new generation. The virus will proliferate as the human lymphocytes it resides in do. The new progeny virions will continually destroy lymphocytes, leading to compromised human immunity.

Negative Impacts of AIDS on Human Society

Only 20 years after the discovery of the first HIV infected patient in 1981, AIDS epidemic has spread all over the world and has become a major public health challenge and social problem. It has great impact on the human society.

Its Impact on the Life Style

The fact that people can contract AIDS by promiscuous sexual behavior and intravenous drug use caused a panic among people. One expert from Global AIDS Special Planning Committee said, "It is effective to prevent AIDS by reducing the number of sex partners, cautiously contacting with homosexuals and avoiding sexual behaviors with bisexually oriented people". This advice awoke people so that some western countries also started to be prudential about sex. One news agency in the USA published a cartoon with an article promoting AIDS prevention, in which a girl told the boy who was expressing his love for her, "Your sexual history and health certificate is preferable to flowers and chocolates." It proved that the westerners have been liberated from the libertine sexual satisfaction and began to reasonably choose his/her sexual partner.

Great Loss in Social Economy

Hening, an economist of the US Health Services and Health Care Technology Assessment Center, pointed out in his research report that the medical costs of each AIDS patient is estimated to be $60,000 during his/her lifetime. Countries with serious AIDS epidemic will be faced with the reduction of foreign investors, and suffer from loss resulting from decline of tourism income. Some poor developing countries also have to assign their limited money to prevent and control AIDS. Therefore, the whole world economy will be negatively affected by these serious problems.

New Problems in Implementing Current Laws

The legal problems caused by AIDS have aroused great public attention in many countries. Many people proposed that it be necessary to enact health law to grant immunity to the medical lawsuits and protect personal privacy. As for the legal problems about blood transfusion, the blood suppliers shall hold accountability since now there are blood screening methods which can technically prevent the contaminated blood from being transfused to patients. Another problem is about the mandatory screening of high risk populations. Although it may violate people's private life and bring on discrimination, there shall be at least some rules to encourage and promote the screening of high risk populations. Under such circumstances, the laws shall balance the individual interests and the public interests. Some regulations should be formulated to arouse AIDS patients' awareness so as to avoid the transmission of the disease. The individual responsibility for AIDS control shall be advocated. The behaviors of the AIDS patients who use the infection as a weapon to harm others deliberately or attempt to harm others is not only a civil tort, but also a crime. Currently, the Soviet Union is the only country in the world where the civil liability and criminal liability of those who deliberately infect others will be investigated.

Effects on Personal Daily Life and International Communications

Some experts predicted that close contacts such as kissing, hugging, shaking hands in social occasions may reduce sharply. In addition, many people may try to avoid going to public bath rooms, assemblies as well as restaurants and even avoid using public transportations. The restrictive measures and requirements of blood testing adopted by many countries to prevent AIDS spreading from overseas will negatively affect immigration, travelling, studying abroad and certain international activities.

Necessities of Studying HIV/AIDS Imaging

The immune system of the HIV-infected patients is extremely suppressed or even destroyed. Under such conditions, various pathogens have the opportunity to attack human body to cause various AIDS-related diseases such as tumors, which in turn impair organ functions to cause organ failure and even death. Therefore, AIDS-related diseases are the common seen causes of death in AIDS patients.

The unclearly defined AIDS associated diseases will result in unreasonable use of antibiotics in the clinic which may delay diagnosis and treatment and ultimately lead to occurrence of death.

Both in specialized hospitals of infectious diseases and general hospitals, HIV-infected patients are commonly unaware of their infections of HIV. Such patients usually have lived through the 5–10 years' incubation period of HIV without any clinic visits until the occurrence of the symptom. Therefore, the radiologists should preferably have knowledge about the spectrum of AIDS-related diseases to reasonably define the diagnosis for HIV infected patients. Based on their primary suspected diagnosis, related laboratory tests can be ordered to confirm the diagnosis. These diagnostic procedures are of great significance for clinical diagnosis of AIDS. We have experienced the cases that the surgical plan had to be changed just before the operation due to the preoperative HIV positive findings in immunologic tests.

The diagnostic imaging on HIV/AIDS plays important role in the diagnosis and differential diagnosis of AIDS-related diseases.

Development and Clinical Application of HIV/AIDS Imaging

In China, the AIDS patients receive the therapies in local primary hospitals in some areas of China. Generally, these hospitals are poorly equipped with health care workers and devices, and the clinicians and radiologists have insufficient knowledge about the diagnostic imaging of HIV/AIDS. In general hospitals, patients with AIDS are usually found HIV positive by routine laboratory tests before the operation or some special examinations. Consequently, the diagnostic imaging results are then retrospectively reanalyzed. It has been appreciated that AIDS is susceptible to missed diagnosis and misdiagnosis due to our insufficient knowledge about the diagnostic imaging of HIV/AIDS. The fact challenges radiologists to expand their knowledge for differential diagnosis. For patients who are unaware of their HIV infections or are unwilling to inform their HIV infections, the radiologists should conduct backward reasoning on the basis of the diagnostic imaging results. Recommendations should be given to the suspected AIDS patients for clinical HIV tests. HIV itself is not life threatening in short term due to its weak virulence. The common death cause of HIV infected patients is the AIDS-related diseases. Because the diagnostic imaging is the major available way for diagnosis and differential diagnosis of AIDS-related diseases, application of the achievements in diagnostic imaging of HIV/AIDS research is of great importance for individualized therapies and rational use of antibiotics. In the developed countries in Europe and America, patients with AIDS have almost the same quality of life as the healthy population. Their deaths from AIDS-related diseases rarely occur. The cause of death is mostly natural failure. Such achievement is closely related with the nationally formulated clinical guidelines for patients with AIDS, effective measures for AIDS prevention, accurate diagnosis of AIDS and AIDS-related diseases, and the focused attention to AIDS. The treatment for AIDS patients include two steps, the first being antiviral therapies and the second being therapies for AIDS-related diseases. For patients with favorable compliance and good economic conditions, the earlier antiviral therapies should be preferably administered. Once the AIDS-related diseases occur, the treatment shall be focused on AIDS-related diseases. The therapeutic plan should be scientific, comprehensive and rigorous based on reasonable differential diagnosis. Therefore, it is advocated to use the diagnostic imaging for early diagnosis of AIDS-related diseases. It is our first responsibility to improve the life quality of AIDS patients, reduce occurrence of AIDS-related diseases and decrease the death rate.

The diagnostic imaging findings that are characteristically HIV/AIDS related include:

1. In the whole course of AIDS, it is common for only one system or one organ to be involved. Concurrent involvement of multiple systems is rarely found.
2. With the gradual decrease of the immunity and the prolonged survival time, the patients' chance of being infected by multiple pathogens increases. Concurrent multiple pathogens cause AIDS-related diseases, which have multiple imaging demonstrations.
3. The diseases occur before the onset of AIDS and the newly emerging diseases after the onset of AIDS should be differentiated to clarify their relationship.
4. The diseases caused by HIV itself and the AIDS-related diseases should be differentiated to clarify their relationship.
5. The diagnostic imaging findings characteristic to AIDS before and after HAART therapies should be differentiated.

Classifications of HIV/AIDS-related diseases:

1. Classification based on the pathogenic factors:
   (1) Diseases caused by HIV itself; (2) AIDS-related opportunistic infections; (3) AIDS-related neoplasms.
2. Classification based on the occurrence rate and locations of lesions:
   (1) Respiratory type; (2) Neural type; (3) Oculopathy type including orbit diseases and ocular fundus diseases; (4) Cardiovascular type; (5) Gastrointestinal type; (6) Musculoskeletal type; (7) Cutaneous type.

The location, size and range of AIDS-related inflammations, tuberculosis and neoplasms can be diagnosed by MR, CT, DR and PET-CT. In combination with immunological indices or pathological analysis, the qualitative diagnosis can be defined. For example, DR and CT are of great value in diagnosing pulmonary AIDS-related diseases for their favorable natural density contrast of the lungs. The ophthalmoscopy and fluorescein angiography (FFA) can be applied to define the range and location of AIDS-related fundus lesions. In combination with laboratory indicators, a qualitative diagnosis can be defined. The gastrointestinal endoscopy and barium meal imaging in combination with biopsy can be applied to define gastrointestinal mycotic inflammation, ulcer, tuberculosis, related lymphoma and KS sarcoma. MR has a favorable natural resolution on neural inflammations, musculoskeletal inflammations and neoplasms, whose definitive diagnosis can be made in combination with histological examinations. The dermatosis can be diagnosed by combined stereological examinations and pathological analysis.

References

1. Yantao Xin. The mystery of the origin of AIDS. Beijing: China Environmental Science Press; 2005. ISBN 9787802092372.
2. Miyazawa T. Infections of feline leukemia virus and feline immunodeficiency virus [J]. Front Biosci. 2002;1(7):d504–18.
3. Gottlied MS, Schroff R, Schanker HM, et al. Pneumocystis carinii pneumonia and mucosal candidiasis in previously healthy homosexual men:evidence of a new acquired cellular immunodeficiency [J]. N Engl J Med. 1981;305(24):1425–31.
4. Centers for Disease Control. Update on acquired immune deficiency syndrome (AIDS) among patients with hemophilia A [J]. MMWR Morb Wkly Rep. 1982;31(48):644–6652.
5. Montagnier L. Lymphadenopathy-associated virus: from molecular biology to pathogenicity [J]. Ann Intern Med. 1985;103(5):689–93.
6. Ginzburg HM, French J, Jackson J, et al. Health education and knowledge assessment of HTLV-III diseases among intravenous drug users [J]. Health Educ Q. 1986;13(4):373–82.
7. Warrell DA, Cox TM, Firth JD. Oxford infections [M]. Oxford University: Oxford University Press; 2003.
8. Montagnier L. Lymphadenopathy-associated virus: from molecular biology to pathogenicity [J]. Ann Intern Med. 1985;103(5):689–93.
9. Ginzburg HM, French J, Jackson J, et al. Health education and knowledge assessment of HTLV-III diseases among intravenous drug users [J]. Health Educ Q. 1986;13(4):373–82.
10. Levy JA, Hoffman AD, Kramer SM, et al. Isolation of lymphocytopathic retroviruses from San Francisco patients with AIDS [J]. Science. 1984;225(4664):840–2.
11. Montagnier L. Lymphadenopathy-associated virus: from molecular biology to pathogenicity [J]. Ann Intern Med. 1985;103(5):689–93.
12. Ratner L, Gallo RC, Wong-Staal F. HTLV-III, LAV, ARV are variants of same AIDS virus [J]. Nature. 1985;313(6004):636–7.
13. Benn S, Rutledge R, Folks T, et al. Genomic heterogeneity of AIDS retroviral from North America and Zaire [J]. Science. 1985;230(4728):949–51.

Molecular Biology of HIV/AIDS and Its Clinical Management

Contents

1.1 Application of Modern Molecular Biology in HIV Research

1.1.1 Recombination DNA Techniques

Gene engineering, also called genetic engineering or recombinant DNA technique, has been a newly emerging technology since 1970s. Its principle is to artificially isolate biological genetic materials (usually DNA) for their being cleaved, incorporated, restructured, transferred and expressed in vitro. Generally, it involves four steps. The first step is the cloning of the target gene to obtain the needed DNA segments. The second step is to obtain the recombinant DNA by connecting the target gene with DNA vector. The third step is to introduce the recombinant DNA into the bacteria or mammalian cells for its proliferation. And the last step is to screen the receptor cells that express the target genes for expression of the corresponding proteins and other products. The recombinant DNA technique is one of the most commonly used technologies in molecular biology, which has been widely applied in scientific research and the clinical detection of HIV.

Two companies, ViroLogic (San Francisco, CA) and Virco (Mechelen, Belgium), are the first two companies that improved phenotypic analysis technology on the basis of recombinant DNA technique for the phenotype drug resistance detection. The improved phenotypic analysis technique skips the procedure of virus isolation, shortens the detection time, automize the detection procedures and saves manpower, and thus ensures the experimental stability and reproducibility. The phenotypic detection technique developed by ViroLogic, Pheno Sense [1], is to obtain HIV-1 protease genes and reverse transcriptase genes from the HIV-infected patients by adopting RT-PCR amplification and to prepare a viral vector containing the recombinant genes segments by recombination DNA techniques. The vector carries a luciferase labelled gene that replaces the HIV envelope gene. The protease and reverse transcriptase genes of the HIV-infected patients are recombined with the vector for the genetic

H. Li (ed.), *Radiology of HIV/AIDS*,
DOI 10.1007/978-94-007-7823-8_1, © Springer Science+Business Media Dordrecht and People's Medical Publishing House 2014

hybridization to form a recombinant virus. The recombinant virus proliferates at the presence of tested drugs, and the expression level of luciferase is concurrently examined. By comparing to the standard virus strain sensitive to drugs, the logarithmic graph of the drug concentrations can be drawn and IC50 value can be calculated. The technique developed by Virco [2] is to insert the amplified protease genes and reverse transcriptase genes into standard HIV strains containing both of the two genes and to transfect a CD4 T cell line for a recombinant HIV strain containing protease and reverse transcriptase genes from HIV-infected patients. Under a light microscope with high resolution, the drug susceptibility IC50 of the recombinant virus to different antiviral drugs can be real-time read by monitoring recombinant virus cultured with different drugs or with the same drug of different concentrations.

1.1.1.1 Development of HIV Vaccine

AIDS genomes contain genes like gag, pol and env. The proteins encoded by these genes possess many important epitopes which stimulate the body to produce various specific antibodies. Some of these antibodies with neutralizing activities can inhibit or partially slow down the invasion of the virus and others can fight against the virus. Years ago some scientists had already used recombinant DNA technique to construct important epitopes of these genes into the expression vector for their recombination and expression in vitro to produce vaccines. Thus effective attacks would be initiated targeting proteins encoded by these genes. In addition, by using genetic engineering/recombinant DNA technique, a pseudovirus, being deprived of pathogenicity with partial HIV activity to encode HIV proteins but being incapable of invasion, can be developed. This discovery builds a technology platform for the manufacture of plentiful, safe and economical AIDS vaccine and for the development of ways to detect drug resistance. Currently in the U. S., an HIV vaccine has been developed to produce HIV antibodies in animals. The experiments on the vaccine are in progress. And its application in clinical practice is expected.

1.1.2   Application of Nucleic Acid Hybridization in HIV Research

Nucleic acid hybridization is one of the most widely applied technique in biochemical and molecular biological studies, which is a powerful tool for the qualitative or quantitative detection on the sequences of the specific RNA or DNA segments. It is developed on the basis of complementary base pairing. The hydrogen bond that holds the double strands can be broken down (denaturalized) and thus the double strands can be separated into two single strands if heated in alkaline conditions or the denaturants are added. At the moment, the heterologous DNA or RNA (single strand) will be put in and insulated in a certain ionic strength and temperature (renaturation). If there are complementary base sequences between the heterologous DNA or RNA, the nucleic acid molecules will be hybridized during the renaturation.

Gene chip is an improved molecular hybridization technique developed in recent years, with rapid development and widespread application in clinical practice. In just a few years, it has been primarily applied to detect the genic mutations and analyze the genetic expressions of the human-related diseases like tumor and genetic diseases. Nucleic acid hybridization has been widely used in HIV clinical research as the following.

1.1.2.1 Application of Gene Chip in Clinical Identification of HIV

Gene chip for HIV detection integrates PCR with molecular hybridization, which can directly detect the virus and considerably improve diagnostic accuracy by analyzing HIV genome and taking the highly conserved sequences of the virus as the identification index. In early 1998, doctors, including Hauser, detected HIV for the HIV-infected patients before the onset of antibody response by using DNA chip. The technique plays an important role in the early diagnosis of AIDS [3].

1.1.2.2 The Application of Gene Chip in HIV Genotyping

The basic principle is to fix the characteristic gene fragments (target gene) of the pathogen on the glass slide to prepare a detecting chip. The HIV RNA extracted from the patients then is amplified and labeled with fluorescence to be hybridized with the detecting chip. The hybridizing signal is scanned by scanner to be analyzed by a computer for a definite diagnosis.

1.1.2.3 The Application of Molecular Hybridization in Detecting Drug Resistance

The methods testing HIV drug resistance can be divided into two types. The first is to sequence the target gene to find out all the possible gene mutations responsible to drug resistance. In other word, that is to amplify the target gene to obtain protease gene and reverse transcriptase gene fragments of the virus directly for gene sequencing, followed by translating gene sequences into amino acid sequences to compare them with the reference sequences in the database. Thus the mutations responsible for drug resistance can be identified and their clinical significance can be clarified. This is the standard test procedures for HIV-1 genotypic drug resistance. And the other type of tests is to identify mutations responsible to drug resistance using molecular hybridization or mutation PCR for specific genomic loci. The molecular hybridization includes the following two techniques [4].

The Linear Probe Assay (LIPA) [5]

The technique is developed by Innogenetics based in Belgium. On the basis of reverse hybridization, wild or mutant oligonucleotide gene probes targeting on HIV-1 reverse transcriptase and protease are firstly fixed on the nitrocellulose membrane. The tested specimen is then amplified by RT-PCR for fragments of the reverse transcriptase gene and protease gene by using biotin labeled primers. The amplified biotinylated fragments are consequently hybridized with oligonucleotide probe fixed on nitrocellulose membrane. Finally, the mutations responsible for drug resistance can be identified based on hybridization between the viral sequence and probe.

Sequencing with Hybridization and Gene Chip

The Gene Chip by Affymerix [6] fixed over 16,000 probes with a coverage of HIV-1 reverse transcriptase and protease on silica slides to prepare a probe array. The HIV RNA in specimens to be tested was synthetized into fluorescent-labelled virus cRNA via transcription in vitro for hybridization with the probe array. A laser scanner was then applied to scan the results. The probe with the best matching with the target sequence will show the strongest fluorescence intensity. The average signal strength was then calculated by using specific software and thus to identify the sequences of target gene and the mutations responsible to drug resistance.

1.1.3   Recent Development of Molecular Biology Techniques in HIV Research

Molecular biology has been widely used in the diagnosis and scientific research of HIV. With the rapid development of molecular biology, its applications in HIV are diverse. In addition to the previously introduced recombinant DNA technique and molecular hybridization technique, the commonly used techniques also include the preparation of HIV pseudovirus. The following is the introduction of HIV pseudovirus and its applications.

HIV is highly pathogenic to human, which constitutes challenges in terms of studies on active virus strains, tests on its pathogenicity in vitro and its drug resistance. However, all these challenges can be fundamentally overcome by using HIV pseudovirus with partial HIV proteins. Currently, the most widely used is HIV pseudovirus with mutated gag protein, which plays an important role in studying the mechanism of HIV attacking human body. The pseudovirus consists of two plasmids, with one containing HIV genome of the mutated gag protein and the other containing genes of the mutated gag protein. When transfecting cells together, the two plasmids can complementarily express HIV proteins for successful package of virions. In addition, due to its incomplete gag genes components, the virus particles after cell transfection fail to be packaged and bud. Their ability to

continue transfection is thus lost. Therefore, the problem of biosafety can be completely solved.

1.1.3.1   Diverse Applications of HIV Pseudovirus

Drug Screening

The pseudovirus system can be applied for rapid and accurate detection of drug concentration and IC50 test of drugs. It can even be applied to judge the corresponding viral infection procedure based on the different time frames of the drug in effects.

Viral Tropism Analysis

The virus strains of different sources are firstly cloned into pseudovirus vectors. The pseudovirus then infects cell lines of different receptors. The expression level of p24 antigen in cellular supernatant is examined to determine the viral tropism.

Tests on Phenotypic Drug Resistance

The tested gene sequence is firstly cloned into HIV pseudovirus vectors. The expression level of the genes can be reported to evaluate the extent of viral drug resistance. This is the most widely applied technique for detection of HIV drug resistance in recent years.

1.2   Mechanism of Genetic Diagnosis for HIV

Nucleic acid is the genetic material of life. Gene diagnosis can be applied for detection of HIV nucleic acid.

1.2.1   HIV Sequence Detection

The detection of HIV sequence can be applied to diagnose, sequence and classify HIV. Due to the extensive heterologous of HIV-1 genomes, different primers including primers of the LTR, gag and env genes can be used to increase the positive rate of the detection. However, it should be noted that detecting HIV sequences is not the way to diagnose HIV/AIDS. The definitive diagnosis of HIV/AIDS can be made based on WB antibody testing.

1.2.1.1   Amplification of Proviral HIV Sequences

The proviral HIV sequences can be detected from the monocytes in the peripheral blood from seropositive HIV-infected patients. In general, HIV diagnosis is mainly directed at detecting the PCR of the relatively conserved sequences, such as gag. The Nested PCR can be applied to amplify the specific sequences of HIV for diagnosis.

1.2.1.2   Amplification of HIV Genome

HIV genome is composed of two positive-strand RNAs. HIV sequences can be amplified in the plasma of the patients by PCR reverse transcription for sequence analysis or diagnosis.

1.2.2 HIV Sequence Detection for Immune Antibody Negative Individuals

There is a lag phase between HIV infection and immune responses, which is seronegative and lasts for 6 weeks to 6 months. The phase may be longer in cases with no antibodies produced. Due to undetectable antibody during this lag period, those seronegative may still be patients infected with HIV.

The diagnosis using PCR to detect HIV-1 among high-risk groups is generally 6 months earlier than the diagnosis based on seroconversion to positive. For a few cases with the initial serial negative findings, PCR can even confirm their HIV infection 24–39 months earlier before the seroconversion to positive. For those with indefinite diagnosis by serology tests, PCR can be applied for further analysis and diagnosis.

1.2.3 HIV Sequence Detection for Newborns

The HIV antibody tests for infants whose mother is HIV infected are usually positive due to the presence of maternal antibodies. But only 20–60 % infants are actually infected with HIV. Therefore, it is very important for the infants to clarify their diagnosis earlier. Now it has been proved that 30–50 % neonates may be infected with HIV during periods of pregnancy, delivery, induced labour and postpartum lactation. But neonates being seropositive are not necessarily HIV infected because their maternal HIV antibody can live in their bodies for 15 months. In general, the infants do not show any symptoms of HIV infection. Therefore, virus cell culture fails to constitute a reliable and applicable way for HIV diagnosis in neonatals. In addition, it is impossible to detect HIV specific IgM antibody in the presence of maternal antibodies. And it is very challenging to detect HIV antigen in serum in the presence of excessive serum antibodies. Therefore, gene diagnosis plays an indispensable role in HIV diagnosis for infants. It can even be considered as a diagnostic basis for the special groups. The conditions progress rapidly in infants with HIV. Therefore, their early diagnosis is of great importance for effective intervention to be adopted to slow down or arrest the progression of HIV infection. The antiviral drugs presently used should not be administered to

seropositive infants but with no HIV infection due to their high toxicity. Antiviral therapies combined with immunity and nutritions improving therapies should be administered after detection of HIV-DNA sequence by PCR.

Detecting HIV-DNA sequence by gene diagnosis plays an important role in defining the diagnosis of AIDS and ARC. But some clinicians believe that PCR is unnecessary for patients with positive findings for HIV antibody, antigen or virus culture. Those with suspected HIV infection but having no sufficient evidence in serology should be strongly recommended for gene diagnosis. Such groups include infants with HIV positive mothers, sexual partners of HIV positive patients, intravenous drug abusers and serologically suspected patients.

1.2.4 Detection of HIV Infected Blood Products and Vaccines

Gene diagnosis is preferably used for primary screening of HIV contaminations on blood products and vaccines because it is time saving, reliable and inexpensive.

References

1. Church JD et al. Comparison of laboratory methods for analysis of non-nucleoside reverse transcriptase inhibitor resistance in Ugandan infants. AIDS Res Hum Retroviruses. 2009;25(7):657–63.
2. Kellam P, Larder BA. Recominant virus assay: a rapid, phenotypic assay for assessment of drug susceptibility of human immunodeficiency virus type 1 isolates. Antimicrob Agents Chemother. 1994;38(1):23–30.
3. Drmanac S et al. Accurate sequencing by hybridization for DNA diagnostics and individual genomics. Nat Biotechnol. 1998;16(1):54–8.
4. Petropoulos CJ et al. A novel phenotypic drug susceptibility assay for human immunodeficiency virus type 1. Antimicrob Agents Chemother. 2000;44(4):920–8.
5. Descamps D et al. Line probe assay for detection of human immunodeficiency virus type 1 mutations conferring resistance to nucleoside inhibitors of reverse transcriptase: comparison with sequence analysis. J Clin Microbiol. 1998;36(7):2143–5.
6. Vahey M et al. Performance of the Affymetrix GeneChip HIV PRT 440 platform for antiretrovital drug resistance genotyping of human immunodeficiency virus type 1 clades and viral isolates with length polymorphisms. J Clin Microbiol. 1999;37(8):2533–7.

An Overview of Clinical Immunology of HIV/AIDS

Contents

2.1 Defense Mechanism of Organisms

2.1.1 Non-specific Immunity

Innate immunity is the first line of defense in infection control. The key to control HIV infection and its progression lies in the host's immune defense. The immunity against infections can be divided into two types, non-specific immunity, also referred to as the innate immunity, and specific immunity, also known as adaptive/acquired immunity.

Innate immunity is already equipped at the time of birth. As the first line of defense, innate immunity has the ability to protect the body rapidly against infection and to trigger adaptive immune responses. The innate immunity consists of skin and mucosal epithelia, phagocytes and NK cells, as well as a series of soluble factors, such as cytokines, chemokines, and small molecular substances, like complements and Mannan-binding lectin (MBL) (see Table 2.1). All these factors constitute the rapid response system to protect human body against infections, whose functions to prevent the spreading of infections.

As antigen presenting cells, dentritic cells and mononuclear cells play roles in both innate and specific immunity. In addition to the natural barrier of skin mucosa, and cells components mentioned above, the innate immunity also includes some soluble factors. These factors either directly involve in fighting microorganisms, such as IFN-α/β or indirectly via reinforcing cell reactions, such as NK cells reaction. The innate immunity also enhances the expression of MHC in effector cells to strengthen the immunity of lymphocytes against pathogens. In addition, innate immunity participates in the activation of intracellular signal bypass, which is achieved by the recognition of the receptors at the surface of antigen presenting cells, namely TLRs (Toll-like receptors). As a result, the NFκB (nuclear factor-activated T cells) are activated to induce the expression of cytokine with different immunologic functions [1].

Other differences between innate immunity and specific immunity include: (1) Innate immunity has a quick response

H. Li (ed.), *Radiology of HIV/AIDS*,
DOI 10.1007/978-94-007-7823-8_2, © Springer Science+Business Media Dordrecht and People's Medical Publishing House 2014

Table 2.1 Components of the innate immunity

Cellular component	Soluble factors
Dentritic cells	Cytokines
Macrophages	Chemokines
Neutrophils	Definsins
NK cells	APOBEC
γδT cells	Complement
NK-T cells	Lectin-binding proteins
Plasmacytoid dendritic cells	Acute-phase reactants
CD8+T cells	Mannan-binding lectin, MBL
B-1 cells	

(within minutes to days), while specific immunity is a delayed reaction (within days to weeks); (2) Innate immunity is a direct reaction against infection, while specific immunity targets at the specific antigen peptide of pathogens; (3) Innate immunity is non-specific, with no immunological memory, which can be repeatedly activated by appropriate factors, while specific immunity has immunological memory, with quicker and stronger responses to the recurrent infections.

2.1.2   Specific Immunity

The primary infection of HIV usually causes a strong specific immune response in human body. The specific immune response can be categorized into humoral immune response and cellular immune response.

2.1.2.1 Humoral Immune Response

Infections of HIV proteins can stimulate the human body to produce antibodies. Generally, after 2–12 weeks of HIV infection, B cells can produce a variety of specific antibodies against HIV proteins. Antibodies to IgM are firstly produced, targeting at the regions of gag and env, but with a brief persistence. Antibodies to IgG are produced slightly later, firstly those targeting at regions of p24, gpl20, gp160 and p41, with a longer persistence. Neutralizing antibodies are produced later on, with only antibodies against envelope proteins having the anti-viral neutralizing activity. With the emergence of large amount antibodies, the viruses are largely cleared; and others are captured by the dendritic cells in lymph nodes. With the decreased virus in blood, the primary HIV infection progresses into chronic infection. Generally, after neutralizing antibodies are produced in virus infections, they can bind to and eliminate the viruses. Therefore, this neutralizing activity is commonly used to assess the anti-viral immunity. But HIV-infected patients largely have low concentration and affinity of neutralizing antibody, which plays a protective role in early phase of infection or in long-term non-progressive infection. Enhancing antibodies are also produced in HIV-infected patients, which contribute to viral infections. And even some

neutralizing antibodies have enhanced activity after diluted. In addition, neutralizing antibodies with the same specificity in different individuals may show a opposite activity to inhibit or enhance HIV infections. Therefore, simple use of antibodies or neutralizing antibodies production cannot sufficiently assess the immunity against HIV.

2.1.2.2 Cellular Immune Response

In HIV infected patients, cell-mediated immune response plays an important role in the control and removal of the infectious agents. Cellular immune responses mainly include CD4+ T lymphocytes immune response, the cytotoxic effect of cytotoxic T lymphocytes (CTL), natural killer cells (NK) immune response and CD8+ cell-mediated non-cytotoxic antiviral effects. Various HIV structures and regulatory proteins (ENV, GAG, POL, NFF and RT) can cause specific cellular immune response. But unlike antibody reactivity, the strength and range of the cellular immune response have obvious individual differences.

2.1.3   Cytokines

In addition to the direct regulation of HIV expression or latency in virus infected cells, cytokines play a more important role in the modulation of immune responses and maintenance of immune balance. Many cytokines can up-regulate the expression of HIV [2, 3]; some cytokines, such as GM-CSFB, can induce the expression of proviral HIV during the incubation period. TNF-α can up-regulate the expression of HIV by means of paracrine and exocrine. TNF-α and IL-6 have a synergistic and promoting effect on the expression of HIV in mononuclear cells. Among the cytokines down-regulating the expression of HIV, IFN-α, IFN-β and IL-10 play definitive roles. But IFN-γ, TCF-β, IL-4 and IL-13 demonstrate two different effects according to the differences in target cells, their activations and differentiations, status of virus infection, as well as interactions between different cytokines [4, 5]. Cytokines have multiple functions in the human body. In addition to increasing the expression of HIV, TNF-α is also an important inflammatory mediator and cachectin, which exerts an important role in pathogenesis of AIDS. In addition to promoting the expression of HIV and inducing cachectin, IL-6 is also related to the hyper-reaction of another immune characterized B cells in HIV infections. Additionally, IL-6 is related to the occurrence of B lymphocytes sarcoma.

2.1.4   Chemotactic Factors (CF)

Chemokine is a class of small molecules belonging to the super-family of cytokines. Chemokines and their receptors play important roles in the occurrence and development of

Fig. 2.1 Chemokine receptors and HIV infection. (**a**) T cells expressing receptors CD4 and CCR5 can be infected by HIV. (**b**) Chemokines can block the binding of HIV with CCR5. (**c**) Failed binding with mutated CCR5, no infection of T cells

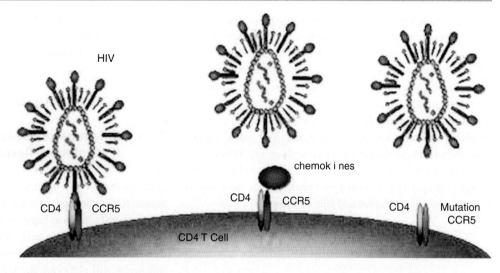

many pathologic and physiologic processes, such as inflammation (including allergic inflammation), removal of the exterior pathogens, development of tissues and organs, the growth and metastasis of carcinomas, and immunodeficiency diseases. It was firstly discovered in 1996 that the chemokine receptor CXCR4 is the facilitative receptor for T-tropic HIV-1 invading T cells [6]. After that, it was discovered that CCR5 is the facilitative receptor for macrophage tropic HIV-1 infecting macrophage. Dean and his colleagues [7] have proved that the genetic mutation of CCR5 is associated with highly exposed and low-level infected populations. Studies in recent years have shown that some chemokines have an anti-HIV effect [8] (Fig. 2.1). HIV infection needs facilitations by chemokines receptors whose genetic mutation may change the susceptibility and the outcomes of HIV infection. On one hand, chemokines block the HIV-1 binding site by binding specifically with facilitative receptors. On the other hand, chemokines can down-regulate the expression of their facilitative receptors on the surface of HIV-1 susceptible cells. Therefore, chemokines and its derivatives are main components of facilitative receptor blockers.

2.2 Mechanism of Immune Response

2.2.1 Antiviral Immune Response

The innate immunity is the first line of defense for the human body to protect itself against HIV. Various innate immune cells and soluble factors play important roles in fighting against HIV infection. Most cytokines and substances from body fluids, such as saliva, tears and milk, are the components of innate immune system. Macrophages and dentritic cells bridge between the innate immunity and the acquired immunity. The non-cytotoxic anti-HIV effects of CD8+ cells have characteristics of innate immune response. Studies have demonstrated that astrocytes, DCs, macrophages, microglial cells and some

soluble factors (like complements and chemokines) can interfere and impact on central nervous system diseases caused by HIV. Inducing the innate immune activities with specific cytokines and their complexes can effectively slow the progression of AIDS. The conventional reaction of the hosts to virus infection is to produce antibodies, which bind with viruses to inactivate them. The major viral proteins associated with neutralization of antibodies locate on the exterior membrane of gp120 and gp41. According to studies, anti-gp120 antibody has selective reactivity to B subtype of HIV-1 and anti-gp41 antibody has reactivity to a wider subtype of HIV-1. The mechanism of antibody-mediated HIV neutralization is not clear yet. The capability of antibody to cover the envelope or to make the envelope protein shed from virion may determine the neutralizing ability of the antibody. Some CD4+ cells have CTL activity specific to virus infected or uninfected CD4+ cells or MHC-II molecules related HIV expressions of polypeptide cells. But its antiviral reaction is at a relatively low level. A majority of cells capable of specifically removing virus-infected cells are CD8+ cells, whose toxicity killing reaction is characterized by HLA restrictions and antigenic specificity. In addition, its toxicity killing reaction requires intercellular interactions. The HIV specific cytotoxicity is mainly achieved by CD8+ effector cells secreted by IFN-γ and TNF-α, especially the cellular subsets expressing perforin and CD107.

2.2.2 Antibacterial Immune Response

Bacterial infection is the common opportunistic infection in patients with HIV/AIDS, and it is also one of the major causes of their clinic visits and death. Mycobacterial disease, bacterial pneumonia, skin and intestinal bacterial infections and tuberculous meningitis are commonly encountered bacterial infections. Neutrophils and phagocytosis of neutrophils, mononuclear cells and macrophages as well as activation of complement system play important roles in eliminating bacteria. Bacterial endotoxin stimulates macrophages and vascular endothelial cells to produce inflammatory factors such as TNF, IL-1, IL-6 and chemokines, which can promote inflammatory responses and facilitate eliminating bacteria. Exocellular bacterial antigen can directly stimulate B cells to induce protective humoral immunity. Responses to main T cells of extracellular bacteria include CD4+ cells' response to MHC-II molecules binding proteins. The main immune responses to extracellular bacteria, such as mycobacterium, are mediated by CD4+ and CD8+ T cells. By producing IFN-γ, macrophages are activated to enhance their activities of phagocytosis, degradation and sterilization.

2.2.3   Antiparasitic Immune Response

CD4 T cell count obviously decreases in patients with HIV/AIDS. Some opportunistic parasites may cause serious and even fatal infections. Opportunistic parasites that cause intestinal infections in patients with AIDS include cryptosporidium, isospora, strongyloides stercoralis and microsporidia. Those cause pulmonary infections include pneumocystis and microsporidia. Those cause eyes infections include toxoplasma gondii, acanthamoeba and microsporidia. Those cause cerebral infections include toxoplasma gondii and acanthamoeba. In addition, toxoplasma gondii, strongyloides stercoralis and microsporidia can also cause general disseminated infections. Parasites gaining access to the blood circulation or tissue can adapt to and resist to the body's innate immunity for their survival and replication. Specific immunity is the principal mechanism for antiparasitic infection. Due to different structures and biochemical properties of different parasites, they induce different specific immune responses, including IgE medicated cytotoxicity depending on eosinophils, granuloma formation and fibrosis, specific CTL response and the effects of cytokines.

2.2.4   Anti-tumor Immune Response

Up to 40 % HIV-infected patients may develop carcinoma. The occurrence of carcinoma in HIV-infected patients is a three-stage process, namely initiation, promotion and transformation. Immunosuppression caused by HIV infection inhibits the normal immunological surveillance and the inhibition of transformative cells growth to initiate the occurrence of malignant tumor. After virus infection, the initiation can be induced by immunity induced cytokines, to promote the proliferation of B cells, endothelial and epithelial cells. High level abnormal secretions of some cytokines lead to secondary malignancies. Probably produced by super-responsive cells caused by immune system disturbance, these cytokines can induce cell proliferation, as well as virus activation. Finally, proliferations stimulated by cytokines or

direct effects of infectious agents cause chromosomal changes, leading to independent cellular growth and transformation, with final occurrence of carcinomas.

2.3   Allergic Response

2.3.1   Inflammatory Reaction Process (Pathological Response)

With the help of CD4 receptor and co-receptor, HIV gains access to human body. Its target cells include CD4 T cells, dendrtic cells, macrophages, CD8+ T cells, natural killer T cells and natural killer cells. Therefore, the tissue distribution of these target cells determines their organ tropism. The following will elaborate the inflammatory responses caused by HIV and its pathological process based on the distribution of these target cells of HIV invasion.

2.3.1.1 Lymphoid Organs
Many studies have demonstrated that HIV viral load in lymphoid organs is higher than that in peripheral blood. In the acute phase of HIV infection, the mucosa is the major locus of HIV infection. Gastrointestinal and other mucosal tissues contain nearly half of the T cells of the human body, predominantly CCR5+ in their active state. In the acute phase of infection, HIV rapidly replicates and proliferates in the mucosal lymphoid structures, resulting in the collapse of the immune system after infection. After the acute phase and during the chronic phase, HIV replication sites begin transferring to other lymphoid organs. High level HIV is concentrated in the lymph node follicular dendritic cells originated from epithelium. They are different from dendritic cells with hematopoietic origin. These cells constitute a reservoir of infectious HIV in the subsequent stage of infection. The viruses replicate in the lymph nodes and the subsequent T cells activation may destruct the structure of the lymph node [9]. Thymus and bone marrow are the major organs generating lymphocytes, also may be the replication sites of HIV. HIV infection in both adults and children can cause thymus degeneration and thymocytes elimination [10].

2.3.1.2 Central Nervous System
Central nervous system diseases caused by HIV infection demonstrate that the virus can persistently exist and replicate in the central nervous system. It has been proved that the viruses exist in brain macrophages, microglia and multinucleated giant cells and the virus can be isolated from the cerebrospinal fluid. So far, it is known that HIV can directly damage the microglia, but the pathogenesis of HIV-related neurological complications is still unknown. It has been speculated that HIV activates Tat factor. With the help of CD91, the Tat factor gains access to neurons, and destroys the integrity of the blood-brain barrier through the neurotoxicity of

nitric oxide [11]. The concentration of antiretroviral drugs in the cerebrospinal fluid is significantly lower than their serum concentration. Drug resistant strains are isolated from both serum and cerebrospinal fluid of the treated patients. These facts indicate that the currently applied anti-viral therapies fail to discontinue the replication of HIV in the central nervous system [12]. The study on HIV-related brain dementia found tiny glial cell nodules in 47 % patients with brain dementia.

2.3.1.3 Genitourinary Tract

Blood-testis barrier fails to prevent HIV from gaining access to sperm. Virus replications have already been observed in the sperm, renal epithelial T cells and macrophages. Kidney biopsy tissues from HIV-infected patients were performed in situ hybridization, which demonstrated that genitourinary tract is the reservoir for HIV virus. At the same time, HIV is also detected in cervical macrophages and lymphocytes. Being same as the central nervous system, it is difficult for anti-retroviral drugs to get access to these areas for an effective therapeutic concentration [13].

2.3.2 Pathophysiological Changes in Stress

In the initiating stage of HIV infection, namely the early stage of infection, the viruses proliferate locally at their access area to develop into viremia. Viremia is then controlled by an immediate strong immune response. Within 2–8 weeks after HIV infection and before positive seroconversion, the patients may show transient (1–12 weeks) clinical manifestations similar to infectious mononucleosis, including fever, lymphadenectasis, pharyngitis, arthralgia, fatigue, rash and sleepiness, occasionally accompanied by acute retroviral syndromes (ARS) like aseptic meningitis. The occurrence of these symptoms is approximately 40.9 % in patients during their acute phase of infection. During this period, the viruses rapidly proliferate in the human body to cause viremia, with plasma viral RNA reaching 10^5–10^8 copies/mL and serum P24 antigen above 100 pg/mL. These indices indicate the high levels of free virus and viral antigens in the blood circulation. But tests of anti-HIV-1 antibody are often negative. With the occurrence and development of immune response to HIV-1 infection, the levels of virus and viral antigen in the blood circulation of most patients significantly drop. In the early stage of infection, CD4+T cells count decreases, sometimes even to the level for occurrence of opportunistic infections [14]. It may be a direct result from virus infection, while it may also be the result of trapped CD4+T cells in peripheral lymphoid organs. After the early infection, with no any antiviral therapy, the level of CD4+T cells can slowly ascend, but still being lower than that before infection. In fact, not only the number of CD4+T lymphocytes declines, its function also undergoes substantial impairment

[15]. In this period, the number of CD8+T cells usually increases, which may be the result of the CTL immune response after infection. Observations indicated that multiple immune mechanisms play their roles in the early stage of HIV-1 infection. In the early stage, it is difficult to detect antibodies with neutralizing activity. Within 2–43 weeks after AIDS onset, anti-HIV-1 neutralizing antibody is detectable in serum and HIV-1-specific CTL may be produced earlier. Both play critical roles in the control of acute HIV-1 infection. In the acute phase of infection, CD8+T cells proliferate in a large scale, which is related to the decline of early viral load [16]. CD8+ T cells can directly kill target cells through dissolution. They can also secrete cytokines and chemokines to indirectly eliminate the virus [17].

2.3.3 Tissues Damage Related to Immune Response

Immune response of the host may also contribute to the occurrence of immune diseases, such as invasion of virus-infected and uninfected CD4 cells and cytotoxic T cells. The autoimmunity of host can also destruct T cells in HIV-infected patients. Antibodies against gp120 and gp41 can cross react with the type II HLA molecules, destroying those uninfected cells with the antibody dependent cellular cytotoxicity. On the one hand, the anti-viral immunity can neutralize the virus in plasma and clear the infected cells. On the other hand, HIV-specific CTL may impair the immune system. This activity can be used to fight against some cells, which make the virus envelope in the circulation bind with CD4 molecules on its surface. Antigen that induced by the virus in the lymphocytes or the autoantibodies of normal cells antigen produced by HIV with immunogenicity may led to immune diseases. These antibodies may also be resulted from the accompanying activation of polyclonal B cells to HIV infection. During infection, they may produce inhibitory gene T cells or other factors to impair the immune system. Finally, the antibodies enhancing virus infection may have effects on infection control against the host. Activated immune system is a manifestation of normal immune system, but persistent activation will cause some adverse consequences. Additionally, other cytokines such as IFN- can cause persistent virus infection, up-regulate the virus growth, and further lead to the activated and damaged immune system.

2.4 Immunity Reconstruction

Immunity reconstruction refers to the use of current medical means to recover the impaired immunity to normal level or close to the normal level. Concerning HIV infection, it is to restore the following immunity indices of HIV infected patients with appropriate therapies: (1) the decreased CD4+T cells count returns to normal and the restored ratio of CD4+/ CD8 to normal; (2) the CD4 T cells restore their normal responses to antigen, namely the newly produced cells have normal immune functions; (3) abnormal immunity is activated to restore normal. The currently applied measures for immunity reconstruction include:

1. Highly active antiretroviral therapy (HAART)

In 1997, Autran et al. [18] firstly reported the impact of HARRT on the immune system of HIV infected patients. After a period of treatment with HAART, T-cell count of the patients increased with a biphasic change, suggesting a successful immunity reconstruction. It decreases occurrence of and death rate from AIDS.

2. Intermittent structural therapy (STIs)

Although HAART successfully controls viremia in most patients with AIDS, some problems still hinder its application, such as drug toxicity, drug resistance and the high cost of treatment. Therefore, a novel therapeutic strategy has been proposed, intermittent structure therapy (STIs). It means application of antiviral drugs like cancer chemotherapy, administering anti-viral drugs for a period of time followed by drugs withdrawal, and then anti-viral drugs use again. By administering anti-viral drugs intermittently, virus replication is expected to be inhibited, leading to improved immunity.

3. IL-1 and IL-7

HAART marks a great progress in the treatment of HIV infection, but some problems exist though. Viremia is controlled in about 70 % patients after HAART administration, but increased CD4+ T cell count fails to occur [19]. Therefore, some novel strategies are still needed. Currently, the use of immunomodulatory agents has attracted great attention, and IL-2 is the most common one. IL-2 itself has no antiviral activity and its combined use with HAART is the common practice in clinical trials. Long-term use of low-dose IL-2, together with HAART can significantly increase the number and function of immature CD4+ T cells within 24 weeks. Meanwhile, the side effects of IL-2 are alleviated and the occurrence of clinical events is reduced [20]

2.5 Pharmacological Basis of Highly Active Antiretroviral Therapy (HARRT)

HE Da-yi, man of the year in 1996 by *Times* magazine, proposed that simultaneous use of three or more antiretroviral drugs, known as the triple therapy or highly active antiretroviral therapy (HAART) change the natural progression of AIDS.

All the antiretroviral drugs inhibit replication of HIV by interfering their lifecycle from their different stages. The drugs can be divided into six categories (see Table 2.2).

Table 2.2 Commonly used antiretroviral drugs approved by American FDA

Drug name	Trade name	Abbreviation	Ingredients
1. Nucleotide and nucleotide related reverse transcriptase inhibitors (NRTIs)			
Combivir	Combivir	CBV	AZT+3TC
Emtricitabine	Emtriva	FTC	Emtricitabine
Lamivudine	Epivir	3TC	Lamivudine
Zidovudine	Retrovir	AZT	Zidovudine
Videx	Videx	ddI	Didanosine
Abunidazole	Trizivir	TZV	AZT+3TC+ABC
Tenofovir	Viread	TDF	Tenofovir
Stavudine	Zerit	D4T	Stavudine
Abacavir	Ziagen	ABC	Abacavir
2. Non-nucleotide reverse transcriptase inhibitors (NNRTIs)			
Delavirdine	Rescriptor	DLV	Delavirdine
Efavirenz	Sustiva/Stocrin	EFV	Efavirenz
Nevirapine	Viramune	NVP	Nevirapine
Combinations	Atripla		EFV+TDF+FTC
3. Protease inhibitor (PIs)			
Tipranavir	Apivus	TPV	Tipranavir
Amprenavir	Agenerase	APV	Amprenavir
Indinavir	Crixivan	IDV	Indinavir
Saquinavir	Invirase500	SQV	Saquinavir
Lopinavir	Kaletra	LPV/r	Lopinavir/Ritonavir
Ritonavir	Norvir	RTV	Ritonavir
Atazanavir	Reyataz	ATV	Atazanavir
Fosamprenavir	Telzir/Lexiva	fAPV	Fosamprenavir
Nelfinavir	Viracept	NFV	Nelfinavir
Kaletra	Kaletra	LPV/r	LPV+RIV
4. Entry/fusion inhibitors			
Enfuvirtide	Fuzen	T-20	Enfuvirtide
5. Integnase inhibitors			
Raltegravir			Raltegravir
6. Co-receptor antagonist			
Celsentri	Celsentri/ Selzentry	MVC	Maraviroc

1. Nucleotide and nucleoside related reverse transcriptase inhibitors (NRTI)

Nucleotide analogue is a modified variant natural cell nucleotide substance. These purines and pyrimidine bases bind to the pentose ring, and then further phosphorylated by enzymes within the cells to be nucleotides, namely basic components of DNA and RNA. Nucleotides can be identified by reverse transcriptase of virus, and thus embedded in the expanded DNA chain. Nucleotides have no hydroxyl end that is necessary to continue the nucleotide spiral, so they are the terminators of the chain. The nucleotide drugs (such as tenofovir) act in a mechanism that is similar to NRTI, with a difference in their access to cells after phosphorylation.

2. Non-nucleoside reverse transcriptase inhibitors (NNRTI)

Via its combination to reverse transcriptase, conformational changes occur to inhibit its functions.

3. Protease inhibitor (PI)

Containing similar parts to important HIV protein fragments, PI can be identified by HIV protease and PI can inhibit the activity of the HIV protease. Therefore, the precursor protein fails to break into the functional structure proteins and enzymes, with consequent inhibition of the viral replication.

4. Entry/fusion inhibitors (EI/FI)

EI/FI are capable of preventing the fusion of HIV with the cell membrane, thus act to inhibit both wild strains and drug-resistant strains

5. Integnase inhibitors (IIs)

IIs acts to prevent the integration of HIV DNA to the host cell DNA, thus inhibit virus replication, new cell infections and the occurrence of virus reservoir.

6. Co-receptor antagonist

Co-receptor antagonist, such as CCR5 antagonist, acts to prevent CCR5-tropic HIV-1 from gaining its access to the target cells. Co-receptor antagonist is an ideal anti-HIV candidate drugs.

References

1. Bogdan C. The function of type I interferons in antimicrobial immunity. Curr Opin Immunol. 2000;12(4):419–24.
2. Fauci AS. Multifactorial nature of human immunodeficiency virus disease: implications for therapy. Science. 1993;262(5136):1011–8.
3. Poli G, Fauci AS. The role of monocyte/macrophages and cytokines in the pathogenesis of HIV infection. Pathobiology. 1992;60(4):246–51.
4. Emilie D et al. Cytokines from lymphoid organs of HIV-infected patients: production and role in the immune disequilibrium of the disease and in the development of B lymphomas. Immunol Rev. 1994;140:5–34.
5. Mikovits JA et al. IL-4 and IL-13 have overlapping but distinct effects on HIV production in monocytes. J Leukoc Biol. 1994;56(3):340–6.
6. Feng Y et al. HIV-1 entry cofactor: functional cDNA cloning of a seven-transmembrane, G protein-coupled receptor. Science. 1996;272(5263):872–7.
7. Dean M et al. Genetic restriction of HIV-1 infection and progression to AIDS by a deletion allele of the CKR5 structural gene. Hemophilia Growth and Development Study, Multicenter AIDS Cohort Study, Multicenter Hemophilia Cohort Study, San Francisco City Cohort, ALIVE Study. Science. 1996;273(5283):1856–62.
8. Oravecz T, Pall M, Norcross MA. Beta-chemokine inhibition of monocytotropic HIV-1 infection. Interference with a postbinding fusion step. J Immunol. 1996;157(4):1329–32.
9. Schacker TW et al. Collagen deposition in HIV-1 infected lymphatic tissues and T cell homeostasis. J Clin Invest. 2002;110(8):1133–9.
10. Haynes BF et al. The role of the thymus in immune reconstitution in aging, bone marrow transplantation, and HIV-1 infection. Annu Rev Immunol. 2000;118:529–60.
11. Liu Y et al. Uptake of HIV-1 tat protein mediated by low-density lipoprotein receptor-related protein disrupts the neuronal metabolic balance of the receptor ligands. Nat Med. 2000;6(12):1380–7.
12. Venturi G et al. Antiretroviral resistance mutations in human immunodeficiency virus type 1 reverse transcriptase and protease from paired cerebrospinal fluid and plasma samples. J Infect Dis. 2000;181(2):740–5.
13. Si-Mohamed A et al. Selection of drug-resistant variants in the female genital tract of human immunodeficiency virus type 1-infected women receiving antiretroviral therapy. J Infect Dis. 2000;182(1):112–22.
14. Gupta KK. Acute immunosuppression with HIV seroconversion. N Engl J Med. 1993;328(4):288–9.
15. Lichterfeld M et al. Loss of HIV-1-specific CD8⁺ T cell proliferation after acute HIV-1 infection and restoration by vaccine-induced HIV-1-specific CD4⁺ T cells. J Exp Med. 2004;6:701–12.
16. Borrow P et al. Virus-specific CD8⁺ cytotoxic T-lymphocyte activity associated with control of viremia in primary human immunodeficiency virus type 1 infection. J Virol. 1994;68(9):6103–10.
17. Cooper DA et al. Acute AIDS retrovirus infection. Definition of a clinical illness associated with seroconversion. Lancet. 1985;1(8428):537–40.
18. Autran B et al. Positive effects of combined antiretroviral therapy on CD4⁺ T cell homeostasis and function in advanced HIV disease. Science. 1997;277(5322):112–6.
19. Autran B et al. Restoration of the immune system with antiretroviral therapy. Immunol Lett. 1999;66(1–3):207–11.
20. De Paoli P et al. Changes in thymic function in HIV-positive patients treated with highly active antiretroviral therapy and interleukin-2. Clin Exp Immunol. 2001;125(3):440–6.

An Overview of Clinical Microbiology of HIV/AIDS

3

Contents

3.1 AIDS Related Pathogenic Microorganisms

3.1.1 Structure and Classification of Pathogenic Microorganisms

Due to compromised immunity and weakened defense function in patients with AIDS, opportunistic infections commonly occur. Nearly 80 % patients suffering from AIDS die from opportunistic infections. The pathogens causing opportunistic infections include the following four types: viruses, bacteria, fungi and parasites.

3.1.1.1 Virus Infection

Herpes viruses include varicella-zoster virus (VZV), cytomegalovirus (CMV), Epstein-Barr virus (EBV), herpes simplex virus type 1 (HSV-1) and herpes simplex virus type 2 (HSV-2). It is believed in literatures that in incidences of AIDS related opportunistic infections, CMV infection is only second to pneumocystis carinii infection. CMV infection is disseminating to infect almost all organs, with the most commonly infected including adrenal gland, lung and digestive tract. Herpes simplex virus (HSV) infections involve the skin and mucous membranes to cause local thin-walled herpes. In HIV infected patients, the incidence of lung diseases caused by herpes simplex virus infection is less than 2.2 %, including interstitial pneumonia with intra-interstitial infiltration of the mononuclear cells. Patients with AIDS have a higher occurrence of EB virus infection, 96 % patients being EBV antibodies positive. The infection rates of human herpesvirus type 6 (HIV-6), human herpesvirus type 7 (HIV-7) and human herpesvirus type 8 (HIV-8) are high in the general population. Their viral antigens can be detected in most AIDS patients, but with no detectable specific pathological changes.

3.1.1.2 Bacterial Infection

About 13–40 % of AIDS patients sustain bacterial infections, including escherichia coli, staphylococcus aureus, pseudomonas aeruginosa, haemophilus influenzae, streptococcus

H. Li (ed.), *Radiology of HIV/AIDS*,
DOI 10.1007/978-94-007-7823-8_3, © Springer Science+Business Media Dordrecht and People's Medical Publishing House 2014

pneumoniae, klebsiella pneumoniae, and mycobacterium. In Europe and America, mycobacterium is the third common opportunistic pathogen attacking patients with AIDS. In AIDS-related tuberculosis, pulmonary tuberculosis is the most common, followed by lymphoid tuberculosis, hepatobiliary tuberculosis and renal tuberculosis.

3.1.1.3 Fungal Infection

Various fungal infections occur in patients with AIDS. In the United States and Africa, during the periods of AIDS-related syndromes and AIDS, 58–81 % patients are fungus infected. By autopsy, the detection rate of fungal infection is 8–40 %. The common fungi are candida albicans, cryptococcus neoformans, aspergillus, mucor, histoplasma, coccidioides, and pneumocystis carinii.

Candida Albicans

Candida infection is the most common infection in patients with AIDS. By autopsy, its detection rate is approximately 25 %. The pulmonary candida infection occurs in 23 % patients with AIDS but a low incidence of brain or kidney candida infection.

Pneumocystis Carinii

In Europe and America, pneumocystis carinii is the most common pathogen causing opportunistic infection in AIDS patients. Its incidence rate is 54–85 % by pathological autopsy for patients with AIDS. Pneumocystis carinii infection causes interstitial pneumonia and alveolar pneumonia. The over proliferation of pulmonary bacteria and exudative lesions lead to its extrapulmonary dissemination along lymph or blood circulation. About 2.5 % patients show involved lymph nodes, bone marrow, spleen, liver, gastrointestinal tract, pancreas and other parts of body.

3.1.1.4 Parasitic Infections

AIDS-related parasitic opportunistic pathogens include toxoplasma gondii, cryptosporidium, isospora, giardia lamblia, entamoebiasis histolytica, microsporidia, strongyloides stercoralis, blastocystis hominis and leishmania donovani. Toxoplasma gondii and cryptosporidium are the most common pathogens.

3.1.2   Characteristics of Pathogenic Microorganisms

3.1.2.1 Protozoon
Toxoplasma

Toxoplasma is an intracellular parasitic protozoan, categorized into the top complexes subphyla, cryptosporidium classis, eucoccidia order. As a zoonotic disease, toxoplasma infection can infect people when HIV infection develops into AIDS, resulting in serious consequences of central nervous system damage and systemic disseminated infection. Toxoplasma infection is primarily an animal infectious disease caused by a parasitic protozoan, mouse toxoplasma. Its transmission routes in human include congenital infection from mother to fetus via placenta and acquired infection caused by eating raw or undercooked meat containing tissue cysticercosis.

Cryptosporidium

Cryptosporidium is a small sized coccidia parasite, surviving in a variety of vertebrates. The diseases caused by cryptosporidium are called cryptosporidiosis, which is a zoonotic disease with a prominent symptom of diarrhea.

3.1.2.2 Virus
Cytomegalovirus

Cytomegalovirus is a herpes DNA virus, with an extensive existence. Most CMV infected patients are asymptomatic. Human CMV homogeneously spreads, with its proliferation in human fibroblasts. But CMV infected patients can excrete the viruses through urine, saliva, feces, tears, breast milk and sperm. Thus, CMV infection can be transmitted via blood transfusion, mother's placenta, organ transplantation, sexual intercourse and breast milk feeding.

Herpes Simplex Virus

Herpes simplex virus is the most common pathogen attacking human body and human is its only natural host. The main transmission routes are direct contact and sexual contact. It also can be transmitted through droplets. The viruses gain their access to the human body via the respiratory tract, mouth, eyes, genital mucosa or lacerated skin. Pregnant woman can pass the virus to her baby during childbirth.

Elzatein-Barn Virus

Elzatein-Barn virus is also known as human herpes virus, commonly infecting the human oropharyngeal epithelial cells and B lymphocytes.

3.1.2.3 Fungus
Pneumocystis Carinii

Pneumocystis carinii had been thought to be a protozoan. Recently, scholars consider it to be a fungus. In its life history, it survives in lungs in two forms, sporozoites and trophozoites.

Candida Albicans

Candida albicans is commonly found in oral cavity of healthy population and is an opportunistic pathogen. It can invade many parts of the human body, including skin, mucous membrane, internal organs and central nervous system.

Cryptococcus

Cryptococcus is also known as torula histolytica, the saprophytes of the soil, pigeons, cow milk, and fruits. It can also survive in human mouth and is an opportunistic pathogen.

3.1.3 Pathogenicity of Pathogenic Microorganisms

The opportunistic infections are caused by conditional pathogenic factors, which cannot cause diseases when human immunity is normal due to their low pathogenicity. However, when the human immunity is compromised, these pathogenic microorganisms have a conditional opportunity to invade human body, causing diseases that are known as opportunistic infections. Therefore, opportunistic infections occur in the special physical situation of the AIDS patients. In fact, opportunistic infections are the major cause of death in AIDS patients. Findings by autopsy indicated that 90 % AIDS patients die from opportunistic infections. The following elaborates the pathogenicity of protozoa, viruses, fungi and bacteria.

3.1.3.1 Protozoa

Toxoplasma Infection

The AIDS patients with toxoplasmosis infection are commonly toxoplasmosis of the nervous system, with an incidence of 26 %. Its clinical manifestations are paralysis, focal neurological abnormalities, convulsions, disturbance of consciousness and fever. CT scanning demonstrated singular or multiple focal lesions. Examinations of histopathological sections or cerebrospinal fluid can find toxoplasma gondii. It is rare (incidence of about 1 %) to find toxoplasmosis with lungs involved.

Cryptosporidiosis

Cryptosporidium is a small protozoan parasitizing in domestic or wild animals. Its invasion of human by attaching to epithelial cells in the small intestine and colon causes malabsorptional diarrhea. The patients sustain large quantities of uncontrollable watery stools, more than 5–10 times daily. And their daily water loss can be up to 3–10 L. The death rate from it is as high as above 50 %. Its diagnosis can be defined by colonoscopic biopsy or by stool examination to find protozoan oocysts.

3.1.3.2 Viruses

Cytomegalovirus Infections

AIDS related cytomegalovirus infection commonly has clinical manifestations of hepatitis, cytomegalovirus pneumonia, cytomegalovirus retinitis, thrombocytopenia and leukopenia, skin rash. Its diagnosis can be defined by finding the inclusion bodies or isolating the virus in biopsy or autopsy specimens. According to autopsy by Guarda et al. on 13 cases of AIDS, the most common diagnosis is cytomegalovirus infections (12 cases), followed by Kaposi's sarcoma (10 cases). Cytomegalovirus infection in all 12 cases is disseminative, with 2 or more organs involved.

Herpes Simplex Virus Infections

Herpes simplex virus infection causes impaired skin and mucous membrane in AIDS patients, with perioral, external vaginal, perianal, back of the hand, esophageal, bronchial mucosa and intestinal mucosa involved. The most common is herpes simplex in lip margin and corner of the mouth. The lesion is a highly dense cluster of small blisters, with a slightly red base. Ulcer usually occurs after blisters scraped. The ulcers are large and deep with pain, accompanied by secondary infection. The symptoms are mostly severe, with a long-term progression. Tissues from the lesion can be cultured to find the herpes simplex virus. By biopsy, typical inclusion bodies can be found.

3.1.3.3 Fungi

Pneumocystis (Carinii) Pneumonia

Studies have proved that PCP is a fungal infection, instead of a protozoan infections. Until now, it is sometimes called as pneumocystis carinii in some documents and literatures. PCP is transmitted via respiratory tract, specifically via air and droplets. After healthy people are infected by HIV, their immunities are compromised. As a result, pneumocystis (carinii) obtains its conditional opportunity to invade human body and there to multiply itself in large amount. The alveoli are filled with exudates and various pneumocystis carinii, resulting in serious damage to the lungs. PCP is a common cause of death in AIDS patients and is the most serious opportunistic infection in more than 60 % AIDS patients. PCP occurs in about 80 % AIDS patients at least once. AIDS related PCP initially has clinical symptoms of progressive malnutrition, fever, general upset, weight loss and lymphadenectasis, followed by cough, difficulty breathing and chest pain. The whole progression lasts about 4–6 weeks. Signs of fever (89 %) and shortness of breath (66 %) are the most commonly found concerning the respiratory system, with lungs rales heard in some patients. PCP is frequently recurrent and serious, being a common cause of death in AIDS patients. The chest X-ray for patients with PCP found extensive infiltration of both lungs. But the chest X-ray of a few patients (about 23 %) may be normal or close to normal. The progression of PCP is acute, sometimes chronic, ended by death from respiratory failure due to progressive difficulty breathing and hypoxia. The death rate from PCP is up to 90–100 %.

Candidal Infection

Candida albicans is an opportunistic pathogenic fungus. When the defense system is weak or dysbacteriosis occurs, candida albicans is pathogenic, leading to candidal infection. Candidal infections can be categorized into cutaneous candidiasis and mucosal candidiasis. The later is commonly specified as thrush, a milky white coating on the oral mucosa, tongue and throat, gums or lips mucosa. The coating is susceptible to peeling off with exposure of its fresh and moist red base. Candidal infection is common in the advanced stage of serious diseases or in HIV-infected patients. For homosexuals with persistent thrush of unknown reasons, it is an indicator of HIV infection or progression into AIDS. Candida esophagitis causes swallowing difficulty and pain, or retrosternal pain. By esophagoscopy, irregular ulcers and white pseudomembrane can be found in esophageal mucosa. Other candida infections include candidal angular cheilitis, candidal vaginitis, candidal balanoposthitis, and organ candidal infection. The diagnosis of skin and mucosal candidiasis depends on clinical manifestations and laboratory tests on fungi.

Cryptococcosis

Cryptococcosis is an acute or chronic deep mycosis caused by cryptococcus neoformans infection. When the immune defense is weak, cryptococcus obtains chances to invade the human body via the respiratory tract, occasionally via the intestine or skin, leading to diseases. Cryptococcal meningitis is a common complication of AIDS, with a high death rate. The clinical manifestations include fever, headache, insanity, and meningeal irritation. Pulmonary cryptococcosis is subacute or chronic, with accompanying cough, thick phlegm, low grade fever, chest pain and fatigue. Chest X-ray findings are non-specific. And its diagnosis can be defined by clinical manifestations and laboratory tests on fungi.

3.1.3.4 Bacteria

Mycobacterium Tuberculosis

Tuberculosis often occurs in patients with HIV infection but no progression into AIDS. Its occurrence may probably due to the stronger virulence of mycobacterium tuberculosis than other AIDS-related opportunistic pathogens, such as pneumocystis carinii. Thus, tuberculosis is more likely to occur in early stage of immunodeficiency. In HIV infected patients with tuberculosis, 74–100 % substain pulmonary tuberculosis, whose signs and symptoms are often difficult to be differentiated from those of other AIDS-related lung diseases. AIDS patients usually have disseminative infections. The characteristic clinical finding of HIV-infected patients with concurrent tuberculosis is the high incidence of extrapulmonary tuberculosis, being up to 70 %. The most common findings of AIDS with extrapulmonary tuberculosis are

lymphadenitis and miliary lesions, with involvements of bone marrow, genitourinary tract and central nervous system.

Atypical Mycobacterium Infection

Atypical mycobacterium infection is one of the important complications of AIDS. It often involves the liver, lung, spleen, kidney, blood, bone marrow, gastrointestinal tract and lymph nodes. The clinical manifestations include fever, weight loss, malabsorption, lymphadenectasis and hepatosplenomegaly. Findings by laboratory tests are non-specific and its diagnosis can be defined by pathogen isolation, culture and biopsy.

Other Common Pathogenic Bacteria Infections

Pseudomonas aeruginosa, escherichia coli, salmonella typhi, and neisseria gonorrhoeae are other common pathogenic bacteria in patients with AIDS.

3.2   Methods of Clinical Specimen Collection

Specimens for AIDS related tests include blood, cerebrospinal fluid, secretions, excretions, and lymph node tissues. Specimen collection is critical for the accuracy and effectiveness of the laboratory tests.

3.2.1   Specimens for Virus Isolation, Nucleic Acid and Antigen Detection Should Be

3.2.1.1   Fresh

Blood samples for HIV immunoassay, such as blood samples for CD4[+] T lymphocyte counts, are required to be stored at room temperature, and to be detected within 24 h.

3.2.1.2   Storage

The virus in vitro is susceptible to death at room temperature. So the collected specimens should be submitted for laboratory tests as soon as possible. Specimens that cannot be immediately tested should be stored in a container with ice or dry ice before submission. Blood or body fluid specimens for HIV nucleic acid test should be stored at a low temperature for a short period of time. Frozen specimens should not be repeatedly thawed and frozen.

3.2.1.3   Uncontaminated

Specimens for HIV diagnosis should be uncontaminated. Specimens for genetic diagnosis particularly cannot be contaminated. Even a minor contamination by virus may result in false positive finding.

3.2.1.4 Biologically Safe

Comprehensive prevention measures should be observed in all operating procedures. Wearing gloves should be strictly observed for all operations. Blood collection from animals or patients should be performed by appropriately trained personnel. For blood collection from vein, specialized vacuum blood collector should be used instead of conventional needles and syringes to ensure the blood directly flow into the transport tube and/or culture tube with plugs.

3.2.2 Specified Procedures for Specimen Collection

3.2.2.1 Blood for Virus or Immunoassay
(1) Clean the surface of the skin for blood culture;
(2) Collect blood with the 5 mL EDTA vacuum collection tube (lavender top);
(3) Flip the test tube several times after collection;
(4) Specimens for immunoassay should not be refrigerated and tests must be performed within 24 h.

3.2.2.2 Body Fluid: Sterile Except for Urine and Cerebrospinal Fluid
(1) Sterilize the skin surface;
(2) Collect fluid with disinfected needles and syringes;
(3) Keep 10 mL fluid for analysis and transport the remaining specimens in sealed syringes;
   - For coexistent aerobic bacteria and anaerobic bacteria, apply anaerobic transporting bottles to ensure the survival of anaerobic microorganisms.
   - Keep 10 mL peritoneal fluid in blood culture bottle. Peritoneal fluid is the only body fluid that can be kept in the blood culture bottles.
   - For virus isolation, 3 mL or less body fluid should be stored in virus transporting media or sterile bottles.
   - Virus samples should be directly submitted at the temperature of 2–8 °C.

3.2.2.3 Cerebrospinal Fluid
(1) Lumbar puncture should be performed aseptically. The physician responsible for collecting specimens must wear a surgical gown, a face mask and gloves.
(2) Collect body fluid in appropriate volume according to the following requirements:
   - Bacteria culture: >1 mL
   - Fungi culture: 8–10 mL
   - Molecules test: >1 mL
   - Mycobacteria culture: 8–10 mL
   - Virus culture: >2 mL

3.3 Detection of Pathogenic Microorganisms in Opportunistic Infections

3.3.1 Pathogenic Tests in Opportunistic Infections

3.3.1.1 Virus Infections
Varicella-Zoster Virus (VZV) Infection
With typical clinical symptoms, VZV infection can be diagnosed with no laboratory tests. The definitive diagnosis of VZV infection can be made on Wright's or Giemsa staining of the tissue fragments at the base of herpes for eosinophilic inclusions. Otherwise, an electron microscope can be used to observe typical herpes virus for definitive diagnosis.

Cytomegaoviyns (CMV) Infection
Examination of cytomegalic inclusion: Giemsa or Wright's staining of the centrifugal precipitates of patient's urine or saliva, followed by microscopic observation of the giant cells of eosinophilic intranuclear inclusions. Giemsa or Wright's staining of the shed cells from tissue biopsy, followed by microscopic observation of the giant cells of eosinophilic intranuclear inclusions.

Virus isolation: after the specimens are inoculated into the human embryonic fibroblasts and CMV can be isolated.

Serological tests: Single serum specimen with anti-CMV antibody titer being 1:8 and positive indicates the examinee has a past history of infection; double serum specimens with anti-CMV antibody titer increasing at least four times have diagnostic significance.

Immunohistochemistry

CMV nucleic acid detection: samples DNA extracted for dot-blot hybridization or Southern Blot hybridization with a probe. PCR applicable.

Epstein-Barr Virus Infection
EB virus is difficult to be isolated and cultured. Serum IgM antibody of anti-Epstein-Barr virus positive indicates recent infection of EB virus. Serum IgG antibody detection has little clinical significance.

HSV-1 and HSV-2 Infections
For definitive diagnosis of HSV infection, herpes fluid or tissues at the base of ulcer should be collected from the herpes or ulcers, followed by their culture in human amniotic cells or human embryonic fibroblast cells or rabbit kidney cells. After culture for 24–48 h, cytopathic effect in the cultured cells can be observed, which indicates HSV infection. The suspected HIS infection can be confirmed by

immunofluorescence technique. After the specimens collection, Wright's or Giemsa staining, Gram staining or direct immunofluorescence staining can be selected for microscopic observation of multinucleated giant cells or eosinophilic intranuclear inclusions. Virus antigens can also be detected.

HHV-6, HHV-7 and HHV-8

In diagnosis of HHV-6 or HHV-7 infection, the blood, saliva, body cavity fluid, or herpes fluid can be cultured for detection of the pathogens. The infected cell lines in vitro can also be used to detect the specific virus antibody in serum of patient by using indirect immunofluorescence assay or ELISA. In addition, viral nucleic acid in the specimen can also be directly detected by using molecular hybridization or PCR.

Using HHV-8 infected B lymphocyte lines, serological tests for HHV-8 infection can be conducted in general population and AIDS patients.

3.3.1.2 Bacterial Infections
Staphylococcus Aureus Infection

After specimens collected from different lesions, smearing and Gram staining are performed for direct microscopic observations on the, arrangement and staining of the bacteria.

Streptococcus Pneumoniae Infection

After smearing, Gram staining and capsule staining of the specimens, spherical or oval Gram stain-positive bacteria can be microscopically observed. These bacteria have capsules, arranged in chains.

Haemophilus Influenzae Infection

The specimen of cerebrospinal fluid, nasopharyngeal secretions, pus or sputum is directly smeared, followed by Gram staining for microscopic observation. In addition, capsular swelling test can be performed with the influenza bacillus specific serum.

Mycobacterium Tuberculosis Infection

It can be detected directly or after bacterial concentrate. After acid-fast staining, bacilli could be found under a microscope. Or after bacterium culture and smear staining, bacilli could be observed. Or PCR or DNA probe can be used to detect the mycobacteria tuberculosis in the specimens.

Mycobacterium Avium Infection

Its microbiological examination is similar to the method for detecting TB bacilli, but the bacterial colony is thin and transparent. In addition, immunoassay can be used to detect the specific antigens in specimens. Frequency pulsed electron capture gas–liquid chromatography can also be used to detect tuberculostearic acid in bacteria.

Last but not least, specific RNA or DNA probe can be used for hybridization test. PCR is also an alternative method.

3.3.1.3 Fungal Infection
Pneumocystis Carinii Infection

To define the diagnosis of pneumocystis carinii infection, the collected sputum, organ secretions or lavage fluid and pulmonary biopsy tissue specimens should be prepared into smears, imprints or tissue sections. After staining and microscopy, definitive diagnosis can be made. The most recent diagnostic methods include antibody test [3]. In addition, by S-adenosylmethionine measurement, the patient with pneumocystis carinii infection has lower level of S-adenosylmethionine [26].

Cryptococcus Neoformans Infection

Suspected cases of cryptococcus neoformans infection should receive cerebrospinal fluid examination. Cryptococcus neoformans antigen titer in patients cerebrospinal fluid is high, and the positive rate by blood culture is also high. In addition, after residues of cerebrospinal fluid is smeared and stained by India ink or Congo red aqueous solution, the fungi can be observed under a microscope.

Histoplasma Capsulatum Infection

In the cultured blood or tissues, histoplasma capsulatum in oval shapes can be observed.

Candida Infection

To define the diagnosis of candida infection, specimens should be collected from the lesion for examination. Biopsy can also be used. To define the diagnosis of fungal esophagitis, hyphae invaded tissues must be observed under a microscope. Positive blood culture can be definitively diagnosed as disseminative candidia infection.

Aspergillus Infections

To define the diagnosis of aspergillus infection, the pathogenic bacteria must be isolated from the tissue of lesion or blood culture.

3.3.1.4 Protozoal Infection
Toxoplasma Gondii Infection

Sabin-Feldman staining exclusion test or indirect fluorescent antibody test can be used to detect the serum toxoplasma specific antibody. DNA probe and PCR amplification can be used to detect the pathogenic nucleic acid.

Cryptosporidium Infection

To define the diagnosis of cryptosporidium infection, patients stool should be examined for eggs of cryptosporidium. In addition, indirect immunofluorescence assay can be used to detect the pathogens in the specimens.

3.4 Quality Control in Microbiology Laboratory

Quality control in laboratories is the basis for interlaboratory quality control, while interlaboratory quality control tests and verifies the quality control in laboratories. Quality is the life of the clinical microbiologic laboratory. An AIDS-related clinical microbiologic laboratory requires the following operations in quality control.

3.4.1 Maintenance of Equipments in Clinical Microbiologic Laboratory

The commonly used equipments in clinical microbiologic laboratory include: bacterial culture instrument, bacterial identification and drug sensitivity testing instrument, microscopes, autoclaves, thermostatic incubator, scales, refrigerators, water bath box, and turbidimeter. The maintenance of these equipments is essential for the quality of the testing results. The maintenance of their functions and the maintenance frequency refer to the users' manual provided by the manufacturer. For unspecified detail about the maintenance of instruments or the lab is incapable of the maintenance, the maintenance should be performed by negotiation with and assistance by the manufacturer at least once a year.

3.4.2 Quality Control of Bacterial Isolation and Identification

3.4.2.1 Quality Control of Culture Media
Two aspects of quality control are requested for the quality of the culture media. The first is aseptic test and known bacteria growth test. Aseptic test is to sample randomly 3–5 % culture media for a culture of 48 h at 35 °C. Each batch of culture media should be performed aseptic test at least once. The prerequisite for known bacteria growth test is that the laboratory has sufficient reserves of known bacteria, including the standard strains (such as ATCC or NCTC standard strain) and the already identified clinical isolates. If possible, standard strains should be used. The expected results of known bacteria growth test should be defined. Each batch of culture media should be performed known bacterial growth test for at least once.

3.4.2.2 Quality Control of Bacteria Staining
The quality of the staining fluid and contamination should be checked daily before use.

3.4.2.3 Quality Control of Reagents
Purchase of new reagents; batch number replacement of the reagents; replacement of the manufacturer; abnormal findings and other unexpected findings should be performed quality control with appropriate standard strains.

3.4.3 Quality Control of Fungi Isolation and Identification

3.4.3.1 Fungi Smear
Specimens smear of sterile body fluid should be conducted centrifugal concentration to increase the positive rate. Mycelium should be definitely detected. Sputum and oral specimens should be quantitatively (colony count) or semi-quantitatively (indicating with a plus sign, rich growth in all the three districts by the partition line is reported as + + +, and two districts growth is + +, one district growth is +) indicated. Tissue specimens should be ground for preparation of smear, but the morphology of the mycelium should be protected. Smears should not be less than three pieces, if possible.

3.4.3.2 Fungi Identification
For yeast-like fungi, such as candidiasis or cryptococcosis, there have been mature methods to detect them in conventional clinical bacterial laboratories. Fungi should be identified with chromogenic media or automation system. Conventional identification of filamentous fungi is mainly dependent on its morphological changes and characteristics in its growth. Therefore, professional short-term training is required for personnel who performs filamentous fungi detection. Laboratories should establish a standardized smears identification method. Yeast-like fungi, filamentous fungi, mucor and spergillus (with top capsule) should be correctly identified. The rarely found fungi reported as contaminating fungi should be cautiously performed.

3.4.4 Quality Control of Drug Sensitivity Test

3.4.4.1 Establishing Reasonable Categories of Routine Drug Sensitivities
Antibacterial spectrum of different antibiotics is different, with different antibacterial strength and different bacterial drug resistance spectrum. Therefore, it is necessary to establish the correct categories of routine drug sensitivities of different pathogenic bacteria. Incorrect reports of drug sensitivities categories may mislead the physicians. According to requirements by CLSI and the drug use routines, the categories of routine drug sensitivities should be established.

3.4.4.2 Quality Control of the Drug Sensitivities to Special Bacteria
For some drug-resistant strains, such as the high-level aminoglycoside-resistant enterococci, oxacillin-resistant staphylococcus aureus and vancomycin-resistant enterococci, the specific procedures of IQC, strains for quality control and expected results of quality control should be referred to in the recent CLSI guidelines. The quality control should be simultaneously performed with clinical strain test.

Extended Reading

1. Autran B et al. Positive effects of combined antiretroviral therapy on CD4$^+$ T cell homeostasis and function in advanced HIV disease. Science. 1997;277(5322):112–6.

2. Autran B et al. Restoration of the immune system with antiretroviral therapy. Immunol Lett. 1999;66(1–3):207–11.

3. Bishop LR, Kovacs JA. Quantitation of anti-Pneumocystis jiroveci antibodies in healthy persons and immunocompromised patients. J Infect Dis. 2003;187(12):1844–8.

4. Bogdan C. The function of type I interferons in antimicrobial immunity. Curr Opin Immunol. 2000;12(4):419–24.

5. Borrow P et al. Virus-specific CD8$^+$ cytotoxic T-lymphocyte activity associated with control of viremia in primary human immunodeficiency virus type 1 infection. J Virol. 2001;68(9):6103–10.

6. Church JD et al. Comparison of laboratory methods for analysis of non-nucleoside reverse transcriptase inhibitor resistance in Ugandan infants. AIDS Res Hum Retroviruses. 2009;25(7):657–63.

7. Cooper DA et al. Acute AIDS retrovirus infection. Definition of a clinical illness associated with seroconversion Lancet. 1985;1(8428):537–40.

8. De Paoli P et al. Changes in thymic function in HIV-positive patients treated with highly active antiretroviral therapy and interleukin-2. Clin Exp Immunol. 2001;125(3):440–6.

9. Dean M et al. Genetic restriction of HIV-1 infection and progression to AIDS by a deletion allele of the CKR5 structural gene. Hemophilia Growth and Development Study, Multicenter AIDS Cohort Study, Multicenter Hemophilia Cohort Study, San Francisco City Cohort, ALIVE Study. Science. 1996;273(5283):1856–62.

10. Descamps D et al. Line probe assay for detection of human immunodeficiency virus type 1 mutations conferring resistance to nucleoside inhibitors of reverse transcriptase: comparison with sequence analysis. J Clin Microbiol. 1998;36(7):2143–5.

11. Drmanac S et al. Accurate sequencing by hybridization for DNA diagnostics and individual genomics. Nat Biotechnol. 1998;16(1):54–8.

12. Emile D et al. Cytokines from lymphoid organs of HIV-infected patients: production and role in the immune disequilibrium of the disease and in the development of B lymphomas. Immunol Rev. 1944;140:5–34.

13. Fauci AS. Multifactorial nature of human immunodeficiency virus disease: implications for therapy. Science. 1993;262(5136):1011–8.

14. Feng Y et al. HIV-1 entry cofactor: functional cDNA cloning of a seven-transmembrane, G protein-coupled receptor. Science. 1996;272(5263):872–7.

15. Gupta KK. Acute immunosuppression with HIV seroconversion. N Engl J Med. 1993;328(4):288–9.

16. Haynes BF et al. The role of the thymus in immune reconstitution in aging, bone marrow transplantation, and HIV-1 infection. Annu Rev Immunol. 1966;118:529–60.

17. Kellam P, Larder BA. Recombinant virus assay: a rapid, phenotypic assay for assessment of drug susceptibility of human immunodeficiency virus type 1 isolates. Antimicrob Agents Chemother. 1994;38(1):23–30.

18. Lichterfeld M et al. Loss of HIV-1-specific CD8$^+$ T cell proliferation after acute HIV-1 infection and restoration by vaccine-induced HIV-1-specific CD4$^+$ T cells. J Exp Med. 2004;6:701–12.

19. Liu Y et al. Uptake of HIV-1 tat protein mediated by low-density lipoprotein receptor-related protein disrupts the neuronal metabolic balance of the receptor ligands. Nat Med. 2000;6(12):1380–7.

20. Mikovits JA et al. IL-4 and IL-13 have overlapping but distinct effects on HIV production in monocytes. J Leukoc Biol. 1994;56(3):340–6.

21. Oravecz T, Pall M, Norcross MA. Beta-chemokine inhibition of monocytotropic HIV-1 infection. Interference with a postbinding fusion step J Immunol. 1996;157(4):1329–32.

22. Petropoulos CJ et al. A novel phenotypic drug susceptibility assay for human immunodeficiency virus type 1. Antimicrob Agents Chemother. 2000;44(4):920–8.

23. Poli G, Fauci AS. The role of monocyte/macrophages and cytokines in the pathogenesis of HIV infection. Pathobiology. 1992;60(4):246–51.

24. Schacker TW et al. Collagen deposition in HIV-1 infected lymphatic tissues and T cell homeostasis. J Clin Invest. 2002;110(8):1133–9.

25. Si-Mohamed A et al. Selection of drug-resistant variants in the female genital tract of human immunodeficiency virus type 1-infected women receiving antiretroviral therapy. J Infect Dis. 2000;182(1):112–22.

26. Skelly M et al. S-adenosylmethionine concentrations in diagnosis of Pneumocystis carinii pneumonia. Lancet. 2003;361(93650):1267–8.

27. Vahey M et al. Performance of the Affymetrix GeneChip HIV PRT 440 platform for antiretroviral drug resistance genotyping of human immunodeficiency virus type 1 clades and viral isolates with length polymorphisms. J Clin Microbiol. 1999;37(8):2533–7.

28. Venturi G et al. Antiretroviral resistance mutations in human immunodeficiency virus type 1 reverse transcriptase and protease from paired cerebrospinal fluid and plasma samples. J Infect Dis. 2000;181(2):740–5.

Part II

General Review on HIV/AIDS in Clinical Medicine

Contents

4.1 Pathogens

In the year of 1983, a special kind of virus was initially isolated from the blood of a patient with AIDS [1]. Later, the virus was named human immunodeficiency virus (HIV). With the enlarged population of AIDS patients globally, the isolated virus showed variances. Thus, the virus was classified into two types, namely HIV-1 and HIV-2. HIV-1 has been known to have a widespread and a earlier identification. With recently advanced molecular biology technology, polymerase chain reaction (PCR) was applied to characterize HIV-1 into seven subtypes, namely A, B, C, D, E, F and G. The following is of the knowledge about HIV-1.

HIV is a membrane-budding retrovirus. Structurally, it is a symmetrically cubic icosahedron spheroid particle with a diameter of 100–140 nm. It grossly is composed of a compact conical core and viral envelope. Its nucleocapsid is composed of P24 Gag viral capsid protein, containing two identical positive single-stranded RNA, transcriptase (P51/P56), integrase (P32) and stromatin (P9 and P6). The viral envelope has a framework of two layers lipid membranes, with a surface containing 72 spikes (glycoprotein compound). Each spike is composed of surface glycoprotein GP120 and one transmembrane protein GP41 trimer. GP120 combines with the cell receptor (mainly CD4 T cell). Stromatin P17 attaches to the inner lipid membrane and links between the membrane and the stroma of the core, for stabilization.

The viral genome consists of totally nine genes, including three structural genes (*gag, pol, env*), three regulatory genes (*tat, rev, nef*), and three virus infectors (*vif, vpr, vpu/vpx*) (*vpx* in HIV-2). Their functions are listed in Table 4.1.

HIV can survive for more than 15 days at room temperature (22–27 °C) in liquid circumstance. However, it is sensitive to heat. Temperature of 56 °C for 30 min deprives HIV of its infectivity to T lymphocytes in vitro and partially inactivates HIV in serum. Commonly, after being at a temperature of 60 °C for 3 h or at a temperature of 80 °C for 30 min, no infectious virus can be detected. As a result, WHO recommends a temperature of 100 °C for 20 min to inactivate

H. Li (ed.), *Radiology of HIV/AIDS*,
DOI 10.1007/978-94-007-7823-8_4, © Springer Science+Business Media Dordrecht and People's Medical Publishing House 2014

Table 4.1 Functions of genes

Category	Gene	Function
Structural Genes	Group specific antigen (gag)	To code the core proteins p24, p17, etc.
	Polymerase (pol)	To code polymerases and integrases.
	Envelope (env)	To code envelope proteins, p120 and gp41
Regulatory Genes	Transactivator (tat)	To positively regulate HIV genes
	Regulator of expression of virion proteins (rev)	To enhance the expression of gag and env for the structural proteins
	Negative factor (nef)	To suppress the multiplication of HIV
Viral Infectors	Virion infectivity factor (vif)	To enhance intracellular multiplication and the infectivity of HIV, assisted by some cytokines
	Viral protein, R (vpr)	To accelerate the production of viral protein
	Viral protein, U (vpu)	To promote the release of HIV-1 from the cell membrane
	Viral protein, X (vpx)	To be required in HIV-2 multiplication in lymphocytes and macrophages; to enhance the formation of virions

the retrovirus. HIV has no resistance to acid, with a pH value of 3.0 decreasing logarithmically the virus titer by 4. However, it is resistant to alkali, with a pH value of 9.0 slightly decreasing the virus titer. It is worthy noting that the virus is quite sensitive to chemicals of disinfectants and decontaminants. In 0.2 % potassium hypochlorite, 0.1 % domestic bleaching powder, 0.1 % glutaric dialdehyde, 0.5 % NP40, 0.5 % paraformaldehyde or 30 % alcoholic solution for 5 min, or in 20 % alcoholic solution for 10 min, HIV can be inactivated.

4.2 Sources of Infections

As far as we know, human is the only host or source of infection of HIV. Chimpanzees are sensitive to HIV and a strain of retrovirus similar to HIV-1 was once isolated from a chimpanzee captured in mid Africa. Evidence so far still is still weak to be persuasive for animals as the source of infection of the disease. HIV has been isolated from blood, sperm, cerebrospinal fluid, saliva, tears, cervical discharge, urine, breast milk, brain tissue and lymph node of infected persons. However, its spreading is via blood, sperm and cervical discharge, from which the virus is the most frequently isolated with the strongest infectivity. The asymptomatic infected persons as well as the infected persons with negative antibody are more epidemiologically dangerous. In order to define the diagnosis of AIDS, the serum should be tested for HIV antibody. The epidemiological studies using such test should pay focused attention to the following cases: (1) false-positive findings caused by serum contents of human leukocyte antigen (HLA), antinuclear antibody, autoantibody or plasmodium antigen and false positive findings caused by heated serum at 56 °C; (2) negative findings in end-stage patients or extremely weak patients; (3) rare occurrence of negative antibody but positive antigen.

4.3 Routes of Transmission and Population Distribution

HIV survives in blood, sperm, vaginal discharge and breast milk of infected persons. Therefore, its transmission routes include sexual contacts (heterosexual, homosexual or bisexual), blood and blood products (sharing the needle for intravenous drug abuse, interventional medical operations), vertical mother-to-child transmission (ante partum, partum, post-partum). Daily life contacts including shaking hands, hugging, etiquette kissing, eating and drinking together, sharing toilets or bathrooms, sharing offices and public transportations and sharing entertaining facilities do not transmit HIV/AIDS.

The susceptible populations of HIV/AIDS refer to male homosexuals, intravenous drug abusers, hemophilic patients, and people receiving blood transfusion or blood products and people having sexual intercourse with person from above mentioned high risk populations.

1. Male homosexuals, including bisexuals is the high risk population due to the anal sex. But homosexual is not equal to AIDS patient.
2. Drug abusers. The intravenous drug abusers account for about 15–17 % in patients with HIV/AIDS. The recurrent use of disinfected or incompletely disinfected syringes, needles is the cause of HIV/AIDS spreading in such populations. Thus, drug abusers constitute the second large population suffering HIV/AIDS. In addition, many drug abusers are simultaneously homosexuals or sexual abusers. The occurrence of AIDS is higher in the population with overlapping of these spreading routes. It has been reported that the women with sexual contacts to male drug abusers has a 30 times higher occurrence of HIV/AIDS than the general populations, indicating the high incidence of HIV/AIDS caused by drug abuse.
3. Hemophilic patients constitute the third largest susceptible population. HIV/AIDS infected hemophilic patients

account for about 1 % in patients with HIV/AIDS. It is related to their infusion of exogenous coagulation factors VII (IX). It has been reported that about 6–8 % blood donors in the U.S. are HIV carriers. As a result, some hemophilic patients are infected by HIV/AIDS via blood transfusion of coagulation factors VII (IX). In addition, based on the analysis for hemophilic patients, slight dysfunction of lymphocytes was found. For such patients with slightly compromised immunity, susceptibility to HIV/AIDS is resulted in.

4. Populations receiving blood or blood products transfusion. In addition to antihemophilic blood products, transfusion of blood or other blood products (concentrated blood cells, platelet and fresh frozen plasma) is related to the spreading of HIV/AIDS.

5. Populations having sexual contacts to high risk populations. The population that has sexual contacts with the above mentioned high risk populations is another susceptible population of HIV/AIDS. It is possible to be infected by HIV/AIDS for people having sexual relationship with homosexuals, hemophilic patients, recipients of blood transfusion and intravenous drug abusers.

4.4 Characteristics of HIV Epidemic

Recent years, the prevalence of HIV/AIDS increases rapidly. In terms of age, HIV/AIDS patients vary greatly, almost found in each age group. But 90 % cases are under the age of 50 years and two age groups see the most frequent occurrence, namely the adult age group with their ages ranging from 20 to 40 years and the infant group. According to a study from the U.S., 21,726 cases of AIDS are mainly young and middle aged. Specifically, 89 % cases are at the age of 20–49 years and 47 % at the age of 30–39 years. A cases study from Zaire found that the average age of patients with AIDS is 33.6 years and three-fourth of them ages between 20 and 39 years, indicating predominantly young patients with AIDS. Previous studies found that the majority of young patients with AIDS are male. But recent data suggested the increasing number of female patients. Their infections at a young age (below 20 years) are mainly due to the use of blood products and as recipients of blood transfusion. It has been reported that 72 % of teenagers aged between 15 and 16 years are infected by HIV/AIDS via blood products use or blood transfusion. However, as they grow up, HIV/AIDS infection caused by blood transfusion is decreasing. At the age of 17–19 years, the infection rate via blood transfusion decreases drastically to 20 %, while the infection rate via sexual behaviors is increasing, from 9 % at age of 13–14 years to 24 % at the age of 17–19 years and 69 % at the age of 17–18 years. More than 90 % of the male patients aged from 20 to 24 years is infected via sexual contacts, with 36 %

due to homosexual behaviors and 7 % due to a history of intravenous drug abuse. In female patients, the most common cause of the infection is heterosexual contacts (about 44 %), followed by intravenous drug abuse (about 28 %). Due to the variance in gender, ethnic group and races, the incidence of HIV/AIDS infection and its causes at a young age vary. In teenagers of U.S.A., at the age of 13–19 years, the incidence of HIV/AIDS infection in males (18 per million) is 4.5 times as high as female patients (4 per million). The incidence in the black (27 per million) is 3.8 times as high as in Caucasians. The incidence in Latin Americans (25 per million) is 3.6 times as high as Caucasians. Among Caucasian teenagers, 50 % is infected via blood products and other 24 % via homosexual contacts. In the blacks, 44 % is infected via homosexual contacts, and other 19 % via heterosexual contacts. In Latin American teenaged patients, 35 % is infected via intravenous drug abuse, and other 29 % via homosexual contacts. Heterosexual contacts and intravenous drug abuse in the black and Latin American teenaged patients outweigh those in Caucasian teenaged patients because the majority of patients in the black and Latin American teenaged patients are females. And, mother patients can transmit HIV/AIDS to their fetus or infants via placenta, birth canal and breast milk. Therefore, their children are also a susceptible population. In terms of geographic distribution, the latest data from UNAIDS indicated that most AIDS-infected patients live in the area south to Sahara in Africa. This area has only 10 % of the global population but 60 % of global AIDS-infected population. In this area, female patients account for 57 % of the AIDS-infected population, causing a high infection rate in infants. In addition, Latin America is one of the most seriously affected areas by AIDS. In recent years, Eastern Europe and central Asia are areas with the fastest growth of AIDS-infected population.

4.5 Epidemiology of HIV/AIDS in China

The prevalence of HIV/AIDS in China is increasingly serious. In terms of age, young and middle aged population is seriously affected by HIV/AIDS. Children patients under the age of 15 include HIV infected children and children with AIDS. Children patients are mostly concentrated in local areas with high prevalence, such as Henan province and Yunnan province.

In terms of gender distribution, most HIV infected is males. Data suggested that the male/female ratio of HIV infected patients in China is 2.6:1. And the male/female ratio in the accumulative patients with AIDS is 1.3:1. It has been noticed that in recent year, the proportion of newly-detected and reported female HIV-infected cases increases annually. The risk of vertical transmission from mother to child transmission is increasingly challenging.

In terms of ethnic distribution, the majority (67 %) of national reported AIDS patients is population of Han nationality, another 30 % is population of minority nationalities and the other is population from overseas or with undefined nationality. In China, HIV/AIDS spread in some minorities has special reasons. As exposed to the same risk factors, different ethnic groups may sustain varied hazards. The risks of HIV/AIDS infection for minorities include: (1) residing in national border areas that produce drugs or in areas along drug trading route; (2) some traditional customs, such as sexual sharing; (3) lower educational level; (4) poor medical facilities, limited knowledge about HIV/AIDS and the resulted higher incidence in the second generation. Therefore, the HIV/AIDS epidemic in minorities should be attentively controlled.

In addition, detection rate of HIV/AIDS patients at the national borders is rapidly growing. The HIV/AIDS infected with foreign nationalities is commonly from southeastern Asia and Africa for traveling, business, study and borderline area trade. The Chinese HIV/AIDS infected commonly works as laborers, businessmen, sailors or borderline personnels. The HIV infected people, both foreigners and Chinese, have caused second generation infection at their habitats. Even HIV-2 infection is found in some regions.

4.6   Seroepidemiology of HIV/AIDS

Since the first reported case of HIV-1 infection in the year of 1985, the prevalence of HIV-1 in China is spreading from high risk populations to general populations [2]. Among HIV-1 related high risk factors, sharing syringe for intravenous drug abuse is the main route of transmission. The HIV-1 infected intravenous drug abusers are more frequently found in the provinces of Yunnan, Guangxi and Sichuan. In 1990s, blood was illegally collected and transfused in some areas of Henan province, which constitutes the second frequently found transmission route in China. Studies have proved that the HIV-1 strains transmitted via intravenous drug abusers and paid blood donors belong to two different virus subtypes. Intravenous drug users in provinces and areas of Yunnan, Guangxi and Xinjiang carry HIV-1 CRF07BC and HIV-1 CRF08BC, while the paid blood donors in Henan province carry HIV-1 B' subtype, similar to B' subtype detected in Thailand. HIV-1 B' subtype may be the main virus subtype attacking paid blood donors in Henan province and some adjacent provinces, including Hubei, Anhui and Shaanxi. HIV-1 B' subtype is obviously different from the subtypes of CRF07BC and CRF08BC that attack intravenous drug users in provinces and areas of Yunnan, Guangxi and Xinjiang. The different distribution of subtypes is closely related the routes of transmission. Hereditary effect is significant in the subtype found in the intravenous drug users in Dehong district of Yunnan province. The B' subtype found in paid blood donors may be transmitted into the central provinces

of China before the various subtypes of chimeric HIV-1 strain dominated Yunnan provinces. The diversity of HIV-1 genotype is challenging in fields of HIV/AIDS surveillance, long-term anti-viral therapy, and effective development of vaccines. Therefore, the analysis of HIV-1 subtypes is of great significance in clinical researches for antiviral drugs and vaccine screening.

4.7   Molecular Epidemiology of HIV/AIDS

According to gene variance, HIV is divided into two types of HIV-1 and HIV-2, sharing 40–60 % homogeneity in amino acid sequences. The currently prevalent HIV is HIV-1, which can be further divided into various subtypes. According to homogeneity of the *env* gene encoding envelope protein and the *gag* gene encoding shell protein, HIV-1 can be further divided into three groups: Group M (main group including 11 subtypes of A, B, C, D, E, F, G, H, I, J and K), Group O (outline group) and Group N (new group, non-M group or non-O group). Group M can be subdivided into 10 subtypes of A, B, C, D, E, F, G, H, I and J. Between HIV-1 and HIV-2, the homogeneity of nucleotide sequences is only 45 %. Within the type of HIV-1, the gene dispersion rate of different subtypes is 20–35 %, while within the same subtype, the gene dispersion rate is 7–20 %. Group O was isolated in Cameroon and Gabon, sharing homogeneity of 50 % nucleotide sequences with Group M. Group N was recently isolated from two patients in Cameroon, which belongs to neither Group M nor Group O in the system tree. In addition, several prevalent recombinant forms have been found in recent years. HIV-2 shares similar biological features to HIV-1, but its infectivity is lower and HIV-2 infection has a slower clinical progression with more slight symptoms. HIV-2 has at least 7 subtypes, namely A, B, C, D, E, F and G. In China, HIV-1 is the major prevalent strain, and has 8 subtypes (A, B, occident B, C, D, E, F and G) and several prevalent recombinants. Since 1999, HIV-2 infected cases have been rarely identified in some areas. Its genes are highly varied due to the following four reasons: (1) high error rate by revertase, whose replication fails to remove the mistakenly introduced nucleotide. Occurrence of an error in each replication cycle gives the virus chance for random variance. (2) Rapid virus replication. It has been estimated that an HIV-infected person produces and eliminates 10 billion virus particles. (3) Immunoselection of the host. Under the pressure of the immunoselection by the host, the variation rate of genome triggering cellular immunity or humoral immunity is higher than the other genomes, such as gp120 V3 hypervariable ring region. (4) Genetic recombination of different virus strains. The classification of HIV biologically marks the research field of molecular epidemiology, based on which we can trace the transmission of HIV and gain knowledge about the global epidemics of HIV. Both HIV-1 and HIV-2 originated from Africa. However, different HIV types and subtypes are not evenly distributed in the world. Groups O and N of HIV-1 and HIV-2 have confined prevalence in some local areas in Africa, while Group M of HIV-1 is globally spreading. Until present, most globally prevalent virus strains are subtype strains of A and C in Group M of HIV-1, followed by B' subtype and then recombinant subtypes of A/E and A/G. Further studies on its molecular epidemiology suggested that almost all HIV subtypes prevail in Africa, predominantly subtypes of A and C. Meanwhile, due to concurrent prevalence of several subtypes in Africa, viral recombinations are commonly found. In North America, Europe and Australia, B' subtype is still the most commonly found subtype, although cases infected by other subtypes in Group M, even subtypes in Group O have been reported. Such cases are mostly immigrants from Africa by further field epidemiological studies. In south America, subtype B dominantly prevails, with spreading of subtypes C and F. In Argentina and Brazil, cases infected by recombinant virus strain B/F are reported. In Asia, different HIV subtypes prevail in different areas, predominant subtype C in India with concurrent prevalence of subtypes A, B and recombinant strain A/C, independent prevalence of subtypes B and E (namely recombinant strain A/E) in Thailand, and predominant prevalence of subtypes B, C and E with spreading of subtypes A and F, HIV-2 in China. The transmission and progression of HIV-1 and HIV-2 infections are obviously different. HIV-2 has a weaker infectivity via sexual behaviors and mother-to-child transmission, with longer latent period of progression into AIDS, comparing to those of HIV-1 infection. However, it is still no inclusive about the variances in transmission and progression of infections by HIV-1 subtypes. Some research reports indicated obvious variances in the transmission and progression of infections caused by different subtypes. A prospective study in female sex service providers in Senegal suggested that the possibility of progressing into AIDS for the female subjects infected with HIV-1A is eight times less than those infected by other HIV-1 subtypes. Another study on HIV-1 positive pregnant females in Kenya also indicated that patients infected with HIV-1C have more virus load and less CD4 count than those infected by HIV-1A or D, both of which are the most important indicators marking the progression of HIV infection. Additionally, other reports indicated that most patients infected by HIV-1C have no facilitative receptors CXCR4, an indicator marking a faster progression of HIV infection, while patients infected by HIV-1B commonly have the receptor in their bodies. However, not all study results are in agreement with these findings. One study conducted in Israel found no variance in progression of HIV-1B and HIV-1C infections. Another research in Sweden also demonstrated identical progression of infections in patients with HIV-1A, B, C and D [3].

Researches on the effects of HIV subtypes on its transmission also have the same conclusion. On one hand, a study in Thailand showed that the sexual transmission rate of subtype E in Thailand is five times as high as that of subtype B in the United States of America. On the other hand, Mastro, Shatter et al. [4] found no difference in the sexual transmission or vertical mother-to-child transmission among different HIV subtypes. Generally, the progression of HIV infection is affected by virus strains, hosts and other factors, with great individual differences. It is quite challenging to evaluate the differences in transmission and progression of infections among patients with different virus subtypes.

4.8 Prevention and Control of HIV/AIDS

1. Reporting of the cases

    Voluntary consultation and voluntary detection for AIDS are encouraged. Once an HIV infection is confirmed, the case should be immediately reported to the local CDC as a state-stipulated B grade communicable disease. Appropriate measures should be taken simultaneously.

2. Medical management

    Secret security principles should be followed. In addition, follow-up visits should be attentively emphasized to provide therapeutic and psychological consultations.

3. Preventive measures

    The preventive measures include promoting healthy and safe sexual behaviors, no drug abuse and no sharing of syringes in drug use, promoting voluntary blood donation and HIV screening for blood donors, enhancing hospital management, strict observation of disinfection in hospitals, controlling hospital cross-infections, preventing occupational exposure to HIV infections, controlling vertical mother-to-child transmission. For spouses and sex partners of HIV/AIDS infected patients, those sharing syringes in intravenous drug use and children of HIV/AIDS infected patients, medical examinations and HIV tests should be performed and consultation services should be provided.

References

1. Valdespino-Gomez JZ, Garcia-Garcia Mde L, del Rio-Zolezzi A, et al. The epidemiology of AIDS/HIV in Mexico: from 1983 to March 1995. Salud Publica Mex. 1995;37(6):556–71.
2. Zheng XW. A report on AIDS surveillance from 1985 to 1988 in China. Zhonghua liu xing Bing Xue Za Zhi. 1989;10(2):65–7.
3. Alaeus A, Lidman K, Bjorkman A, et al. Similar rate of disease progression among individuals infected with HIV-1 genetic subtypes A–D. AIDS. 1999;13(8):901–7.
4. Masro TD, Kunanusont C, Dondero TJ, et al. Why do HIV-1 subtypes segregate among persons with different risk behaviors in South Africa and Thailand? AIDS. 1997;11(1):113–6.

Pathogenetic and Pathological Mechanism

5

Contents

5.1 Pathogenetic Mechanism

5.1.1 Process of Virus Infection

5.1.1.1 Primary Infection

Assisted by surface receptors of susceptible cells, HIV can successfully get access to cells, including the first receptors and the second receptors. Firstly, envelope glycoprotein gp120 of HIV-1 binds to the first receptors, followed by its binding to the second receptors. Its structural changes cause its detachment from gp41, resulting in fusion of HIV and host cellular membrane and its successful access to host cells. Within 24–48 h after its access, HIV reaches the local lymph nodes. At d 5, HIV components can be detected in the peripheral blood. The attack of HIV causes viremia, leading to acute infection.

5.1.1.2 Process of HIV Infection in Human Cells
Attachment and Penetration

After successful access to human body, HIV selectively adheres to CD4 receptors of the target cells. Assisted by the facilitative receptors, it gains successful access to the host cells.

Cyclization and Integration

The virus RNA is transformed into cDNA, with contributions from reverse transcriptase, followed by its further transformation into double-stranded DNA with contributions from DNA polymerase. The newly-formed non-covalent-interacted double-stranded DNA integrates with chromosome DNA in host cells to form the viral double stranded DNA, also known as provirus.

Transcription and Translation

The provirus is then activated to transcribe itself with the virus DNA transcribed into RNA. Some RNAs are capped and tailed as the RNA of the filial generation genome. Some other RNAs are spliced as virus mRNA. It is then translated into structural and non-structural proteins of the virus on Palade's granule. The synthesized virus protein is saccharified

H. Li (ed.), *Radiology of HIV/AIDS*,
DOI 10.1007/978-94-007-7823-8_5, © Springer Science+Business Media Dordrecht and People's Medical Publishing House 2014

and processed in ribosomes of endoplasmic reticulum, followed by splitting contributed by protease to produce the protein and the enzyme of the filial generation virus.

Assemblage, Maturation and Pullulation
Gag protein and virus RNA are assembled into nucleocapsid. The virus envelope is obtained during the release of budding from serolemma. Thus a mature virus particle is formed.

5.1.1.3 Three Types of Clinical Outcomes After HIV Infection
Because the human immune system cannot eliminate all the virus, chronic infection occurs. Clinically, the infection has three types of clinical manifestations, typical progression, rapid progression and long term no progression. The factors influencing the progression of HIV infection include virus itself, host immunity and genetic background.

5.1.2 Anti-HIV Immune Responses

Anti-HIV immune responses include specific immune response and nonspecific immune response. Specific immune response more commonly occurs.

5.1.2.1 Specific Humoral Immunity
Within 2–12 weeks after access of HIV to human body, the human immune system produces various specific antibodies targeting HIV proteins. Only neutralizing antibody has antiviral effects.

5.1.2.2 Specific Cellular Immunity
The specific cellular immunity includes specific CD4 T lymphocytes responses and specific cytotoxic T lymphocytes responses. CD4 T lymphocytes, as the central cells in human immune system, play critical roles in specific immune responses. By secreting various cytokines, it induces B cell to produce anti-HIV antibody. By promoting the production and maturation of specific anti-HIV CD4 T lymphocytes, it activates macrophage and NK cells. CD8+ T lymphocytes, the effector cells of specific cellular immunity, inhibit the replication of HIV directly or indirectly via secretion of various cytokines, such as tumor necrosis factor and interferon.

5.2 Pathophysiology

5.2.1 A Drop of CD4 T Lymphocyte Count

After HIV infection, CD4 T lymphocyte count keeps decreasing. The acute phase of HIV infection is characterized by a transient rapid decrease of CD4 T lymphocyte count during a short period of time. For most patients infected by HIV, their CD4 T lymphocyte counts can voluntarily regain normal without any therapeutic interventions. The asymptomatic phase is characterized by a continuous slow decrease in CD4 T lymphocyte count (usually 800–350/μl). The duration of this phase varies from several months to several years, with a mean of 8 years. In symptomatic AIDS phase, CD4 T lymphocyte count drops dramatically again, being below 350/μl in most patients with AIDS. For some patients in their advanced stage, the CD4 T lymphocyte count may quickly decrease to the level of below 200/μl. The drop in the CD4 T lymphocyte count can be attributed to several factors, including increased damages to CD4 T lymphocytes, decreased manufacture of CD4 T lymphocytes, strapped CD4 T lymphocytes in peripheral blood by lymphoid tissues.

5.2.2 Dysfunction of CD4 T Lymphocytes

The main manifestation of dysfunction of CD4 T lymphocytes is the substitution of T helper 1 (Th1) by T helper 2 (Th2), impaired function of antigen presenting cells, decreased production of interleukin-2 and the incapability to activate antigen reaction. Under such conditions, patients with HIV/AIDS are susceptible to various infections.

5.2.3 Abnormal Immunity Activation

Abnormal activation of immune system is another immunologically pathologic change after HIV infection. The levels of immunity activation markers, such as CD69, CD38 and HLA-DR expressed by CD4 T and CD8+ T lymphocytes abnormally increase. And the levels of these biomarkers also have favorable correspondence with HIV virus load in blood plasma. With the progression of the infection, the level of cells activation is increasing. Therefore, the abnormal immunity activation marks changes of plasma virus loading and can be used to predict the decrease of CD4 T lymphocytes.

5.2.4 Immunity Reconstruction

It has been proved that HAART promotes the immunity reconstruction, which is recognized as one of the important breakthroughs in AIDS researches. It also greatly impacts on the treatment and research of AIDS. The immunity reconstruction in patients with AIDS refers to the compromised immunity in patients can regain normal or be close to normal after the anti-viral therapies. That is to say, (1) the decreased CD4 T lymphocytes regain to normal level; (2) CD4 T lymphocytes regain its reactivity to the stimulations by remembered antigen; (3) abnormal human immunity activation regains to normal level. In addition, successful immunity reconstruction also refers to the lower incidence of AIDS-related opportunistic infection and neoplasms after anti-viral therapies, the lower incidence of AIDS and the lower death rate from AIDS. However, HAART therapy has its limitations, including (1) HARRT fails to successfully reconstruct all patients' immunity; (2) HARRT fails to rebuild specific anti-HIV CD4 T lymphocytic immune response and decreases the specific anti-HIV CD 8+ lymphocytic immune response, which means a long-term medication.

5.3 Pathology of HIV/AIDS

AIDS is a systemic disease with involvement of multiple organs. HIV infection causes pathological changes of immune system, opportunistic infections (including protozoan, virus, bacteria and fungus infections) of multiple systems, and malignant tumors (including Kaposi's sarcoma, malignant lymphoma and cervical carcinoma). Thus, AIDS is pathologically complex.

5.3.1 Common Opportunistic Infections and Malignant Tumors

5.3.1.1 Pulmonary Coccidioidomycosis

Pulmonary coccidioidomycosis commonly causes pneumocystis carinii pneumonia. By diagnostic imaging, both lungs are demonstrated to be diffusively involved, with parenchymal changes, increased weight and obviously decreased gas contents. After being fixed by formalin, the pulmonary sections appear to be coarse spongiform. The alveolar cavities see characteristic honeycomb exudates, which are foam liked, red stained and non-cellular exudates. The alveolar epithelia proliferate into cuboidal.

5.3.1.2 Toxoplasmosis

Although disseminating toxoplasmosis can also involve eyes, lungs, heart and gastrointestinal tract, most patients with HIV/AIDS sustain toxoplasmic encephalitis. The cerebral lesions could be local or diffusive abscesses in basal ganglia or cerebellar cortex, which can also be found in the cavum subarachnoidale. Toxoplasmic cerebral abscess is characteristically demonstrated by enhanced CT scanning, including singular or multiple lesions in gray matter, which is circumferentially cystoid. Coagulation hemorrhagic necrosis occurs in local brain tissues, with rare toxoplasmas in necrotic areas. Surrounding the necrotic area, a proliferative zone of vascular endothelia can be found with congestion, inside which severe inflammatory infiltration occurs with many toxoplasm tachyzoites and pseudocysts containing bradyzoites. The tachyzoite in brain tissue is round or oval in shape instead of crescentiform in other tissues. In the sections of other tissues, crescentiform tachyzoite (2–5 μm) and cyst/pseudocyst (50 μm) can be clearly observed after HE staining. In addition, increased serum antibody titer is a diagnostic indicator for toxoplasmosis.

5.3.1.3 Candida Albicans Disease

In patients with AIDS, recurrent candida albicans disease is the most common opportunistic fungal infection. Concerning patients with oral cavity involved candida albicans disease; their tongue surface shows white diffusive plaques or even thick dark brown cover due to the coverage of exudates. Oral cavity involved candidiasis indicates that HIV infection has progressed into AIDS. Any part of the gastrointestinal tract can be involved, with esophagus as the most common involved part. Gray pseudomembrane, composed of fibrin and necrotic tissue with network of pseudohypha, and irregular ulcer can be found on the mucosal surface. Disseminated oral candidiasis usually involves multiple organs, such as kidney (about 80 %), brain (about 50 %) and heart (about 58 %). Multiple abscesses occur in the involved organs. Histologically, candida albicans is composed of yeast-like spore or blastospore (in round or oval shapes with a diameter of 3–4 μm) and pseudohypha (rosary spore).

5.3.1.4 Mycobacteriosis

Mycobacteriosis is common in patients with AIDS, including tuberculosis and mycobacterium avium infection. Tuberculosis occurs in either early stage or advanced stage of AIDS, with the most common occurrence of extrapulmonary TB. It is more invasive and may spread throughout the body. Under a microscope, patients with AIDS have atypical tuberculosis granuloma, obvious cheesy necrosis and less epithelioid/giant cells. Pulmonary tuberculosis is characterized by exudative lesions, parenchymal changes of gas cavities with inside fibrin, neutrophile granulocyte and histocyte, extensive necrosis and more anti-acid tubercle bacillus. Mycobacterium avium infection occurs in the advanced stage of AIDS, with CD4 T lymphocyte count being less than 100/mm^3. It commonly causes disseminated mycobacteriosis. Miliary granuloma sometimes can be observed on the sections of spleen, liver, lymph nodes, heart and kidney. Under a microscope, local structure is replaced by the tissue cellular mass; highly swollen histiocytes are in striation or foam liked; yellow stained or blue stained endochylema with deeper staining of nucleus, rare formation of giant cells, rare or no necrosis, no calcification and fibrosis. Acid-fast staining demonstrates swollen macrophages, filled with mycobacteria avium.

5.3.1.5 Cytomegalovirus Infection

Cytomegalovirus infection in patients with AIDS can cause gastrointestinal tract ulcer, interstitial pneumonia, glomerular nephritis and amphiblestritis. Cytomegalovirus infection can also involve any part of brain and spinal cord, including spinal nerve root and cranial nerve. By autopsy, it has been found that adrenal gland and respiratory system are commonly involved. Under a microscope, some large cells can be observed, with obvious and well defined inclusions in the intranuclear and endochylema inside them. In all human virus, cytomegalovirus has the biggest inclusion, visible in both nucleus and cytoplasm of the infected cells. The inclusion of cytomegalovirus is characterized by (1) intranuclear amphochromophil inclusion surrounded by a transparent halo like an owl eye, referred to as the owl eye sign; (2) cytoplasmic amphochromophil or eosinophilic inclusion; (3) inclusions in epithelium, endothelium, macrophage and smooth muscle cell. Immunohistochemistry, DNA in situ hybridization and PCR are facilitative for the definitive diagnosis.

5.3.1.6 Kaposi's Sarcoma

Kaposi's sarcoma is the most common neoplasm in patients with AIDS. Epidemic Kaposi's sarcoma or other AIDS-related Kaposi's sarcoma are different from other types in the following aspects: (1) common in homosexual or bisexual males and in intravenous drug users; (2) multicentered lesions that are more aggressive to involve skin and organs (about 75 %). The frequently involved organs are lungs, lymph nodes, gastrointestinal tract, liver and urogenital system and the rarely involved organs are adrenal gland, heart and spleen. Kaposi's sarcoma of skin appears red or prunosus, being in flat spot in its early stage and progressing into prominent plaques and finally nodules, with possible occurrence of erosion and ulcer. The tumor consists of spindle cells that are capable of forming vascular fissure. Erythrocytes can be observed in the tumor, whose cells share some common features with endothelium and smooth muscle cells. Human herpes virus-8 is related to the occurrence of Kaposi's sarcoma.

5.3.2 Pathological Changes of the Immune System

5.3.2.1 HIV-Related Lymph Nodes Diseases

HIV related lymph nodes diseases can be divided into four types, namely follicular hyperplasia with follicle breaking, follicular hyperplasia without follicle breaking, follicle degeneration and follicle exhaustion. Patients have persistent systemic lymph node diseases before HIV infection progressing into AIDS. Swollen lymph node is normally no more than 3 cm in diameter. Most HIV-infected patients have follicular hyperplasia of lymph nodes histologically. The lymph nodes in patients with AIDS are small in size, with occurrence of follicle degeneration or exhaustion.

5.3.2.2 Pathologic Change of Spleen

Splenomegaly is common clinical symptom for patients with AIDS. When an adult patient's spleen weighs more than 400 g, it often indicates the occurrence of intrasplenic opportunistic infections and malignant neoplasms. The pathologic changes of spleen in patients with AIDS is highly exhausted lymphocytes, less or exhausted white pulp. The pathologic changes of spleen in children with AIDS are obviously exhausted lymphocytes, engulfed erythrocytes and Kaposi's sarcoma (in about 50 % cases).

5.3.2.3 Pathologic Changes of Thymus

No notable pathologic changes occur in thymus of adult patients with AIDS while B cell follicular hyperplasia sometimes occurs. Premature degeneration of thymus occurs in children with AIDS. HIV impairs thymus epithelia to induce atrophy and exhaustion of lymphoid tissues, with noticeable plasmocytes infiltration and multinucleus giant cells formation. The thymus has corpuscles cysts.

5.3.2.4 Pathologic Change of Bone Marrow

In the early stage, three-fourth cases have cellular proliferation, predominantly granulocytes and megakaryocytes. In the advanced stage, failure occurs with decreased marrow cells, immature dysplastic precursor cells, concentrated lymphoid cells, atypical megakaryocytes, fine network of necrosis, mild vascular hyperplasia, histocytic hyperplasia and Hemosiderin deposition.

Clinical Manifestations of HIV/AIDS Infection

Contents

6.1   Incubation Period

After successful invasion of HIV into the human body, HIV antibody occurs within 4–8 weeks, followed by its incubation period lasting 2–10 years. During this period, HIV still replicates incessantly to compromise the immune system, with gradually decreasing CD4 T lymphocytes and infectivity. Even though the patients show no clinical symptoms, they, as HIV carriers, can spread the virus via various transmission routes.

6.2   Clinical Characteristics

The progression of HIV infection is a long-term natural developing process. The patients' survival duration depends on the quantity of HIV in the body, individual health difference, nutritional status and the effectiveness of the therapies. HIV induces exhaustion and death of T cells, which is demonstrated by decreased CD 4T lymphocytes count. Clinically, the progression of HIV infection can be divided into three stages, namely acute stage, asymptomatic stage and AIDS stage.

6.3   Clinical Symptoms and Signs

6.3.1   Acute Stage

After preliminary HIV infection, the HIV infection progresses into acute stage in 2–4 weeks. Some patients show symptoms of HIV related viraemia and acute immunity impairment. Most patients have slight clinical symptoms that are relieved after 1–3 weeks. The most commonly found symptom is fever, with accompanying sore throat, muscle pain, headache, nausea, vomiting, skin rash, thrush, arthralgia, splenohepatomegaly, enlarged lymph nodes, weight loss and nervous system symptoms. Some patients may also have slight leukocytopenia, thrombocytopenia or liver malfunction.

H. Li (ed.), *Radiology of HIV/AIDS*,
DOI 10.1007/978-94-007-7823-8_6, © Springer Science+Business Media Dordrecht and People's Medical Publishing House 2014

6.3.2 Asymptomatic Stage

During the stage, no clinical manifestation can be found, while 40–60 % patients may have specific lymphadenectasis, predominantly axillar lymph nodes. The persistent general lymphadenectasis is defined as the following:

1. Lymphadenectasis occurs in at least two parts of the body in addition to groin;
2. Lymph node is larger than 1 cm in diameter, with no tenderness and adhesion;
3. Lymphadenectasis lasts at least 3 months;
4. Exclusion of other etiologic factors.

6.3.3 AIDS Stage

AIDS stage is the final stage of HIV infection. The patients usually have obviously decreased CD4 T lymphocytes count of lower than 200/μl, obviously increased HIV virus load in plasma. During this period, the clinical manifestations include HIV-related symptoms, various opportunistic infections and neoplasms.

1. Persistent irregular fever of above 38 °C for more than 1 month, with no cause found;
2. Diarrhea (bowel movement more than three times daily), persistent more than 1 month;
3. Weight loss over 10 % in 6 months;
4. Recurrent attacks of oral candidiasis albicans;
5. Recurrent attacks of herpes simplex virus infection or herpes zoster virus infection;
6. Pneumocystis pneumonia (PCP);
7. Recurrent bacterial pneumonia;
8. Active tuberculosis or nontuberculous mycobacteria;
9. Deep fungal infections;
10. HIV-related dementia;
11. Progressive multifocal leukoencephalopathy;
12. Active cytomegalovirus infection;
13. Cerebral toxoplasmosis;
14. Penicillium infection;
15. Recurrent septicemia;
16. Kaposi's sarcoma and lymphoma in skin mucus and organs;
17. Chronic isosporiasis;
18. Coccidioidomycosis and histoplasmosis;
19. Invasive cervical cancer.

6.4 Clinical Classification

According to the clinical manifestations, AIDS can be divided into the following five types:

6.4.1 Pulmonary Type

Pulmonary type is the most common type of AIDS, with symptoms of dyspnea, hypoxemia and chest pain. Chest X-ray demonstrates pulmonary diffusive infiltration and decreased pulmonary functions. The most common deadly infection is pneumocystis pneumonia (PCP).

6.4.2 Central Nervous Type

Central nervous type can be found in 30 % patients with AIDS. HIV itself can attack brain issue to cause encephalitis liked symptoms. Toxoplasma gondii and cryptococcus can attack central nervous system to cause cerebral abscess, diffusive encephalitis and encephalomeningitis. The symptoms include headache, vomiting, consciousness impairments, spasm, dementia and relevant symptoms of space-occupying lesions. The diagnosis can be defined by cerebrospinal fluid smear and culture as well as brain CT scanning.

6.4.3 Gastrointestinal Type

Patients with gastrointestinal type AIDS have diarrhea and weight loss. For serious cases, the symptoms also include malabsorption and cachexia. Cryptozoite infection is the common cause of AIDS related gastrointestinal infection, with symptoms of chronic diarrhea and watery stool for months. It is also the common cause of death in patients with AIDS. Infections of other pathogens, such as cytomegalovirus, salmonella, bacillus dysenteriae and Amoeba trophozoite, also contribute to symptoms of enteritis including diarrhea, abdominal pain, tenesmus, purulent and bloody stool and malabsorption. Candida albicans caused esophagitis and glossitis can be definitively diagnosed by gastroscopy.

6.4.4 Fever of Unknown Causes

Due to infection of pathogens, high fever, upset, fatigue and general lymphadenectasis occur.

6.4.5 Neoplasm Type

Kaposi's sarcoma is the most common AIDS related neoplasm, with no discoloration under finger pressure but tawny ecchymosis surrounding it and rapid progression. The skin lesions can be found in face and neck, spreading to oral cavity, lungs and alimentary tract, to cause bleeding and death.

Pathological biopsy can be applied for definitive diagnosis. Other malignant neoplasms include lymphoma, liver carcinoma, and pulmonary squamous cell carcinoma.

6.5   Characteristics of Children with HIV/AIDS

Most clinical manifestations of children with AIDS are similar to those of adult patients, except that lymph nodes lesions, Kaposi's sarcoma and opportunistic infections do not occur in children with AIDS. Almost all children with AIDS sustain splenohepatomegaly, interstitial pneumonia and developmental impairments. After HIV infection, children have a shorter incubation period but fast progression. Both the survival rate and clinical manifestations are correlated with age. About 50 % children with AIDS survive 12 months after their definitive diagnosis. The 1 year survival rate of children suffering from PCP and being younger than 12-month-old is only 30 %. The 1 year survival rate of elder children with PCP is 48 %. The 1 year survival rate of elder children with other AIDS related diseases is 72 %. The characteristic clinical manifestations occur in early childhood. PCP, HIV wasting syndrome and encephalopathy occur in children aged 4–8 months. Concerning opportunistic infections, children patients are different from adult patients in occurrence of bacterial infections and Kaposi's sarcoma. Children with AIDS have a higher occurrence of bacterial infections, such as otitis media, encephalomeningitis and pneumonia, but a rare occurrence of Kaposi's sarcoma.

Common opportunistic infections in children with AIDS include:
1. Pneumocystis pneumonia (PCP)
2. Lymphocytic interstitial pneumonia (LIP)
3. Toxoplasma gondii infection
4. Diarrhea
5. Pediatric tuberculosis
6. Disseminated mycobacterium avium infection (MAC)
7. Recurrent bacterial infection
8. Candida infection
9. Pediatric cytomegalovirus infection (CMV)

6.6   Characteristics of Women with HIV/AIDS

The physiological structures of men and women are different. Therefore, symptoms of AIDS in female patients are different from those in male patients. The characteristics of female patients with AIDS are as the following:

1. Cervical dysplasia of papilloma virus infection is common in women, which would cause cervical carcinoma.
2. Occurrence of Kaposi's sarcoma is 1 % in women and 3 % in men. Occurrence of PCP is lower in women than in men.
3. Occurrence of anemia is more common in women than in men.
4. Occurrence of urinary tract infection is higher in women than in men.
5. Occurrence of lower genital tract infections is higher in women, such as herpes genitalis, candida infection, trichomonas vaginitis and pelvic inflammation.

In the advanced stage of HIV/AIDS infection, women may develop following gynecological complications:
1. Menstruations, including hypermenorrhea, hypomenorrhea or amenorrhea.
2. External vaginal infection, including occurrence of candida infection in early stage with multiple attacks yearly or intermittent exacerbation, occurrence of herpes simplex virus infection with stubborn and recurrent attacks to external vagina, vaginal tract and anus.
3. Cervical epithelial neoplasms, its incidence being ten times as high as that in general female population, with human papilloma virus playing a crucial role in its pathogenesis.
4. Pelvic inflammatory diseases (PID), with involvement of Fallopian tubes, uterus and cervix. It has various pathogenic bacteria including chlamydia trachomatis and diplococcus reniformis, with tuberculous Fallopian tube and ovarian abscess being the most common infections.

6.7   Diagnostic Criteria and Treatment Guideline for HIV/AIDS in China

The diagnosis of HIV/AIDS can be defined based on the combination of epidemiological history (unsafe sexual behaviors, intravenous drug use, receiving blood or blood products with no test on HIV antibody, children of HIV positives and vocational exposure), clinical manifestations and results of laboratory tests. The diagnosis of HIV/AIDS should be firstly based on positive findings of HIV antibody test (confirmed by definitive tests), while tests on HIV RNA and P24 antigen facilitate the diagnosis of HIV/AIDS. The diagnosis of HIV infection is especially important for infants, which helps shortening the window period of HIV antibody and early detection of HIV infection.
1. Diagnostic criteria
   1.1. Acute HIV infection
      1.1.1. Epidemiological history

1.1.1.1. History of multiple homosexual/heterosexual partners, or spouse or sexual partners with positive anti-HIV antibody

1.1.1.2. History of intravenous drug abuse

1.1.1.3. History of receiving imported blood products, such as VII-factor.

1.1.1.4. History of close contacts with HIV/AIDS patients

1.1.1.5. History of sexually transmitted diseases such as syphilis, gonorrhea, nongonococcal urethritis.

1.1.1.6. History of travelling abroad

1.1.1.7. Children whose bio-parents are anti-HIV positive

1.1.1.8. Receptors of blood with no test on anti-HIV antibody

1.1.2. Clinical Manifestations

1.1.2.1. Upper respiratory tract infections with symptoms of fever, fatigue, sore throat and general upset

1.1.2.2. Occasional cases of headache, skin rash, encephalomeningitis or polyneuritis.

1.1.2.3. Lymphadenectasis in neck, axilla and occiput similar to mononucleosis

1.1.2.4. Splenohepatomegaly

1.1.3. Laboratory tests

1.1.3.1. Decreased WBC count and lymphocyte count in peripheral blood after the onset of disease, then increased lymphocyte count with detectable abnormal lymphocytes

1.1.3.2. CD4/CD8 ratio exceeds 1

1.1.3.3. Conversion of anti-HIV antibody from negative to positive. During the window stage of HIV infection, the HIV antibody is negative. It usually takes 2–3 months and sometimes up to 6 months for HIV antibody to convert positive.

1.1.3.4. Rare cases of positive serum P24 antigen in the early stage.

1.2. HIV infection with no symptoms

1.2.1. Epidemiological history
The same as acute HIV infection.

1.2.2. Clinical Manifestation.
Commonly no symptoms or signs

1.2.3. Laboratory tests

1.2.3.1. Anti-HIV antibody test positive, defined by confirmative laboratory tests.

1.2.3.2. CD4 T lymphocytes count normal and the ratio of CD4/CD8 over 1

1.2.3.3. Serum P24 antigen negative

1.3. AIDS

1.3.1. Epidemiological history, the same as Acute HIV infection

1.3.2. Clinical Manifestations

1.3.2.1. Compromised immunity of unknown causes

1.3.2.2. Persistent lymphadenectasis of unknown causes (lymph nodes being larger than 1 cm in diameter)

1.3.2.3. Chronic diarrhea of 4–5 times daily, weight loss more than 10 % within 3 months

1.3.2.4. Concurrent oral candida infection, PCP, cytomegalovirus (CMV) infection, toxoplasmosis, cryptococcal meningitis, active pulmonary tuberculosis with rapid progression, Kaposi's sarcoma of skin mucus and lymphoma.

1.3.2.5. Dementia occurs in young and middle-aged patients

1.3.3. Laboratory tests

1.3.3.1. Anti-HIV antibody positive, defined diagnose by the confirmative laboratory tests

1.3.3.2. P24 antigen positive (confirmative diagnosis recommended if conditions permit)

1.3.3.3. CD4 T lymphocytes count less than 200 or 200–500/µl

1.3.3.4. The ratio of CD4/CD8 being less than 1

1.3.3.5. Decreased WBC and Hb in peripheral blood

1.3.3.6. Increased β2 microglobulin level

1.3.3.7. Etiological basis can be found for above mentioned complications or pathological basis of neoplasms can be found.

1.4. Cases classification

1.4.1. Definitely diagnosed cases

1.4.1.1. HIV infection is demonstrated by positive findings of anti-HIV antibody test. Acute HIV infection refers to anti-HIV antibody converts to positive during the follow-up for high risk populations.

1.4.1.2. Cases of AIDS: person with either 1.3.1 or 1.3.2 and with 1.3.3.1, 1.3.3.3 and 1.3.3.7.

2. Prevention principles against HIV/AIDS

HIV can be isolated from blood, sperm, saliva, tear, cerebrospinal fluid, cervical secretions and milk of patients with AIDS. Mostly, the virus is spreading via blood and sperm. HIV infection cannot be transmitted via daily hand shaking, social life and contacts.

2.1. Propagation and education. The public should thoroughly know the risks and transmission routes of HIV/AIDS by propagation and health education via TV shows, booklets and health lectures.

2.2. In addition to providing therapies for sexually transmitted diseases (STD), STD clinics and STD control departments should also offer tests for HIV antibodies to the patients and spouses or sexual partners of the patients. Health education should also be simultaneously performed.

2.3. Knowledge about HIV/AIDS should be transmitted to high-risk populations, such as prostitutes, homosexuals and intravenous drug users.

2.4. Abortion should be immediately performed for pregnant women with HIV/AIDS.

2.5. Blood donors should be tested for HIV antibody before donating their blood, which should be conducted from big cities as the beginning. Persons with positive HIV antibody are not allowed to donate their blood and should receive epidemiological investigation.

2.6. Needles and syringes should not be used repeatedly in any medical unit. Syringes and needles should be disinfected strictly for repeated use according to the disinfection regulations in medical units with no disposable syringes and needles. And the disinfection for medical instruments, especially the dental instruments and endoscopes, should be reinforced.

2.7. Education and regular follow-up should be offered to patients with definitely diagnosed HIV/AIDS. And their family members, especially the spouse or sexual partner, should be provided with guidance or even HIV antibody test if practicable.

2.8. Intravenous drug users should be educated. Together with their family members, they should be persuaded to go to rehab for drug quitting. Due to the high relapse rate, the severe consequences of HIV/AIDS and its transmission routes should be propagated to the intravenous drug users and their family members.

2.9. Suspected case should be sent to local CDC for blood HIV antibody test. The definitely diagnosed cases should be reported to the Ministry of Health according to *Law of the PRC on the Prevention and Treatment of Infectious Diseases* and *Implementation Measures for Prevention and Treatment of Infectious Diseases, People's Republic of China*.

3. Treatment principles of HIV/AIDS

For patients with acute HIV infection or with asymptomatic infection, no special medical treatment is necessary. They should pay close attention to well resting, improving nutrients intake and well balancing jobs and entertainments. Moreover, their HIV infection should be avoided to transmit to others. The patients with AIDS should receive therapies targeting to the pathogens and complications. Other therapies including supportive therapies, immunoregulations, and psychotherapies should also be provided. For cases with positive P24 antigen and CD4 T lymphocyte count being less than 350 μl, drugs for inhibiting HIV reverse transcriptase can be administered to reduce the replication of HIV.

3.1. Rest

Patients with HIV infection can work and study as usual. But patients with slight symptoms including low-grade fever, diarrhea, or various infections should take a good rest.

3.2. Nutrients intake

Due to fever, oral candidiasis or herpes virus infections, patients with AIDS cannot eat well. As a result, high-protein diet is recommended to avoid the complications caused by dystrophy and compromised immunity, such as tuberculosis.

3.3. Therapies targeting at pathogens

The standard first-line therapy is recommended: Zidovudine (AZT) or Stavudine (d4T) + lamivudine (3TC) + Nevirapine (NVP) or Efavirenz (EFV) Domestic drugs for anti-retroviral therapy include NNRTIs, NRTIs, PIs and the fourth category of integrase inhibitor, in total of 12 kinds. Combined administration could be chosen.

3.4. Immunoregulatory drugs

3.4.1. Interferons

Interferons have antiviral and immunoregulatory effects. It should be injected intramuscularly in a dose of 3 Miu, 3 times per week, for a period up to 3–6 months.

3.4.2. Interleukin II (IL-II)

IL-II can increase the lymphocytes count and enhance the immunity. Currently, recombinant IL-II is mostly applied (Interferons and IL-II have the side effect of fever).

3.4.3. Gamma globulin

Patients with AIDS are susceptible to various bacterial infections due to their compromised humoral immunity. As a result, regular administration of gamma globulin can reduce the occurrence of bacterial infections.

3.4.4. Chinese medicinals, such as lentinan, Salvia miltiorrhiza, radix astragali and glycyrrhizin can also enhance immunity. Currently, it has been found that some Chinese medicinals can inhibit HIV *in vitro*, which is prospectively promising in further clinical application.

3.5. Treatment of various complications

3.5.1. Oral candida infection

Patients with AIDS usually have recurrent oral candida infection, sometimes with involvement of tonsils and retropharyngeal wall. For such cases, mycin and glycerin can be applied locally; mycin and glycerin may be mixed into pellets for slow swallowing; itraconazole or fluconazole can be taken orally.

3.5.2. Pneumocystis pneumonia (PCP)

Clinical manifestations include dyspnea and obviously low PO2 (about 70 mmHg). When chest X-ray demonstrates not serious lesions, PCP should be considered based on combination of case history and positive HIV antibody. Oral intake of SMZ-TMP is recommended for treatment. Intake at regular interval is recommended to prevent recurrence. Patients with long-term intake should receive examinations for hemogram and renal functions. Internationally, Pentamidine is prepared for oral intake and aerosol spray.

3.5.3. Bacterial infection

For cases with recurrent saimonella infection and positive findings by blood culture, Du-6859a is recommended for oral intake. It has been reported in the United States that the incidence of tuberculosis and atypical mycobacterial infection is high in patients with AIDS and their progressions are rapid. 3-drug or 4-drug regimen can be selected. During the medication, the functions of liver and kidneys should be monitored.

3.5.4 Cryptococcal meningitis

Its treatment principle is encephalic depressurization. Either 20 % mannitol or ventricular drainage can be applied. Regarding to antibiotics, fungizone or fluconazol can be used. After the conditions are stabilized, fluconazol can be applied for oral intake.

3.5.5 Herpes virus infection

For cases of skin shingles, acyclovir can be prescribed for oral intake. For cases of mucosa herpes simplex or cytomegalovirus infection, oral intake of acyclovir or administration of interferon is recommended.

3.5.6 Toxoplasm

Oral intake of sulfadiazine and pyrimethamine is recommended. The substitutive therapy is SMZ-TMP in combination with clindamycin or azithromycin for 6 weeks.

3.5.7 Cryptosporidiosis

Its manifestation is diarrhea. No specific treatment is available now. In addition, both Isospora and Micro-sporidia can induce diarrhea and intestinal malabsorption. Consequently, special staining and electron microscopy for stool smear should be performed for diagnosis. The therapies are to supplement fluid and electrolytes as well as to regulate the immune functions.

3.5.8 Neoplasms

For Kaposi's sarcoma with rapid progression, combined administration of leurocristine (or vinblastine) and bleomycin or azithromycin can be applied. Interferon is another choice for treatment. Administration for 0.5–1 year has the favorable outcomes. Local radiotherapy can be the other choice for the treatment.

Laboratory Test and Special Examinations

7

Contents

7.1 Routine Examination

The patients or suspected cases of HIV/AIDS should receive the following laboratory tests:

1. HIV antibody test

   HIV antibody can be tested with ELISA, Western hybridization, or rapid method with golden standard. The sensitivity of the 3 tests is all above 99 %;

2. Virus isolation and culture

   The peripheral lymphocytes are commonly used for virus culture, with a positive rate of above 95 %.

3. Anti-HIV antibody positive proved by confirmative test

   Enzyme linked immunosorbent assay (ELISA) and Western blotting are commonly used for antibody detection. ELISA has favorable sensitivity and specificity, appropriate for early screening. Twice tests positive can be defined as the positive. Western blotting has a higher specificity in determining virus protein, appropriate for confirmative test.

4. Serum P24 antigen positive.

   ELISA is commonly used to detect virus antigen including P24 antigen.

5. Characteristic drop of TH cells.

   The TH cell percentage in healthy persons is 40–70 %, with an absolute count of 500–1,600/mm^3. For diagnosis of HIV/AIDS, the ratio of TH/TS is less than 1.0, being 1.75–2.7 in healthy persons.

6. Delayed hypersensitive skin test.

   Skin tests against DNCB (dinitrochlorobenzene), trichothecin and candidin are negative.

7. T cell conversion test

   T cell conversion test shows a decreased result, with e-rosette being less than 65.

8. Increased β_2 microglobulin

   After HIV infection, monocytes are activated or destroyed to increase the serum β_2 protein level (>3–5 mg/l). Radio

H. Li (ed.), *Radiology of HIV/AIDS*,
DOI 10.1007/978-94-007-7823-8_7, © Springer Science+Business Media Dordrecht and People's Medical Publishing House 2014

immunoassay or enzyme immunoassay are commonly used to detect it.

9. Pathogen examination

   Tests for opportunistic pathogens include carinii, candida albicans, cryptococcus neoformans and toxoplasma.

7.2 Autopsy

By autopsy, the various conditions of the dead can be comprehensively understood, including the lesion location, the range, the property and the type. Blood tests of autopsy can be applied for detection of various pathogens. It is possible to find some rare or unexpected diseases by blood tests of autopsy. Autopsy findings of patients with AIDS enrich and extend our knowledge to AIDS related diseases. The precautions in autopsy include: Exposure to the blood, body fluid, secretions and organ tissues of the death case should be in great precausion. There should be specialized room or specialized operating table for autopsy of AIDS cases. All items on the operating table should be prominently marked. The autopsy room should be equipped with facilities of bathing, sanitary equipment, air-conditioner and heating installation. In the autopsy room, there should be specialized clothing, devices and equipments, with efficient disinfectant and fixing fluid. The autopsy room should also be equipped with specialized sewage system. And the above mentioned devices, equipments and installations should be managed by a specific personnel. Safety should be guaranteed for personnels performing autopsy and during autopsy, following precautions should be paid focused attention:

1. Take initiatives to understand the related clinical data and physicians requirements to have a definite aim in autopsy. For suspected cases of AIDS, the preventive measures should be reinforced for favorable disinfection and quarantine.

2. Autopsy generally follows routine operational procedures, including the brain. If necessary, blood can be collected after thoracotomy for use (e.g. pathogen as well as antigen and antibody tests). Specimens that require specialized processing should be prepared in advance.

3. AIDS patients often have KS, manifested as bleeding plaques or nodules in skin, mucosa, lymph node or organs. Close attention should be paid during examinations on the body surface and organs for appropriate sampling.

4. AIDS patients commonly have obvious lesions in lungs, gastrointestinal tract and brain. Sometimes multiple lesions mix together, which needs special attention. The examiner in chief should well know the disease spectrum of AIDS. The suspected lesions should be more sampled to avoid missing diagnosis of important diseases.

5. Lymph node may have HIV-induced lesions, with possible occurrence of infections and neoplasms. The autopsy should be performed for the whole body and specimens collected from multiple lesions (including superficial lymph nodes and thoracic and intraperitoneal lymph nodes). The shrunk lymph nodes also needs examining.

6. AIDS patients often have histories of intravenous drug abuse, homosexuality and sexually transmitted diseases. The upper arm, perineum and anus should be performed examinations during autopsy for clues of diagnosis.

7.3 Pathological Examinations and Immunohistochemistry

7.3.1 Pathological Examinations

7.3.1.1 Biopsy

Surgical removal of the pathological lesions for biopsy can be used for patients with lesions in skin, mucous membranes and superficial lymph nodes. Endoscopic forceps for biopsy can be used for patients with lesions in the digestive tract and respiratory tract. If necessary, imaging guided puncture or open biopsy can be applied to harvest the diseased lesions. Due to the compromised immunity of the patients, the trauma should be possibly avoided and biopsy is a favorable choice. In addition to the routine histological examinations, histochemistry, immunohistochemistry, electron microscopy, PCR and in situ hybridization can also be considered for use. The application of cell culture, animal inoculation and other means of detection can also be applied to determine the pathogens.

Biopsy and specimens collection

1. Try to avoid scratched, lacerated and needle-stuck skin by sharp instruments. Be cautious of preventing spillage of blood and body fluid from patients. The fixed specimens may still have active HIV in them. Therefore, the contacts to skin and mucous membrane as well as specimens collection should be cautiously performed.

2. The focal, plaque and nodular lesions should be completely removed. For diffusive lesions, sampling from different sites should be performed and the lesion for sampling should be from lesions with different manifestations. For lesions with uncertain definitions, the specimens should be possibly collected more to reduce the chances of another exposure.

3. The organs should be examined carefully, including blood vessels, bronchus, interior organs and coating membranes. Any abnormalities should be cautiously attended. Some lesions occur in the connective tissues. Pathogens may exist in blood vessels and bronchus, which should be incised in great caution. Fast irrigation with running water should be avoided due to the possibilities of flushing pathogens out.

4. The collected specimens should be carefully marked with the collection site, which would facilitate the diagnosis of

lesions and their ranges. Specimens from AIDS patients should be processed separately. For special considerations, specimens from AIDS patients should be processed respectively.

7.3.1.2 Cytology

Cytological examination is a noninvasive method with simple operations and favorable reception by patients. It can be repeatedly performed, sometimes with favorably definitive diagnosis. However, it has low positive and accurate rates.

7.3.2   Immunohistochemistry

HIV antibody is produced gradually in human body several weeks after HIV infection and can exist in the human body persistently for a lifelong time. Serologic tests include preliminary screening and confirmative test. The most commonly used screening test and confirmative test are enzyme-linked immunosorbent assay and Western blotting (WB). Conventional experimental methods include ELISA, Western blotting and indirect immunofluorescence assay (IFA). The methods for rapid detection include gelatin particle agglutination test, dot immune-node test, P24 antigen detection, molecular biological methods, RT-PCR assay, real-time fluorescence PCR, the branched chain DNA (bDNA), the enzyme enzymatic chain reaction (LCR), nucleic acid sequence dependent amplification (NASBA) and transcription-mediated amplification (TMA).

7.3.2.1 Enzyme-Linked Immunosorbent Assay (ELISA)

The basic principle of ELISA is that immune reactants chemically or immunologically change into enzyme conjugates. These enzyme conjugates are capable of binding to the corresponding antigen or antibody in the samples to be assayed to form immune complexes. The subsequently added colorless enzyme substrate is stained through enzyme catalysis or hydrolysis for observations by naked eyes and spectrophotometer. The HIV ELISA reagents for preliminary screening have been developed to the fourth generation. The first generation of reagents detects the antibody in serum with viral lysates or partially purified virus antigen coating reaction plate. Due to the defective purity of the coating antigen, the false positive rate is high. The second generation of reagents applies gene engineering to obtain recombinant antigens and synthetic peptide coated reaction plate. Due to the use of purified antigen, the specificity has been greatly improved. The third generation of reagents applies double antigen sandwich assay for the detection of antibodies to further improve the sensitivity. On the basis of the third generation, the fourth generation of reagents further improves the detection of P24 antigen. Simultaneous HIV antigen and anti-P24 antibody coated plate enables simultaneous detection of serum HIV antibody and P24 antigen.

7.3.2.2 Western Blotting

Western blotting is commonly used for confirmative test. Its basic principle is that SDS-PAGE electrophoresis of HIV virus antigen used to separate proteins of different molecular weights. The separated proteins are then transferred to nitrocellulose membrane for being sectioned into strips. Therefore, each nitrocellulose membrane strip contains the HIV virus antigens separated by electrophoresis. Subsequently, serum samples to be tested are diluted with diluents into 1/100 solution, which is then added to the nitrocellulose membrane for oscillation at a constant temperature for thorough contact and reaction. The anti-HIV antibodies in the serum would bind to the antigen on the nitrocellulose membrane. At this time, the addition of anti-human IgG-peroxidase and substrate, the reacting antigen-antibody binding strip would be in color of show purple brown. According to the demonstrations on strip, testing results can be obtained. It has been reported that Western blotting has an unfavorable specificity, with a false positive rate of about 2 % false positive rate. However, it is still the most commonly used confirmative test for HIV infection.

7.3.2.3 Immunofluorescence Assay (IFA)

The basic principle of IFA is to use H9 or HUT78 cell culture as the carrier for HIV-infected cells that contain HIV antigen. The HIV-infected lymphocytes are then smeared on a glass slide. After its fixing, the antigen section is prepared. Then the serum to be tested is added for its anti-HIV antibody to bind with the antigen, followed by its binding with fluorescence-labeled anti-human Ig. Therefore, yellowish green fluorescence can be observed within the cells under a fluorescence microscope.

7.3.2.4 Gelatin Particle Agglutination Test (PA)

The basic procedure of PA is to dilute the sample firstly, followed by respective addition of the antigen sensitized and non-sensitized gelatin particles for thorough mixing and its preserving at a constant temperature (usually at room temperature). When the HIV antibodies do exist in the serum, reaction occurs between the antigen sensitized gelatin particles and the antibody. According to the gelatin particles agglutination in the hole, testing results can be obtained. PA is advantageous in its simple operations, no need of special equipment and being appropriate for small amounts of samples.

7.3.2.5 Dot Blotting (Immunochromatography or Infiltration)

In dot blotting, nitrocellulose membrane is used as the solid phase carrier to coat HIV antigens. The specimen to be tested (usually serum, plasma, urine and other body fluids) is added.

After reaction at a certain temperature, residue specimen with no binding to the solid phase carrier is washed away. The coated antigen binds with antibody in serum to be tested, which is then connected to staphylococcal protein A with substitution of substrate by colloidal gold (or colloidal selenium). The gold labeled protein A is capable of binding with human Ig, thus can bind with the captured HIV antibody. The specimen with HIV antibodies would show an orange-red spot (or line) on the nitrocellulose membrane within 3–10 min, with favorable specificity. The test is more appropriate for tests before clinical use of blood in remote area. However, it is inappropriate for screening blood donors in urban areas.

7.4   Molecular Biological Test

With the development of biotechnology, nucleic acid detection has gained more and more attention. It can be used for directly examining HIV-RNA. And it can also be used to detect HIV infection before its serological changes, with more favorable sensitivity than P24 antigen detection.

7.4.1   Polymerase Chain Reaction (PCR)

The basic principle of the PCR technique is similar to natural DNA replication process, which has specific dependence on the oligonucleotide primers of complementary ends of the target sequence. PCR includes three basic reaction procedures, namely degeneration, annealing and extension.

7.4.1.1 Template DNA Degeneration
After heating for a period of time to 93 °C, the double strands of the template DNA or double-stranded DNA amplified by PCR is separated into single strands. The separation facilitates its binding with the premier for the reaction of the next round.

7.4.1.2 Annealing of the Template DNA and Prime
After the degeneration of the template DNA into single strands and the drop of temperature to about 55 °C, the primer and the complementary sequence of the template DNA single strand match in pairs.

7.4.1.3 Primer Extension
DNA template-primer conjugates, under effects of TaqDNA polymerase and with dNTP as the reactants, the target sequence as the template, synthesize a new semiconservative replication chain complementary to the template strand of DNA based on the principle of base pairing and semiconservative replication. Repeated cycle of degeneration, annealing and extension may produce more semiconservative replication chain. The new chain is then the template for the next cycle. Each cycle takes about 2–4 min and within 2–3 h, the target gene can be amplified to millions of times. To detect the RNA of HIV, RNA is firstly transcribed into cDNA via reverse transcription reaction, followed by PCR amplification with cDNA as the template. The reaction is known as RT-PCR.

7.4.2   Real-Time Fluorescence Quantitative PCR

Real-time fluorescence quantitative PCR refers to the addition of fluorescent moieties in the PCR reaction system, which is used for the real-time monitoring of the whole PCR process for qualitative analysis of the unknown template with the standard curve.

Its principle is to label probe with fluorescent moieties, with the end of 5′ to label fluorescent moiety of R and with the end of 3′ to label the quenching moiety Q. Without PCR amplification, the fluorescent moiety is spatially close to the quenching moiety to quench the fluorescent moiety, resulting in the failure of showing fluorescence. In PCR amplification, the primier and the fluorescence labeled specific probe conjugate in the template. The binding site of the fluorescence labelled probe and the template is between the upstream and downstream primers. By using 5′3′ exonuclease activity of Taq enzyme, the fluorescent probes are hydrolysed to release fluorescent moieties. Due to its spatial separation from quenching moiety, the fluorescence is shown. The emitted fluorescence can be detected by fluorescent probe. Test is performed while PCR amplifies for real-time detection. The technique improves PCR from semiquantitative to quantitative. Compared to routine PCR, it has favorable specificity and automation, which effectively solves the problem of PCR contamination.

7.4.3   branch DNA Assay (bDNA)

bDNA is a method for quantitative detection of plasma HIV-1 RNA. bDNA refers to an artificially synthesized DNA segments with a side chain and each side chain can be labeled with the stimulated marker. The RNA is released from HIV viral particles by centrifugation and then is captured to microspores by capture probe 1. The capture probe 2 binds to another part of viral RNA specifically, also to the pre-amplification probe, with the latter hybridizes with amplification probe namely bDNA. Two sets of target probes bind with different regions of the viral RNA pol gene respectively and specifically to form HIV-RNA oligonucleotide complexes in the microspores. The following addition of a chemical fluorescence substrate can amplify the chemical fluorescence signal after incubation. Based on the fluorescence intensity, quantification can be achieved due to the fluorescence intensity is positively related to the HIVRNA content in the samples. Cross infection of amplification does not occur in bDNA, which is a great progress compared to PCR. bDNA has dozens of probes covering the entire genome and can detect some mutants of HIV at convenience. But it is less sensitive than PCR, which is a challenge to be solved.

7.4.4 Nucleic Acid Sequence Based Amplification (NASBA)

NASBA is a new technology for RNA isothermal amplification of nucleotide sequence with in vitro specificity mediated by a pair of primers continuously and uniformly. Reaction occurs at 42 °C, which amplifies the RNA template for 109 times within 2 h. The principle of NASBA is to extract viral RNA, followed by addition of AMV reverse transcriptase, RNA enzyme H, T7 RNA polymerase and primer for amplification. The whole process can be divided into non-cyclic phase and cyclic phase. In non-cyclic phase, primer and the template RNA are synthesized into cDNA to form heterozygote of RNA and DNA after annealing under the effects of the AMV reverse transcriptase. After that, RNaseH degrades RNA; the primer II and cDNA annealing occurs. The second complementary DNA strand is synthesized with contributions from the reverse transcriptase. The double-stranded DNA transcribes RNA initiated by the promoter sequence, with T7 RNA polymerase playing a role. RNA is then reversely transcribed into DNA, with the reverse transcriptase playing a role, to enter the cyclic phase. During the cyclic phase, the template is amplified in large amount.

7.4.5 Transcription Mediated Amplification (TMA)

Technical principle of TMA and NASBA are basically the same. The slight difference is that in TMA, both MMLV reverse transcriptase and T7RNA polymerase are used. And MMLV reverse transcriptase has the activities of both reverse transcriptase and RNA enzyme H. The reaction occurs at 41.5 °C with 10^9 times amplification of RNA template within 1 h.

7.4.6 Ligase Chain Reaction (LCR)

LCR is a probe amplification technology based on the interconnection of target molecule dependent oligonucleotide probes. It is a recently developed in vitro amplification technology following the PCR with promising prospects. Its principle is the hybridization of two segments of single-stranded oligonucleotide DNA probes and the target sequence. After annealing of the two segments of DNA probe and non-mutated template, the two adjacent probes with no partition by nucleotide can be connected with ligase playing a role. The connected new chain acts as the new template to introduce the connection of the next cycle for generation of a new sub-chain. The nucleotide gene mutation in the connecting section fails the connecting reaction to terminate the amplification.

7.5 Bronchoscopy

Bronchofiberscopy examination is the direct observation of the bronchus by inserting the flexible bronchofiberscope into the trachea and bronchus via nasal cavity to detect the lesions. The practitioner also can use the clamp to harvest tissues from the lesion for pathological biopsy. Alternatively, a specialized brush can also be used to wash the lesion site, followed by examination of the washing liquid for detection of pathogens or cancer cells. Sometimes, irrigation therapy is applied for some pulmonary diseases to unclog minor bronchi and bronchioles, followed by introducing drugs by bronchoscope. Access of foreign particles to trachea or bronchus can be relieved by clamping them out with bronchoscopy.

Bronchoscopy is used primarily for etiological examination and culture in the diagnosis of pulmonary infections, including bronchial lavage, bronchoalveolar lavage fluid, brush and pulmonary biopsy. For patients with lower respiratory tract bacterial infection, bronchoalveolar lavage (BAL) or protective brushing can be applied. The cases with bacteria amount in BAL washing fluid exceeding 103 cfu/ml have 75 % chances of suffering from pneumonia. It also helps to find pneumocystis jiroveci in the washing fluid for the diagnosis of AIDS. The cases with the bacteria amount exceeding 104 cfu/ml in BAL washing fluid can be defined as lower respiratory tract bacterial infection positive. For patients with mycobacterium infection, the accurate diagnosis rate of tuberculosis by bronchoscopy is 58–96 %, with a mean of 72 %. About 5 % cases can only be confirmatively diagnosed by bronchoscopy. About 45 % patients with acute pulmonary tuberculosis obtain their diagnosis by bronchoscopy. The diagnosis rate by conventional bronchoscopy is only 10 %, while its combination with brush, irrigation or biopsy has a diagnosis rate of above 80 %. The diagnosis of bronchial tuberculosis is often missed, which is commonly found when tracheal/bronchial stenosis develops to a certain degree and causes shortness of breath. At this time, the golden time for therapeutic intervention is missed. For AIDS patients with respiratory fungal infection, bronchoscopy also plays an important role in both diagnosis and fungus identification. For immunity inhibited host patients, the chance of pulmonary infection defined by bronchoscopy is 90 %. For patients with AIDS, the sensitivity of pathogen diagnosis by BAL and TBLB are the same, both above 90 %. Bronchoscopy can also be applied for the etiological diagnosis of diffusive pulmonary diseases such as sarcoidosis. The bronchoalveolar lavage during bronchoscopy is also a favorable tool for the clinical epidemiological investigation of AIDS patients with respiratory tract opportunistic infections.

7.6   Gastrointestinal Endoscopy

The advantages of gastroscopy and colonoscopy (collectively, gastrointestinal endoscopy) include direct observation of the upper digestive tract (including esophagus, stomach and duodenum) and lower digestive tract (including the rectum, sigmoid colon, descending colon, ascending colon and the ileocecal junction) with the naked eyes of the physician, findings of severe lesions such as ulcers, tumors, polyps and diverticulitis, and detections of minor changes such as congestion, edema and color change of mucous membrane. Tissues from the suspected lesions can be clamped and harvested for pathological biopsy. It can also define the occurrence of helicobacter pylori infection that is closely related to chronic gastritis, gastroduodenal ulcer and gastric cancer. Its disadvantages include nausea or upset when the gastroscope is passing through pharynx, and abdominal pain of varying degrees at the access of the colonoscope to the intestinal lumen.

A series of complications may occur during the middle-advanced stage of AIDS. Due to the direct contact of digestive tract to the external environment as well as the importance of mucosal immune system in the prevention of infections, gastrointestinal tract is one of the vulnerable organs in the process of HIV infection. Diarrhea is the most common clinical manifestation and about 30–80 % AIDS patients have diarrhea. In them, about 64 % suffers from chronic diarrhea and about 50 % has their pathogens defined, including candida albicans and cytomegalovirus. Another common manifestation of the digestive system is fungal infections, with an occurrence of 59 % in AIDS patients. About 46 % cases of fungal esophagitis is caused by candida albicans infection. Clinically, diagnosis of patients with chronic diarrhea and esophageal fungal infection should be considered AIDS. Early HIV antibody detection and other immunological

examinations such as CD4/CD8 should be performed for timely diagnosis and treatment. AIDS patients have some characteristic manifestations in gastrointestinal endoscopy. For AIDS patients with fungal esophagitis, scattered or fusion of yellowish white plaques can be found, sometimes even with involvement of the whole esophagus and gastrointestinal tract. The definitive diagnosis can be made based on the brushing and smearing for fungi detection and mucosal biopsy. Gastrointestinal lesions caused by cytomegalovirus are usually singular/multiple ulcers or diffusive erosions with clearly defined borders under the gastrointestinal endoscope. The mucosa between lesions is normal. Colonic lesions are mostly continuous, originating from the distal colorectum and extending to the proximal colon. Sometimes only the right colon or the distal colon is involved, which should be differentiated from inflammatory bowel diseases. Due to the absence of cytomegalovirus in esophageal squamous epithelium, it can be detected only in the submucosal tissue. Therefore, for esophageal ulcer biopsy, specimen should be harvested from the base of the ulcer. CMV in the stomach and duodenum is present in columnar epithelium around ulcer and deep tissues of the ulcer base. Therefore, the specimen for biopsy should be harvested from the surrounding tissues of ulcer and the base of ulcer. When specimen for biopsy is insufficient or the pathogenic effect of virus is atypical, the diagnosis can be missed. For some patients, the endoscopy demonstrates no characteristic findings, but findings of mucosal congestion and edema as well as erosion. Due to the limitations of the examinations, endoscopic findings about intestinal mucosa in AIDS patients are rarely reported. The definitive diagnosis of gastrointestinal cytomegalovirus infection requires endoscopic biopsy for pathological examination. During endoscopy, mucosal biopsy and brushing biopsy are direct ways for the diagnosis of AIDS related gastrointestinal tract infection and for the exclusion of other concurrent causes.

7.7   CT-Guided Puncture for Biopsy

CT guided percutaneous lung biopsy is relatively safe for the early diagnosis of the disease. Exposure to infection during operation should be strictly prevented.

Diagnostic Imaging

Contents

8.1 Imaging

Due to the compromised immunity in AIDS patients, the complicated opportunistic infections and malignant neoplasms seriously threaten their lives. Diagnostic imaging is the important way for the diagnosis of AIDS-related diseases. We have already gained much knowledge about diagnostic imaging of AIDS.

8.1.1 Diagnostic Imaging Provides Valuable Information for Diagnosis of AIDS Related Diseases

Human immunodeficiency virus (HIV) infection compromises immunity of human body and the complicated opportunistic infections and AIDS-related malignant neoplasms are common causes of death in patients with AIDS. The diagnostic imaging can help to define AIDS-related diseases timely, which is important for timely therapeutic interventions and decreasing death rate. AIDS related diseases can involve the central nervous system, respiratory system, digestive system, bones and soft tissues, which is in different fields of diagnostic imaging. The diagnosis of opportunistic infections is an important field in diagnostic imaging. The pathogens include bacteria, viruses, fungi and protozoa. Pneumocystis carinii often involve lungs; cytomegalovirus invades lung and brain; herpes simplex virus and toxoplasma gondii cause intracranial infection; tuberculosis can simultaneously involve multiple sites. Opportunistic infection is most commonly found in lungs, with chest X-ray and CT scanning demonstrating morphologically different imaging findings. There are imaging demonstrations of ground glass liked density, parenchymal changes, nodules, cavities and lymphadenectasis. The opportunistic infections of the nervous system can be diagnosed by CT scanning and MRI imaging. HIV can cause AIDS related encephalopathy by passing through blood brain barrier, which may develops into progressive brain atrophy. Gastrointestinal tract and abdominal organs are also susceptible to a variety of pathogenic infections. Soft tissues infection of extremities are commonly caused by group A streptococcus and staphylococcus aurous, leading to purulent lesions such as cellulitis. Infections of bones and joints include osteomyelitis and septic arthritis. AIDS related malignancies can be demonstrated a space-occupying effect by the diagnostic imaging of the corresponding tissues or organs, in which Kaposi's sarcoma and Non-Hodgkin's lymphomas are the most common. The incidence of other neoplasms is also higher than the general population. For instances, in the low age group sustaining HIV infection, the occurrence of pulmonary carcinoma increases. Some diseases have obviously higher occurrence in patients with AIDS than in the general population, which can be used as the indicator disease of AIDS, such as penicilliosis marneffei, Kaposi's sarcoma and non-Hodgkin's lymphoma. Some imaging findings are common in AIDS related diseases, such as the diffusive lesions in lungs and brain, multiple enlarged lymph nodes, multiple organs lesions and imaging findings that are less common in the general patients. When these diseases or imaging findings are found, HIV infection should be considered in the differential diagnosis. The appropriate diagnostic imaging is favorable for timely detection and diagnosis of diseases. Due to the limited value of chest X-ray in the early detection of pulmonary opportunistic infections, clinical symptoms with negative chest X-ray findings should be further examined by CT scanning. CT scanning can facilitate the demonstrations of intra-pulmonary ground-glass density shadows, small nodules and enlarged lymph nodes. CT scanning can help to further analyze the non-specific changes demonstrated by chest X-ray. And CT scanning with high resolution is necessary for the differential diagnosis of intrapulmonary small lesions and diffusive lesions. Lesions in the brain can be diagnosed with CT scanning as the first choice, but MRI has more favorable sensitivity to lesions. Based on these diagnostic imaging, some special techniques are sometimes needed, such as MR spectroscopy, single photon emission computed tomography (SPECT) and magnetic transfer contrast imaging, for facilitative examinations and early diagnosis of AIDS. MRI can favorably show the range and depth of soft tissue infections, and necrosis; multislice spiral CT and its restructuring techniques contribute to findings and diagnosis of the chest and abdomen diseases; digitized X-ray has improved demonstrations of chest X-ray films and gastrointestinal radiography.

8.1.2 Diagnostic Imaging Provides Information for Differential Diagnosis of AIDS Related Diseases

Due to compromised immunity of patients with AIDS, the imaging demonstrations of AIDS-related diseases are different from those of common diseases. Pulmonary tuberculosis is one of the AIDS-related diseases, occurring in 20 % patients with AIDS related pulmonary infections. In patients with severely compromised immunity and the CD4 count being less than 200/ul, AIDS related pulmonary tuberculosis has different imaging findings from common secondary TB in adults, but similar to primary TB. AIDS related TB commonly causes intra-thoracic lymphadenectasis. In addition, AIDS related TB has more atypical demonstrations in lesions locations and morphology, with more common findings of blood dissemination and bronchial dissemination. For AIDS related TB, extrapulmonary occurrence is up to 50 %, with involvement of peritoneum, liver, spleen, pancreas and gastrointestinal tract. However, in patients with non AIDS related TB, the occurrence of extrapulmonary TB is only 10–15 %, with primary manifestations of systemic lymph nodes tuberculosis including lymphadenectasis of superficial, pulmonary hilus, mediastinum and abdominal cavity. AIDS related bacterial pneumonia can have atypical manifestations, such as diffusive lesions in both lungs by diagnostic imaging. AIDS related neoplasms occur in multiple locations, with occurrence of Kaposi's sarcoma in lymph nodes, gastrointestinal tract and lungs, occurrence of non-Hodgkin's lymphoma in 75 % AIDS patients during the progressive stage. Extracapsular extension is commonly seen in the central nervous system, gastrointestinal tract and bone marrow. Pulmonary manifestations are multiple nodules, parenchymal changes and pleural effusion. Differential diagnosis of AIDS related diseases is the premise for administration of a specific therapy. For the diagnostic imaging, infections should be firstly differentiated from neoplasms. Many scholars have focused attention on the image findings of these diseases and a comprehensive analysis of the imaging signs will facilitate the defining of the lesions range. Due to the multiple pathogens to cause infections, their imaging manifestations are mostly similar, presenting challenges for the differential diagnosis. It is therefore important to combine the diagnostic imaging and the clinics (including transmission route of HIV, clinical manifestations and signs, laboratory tests, immunity and therapeutic outcomes) to diagnose and differentially diagnose AIDS related diseases. CD4 count is an indicator of immunity. Different CD4 counts indicate the hosts susceptible to different diseases with different manifestations. Before etiological and histological examinations findings, the preliminary diagnosis can be made based on clinics and the diagnostic imaging, which will facilitate the early therapeutic intervention.

8.1.3 Application of Diagnostic Imaging in the Observation of Therapeutic Effects During Follow-Ups

8.1.3.1 Therapeutic Effects Against HIV/AIDS Related Diseases

Diagnosis of AIDS related diseases by diagnostic imaging is mostly confirmed by the clinical course. Therapeutic outcomes are an important factor to verify the diagnosis made by diagnostic imaging. The observation of therapeutic effect can provide an opportunity to correct the diagnosis made by imaging. The dynamic changes of imaging manifestations are related to the severity of compromised immunity, multiple infections, drug sensitivity and the occurrence of neoplasm and inflammation. AIDS complicated by infections can be alleviated or cured after treatment. After proper treatment, the obviously progressive deterioration of lesions by diagnostic imaging indicates unfavorable prognosis.

8.1.3.2 Follow-Ups of Anti-HIV Therapies

Patients receiving the highly active anti-retroviral therapy (HAART) may suffer from immune reconstitution inflammatory syndrome (IRIS). The occurrence of IRIS means restored ability of the immunity to recognize pathogens and antigens after the anti-viral therapy. Clinically, its manifestations include deteriorating opportunistic infections, atypical manifestations of infections, or autoimmune diseases. IRIS is the most common in cases of mycobacterium tuberculosis and cryptococcal infection, accounting for about 30 % of the respective infection. IRIS peaks several months after HAART treatment, with chest X-ray demonstrations of progressively deteriorating pulmonary lesions. It has been reported that the incidence rate of IRIS is 36 % in the AIDS patients complicated by pulmonary TB and receiving combined anti-tuberculosis therapy and HAART. According to imaging analysis of IRIS based on a group of 11 patients, lymph node is the most commonly involved (73 %), especially in the abdominal, axillary and mediastinal lymph nodes. Diffusive pulmonary nodules occur in 55 % patients, with pleural fluid and ascites. About 36 % patients have newly emerging or worsening abscess. During follow-ups for patients with opportunistic infections, the effect of IRIS on the therapeutic efficacy should be taken into account. The diagnosis of AIDS related diseases is difficult with the diagnostic imaging. Therefore, it is necessary to comprehensively understand clinical AIDS and the diagnostic imaging for the application of the diagnostic imaging in the diagnosis of AIDS related diseases.

8.2 X-ray

8.2.1 Chest Examinations

X-ray is the most commonly used imaging technique in clinical practice. Chest X-ray can help to know the development of thymus and pulmonary infections. Anterioposterior and lateral chest X-ray for children under 12 months old can find thymus shadow on the surface of major blood vessels in unilateral or bilateral mediastinum. Lateral observation can find that thymus shadow is immediately behind the sternum, inside the anterior mediastinum and upper mediastinum.

For children under 12 months old, invisible thymus shadow by chest X-ray indicates severe cellular immunodeficiency or combined immunodeficiency. But for children aged above 12 months or elder, chest X-ray bears unfavorable findings. Instead, special examinations such as mediastinal pneumography, mediastinal ultrasonography, CT scanning, MRI imaging and isotope scanning can be used to examine the development of the thymus. Chest X-ray may find the abnormalities in patients with pulmonary infections, such as bronchiectasis, interstitial pneumonia and lobular pneumonia. Pneumocystis carinii pneumonia is common disease in patients with AIDS or with severe immunodeficiency. By chest X-ray, the demonstrations are symmetrical blurry infiltration shadows surrounding pulmonary hila. For serious cases, the lesions can involve the middle lateral areas of both lungs. In patients with AIDS, the lungs can be obviously abnormal or close to normal in the early stage, with following occurrence of (1) lobar or lobular parenchymal lesions; (2) ground glass liked lesions; (3) singular or multiple nodular lesions; (4) cavitations; (5) hilar lymphadenectasis; and (6) pleural effusion. The lesions above can be concurrent. For some commonly seen diseases with unknown causes, AIDS related diseases or immunodeficiency should be considered.

8.2.2 Gastrointestinal Examinations

For cases of immunodeficiency with accompanying esophageal candida infection, esophageal mucus is rough with unsmooth border. Esophagus is susceptible to cytomegalovirus infection. In such cases, esophageal mucosal folds are thickened, filling with defects and have occurrence of erosion or ulceration. Gastric cytomegalovirus infection may show lesions of stomach stenosis, granuloma, erosion or ulceration, thickened and stiff intestinal wall. Kaposi sarcoma and lymphoma occur commonly in gastrointestinal tract, with polypoid, ulcer-like, plaque or nodule-like lesions in sizes of several millimeters to several centimeters. The lesions have no significant specificity, whose definitive diagnosis should be based on barium meal, in combination with gastrointestinal endoscopy and pathological biopsy if necessary.

8.3 Computerized Tomography (CT) and Magnetic Resonance Imaging (MRI)

Due to the invasion and replication of HIV in lymphoid CD4 cells, CD4 cells are destroyed to compromise the immunity of the patients, who are then susceptible to various opportunistic infections. Chest, digestive system and the nervous system are commonly involved. The demonstrations by CT scanning include:

8.3.1 Chest Imaging Demonstrations

8.3.1.1 Pneumocystis Pneumonia

Its CT manifestations can be divided into the following five types: (1) symmetrical diffusive shadows with ground glass density with hilus as the center in both lungs; decreased transparency of both lungs with demonstrations of overlapping pulmonary vascular shadows; pulmonary lobular lesions by HRCT with fusions; gas containing transparent regions between lungs and at pulmonary borders with map liked irregular margin. (2) scattered multiple linear and reticular shadows in both lungs, with thickened pulmonary markings; interlobular septal and intralobular interstitial thickening and thickened bronchovascular bundle by HRCT with confined ground glass liked density and no nodular shadows. (3) obviously increased pulmonary markings in both lungs, with possible multiple wire reticular shadows and diffusive small nodular shadows; no foci found in both lungs after administration of SMZ therapy. (4) multiple parenchymal shadows in both lungs, with increased pulmonary markings in middle and lower lungs fields and with blurry flaky shadows. (5) pulmonary interstitial fibrosis in strip liked shadows of increased density in the advanced stage, with demonstrations of emphysema and pneumothorax.

8.3.1.2 Kaposi's Sarcoma

X-ray finding is extensive, in bilateral interstitial or parenchymal shadows. Occasionally, there are confined shadows or blurry nodular shadows. Hilar and mediastinal lymphadenectasis have an occurrence of 10–21.9 %, pleural effusion 30 %, mostly bilateral. CT and HRCT findings are characteristic. The typical findings are dense and parenchymal hilus, flaky dense shadows surrounding bronchi and blood vessels with blurry borders.

8.3.1.3 AIDS-Related Tuberculosis

The imaging findings include: (1) atypical locations of the lesions. Generally, tuberculosis commonly occurs in the superior lobe, posterior-apical segment and dorsal segment of the inferior lobe, with confined range of lesions. It usually involves 1–2 pulmonary fields, with low occurrence of caseous pneumonia. In contrast, AIDS-related tuberculosis usually involves 2–6 lung fields with diffusive distribution. It involves the superior lobes of both lungs or inferior lobes of both lungs, and even concurrent involvement of both inferior lobes and both superior lobes. Involvement of singular lobe is rare and there is no commonly invaded location. (2) the nature and morphology of lesions are varied, with imaging findings generalized into 3 multiple and 3 less, namely multiple natures (exudates, proliferation and cavity) of lesions coexist, with multiple morphologies and multiple distributions

in multiple lobar segments, but less commonly seen shadows of fibrosis, calcifications and masses. (3) Lesions are susceptible to cavities, singular or multiple; multiple cavities are more common, with thin wall and sometimes liquified level. (4) high incidence of hilar and mediastinal lymphadenectasis. (5) complication of pleuritis is common.

8.3.1.4 Other Infections

Other infections in AIDS patients include infections of catenabacteria, influenza bacillus and legionella. The common manifestation is purulent change, but imaging findings not characteristic.

8.3.2 Imaging Demonstrations of the Digestive System

8.3.2.1 Non-specific Inflammatory Lesions

CT scanning of the digestive system demonstrates mesenteric and peritoneal nodules, enlarged lymph nodes to form local masses with central changes of low density changes, enlarged liver and spleen with ascites. AIDS related gastric and intestinal cryptosporidiosis has manifestations of prominent mucosal folds, narrowed and stiff gastric antrum, and dilation of partial or whole small intestine. CT scanning demonstrates thickened mesentery and peritoneum, with nodular lesions, blurry strip shadows and accompanying large amount ascites. For homosexuals, proctitis is common, leading to extensive stenosis of rectum and ulceration.

8.3.2.2 Kaposi's Sarcoma

Kaposi's sarcoma commonly occurs in the stomach and small intestine, with mucosa and submucosa lesions in intraluminal polypoid changes. At the center of esophageal polypoid lesion, some barium accumulates, referred to as bull's eye sign. Stomach and duodenum may have thickened mucosal folds and irregular ulceration. Polypoid changes are common in the colon, scattered and discontinuous, gradually develop and fuse to involve the intestinal wall and result in stenosis and stiffness. Kaposi's sarcoma can also present as granuloma-liked jumping infiltration lesion, common in rectum with obvious stenosis, filling defect and fistulation. Abdominal CT scanning demonstrates retroperitoneal nodular changes, rectal posterior wall tumor infiltration and thickening, mesenteric and retroperitoneal lymphadenectasis. Hepatic and splenic CT scanning demonstrates intraparenchymatous round shaped low density area with clearly defined border.

8.3.2.3 Lymphoma

Abdominal CT scanning demonstrates abdominal lymphadenectasis and their fusion into mass, especially in patients with Burkit's lymphoma. Abdominal, pelvic and intestinal mesenteric masses may occur with enlarged liver and spleen, in which low density foci are visible. Invasion of gastrointestinal tract has demonstrations of irregular thickened mucus and nodular changes. Kidneys and joints are possibly involved with enlarged and deformed kidneys, in which low density mass shadows are visible or with multiple nodular changes. For cases with involvement of ilium and hip joint, irregular low density area and bone destruction occur, with accompanying soft tissue mass shadows.

8.3.3   Imaging Demonstration of the Nervous System

8.3.3.1 HIV Encephalitis
CT scanning demonstrates normal or only mild brain atrophy, sometimes serious brain atrophy. Occasionally, diffusive low density area in the white matter is visible. MRI T2-weighted imaging demonstrates high signal area in the white matter.

8.3.3.2 Conditional Pathogenic Virus Infection
Progressive Multiple Leukoencephalopathy
CT scanning demonstrates low density areas in the involved white matter, mostly in parietal occipital lobe, 10 % in the frontal lobe, brainstem or cerebellum and rare involvement of the gray matter. MRI favorably demonstrates these lesions as long T1 and T2 signals.

Cytomegalovirus Encephalitis
CT scanning and MRI imaging demonstrate encephalitis as local edema and space occupying effect. Enhanced CT scanning demonstrates diffusive enhancement within the chamber tube. MRI demonstrates periventricular high signals.

8.3.3.3 Non-viral Infection
Cryptococcus Neoformans Infection
It belongs to subacute meningitis, with normal demonstrations by CT scanning and MRI imaging. Lesions in the basal ganglia and ventricle are rarely found.

Toxoplasmosis
It is a common infection in brain parenchyma of patients with AIDS. Plain CT scanning demonstrates low density areas within the brain parenchyma. Enhanced CT scanning demonstrates irregular nodular or ring shaped enhancement. For cases with diffusively distributed lesions, lesions are commonly found in the deep gray matter of the brain, with basal ganglia involvement in 75 % patients. MRI T1 weighted imaging demonstrates low signal areas with unclearly defined borderline, which are high signal areas with surrounding

high signal edema areas by T2 weighted imaging. Enhanced T1 weighted imaging demonstrates irregular nodular or ring shaped enhancement and space occupying effect. With the development of AIDS therapies, the clinical symptoms are masked with overlapping imaging demonstrations. The typical imaging findings are in a decreasing trend, which present challenges to the imaging diagnosis. The etiological diagnosis should be based on clinical examinations and laboratory tests. A full understanding of imaging demonstrations can facilitate the radiologists to propose diagnostic suggestions.

8.4   Positron Emission Tomography-Computed Tomography (PET-CT)

PET-CT is an abbreviation for positron emission tomography/computed tomography. This imaging technique is to inject extremely small amounts of positron tracer into the human body, which are mostly isotope with ultrashort half-life in the basic elements of the human body or radionuclide that is very similar in nature, such as carbon (C), nitrogen (N), oxygen (O) and fluorine (F). Tracers that carrying these positrons are the basic materials of life, such as glucose, water, amino acids, or commonly used drugs to treat diseases such as anti-cancer drugs. Therefore, by using different contrast agents, PET scanning can be performed as different functional tests and its clinical use is very extensive. Since tracer substances used in PET imaging is closely related to life metabolism, PET imaging findings demonstrate the dynamic changes of a specific metabolite (or drug) in the human body. Since CT can provide anatomic images with high resolution, PET-CT imaging integrates anatomic structures for imaging of metabolic functions, and demonstrates subtle physiological or pathological changes at the molecular level in the human body. PET-CT imaging can be a continuous imaging for whole human body for a 3D demonstration of whole human body to assess functions and metabolic status of systemic tissues and organs (especially systemic lesions or metastatic lesions). Therefore, neoplasms can be accurately staged. Many diseases (such as cancer and Alzheimer's disease) have undetectable pathologically metabolic changes in some tissues and organs initially, which gradually develop into a substantial lesion and finally obvious clinical symptoms. When the clinician can confirm the diagnosis, the diseases may have developed into its advanced stage. The opportunity for an early cure has then been missed. As a metabolic imaging technique with sensitivity and accuracy, PET-CT scanning can be performed for early detection of such diseases by a quantitative analysis of metabolic changes of tissues or lesions using complicated computer technology.

PET-CT imaging can be presently applied for the diagnosis of following conditions:

8.4.1   Neoplasms

PET-CT imaging can be applied for the differential diagnosis of most benign and malignant neoplasms in human body, neoplasms staging, assessment of the systemic condition, assessment before and after therapeutic interventions for therapeutic outcomes (including post-operative residual tumor, differential diagnosis of recurrence and scar tissue, changes of the tumor lesions before and after radiotherapy and chemotherapy, differential diagnosis of radiation pneumonia and recurrence of tumor) and systemic monitoring of tumor metastases. The applicable neoplasms include various pulmonary malignant tumors, brain tumor, colorectal cancer, lymphoma, esophageal carcinoma, metastatic liver cancer, pancreatic cancer, melanoma, breast cancer, ovarian cancer, pheochromocytoma, thyroid carcinoma, parathyroid carcinoma and multiple myeloma. For other neoplasms, PET-CT imaging is applicable for assessing metastatic neoplasms and their therapeutic outcomes, searching for unknown primary site of metastatic tumors and assessing their systemic metastasis. The development of PET-CT imaging techniques further promotes the radiotherapy for tumors. The present PET-CT technology allows radiologists understand the metabolism of the lesions for formulation of new therapeutic plan and treat the tumors according to their biological targeting areas. The PET-CT imaging demonstrates hypoxia of tumors and their cells proliferation status to guide adjustments to the therapeutic plan.

8.4.2   Neurological and Psychiatric Diseases

PET-CT imaging can be performed preoperatively for patients with epilepsy to lateralize and localize the lesion. It is also applicable for the diagnosis of Alzheimer's disease (senile dementia), assessment of mental illnesses, assessment of drug addiction, assessment of therapies for drug abuse quitting, assessment of cerebral metabolic status after brain traumatic injury, assessment of other brain metabolic dysfunctions (such as CO poisoning), early diagnosis of cerebral ischemic diseases, cerebral oxygen metabolism imaging, brain receptor imaging in Parkinson's disease (^{18}F-FP-CIT imaging), metabolism imaging of amino acid, metabolism imaging of choline.

8.4.3   Cardiovascular Diseases

PET-CT imaging can simultaneously performed with 16-slice CT coronary angiography, calcification scoring and PET myocardial perfusion imaging for understanding of vascular hardening in the heart and myocardial ischemia for the early diagnosis and assessment of coronary heart disease. By myocardial FDG-PET imaging, the radiologists and physicians can assess the myocardial viability, evaluate the efficacies of cardiac surgery, assess the severity of coronary artery disease, predict the prognosis of dilated cardiomyopathy, and make the early diagnosis of coronary heart disease.

Due to the compromised immunity of patients with AIDS, the complicated opportunistic infections and malignancies are seriously life-threatening, with common involvement of chest, digestive system and nervous system. PET-CT imaging has an extensive application, applicable for the diagnosis and monitoring of various diseases and their therapeutic efficacies. It can define the lesions in the tissues and organs of AIDS patients, especially having significance in the early diagnosis of these diseases.

8.5   Ultrasonography

Ultrasonographic organs demonstrations in patients with AIDS are described as the following:

8.5.1   Ultrasonographic Organs Demonstrations in Patients with AIDS

8.5.1.1 Ultrasonographic Heart Demonstrations
The vascular and cardiac impairments in patients with AIDS commonly occur in the advanced stage of AIDS. According to the report, the occurrence of cardiac lesions in patients with AIDS is less than 7 %, including pericardial effusion, endocarditis and myocarditis.

Pericardial Effusion
Autopsy indicated that 50–60 % patients with AIDS have pericardial lesions, with the most common occurrence of pericardial effusion. Both specificity and sensitivity of ultrasonography to pericardial effusion and pericardial filling are high. Occurrence of pericardial effusion is a predictor for the terminal stage of AIDS, which is related to the shortened survival period.

Endocarditis
Autopsy indicated that occurrence of endocarditis is 3 % in patients with AIDS, with most common occurrence of non-bacterial endocarditis or healed bacterial endocarditis. By echocardiography, the findings include valvular neoplasm (being sensitive to transesophageal ultrasound), nodular thickening of the valves, perforation, adhesions, interventricular septal perforation and papillary muscle lesions.

Cardiomyopathy
Autopsy indicated that the occurrence of cardiac abnormalities in patients with HIV infection is 25–75 %, in which

cardiomyopathy is the most common with an occurrence of up to 90 %. However, cardiac involvement is rarely found during their lifetime (29 %). This is mainly because clinicians often ignore the concealed clinical cardiac manifestations of HIV infection. By echocardiography, the findings include low motion of left ventricular wall, enlargement of both ventricles and mitral regurgitation.

8.5.1.2 Ultrasonographic Liver Demonstrations

As a part of the reticuloendothelial system, liver is the main organ responsible to eliminate HIV infected cells and also an organ for HIV replication, therefore being susceptible to opportunistic infections. It is also a window for the diagnosis of systemic opportunistic infections. Data indicated that almost all patients with HIV infection have varying degrees of liver dysfunction, but liver disease is not a major cause of death in patients with HIV infection.

By ultrasonography, the findings include enlarged liver, disproportional liver and decreased liver density. For cases with complicated opportunistic infections, the ultrasonographic findings also include local nodules, thickened bile duct wall, intrahepatic space occupying lesions.

8.5.1.3 Ultrasonographic Biliary Demonstrations

There have been increasingly reports about biliary impairments in patients with AIDS, commonly occurring in 1–8 months after the incidence of AIDS.

By ultrasonography, the findings include enlarged gallbladder with thickened wall, dilated common bile duct, irregular and unobvious intrahepatic bile duct dilatation with different demonstrations in different parts of liver (indicating the irrelevance of intrahepatic bile duct dilations) and enhanced ultrasound from intrahepatic bile duct (indicating sclerotic cholangitis or malignancies).

8.5.1.4 Ultrasonographic Pancreas Demonstrations

AIDS patients are vulnerable to pancreatic diseases. Reports from autopsy indicated that occurrence of pancreatic diseases in patients with AIDS is 10 %. But it is often ignored by clinicians due to the unobvious symptoms. Pancreatic disease occurs in patients with AIDS who are intemperant or drug abusers, manifested as acute and chronic pancreatitis.

By ultrasonography, the findings include enlarged pancreas, pseudocyst formation in patients with acute pancreatitis; pancreatic calcified plaque, pancreatic stones, changes of common bile duct in patients with chronic pancreatitis.

8.5.1.5 Ultrasonographic Spleen Demonstrations

As a part of the lymphoreticular tissue, spleen can be involved in each stage of AIDS. In the acute stage, some patients may have splenomegaly and moderate splenomegaly has a most common occurrence, with a few cases of massive splenomegaly. Spleen lesions are in consistency with systemic lymphocytic changes.

By ultrasonography, the findings include obviously enlarged spleen with some cases of massive splenomegaly, hypoechoic nodules in the spleen with clearly defined peripheral parts and some with calcified plaque. Enlarged spleen is often the early sign of HIV infection.

8.5.1.6 Ultrasonographic Kidney Demonstrations

HIV related kidney diseases include acute renal failure and chronic glomerular lesions. The former is generally caused by the renal toxicity of drugs, including drugs to treat HIV and related infections while the latter is related to HIV infections.

By ultrasonography, the findings include enlarged kidneys, unclearly defined cortex/medullar interface. The differences from those demonstrations of chronic renal failure are that the ultrasonic echo intensity and the kidneys enlargement are disproportional to the degree of renal lesions. In the advanced stage, the kidneys still enlarge. For cases with infection caused renal abscess, demonstrations include space occupying effect, hypoechoic nodules or no ultrasonic echo in the early stage.

8.5.1.7 Ultrasonographic Eyes Demonstrations

Incidence of AIDS-related eye diseases is relatively high among the sensory organs. In patients with AIDS, more than 90 % have opportunistic infections related ocular manifestations and more than 70 % have accompanying signs of eye diseases.

By ultrasonography, the findings include vitreous opacities, which is the most common with an occurrence of more than 50 % in a randomized sample of 10 hospitalized patients; followed by thickened retrobulbar wall and space occupying effect, which may be related to AIDS complicated by cytomegalovirus infection and T. gondii infection. Ocular lesions often require specialized examinations, such as retinal optical imaging and CT scanning. As a non-invasive examination, ultrasonography is convenient and fast, thus a favorable way for early detection. During the operation, attention should be given to probe distance and staff protection (tears).

8.5.1.8 Ultrasonographic Lymph Nodes Demonstrations

Lymph node lesions can be detected in the early stage of AIDS, with demonstrations of transient general superficial lymphadenectasis 2–6 weeks after HIV infection. As the disease progresses, atrophy of lymph nodes occurs. In the stages of pre-AIDS and AIDS, sustained systemic lymphadenectasis occurs with lymphadenectasis of another two regions in addition to inguinal lymphadenectasis.

By ultrasonography, the findings include superficial or abdominal lymphadenectasis, normal structures and morphology of lymph nodes, visible lymphoid hilum, clearly defined cortex and medulla of lymph nodes, and infusion of lymph nodes into mass in the advanced stage.

8.5.2 The Value of Ultrasonography in Diagnostic Imaging of AIDS

Due to advantages of ultrasonography, namely non-invasive, repeatable, wide range of detection, low cost and favorable tolerance by patients, it has an extensive application in the clinical practice, especially applicable for patients with AIDS. It can be used for quick and accurate assessment of the substantive organs and thus provides references for clinical physicians. It is especially applicable for patients with AIDS who are drugs abusers, because it is challenging for them to receive other examinations and tests, such as blood sampling difficulty due to the serious vascular damage, their difficulties for standing and other postures for radiological examinations due to their poor compliance. Ultrasonography provides first-hand information quickly and accurately for clinical use. It facilitates assessments for organs sizes, internal structural changes, relationship with adjacent organs, and some organs functions. As accumulated experience by radiologists, ultrasonography can provide more clinical information. For example, before occurrence of death, patients with AIDS commonly have enlarged liver, with intense and enhanced ultrasound echo, blurry network structure like serious fatty liver; but no attenuated posterior echo; enlarged kidneys similar to chronic renal failure, indicating organ failure, which has been retrospectively verified. Based on our experience and knowledge, we found the organs impairments are in line with the following changes: superficial lymphadenectasis → hepatosplenomegaly → eye vitreous opacity → organ changes including gallbladder, pancreas, kidney, pericardium and other organs. In the future, we will further summarize our experience and gain knowledge in this field to provide valuable diagnostic information for clinical application.

8.6 Implications of HIV/AIDS Infection for Health Care Staffs

World AIDS Report 2006, issued by UNAIDS and WHO (World Health Organization) on Nov. 21, 2006, indicated that the newly emerging patients with HIV infection are 4.3 million in the year of 2006, so that patients with HIV/AIDS have reached 39.5 million. In the year of 2005, occurrence of death in patients with AIDS was nearly 2.9 million. On Nov. 25, 2006, the Chinese Ministry of Health, the UNAIDS and the WHO made a joint announcement that China has about 0.65 million patients with HIV/AIDS. With the spread of the disease, more and more patients with HIV/AIDS paid their visits to the clinics and the medical staffs are increasingly exposed to HIV/AIDS. With more serious occupational exposure to HIV/AIDS, the awareness of their occupational protection should be raised.

8.6.1 Occupational Exposure to AIDS in Medical Care

8.6.1.1 The Concept of Occupational Exposure

Occupation exposure to HIV/AIDS refers to the possibility of HIV infection by medical staffs during the prevention and treatment. Specifically, their defect skin or non-gastrointestinal mucus is contaminated by blood or body fluid of patients with HIV/AIDS; their skin is stabbed by needles or other sharp instruments by HIV containing blood or body fluid.

8.6.1.2 The Status of Occupational Exposure

The cases of occupational exposure to HIV/AIDS were totally 100 cases in the year of 2002. CDC of the U.S.A estimated that the totally number of occupational exposure to HIV/AIDS is 5,000 cases each year worldwide. Research reports indicated that the occupational exposure rate of HIV/AIDS in China is 62.8–98.0 %, while the occupational exposure rate of HIV/AIDS worldwide is 22.5–73.0 %.

8.6.1.3 Reasons of Medical Occupational Exposure

Weak Awareness of Self-Protection in Medical Staffs
Since 1990s, in the field of medicine, occupational protection against HIV/AIDS has gained focused attention. But it has been reported that the understanding of standard prevention principles against HIV/AIDS by medical staff is not sufficient, and their awareness of self-protection against HIV/AIDS is poor. To ensure occupational safety, the CDC of the U.S.A. proposed the concept of standard prevention, which has been implemented in the U.S. since 1996. By standard prevention, the blood, body fluids, excretions and secretions of patients with HIV/AIDS are infectious; people who have exposure to these should be performed quarantine and preventive measures, no matter whether there is obvious blood contamination or whether there is contact with non-intact skin and mucous membranes. In China, the concept of standard prevention has been incorporated into the *Guideline for Hospital Infections Management (for Trial Implementation)* issued by the Ministry of Health in 2000. Studies indicated that medical staffs fail to strictly observe the regulations like wearing gloves, goggles and other protective devices and they tend to ignore the correct operation, with poor awareness in occupational protection. Odujinrin et al. [1] reported that during the whole process of exposure to blood from

patients with HIV/AIDS, 69 % medical staffs always observe the standard prevention principles and 29 % sometimes observe the standard prevention principles. Odubuyide et al. [2]. reported that more than 90 % interviewees of medical staffs had experienced stab injuries by needles or sharp instruments, 3/4 interviewees of medical staffs observes standard preventive measures in half or less operations. A study from China reported that 52.9 % medical staffs stab their fingers once every 3 months on average. During injection, fluid transfusion and blood sampling operation, only 7.7 % nurses reported to often wear gloves and 22.1 % occasionally wear gloves.

Management Factors
Insufficient systemic occupational prevention training against AIDS is another important reason for the high incidence of occupational exposure to HIV/AIDS. In addition, insufficient occupational protective facilities for medical staffs are still another reason for occupational exposure. No complete reporting system for supervision is the other problem that hinder occupational protection against HIV/AIDS.

8.6.1.4 High Risk Populations of Occupational Exposure
All medical staffs in medical environments have the risk of HIV infection. Medical staffs working in different departments have different risks of occupational exposure. According to an international report, occurrence of injuries by sharp instruments is the most frequent in nurses, about 1/3 injuries by sharp instruments in the U.S. occur in nurses. Surgeons in departments of surgery, obstetrics and gynecology, and dental are susceptible to HIV infection during surgical procedures. Department of laboratory tests is also a department that susceptible to iatrogenic infection. Medical staffs working there are possibly infected during the processes of blood sampling, samples centrifuging, managing tests equipments. Medical staffs working in the department of pathologic diagnosis are responsible to deal with the lesions tissues from patients with AIDS and their skin and mucus exposure may cause them susceptible to HIV infection. The above mentioned studies indicate that the occupational exposure rate of HIV/AIDS is high in nurses. The population of nursing workers deserves focused attention because they are susceptible to stab injuries when processing the medical disposals. Nursing workers should receive focused attention and training for awareness of self-protection against HIV/AIDS.

8.6.1.5 The Routes and Ways of Occupational Exposure
A research team from the U.S. interviewed 1,202 medical staffs and found that in the occupational exposure to HIV/AIDS, 80 % are needle stab injuries, 8 % are injuries by

sharp instruments and 7 % are open wound infection, which are in consistency with the study results from China. The occupational exposure to HIV/AIDS is mostly via defective skin, wounds, mucosa, dressing change, disposal of excretions, vomiting, secretions and drained fluid, emergency treatment of trauma and massive bleeding. Physicians, nurses and practitioners of laboratory tests are susceptible to scratches or stabs by contaminated sharp equipments during surgical procedures, injections, punctures and equipments cleansing. They may also be occupationally exposed to blood or other body fluids from HIV-infected patients via defective skin or mucous membrane. Other body fluids include sperm, vaginal secretions, cerebrospinal fluid, synovial fluid, pleural effusion, ascites, pericardial fluid, amniotic fluid and other body fluids from HIV infected patients. The main reason for occupational injuries by sharp instruments is that the medical staffs fail to observe the operating procedures. Occupational infection of HIV/AIDS via occupational exposure is mostly caused by stabs and scratches by contaminated needles and other sharp instruments. These occupational injuries are commonly caused by their carelessness and inappropriate operations. *The Universal Protection Principles* recommended by the WHO is a guideline for safe operations by medical staffs. Due to the high probability for first line clinicians and medical staffs to be occupationally exposed to blood and body fluids from patients with HIV/AIDS, their failed observation to *The Universal Protection Principles* during medical operations will increase the risks of occupational infection.

8.6.1.6 Occupational Exposure Risks
Concerning the occupational exposure risk of HIV infection, the probability of occupational exposure via defective skin is 0.3 %, via mucosal contact 0.09 %, whereas the probability of occupational exposure via large volume blood and (or) blood with high viral load is above 5 %. The mean probability of occupational infection after epidermal contacts to HIV contaminated blood is less than 0.1 %. Although studies have shown that the occupational exposure risk of HIV/AIDS is low but it persistently exists. Therefore, the probability of occupational infection should be indicated with the index of accumulative risk.

8.6.2   Occupational Protection Against HIV/AIDS in Medical Care

8.6.2.1 Management and Supervision
For prevention and control of iatrogenic HIV/AIDS transmission, the Chinese Ministry of Health has issued a series of regulations such as the *Guideline for Hospital Infections Management (for trails implementation)* and *Guidelines for Protection of Medical Staffs against Occupational Exposure*

to HIV/AIDS (for trails implementation). The medical institutions should strictly implement these regulations. Government agencies for health and medicines should reinforce the management of blood sampling and supplying. Medical institutions should be intensively supervised and inspected for their implementations in control of iatrogenic infections.

8.6.2.2 Education and Training

Weak awareness of medical staffs in self-protection against iatrogenic infections also contributes to the iatrogenic infections. Therefore, the medical institutions should strengthen the education and training to medical staffs about the knowledge of iatrogenic HIV infection. Their enhanced awareness in self-protection will affect their behaviors in adopting standard preventive measures.

8.6.2.3 Equipments Disinfection

Various medical instruments and equipments should be strictly disinfected and sterilized. Disposable instruments and equipments should be selected if possible. For some complicated instruments and equipments, such as endoscopes, dental or gynecological instruments, and surgical instruments, the recently recognized methods should be applied for their disinfection and sterilization.

8.6.2.4 Standardized Preventive Measures

With increasing number of asymptomatic cases in clinical practice, the only strategy for safety is to implement the standard preventive measures, which require the treatment of blood and other body fluids from patients as potentially infectious blood-borne pathogens.

8.6.2.5 General Protective Measures

Firstly, the skin of the medical staffs should be kept intact. When exposed to blood, body fluids, mucous membranes or defective skin of patients with AIDS, the medical staffs should wear gloves. Before and after contacts to patients with HIV/AIDS, hands should be carefully washed. Once the gloves are taken off, the hands also should be thoroughly washed. When medical operations are performed with possible splashes of blood and/or body fluids, protective gloves, mask and glasses should be worn, with impermeable protective clothing if necessary. To reduce injuries by sharp instruments is the main preventive measure against occupational exposure. The used sharp instruments should be put into a specified tool box that cannot be penetrated. Recapping the used needle is prohibited to avoid direct contacts to the used needles and blades.

8.6.2.6 Treatment After Exposure
Emergency Treatment
The contaminated regions should be washed with soap and running water. For cases of contaminated eyes mucus, the eyes should be repeatedly flushed with large amount of saline. For cases with wound, the blood should be possibly squeezed out from the wound, and the wound should be washed with soap and running water. The wound should then be disinfected and sterilized with 75 % ethanol and 0.5 iodophor, followed by dressing.

Preventive Medication After Exposure
Preventive medication after exposure should be preferably within 24 h after the exposure. For cases of more than 24 h after the exposure, preventive medication is also recommended. The basic medications include two retroviral inhibitors in conventional doses, oral intake of dipeptide Chi (zidovudine plus lamivudine) for 28 days. The supplementary medication is the addition of a protease inhibitor based on the basic medication.

Reports and Follow-Ups After Exposure
The occupational exposure should be recorded in details and reported. The main contents of reporting include the type of exposure, relation to sharp instruments, depth of stabs, defective severity of the skin and mucus, substances exposed to, duration of exposure, management after exposure, preventive medications and the initial medication. Based on these details, the severity of the exposure and the possibility of HIV infection are estimated. According to the standard requirements, the cases of occupational exposure should receive HIV antibody tests. Therefore, for cases of occupational exposure, serum samples should be collected as soon as possible for detection of HIV antibody. If negative, the seral HIV antibody should be tested at week 6, 12 and 24 after the exposure. Despite of the small risk of HIV infection by occupational exposure in medical staffs, the HIV infection after occupational exposure can be very serious due to the insufficiency of effective medications. However, it is unnecessary to be panic to occupational exposure. A comprehensive knowledge about preventive measure against occupational exposure to HIV/AIDS, strict observation of the operational guidelines for safety and careful operational procedures can greatly decrease the risk of occupational exposure and infection rate of HIV infection caused by occupational exposure.

8.7   Relationship Between AIDS and Clinical Medicine

8.7.1   AIDS and Internal Medicine

Since the recognition of AIDS, scientists have dedicated to the research for the development of anti-HIV drugs and therapies. Therapies of the internal medicine include antiviral therapy, immunotherapy, gene therapy and the therapy of traditional Chinese medicine. In the year of 1987, the nucleosides, such as AZT, were firstly applied to treat AIDS [3]. In the year of 1994, protease inhibitors were applied for treatment of AIDS [4]. Both therapies showed poor outcomes. In the year of 1995, Chinese American Dayi HE proposed the application of combined medication of 3 drugs from the above two types of drugs, which is now known as highly active antiretroviral therapy (HAART) [5]. Thereafter, the antiretroviral therapy is developed and advanced. In the year of 1997, the combination of two nucleosides with a protease inhibitor/a non-nucleotide reverse transcriptase inhibitor to inhibit retroviral replication showed significant therapeutic efficacy [6]. Such timely and reasonable choice of multiple drugs for a combination therapy can suppress viral replication and reduce the mortality and morality of AIDS-related opportunistic infections and neoplasms, which is one important breakthrough in AIDS therapies. But even viral replication has been completely suppressed in patients after the treatment, their plasma levels of HIV virus DNA concentration decrease very slowly and replication-competent HIV can be separated from the blood. A rapid rebound of viral replication also may occur in such patients. Therefore, long-term administration of the therapy is recommended.

8.7.1.1 Antiretroviral Therapy

Drugs Classification

1. Integrase inhibitor, Fuzeon (T20), that prevents HIV binding to the cell surface receptor;
2. Nucleoside reverse transcriptase inhibitors (NRTI) and non-nucleotide reverse transcriptase inhibitors (NNRTI) that inhibit the activity of virus reverse transcriptase; NRTI including Azidothymidine (AZT), Didanosine (DDL), Stavudine (D4T), Lamivudine (3TC), Abba Cabey (ABC), Combivir, Zalcitabine (DDC), Tenofovir (Viread), Emtricitabine (FTC) and Trizivir (ABC + AZT + 3TC) and NNRTI including efavirenz (EFV), nevirapine (NVP) and Delavirdine (DLV);
3. Integrase inhibitors that prevent the integration of virus DNA into cellular DNA;
4. PIs that inhibit the assembly of viral proteins including indinavir (IDV), ritonavir (RTV), Nelfinavir (NEV), saquinavir capsules (SQV), Agenerase (APV), Atzanavir, Fosamprenavir (f-APV), Kaletra (Lopinavir plus Ritonavir) and Lopinavir (LPV).

The Opportunity for Receiving Therapies

Due to the adverse reactions and drug resistance of antiviral drugs for AIDS, the selection for therapeutic opportunity is very important. Early treatment suppresses the virus earlier, with advantages of restoring immunity and inhibiting the spread of the virus but disadvantages of decreased quality of life caused by their adverse reactions, the secondary severe toxic and side effects, early emergence of drug resistance and limited subsequent drugs selection. Late administration of drug therapies can avoid the decrease of life quality caused by adverse reactions, delay the occurrence of drug resistance and reserve more options for drugs use. However, a serious unrecoverable immune dysfunction may be caused, as well as the increased difficulty in anti-HIV and increased risks of HIV spreading. Generally speaking, for patients with their CD4 count being below 200/μl should immediately receive antiviral therapy, which has no controversy. Patients with their CD4 count being between 200 and 350/μl should also receive the antiviral therapy immediately, but controversy still exists. The anti-viral therapy for patients with their CD4 count being above 350/μl should be based on their viral load (VL). According to the recent guideline from the United States Department of Health and Human Service (DHHS), patients with CD4 count being above 350/μl and VL being above 55,000 (by RT-PCR or bDNA) should immediately receive the antiviral therapy. Currently, it has been recognized that the indicators for antiviral therapy include VL being above 55,000/μl or CD4 being less than 350/μl or the decrease of CD4 count being more than 300/μl within 2–18 months or occurrence of AIDS related diseases and symptoms.

Therapeutic Planning

With the development of drugs and occurrence of drug resistance, the therapeutic planning should be changed accordingly. Till the year of 2004, there have been 24 anti-viral drugs approved for clinical use, including 10 NRTIs, 3 NNRTIs, 10 PIs and 1 integrase inhibitor (T20). In China, 5 anti-viral drugs can be manufactured including 1 Pi. Different combinations of anti-viral drugs for different therapeutic planning can be formulated. The most commonly used combination is 2 NRTIs plus 1 NNRTI.

8.7.1.2 Immunotherapy

Not all cases of HIV infection develop into AIDS. For some patients, HIV is static in their bodies. Therefore, it is promising for them to control HIV through the reconstruction of their immunity by therapies to generate immunity compensation. In addition, opportunistic infections and malignancies occur in patients with AIDS due to their compromised immunity. To control these complications, immunity should be improved. Therefore, the therapy for immunity reconstruction is important for patients with AIDS. But immunity reconstruction depends largely on the suppression/clearance of HIV. Therefore, combination of anti-HIV therapy with immunity reconstruction should be concurrently applied to effectively suppress HIV/AIDS.

The immunotherapies include:

1. Immunocyte replacement

    Immunocyte replacement can be performed by bone marrow transplantation, thymus transplantation, lymphocytes transfusion to improve immunity of human body, increase the CD4 counts and cause delayed skin hypersensitivity. But these therapies have transient therapeutic efficacy due to allergic reactions and rejections.

2. Immunomodulators

Interferons have broad spectrum antiviral effect and one interferon works against several different viruses. A large dose of interferon inhibits humoral and cell immunity while a small dose of interferon improves immunity. Among interferons, alpha interferon has the strongest effects, which can be applied to treat HIV infection, increase the lymphocytes and CD4 count and reduce the occurrence of opportunistic infections. Interleukin 2 is a T cell secreted lymphokine, which reversely acts on the proliferation of T cells. Patients with AIDS have decreased CD4 count and monocytes in their peripheral blood. The release of interleukin 2 and its receptor are concurrently reduced, resulting in decreased activity of cytotoxic T lymphocytes and natural killer cells. Due to the decreased release of lymphokine, defense mechanism is compromised to provide opportunities for occurrence of opportunistic infections. This drug acts to increase the number of peripheral lymphocytes in patients with AIDS and thus improve their immunity. Granulocyte-macrophage colony stimulating factor (GM-CSF) and granulocyte colony stimulating factor (G-CSF) act to increase the granulocytes and macrophages in the peripheral blood. And the underlying mechanism is to stimulate the blood manufacturing by bone marrow and accelerate the cells maturation and release. Granulocyte colony stimulating factor (G-CSF) only contributes to the increase of granulocytes. But both contribute to the increase of white blood cells in the peripheral blood and thus improve the body's defense mechanism to fight against the opportunistic infections, which are especially applicable for patients with bone marrow depression caused by the use of AZT. Thymosin contributes to the transformation of bone marrow stem cells into T lymphocytes to participate in regulating the immunity and improving the cellular immunity. Gamma globulin contributes to improving the immune status and clinical course for children with AIDS and patients with AIDS-related syndrome. T peptide is a constituent of vascular intestinal peptide (VIP) and also a segment of HIV envelope glycoprotein, gp120. Containing pentapeptide, it can block HIV to bind with lymphocytes and CD4 receptors of brain cells, thus preventing HIV from its access to cells and its replication in lymphocytes.

Immunopotentiators

Inosine, as the main component of isoprinosine, acts to stimulate bone marrow stem cells to produce new granular lymphocytes, increase the count and activity of killer cells and CD4 lymphocytes. Lentinan acts to improve the general condition of the patients and increase the production of interferons.

Vaccines

Vaccines against HIV/AIDS include recombinant gp160 plus incomplete Freund adjuvant and inactivated HIV.

8.7.1.3 Gene Therapy

Gene therapy is to introduce anti-viral genes into the cells of the patients to strengthen their defense mechanism. Gene therapy is applied for patients with AIDS because AIDS is an acquired disease caused by integration of HIV gene with the chromosomes and the inhibition of such integration can prevent the progression of HIV infection into AIDS. AIDS is a disease of lymphoid system, which defines the target cells for gene therapy. Compared to impaired lymphocytes by HIV, lymphocytes produced by anti-HIV gene therapy have more powerful proliferative ability. Even introduction of HIV resistance gene into partial lymphocytes is also expected to achieve curative effect. The application of gene therapy for patients with AIDS is based on the fact that binding of HIV tat and rev with their target genes RNA to form a functional complex, which plays its pathogenic role. Therefore, factors to interfere the formation of the functional complex hold important significance to interfere HIV replication and the progression into AIDS.

8.7.1.4 Traditional Chinese Medicine

Traditional Chinese medicine (TCM) is an effective weapon in fights against illnesses for thousands of years in China. Much experience and knowledge in traditional Chinese medicine have been gained to form a theoretical system. In the treatment of AIDS, TCM plays the roles of improving the immunity, controlling the opportunistic infections by differential syndrome and therapy, improving the quality of life for patients with AIDS, inhibiting HIV and decreasing the toxic and side effects of chemical therapies. Is has been known that acupuncture, shadow boxing and herbs including ginseng, glossy ganoderma, astragalus root and Chinese angelica act to improve the immunity of human body. And some herbs act to inhibit HIV, such as trichosanthin and glycyrrhizin.

8.7.2   AIDS and Surgery

Apart from various opportunistic infections and neoplasm, AIDS can also be complicated by some surgical diseases and the diagnosis of some complications needs to harvest specimens by surgical operations. Therefore, sometimes it is necessary for patients with AIDS to be surgically managed. Due to some special problems caused by immunodeficiency in AIDS patients, surgical indications should be strictly chosen, with more detailed surgical planning. Due to the common occurrence of spinal cord lesions, AIDS patients should not receive spinal anesthesia and epidural anesthesia. And the surgical outcomes in patients with AIDS are generally poorer than patients with other diseases, with more occurrence of complications and high death rate. During the surgical procedures, the surgeons are susceptible to occupational exposure caused by skin injuries of the surgeons.

Common surgery related complications of AIDS include AIDS-related lymphadenectasis, splenomegaly; AIDS related malignancies; brain abscess caused by opportunistic infections of toxoplasmosis, candida infection and cryptococcosis; increased intracranial pressure caused by space occupying lesions of tumor; bleeding, perforation and toxic megacolon caused by cytomegalovirus; avian mycobacterium induced intestinal obstruction and intra-abdominal inflammatory swelling; gastrointestinal bleeding, intestinal obstruction and intussusception caused by Kaposi's sarcoma; anal condyloma; appendicitis and cholecystitis caused by opportunistic infections or neoplasms; pancreatitis caused by infection or medications.

8.7.2.1 Common Surgical Treatments for Patients with AIDS

Minor operations include:

1. Catheterization of a silicon rubber tube into superior vena cava for indwelling for cases receiving long-term intravenous therapy for venous access.
2. Biopsy of lymph nodes and muscles
3. Abscess drainage
4. Surgical removal of cystoid swelling
5. Hernioplasty
6. Surgical operations on anus and rectum to treat hemorrhoids, anal fistula and abscess
   Major operations include:
1. Surgical explorations: emergency operations for appendicitis, cholecystitis, obstruction, bleeding and perforation of the gastrointestinal tract caused by opportunistic infections and tumors; abdominal symptoms caused by organ masses, retroperitoneal lymphadenosis.
2. Emergency operations: acute inflammation caused by blockage or obstruction of gallbladder, bile duct and appendix; gastrointestinal bleeding, perforation and toxic megacolon caused by cytomegalovirus; acute abdominal illnesses caused by various reasons.

Early Diagnosis and Treatment

Early diagnosis and treatment is important for AIDS related acute abdominal illnesses. In principle, the precautions include: removing the key pathogenic cause of acute abdominal illness; minimizing surgical damages to the human body; treating opportunistic infections; strengthening nutritional support. Surgical treatments for other diseases include acute pancreatitis, tumor, and spleen resection. The occurrence of complications and death in patients with AIDS after surgical operations depends mainly on the patients' immunity and other contributing factors include general condition, nutritional status, therapeutic opportunity and the complicated diseases.

8.7.2.2 The Risks of HIV Infection in Surgical Operations

During surgical procedures, surgeons use sharp instruments and contact to blood and body fluids of AIDS patients. Therefore, there is certain risk of HIV infection. Surgeons should have general knowledge about AIDS prevention and treatment and be aware of iatrogenic infection. The patients with AIDS should be attended with warm-heartedness and awareness of preventing iatrogenic transmission of HIV. Surgeons should also adopt appropriate protective measures during surgical operations for patients with AIDS.

References

1. Odujinrin MT, Adebajo SB. Social characteristics, HIV/AIDS knowledge, preventive and risk factors elicitation among prisoners in Lagos, Nigeria [J]. West Afr J Med. 2001;20(3):191–8.
2. Odubuyide IO. Doctors at risk of hepatitis B and HIV infection from patients in Nigeria [J]. J R Soc Health. 1996;116(3):157–60.
3. Yarchoan R, Broder S. Development of antiretroviral therapy for the acquired immunodeficiency syndrome and related disorders. A progress report [J]. N Engl J Med. 1987;316(9):557–64.
4. Katz RA, Skallka AM. The retroviral enzymes [J]. Annu Rev Biochem. 1994;63:133–73.
5. Finzi D, Hermankova M, Carruth LM, et al. Identification of a reservoir for HIV-1 in patients on highly active antiretroviral therapy [J]. Science. 1997;278(5341):1295–300.
6. Sorg T, Methali M. Gene therapy for AIDS [J]. Transfus Sci. 1997; 18(2):277–89.

Contents

9.1   Tasks of Evidence Based AIDS Imaging

Evidence based medicine (EBM) is a concept combining clinicians' personal professional knowledge, the optimal clinical evidence available, and the choice of patients to guide clinical practice and make the best clinical decision. The core idea of EBM is to seriously and cautiously apply the latest and optimal information gained from clinical studies to diagnose and treat patients. The three fundamental factors of EBM are to seek, evaluate and correctly use evidence. The significance and necessity of evidence in decision-making is emphasized. The rapid development of new techniques and methods of modern medical imaging provides more and more information for clinical practice. The symptoms of AIDS patients are complex, usually with involvements of multiple systems, multiple organs, and diverse pathogens simultaneously or successively. Therefore, the diagnosis of AIDS patients depends on various investigations, in which diagnostic imaging is the primary method to obtain clinical evidence. How to start from clinical symptoms to select appropriate diagnostic imaging methods for persuasive evidence of HIV/AIDS is a new subject for radiologists. The method and thinking way of EBM offers essential reference for HIV/AIDS imaging in clinical practice.

9.2   Relationship Between AIDS Imaging and Evidence Based Medicine

Evidence based medicine (EBM) is a practical pattern and thinking methodology for clinical medicine rather than a specific method or technique to solve a clinical problem. The three principles of EBM are optimal evidence available as the basis of decision-making; clinicians' personal professional knowledge as professional support; patients' benefits and needs as the supreme goal. The five steps of EBM include: (1) evidence retrieval; The primary evidence is from original research articles including experimental research

H. Li (ed.), *Radiology of HIV/AIDS*,
DOI 10.1007/978-94-007-7823-8_9, © Springer Science+Business Media Dordrecht and People's Medical Publishing House 2014

articles and observational research articles. The secondary evidence is from comprehensive analysis and reviewing based on the original research articles, including Meta-analysis, systematic review, reviews, commentaries and case histories correctly collected as the first-hand clinical data. (2) questions raising; Based on the clinical data and imaging findings of patients, one or several questions with potentials to be resolved are raised to establish the research key terms. Data being closely related to the clinical questions is then retrieved in authorities literatures for further review and analysis. (3) evidence assessment; It is mainly based on the authenticity and clinical importance (assessed by clinical epidemiology and the principles of EBM). (4) evidence application; The clinical cases vary in terms of gender, age, HIV/AIDS related diseases, the severity and course of these diseases, patients' compliance, social factors, cultural backgrounds, biological and clinical characteristics. Authentic and reliable evidence with clinical value is not necessarily appropriate to all patients. Rather, comprehensive analysis is necessary to combine professional clinical knowledge, physical and mental conditions of each patient, selections of the patients. The application of the evidence should be adjusted accordingly to assess the reliability and authenticity of the evidence using epidemiologic and EBM standards. (5) Intervention outcomes assessments. The discrepancies between the real intervention outcomes and expected intervention outcomes should be assessed. The reasons for the discrepancies should be analyzed to improve the standardization of clinical decision making. The optimal clinical evidence should be applied to guide the clinical practice.

The three principles of EBM are the codes for radiologists. The five steps are the procedures for them to observe in diagnostic imaging. HIV/AIDS imaging is inherently related to EBM. HIV/AIDS diagnostic imaging focuses not only on accumulation of personal clinical experience, but also on the collection and systematic review of medical literatures. The increase of related medical literature is essential to the development of HIV/AIDS imaging. The importance of medical publications is emphasized in the clinical diagnosis and treatment, which is consistent to the principles of EBM in guiding clinical decision making by systematically synthesized and analyzed information obtained from medical literatures.

Due to compromised immunity in patients with AIDS, their organs are susceptible to direct HIV invasion as well as multiple complications. Compared to the imaging findings in healthy populations, there are many findings in common. However, the imaging findings of patients with AIDS are characteristic. Therefore, in clinical practice of HIV/AIDS imaging, the specific imaging should be correctly chosen based on the EBM principles and clinical symptoms. The data obtained should be integrated to the numerous related literatures for assessment, with resulted optimal objective

evidence. The core of EBM is to obtain the most recent and powerfully persuasive evidence in the development of medical sciences based on personal clinical experience to continuously improve the quality of clinical diagnosis and treatment. The nature of EBM is a new and effective lifelong learning for clinicians, with a focused emphasis on evidence obtaining and assessing. But how should we obtain correct evidence? The method is the key. Only by selecting the most appropriate imaging examination can we obtain the most powerfully persuasive evidence. EBM also stresses the importance of analysis and synthesis of the information. The diagnosis and differential diagnosis of HIV/AIDS imaging are actually based on the theoretical systems of X-ray, B-ultrasonography, CT scanning and MRI imaging. All of these implicate the inherent correlation between EBM and HIV/AIDS imaging in terms of diagnosis, treatment and reasoning methodology. The diagnostic pattern and reasoning of HIV/AIDS imaging would also develop with the development of EBM.

9.3 Necessity of Evidence in AIDS Imaging

The wide application of EBM requires radiologists to learn more knowledge, establish rigorous reasoning, and correctly apply various imaging examinations for their clinical service. Therefore it is essential to develop evidence based reasoning for clinical diagnosis and treatment.

For evidence based imaging diagnosis of HIV/AIDS, a technique guideline should be established according to the features of AIDS. Two or more imaging examinations should be assessed for their practicality and specificity to find an optimal imaging examination for the diagnosis of AIDS related diseases. For example, for the diagnosis of AIDS related pulmonary diseases, chest X-ray, CR, DR, CT scanning, MRI imaging and bronchoscopy are the commonly used imaging examinations. Chest X-ray provides dynamic imaging from all perspectives for patients with AIDS. CR and DR can effectively display pathological changes of thorax and lungs, but fail to define minor lesions or pathological changes overlapping with organs (such as interstitial pneumonia, mediastinal lymph nodes and retrocardiac lesions). CT scanning can compensate the disadvantages of CR and DR. Chest X-ray preferably demonstrates organs functions to CR, DR and CT scanning. Bronchoscopy is favorable in demonstrating intraluminal lesions by direct observation and pathological biopsy. MRI imaging demonstrates the 3-dimensional morphology and tissues signaling of pulmonary diseases and functional imaging techniques can be applied for qualitative and quantitative assessments of pulmonary diseases (such as spectral analysis and diffusion tensor imaging (DTI). According to EBM concepts, chest X-ray,

CR/DR, CT scanning can be firstly chosen for the diagnostic imaging of HIV/AIDS, whose failed definitive diagnosis should be further clarified by MR imaging. The comparison and assessment on the imaging examinations for the diagnosis of HIV/AIDS suggest that evidence based HIV/AIDS imaging has great clinical significance. Based on continuously improved clinical practice, radiologists can scientifically and appropriately select optimal imaging examination, formulate more effective imaging plan and avoid misuse and overuse of imaging examinations. All of these will improve the levels of the diagnosis and treatment, reduce the costs and protect patients with HIV/AIDS against excessive exposure to radioactive rays.

9.4 Methods and Thinking Way for Evidence in HIV/AIDS Imaging

Integration of EBM with HIV/AIDS imaging still has some difficulties. (1) Application and benefits of clinical guidelines as well as automatic electronic database retrieval have some limitations. (2) The clinical trials with prospective design, sufficient randomized sampling and size in HIV/AIDS are far less enough. (3) There is limited funding in the applicable basic science research in HIV/AIDS, but there are excessive small-scale and low-funded researches in HIV/AIDS. (4) Researches in HIV/AIDS are heterogeneous, with different criteria for recruitment of subjects. Therefore, the results are in disagreement. (5) Many scholars and clinicians have insufficient understanding and knowledge about their jobs in HIV/AIDS. (6) The routes for evidence are not sufficiently diverse. The related research focuses on one research question that is not systematic, leading to insufficient evidence for the diagnosis of some difficult and rarely occurred diseases. Many studies have proved that systematic review has irreplaceable effects comparing to individual studies.

To develop evidence based diagnostic imaging of HIV/AIDS, EBM related research institutes should be established and database for systematic assessment of HIV/AIDS imaging should also be established. Currently, national research resources can be integrated for HIV/AIDS imaging studies in terms of X-ray, B-mode ultrasonography, CT scanning, MRI imaging and PET-CT. Such integration will largely promote the quality of researches in HIV/AIDS imaging and even may achieve breakthroughs in the basic theoretical research in HIV/AIDS imaging. Publications about evidence based HIV/AIDS imaging and the systematic reviews should be encouraged to promote the application of EBM and systematic review in the field of HIV/AIDS imaging. To develop the field of evidence based HIV/AIDS imaging, radiologists need to know more about epidemiology, computer skills and clinical statistics apart from accumulating clinical experience. In addition, radiologists should have improved awareness and skills in searching, assessing, synthesizing and analyzing information. For example, knowledge and skills to retrieve information in Cochrane Library should be obtained by radiologists.

Academic journals on HIV/AIDS imaging should pay focused attention on research articles about the randomized controlled trial (RCT) to improve the reliability of evidence. According to EBM, the reliability and importance of evidence must be guaranteed. If the original materials including published research articles and unpublished research articles for systematic review are poor in quality, the evidence obtained by systematic review is less reliable, resulting in biased or even wrong conclusion by systematic review. Diagnostic imaging reports writing is one of the important work of radiologists and is also the foundation of evidence based HIV/AIDS imaging. The quality of a diagnostic imaging report not only demonstrates the diagnostic competence of a radiologist, but also is related to the diagnosis and treatment for patients. In the practice of EBM, department of diagnostic imaging, as one of the departments having the most diagnostic and therapeutic information, is facing more challenges. The requirements for reports writing in diagnostic imaging include: coincidence rate of diagnostic localization should be above 95 %; the diagnostic information about lesions should be authentically, comprehensively and accurately provided; the diagnostic conclusions should be logic, stratified and insightful; language use in writing should be formal, fluent, focused and specific; the direction of further examinations should be recommended if necessary. In the whole course of HIV infection and AIDS, the degree of immunodeficiency and the pathological findings vary, with singular occurrence of complications, co-existence of multiple pathogens or different manifestations of the same disease. The complex variations of HIV/AIDS manifestations require the radiologists to understand the features of HIV/AIDS imaging. And the writing of diagnostic imaging reports is a process of improving basic skills and professionalism. The reports should begin with description of positive signs, followed by signs for differential diagnosis and important negative signs. For the description of positive signs, the main or primary signs should be firstly reported, followed by less important or secondary signs. In primary and secondary changes, the main, serious and important signs changes should be firstly reported, followed by the less important and mild changes. The diagnostic conclusions should be based on the imaging analysis and generalization as well as clinical demonstrations. (1) The imaging diagnosis should possibly include name, location, degree and complications of the disease. (2) For cases with concurrence of several unrelated diseases, the diagnosis can be listed in the order of the importance and the relationship with the current clinical manifestations. (3) The diseases with cause and effect relationship must not be reported as several independent diseases.

Modern medical imaging technique is rapidly developing and evidence based HIV/AIDS imaging should keep up its steps with the modern medical imaging technique. The EBM is innovative for the optimal evidence is updated with the development of science and technology.

HIV/AIDS imaging is challenging for imaging diagnosticians in terms of differential diagnosis of the complex imaging findings in patients with AIDS from those in patients without AIDS. The imaging diagnosticians should know how to find objective and rational evidence in literatures and evaluate their reliability and validity. They should follow the trend of medical development, cultivate proper diagnostic reasoning and master the assessment method of EBM. In addition, EBM does not reject personal skills and experience but encourages integration between evidence and personal experience for decision making. For various evidences, the clinicians should assess and screen according to their own experience and knowledge. Evidence by RCT should be respected but should not be blindly believed. Patients and physicians related conditions should be taken into consideration for independent and scientific reasoning. In such way, the benefits of evidence can be maximally achieved.

Contents

10.1 Development of Therapeutic Medication Against HIV/AIDS

Highly Active Antiretroviral Therapy (HAART) has been applied since the middle of 1990s. It combines medications against the replication of HIV in different stages to maximally inhibit the replication of HIV, which has been proved to be the most effective therapy targeting on the etiological factors of HIV/AIDS. In the year of 1987, the first antiretroviral medication, AZT, was developed. So far, there has been totally more than 30 medications (categorized into six types) against HIV/AIDS, including Nucleoside Reerse Transocriptase Inhibitors (NRTIs), Non Nucleoside Reverse Transcriptase Inhibitors (NNRTIs), Protease Inhibitors (PIs), Integrase Inhibitors (IIs), Entry/Fusion Inhibitors (EIs/FIs) and CCR5 inhibitor (maraviroc). Since Chinese government began to promote antiviral therapy free of charge in the year of 2003, the death rate has obviously been decreased and the quality of life in patients with AIDS has been greatly improved. In China, four types of antiretroviral medications are administered, namely NNRTIs, NRTIs, PIs and IIs with a total of 12 drugs.

10.2 Therapeutic Efficacy and Adverse Effects of Highly Active Antiretroviral Therapy (HAART)

The efficacy of HAART is assessed by three criteria, including virological indicators, immunological indicators and clinical symptoms, among which virological indicators are the most important.

10.2.1 Virological Indicators

After HAART is administered, most patients with AIDS may have decreased viral load (VL) by more than 1 log within 4 weeks. After HAART is administered for 3–6 months, the viral load is undetectable.

H. Li (ed.), *Radiology of HIV/AIDS*,
DOI 10.1007/978-94-007-7823-8_10, © Springer Science+Business Media Dordrecht and People's Medical Publishing House 2014

10.2.2   Immunological Indicators

After HAART is administered for 3 months, the CD4 T lymphocyte count increases by 30 %. And after HAART is administered for 1 year, the CD4 T lymphocyte count increases to 100/µl. Both indicate effective treatment by HAART.

10.2.3   Clinical Symptoms

One of the most sensitive indicators for the efficacy of HAART is the weight gain, while for children the sensitive indicators include height, nutritional status and development. After the administration of HAART, the cases with alleviated clinical symptoms could have decreased occurrence of opportunistic infections and decreased death rate from AIDS. During the initial 3 months after HAART, the occurrence of opportunistic infections should be differentiated from immunity reconstruction inflammatory syndrome (IRIS). The adverse effects and patients' tolerance to HAART are factors influencing the medication compliance of patients and further influencing the therapeutic efficacy of HAART. Therefore, proper tolerance monitoring and management of adverse effects of medication are crucial to the therapeutic efficacy of HAART.

10.2.3.1 Nucleosides and NRTIs

NRTIs can suppress DNA polymerase of cellular mitochondrion and cause untoward reaction like acidosis, fatty degeneration, peripheral neuropathy and pancreatitis. Acidosis and pancreatitis can directly cause death. Acidosis is an adverse effect commonly found in all NRTIs-related medications, with different toxicity levels. D4T, DDI and AZT are highly toxic while 3TC and DDC are less toxic. Other adverse effects are caused by some of the NRTIs drugs, such as bone marrow depression (BMD) caused by AZT, peripheral neuropathy caused by D4T and DDI, pancreatitis caused by DDI and D4T, and hypersensitivity reaction caused by ABC.

10.2.3.2 NNRTIs

The toxic reactions of NNRTIs include rash and anaphylaxis. Commonly used medications like Efavirenz can also induce lesions of central nervous system and Nevirapine can induce hepatic impairments.

10.2.3.3 PIs

Untoward reactions of PIs include fat redistribution, abnormal blood lipid level, insulin resistance (with rare occurrence of diabetes), increased bleeding episodes in patients with hemophilia, and Indinavir induced kidney stones.

10.3   Clinical Practice of Anti-opportunistic Infections Therapies

Occurrence of HIV/AIDS related opportunistic infections is related to the virulence of the pathogenic bacteria and immunosuppression level of patients. Currently, CD4 T lymphocyte count is the most important indicator showing the risk of opportunistic infections. Related studies have demonstrated that cases with CD4 T lymphocytes count being lower than 200/µl have 33 % chance of suffering from opportunistic infection within 1 year and 58 % chance within 2 years. Clinical and epidemiological studies have demonstrated that the most common HIV/AIDS related opportunistic infections are bacterial infections, PCP, cerebral toxoplasmosis, CMV, MAIC and fungal infections.

10.3.1   Bacterial Infections

Antibiotics are selected for treatment according to drug sensitivity test. Before the test, empirical therapy is generally administered.

10.3.2   Fungal Infections

Fluconazol, amphotericin B and Itraconazole are applicable.

10.3.3   Mycobacterial Infections

10.3.3.1 Mycobacterial Tuberculosis

The first-line anti-TB drugs include isoniazid (INH), rifampicin (RFP), pyrazinamide (PZA), ethambutol (EMB) and streptomycin (STM).

10.3.3.2 Mycobacterium Avium Complex (MAC)

The preferred medication is Clarithromycin or Azithromycin plus Ethambutol.

10.3.4   Viral Infections

Ganciclovir is the first choice medication for CMV infection. Other antiviral drugs applicable are Foscarnet Sodium and Aciclovir.

10.3.5   Pneumocystis Pneumonia (PCP)

The first choice medication is Trimethoprim, namely Sulfamethoxazole. For moderate and severe cases, Prednisone can be concurrently administered. Patients with obvious progressive dyspnea can be artificially facilitated for ventilation.

10.3.6   Toxoplasmosis

The first choice medication is Pyrimethamine plus Sulfadiazine and the second choice medication is synergic Sulfonamides plus Azithromycin. Leucovorin can be concurrently administered to reduce the untoward reactions of hematological system.

10.4   Treatment of HIV/AIDS Related Tumor

The commonly found HIV/AIDS related neoplasms are lymphoma and Kaposi's sarcoma, whose definitive diagnosis depends on biopsy. Individualized comprehensive treatment should be administered to patients according to their immunity, including surgical operation; chemotherapy and radiotherapy (see detail instructions in related guidance). Doses of chemotherapeutics and radiation should be adjusted according to patients' immunity. The therapeutic plan is as the following:

1. HAART
2. Chemotherapy
   According to the medical history, CD4 T cell counts and general conditions of patients, full dose or partial dose of chemotherapeutics should be administered.
3. Symptomatic supportive treatments
4. Other treatments
   Kaposi's sarcoma and primary effusive lymphoma (PEL) can be treated with anti-human herpes virus-8 (HHV-8) therapy.
5. Drugs interactions
   Concurrent administration of chemotherapy and HAART should possibly avoid the adverse effects, such as overlapping bone marrow involvement of antiviral medication and chemotherapeutics.

Introduction to Assessment and Monitoring of Critical AIDS

11

Contents

11.1 Overview

Critical medicine is a newly emerging branch of modern medicine and is an important symbol of medical progress. In China, critical medicine started late. However since 1980s, with the advance in medicine, more and more hospitals have been establishing comprehensive or specialized intensive care unit (ICU). More and more professional ICU staffs have been improving their diagnostic and therapeutic ability through education and practice.

In China, patients with communicable diseases are required to be treated in local hospitals specialized in infectious diseases. In these specialized hospitals, establishment and development of ICU are later than those in the comprehensive hospitals. Due to the lack of specialized staffs in respiratory, renal, hematological and cardiovascular fields and the lack of common facilities such as breathing machine, bedside hemofiltration, hemodynamic monitoring, it is difficult for specialized hospitals to launch critical medicine. Nevertheless, with the development of modern medicine and the growing demand for health care, specialized hospitals in infectious diseases need to provide services in critical medicine, which should be supported by related research. Undoubtedly, patients with AIDS are the most important and special group demanding intensive care services in specialized hospitals of infectious diseases.

AIDS was firstly found in patients with pneumocystis pneumonia and Kaposi's sarcoma. Both are still AIDS-related diseases threatening the life of patients. In addition, many other opportunistic infections and malignant tumors caused by AIDS are also being life-threatening. In the past 50 years, with the development of antiviral therapy, HIV infection has changed from a deadly infectious disease to a controllable chronic disease. More and more patients with HIV/AIDS are able to work and live as healthy population and the progression of the disease is increasingly slowed. Moreover, with the development of intensive care techniques, the survival rate of patients in ICU is notably increased. However, with prolonged life expectancy, life-threatening causes of advanced

H. Li (ed.), *Radiology of HIV/AIDS*,
DOI 10.1007/978-94-007-7823-8_11, © Springer Science+Business Media Dordrecht and People's Medical Publishing House 2014

AIDS are becoming increasingly complex. In this chapter, assessment and monitor of critical illnesses threatening the life of patients with AIDS are described and discussed.

11.2   HIV/AIDS Related Critical and Severe Opportunistic Infections

Most HIV-infected patients are unaware of their infection until the infection progresses into the stage of AIDS. Commonly, most patients are diagnosed as having HIV infection after the occurrence of opportunistic infections. Some patients are even diagnosed when they sustain a life-threatening condition caused by critical opportunistic infections. When AIDS was initially acknowledged, the death rate in patients with AIDS receiving intensive care was up to 90 % due to their severely compromised immunity. But recently, the death rate in patients with AIDS receiving intensive care has dropped to less than 50 %. In China, opportunistic infections have always been the main cause of death in HIV-infected patients, and clinicians treating patients with HIV/AIDS need more knowledge about the related critical and severe opportunistic infections.

The CD4 T cell count in HIV infected patients is closely related to the types of opportunistic infections as well as the location and involved range of neoplasms. When CD4 T cell count is above 500/μl, patients are susceptible to acquired pneumonia and have more frequent occurrence o tuberculosis than non-HIV-infected subjects, but with basically the same diseases spectrum as the non-infected group. When CD4 T cell count is below 500/μl, opportunistic infections may occur and recur, including esophageal candidiasis, herpes simplex virus infection, and zoster virus infections. In addition, they also have a higher incidence of pneumococcal infection than populations with normal immunity. When CD4 T cell count is below 200/μl, the incidence of pneumocystis pneumonia (PCP) increases significantly. When CD4 T cell count is below 50/μl, disseminated infections tend to occur, such as cytomegalovirus infection and cryptococcus infection. In addition, such patients have a higher occurrence of central nervous system infections.

Pneumocystis pneumonia (PCP) is the most common opportunistic infection and is the main cause of death during early days HIV epidemic. In the year of 1988, the pathogen was proved to be fungus and later specified to be pneumocystis carinii (PC) [1]. Most HIV-infected patients are not aware of their infection until the onset of symptoms. Their symptoms like fever and cough are commonly misdiagnosed as common respiratory infection and are treated with common anti-infection therapies that are ineffective for PCP. Consequently, many patients are only accurately diagnosed after the occurrence of tachypnea or even respiratory failure. Therefore, most patients with PCP receive oxygen therapy or even mechanical ventilation. Nowadays, PCP is still the main cause of death in HIV-infected patients for its high case fatality rate.

Since toxoplasma gondii has an affinity to the central nervous system, toxoplasmic encephalitis is a life threatening opportunistic infection. Even after timely appropriate treatment, sequelae occur, including focal neurological deficits, hemiplegia and epilepsy. The severity of toxoplasmic encephalitis is related to the location of lesions. It is characterized by acute onset and rapid progress. Without timely appropriate therapies, it is life-threatening.

Despite of slow progression of tuberculosis, its case fatality rate is significant, as its occurrence in HIV-infected patients. The occurrence of tuberculosis in HIV-positive population is 8 times higher than that in HIV-negative populations. Meanwhile, HIV infection accelerates multi-drug resistance to tuberculosis, leading to increased difficulties in treating tuberculosis. Tuberculosis rarely causes death in patients but aggravates existing illnesses and accelerates the decline of immunity to cause their susceptibility to other opportunistic infections. Therefore, it is necessary to administer drug sensitivity monitoring for patients with AIDS complicated by tuberculosis.

Atypical mycobacteriosis is one of the main reasons for the symptoms of fever, diarrhea and weight loss in HIV-infected patients. Without timely appropriate treatment, it could cause deterioration of the clinical conditions.

Progressive multifocal leukoencephalopathy (PML) is a serious demyelinating disease of the central nervous system. It is caused by JC virus, a polyoma virus, which is the second most common opportunistic infection of the nervous system in patients with AIDS, following toxoplasmosis. Its clinical symptoms include cognitive impairment and focal neuropathy and hemiplegia, language disorder or visual disorders are the most common. Clinically, there is no specific therapy against it.

Bacterial pneumonia occurs in any stage of HIV/AIDS, whose occurrence is not obviously related to the decrease of CD4 T cell count. However, the promotion of ART treatment does not significantly reduce its incidence and its treatment is similar to those for non-HIV-infected patients.

Cryptosporidiosis is an intestinal parasitosis with a spreading route of faecal-oral transmission. Death may occur in such patients with severely compromised immunity due to fluid and electrolytes loss caused by long-term diarrhea.

Cryptococcus neoformans infection is commonly transmitted by bird faeces, commonly involving lungs and central nervous system. Without timely definitive diagnosis and appropriate treatment, it may invade the central nervous system, followed by a rapid progression. Such patients may have fever, headache and conscious disturbance, cranial nerve palsy, severe headache caused by increased intracranial pressure. Its definitive diagnosis depends on microscopic examination after India ink staining of cerebrospinal fluid (CSF) obtained by lumbar puncture.

11.3 HIV/AIDS Related Advanced Cancer

The most common HIV/AIDS related tumors are Kaposi's sarcoma (KS) and lymphoma. KS is related to human herpes virus 8 (HHV-8), spreading by sexual contacts, blood and saliva and is an indicator of AIDS. The patients in advanced stage of AIDS with no history of therapies usually have a rapid progression of KS, with an average survival period of less than 1 year. Even death may occur within several weeks in cases of rapid progression. Unlike cases of non-HIV-infected patients, KS in HIV-infected patients occurs at varying locations, including skin, oral cavity, alimentary canal, genital organ and ocular region. And the lesions range from painless skin lesion to invasive and disseminated lesions with lymph nodes and internal organs involved.

KS is conventionally diagnosed based on the following clinical findings on the skin or mucous membranes:
1. Purple plaques or nodules;
2. Lesions distributing along dermal texture;
3. Yellowish green skin surrounding the lesion of tumor hemorrhage;
4. Peripheral edema;
5. Disseminated lesions, with possible involvement of skin mucosa.

Definitive diagnosis can be made based on biopsy of the focal tissues. KS can be self alleviated or alleviated after treatment. But due to hemosiderin deposition caused by erythrocyte exudation, brown or light brown pigmentation may present for several months or several years. For the cases of initial KS diagnosis, following examinations should be regularly performed for monitoring, the clinical staging and corresponding treatments:
1. General examination of skin mucosa;
2. Ultrasonography of lymph nodes;
3. Abdominal ultrasonography;
4. Upper gastrointestinal endoscopy;
5. Lower gastrointestinal endoscopy;
6. Chest X-ray;
7. CT scanning.

Simultaneously, CD4 T cell count and HIV virus load should be monitored for decisions about administration of antiviral therapy. Both indicators are valuable in predicting the prognosis.

Compared to healthy subjects, HIV-infected patients are more susceptible to lymphomas, among which invasive B cell Non-Hodgkin's lymphoma (B-NHL) is the most dangerous. Currently, lymphoma has a higher incidence than KS, ranked the first in occurrence of HIV/AIDS related malignancies. Its symptoms include lymphadenectasis and immo-

bile hardened painless masses. The patients may sustain fever, night sweating and/or weight loss. General upset and physical deterioration are also common.

Since chemotherapy is the most commonly used therapy, electrocardiography (ECG) and ultrasonic cardiography (UCG) should be regularly performed to assess the cardiac toxicity caused by chemotherapy. In addition, pulmonary function should be examined before and during therapies containing medication of bleomycin. During chemotherapy, assessment should be performed every other therapeutic course for clinical staging and efficacy evaluation. After the chemotherapies are finished, bone marrow biopsy and CT scanning should be performed for a general clinical staging. For cases of complete remission, follow-up clinical staging should be performed every 3 months during the first year, every 6 months after 1 year and every 12 months after 2 years. During the follow-up period, cerebrospinal fluid test should be ordered regularly to exclude meningeal involvement.

11.4 HIV/AIDS Related Multiple Organ Failure (MOF)

One organ could be involved due to opportunistic infection in HIV-infected patients, which could lead to multiple organ failure (MOF) if such patients cannot receive timely appropriate treatment. Meanwhile, due to compromised immunity, multiple organs infections may occur simultaneously, leading to multiple organs impairments. In conclusion, multiple organs impairments in patients with HIV/AIDS can occur and gradually progress to MOF because of the involvement of one organ or concurrent involvement of multiple organs.

Lymphoma and KS can involve multiple organs simultaneously and lead to multiple organs dysfunction syndrome (MODS) or even multiple organ failure (MOF).

Therefore, for patients with compromised immunity, the monitoring of impaired organ should be performed together with the monitoring of other organs, so as not to delay the treatment of pathological changes of other organs. When receiving antiviral treatment, patients should be aware of impairments to liver and kidney due to medications for complications. Improper combined use of drugs and accumulation of drug toxicity could cause liver and kidney dysfunction and MODS.

11.5 HIV/AIDS Related Severe Malnutrition

The cause of HIV/AIDS related malnutrition is commonly long-term diarrhea caused by gastrointestinal infections. Therefore, for patients with malnutrition, occurrence of infection should be firstly considered and the pathogenic factors should be carefully traced.

Because weight loss is a dangerous factor influencing case fatality rate, body weight should be monitored for HIV-infected patients. The risk of death in AIDS patients with weight loss of more than 10 % is 4–6 times higher than AIDS patients with steady body weight. Those with malnutrition have an obviously increased risk of opportunistic infections.

HIV related lipodystrophy syndromes include metabolic complication and lipid redistribution, which are the adverse effects of antiviral therapy. Clinical symptoms are characterized by local or systemic loss of subcutaneous fat. Patients receiving antiviral therapy of protease inhibitor are subjected to fat redistribution and metabolic disturbance. Metabolic changes include insulin resistance (IR), impaired glucose tolerance (IGT), hypertriglyceridemia (HTG), hypercholesterolemia (HC), increased free fatty acid (FFA) and decreased high density lipoprotein (HDL). These metabolic disorders may occur before fat redistribution. As a result, regular monitoring of above indicators should be performed for HIV-infected patients, especially for those receiving antiviral therapy.

11.6 HIV/AIDS Related Intensive Care

Patients in critical condition should receive intensive care in a quarantined unit. Their monitoring and treatment could refer to diagnostic and therapeutic routines of the unit. However, due to the compromised immunity, their diseases spectrum is different from that of non-HIV-infected patients. For those with seriously compromised immunity, invasive diagnosis and treatment should be avoided. Some noninvasive bacteria for healthy population may cause opportunistic infection in patients with compromised immunity. For patients with AIDS, some common nosocomial infections could occur out of the hospital. For instance, pseudomonas aeruginosa infection, which is commonly recognized as a nosocomial acquired infection, could occur out of the hospital in HIV-infected patients. In recent years, the incidence of pseudomonas aeruginosa infection in AIDS patients has been gradually rising, with a death rate of up to 48–75 %. Therefore, immunity compromised patients possibly sustain various bacterial infections. Precautions should be especially paid to those serious nosocomial infections, which are usually life-threatening.

Patients with different immunity may have different spectrum of diseases and thus different intensive care programs. Compared to non-HIV-infected individuals, intensive care of seriously ill patients with AIDS needs strict observation of procedures for isolation and sterilization. Patients with different complications demand different focuses in intensive care. For instance, for cases of AIDS complicated by HBV/HCV, liver functions should be focused in intensive care;

especially cases of hepatic cirrhosis should not be excluded. Because the following medications of antiviral therapy and opportunistic infection treatment may aggravate liver dysfunction. PCP is the most common reason for respiratory failure in HIV-infected individuals. Patients with PCP are susceptible to bacterial infections; therefore, blood samples and respiratory secretions should be collected and cultured regularly for tests.

Due to compromised immunity in patients with AIDS, the critically ill patients receiving intensive care should avoid cross infections. Meanwhile, invasive operations should also be reduced. Once nosocomial infection occurs, the risk of death would be noticeably increased.

After the intensive care is performed for patients with AIDS, their critical and serious condition should be assessed. Clinically, the acute physiology and chronic health evaluation (APACHE II) and APACHE III are commonly used as the scoring systems. Some important symptoms, signs and physiological indices should be weighted and encoded to quantitatively evaluate the critical and serious conditions. Therefore, the risks of death or serious complications can be evaluated objectively. In addition, the therapeutic efficacy, resources utilization and quality control of ICU can be assessed. The scoring of critical and serious conditions should be performed soon after the patients receiving intensive care.

11.7 HIV/AIDS Related Respiratory Function Monitoring

HIV/AIDS related respiratory diseases include some typical HIV-related diseases such as tuberculosis, pneumocystis carinii pneumonia (PCP), bacterial pneumonia and lymphoma. HIV/AIDS related respiratory diseases also include some common diseases like acute bronchitis, asthma, chronic obstructive pulmonary disease (COPD) and respiratory neoplasms. In China, tuberculosis and PCP are the most common and constitute the leading causes of death in patients with AIDS.

Since PCP is life threatening, it is recommended for patients with their CD4 T cell count being less than 200/μl to receive sulfamethoxazole (SMZ) therapy for prevention. For patients not receiving antiviral therapy but with a decreasing tendency of CD4 T cell count, their CD4 T cell count should be closely monitored because CD4 T cell count is an optimal indicator assessing the risk of opportunistic infections. Patients with CD4 T cell count being above 200/μl have quite low probability of suffering from opportunistic infection. In conclusion, detection of CD4 T cell count is critically important for patients with AIDS.

For patients who suspected diagnosis of PCP, detected eight sporozoite cysts from specimens of respiratory or lung tissues is the evidence for its definitive diagnosis. Since patients cannot cough up pneumocystis carinii with their sputum, natural sputum test only has a sensitivity of about 10–30 % sensitivity in detecting pneumocystis carinii. However, the induced expectoration of sputum and transbronchial lung biopsy has higher sensitivities. In fact, bronchoalveolar lavage and transbronchial lung biopsy can clarify almost all pathogens infections. Occasionally when bronchoalveolar lavage fails to provide definitive diagnosis, percutaneous puncture should be employed to obtain lung tissue for further examination. Grocott's methenamine silver (GMS) staining is favorably used to test cysts resembling to crushed ping-pong balls. The diagnostic imaging is not specific for the diagnosis of PCP. Chest X-ray demonstrates bilateral diffuse infiltration in pulmonary parenchyma and/or pulmonary interstitium, stretching from pulmonary hilum for fusion. The lesions distribute mainly in perihilar regions, with rare involvements of the apex and the pulmonary base. Such lesions may be caused by centrifugal spreading of the pathogen along with bronchi. Typical findings by CT scanning are the ground-glass liked shadows in both lungs. For patients with definitive diagnosis of PCP, hormone therapy should be administrated according to the severity of the conditions. The indications of hormone therapy include arterial partial pressure of oxygen (PO_2) being less than 70–80 mmHg or alveolar-arterial PO_2 difference (A-a gradient) being above 35 mmHg. The alveolar-arterial PO_2 difference is the discrepancy between measured arterial PO_2 (PaO_2) and calculated alveolar PO_2 (PAO_2) and is an indicator of oxygen uptake in pulmonary capillaries. Specifically, in normal breathing, it should be less than 15 mmHg and above 30 mmHg in elderly population; in 30 % oxygen breathing, it should be less than 70 mmHg; in pure oxygen breathing, it should be less than 100 mmHg. An increased A-a gradient indicates lowered ventilation-perfusion (quotient) ratio (V/Q) and occurrence of diffusion dysfunction. Therefore, arterial blood gas should be monitored when PCP is suspected or treated. Meanwhile, since PCP is commonly complicated by pneumothorax, lung signs and chest-X-ray should also be closely observed. For cases with PCP complicated by pneumothorax, tracheal intubation (TI) needs to be performed after pneumothorax is firstly managed. In patients with AIDS complicated by PCP, the lactic acid dehydrogenase (LAD) level is increased in 90 % patients, with high sensitivity but low specificity as an indicator for the diagnosis.

Diseases like cytomegalovirus pneumonia, toxoplasmic pneumonia, tuberculosis and pulmonary infection caused by cryptococcus neoformans cause symptoms of cough and dyspnea in patients. But the definitive diagnosis depends on the etiological evidence. To improve the positive rate of the diagnostic examinations, pulmonary alveolar lavage fluid (PALF) can be used to seek the pathogen.

Studies have shown that HIV can cause pulmonary hypertension (PH), but its underlying mechanism remains unknown. Cases with resting PAP being above 25 mmHg are diagnosed as having PH and such patients may have dyspnea. Obviously decreased resting cardiac output indicates an increased load of the right ventricle caused by serious PH and such patients should avoid physical activities. To define the diagnosis of PH and understand its severity, right heart catheterization for pulmonary hemodynamics is believed to be the golden standard for detecting the changes of lung resistance that have not yet initiate the increase of the pulmonary artery pressure. In the obvious PH stage, the reversibility of vasoconstriction should be examined to find the patients' responses to the vasodilator therapy. In addition, ECG can detect PH; chest-X-ray can show typical changes like dilation of right descending pulmonary artery (the diameter being above 20 mm); ultrasonic cardiogram can recognize the dilated right ventricle, assess pulmonary arterial pressure (PAP) during systole and examine the sizes and functions of cardiac chambers. Pulmonary ventilation/perfusion scanning, pulmonary angiography and CT scanning can recognize or exclude chronic thromboembolic pulmonary hypertension (CTEPH) and the findings can facilitate the formulation of further therapeutic plans. HIV-infected persons with a history of substance abuse are susceptible to repeated episodes of thromboembolism.

11.8 HIV/AIDS Related Renal Function Monitoring

HIV itself can cause pathological changes of renal glomerulus and renal tubules, while HIV/AIDS related renal diseases can cause rapid decline of renal functions. In patients receiving antiviral therapy, long-term use of antiviral drugs has adverse effects on kidney and may cause impaired renal functions. Since kidney impairments can progress into kidney failure within 1–4 months in many patients with HIV-infection complicated by renal diseases, routine monitoring of renal functions should be performed.

For HIV-infected populations, renal functions and blood electrolytes should be tested every 3 months, as well as urine glucose, urine protein, white blood cells (WBC) and red blood cells (RBC) in urine. Patients with obvious proteinuria or elevated serum creatinine should receive general examinations should be performed to identify the pathogen. Renal biopsy should also be performed when necessary.

Glomerulonephritis (GN) is the common HIV related renal disease. Cases with edema, hypoproteinemia, hyperlipemia and daily urine protein above 3.5 g can be diagnosed as having renal syndrome. Proteinuria and hematuria are characteristically GN, whose definitive diagnosis can be made by urinary sediments. In the early period of increasing serum creatinine, creatinine clearance rate (CCR) is detected to assess the renal dysfunction.

Like any other medication, antiviral therapy impairs renal functions that progresses into renal failure. Therefore, monitoring of renal functions is necessary during the antiviral therapy. Retesting of renal functions is required each time when any drug is changed. Application of DDI, D4I and 3TC can cause renal tubular dysfunction (RTD), while the effects of IDV on the renal functions range from asymptomatic urinary crystal to kidney failure. More than 10 % patients report to have kidney stones. The use of TDF can lead to renal tubular dysfunction and the patients with a past history of proteinuria, nephrotic syndrome, hepatic cirrhosis and metabolic disorder of lipoprotein should avoid such nephrotoxic drugs. TDF is mainly metabolized through kidneys and the common renal complication of TDF medication is Fanconi syndrome, which occurs averagely after 7 months administration and whose diagnosis is dependent on hypophosphatemia, elevated urine glucose and slight proteinuria. After receiving antiviral therapy containing TDF, even patients with normal renal function should receive renal function monitoring every month during the first year of treatment, and every 3 months thereafter. For patients with concurrent use of other nephrotoxic drugs like aminoglycosides, amphotericin B, ganciclovir or vancomycin, it is recommended to monitor the renal functions weekly. For patients with already impaired renal function, drug doses should be adjusted according to CCR when any antiviral medication and other medication is administered.

11.9   HIV/AIDS Related Cardiovascular Function Monitoring

HIV seldom impairs the cardiovascular system directly but antiviral medication can cause metabolic disorder. Thus, in patients with long-term use of antiviral therapy, the risk of cardiovascular diseases is increasing. Studies have demonstrated that occurrence of atherosclerotic plaque in HIV patients has been increasing in recent years. The increased risk of cardiovascular diseases may reduce the benefits from antiviral medication.

Patients receiving antiviral medication should be monitored for their blood lipid level and blood glucose level, because the therapy can cause hyperlipemia (HL) and insulin resistance (IR). ECG should be performed for such patients every year and for patients with cardiovascular symptoms other related examinations should also be performed including stress ECG, ultrasonic cardiogram (UCG) and coronary angiography (CAG).

In more than 8 % patients with AIDS, UCG demonstrates dilatated myocardium and subclinical decreased cardiac function. Thus it is necessary for HIV-infected populations

to receive cardiovascular monitoring by UCG. Occasionally, HIV or other viruses may directly invade cardiac muscle cells to cause myocarditis and the serious cases may show cardiac dysfunction or even heart failure. In the early stage, patients may suffer from reduced exercise tolerance, which can be tested by 6-min walking test. Cases with occurrence of dyspnea and edema in the test have cardiac dysfunction by ECG, chest X-ray and UCG. BNP can be used to differentiate cardiac dysfunction from pulmonary dysfunction.

HIV/AIDS related tuberculosis (TB) can cause tuberculous pericarditis, which is more common in areas with high TB prevalence. In these areas, UCG should be performed early for HIV-infected populations with related symptoms to facilitate the diagnosis. HIV/AIDS complicated by bacterial infections or fungal infections can cause valvular disease of heart (VDH). In HIVE infected populations, 40 % cases of endocarditis is caused by staphylococcus aureus infection and other pathogens include streptococcus pneumoniae and haemophilus influenzae. The pathogens of fungal endocarditis are commonly aspergillus, candida albicans or cryptococcus and its prognosis is commonly poor. Its monitoring depends on periodic physical examination and auscultation to find the cardiac murmur. Fever of unknown causes implicates endocarditis and VDH, whose diagnosis is dependent on repeated blood cultures and transesophageal echocardiography. The antibiotic therapy should be administered early.

11.10   HIV/AIDS Related Central Nervous System Function Monitoring

HIV/AIDS related central nervous system (CNS) impairments could be primary or secondary. HIV can infect CNS to cause HIV encephalopathy (HIVE), including AIDS dementia complex (ADC), AIDS-associated dementia (AAD), HIV-associated dementia (HAD) and HIV-associated motor/cognitive complex. However, HIVE only occurs in the advanced period of infection, usually with CD4 T cell count less than 200/µl. Such patients have high virus load in the cerebrospinal fluid and brain parenchyma, whereas the level of virus load is not significantly related to the illness conditions. Before effective antiviral therapy, ADC is a main cause of death in patients with AIDS.

Generally, HIVE develops slowly, commonly with symptoms of dementia, such as declined memory, retarded thinking, difficulty concentrating and affective disorder found by their family members. HIVE has no specific laboratory tests and imaging examinations for its diagnosis, therefore, its clinical monitoring only can be performed by observations and judgements by people socializing with the patients. It can be assessed by international criteria for HIV associated dementia and its severity could be evaluated by relevant scales. Patients with ADC or HIVE seldom have completely normal cerebrospinal fluid, mostly with elevated protein level and 25 % with increased mononuclear lymphocytes. In some patients, HIV nucleic acid can be detected from their cerebrospinal fluid, which is the evidence of HIV/AIDS related encephalopathy. For patients with CD4 T cell count less than 200/μl, the virus load in cerebrospinal fluid is related to the severity of the conditions. Imaging examinations lack specificity for the diagnosis of ADC. Therefore, for HIV infected populations with accompanying memory and intelligence changes should be assessed and monitored for their memory, intelligence and attention as well as other mental status.

Impairments of central nervous system caused by other complications could mostly be diagnosed and analysed by cerebrospinal fluid examination and imaging examinations. Generally, patients with AIDS complicated by central nervous system impairments are in demand of intensive care.

1. CMV encephalitis
   CMV infection is a common opportunistic infection in AIDS patients. Such patients mostly have accompanying retinitis, colonitis, pneumonia or esophagitis. Thus patients with CMV infection in the above body parts are also necessary to be monitored for their nervous system. Routine cerebrospinal fluid (CSF) analysis and biochemical tests could find increased CSF cell count, dropped glucose level and elevated total protein level. By PCR, CMV in cerebrospinal fluid can be detected; CMV-DNA or CMV antigen (pp65) can be detected in blood. In addition, blood and cerebrospinal fluid are both positive for CMV antigen.

2. Toxoplasmic encephalitis
   Imaging examinations can help to define toxoplasmic encephalitis. Specifically, CT scanning and MR imaging can demonstrate the singular and multiple lesions commonly in basal ganglia and thalamus, with space occupying effect and edema and accompanying flaky or ring liked enhancement shadows. Blood and cerebrospinal fluid tests could find toxoplasma gondii antibody (Tox-ab).

3. Primary central nervous system lymphoma
   By CT scanning or MR imaging, singular or multiple lesions can be found adjacent to cerebral ventricles, with space occupying effect and edema. They are commonly demonstrated as flaky or ring liked high density shadows.

4. Varicella-zoster virus (VZV) encephalitis
   Most patients are suffering from or have a past history of skin lesions caused by herpes zoster virus. Their cerebrospinal fluid shows inflammatory changes, with specific antibody positive. By PCR, VZV can be detected.

5. Cryptococcal meningitis
   Positive findings by India ink staining of CSF, increased intracranial pressure, positive findings by fungi culture of blood and cerebrospinal fluid can define the diagnosis of cryptococcal meningitis. Detection of cryptococcus antigen in serum or CSF (Titer above 1:4 is considered significant.) has more than 95 % sensitivity and specificity for the diagnosis of cryptococcal infection, which can be the basis for the definitive diagnosis. For HIV-infected populations with symptoms of nervous system should routinely receive tests for cryptococcus. CT scanning has a low specificity for cryptococcus. However, MR imaging is more sensitive to singular or multiple enhanced nodules in cerebral parenchyma, meninges, basal ganglia and midbrain. In addition, MR imaging also can be applied for its differential diagnosis from toxoplasmic encephalitis and central nervous system lymphoma. In well facilitated hospitals, MRI should be performed for AIDS patients with nervous system symptoms. For patients with confirmative diagnosis of cryptococcal meningitis, routine blood test, hepatorenal functions and electrolytes should be re-examined every 1–2 weeks to monitor the adverse effects of the therapy during the medication. A small portion of patients with serious renal impairments may have to discontinue or change their therapeutic plan. For patients with initially definitive diagnosis of cryptococcal meningitis, lumbar puncture should be performed to test CSF pressure. For cases with high CSF pressure and severe headache, it is recommended to drain CSF of 20–30 ml for alleviation of symptoms. During therapy, CSF pressure should be monitored according to patients' condition and drainage of CSF should be performed again to alleviate symptoms when necessary.

6. Tuberculous meningitis
   Pulmonary or extrapulmonary tuberculosis do not necessarily concur. CSF culture and PCR examination can help to find mycobacterium tuberculosis.

7. Progressive multiple leukoencephalopathy
   MR imaging can help to find singular or multiple lesions of leukoencephalopathy, with no space occupying effects and edema. The test of CSF can help to find JC virus.

11.11 HIV/AIDS Related Digestive System Function Monitoring

After HIV infection, opportunistic infections may occur in the digestive system, including fungal, bacterial and viral infections. Symptoms may range from ulcer and diarrhea to hepatic impairment and hepatocirrhosis. Administration of antiviral drugs or medications for other complications may cause side effects such as nausea and vomit, as well as negative events like drug-induced liver impairment.

Ulcer and diarrhea are the most common symptoms of digestive system infections. For patients with long-term fever and diarrhea, the possibility of HIV/AIDS related digestive system infections should be considered. Etiological examinations of feces or blood can help to clarify the pathogens. But sometimes it is necessary to receive gastroscopy or enteroscopy to understand the severity and the range of pathological changes. And sometimes biopsy is needed to confirm the nature and pathogen of the lesions. Chronic diarrhea often causes emaciation, dehydration, electrolyte disturbance and acid-base disturbance. Therefore, it is necessary to monitor electrolytes and acid-base balances. Antiviral drugs, especially protease inhibitors, can cause digestive manifestations such as nausea, vomiting and diarrhea, and may cause electrolyte disturbance and increased lactic acid level. Therefore, blood gas analysis and lactic acid level should be monitored. For cases with suspected gastrointestinal conditions, the following routine examinations should be performed: (1) Color, shape and frequency of bowel movements. Patients with gastrointestinal catheterization in ICU should regularly receive bacterial and fungal cultures. (2) Feces occult blood (FOB) test. It is performed to understand bleeding of alimentary tract. (3) pH value of gastric mucosa. The physiology of circulation indicates that gastrointestinal blood perfusion is "the first response" but "the last cured" after pathogenic attacks to the circulatory system. Deficiency of blood perfusion can cause local tissue hypoxia and acidosis and monitoring of gastric mucosal pH value can precaution the ischemia and hypoxia of the body tissues. (4) gastrointestinal endoscopic examinations. Gastrointestinal endoscopy can be applied to understand the nature and scope of the lesions. It can also be used to collect specimens for biopsy.

Another most common and possibly the most serious problem of digestive system is hepatic function impairment. It could be caused by various complications and also could be induced by medication. HIV infection complicated by HCV infection is very common, especially in western countries, probably because both viruses have the same route of transmission. HBV is highly prevalent in China, and therefore HIV infection complicated by HBV infection is more common in China. In HIV-infected individuals, up to 95 % have a history of HBV infection and about 10–15 % sustain chronic hepatitis B. Therefore, it is recommended to routinely monitor antibodies against HBV and HCV in HIV infected patients. For cases with HBV infection, antiviral therapy against HBV/HCV should be considered based on DNA/RNA of the patients. For patients with HIV infection complicated by HCV infection, interferon and antiviral therapy is administered and autoantibodies series should be tested before the therapy application, including antinuclear antibody, anticardiolipin antibody, antismooth muscle antibody and liver-kidney microsomal antibody. In addition, thyroid functions, TSH level, blood glucose level, and mental status should be assessed before the use of interferon and antiviral therapy. During the antiviral therapy, blood routine and renal function should be examined every 2–4 weeks; HCV-RNA or HBV-DNA test every 12 weeks, CD4 T cell count test every 12 weeks, and TSH level detection every 12 weeks. Patients with HIV infection complicated by HBV infection should regularly receive renal function test and HBV-DNA level examination. For cases with ALT level being twice of the normal level, but with DNA level being in line with antiviral indications, anti-HBV therapy should be administered.

During antiviral therapy against HIV and other complications, the possibility of drug-induced hepatic injury should be considered and the hepatic function should be monitored with focused attention to the following indicators:

1. Protein metabolism
   Liver is the main organ for protein metabolism. Albumin, glycoprotein, lipoprotein, blood coagulation factor, fibrinolytic factors and various transport proteins are all synthesized by hepatocytes. The levels of proprotein, albumin and choline esterase as well as prothrombin time (PT) are all indicators demonstrating the hepatic reserving function. The decreased levels of these indicators implicate reduced protein synthesis ability. Persistent decline of choline esterase activity with no signs of recovery indicates a poor prognosis.

2. Monitoring of glycometabolism
   Liver is the main organ for glycometabolism and plays an important role in maintaining blood glucose level. Monitoring of glycometabolism provide evidence for the nutritional status of critically and seriously ill patients and further for the formulation of the nutritional supporting plan.

3. Lipid metabolism
   In liver, endogenous cholesterol and fatty acid are synthesized. Meanwhile, liver can also intake exogenous lipid and free fatty acid from decomposed adipose tissue. Hypercholesteremia in patients with jaundice indicates obstructive jaundice, while liver impairment could cause decreased cholesterol level.

4. Bilirubin metabolism
   Various bilirubin criteria can be used to identify the causes of jaundice, evaluate the severity of hepatic impairment and serve as an important prognostic indicator.

5. Monitoring of hepatic enzyme
   Hepatic enzyme can sensitively demonstrate the severity of impaired hepatocytes. An increasing bilirubin but decreasing aminopherase indicates hepatic necrosis.

Reference

1. Mileski GJ, Bumpus JA, Jurek MA, Aust SD. Biodegradation of pentachlorophenol by the white rot fungus Phanerochaete chrysosporium [J]. Appl Environ Microbiol. 1988;54(12):2885–9.

HIV Related Effect Factors

12

Contents

12.1   Blood and HIV Infection

Blood is most closely related to HIV infection. Firstly, blood provides an environment for survival of HIV. After HIV gains access to the blood, it attacks the CD T lymphocytes. With the decrease of CD T lymphocyte count, HIV infection gradually progresses into AIDS. Meanwhile, the static CD T lymphocytes constitute reservoir for incubation of HIV. The incubated HIV fails to be eliminated by ART treatment.

Secondly, blood transmission is one of the three routes of HIV transmission, including spreading via blood transfusion, blood products use, intravenous drug abuse and iatrogenic transmission due to no or incomplete sterilization of syringes, needles, surgical instruments, oral instruments or obstetric instruments. In daily life, incomplete sterilization of hairdressing instruments, beauty instruments and pedicure knives in bathroom, or sharing razors, toothbrushes with others could also transmit HIV.

As modern medicine develops, the application of blood transfusion and blood products is being increasingly extensive, which saves numerous lives. However, transfusion of HIV contaminated blood or blood products indicate that HIV is directly transfused into recipients' blood circulation. Blood constituents like coagulation factor VII are extracted from plasma of donors' blood, with higher risk of being contaminated by HIV. In some countries, blood safety is not secured and the blood recipients thus have higher risks of HIV infection. HIV infection via blood rapidly progresses into AIDS, with a mean of 3–5 years (in children, about 2 years). In the early 1980s, coagulation factor VII produced in the United States caused worldwide HIV infection in patients with hemophilia. A blood sampling centre in France was once contaminated by HIV and caused thousands of healthy recipients were infected. In 1990s, blood donation and supply was managed privately in some local areas of China and caused HIV infection in some blood donators. These cases have taught us a lesson. Currently, screening of blood donors has been strengthened in developed countries. In China, the management of blood donors and blood products has been strengthened.

H. Li (ed.), *Radiology of HIV/AIDS*,
DOI 10.1007/978-94-007-7823-8_12, © Springer Science+Business Media Dordrecht and People's Medical Publishing House 2014

To reduce HIV transmission via blood transfusion, screening of blood and blood products should be the starting point. In addition, unnecessary and inappropriate blood transfusion should be greatly reduced and prohibited.

12.2   Drug Abuse and HIV Infection

Drugs include opium, heroin, morphine, marijuana, cocaine and other narcotic and psychotropic drugs which could cause serious drug dependence. In China, some common drugs nowadays include heroin, opium, marijuana, crystal meth and ecstasy. Drug abuses include oral, inhaling and intravenous uses of drugs for non-medical purposes.

Drug abuse is one of the main routes for AIDS transmission, because:

1. Drug users often share needles and syringes. HIV infected one such drug user can spread HIV via instruments sharing in drug abuse.
2. Sexual promiscuity is common among drug users, which could induce sexually transmitted HIV infection.
3. Physical deterioration in drug users causes their decreased immunity, which provides opportunity for HIV infection.

Intravenous drug users (IDU) account for 15–17 % of the total patients with HIV/AIDS. The reason for the spreading of HIV in such population is that they repeatedly use syringes and needles with no or incomplete sterilization. The HIV contaminated syringes and needles cause the prevalence and transmission of HIV infection in such a population. And intravenous drug abuse constitutes the second common risk of HIV infection. Abuse of addictive drugs is an important cause for frequent occurrence and prevalence of AIDS. Quite a few drug users are also homosexual or sexually promiscuous and AIDS occurs more frequently in the population with overlapping risk factors. In the United States, about 0.4 million drug users are HIV positive, with males being twice as many as females. Other reports indicate that women with a history of sexual contact with male drug users have an incidence of AIDS 30 times higher than the general population. This finding suggested the high incidence of AIDS due to drug abuse. Via unsterilized needles, drug users may also be subjected to other infectious diseases such as hepatitis B and hepatitis C, and may have direct impairments to their immunity. Therefore, the drug abusers are more susceptible to HIV infection. Meanwhile, interactions among diseases could accelerate the progress of HIV infection, which negatively affects the therapeutic efficacy of the following antiviral therapy. Interaction between antiviral medication and replacement drugs for drug users such as methadone is a factor influencing the therapeutic efficacy and medication option, which is closely related to the prognosis of HIV-infected patients.

12.3   Sexual Behaviors and HIV Infection

Worldwide, sexual behavior is the leading route of HIV transmission. HIV can spread through sexual intercourse between males or between male and female. The more sexual contacts bring about the greater risk of HIV infection. With the social development, traditional sexual belief that the sex serves the goal of reproduction is changed among some young people. Instead, they believe that sex has its independent value. The change of the sex belief has greatly generated more common premarital and extramarital sexual behaviors. Once one person is HIV infected, he/she may transmit it to more heterosexual partners.

In China, the incidence of HIV/AIDS infection in male homosexuals ranks second among the high risk populations. It is estimated that there are five to ten million male homosexuals in China. The reasons for the high incidence of HIV infection in this population are multiple sexual partners, low rate of condom use and their peculiar sexual behaviors. Among male homosexuals, 60–70 % have heterosexual partners or even have their own families, which is a route of HIV transmission to healthy persons. Currently, HIV/AIDS infection transmitted by homosexual behavior amounts to 32 %, whereas that by heterosexual behavior amounts to 40 %. In the year of 2008, professionals conducted a survey among homosexual individuals in 61 cities in China. It was found that on average, 4.8 % homosexuals have HIV/AIDS and the maximum reaches up to 18 %. In China, the incidence of HIV infection in male homosexuals is 45 times higher than that in general population. Individuals who have sexual behaviors with homosexuals, hemophilics, blood recipients, intravenous drug abusers could be infected by HIV and will constitute susceptible population of AIDS. Therefore, observation to sexual ethnics is the fundamental measure to prevent sexually transmitted HIV infection. Governments of many countries have paid their focused attention to the prevention of sexually transmitted HIV infection in the first place. The most important preventive measure against sexually transmitted HIV infection is to lead a healthy sexual life with only one sexual partner, and to refuse sexual contacts with HIV/AIDS patients or high risk populations. Heterosexual contacts with a person of unknown healthy conditions should also be avoided. Condom use can prevent HIV infection in sexual life. However, because condom could be torn, the condom use cannot completely avoid accidental HIV infection.

Chinese traditional custom and ethnics emphasizes the maintenance of a healthy sexual life, which is helpful to prevent sexually transmitted HIV infection. However in recent years, with increasing international communications, the sexual belief is changed and the possibility of HIV/AIDS infection is also increasing. Personally, it is advisable to lead a healthy sexual life, avoid voluntary inappropriate sexual contacts and use qualified condoms properly.

12.4 Mental Health and HIV Infection

Mental health means individuals can adapt to the ever developing environment with integrative personality traits, and can think, feel and respond in a positive way with normal regulating ability. In real life, mentally healthy person has a proper self-understanding and self-control and is able to properly respond to stress from external environment to keep a well-balanced mental state. Psychological well-being is an important component of a person's physical and mental health. It is also beneficial to the normal development of physical health. Without mental health, various physical problems may occur. China is now in the period of social transformation, which impacts on families and the society. Numerous social, interpersonal and psychological conflicts occur, and some individuals are self-lost, with occurrence of various psychological problems. Drug abuse and unhealthy sexual behaviors are ways they used to transiently evade from the psychological problems. However these behaviors are also the high risk factor of HIV infection. In conclusion, it is beneficial to reducing HIV transmission with a psychological well-being and a healthy sexual life.

On the other hand, HIV infected persons have serious psychological problems. HIV spreading is not only a medical issue, but also has great impacts on psychological and social health. Some symptoms of HIV infection are caused by the social impacts. Symptoms like perspiration, insomnia, diarrhea and weight loss are not related to the severity of disease. Instead, hypochondriasis and somatization occur due to insufficient care or even rejective attitudes to patients with HIV/AIDS. After HIV infection, the patients change their relationship with the outside world, their personality and their self-esteem. In addition, some symptoms are caused by organic changes after invasion of HIV to the brain and the nervous system, with either excited manifestations or dementia manifestations.

It is common that HIV-infected persons have some psychological problems like anxiety, interpersonal sensitivity, depression, hostility and more serious phobia. Factors like adverse drug reactions, physical symptoms, being discriminated, loneliness, uncertain illness and economic burden lead to the varying degree of affective disorder in HIV-infected patients, with an incidence of depression and anxiety being about 2–21 % higher than that of the general population. In addition, the incidence of serious depression in HIV infected population is 22–36 %. All these psychological problems play negative role in the treatment, life quality and survival of patients with AIDS.

Studies have demonstrated that anxiety in AIDS patients infected via sexual behaviors is significantly obvious than that in AIDS patients infected via intravenous drug abuse, while depression in AIDS patients infected via intravenous drug abuse is more serious. Paid blood donors infected by HIV commonly have negative emotions such as depression, anxiety and stress and are more vulnerable to suicide. Risk factors for the above negative emotions include severe discrimination and negative impacts of the illness on daily activities, while favorable social support can greatly reduce the risks of such negative emotions. Depression in paid blood donors infected by HIV plays important role in their committing suicide, whereas the factor of friendly family could help to eliminate their decisions about committing suicide. Most HIV-infected individuals are willing to receive psychological support services and to communicate with other AIDS patients, families and friends. They are also willing to consult physicians for health.

It is reasonable to provide care and support for HIV-infected persons, since they are the victims of HIV/AIDS and deserve humanitarian help. The family and community should create a friendly, understanding and healthy environment for AIDS patients and HIV-infected individuals at work and in daily life. The patients with HIV/AIDS should be encouraged to adopt a positive attitude toward life. Their high-risk behaviors should be changed and they should have favorable compliance to recommendations by physicians. All of these are beneficial to prolonging their life expectancy and improving their quality of life. Meanwhile, these are also beneficial to the prevention and control of AIDS as well as to the social stability.

Above all, care, assistance and respect to AIDS patients and HIV-infected persons is an integral part of HIV/AIDS prevention and control.

12.5 Social Customs & Ethics and HIV Infection

The incidence of HIV infection varies from place to place due to the various social culture, customs and life styles.

In some remote mountainous areas of China, there used to be no AIDS epidemic, but later it occurred and has been gradually increasing in recent years. These places are scarcely inhabited, with poor economy and poorly developed culture. The residents there have insufficient consciousness about sanitation. In some areas with residence of minorities, sexual behaviors are voluntary due to traditional customs and habits. As a result, premarital and extramarital sexual behaviors are more common. Therefore, the high risk population is increasing year by year, with a more serious HIV/AIDS epidemic than other areas.

In terms of drug use and prostitution, Chinese people have different beliefs and opinions from western countries. In many countries, sexual tourism is officially permitted. Prostitutes are managed and able to receive regular medical examinations and related education in the red-light district. In China, however, prostitution is illegal and red-light district is forbidden, but with commercial sexual dealings underground. In some recreational places, including dance halls, KTV rooms, bath centers and hotels, the commercial sexual behaviors cause the spread of HIV/AIDS and other sexually transmitted diseases (STDs).

In addition, in some African countries, religions and national customs encourage the practice of injuring vaginal tissues, for no man would marry a woman without such injuries. Other traditions like child marriage can also lead to impairments of female sex organ. Such sexual behaviors in Africa accelerate HIV transmission among heterosexuals and cause a higher incidence of female HIV infection than other countries.

The attitudes towards homosexuality vary in different countries and regions due to different economic status, cultures, customs and ethnics. Currently, homosexuality culture could only coexist with mainstream heterosexuality culture in a few Nordic countries. In most countries and regions, homosexuality is considered against traditional ethnics or even as paraphilia. Some countries have special laws prohibiting homosexuality. These various customs, habits and ethnics have impacts on homosexual behaviors. In countries with unrecognized homosexuality, the homosexuals tend to live a secret life, or even marry heterosexually to follow the mainstream culture while keeping homosexual behaviors. In such way, more HIV infection may occur due to heterosexual behaviors.

HIV/AIDS Related Nervous System Diseases

13

Contents

13.1 An Overview of HIV/AIDS Related Nervous System Diseases

HIV is lymphotropic to CD4+ lymphocytes and neurotropic. It selectively infects and destroys the CD4 T lymphocytes of its hosts, causing seriously compromised cellular immunity, which in turn leads to their increased susceptibility to opportunistic infections and AIDS defining neoplasms.

HIV infected monocytes and giant cells pass through the blood–brain barrier and directly attack brain parenchyma, especially colloid cells, stellate cells and even microglial cells, to involve the central nervous system. Clinically, 40–50 % patients with AIDS have central nervous system symptoms and about 10 % show their central nervous system symptoms as the initial symptom of AIDS. By autopsy, about 75 % patients with AIDS have pathological changes in central nervous system. HIV is also a neurotropic virus, which can be phagocytized by macrophages to pass through the blood–brain barrier. As a result, brain tissue and cerebrospinal fluid (CSF) are invaded for its replication. HIV has been isolated from specimens of brain tissues, spinal cord, peripheral nerves and CSF in patients with AIDS. By electron microscopy, immunohistochemistry (IHC) and in situ hybridization, HIV has been proved to invade the mononuclear cells and multinuclear cells. We have detected HIV-1 DNA sequence in the brain tissues of patients with AIDS by PCR. And we also have proved that DNA copy number of HIV is significantly associated with pathological changes caused by HIV/AIDS.

Nervous system involvement is common in patients with HIV/AIDS related infections, which is one of the main reasons for increased death rate in patients with AIDS.

Pathogens of HIV/AIDS related nervous system infections include parasite, fungus, mycobacteria, virus and bacteria. Among patients with AIDS, 10–20 % initially shows symptoms of the nervous system, 30–50 % adult patients and 70–80 % children patients have clinical manifestations of nervous system dysfunction. According to an international report, 80 % patients were found to have neuropathological lesions by autopsy. The complexity of HIV/AIDS related nervous system infections includes: (1) During the whole course of the disease, AIDS patients show predominantly complications of one system/organ, or with involvement of multiple systems/organs; (2) With the decreased immunity and prolonged survival time, incidence of complex infections of nervous system has increased, which is characterized by multiple pathogens, complex pathological changes and diverse imaging demonstrations; (3) Relationship between pathological changes before and after the onset of AIDS; (4) Relationship between pathological changes caused by HIV itself and by HIV/AIDS related nervous system infections; (5) Clinical and imaging demonstrations before and after HARRT.

According to the origin, location and spectrum of diseases, HIV/AIDS related nervous system diseases can be categorized into following five types: (1) HIV/AIDS related impairments, such as HIV encephalitis and aseptic meningitis; (2) opportunistic infections of nervous system, such as toxoplasmic encephalitis, cytomegalovirus (CMV) encephalomyelitis, herpes viral encephalitis, progressive multifocal leukoencephalopathy, cryptococcal meningitis and tuberculosis infection; (3) neoplasms of the nervous system, including non-Hodgkin lymphoma, occasionally with focal lesions caused by Kaposi's sarcoma; (4) cerebrovascular diseases, such as cerebral vasculitis, cerebral hemorrhage, encephalatrophy and cerebral infarction; (5) peripheral neuropathy.

13.1.1 HIV-Related Brain Lesions

13.1.1.1 HIV Encephalitis

HIV encephalitis is caused directly by HIV, showing related neuropsychiatric symptoms. Its main manifestation is dementia, which is referred to as HIV encephalitis or AIDS dementia complex (ADC). It is now believed to be an HIV related disease in its advanced stage. The pathogenesis is as following: (1) HIV infects vascular endothelial cells (VEC) of the nervous system to impair the blood–cerebrospinal-fluid barrier. In addition, microvascular changes could also cause impairments to the nervous system. (2) The neurotropism of HIV has less negative impacts on nerve cells and neurons. (3) HIV produced envelope protein gp120 is neurotoxic. (4) HIV-infected microglial cells and macrophages are also toxic and could cause indirect injury to nerves. (5) HIV could induce autoimmune response. (6) Children

with AIDS are more susceptible to HIV infection due to their developmental immatureness. The pathological changes include: no morphological changes in the early stage of HIV encephalitis, but brain atrophy of varying degrees with its progression with higher occurrence of local encephalatrophy, especially atrophy of the frontal lobe and the temporal lobe. In the advanced stage, ventricular dilation could be found with decreased brain volume. HIV encephalitis could involve the white and gray matter of the brain. Pathological changes are more serious in the deep gray matter (basal ganglia and brain stem nuclei). Focal or massive necrosis of brain tissue could also be found. Microscopically, two types of HIV encephalitis could be found, including multinuclear giant cell encephalitis and nodular encephalitis, which are characterized by widespread microglial nodules infiltration. Microglial cells proliferate and aggregate into nodules. In general, multinuclear giant cells and microglial nodules are believed to be pathological markers of HIV encephalitis. HIV encephalitis is clinically characterized by progressive dementia, with manifestations of decreased intelligence, cognitive dysfunction, motor impairments, behavioral problems, retarded response, reluctant expressions, decreased memory ability and dystaxia. Its clinical diagnosis is based on the following evidences: (1) definitive evidence of HIV infection; (2) progressively decreased intelligence and motor ability, persisting for several months; (3) CSF test excluding other infections or neoplasms; (4) MRI demonstrations of diffusive or focal white matter abnormalities, with flaky long T1 and long T2 signals, widened cortical sulci, dilated brain ventricle and reduced or normal brain volume.

13.1.1.2 HIV/AIDS Related Aseptic Meningitis

Aseptic meningitis occurs in some HIV infected patients, with manifestations of acute onset of headache, photophobia, fever and meningeal irritation. The cranial nerves VII are the most commonly involved, followed by cranial nerves V and VII involvement. Mental status can be also changed. Because its clinical manifestations and imaging demonstrations are neither specific nor characteristic, the differential diagnosis should be made based on comprehensive analysis of the clinical data.

13.1.2 HIV/AIDS Related Opportunistic Infections

13.1.2.1 HIV/AIDS Related Toxoplasmic Encephalitis

Toxoplasmic encephalitis is the most common HIV/AIDS related parasitic infection. In immunocompetent hosts, toxoplasmic infection is a subclinical and self-healing disease. However, in immunocompromised hosts, acute or occult toxoplasmic infection could reoccur to cause disseminated infections. The most commonly involvements include brain, spinal cord and heart. Especially when CD4 count is less than 100/μl, the occurrence of toxoplasmic infection is notably increasing. Toxoplasmosis is an AIDS-defining disease and is main cause of death in AIDS patients. Its pathogenesis is that access of toxoplasma parasites to the vascular and lymphatic vessels via gastrointestinal tract to cause parasitemia, followed by their access to organs of brain, heart and lungs along with blood flow or to local lymph nodes along with lymphoid flow, to parasitize in various karyocytes. They proliferate in host cells and lead to cellular necrosis and histoclasia. Meanwhile, soluble antigens released from cells cause inflammatory responses of their surrounding tissues. The pathological changes of toxoplasmic encephalitis include multiple abscesses, most commonly involving the interface of cerebral cortex and cerebral medulla, as well as basal ganglia. Brain stem and cerebellum could also be involved, with occasional involvement of the spinal cord. In brain tissues, multifocal necrosis can be found, with degeneration, necrosis and disappearance of nerve cells in the center of the focus. Its peripheral vascular vessels are congested, with accompanying lymphocytes infiltration and microglia proliferation. At the margin areas, pseudocysts and free tachyzoites (trophont) of toxoplasma gondii could be observed. The clinical manifestations include systemic symptoms such as fever, lymphadenectasis and hepatosplenomegaly. In cases with the nervous system involvement, neuropsychiatric symptoms can be found including headache, vertigo, mental disorder, loss of memory, coma and other diffuse cerebral symptoms. Focal symptoms include limb weakness, numbness, pain, convulsion, hemiplegia, gatism, ataxia and possible occurrence of meningeal irritation. The imaging demonstrations include T1WI low signal and T2WI moderate signals of the foci by MRI; high signals in the surrounding edema areas; high signals of foci after injection of the contrast agent (Gd-DTPA) with no enhancement of the edema areas.

13.1.2.2 HIV/AIDS Related Cytomegalovirus (CMV) Encephalomyelitis

HIV/AIDS related cytomegalovirus (CMV) encephalitis could be either congenital infection or acquired infection. Congenital CMV encephalitis often spreads via mother-infant vertical transmission and is the important reason for congenital malformation and infant intellectual disturbance. Its occurrence in adults sees in those with deficiency in cellular immunity. The natural history of CMV encephalitis is complex. After primary infection, the toxin is expelled for weeks, months or even years, followed by its transformation into incubation period. Its recurrence and recurrent toxin expelling are common. Even many years after primary infection, the latent virus could be reactivated. Possibly, re-infection could also be caused by virus strain with different pathogenicity. The clinical manifestations of CMV encephalomyelitis are varied according to the patients' immunity and age. The symptoms and signs are varying in patients infected by vertical, parallel or nosocomial transmission routes. As to acquire CMV brain infection, deficiency in immunity leads to occurrence of vasculitis, omentitis, pneumonia and gastrointestinal infections, with involvements of lungs and brain. The pathogenesis is that CMV, the DNA virus, induced decreased immunity to cause the decreased cellular immunity in patients with HIV/AIDS related CMV encephalitis. Brain CMV infection has significant impacts on thymus development and the functions of splenocytes, mononuclear phagocytes, NK cells and CTL cells. The pathological changes are enlargement of infected cells, acidophilic inclusion bodies in the nuclei, basophilic inclusion bodies in the cytoplasms. CMV encephalitis is common in advanced stage of HIV infection, with CD4 T count being less than 50/μl. The clinical manifestations include fever, symptoms of respiratory tract, nervous system and hematological system. The body temperatures could range from low-grade fever to 40 °C. The nervous system symptoms include lethargy, coma, convulsion, dyskinesia, cerebral palsy, and occasional symptoms of hydrocephalus, hypophrenia and retinochoroiditis. MRI demonstrations include flaky long T1 and T2 signals in periventricular white matter. After contrast enhancement, ependyma can be enhanced with no enhancement of the brain parenchyma.

13.1.2.3 HIV/AIDS Related Herpes Viral Encephalitis

HIV/AIDS related herpes simplex virus often causes infection of skin and mucosa and rarely causes viral encephalitis. The pathological changes include the compromised immunity induced reactivation of herpes simplex virus and its spreading to the brain. The lesions are asymmetrically distributed, with obvious foci in medial temporal lobe, hippocampus, and orbital surface of frontal lobe, parietal lobe and cingulate gyrus. Hypothalamus, medulla oblongata and pons could also be involved. The pathological changes include asymmetric bilateral frontal lobe necrosis by naked eyes, with possibly accompanying hemorrhage. Microscopically, hemorrhage, necrosis and liquification of brain parenchyma can be found, diagnosed as acute necrotic hemorrhagic encephalitis. The clinical manifestations include neuropsychiatric symptoms such as headache, fever and epilepsy, and other symptoms like weakness, lethargy, ataxia and aphasia. Imaging findings include foci in cerebral gray matter, with flaky and round shaped or mass liked long T1 and T2 signals in frontal lobe, temporal lobe and parietal lobe. Local brain tissue edema is obvious, but generally with no involvement of the gray matter such as putamen, which is characteristic.

13.1.2.4 HIV/AIDS Related Multifocal Leukoencephalopathy

HIV/AIDS related multifocal leukoencephalopathy is often caused by JC virus, with a rare occurrence of about 10–25 %. It usually occurs in advanced stage of AIDS, with CD4 T count being less than 50/μl. Its pathogenesis is that HIV/AIDS related progressive multifocal leukoencephalopathy (PML) always occurs in patients with deficient cellular immunity. By electron microscopy, large amount of inclusion bodies composed of numerous papova virus particles in some colloid cells. The isolated virus is mostly JC virus. The pathological changes include that oligodendrocytes neural cells are selectively destroyed by JC virus to cause demyelination, with their fusion formed by multifocal lesions in the white matter. Cerebral hemisphere is more easily involved than cerebellum, especially subcortical gray-white matter interface. By autopsy, granular yellow softening lesions can be found in the brain white matter, with diffusive asymmetrical foci fusion into an area in size of several centimeters. Histopathologically, deeply stained oligodendrocytes are occasionally found in the surrounding areas of multifocal demyelination area, with swollen nucleus and intranuclear acidophilic amorphous viral inclusions. By transmission electron microscopy (TEM), the viruses are in crystal liked arrangement in size of 33–39 nm; gigantic deformed stellate cells could be seen with polymorphic segmented nucleus, mostly deformed; large amount of foamy macrophages and tissue necrosis can be observed. The clinical manifestations include progressively decreasing memory, hemianopsia, and hemiplegia and language disorder. The early symptoms could also be memory and language disorders, personality change. Occasionally, patients may show difficulty concentrating their mind, impaired sense of balance and cerebellar ataxia. Progressive multifocal leukoencephalopathy is mainly characterized by multifocal neural defects, with rapid progression. Death occurs in most patients within 6–12 months after the onset of symptoms and a few may survive for a longer period. CT scanning demonstrates that multiple foci are far from ventricular system, localizing in subcortical white matter and mostly in semi-oval center with an uneven distribution; the early foci are round or oval in shape and gradually fuse and enlarge; lesions are demonstrated as low density shadows, with unclearly defined boundary and no space occupying effect. The enhanced scanning demonstrates no enhancement of most foci; rarely found enhancement of foci; encephalatrophy can be found in the advanced stage. MR imaging demonstrates lesions mostly in frontal-parietal lobe and white matter in temporal lobe, with involvement of deep gray matter. Foci show long T1 and T2 signals, with asymmetrical distribution, sometimes in symmetrical distribution with well-defined boundary.

13.1.2.5 HIV/AIDS Related Nervous System Tuberculosis

The spread of HIV leads to increased occurrence of tuberculosis, mostly in the early stage of HIV infection with an incidence rate of about 5–10 %. It usually occurs when CD4 T count is 350–400/μl, with involvements of meninges and cerebral parenchyma. Its pathogenic mechanism is as following: most cases of nervous system tuberculosis are caused by mycobacterium, spreading from its primarily infected site to meninges and/or brain parenchyma along with blood circulation. After the hematogenous dissemination of primary tuberculosis terminates, many tubercle bacillus could survive in the central nervous system. Once cell-mediated immunity changes, tubercle bacillus transforms into nodules, which develop in cerebral parenchyma to form tuberculomas of different sizes surrounded by dense fibers. The tuberculomas are in sizes of less than 1 cm, with caseous necrosis or granulation tissues at their centers. Complete calcification occurs in patients with strong immunity, but it rarely occurs. In the advanced stage, intra-cerebral tubercle bacillus infection manifests as tuberculous meningitis due to deficiency of cell-mediated immunity caused by immunosuppression. The pathological changes include typical tubercles and caseous necrosis. The tubercles are composed of epithelial cell and Langhans' cells, with central caseous necrosis, surrounded by fibroblasts and lymphocytes. The clinical manifestations are as the following: (1) tuberculosis sings of low-grade fever, night sweat, emaciation and rapid blood sedimentation; (2) symptoms of intracranial hypertension and local cerebral lesions, showing as headache, vomiting, papilla optical edema, hemiplegia, aphasia, epilepsy, as well as cerebellar lesions like nystagmus and extremities ataxia. The imaging findings include meningeal exudation and thickening in basal cistern and sylvian cistern in cases with meninges involvement; contrast-enhanced MRI demonstrates significant abnormal enhancement; multiple round liked long T1 and T2 signals by MRI in cases with cerebral parenchymal involvement; obvious finger liked long T1 and T2 signals of surrounding edema with space occupying effect.

13.1.2.6 HIV/AIDS Related Non-Hodgkin's Lymphoma

HIV/AIDS related non-Hodgkin's lymphoma has an occurrence of 5–10 % and is the defining neoplasm of AIDS. Most scholars believe that lymphoma can be originated from undifferentiated multi-potential mesenchymal cells or stem cells in intracranial vascular vessels. Therefore, lymphoma is closely related to blood vessels. Recently, studies by electron microscopy and immunology found that lymphoma belongs to neoplasms of immune system, originating from mesenchymal cells in the human body. Simon believed that in the brain tissue, the specially approved location by immunity, the latent herpes virus can activate B cells to escape from the surveillance of the immunity for the development of lymphoma. The pathological changes include invasion of cerebral base, frontal lobe, temporal lobe, parietal lobe and adjacent tissues of the paracele by non-Hodgkin's lymphoma. The lesion is usually a confined singular mass, with rare occurrence of multi-centered growth to involve bilateral cerebrum. The lesions usually have sufficient blood supply, with occurrence of hemorrhage and necrosis. For cases with involvement of cerebral meninx and ventricles, the extensive infiltration occurs, sometimes within the cerebral ventricles. The pathological changes include: (1) Accumulation of the tumor cells around the blood vessels in arrangement resembling to a sleeve sheath and the demonstrations resembling to vasculitis; (2) Comparatively uniform morphology of the tumor cells with deep nucleus staining and infiltration of tumor cells into surrounding tissues; (3) Scattered phagocytes between tumor cells like stars in the sky and obvious phagocytosis; (4) Congestion, edema, bleeding, degenerative necrosis and accompanying grid cells and colloid cells proliferation in the brain tissues around the tumor. The clinical manifestations are as the following: headache, vomiting, decreased memory, unconsciousness, irritation, gatism and lower extremities paralysis. The onset of these symptoms is in patients with CD4 T count being less than 50/μl. And the imaging demonstrations include: for cases with lymphoma manifested as periventricular infiltration, meninx and ventricles enhanced imaging demonstrates obviously enhancement of the ependyma; for cases with space occupying lymphoma, MR imaging demonstrates long T1 and T2 signals; and enhanced imaging demonstrates heterogeneous enhancement of the mass, with no central enhancement, obviously abnormal enhancement of map liked margins and obvious space occupying effects.

13.1.2.7 HIV/AIDS Related Cerebral Atrophy and Infarction

About 12–20 % AIDS patients have the complication of encephalatrophy. The most common is singular or multiple focal cerebral infarctions, with manifestations of cerebral hemorrhage and transient cerebral ischemic attack. Vascular lesions approximately fall into five categories: (1) non-specific congestion of brain tissue, edema and hemorrhage; (2) cerebrovascular thrombosis and embolism as well as the resulted cerebral infarct; (3) acute granulomatous cerebral vasculitis; (4) certain opportunistic infections induced vascular lesions; and (5) tumorous vascular lesions.

Pathogenesis

HIV related cerebral infarct is caused by endovasculitis that is attributed to vascular endothelial lesions due to angiotropic HIV, opportunistic infections and complications of drug abuse. Tuberculosis, cryptococcal meningitis and cerebrovascular syphilis are the most common opportunistic infections in terms of the frequency of vascular involvement. Those with predominant vascular lesions also include toxoplasmosis encephalopathy, mycosis and herpes virus infections. It is a cerebrovascular disease of the nervous dysfunction caused by the exacerbation or complete occlusion of arteriostenosis due to multiple reasons, which further results in ischemia, anoxia and necrosis of brain tissue.

Pathological Changes

1. Within 6 h after HIV related cerebral artery occlusion, the brain tissue damages are not obvious. After 8–48 h, the ischemic tissues show manifestations of malaria, swelling and necrosis. The interface between grey and white matters is blurry, with occurrence of cerebral infarct. Under a microscope, the tissues structures are cloudy, with degeneration and necrosis of neurocytes and gliocytes, and slight dilation of capillaries. Exudation of fluids or erythocytes of surrounding tissues can be found. After 2–3 days, the surrounding edema is obvious, and after 7–14 days, the lesions are obviously softened, with absence of neurocytes, liquefaction of brain tissue and occurrence of large amounts phagocytes, and proliferations of stellate cells. After 21–28 days, gliocytes and capillaries proliferate, with the small lesions showing glial scars, and big ones into malaria foci.

2. The lesions of AIDS related cerebral watershed infarction are mostly located in the watershed zone between the blood supplying area of neighboring blood vessels, or in their marginal zone. It is generally believed that cerebral watershed infarction results mostly from hemodynamic disturbance.

3. AIDS related lacunar infarction occurs mostly in deep perforating arteries 100–400 pm in diameter. Therefore, the foci are mostly located in the putamen, caudatum, capsula interna, the basal part of pons, and corona radiata, with the diameters ranging from 0.2–15 mm. The softened necrotic tissues were phagocytized, with the remaining small chambers whose agglutination forms the lacunal status, frequently current. Its clinical manifestations are related to the location and severity of the cerebrovascular embolism and infarct. Many factors contribute to the occurrence of cerebrovascular accidents in AIDS patients. For instance, vascular endothelial damages due to HIV infection can induce thrombosis or non-agglutinated immune complex, leading to vascular stenosis. Vascular factors contribute to proliferation of vascular smooth muscle and fibroblasts, which may also cause vascular stenosis.

Imaging Demonstrations

CT scanning demonstrates spots and flakes of low density shadows, no space occupying effect, and slight edema effect. By enhanced scanning, there is no enhancement. By MR imaging, there are spots and flakes of long T1 and T2 signal. The enhanced imaging demonstrates no enhancement or line shaped enhancement of the focal margins.

13.1.3 HIV/AIDS Related Nervous System Diseases in Infants

Central nervous system diseases occur characteristically in infants and children with HIV infection. The immaturely developed nervous system is especially vulnerable to HIV, with an incubation period ranging from 6 months to 2 years, and occasionally up to 5 years. HIV/AIDS related central nervous system diseases include HIV encephalitis, HIV leukoencephalopathy and diffuse gray matter atrophy. Their clinical manifestations include microcephalus, cognitive impairment, retarded development, motion dysfunction, ataxia, tractus pyramidalis illness as well as convulsion, coma, hemiplegia, aphasia and blindness, resembling to those of dementia in adults. The pathological changes include infiltration of HIV infected macrophages and multinucleated cells, edema of the brain white matter, absence of neurons, defect neural dendrites in neocortex, increased diffuse stellate glial cells, calcified basal ganglia with accompanying minor vascular mineralization, the latter being a change characteristically in HIV infected children. The rarely found primary central nervous system (CNS) lymphoma occurs in brain of infants and children with AIDS. And secondary CNS lymphoma may occur on the basis of systemic lymphoid proliferative diseases. Compared to adult patients with AIDS, infant and children patients have a decreased incidence of opportunistic infections, which may be related to their short survival period and therefore reduced risks for such infections. During the course of HIV infection in children, cerebral infarction and cerebral hemorrhage may occur, with the most common clinical symptoms of hemiplegia and accompanying epilepsy. Cerebral hemorrhage tends to occur based on immunologic thrombocytopenia.

13.1.4 Clinical Manifestations of HIV/AIDS Related Brain Lesions

13.1.4.1 Headache
Headache is a commonly found symptom in patients with HIV/AIDS.

13.1.4.2 Epileptic Seizure
In the advanced stage of AIDS, complications such as opportunistic infections of CNS and neoplasms could cause epileptic seizure.

13.1.4.3 Dementia

13.1.4.4 Mental Changes
Patients with HIV infection commonly sustain mental changes, including anxiety, depression, and pessimism. Especially in the advanced stage, confusion and disorientation could occur, mostly caused by opportunistic infections.

13.1.4.5 Dyskinesia
About 80 % of HIV infected patients have dyskinesia.

13.1.4.6 Neuropsychologic Disorders
Neuropsychologic disorders are the important indicators for AIDS complicated by nervous system diseases.

13.1.4.7 Vision Changes
Some patients with AIDS may have loss of the visual field, diplopia, visual deprivation and other vision changes.

13.1.5 Clinical Application of HIV/AIDS Related Nerve Imaging

HIV/AIDS related inflammations, nodules and neoplasms of nervous system can be assessed by MR imaging and CT scanning for the size, shape, number, location and the relationship with surrounding tissues. The qualitative diagnosis can be made in combination with immunologic indices or pathological analysis for HSV encephalitis, CMV infection induced encephalitis, tuberculosis, Toxoplasmosis abscess and lymphoma. DR and CT are highly favorable in diagnosing respiratory diseases due to their favorable demonstrations for density discrepancy, including pulmonary TB, fungal pneumonia, bacterial pneumonia, viral pneumonia, protozoa (PCP, TOX) pneumonia and KS sarcoma. In combination to the laboratory indices or biopsy, their diagnosis can be made. FFA can define the location and range of ocular fundus lesion and can, in combination with the lab indices, define the qualitative diagnosis. Gastrointestinal endoscopy and barium meal radiography in combination with biopsy can conclusively diagnose gastrointestinal mycotic inflammation, ulcer, TB, lymphoma and KS sarcoma.

MR imaging has favorable spatial resolution for HIV/AIDS related soft tissue inflammation and tumor, with widespread clinical applications. The basis of DW imaging is the random motion of free water molecules. The random motion of such molecules is determined by their environment. The histiocytic shape, size, arrangement, distribution and permeability as well as the extracellular space and amount of fluid have a direct impact on the degree of tissue diffusion. Varying with the histological structure changes such as cellular swelling or damage, cellular nucleus deformity, permeability abnormality as well as the distribution changes of intracellular and extracellular fluid, the degree of diffusion is different from that of the normal tissue. HIV/AIDS related neoplasms and inflammations have different values of ADC, which provides the basis for the differential diagnosis. Diffusion and the wave-spectrum features demonstrated by DWI can identify HIV/AIDS related malignancies from benign neoplasms. For instances, MR wave spectrum demonstrations of increased Cr and decreased NAA suggest infectious changes. It can also be used to differentiate the cystic and parenchymal changes of the neoplasm from the peripheral edema of neoplasm. Its application also extends to determine ADC value of brain parenchyma, Cho/Cr, NAA/Cr and NAA/Cho for diagnosis, differential diagnosis and evaluation of the therapeutic efficacy. In addition, DWI can provide accurate information for the diagnosis of HIV/AIDS related cerebral infraction. DWI demonstrates, via MRI, the blood flow perfusion of capillaries, to assess the activity and capability of local tissues. This technology can assess the hemodynamic changes in capillaries of HIV/AIDS related encephalopathy. DTI is a newly developed MR technology, which has gained widespread application in clinical practice and scientific research of leukoencephalopathy. In China, Prof. Hongjun Li from Beijing YouAn Hospital affiliated to the Capital Medical University has, together with his team, initially applied BOLD and DTI into clinical practice and scientific research of HIV/AIDS imaging. They observed the fiber bundles of the white matter of the diseased region for patients with leukoencephalopathy, detected their FA values and analyzed the effects of the fiber bundles border of the white matter. Their findings have been applied for the early detection of compression and migration of the surrounding white matter fiber bundles of the neoplasm, which has gained favorable therapeutic efficacy. PET-CT image and PET-MR image is the integration of PET image with CT and MR image, respectively, which can simultaneously demonstrates pathophysiological changes and morphology of the lesion. Therefore, concurrent localization and qualitative diagnosis of the lesions as well as reference therapeutic plan can be provided. The diagnostic accuracy and the rationality of the therapeutic planning can be greatly improved. Their applications into HIV/AIDS related diseases have been internationally reported through publications of original research papers. The publications especially emphasize their value in differential diagnosis of HIV/AIDS related nervous system diseases and neoplasms, including the differential diagnosis of cerebral toxoplasmosis and lymphoma, the differential diagnosis of somatic infectious diseases and neoplasms, and morphologic and functional assessment of the general lymph nodes in patients with AIDS.

13.1.6 Application and the Future Development of Newly Emerging Imaging Technologies

With the development of imaging technology, we gain more knowledge about diseases and their pathogenesis, such as the application of ESysfMRI and DynaSuite technologies on the nervous system, and the future application of Torso Coil for more valuable information to diagnose organic lesions, the more accurate and humane diagnosis and puncture of breast diseases by Breast Coil and DynaCAD. The application of these new technologies in the current research will be gradually extended to clinical practice. On the basis of the original functions of MR, the clinical applications of the new technologies will be faster, more convenient and accurate in early and differential diagnosis of the diseases. This represents the most recent standards in development of imaging technology, integrating advantages of functional imaging and anatomical imaging and taking the lead in today's diagnostic imaging technology.

13.1.7 Prevention and Treatment of the HIV/AIDS Related Nervous System Diseases

HIV/AIDS related nervous system diseases are directly or indirectly caused by HIV infection. Therefore, we should firstly protect the susceptible populations to terminate the spreading and epidemic of HIV. Secondly, we should perform positive and comprehensive treatment for HIV infected population and patients with AIDS to improve their immunity and reduce the incidence of the opportunistic infections. Therefore, their life quality can be improved and their life expectancy can be prolonged. At the same time, we should further explore and establish the standard treatment guidelines for HIV/AIDS related nervous system diseases, their types and their pathogenesis as soon as possible, thus revealing the characteristics of HIV/AIDS related nervous system diseases. Additionally, we should strengthen the professional training for clinical staff to improve the diagnosis and treatment of HIV/AIDS related nervous system diseases.

Generally speaking, HIV/AIDS related nervous system diseases are important in the disease spectrum of HIV/AIDS imaging. Diagnostic imaging is an important examination for the nervous system infections, playing an irreplaceable role. Early diagnosis is the key to improve the life quality of patients and prolong their lives. However, the complexity and multiplicity of HIV/AIDS related nervous system diseases present challenges for our clinical practice. The categorization of HIV/AIDS related nervous system diseases is the basis for accurate diagnosis and differential diagnosis. A targeted and personalized diagnosis is our goal to serve the clinical practice.

13.2   HIV/AIDS Related Encephalopathy

13.2.1 HIV Related Encephalitis and Dementia

13.2.1.1 Pathogens and Pathogenesis

The HIV infection of the nervous system is mainly initiated from access of HIV carried by macrophages to the brain parenchyma or direct HIV infection of the vascular endothelial cells to attack the brain. Their target organs are major macrophages and microglia cells, with rare invasion to neuronal cells. HIV proteins can cause oxidative stress to damage cellular activity and to destroy the close interconnection of endothelial cells, leading to damages and apoptosis of nerve cells. HIV accumulates in the glial cells or perivascular macrophage for virus replication and eventually leads to encephalopathy. Although neural cells do not have CD4 receptor molecules, the cerebrosides or other glycolipid on the surface of the neural cells may constitute the alternative receptor binding site. HIV antigen is commonly found in macrophages, multinucleated giant cells, vascular endothelial cells, and microglia cells. Microglia cell is considered to be the target c cell of HIV infection. Researchers from California, US pointed out that patients with HIV/AIDS related dementia seem to have decreased level of lysozyme secreted by macrophages and failed secretion of lysozyme by monocytes. But lysozyme is the main defense protein of macrophages and the protein secreted by normal macrophages and monocytes can protect the human body from bacterial and viral invasion. Macrophages and monocytes can also produce other defensive cytokines. Some other researchers found that the severity of AIDS related dementia is closely related to large amounts of macrophages in the brain, but has a little relationship with the amount of HIV infected cells (by immunohistochemical staining of antibody gp41) in the brain. By macrophages and astrocytes culture, it was found that the HIV pathogenic nitric oxide synthase (iNOS) largely increases. The long term exposure to large amount of nitric oxide (NO) can explain the mechanism of damages to the central nervous system. In other words, the neurons and glial cells in the state of AIDS related encephalopathy are not infected by HIV. The damage to the central nervous system is the process of the cytokines and virus being released by the infected macrophages and microglia cells which leads to brain cell damage.

It has been proved that HIV is a neurotropic virus. Boni et al. detected HIV-1 DNA sequence in the brain tissues of AIDS patients by autopsy with PCR, with a finding about the positive rate of 64 % [15]. It has been also found that the number of viral copies is significantly correlated with the pathological changes. Jiao et al. [63] from China reported a positive rate of 60 % by a duplicating experiment in Chinese patients, the results being in agreement. As shown in Fig. 13.1a–c, studies suggest that several pathological

mechanisms may contribute to HIV/AIDS related nervous system dysfunction: (1) HIV infection of vascular endothelial cells of the central nervous system (CNS) leads to the damage to blood–brain barrier system, and microvascular lesions cause impaired nerves; (2) HIV mostly infecting glial cells, but rarely infecting neurons; (3) HIV produced gp120 envelope protein is toxic to the cells of the nervous system; (4) HIV infected microglia cells and macrophages release some cytotoxic substances or cytokines that also have a toxic effect to indirectly impair the nerves; (5) HIV infection induces autoimmune response; (6) Synergic effects of other opportunistic pathogens; (7) Children are more susceptible to nervous system impairments, which may be related to their immature development and thus more vulnerable to HIV invasion.

13.2.1.2 Pathophysiological Basis

Pathological changes fall into two categories. One is inflammatory lesions caused directly by virus and the other is abnormal immune functions induced by virus infection. The pathological features include scattered microglia nodules in white matter and gray matter, multinuclear giant cells infiltration, loose and large flakes of white matter, demyelination and brain atrophy. The infections directly induced by HIV are commonly slight, with short duration. However, opportunistic infections caused by immune dysfunction due to virus infection have long durations, with poor prognosis. The foci of HIV encephalitis distribute in the cerebral white matter and gray matter. The lesions in the deep gray matter (basa, ganglia, brainstem, and nuclear group) are commonly serious, with lentiform nucleus the most commonly involved, followed by thalamus, caudate nucleus, hypothalamus, brainstem and cerebellum. Focal or large flakes of necrosis occur in the brain tissue in some seriously ill patients.

13.2.1.3 Clinical Symptoms and Signs

HIV can impair the nervous system to cause various clinical symptoms. About 10 % patients show early symptoms of cognitive impairment, such as impaired concentration, delayed mental activities, poor memory, and impairment of rapid functional area and motion abnormalities. In the early stage, decreased concentration and memory and emotional changes (such as depression and upset) occur, which will gradually progress into low intelligence, loss of motor function and even loss of self care ability. The behavioral disorders are mainly manifested as loss of interests, emotional reluctance, declined social skills or social activities. The nervous system symptoms include bradykinesia, noncoordination, declining muscular strength, reflectional hyper function and positivity for protractor foot plantar reflection. With the progress of the disease, the consciousness of such patients can be intact, but their language ability is markedly weakened, with demonstrations of characteristic

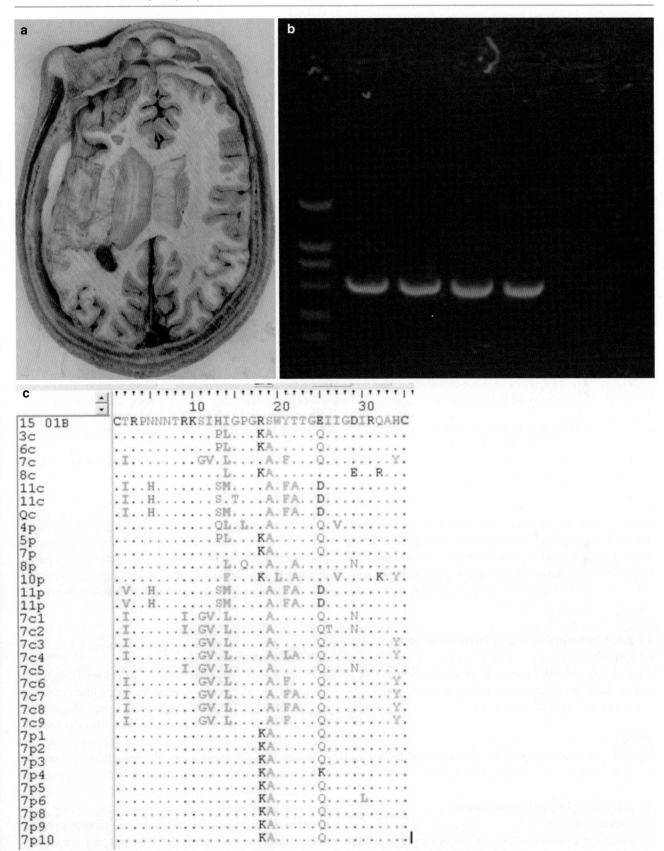

Fig. 13.1 (a) Cross sectional specimen demonstrates liquefaction necrosis and hematoma in the right brain tissue. (b) Autopsy by PCR amplification for integrated HIV-ENV gene V3 sequence in the brain tissue, amplified HIV-ENV gene V3 sequence within 60 % tissues. (c) V3 loop amino acid analysis: two types of V3 loop motif, GPGR and GPGK

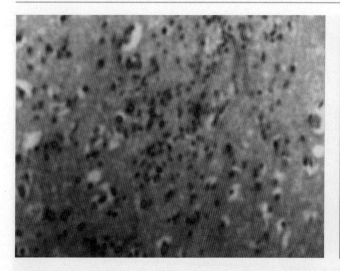

Fig. 13.2 Microglia cell proliferation, accumulating into nodules

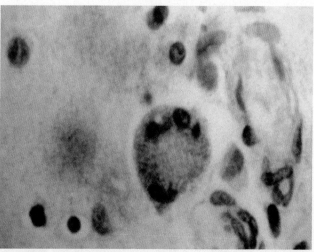

Fig. 13.3 Multinuclear giant cells in HIV encephalitic brain tissue (The figure comes from McGee et al. [101])

Clinical staging and feature of HIV/AIDS related dementia

Staging		Clinical manifestations	
0	Normal functions, no obvious clinical symptoms	Minor neurological symptoms	Minor symptoms
I	Being able to work and self care	Evidence proved functional, intelligence or motion impairments	Being able to walk independently
II	Being unable to work and demanding daily activities	Being able to self care in daily life	Being able to walk with help
III	Impaired intelligence and disability		
Terminal	Vegetative state, low intelligence, decreased social skills and understanding ability	Paraplegia or paralysis of limbs	Incontinence of urine and feces

mono-syllable language or silence. Abnormal motion ability in the advanced period has manifestations of persistent vegetative state, disability to walk, and incontinence of urine and feces. Generally, the survival period is no more than 2 years. Other neurological symptoms include anxiety, panic attack and depression. Acute psychosis is rarely found.

13.2.1.4 Examinations and Their Selection
CT and MRI
CT scanning and MR imaging is the diagnostic imaging of choice. Both can directly demonstrate the size, shape, density, range and ADC of the lesions.

PET-CT
PET-CT can reveal the glucose metabolism of lesions and reveal the anatomical structure of the lesions.

13.2.1.5 Imaging Demonstrations
CT Demonstrations
Symmetric or asymmetric flakes of low density area in bilateral white matter of the brain can be found, commonly around the lateral ventricle angle at the interface of the cortex and medulla. It can also be a local flake of low density area. In the

early stage, brain edema occurs, with no space occupying effect. Enhanced scanning demonstrates on enhancement. In the middle and advanced stages, the total brain volume decreases, with decreased cortex and basal ganglia gray matter. The sulci can be deepened and widened, with enlarged Sylvian cistern and the ventricle. Local lesions are mainly manifested as reduced local brain tissues and thinner gyri.

MRI Demonstrations
Symmetric spots, large flakes long T1 and long T2 signals in bilateral white matter surrounding the lateral brain ventricles can be found. In the early stage, brain tissue edema is not obvious and the space occupying effect is also not obvious. Enhanced imaging demonstrates no enhancement. In patients of middle and advanced stages, the brain tissue volume can be decreased, with obvious decrease of the gray matter. There are deepened and widened sulci, enlarged Sylvian cistern and brain ventricles. Local lesions are mainly manifested as reduced local brain tissues and thinner gyri with long T1 and long T2 signals. By DWI imaging, the cerebral white matter surrounding bilateral ventricle is demonstrated to have symmetric spots and flakes of high signals. MRS lactic acid peak is found to increase.

Case Study 1

A male patient aged 32 years was confirmatively diagnosed as having AIDS by CDC. He complained of poor sleep, slow response, decreased memory, headache and nausea. His CD4 T cell count was 120/μl.

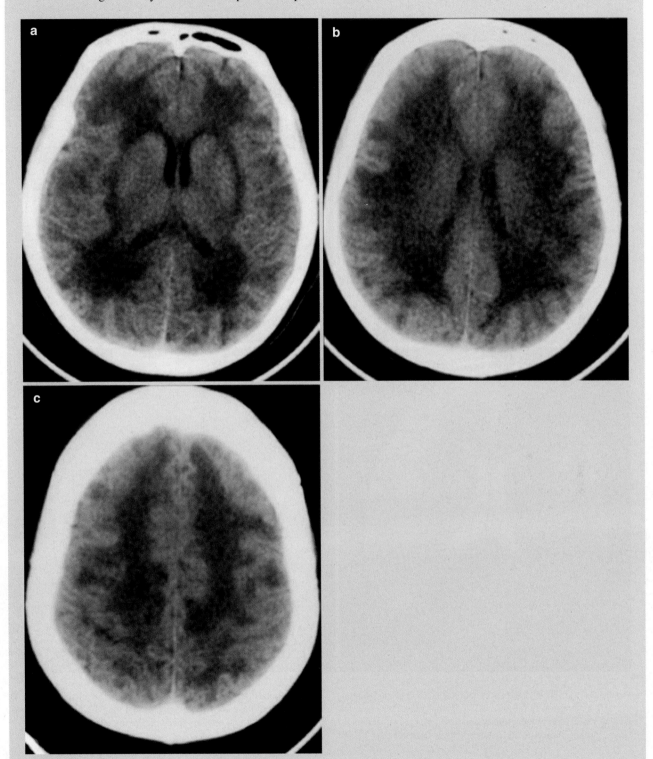

Fig. 13.4 (a–c) HIV related encephalitis and AIDS related dementia. Symmetric large flakes of low density areas in bilateral brain white matters, commonly around the lateral ventricle angle at the interface of cortex and medulla. It can also be local flakes of low density areas. In the early stage, edema of brain tissue can be found, with unobvious space occupying effect. Enhanced scanning demonstrates no enhancement. In patients of middle/advanced stage, their total brain volume can be decreased, with deepened and widened sulci, enlarged Sylvian cistern and brain ventricles. Local lesions are manifested as local decrease of brain tissues and thinner gyri

Case Study 2

A male patient aged 29 years was confirmatively diagnosed as having AIDS by CDC. He complained of slow response and memory loss. His CD4 T cell count was 5/μl.

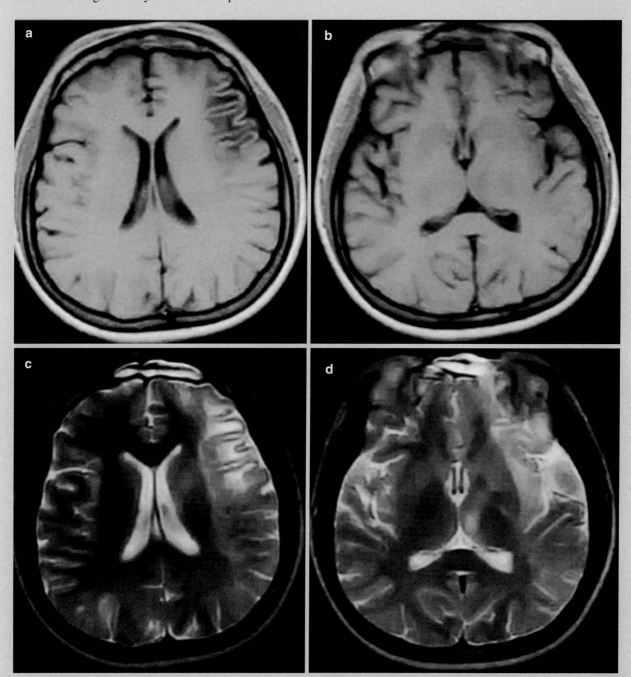

Fig. 13.5 (a–f) HIV related encephalitis and AIDS related dementia. MR imaging of T1WI and T2WI demonstrates deepened and widened local sulci of the left temporal lobe, enlarged subarachnoid space, local atrophy of brain tissues and large flakes of long T1 and long T2 signals (pointed by *black arrow*). (d, e) MR imaging demonstrates small flakes of slightly long T1 and long T2 signals in the left thalamus, with no obvious space occupying effects

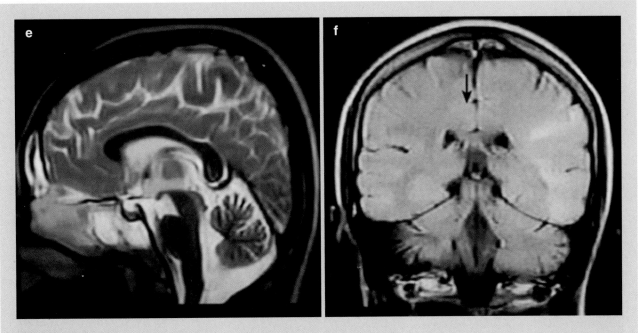

Fig. 13.5 (continued)

Case Study 3

A male patient aged 41 years was confirmatively diagnosed as having AIDS by CDC. He had a history of paid blood donation between the years of 1994 and 1995. By screening test for blood donors, he was definitively diagnosed as HIV positive. His CD4 T cell count was 600/μl.

He complained of fever, cough, and diarrhea and weight loss. In Oct. 2006, his CD4 T cell count was 217/μl and he received HAART. On March 15th, 2007, he complained of headache, dizziness, poor sleep, slow response and memory loss. His CD4 T cell count was 132/μl.

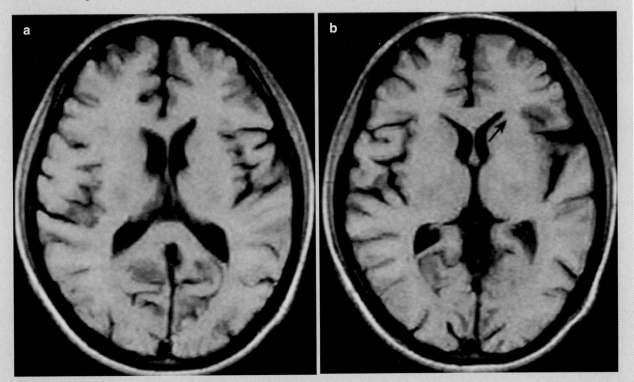

Fig. 13.6 (a–d) HIV related encephalitis and AIDS related dementia. Deepened and widened bilateral brain sulci, obviously enlarged Sylvian cistern especially the left Sylvia cistern and enlarged ventricular system

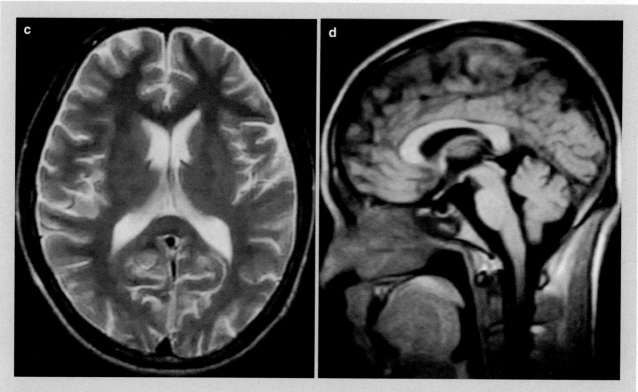

Fig. 13.6 (continued)

Case Study 4

A male patient aged 39 years was confirmatively diagnosed as having AIDS by CDC. He is a drug abuser for a long time, with alcoholism, dementia and ataxia. His CD4 T cell count was 15/μl.

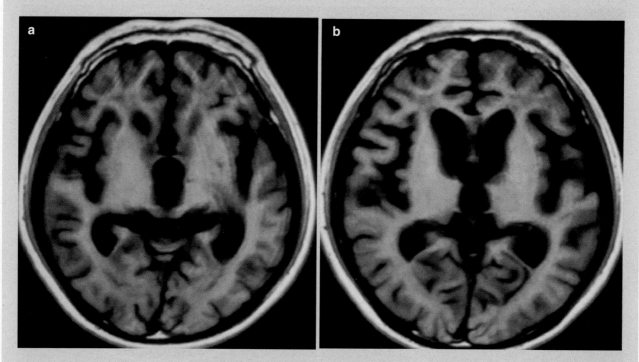

Fig. 13.7 (a–d) HIV related encephalitis and AIDS related dementia. Symmetric deepened and widened sulci of bilateral brain, enlarged ventricular system in long T1 and long T2 signals, widened subarachnoid space and obviously decreased total brain volume

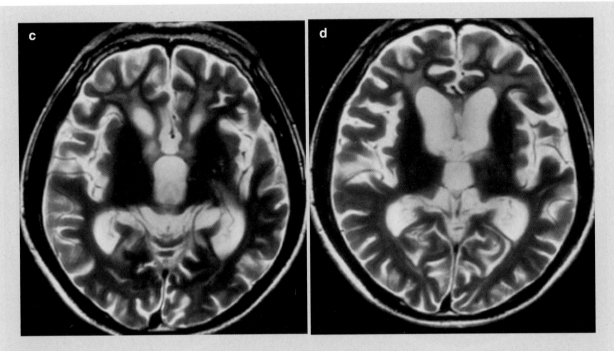

Fig. 13.7 (continued)

Case Study 5

A male patient aged 37 years was confirmatively diagnosed as having AIDS by CDC. He had a history of paid blood donation and he sustained progressive memory loss, dementia and ataxia. His CD4 T cell count was 10/μl.

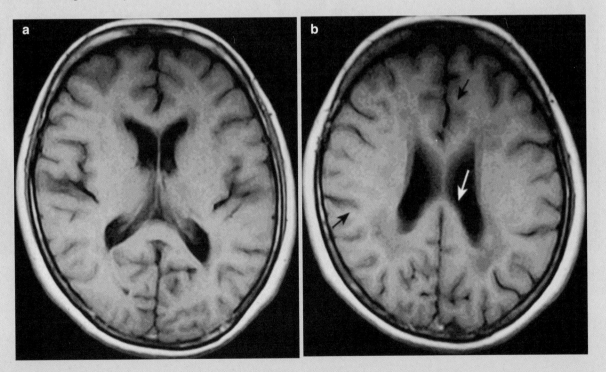

Fig. 13.8 (a–i) HIV related dementia and AIDS related dementia. (a–c) MR imaging demonstrates symmetric spots and flakes of long T1 and long T2 signals in areas surrounding bilateral lateral ventricles and basal ganglia. (d, e) FLAIR demonstrates symmetric spots and flakes of high signals in areas surrounding bilateral lateral ventricles and basal ganglia (pointed with *arrow*). (f–h) IV-Gd-DTPA demonstrates no obvious enhancement of the areas surrounding ventricles and basal ganglia. (i) Sagittal IV-Gd-DTPA demonstrates worm bitten liked long T1 signal of the callosum, with blurry borderline

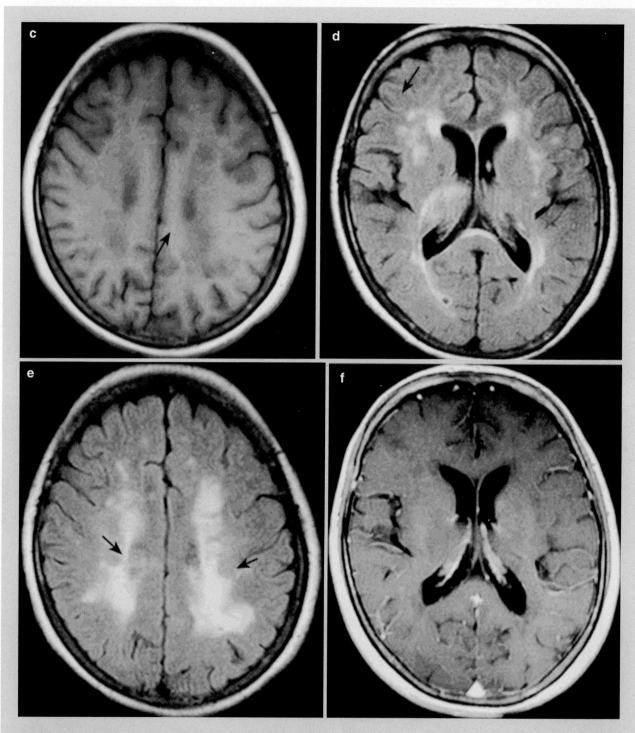

Fig. 13.8 (continued)

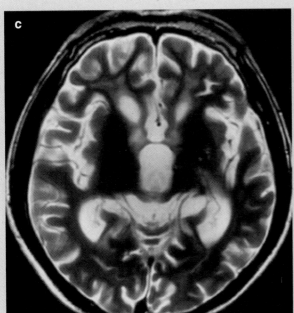
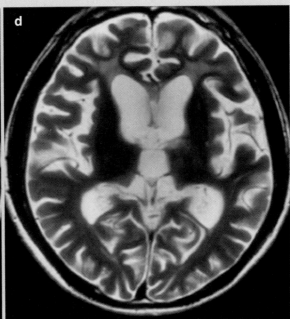

Fig. 13.7 (continued)

Case Study 5

A male patient aged 37 years was confirmatively diagnosed as having AIDS by CDC. He had a history of paid blood donation and he sustained progressive memory loss, dementia and ataxia. His CD4 T cell count was 10/μl.

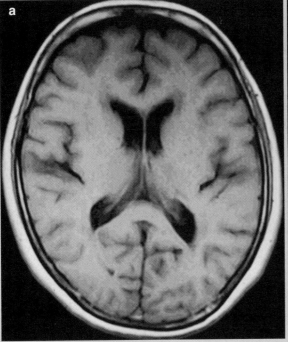
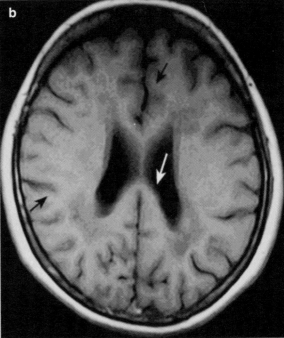

Fig. 13.8 (**a–i**) HIV related dementia and AIDS related dementia. (**a–c**) MR imaging demonstrates symmetric spots and flakes of long T1 and long T2 signals in areas surrounding bilateral lateral ventricles and basal ganglia. (**d, e**) FLAIR demonstrates symmetric spots and flakes of high signals in areas surrounding bilateral lateral ventricles and basal ganglia (pointed with *arrow*). (**f–h**) IV-Gd-DTPA demonstrates no obvious enhancement of the areas surrounding ventricles and basal ganglia. (**i**) Sagittal IV-Gd-DTPA demonstrates worm bitten liked long T1 signal of the callosum, with blurry borderline

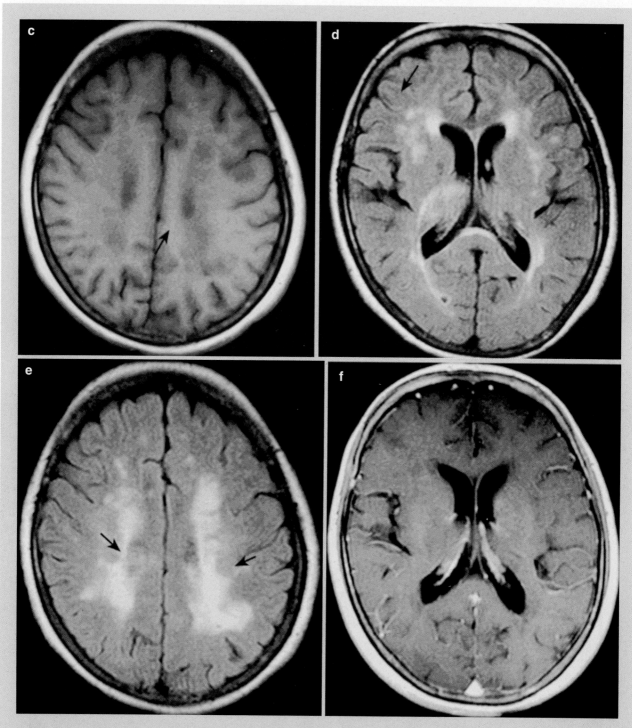

Fig. 13.8 (continued)

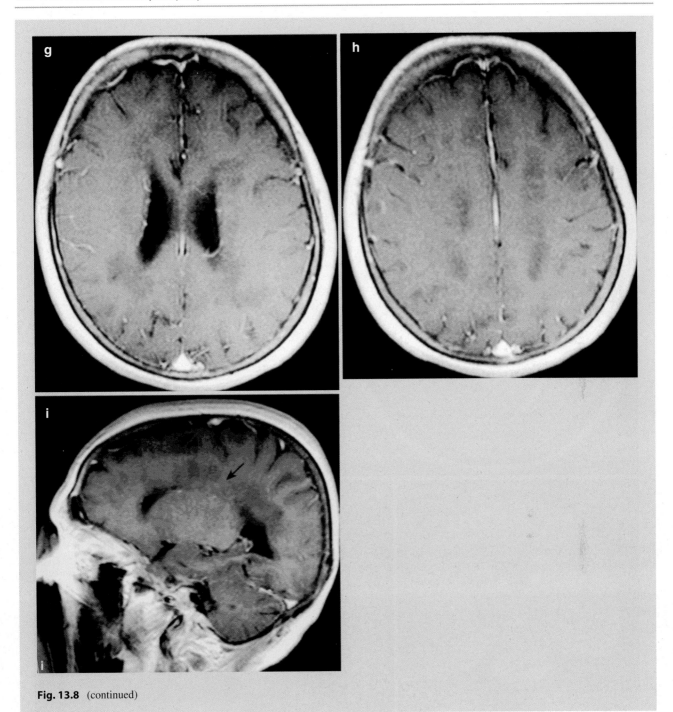

Fig. 13.8 (continued)

Case Study 6

A male patient aged 37 years was confirmatively diagnosed as having AIDS by CDC. He sustained three times epilepsy attacks and had a long history of cocaine abuse for above 12 years in doses of three to six times daily and 2–4 g each time. He was likely to be diagnosed as having cocaine encephalopathy. He had a past history of memory loss, especially recent memories. His CD4 T cell count was 500/μl.

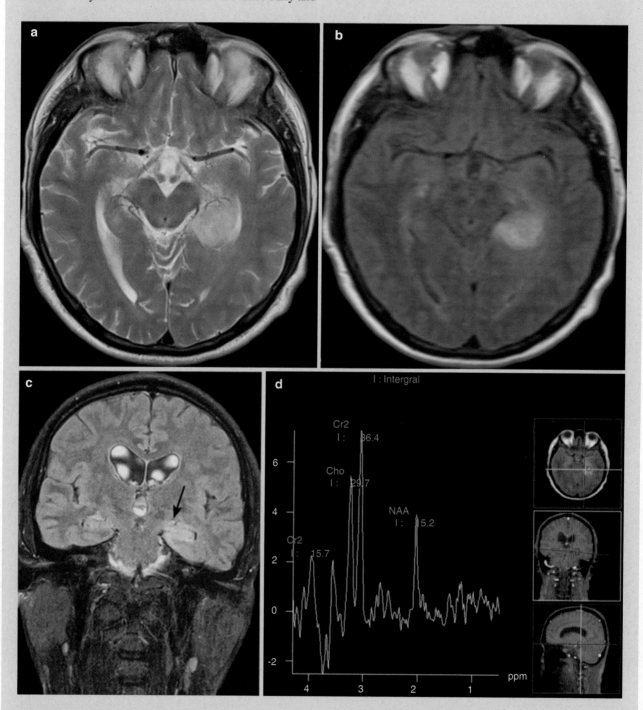

Fig. 13.9 (**a–d**) HIV related dementia and AIDS related dementia. MR imaging demonstrates flaky long T2WI in hippocampal gyrus of the left temporal lobe, with no obvious edema and space occupying effect. (**c**) IR T2WI demonstrates abnormal high signals in left hippocampal gyrus and parahippocampal gyrus, deepened and widened sulci in the temporal lobe. (**d**) MRS demonstrates the lesions with obviously decreased NAA peak, decreased inferior peak area and decreased ratio value of NAA/Cr

Case Study 7

A male patient aged 38 years was confirmatively diagnosed as having AIDS by CDC. He sustained ataxia of HIV encephalopathy, a long history of drug abuse, progressive memory loss and esophageal candidal infection. His CD4 T cell count was 115/μl.

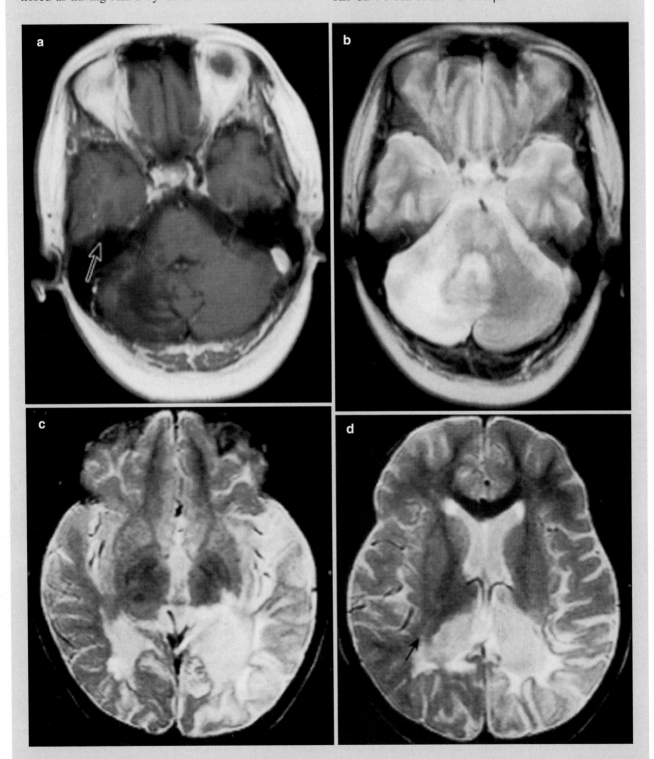

Fig. 13.10 (a–e) HIV related encephalitis and AIDS related dementia. (**a, b**) MR imaging demonstrates large flaky long T1 and long T2 signals in the right cerebellum, decreased volume of the brain tissues, widened and deepened sulci (pointed by *black arrow*). (c–e) Symmetric cap liked and flaky long T2 signal in bilateral lateral ventricle occipital angles, deepened and widened sulci and enlarged posterior angle of the lateral ventricle

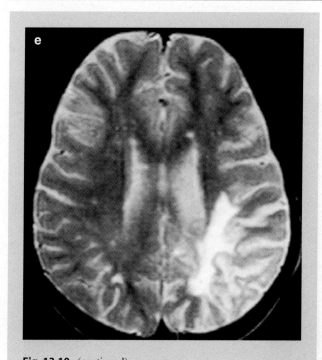

Fig. 13.10   (continued)

13.2.1.6 Criteria for the Diagnosis

1. Confirmatively diagnosed patient with HIV infection by CDC.
2. Neurological symptoms, including memory loss, weak consciousness, and even psychiatric and neurological symptoms.
3. Laboratory test
   HIV-1 RNA level is not important for the diagnosis of AIDS related dementia, but can be a predictor of its severity. In case of poor compliance to RT treatment, isolated viruses in the central nervous system can, when the plasma level is low, result in a high concentration of HIV-1 RNA, which is known as the loss of ESF.
4. CT and MRI demonstrations
   CT scanning demonstrates symmetric focal or whole brain low density areas, with no obvious edema and space occupying effect. MR imaging demonstrates flaky long T1 and long T2 signals, with no obvious edema and space occupying effect. Infarction, malacia, brain atrophy, reduced DWI cerebral perfusion coefficient, increased lactate peak of MRS and decreased NAA occur. There are also increased Cho/Cr ratio of deep gray nuclei; BOLD demonstrations of impaired functional areas, and DTI demonstrations of the morphology, running and defects of the nerve fiber bundles. CT scanning and MR imaging are not sensitive to early lesions, failing to detect microglial nodules, perivascular lesions and small granulomas. Imaging diagnosis is often delayed to the clinical diagnosis. Guided 3D localized biopsy has a diagnostic rate of 90 %.

5. Application of fluorodeoxyglucose labeled PET-CT scanning
   In the early stage of AIDS related dementia syndrome, the metabolism increases in the subcortical area, especially the brain basal ganglia area. In the advanced stage of AIDS, with the progress of dementia, glucose metabolism in the cortex and subcortical regions progressively decreases. The nature of these metabolic changes is still unknown, but may be associated with infection of human immunodeficiency virus.

13.2.1.7 Differential Diagnosis
Differentiation from Acquired Immunodeficiency of Other Causes
In combination of case history, acquired immunodeficiency diseases of other reasons, such as organ transplantation, long-term hormone therapy, and blood and tissue malignancies should be differentiated for the differential diagnosis.

Differentiation from Subacute Spongiform Encephalopathy
Subacute spongiform encephalopathy (BSE) is also known as cortex-striatum-spinal degeneration. It is a rarely sporadic central nervous system disease caused by prion infection. It is clinically characterized by dementia, ataxia, myoclonia and periodic EEG changes, which is a progressive fatal infectious disease. The pathological changes include spongy degeneration of the cerebral cortex, basal ganglia, cerebellum and spinal cord, shedding and necrosis of nerve cells, severe hyperplasia of glial cells and pore liked vacuolization. The qualitative diagnosis depends on biopsy. CT scanning demonstrates diffuse swelling of the brain tissue, shallow sulci, and unclear corticomedullary interface. MR imaging demonstrates multiple scattered flaky long T1 and long T2 signals in the bilateral frontotemporal lobe, double basal ganglia, with no obvious space occupying effect. Enhanced imaging demonstrates no enhancement. In the chronic stage, brain atrophy predominantly occurs.

Differentiation from Cytomegalovirus Encephalitis
The natural history of cytomegalovirus infection is complex, and such viruses can be discharged from saliva, semen, urine, breast milk and cervical secretions. Sexual intercourse with patient of cytomegalovirus infection, who is in the detoxification period, is a route of transmission. Infected pregnant women via sexual behaviors can cause fetal infection and perinatal infection. CMV infection can compromise the immunity of human body, especially the cellular immunity. Pathologically, it commonly involves cortical microglial nodules. The incidence of the involved cortical microglial nodules has been internationally reported to be 48 % by autopsy, among which 40 % with accompanying ependymal meningitis. Cytomegalovirus encephalitis rapidly develops,

with symptoms of confusion and dementia, declined consciousness, fever, cranial neuropathy and convulsions. MR imaging demonstrates periventricular focal necrosis, increased levels of CSF protein, and possible amplification of cytomegalovirus DNA by PCR.

Differentiation from Subacute Sclerotic Panencephalitis

Subacute sclerosing panencephalitis (SSPE) is a rarely found disease with a slow progression caused by persistent infection of variant measles virus to the central nervous system. In brain tissues, measles viruses are confirmed by electron microscopy and measles antigens are found by fluorescent antibody technique. The clinical manifestations of SSPE are considerably different. Some patients have typical EGG changes of paroxysmal multiple high waves and concurrence of two phase waves per second. Cerebrospinal fluid pressure is lower than normal, with significantly increased globulin, accounting for 20–60 % of the total cerebrospinal fluid proteins. Several months to several years (usually several years) after measles, progressive and fatal nervous system (Cerebrum) disorder occurs with accompanying typical intellectual impairments, paroxysmal muscular spasms and epilepsy. CT scanning demonstrates a wide range of cortical atrophy or low density areas in white matter. MR imaging demonstrates bilaterally symmetric long T1 long T2 signals, with no edema and space occupying effect.

13.2.1.8 Discussion

AIDS dementia complex (ADC) is different from HIV related dementia (HIVD). ADC can occur in any stage of the HIV infection. Its incidence rate is 0.4 % in asymptomatic period of HIV infection, while in the symptomatic period the incidence rate is 3 %. In the advanced stage of AIDS, in cases with significantly decreased CD4 T cell count and increased HIV-1 RNA, the incidence of cognitive impairment is up to 30 %, including 15 % with obvious dementia. Those receiving HAART show a decreased incidence. Patients with their CD4 T cell count being lower than $100/\mu l$ show a rapid progression, the untreated such patients have an average survival period of 6 month. The imaging demonstrations of ADC include cortical diffuse atrophy and deep white matter abnormalities. The opportunistic infections are commonly demonstrated as focal lesions (such as local brain atrophy in cases of viral encephalitis), and the severity of brain atrophy is not consistent with clinical symptoms. CT scanning demonstrates basal ganglia degeneration or periventricular low density shadow in children. MR imaging demonstrates brain shrinkage, decreased total brain contents, spots and flaky high signals in the white matter, caudate nucleus atrophy and diffuse gray matter atrophy. The application of functional imaging contributes to the early diagnosis of ADC. For instance, decreased DWI cerebral

perfusion coefficient and increased MRS lactate peak that are related to the inflammation can provide early assessment of the brain impairments. Decreased NAA is related to the neuronal loss and dendritic impairment. In terms of cognitive functions, increased Cho/Cr ratio of deep gray nuclei is consistent with pathological findings of infiltrations of foamy macrophages, microglia and lymphocytes. BOLD demonstrates impairments of the function areas, and DT1 demonstrates the morphology, running and defects of the nerve fiber bundles. The molecular imaging PET-CT demonstrates active subcortical metabolism in the early stage of ADC, suggesting possible HIV leukoencephalopathy, which facilitates the diagnosis of HIV encephalitis and AIDS related dementia.

13.2.2 Aseptic Meningitis

13.2.2.1 Pathogens and Pathogenesis

HIV is neurotropic and can directly infect the central nervous system and cause aseptic meningitis. Virus induced aseptic meningitis is a result of systemic infection spreading to the central nervous system along with blood flow. Although most cases are caused by viruses, it can also be caused by other pathogens or some non-infectious diseases. In addition to virus infection, other factors that cause aseptic meningitis include: (1) infection, such as that of mycoplasma pneumonia and chlamydia trachomatis; (2) autoimmune diseases, such as systemic lupus erythematosus, juvenile rheumatoid diseases, Kawasaki disease and Behcet's disease; (3) systemic medication, such as Azathioprine, a non-steroidal anti-inflammatory drug and carbamazepine; (4) intrathecally injected medication, such as myelography agent, chemotherapy drugs and some antimicrobial drugs; (5) brain tumors and leukemia; (6) heavy metal poisoning. Among all viruses which cause aseptic meningitis, intestinal virus is the most common, followed by HSV-2, and others such as adenovirus, VZV, CMV, EBV, rubella virus, measles virus and rotavirus have also been reported.

13.2.2.2 Pathophysiological Basis

Clinical aseptic meningitis is also known as serous meningitis, lymphocytic meningitis, or viral meningitis. It is a common manifestation of a variety of viral infections of the nervous system. The basic concept of aseptic meningitis refers to meningitis due to pathogenic factors except of bacteria and fungi. It is characterized by meningeal irritation and increased cell count in CSF. HIV/AIDS related aseptic meningitis occurs in any stage of AIDS (except of the advanced stage of AIDS). A class of virus infection mainly causes inflammation of the meninges, choroid plexus, and ependyma, while another class of virus tends to infect neurons and glial cells to cause encephalitis.

13.2.2.3 Clinical Symptoms and Signs

HIV/AIDS related aseptic meningitis occurs in any period of AIDS, except of the advanced stage of AIDS. It commonly involves the seventh, fifth and eighth pair of cranial nerves. The clinical manifestations have rapid onset, with fever (body temperature up to 38–40 °C), severe headache that is more serious than other factors induced fever accompanying headache, mild mental disorder including lethargy, drowsiness or irritability, stupor or coma, neck stiffness, photophobia, pain during the eyeball movement and myalgia. Generally the manifestations can recede in 2–4 weeks, while patients with chronic illness may have recurrent symptoms. It has been reported that some patients with HIV-1 infection can have Guillian-Barre syndrome in the early stage, with manifestations of distal symmetric extremities numbness, loss of sensation, and then progressive paralysis and weakened muscular strength.

13.2.2.4 Examinations and Their Selection

Laboratory Tests

1. Slightly increased CSF cell count and protein, and possibly detected HIV antigens in the acute stage in some patients.
2. Serum HIV antibody positive, but may be negative for cases of acute infection in window period.
3. Isolation of HIV by cerebrospinal fluid culture.

EEG

EEG demonstrated increased diffuse waves, and occasionally findings of epileptic discharges. As the condition improves, EEG demonstrates normal gradually.

Diagnostic Imaging

CT scanning and MR imaging are the imaging examinations of choice. Plain and enhanced CT scanning and MR imaging can help to understand edema, thickening and abnormal enhancement of meninges.

13.2.2.5 Imaging Demonstrations

CT Demonstrations

The foci can be found in the cerebral tentorium and cerebellar tentorium, in strips liked thickening. Enhanced scanning demonstrates linear or strips liked abnormal enhancement. In the chronic stage, the demonstrations include hydrocephalus and expansion of the supratentorial cerebral ventricle.

MRI Demonstrations

The foci can be found in the cerebral tentorium and cerebellar tentorium, in strips liked thickening as well as long T1 and long T2 signals. Enhanced imaging demonstrates linear or strips liked abnormal enhancement.

13.2.2.6 Criteria for the Diagnosis

1. HIV infection confirmed by CDC.
2. Slight increase of CSF cell counts and protein.
3. Increase of the diffuse waves in EEG, with occasional findings of epileptic discharges.
4. Mostly having neurological symptoms, such as memory loss, weak consciousness, and even neuropsychiatric symptoms.
5. Enhanced CT scanning and MR imaging demonstrate abnormal strip or linear enhancement of meninx and ependyma. The finding of dilated ventricles contributes to the diagnosis of HIV/AIDS related aseptic meningitis. The definitive diagnosis depends on brain tissue biopsy.

13.2.2.7 Differential Diagnosis

HIV viruses can cause aseptic meningitis, which can also be caused by other pathogenic infection or certain non-infectious diseases. In addition to viral infections, it should also be differentiated from the following diseases: (1) infections, such as mycoplasma pneumoniae and chlamydia trachomatis; (2) autoimmune diseases such as systemic lupus erythematosus, juvenile rheumatoid diseases, Kawasaki disease and Behcet's disease; (3) brain tumor and leukemia; (4) heavy metal poisoning. Among the viruses causing aseptic meningitis, enteric viruses are the most common, followed by HSV-2. Other viruses such as adenovirus, VZV, CMV, EBV, rubella virus, measles virus, and rotavirus have also been reported.

13.3   HIV/AIDS Related Intracranial Opportunistic Infections

13.3.1   HIV/AIDS Related Intracranial Fungal Infections

13.3.1.1 Cryptococcus Neoformans Meningitis

Pathogens and Pathogenesis

Cryptococcus neoformans is a conditional pathogenic bacteria. Immunodeficiency is an important risk factor for its infection. Cryptococcus neoformans meningitis is caused by the infection of cryptococcus neoformans to meninges and brain parenchyma. The central nervous system infection caused by cryptococcus neoformans can occur in immunocompetent populations, but the infection is the most common in patients with AIDS. The incidence of cryptococcus neoformans meningitis in AIDS patients accounts for about 5–10 % in HIV/AIDS related opportunistic infections, and 11.3–13.8 % in autopsy of AIDS cases, with poor prognosis. It is listed as one of the defining diseases of AIDS by CDCs in Africa and the United States. Cryptococcus neoformans is round or oval, enveloped by cellular wall and capsule and can be found widely in soil, vegetables, milk, grassland, honeycomb and pigeon feces. Cryptococcus neoformans is commonly inhaled via respiratory tract to produce an extracellular phospholipase B, a substance which destroys the alveolar surfactant to cause physical properties changes of lung tissues. Therefore, the intrapulmonary lesions occur to cause inflammatory responses via blood flow to the brain or meninges within months. Cryptococcosis polysaccharide capsule is the major component for capsular virulence, which functions to mediate the inhibition of phagocytes and reduce induced specific T lymphocyte responses. Studies found that capsular thickness is positively correlated with its antiphagocytic ability, and is related to the high molecular weight fragments of polysaccharide capsule. By activating the alexins and inhibiting the phagocytes from releasing cytokines IL-6 and IL-1β, polysaccharide capsule inhibits the immune responses of human body and causes diseases by rendering pathogenic bacteria escaping from the hosts defense system. Melanin is another important pathogenic factor of cryptococcus infection. The synthesized melanin binds to the membrane associated phenoloxidase in the cellular wall. As the abundant catecholamines in the brain can be used as its important reaction substrates, melanin is presumably one of the reasons for the high affinity of cryptococcus to the central nervous system. The main toxic effect of melanin is against free radicals. It has been internationally reported that melanin synthesized from one cryptococcal cell is sufficient to clear a large number of cellular oxidants produced by activated macrophages. By clearing superoxide and other oxides from the body, melanin protects the yeast cell against the destruction by the oxides produced by the host cell. In addition, melanin also has the antifungal effect of resisting ultraviolet rays and plays the role of reducing the sensitivity of amphotericin B. These effects may be one of the reasons why cryptococcus persistently spreads in the body and its infection is formidable to cure. In recent years, with the extensive or unreasonable use of broad-spectrum antibiotics, hormones, immunosuppressive drugs, as well as the increasing incidence of immunodeficiency diseases and the increasing number of patients receiving organ transplantation, the prevalence of this disease is on the rise. Generally speaking, cryptococcus polysaccharide capsule is an important pathogenic substance which can inhibit the immune responses. As the antibodies and alexins against cryptococcus fail to directly kill cryptococcus but indirectly kills it by regulating phagocytosis of macrophage. The absence of these antibodies and alexins in the cerebrospinal fluid renders it difficult to prevent cryptococcosis infection. Therefore, cryptococcus meningitis commonly is in progressive deterioration to cause death.

Pathophysiological Basis

Cryptococcal meningitis has an occult onset in a chronic or subacute process and acute cryptococcal meningitis is rare. It commonly involves meningeal tissues. By naked eyes observation, early lesion is yellowish white jelly liked appearance, with nodular surface of the brain granuloma. Some brain granulomas are cystic, transparent, yellowish white and hardened. On the sectional surface, the fibers intersect in color of grayish white and yellowish white, with semitransparent microcysts among the fibers. Cryptococcal mostly accumulate in Willis arterial ring to cause thrombosis of the basilar artery, multifocal infarction or hemorrhage. With the extension of survival time, cryptococcal continue to proliferate within phagocytes to cause inflammatory responses, leading to granulomas or necrosis, which can fuse into cryptococcal granuloma. It is manifested as unilocular cyst. In patients with a longer course of the disease, space occupying effects of multiple granulomas or multilocular cysts can be found. Under a microscope, the recently developed lesions are composed of a large population of cryptococcus and the resulted inflammatory cell infiltration. The infiltrated inflammatory cells are monocytes, epithelial liked cells, lymphocytes and plasma cells, sometimes with hyperplasic macrophages and small focal granuloma. Cryptococcuses accumulate in Willis arterial ring to cause thrombosis of the basilar artery, multifocal infarction or hemorrhage. The unilocular or multilocular cysts contain a large number of cryptococcus, and are composed of monocytes, epithelioid cells and multinucleated giant cells. In the involved brain, cerebellum, midbrain, medulla oblongata, and subarachnoid space, hyperplasia and hypertrophy of stellate cells occur, with possible occurrence of toxoplasma infection or other bacterial infections. Chronic cryptococcal meningitis commonly involves the base of the soft meninges, where reactive hyperplasia and thickening of the connective tissue occur to cause stenosis of midbrain aqueduct, with supratentorial hydrocephalus and symmetric enlargement. (Figs. 13.12, 13.13, 13.14, and 13.15)

Morphology of Cryptococcus neoformans in the pathological sections and its variants include: clearly defined spores of Cryptococcus neoformans by Alcian blue staining, PAS staining or GMS staining. By PAS staining, both thallus and capsule are stained red. Generally, Cryptococcus neoformans is in round or oval shape, with a diameter of 2–20 mm, commonly piling up with some scattering in the tissues. By H&E staining, there is a space in size of 3–5 mm out of the cellular wall, which is resulted from unstained colloid capsule of the thallus. Light red staining of some capsules can also be found (Figs. 13.12, 13.13, 13.14, and 13.15).

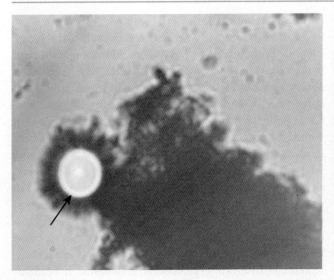

Fig. 13.11 Morphology of Cryptococcus neoformans in cerebrospinal fluid under a microscope after ink staining

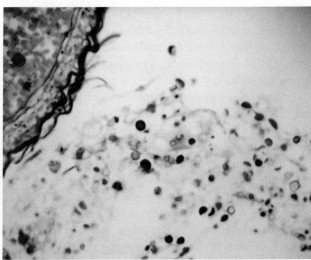

Fig. 13.13 Cryptococcus neoformans in the pathological section of brain tissue after GMS staining, with black spores, 1000 (Provided by Lang ZW)

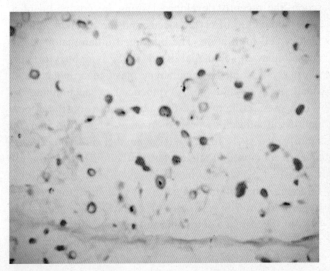

Fig. 13.12 Cryptococcus neoformans in the pathological section of brain tissue, with red spores, PAS1000 (Provided by Lang ZW)

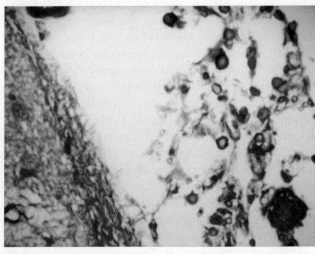

Fig. 13.14 Cryptococcus neoformans in the pathological section of brain tissue, with green spores by Alcian blue staining, 1000 (Provided by Lang ZW)

Clinical Symptoms and Signs

Its clinical manifestations include: (1) mostly chronic onset, occasionally acute; (2) Progressively severe headache, mental disorder, irritation and even disturbance of consciousness of different degrees; (3) Common optic nerve impairments, followed by impairments of VII, VII and VI cranial nerve; (4) Meningeal stimulation such as increased intracranial pressure is the common positive signs in early stage, and fundus papillary edema, pyramidal sign in the advanced stage; (5) Slight hemiparalysis.

Examinations and Their Selection

Pathogenic Examinations

In various specimens, the finding of cryptococcus neoformans is decisive for the diagnosis. The blood routine tests may bear results of slightly/moderately increased white blood cell count, mostly between $(1-2) \times 10^{10}$/L and rarely up to above 2×10^{10}/L; accelerated ESR in some cases; decreased hemoglobin and red blood cell in the middle and advanced stages. The lumbar puncture may find increased pressure of CSF, increased monocytes, slightly/moderately increased protein, slightly low or normal sugar level. A definitive diagnose can be made in cases of finding cryptococcus by CSF centrifuged smear after India ink staining.

Antigen Examination

Latex coagulation test is applied to detect polysaccharide antigen of cryptococcus neoformans capsule in the cerebrospinal fluid. Cryptococcus culture is also a recommended examination. Both are effective laboratory tests for the diagnosis of cryptococcus meningitis.

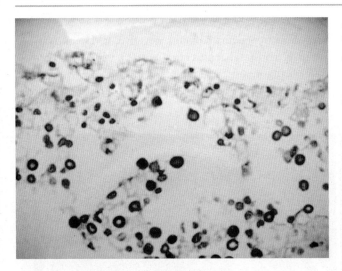

Fig. 13.15 Cryptococcus neoformans in the pathological section of brain tissue after mucous tissue red staining, with red spores, 1000 (Provided by Lang ZW)

Antibody Examination

Detecting Cryptococcus neoformans antibody in the cerebrospinal fluid can facilitate the diagnoses and understand the changes of conditions. The increase of antibody titer indicates improved conditions. Tests include agglutination test, indirect immunofluorescence test, complement fixation test, indirect hemagglutination test and enzyme immunoassay, but with low positive rates.

Diagnostic Imaging

CT scanning and MR imaging are the imaging examinations of choice. They can facilitate to define the size, shape, number, density and location of the intracerebral foci as well as their relationship with the surrounding tissues. They can also be applied to assess the therapeutic efficacy. Enhanced CT scanning and MR imaging can further define the nature of the lesions.

Imaging Demonstrations

According to pathomechanism and imaging demonstrations, Li et al. categorized intracerebral cryptococcus infection into four types, namely Type I of meningoencephalitis, Type II of cerebral infarction (colloid capsule), Type III of cerebral infarction and Type IV of granuloma [30].

Type I of Meningoencephalitis

CT demonstrations include lesions in the cerebral tentorium and cerebellar tentorium, and sometimes in cistern. There is aqueduct stenosis of the midbrain, symmetric enlargement of supratentorial ventricle, nodular or linear shaped enhancement of meninges by enhanced scanning, sometimes with no abnormal enhancement. In the acute phase, there are multiple spots of long T1 and long T2 signals in the cerebral parenchyma, with rare abnormal enhancement by enhanced scanning. In the middle and advanced stages, the commonly found hydrocephalus usually causes slight/moderate symmetric ventricular enlargement, commonly enlargement of lateral ventricle or supratentorial ventricle.

Type II of Cerebral Infarction (Colloid Capsule)

CT scanning demonstrates lesions in the deep cerebral parenchyma, with multiple symmetric spots in the basal ganglia as well as small flakes and worm bitten liked low density shadows but no edema and space occupying effects. The lesions are clearly defined and no obvious abnormal enhancement by enhanced scanning. MR imaging demonstrates multiple oval cysts, with clearly defined boundaries. T1W1 demonstrates slightly lower or homogeneous signal and T2W1 demonstrates high signals. Enhanced imaging demonstrates slight or obvious enhancement, but with no edema and space occupying effect. T2FLAIR demonstrates complex signals and DWI demonstrates partial foci to be diffuse and confined, with multilocular or monolocular cystic space occupying effect. MR imaging demonstrates long T1 long T2 signals, with obvious space occupying effect and surrounding edema. By enhanced imaging, the cystic wall is demonstrated as obviously ring shaped enhancement, with multilocular space occupying effect in typical daisy petals shaped enhancement.

Type III of Cerebral Infarction

CT scanning demonstrates multiple worm bitten liked blurry low density shadows in the bilateral basal ganglia, with no obvious edema or space occupying effect. By enhanced imaging, no obvious abnormal enhancement can be found. MR imaging demonstrates multiple spots or flaky long T1 long T2 signals mainly in bilateral basal ganglia and also in frontal, temporal and parietal lobes. By enhanced imaging, no obvious abnormal enhancement of the lesions can be found, with occasional thin wall ring liked abnormal enhancement.

Type IV of Granuloma

CT scanning demonstrates intracerebral singular or multiple large flakes of low density shadows, with edema and space occupying effect. Enhanced scanning demonstrates multilocular ring shaped abnormal enhancement. MR imaging demonstrations are not specific, with multiple intracerebral singular or multiple foci in round or oval shape. T1W1 demonstrates slightly lower or equal signal and T2W1 demonstrates equal or high signal, all being homogeneous. Enhanced scanning demonstrates nodule and ring shaped abnormal enhancement. In cases of perivascular lesions, enhanced imaging demonstrates beads string liked or grapes cluster liked demonstrations. There are also cranial damage, space occupying effects of compressed ventricles and cisterns, granuloma formation in ventricles, obstructive hydrocephalus and ring shaped enhancement of foci.

Case Study 1

A female patient aged 13 years was confirmatively diagnosed as having AIDS by CDC. When she was 2-year-old, she was admitted to a hospital to receive blood transfusion for fever and was infected by HIV. Laboratory tests show treponema pallidum negative, CMV antibody negative, acid-fast bacillus negative, total white blood cell count being 4.66/L, neutrophils being 41.5 %, lymphocytes being 45.9 % and platelets being 361/L. Her CD4 T cell count was 88/μl.

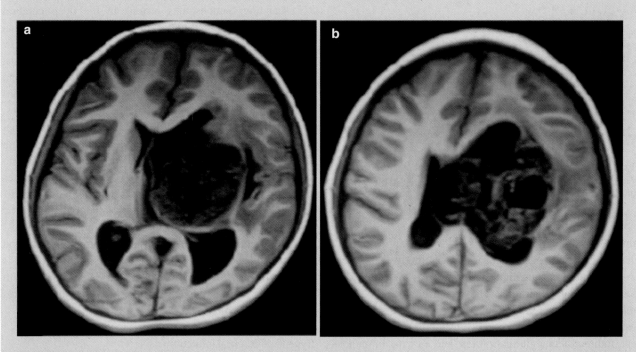

Fig. 13.16 (**a–f₁**) HIV/AIDS related intracerebral cryptococcus infection. (**a–d**) Axial MRI demonstrates multilocular cystic long T1 long T2 signals in the left basal ganglia, with surrounding brain tissue edema and obvious local space occupying effect, compressed left lateral ventricle with obvious displacement and rightward migration of the midline. (**e, f**) Sagittal MRI demonstrates multilocular cystic long T1 long T2 signals in the left basal ganglia, with surrounding brain tissue edema, obvious local space occupying effect, compressed corpus callosum migrating downwards, compressed and deformed ventricle, local gray matter edema in finger liked shape. (**g, h**) Diffusion-weighted imaging demonstrates uniform signal of cystic tissues, the surrounding edema strips in long T2 signal, with clearly defined boundaries. (**i, j**) IV-Gd-DTPA enhanced imaging demonstrates multilobular abnormal enhancement of the left basal ganglia, with obviously compressed surrounding tissues. (**k–p**) MRI reexamination after treatment for 1 month demonstrates slightly shrunk space occupying effect in the left basal ganglia, alleviated surrounding edema, and shrunk range of lesions.

There are also increased liquefied compositions in cystic tissues and increased strain. Water suppressing imaging clearly demonstrates the contour and internal structures of the cystic and parenchymal space occupying effects in the left basal ganglia. (**s–v**) Enhanced MR IV-Gd-DTPA imaging demonstrates cyctic and parenchymal obvious abnormal enhancement of changes including thin wall, multilocular and increased strain of the left basal ganglia, obviously compressed surrounding brain tissues with clearly defined boundaries. (**w–z**) MRS imaging demonstrates increased lactic acid peak. (**a₁–d₁**) Reexamination after anti-cryptococcus therapy for 3 months by enhanced MR IV-Gd-DTPA imaging demonstrates obvious shrinkage of the lesions in terms of thin wall, multilocular cystic and parenchymal space occupying effects in the left basal ganglia. There is obvious enhancement, but alleviated edema of surrounding brain tissues. (**e₁**) Gram staining demonstrates purple bacteria, with central ring shaped transparent unstained area. (**f₁**) Immunofluorescence demonstrates yellowish green transparent lesion, surrounded by ring shaped "lunar aureole"

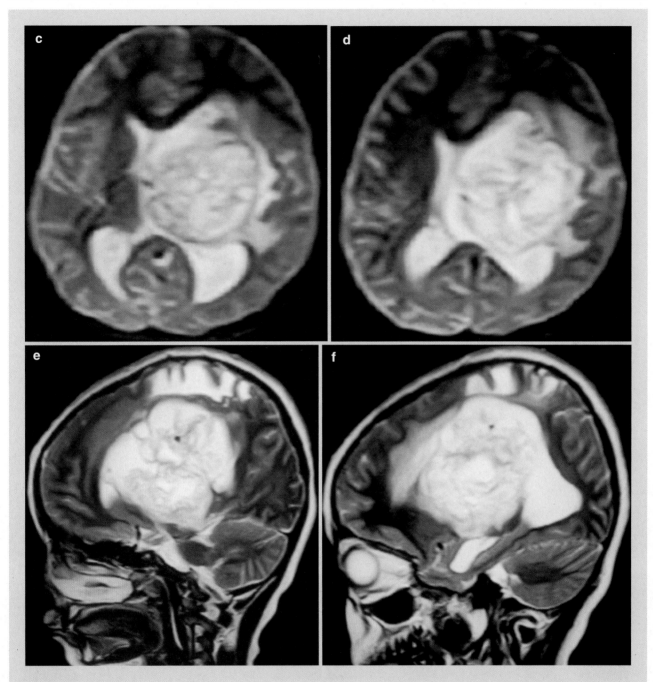

Fig. 13.16   (continued)

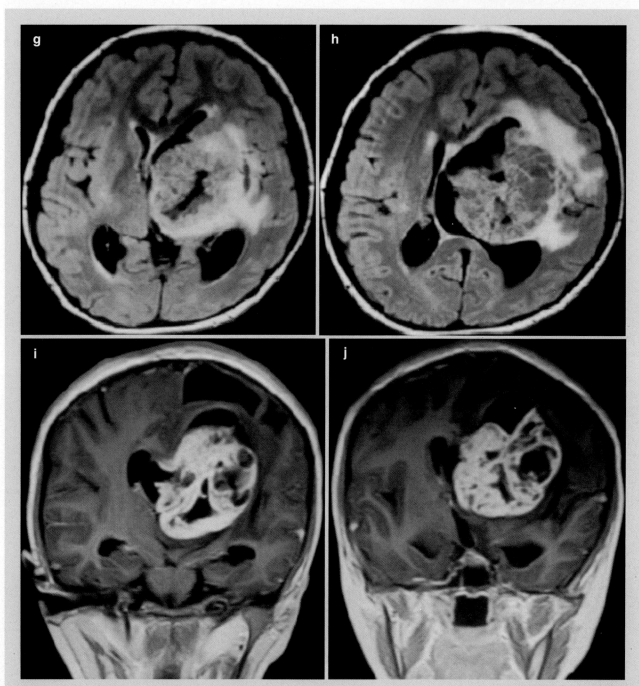

Reexamination findings after receiving antifungal therapies for 2 month

Fig. 13.16 (continued)

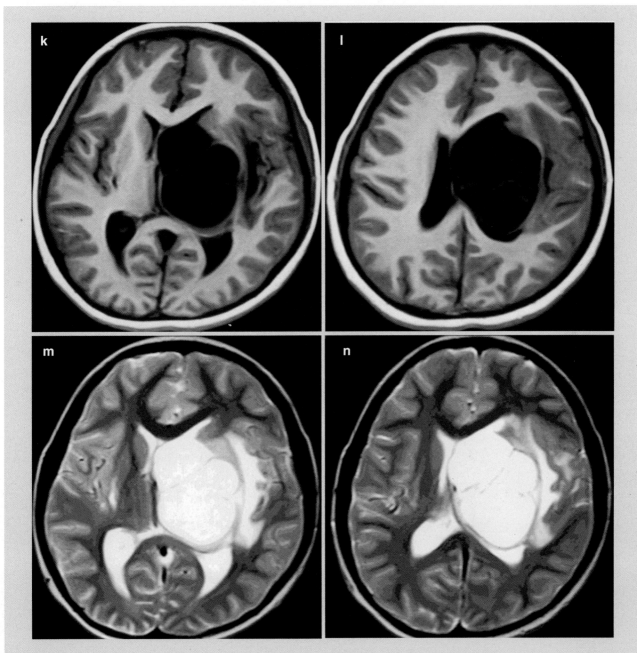

Fig. 13.16 (continued)

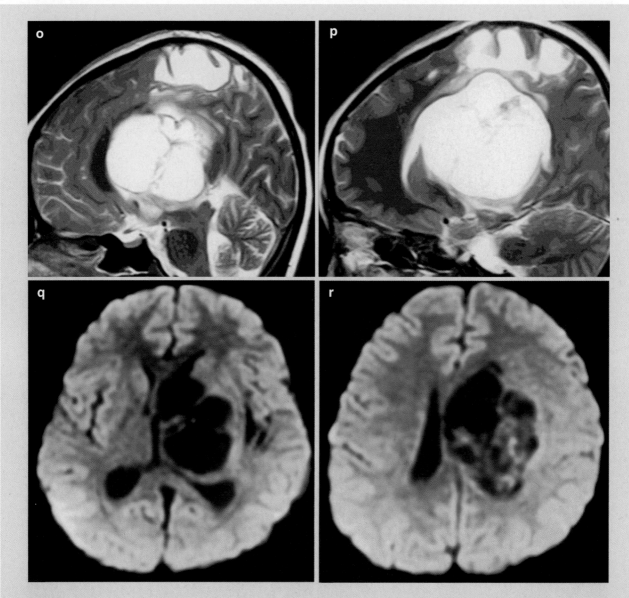

Fig. 13.16 (continued)

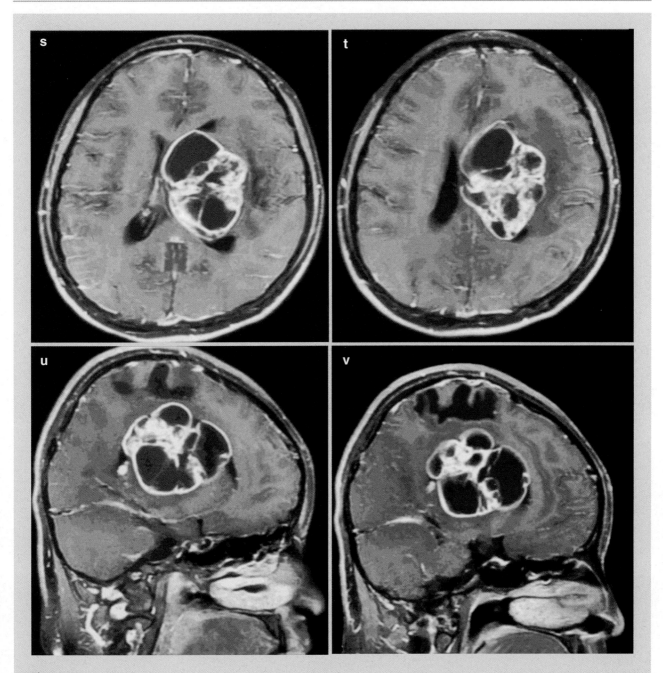

Fig. 13.16   (continued)

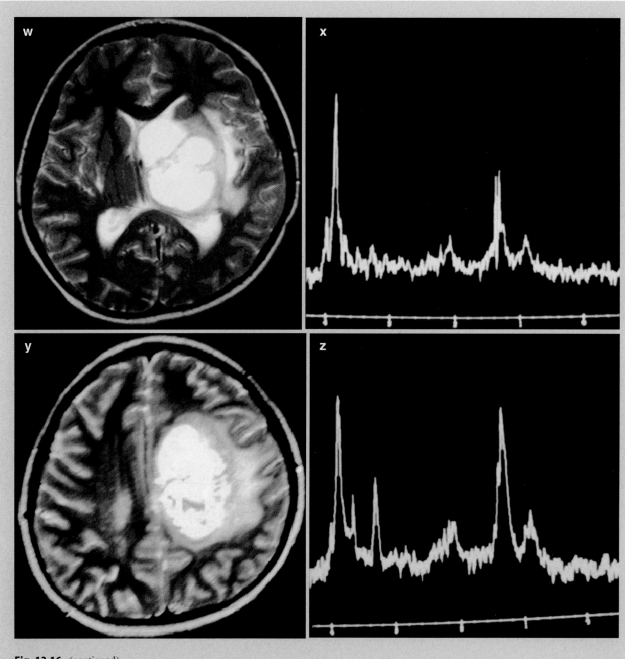

Fig. 13.16 (continued)

Reexamination findings after receiving therapies for 3 months:

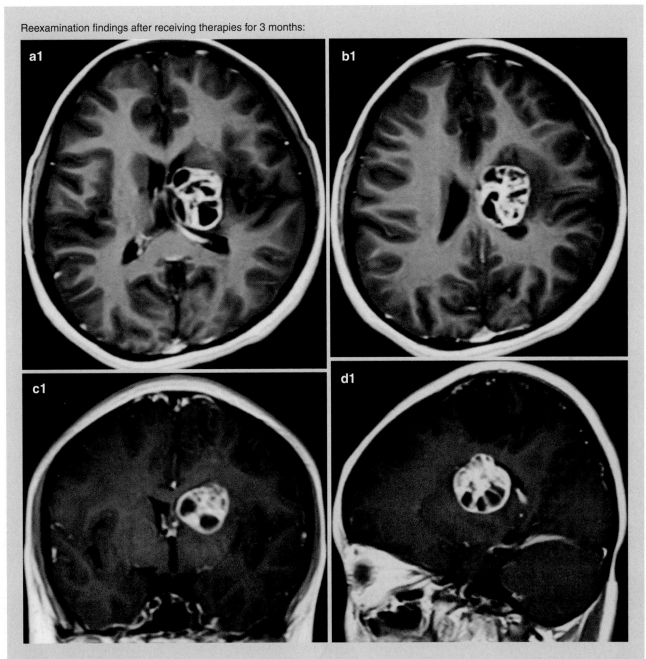

Fig. 13.16 (continued)

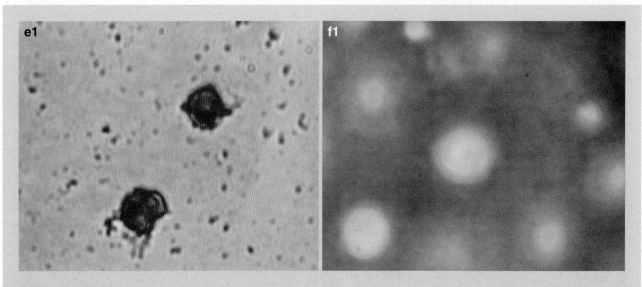

Fig. 13.16 (continued)

Case Study 2

A male patient aged 42 years was confirmatively diagnosed as having AIDS patients by CDC. He had a history of drug abuse and complained of intermittent headache, dizziness, nausea and vomiting for over 2 months. His CD4 T cell count was 67/μl.

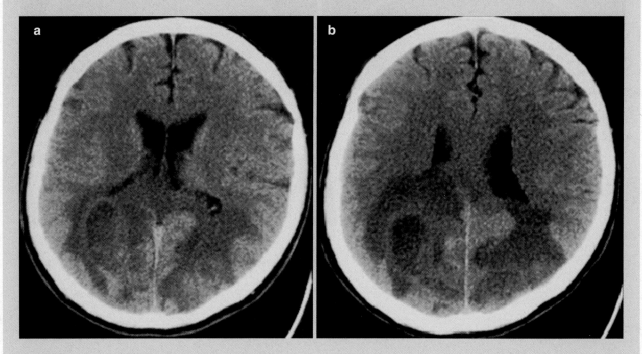

Fig. 13.17 (a–m) HIV/AIDS related intracerebral cryptococcus infection. (a, b) Plain CT scanning demonstrates cystic low density foci in bilateral occipital lobes, with clearly defined boundaries and surrounding large flakes of edema strips; compressed posterior horn of the bilateral lateral ventricle that migrates upwards in deformity. (c–f) Axial MR T1W1 imaging demonstrates multiple round liked long T1 long T2 signals in the bilateral occipital lobe, with obvious space occupying effect and clearly defined boundaries; surrounding strips of edema in finger liked long T1 and long T2 signals. (g–l) Axial, sagittal and coronal enhanced MR IV-Gd-DTPA imaging demonstrates multiple round liked thin-wall cystic foci in the occipital lobe, with ring shaped enhancement. The wall is homogeneous in thickness and is smooth, with some cystic wall fused. (m) Ink staining demonstrates round wheel liked cryptococcus

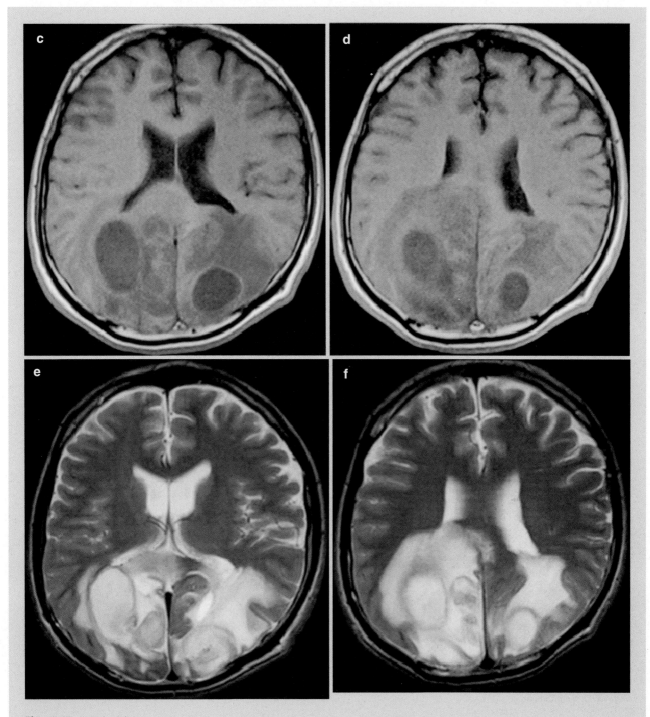

Fig. 13.17 (continued)

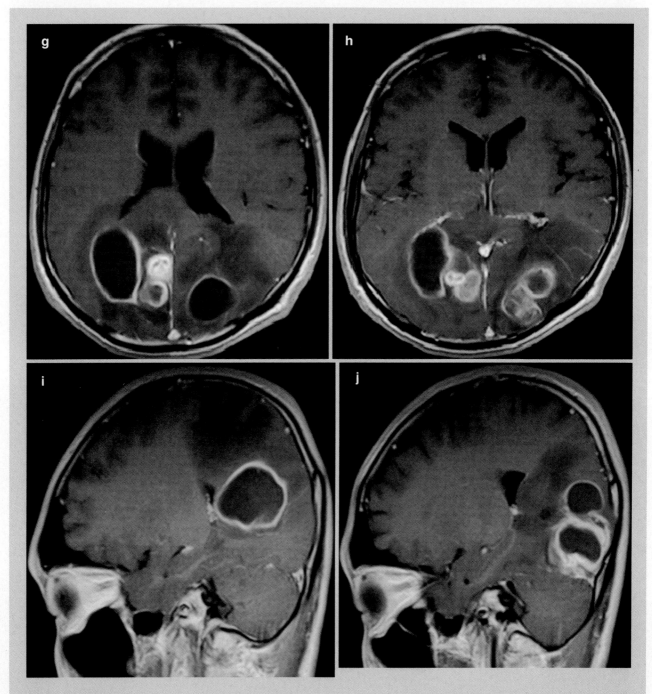

Fig. 13.17 (continued)

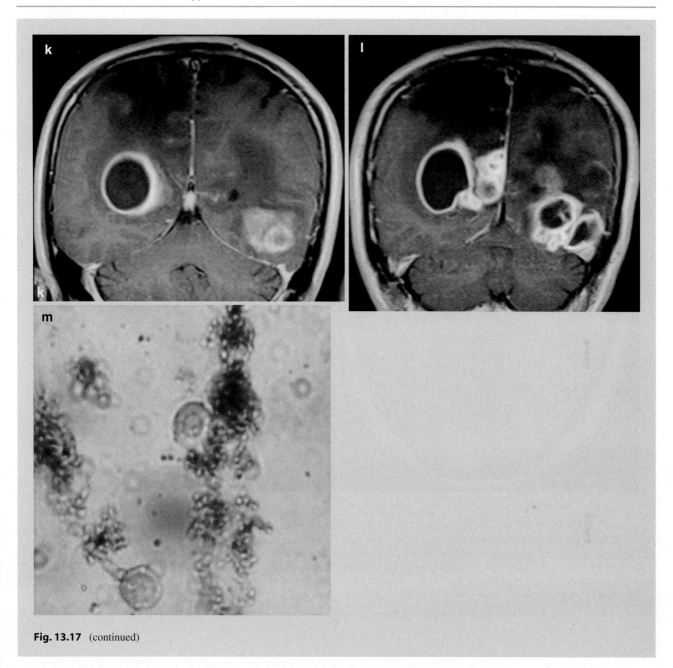

Fig. 13.17   (continued)

Case Study 3

A female patient aged 38 years was confirmatively diagnosed as having AIDS by CDC. She was infected via sexual behaviors and complained of intermittent headache, decreased memory, blurry vision, dizziness, nausea, vomiting and irritation for over 1 month. Her CD4 T cell count was 47/μl.

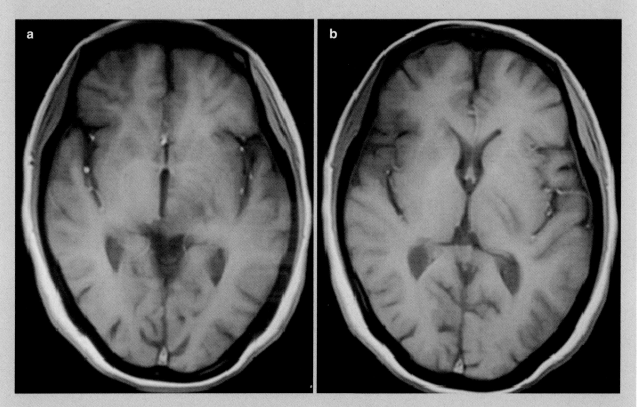

Fig. 13.18 (a–l) HIV/AIDS related intracerebral cryptococcus infection. (**a, b**) MR T1WI demonstrates patchy slightly long T1 signal in the left brachium pontis, bilateral basal ganglia and hippocampal gyrus of the left temporal lobe. (**c, d**) MR T2WI demonstrates patchy long T2 signal in the bilateral basal ganglia, the left brachium pontis, and hippocampal gyrus of the left temporal lobe, with blurry boundaries. (**e, f**) Diffusion-weighted imaging demonstrates patchy foci in high signals in the left brachium pontis, bilateral basal ganglia, and hippocampal gyrus of the left temporal lobe. (**g–l**) Axial, sagittal and coronal enhanced MR IV-Gd-DTPA imaging demonstrate spots liked abnormal enhancement in bilateral basal ganglia, ring shaped enhancement of the left brachium pontis, and central non-enhanced spots

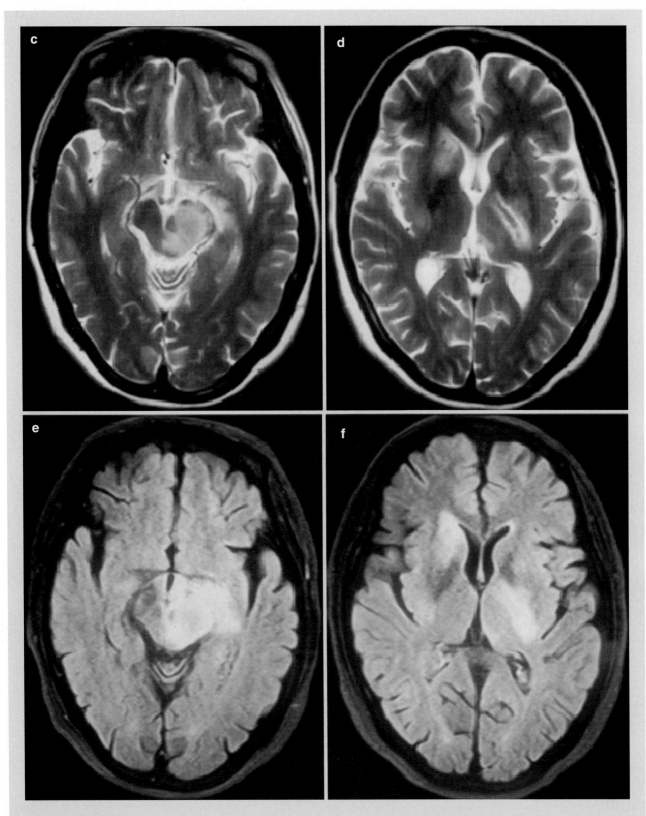

Fig. 13.18   (continued)

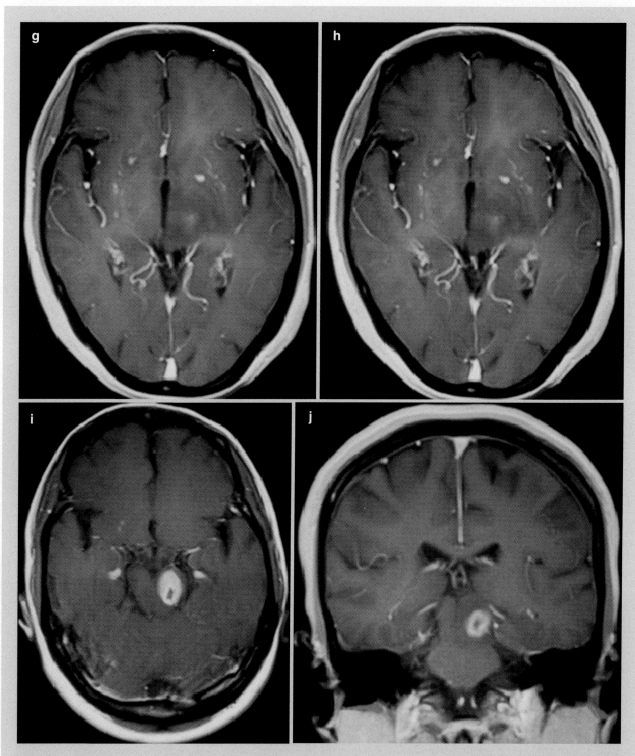

Fig. 13.18 (continued)

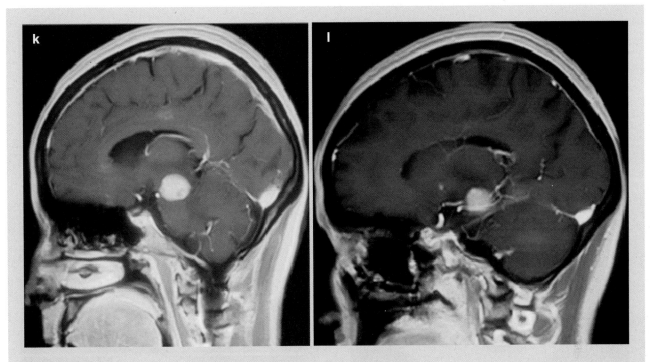

Fig. 13.18   (continued)

Case Study 4

A male patient aged 35 years was confirmatively diagnosed as having AIDS by CDC. He had a long history of drug abuse and complained of intermittent headache, dizziness and irritation for over 2 months. His CD4 T cell count was 21/μl.

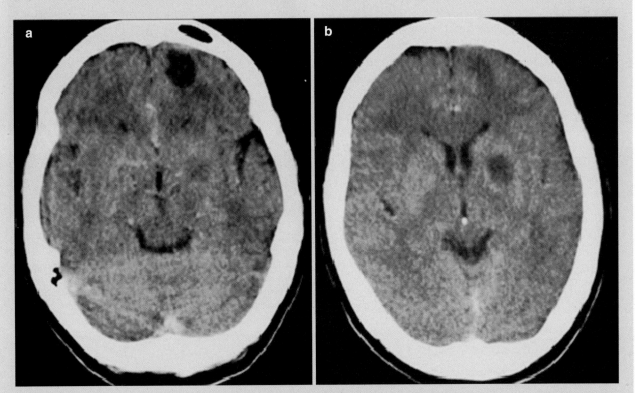

Fig. 13.19   (a–c) HIV/AIDS related intracerebral cryptococcus infection. Plain CT scanning demonstrates flaky low density area in the bilateral frontal lobe and in the left basal ganglia, with no obvious edema and space occupying effect

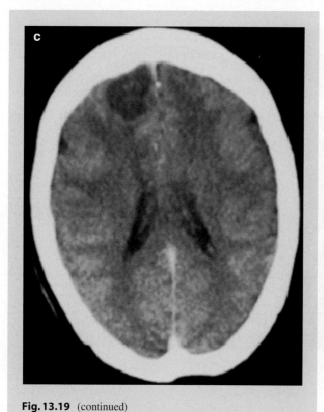

Fig. 13.19 (continued)

Case Study 5

A female patient aged 38 years was confirmatively diagnosed as having AIDS by CDC. She had a history of paid blood donation in the year of 1995. In Apr. 2006, she complained of intermittent fever, diarrhea, weight loss, disturbance of consciousness and left extremities paralysis, urine retention and difficulty breathing. In May, 2005, she was defined as HIV carrier, with obviously increased intracranial pressure. Her CD4 T cell count was 67/μl. In Jul. 2007, she gave up therapies, followed by occurrence of death.

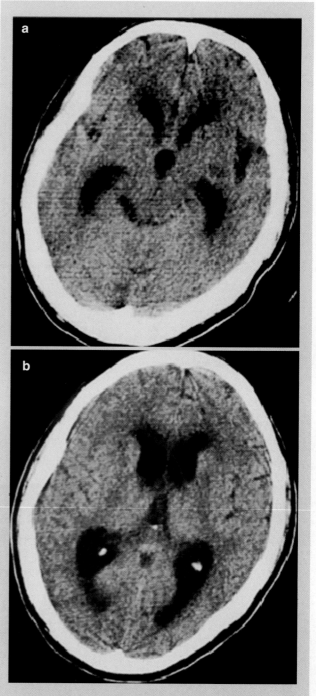

Fig. 13.20 (a–c) HIV/AIDS related intracerebral cryptococcus infection. (a, b) Plain CT scanning demonstrates flaky low density area in the left basal ganglia with unclearly defined boundary, no obvious edema and space occupying effect; symmetric enlargement of the supratentorial ventricles. (c) Ink staining of ESF smear demonstrates cryptococcus thallus (pointed by a *black arrow*)

Fig. 13.20 (continued)

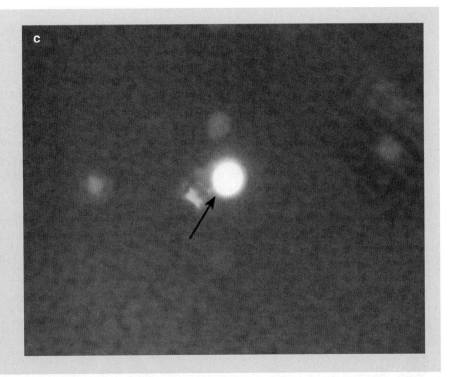

Case Study 6

A male patient aged 31 years was confirmatively diagnosed as having AIDS by CDC. He had a long history of drug abuse and sustained obviously increased intracranial pressure and disturbance of consciousness for 2 weeks. His CD4 T cell count was 17/μl.

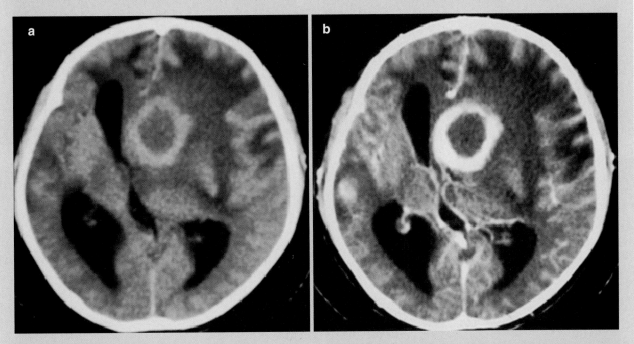

Fig. 13.21 (**a**, **b**) HIV/AIDS related intracerebral cryptococcus infection. Enhanced CT scanning demonstrates obviously abnormal enhancement of ring shaped thick wall in the left basal ganglia, with no central enhancement; surrounding large flaky low density area in the surrounding, with unclearly defined boundary, obvious edema and obvious space occupying effect in the brain tissue; rightward migration of the brain midline, compressed and occluded frontal angle of the left lateral ventricle; obviously abnormal flaky enhancement in the right temporal lobe, with surrounding low density edema strip

Case Study 7

A male patient aged 47 years was confirmatively diagnosed as having AIDS by CDC. He was diagnosed as having cryptococcus encephalitis. He had a long history of drug abuse and complained of intermittent headache, dizziness and irritation for 2 months. Her CD4 T cell count was 21/μl.

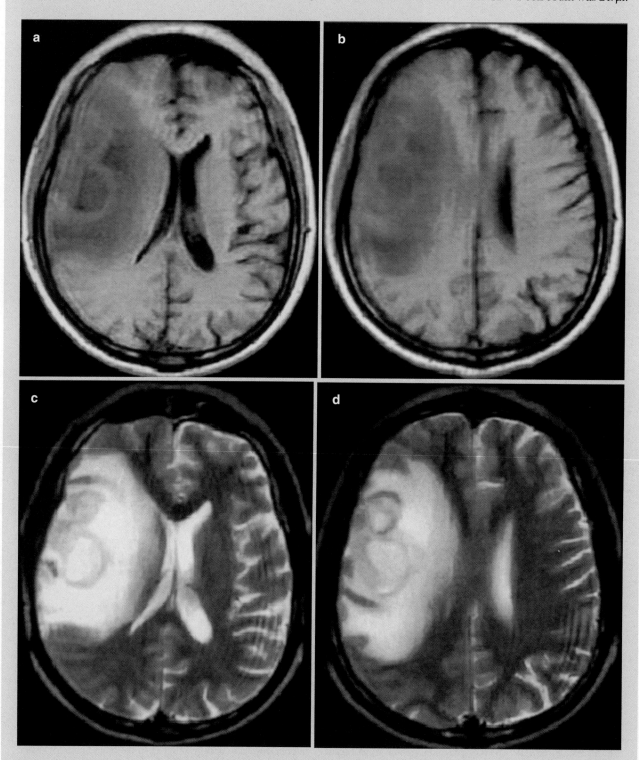

Fig. 13.22 (a–h) HIV/AIDS related intracerebral cryptococcus infection. (a–e) Axial and sagittal MR imaging demonstrate large flaky long T1 long T2 signal in the right temporal lobe, obvious space occupying effect and edema, narrowed right lateral ventricle due to compression. (f–h) It is demonstrated to have obviously abnormal enhancement of multilocular, ring shaped and thick wall of the right temporal lobe in petal shape; surrounding edema stripes in low signaling, obvious space occupying effect and narrowed right ventricle due to compression

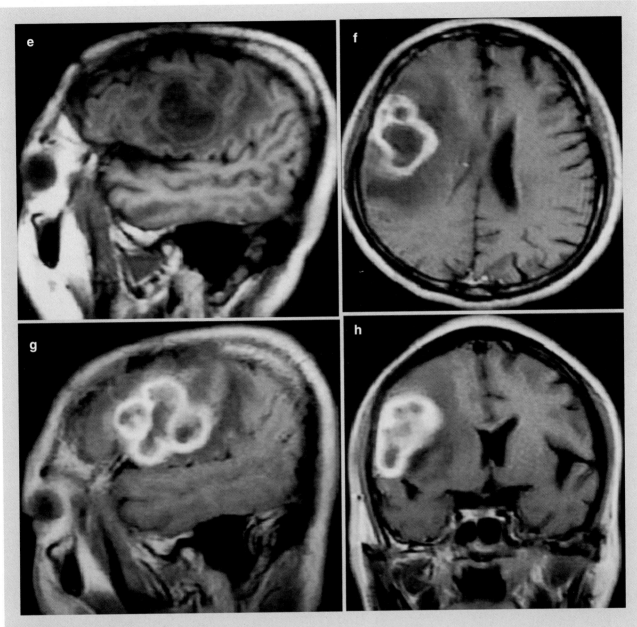

Fig. 13.22 (continued)

Case Study 8

A male patient aged 28 years was confirmatively diagnosed as having AIDS by CDC. He had a history of extramarital affairs and had chief complaints of recurrent headaches for more than 4 months. He was found to have blepharoptosis of the right eye, with slightly worse vision than the left eye. His CD4 T cell count was 21/μl.

History of present illness: Approximately 4 months ago, the patient suffered from episodic headaches of no known reasons, especially severe in bilateral temporal sides. The pain is obvious at night, with no effective way for alleviation. He also had decreased vision of the right eye and occasional vomiting, commonly after meals.

By laboratory tests, he was found to have quantitative protein of cerebrospinal fluid by lumbar puncture 400 mg/L, glucose 3.13 mmol/L, chloride 128 mmol/L, decreased lactate dehydrogenase to 55.7U/L; decreased monocytes to 0.7 %. The cerebrospinal fluid was light yellow in color, which was transparent, with no coagulation and Pandy's test positive. His WBC was 0.1×10^9/L; decreased segmented cell count to 0.3. In Jan. 2009, his headache worsened, with numb fingers and inconvenience in unilateral extremities. The reexamination found intracranial space occupying effect by CT scanning and was hospitalized. One day later, death occurred.

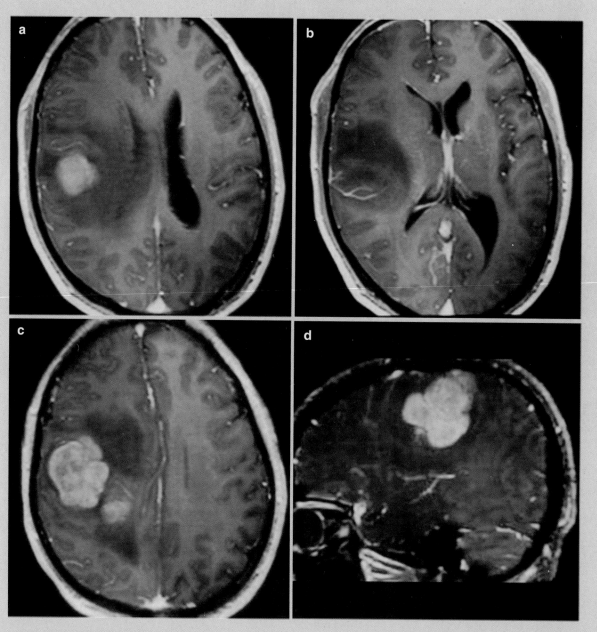

Fig. 13.23 (**a–d**) HIV/AIDS related intracerebral cryptococcus infection. (**a**, **b**) Axial and sagittal enhanced IV-Gd-DTPA MR imaging demonstrates obvious space occupying effect and edema, narrowed right lateral ventricle due to compression. (**c, d**) Obviously abnormal enhancement of multilocular, ring shaped and thick wall in the right temporal lobe in petal shape; surrounding low signaling strip of edema, obvious space occupying effect; narrowed right lateral ventricle due to compression

Case Study 9

A female patient aged 35 years was confirmatively diagnosed as having AIDS by CDC. She had a history of intravenous drug abuse, recipient of blood transfusion and blood products. She was found HIV antibody positive for 10 years and complained of headache for 15 days. She was admitted to hospital on Aug. 31st, 2010. About 10 years ago, the patient was found HIV antibody positive in the physical examination, with her CD4 T cell count being 300/μl and viral load of 40,000 copies/ml, untreated. In the year of 2006, she paid clinical visit due to herpes zoster, with a CD4 T cell count of 159/μl, and received antiviral therapy. During the medication, she subjectively felt weak and poor appetite, with an increased CD4 T cell count of 370/μl. Then she discontinued the medication by herself for half a year, and began the previous antiviral therapy. In Oct. 2007, her CD4 T cell count was 94/μl and she discontinued the medication hereafter. In Aug. 2009, she was admitted to hospital again and the cytomegalovirus test showed IgM positive, with suspected diagnosis of cytomegalovirus retinitis. But she refused to receive further treatment. The CD4 T cell count was 74/μl, but with no antiviral treatment. In Apr. 2010, she was hospitalized for the third time for the diagnosis of AIDS, TB, C type of hepatitis and cirrhosis, with a CD4 T cell count of 57/μl. After treatment of tuberculosis, she started to receive antiviral therapy, but failed to regularly intake the antiviral drugs. During her third time hospitalization, she complained of headache, followed by nausea and non-ejective vomiting of gastric contents. The headache could be slightly relieved by taking pain killer by herself. By laboratory tests, her CD4 T cell count 82/μl, blood CMV-IgM antibody positive, CMV-DNA quantification less than 500 copies/ml. By CSF routine test after lumbar puncture, CSF in color of light yellow, transparent, Pandy's test positive, total cell count 0.006E + 9/L, WBC 0.003E + 9/L, CSF-TP 1.4 g/L, Glu 4.66 mmol/L, C 1125.3 mmol/L; CSF-Cryptococcus neoformans antigen negative, both CSF-CMV and EBV antibodies negative; conventional bacteria smear, acid fast staining and ink staining negative. Cranial CT scanning on Sep. 2, 2010 demonstrated round liked slightly lower density foci in the right temporal lobe and right occipital lobe, with clearly defined boundaries in diameters of 18 and 19 mm respectively; surrounding finger liked edema in the whiter matter; compressed right lateral ventricle, the third ventricle and the midbrain; leftward migration of the midline. Enhanced scanning demonstrates ring shaped enhancement of the foci and slight enhancement of the meninges. After symptomatic treatment to reduce intracranial pressure and protect the liver, the headache was comparatively relieved. Reexamination on Sep. 13, 2010 by cranial CT scanning demonstrates round liked low density shadows in the right temporal lobe and the right occipital lobe in size of approximately 13×20 mm, with an average CT value of 24 HU; obvious surrounding edema, leftward migration of the midline. Enhanced CT scanning demonstrates thin wall enhancement of the space occupying boundary, with no central enhancement. The patient was suspectively diagnosed as intracerebral cryptococcus infection. After an experimental anti-toxoplasmic treatment for 2 weeks, the diagnostic imaging demonstrated no improvement of the conditions. In combination to the CT scanning demonstrations, the cerebral abscesses were suspected to be related to cryptococcus infection. Fluconazole antifungal therapy was then added into the treatment. The reexamination by CT scanning later demonstrated shrinkage of the foci.

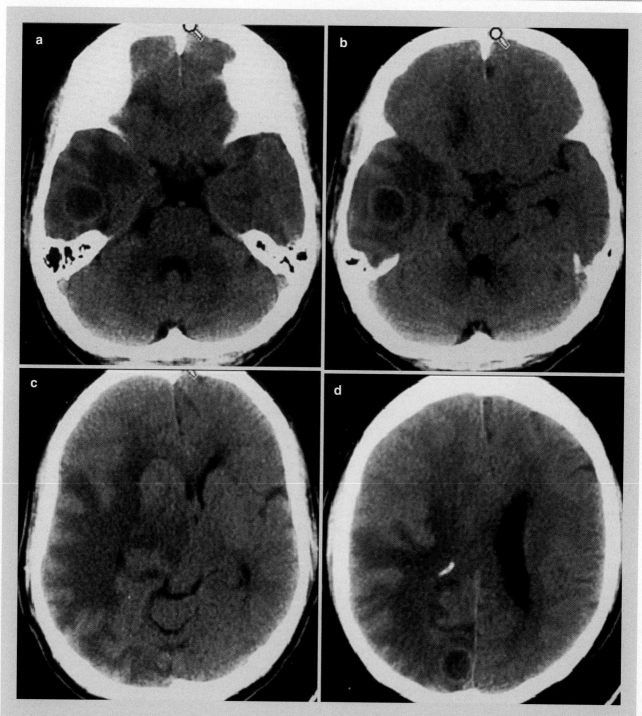

Fig. 13.24 (**a–d**) CT plain scanning demonstrates large flaky low density shadows with ring shaped lower density shadows in the right temporal horn; large flaky low density shadows in the temporal and parietal lobes with obvious space occupying effect; ring shaped low density shadows in the right occipital lobe. (**e–h**) Enhanced CT scanning demonstrates slightly abnormal enhancement of ring shaped and thin wall liked in the right temporal lobe and the right occipital lobe, with no central enhancement; surrounding large flakes of low density area with blurry boundary, obvious edema of brain tissues and obvious space occupying effect; leftward migration of the brain midline; compressed and occluded right lateral ventricle. (**a–m**) HIV/AIDS related intracerebral cryptococcus infection. (**i–k**) CT scanning demonstrates flaky low density shadows in the right temporal horn with ring shaped lower density shadows; flaky low density shadows in the temporal and parietal lobes, with alleviated space occupying effect compared to previous imaging findings; ring shaped lower density shadows in the right occipital lobe. (**l, m**) Enhanced CT scanning demonstrates slightly abnormal enhancement of ring shaped and thin wall liked in the right temporal lobe and the right occipital lobe, with no central enhancement; surrounding large flaky low density area; alleviated edema of brain tissues and alleviated space occupying effect compared to the previous imaging findings; less compressed and greatly improved conditions of the right lateral ventricle compared to the previous imaging findings

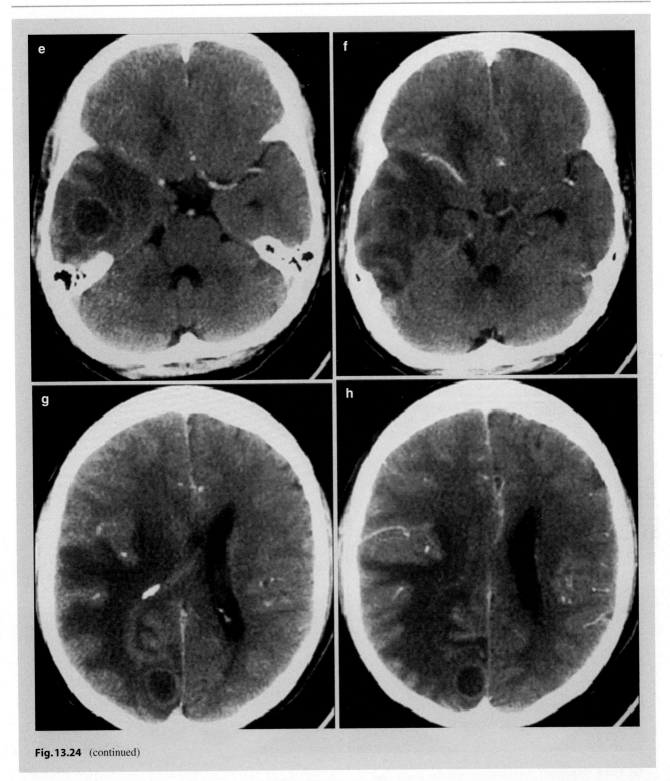

Fig. 13.24 (continued)

Reexamination findings after treatment:

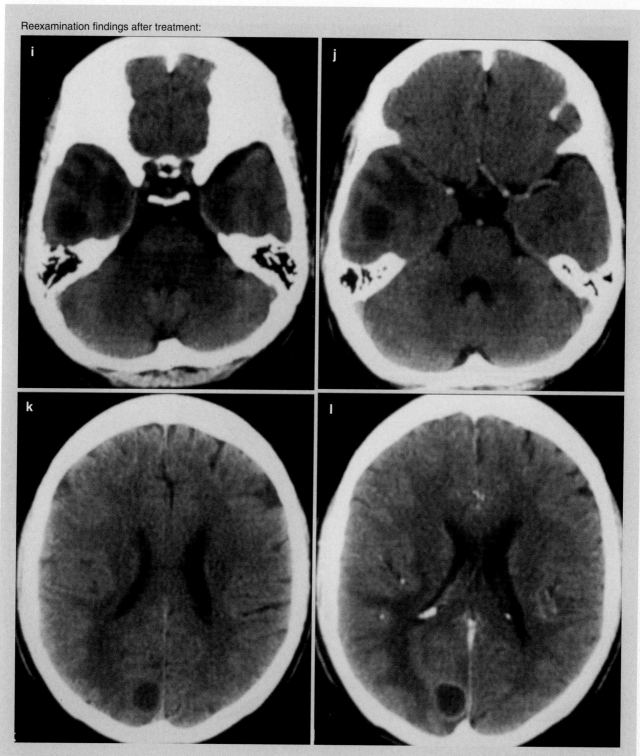

Fig. 13.24   (continued)

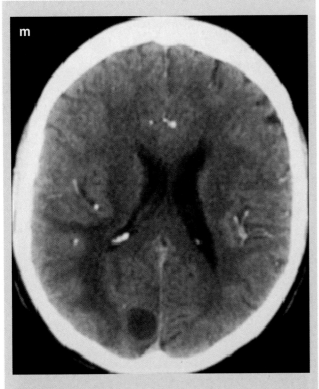

Fig. 13.24 (continued)

Case Study 10

A female patient aged 31 years was confirmatively diagnosed as having AIDS by CDC. She complained of headache for 20 days and had a history of HIV antibody positive for 8 years. Her CD4 T cell count was 12/μl.

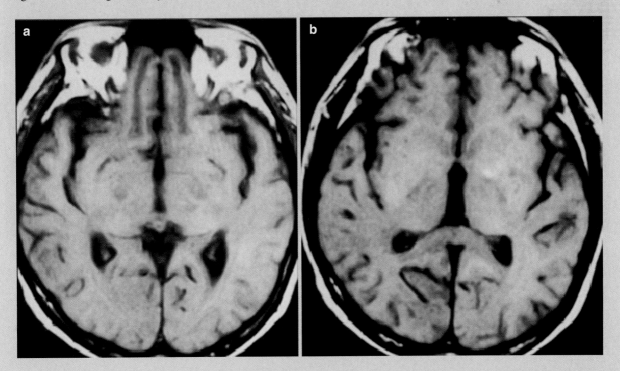

Fig. 13.25 (**a–h**) HIV/AIDS related intracerebral cryptococcus infection. (**a–e**) Axial MR imaging demonstrates multiple spots and flaky long T1 long T2 signals in bilateral brain in different sizes with no edema and no space occupying effect; deepened and widened sulcus and enlarged sylvian cistern. (**f–h**) It is demonstrated to have multiple nodular abnormal enhancement of different sizes in the cerebral parenchyma

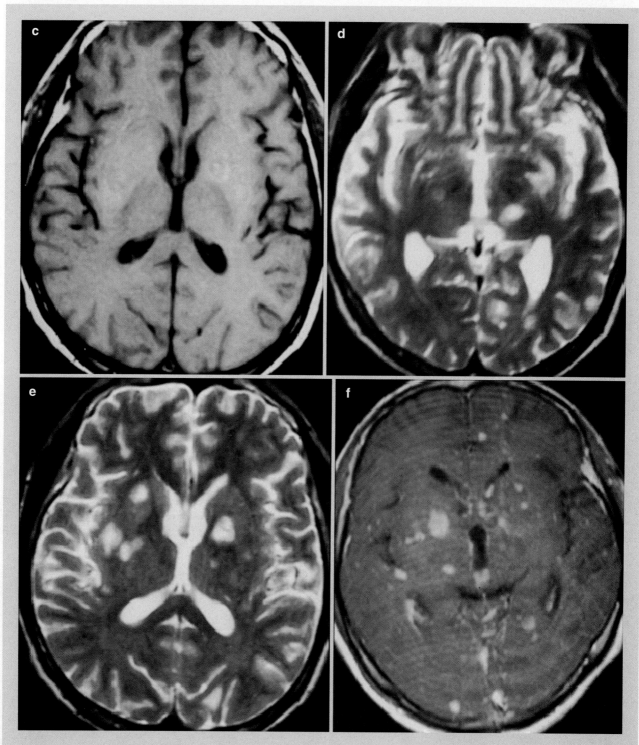

Fig. 13.25 (continued)

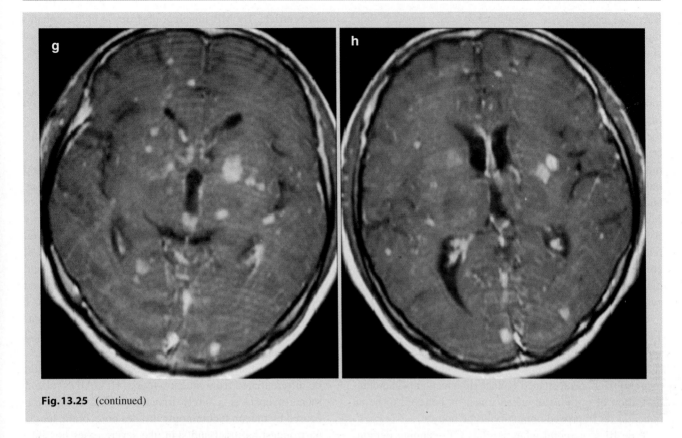

Fig. 13.25 (continued)

Criteria for the Diagnosis

1. AIDS patient confirmatively diagnosed by CDC, with a long history of applying large doses of antibiotics, immunosuppressive drugs and immunocompromised conditions, such as AIDS, lymphoma, leukemia, organ transplantation.
2. Subacute or chronic progressive headache, meningeal irritation, increased quantitative protein, decreased chloride and decreased glucose in cerebrospinal fluid.
3. India ink staining and culture of cerebrospinal fluid for qualitatively defining of the pathogen and finding of cryptococcus neoformans. Serum cryptococcus polysaccharide antigen latex coagulation test has both high sensitivity and specificity in the diagnosis of cryptococcus neoformans infection. Cases with serum cryptococcus antigen titer being higher than 1:8 can be suspectively diagnosed as having cryptococcus infection. The culture finding of cryptococcus in tissues of any body parts is significant.
4. CT scanning and MR imaging demonstrations: According to categorization by Chen et al. [30], HIV/AIDS related intracerebral cryptococcus infection can be divided into 4 types, namely Type I of meningoencephalitis, Type II of cerebral infarction (colloid capsule), Type III of cerebral infarction and Type IV of granuloma.

Type I meningoencephalitis has CT scanning demonstrations of common lesions in the cerebral tentorium and cerebellar tentorium and rarely found lesions in the cistern; midbrain aqueductal stenosis and symmetric enlargement of supratentorial ventricles. It is possibly due to cerebrospinal fluid circulation disorder caused by subarachnoid space inflammatory adhesion during the chronic phase. There is sometimes no enhancement of meninges, primarily due to compromised immunity and the lack of immune mediated inflammatory responses. There are also thickened strips of meninges in linear or strip liked abnormal enhancement by enhanced scanning, sometimes no enhancement and symmetric enlargement of supratentorial ventricle. Demonstrations of diffusive encephalitis in the acute phase include brain edema, multiple patchy long T1 and long T2 signals in cerebral parenchyma. Enhanced CT scanning rarely demonstrates abnormal enhancement but hydrocephalus induced slight/moderate symmetric ventricular enlargement in the middle and advanced stages, with commonly enlarged lateral ventricles and supratentorial ventricles.

Type II of cerebral infarction (colloid capsule) has CT scanning demonstrations of commonly found lesions in deep cerebral parenchyma, multiple symmetric spots, small flaky or worm bitten liked low density shadows in the basal ganglia, no edema and no space occupying effect, and clearly defined boundary. Enhanced scanning demonstrates no obvious abnormal enhancement. MR imaging demonstrates multiple oval shaped cysts with clearly defined boundaries.

Because cryptococcus neoformans can produce acid mucopolysaccharides materials to shorten the duration of T1 signaling, MR T1W1 imaging demonstrates slightly lower or uniform signal, while T2W1 demonstrates high signal. Enhanced imaging demonstrates slight or obvious enhancement, with no obvious edema or space occupying effect. Signals by T2FLAIR are complex, with high signals due to the relatively more mucopolysaccharides materials secreted by focal cryptococcus. In cases with similar percentage of mucopolysaccharides and water content, the foci are demonstrated in equal signal. Foci with high signaling margin and central low signaling are due to the increased protein caused by surrounding inflammatory responses of the foci. By DWI, some foci are diffuse and confined, which may be related to the increase of mucopolysaccharides content in the colloid pseudocapsules. With the progression of the illness, multiple small cystic foci fuse into each other to form large cystic focus, with multilocular or monolocular cystic occupying space effect. MR imaging demonstrates multiple long T1 long T2 signal, with obvious space occupying effect and surrounding edema. Enhanced scanning demonstrates ring shaped obvious enhancement, obvious enhancement of the foci and daisy petal shaped typical enhancement. The demonstration of cystic wall enhancement is believed to be an indicator for improved immunity of the body.

Type III of cerebral infarction has CT scanning demonstrations of multiple worm bitten liked blurry low density shadows in the bilateral basal ganglia, with no edema and space occupying effect. Enhanced scanning demonstrates no obviously abnormal enhancement. MR imaging demonstrates multiple spots or flaky long T1 long T2 signal mainly in bilateral basal ganglia and also in frontal, temporal and parietal lobes. Enhanced imaging demonstrates no obvious abnormal enhancement of the foci, occasionally with thin wall and ring shaped abnormal enhancement.

Type IV of granuloma has CT scanning demonstrations of intracerebral singular or multiple large flaky low density shadows, with edema and space occupying effect. Enhanced scanning demonstrates multilocular ring shaped abnormal enhancement. MR imaging demonstrations are lack of specificity, with intracerebral singular or multiple round or oval shaped foci, with slightly lower or equal signaling by T1WI and equal or higher signaling by T2WI. The signaling is heterogeneous. Enhanced MR imaging demonstrates nodular and ring shaped abnormal enhancement. In cases with perivascular foci, enhanced imaging demonstrates beads string sign or grapes cluster sign. In cases with brain surface foci, the cranium can be defective. Cases with large foci may have accompanying space occupying effects like compressed ventricle or cistern. In cases with invasion of cryptoccocus along ependyma, granuloma may occur in the brain ventricle. By MR imaging, obstructive hydrocephalus and ring shaped enhanced foci are revealed, with fusion of the foci and surrounding edema.

Differential Diagnosis
1. HIV/AIDS related cerebral cryptococcus infection should be differentiated from tuberculous meningitis. The two conditions are extremely similar and should be differentiated based on pathogenic evidence.
2. HIV/AIDS related cerebral cryptococcus infection should be differentiated from cerebral aspergillosis infection. HIV/AIDS related cerebral aspergillosis is a group of chronic fungal diseases caused by aspergillus, commonly with acute onset. The common symptoms include fever, headache, nausea, vomiting and epileptic seizure as well as possible occurrence of hemiplegia, aphasia, ataxia and visual field defects. In severe cases, there may be increased cerebral pressure, leading to fatal cerebral herniation. CT scanning or MR imaging commonly demonstrates singular or multiple brain abscesses, cerebral infarction and hemorrhagic infarction.
3. HIV/AIDS related cerebral cryptococcus infection should be differentiated from mucormycosis. HIV/AIDS related mucormycosis is a rarely found fatal fungal infection caused by mucor. It commonly invades nose, brain, lungs, gastrointestinal tract and skin, the severe cases possibly with general spreading of mucor via blood flow. The most commonly condition is cerebral mucormycosis. The infection initially occurs in nasal turbinate, paranasal sinuses or pharyngeal tissues to cause cellulitis, followed by invasion of orbit, brain, meninges. It might also invade local blood vessels, spreading from the internal carotid to the brain and rapidly leading to encephalitis and meningitis. CT scanning or MR imaging demonstrates brain abscess, cerebral infarction, sinus turbidity, bone destruction and occasional occurrence of cerebral hemorrhage.

Discussion
HIV/AIDS related cerebral cryptococcus infection is the most common fungal infection of the central nervous system in patients with HIV/AIDS, and ranks the second in occurrence of HIV/AIDS related opportunity infections, with an incidence rate of 5–7 %. It is mostly secondary infection of the central nervous system followed by pulmonary infection. Since the cerebrospinal fluid is lack of antibody and complement system, and its dopamine content encourages the growth of cryptococcus neoformans. Therefore, the cryptococcus neoformans in CSF has high affinity with the central nervous system. In spite of many reports on HIV/AIDS related cerebral cryptococcus neoformans infection by domestic and international scholars, they failed to categorize

the diverse MRI demonstrations of the illness. Chen et al. [30] categorized the illness into four types based on its MR imaging and pathomechanism, namely type I of meningoencephalitis, type II of cerebral infarction (colloid capsule), Type III of cerebral infarction and type IV of granuloma. With the long term progression of cerebral cryptococcus neoformans infection, multiple pathogenic infections may occur to complicate the pathological condition, such as toxoplasmosis encephalitis and cytomegalovirus encephalitis. The resulted complex MR imaging demonstrations should be sufficiently understood in the diagnosis.

13.3.1.2 HIV/AIDS Related Cerebral Aspergillosis Infection

Pathogens and Pathogenesis

Aspergillus spores are tiny and may gain its access to the human body via respiration. They adhere to the host tissue cells via mediation of fibrin, laminin and fibrinogen to germinate hyphae and thus cause the disease. Aspergillus has antigen fragments with cytotoxicity, which can specifically bind to IgG and IgE in patients with allergic pulmonary aspergillosis to cause disease via its cytotoxicity and allergic reaction. Other glycoprotein antigens with elastase liked activities might also play a role in the pathogenesis of the disease. The defense ability of hosts mainly depends on effector cell. Mononuclear cells and lung macrophages can kill the conidia that invade the respiratory tract. Lymphocytes can kill inflated spores and hyphae. Especially the neutrophils can destroy the hyphae via the oxidizing and non-oxidizing mechanisms. Cytokines, such as tumor necrosis factor, interleukin, interferon, human granulocyte/macrophage colony stimulating factors participate in this process. They activate macrophages and neutrophils to enhance their ability to migrate and cluster and to promote the release of sterilizing active substances, such as lysosomal enzymes and oxygen free radicals and nitric free radicals. Therefore, the release of phagocytic NADPH oxidase can be increased, and specific receptor expression of mononuclear cell can be up-regulated to further eliminate of the infection. Hosts with suppressed and compromised immunity, especially hosts with insufficient neutrophils, are vulnerable to aspergillus infection.

Pathophysiologic Basis

The histopathology organization of HIV/AIDS related invasive aspergillosis generally manifested as mixed, purulent and necrotic inflammatory responses. Necrosis is caused by the vascular embolization and aspergillus toxin effect. Chronic invasive pulmonary aspergillosis has histopathological manifestations of confined granuloma. The pathological findings include colorless and separated hyphae of aspergillus directing in one direction or with radiating growth from the center to the surrounding, like sunshine, which is a characteristic finding. Giant cells, neutrophils and eosinophils might also show fibrosis, with gradual aggravation. The isolated lesion is surrounded by granulomatous reaction, with contents of Langhans giant cells similar to tuberculosis. There may be central necrosis of granuloma, with rare occurrence of cavities due to calcification or liquefaction in patients with HIV/AIDS. Almost all cases of aspergillosis have primary lesion in the lungs. Aspergillus hypha commonly invades vascular vessels, and might invade the vascular wall to form embolism. Involvement of major blood vessels may cause bleeding, infarction and necrosis.

Examinations and Their Selection

1. Findings of aspergillus hyphae by biopsy or cerebrospinal fluid test.
2. CT scanning and MR imaging are the diagnostic imaging of choice, which can facilitate to define the size, shape and location of the foci and to assess the therapeutic efficacy.

Clinical Symptoms and Signs

Clinical symptoms include gradually aggravated headache, mental problem and irritation. In severe cases, there are psychiatric and neurological symptoms like conscious disturbance of different degrees as well as increased intracranial pressure.

Case History and Clinical Manifestations

Case Study 1

A male patient aged 33 years was confirmatively diagnosed as having AIDS by CDC. He was detected to be HIV antibody positive 9 years ago and complained of paroxysmal spasm of hands and feet with accompanying transient loss of consciousness and headache for over 1 month. His CD4 T cell count was 24/μl.

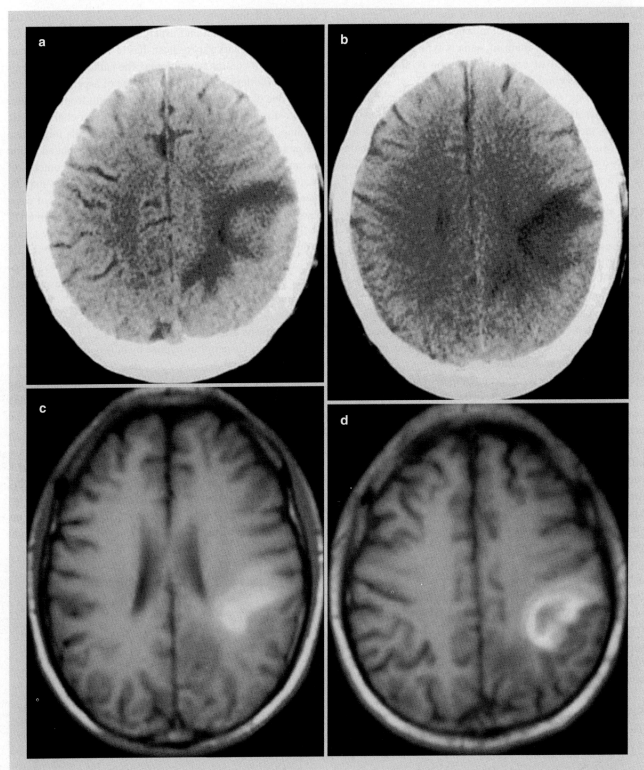

Fig. 13.26 (a–h) HIV/AIDS related cerebral aspergillosis infection. (a, b) CT scanning demonstrates large flaky low density area in the left parietal lobe. (c, d) Ring shaped and flaky high density shadows in the left parietal lobe, with central low density shadow and surrounding edema. (e, f) Large flaky high density shadow and ring shaped high density shadow (spontaneous bleeding) in the left temporal lobe; deepened and widened sulci. (g, h) HE staining demonstrates large amount growth of aspergillus spores and hyphae under a microscope of low and high magnification

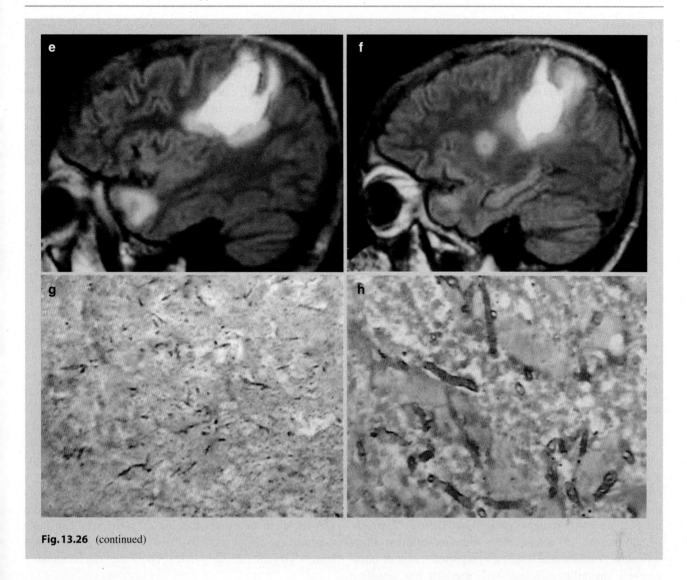

Fig. 13.26   (continued)

Criteria for the Diagnosis

1. Aspergillosis is rarely found in clinical practice, with cerebrospinal fluid demonstrations being similar to those of other fungal infections. Culture with Sabouraud medium may obtain positive finding.
2. CT scanning and MR imaging demonstrate intracerebral granuloma, abscess and hemorrhagic infarction. In addition, it may has following characteristic demonstrations. MR imaging of most patients demonstrates multifocal and polymorphous lesions in the brain parenchyma, with common occurrence of cerebral abscesses, cerebral infarction, cerebral hemorrhage, intracranial granuloma, meningitis and encephalitis. Sometimes, these lesions may have concurrent local epidural abscesses, with accompanying enhancement of endocranium as well as enhancement shadow of surrounding paranasal sinus tissues and orbital soft tissues. Aspergillus abscess shows low signals by T1WI, but high signal by T2W1. The ring shaped enhancement of aspergillus abscess shows thick ring wall. Other molds are of various kinds, whose infections are manifested as similar pathological changes and identical clinical signs. However, the same kind of mold might cause considerably different clinical manifestations due to the diversity of lesion features and locations. Therefore, the diagnosis is difficult and clinically depends on biopsy or cerebrospinal fluid test to find the pathogenic molds.

Differential Diagnosis

HIV/AIDS related cerebral aspergillus infection should be differentiated from bacterial and parasitic cerebral abscess, hemorrhagic infarction and cerebral hemorrhage. It is of most significance for definitive diagnosis to find the pathogenic bacteria by histopathology.

Discussion

Cerebral aspergillus infection is a rarely found disease, with an increased occurrence in patients with AIDS. The most common pathogenic bacteria include aspergillus fumigatus and aspergillus flavus. Aspergillus invades the human body into the brain via the following routes: (1) the most common route of respiration; (2) direct infection of paranasal sinuses, middle ear and mastoid process to invade the brain by destroying bone wall with thin septum to the brain; (3) rare route of surgical and traumatic wounds to cause intracranial infection. Simple intracranial aspergillus infection of brain parenchyma has no clinical manifestations of high specificity, with no aggressive general reactions. Headache is commonly initial symptom of various cerebral aspergillus infections. MR imaging demonstrations of intracerebral aspergillus infection have been rarely reported in literature. In addition to the imaging demonstrations of common brain parenchymal abscess, there are also following two features in MR imaging demonstrations. MR imaging of most patients demonstrates multifocal and polymorphous lesions in the brain parenchyma, with common occurrence of cerebral abscesses, cerebral infarction, cerebral hemorrhage, intracranial granuloma, meningitis and encephalitis. Local epidural abscess occurs with enhancement of endocranium. By MR imaging, aspergillus abscess shows low signal by T1WI, but high signal by T2WI. The ring shaped enhancement of aspergillus abscess has thick ring wall. Yamada et al. [163] argued that enhanced MR imaging demonstrates obvious abnormal enhancement of cerebral abscess in immunocompetent patients but slightly blurry abnormal enhancement of cerebral abscess in immunocompromised patients. Different demonstrations of enhancement indicate different hosts immunity. Yamada et al. [163] also reported 1 case of intracerebral aspergillus infection, with irregular low signaling between the abscess wall and central necrotic focus by T2WI. Pathologically, paramagnetic imaging due to iron is demonstrated, which is necessary for the growth of aspergillus. The low signal indicates that the reproduction of aspergillus is in its active phase. The characteristic low signaling is facilitative for the diagnosis of intracerebral aspergillus infection.

13.3.2 HIV/AIDS Related Intracerebral Parasitic Infections

13.3.2.1 HIV/AIDS Related Toxoplasmic Encephalitis

Pathogens and Pathogenesis

In cases with acquired toxoplasmosis, the involvement of the central nervous system mostly occurs in immunodeficient patients. Toxoplasma selectively invades the cerebral tissues, which has been attributed to the local compromised immunity. Toxoplasmic encephalitis (TE) is a zoonotic disease caused by toxoplasma, with 140 kinds of mammals being able to carry the pathogen in their bodies. The pathogen commonly invades the human body via the digestive tract. Firstly, sporozoites or trophozoites invade the intestinal mucosal cells and reproduce there, leading to rupture of intestinal mucosal cells. The trophozoite spreads along with blood or lymph flow to cause parasitemia. Its further invasion to the brain tissue and rapid proliferation in the tissue cells destroy the host cells, followed by invasion to adjacent cells. Such a process recurs to cause histocytes necrotic foci and acute inflammatory reactions, predominantly mononuclear cells infiltration. Animal experiments have demonstrated those 5 days after peritoneal injection of tachyzoite, tachyzoites can be found in the brain, with subsequent occurrence of perivascular mononuclear cells inflammation. Mononuclear cells can be found to agglutinate to form microglia nodules containing toxoplasma gondii antigen. Tachyzoite infected cells cause multiple small necrotic foci.

Pathophysiologic Basis

In cases of toxoplasmosis, the central nervous system is the most commonly involved. Toxoplasmic encephalitis may have manifestations of focal or diffuse meningoencephalitis, with accompanying necrosis and microgliacyte nodules. Gross observation by naked eyes may find swelling of the brain with congestion and locally softening on the surface. On the cross section, there are necrotic foci. Under a microscope, necrotic foci and infiltration of mononuclear cells, lymphocytes and plasmacytes in the surrounding vascular necrotic foci to form multiple abscesses liked foci. They are commonly found in the interface of the cortex and medulla as well as in the deep gray nuclei. In some cases, they may involve cerebellum, brain stem and the spinal cord. By biopsy or autopsy, toxoplasma pseudocysts and free tachyzoite (trophozoite) can be found.

Clinical Symptoms and Signs

HIV/AIDS related toxoplasmic encephalitis has a sub-acute onset, with non-specific clinical manifestations and imaging demonstrations. Clinical signs and symptoms include fever, headache and lethargy that may progress into coma or even death within a few days or weeks. For cases with meningeal involvement, there is the symptom of transient intracranial hypertension, known as the symptom of false brain tumors. Imaging findings are often space occupying effect being similar to those of tumors or abscesses. There are also neuropsychiatric signs and symptoms including paralysis, seizure episodes, visual disturbances, consciousness disorders, amentia and even coma as well as signs of brain stem and spinal cord involvements. Fever and meningeal irritation are rarely found.

Examinations and Their Selection

Pathogenic Examinations

The commonly applied pathogenic examinations include routine staining or immunocytochemical assays to find trophozoites or cysts of toxoplasma. Application of PCR to

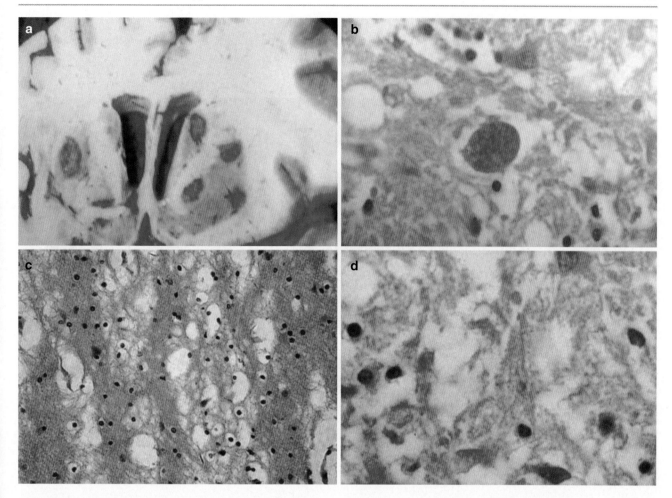

Fig. 13.27 (**a–d**) HIV/AIDS related intracerebral toxoplasma infection. (**a**) Gross observation by autopsy demonstrates multiple abscesses foci in the basal ganglia. (**b**) It is demonstrated to have toxoplasma cysts in the brain tissues. (**c**, **d**) Brain tissue section demonstrates scattering toxoplasma tachyzoites in particles of different sizes, small quantity of infiltration of inflammatory cells and cystic toxoplasma in the necrotic foci (Figures are provided by D. C. Lin)

detect toxoplasma DNA in CSF is of great significance for the diagnosis of cerebral toxoplasmosis.

Immunological Assays

The synthesis of toxoplasma specific IgG, IgM or IgA can be confirmed by Western blot or enzyme-linked immunosorbent assay. PCR can be applied to detect toxoplasma DNA in various clinical specimens.

CSF Test

Patients with toxoplasmic meningitis mostly have normal CSF pressure, yellow CSF, globulin test positive, and slightly increased cell count.

Diagnostic Imaging

CT scanning and MR imaging are the imaging examinations of choice, which help to understand the size, morphology and localization of the intracerebral foci. They can be also applied to assess the therapeutic efficacy.

Imaging Demonstrations

CT Scanning

The foci can be commonly found in the basal ganglia and interface of cortex and medulla, sometimes in cerebellum and brainstem, even in cerebral ventricles. The focus is singular or multiple. By enhanced scanning, there are ring shaped, spiral or nodular abnormal enhancements in diameters of less than 2 cm, occasionally with irregular ring shaped abnormal enhancement in diameter of 3–5 cm.

MR Imaging

The demonstrations include multiple flakes of long T1 long T2 signals. Enhanced imaging demonstrates multiple ring shaped, spiral and nodular obvious abnormal enhancements, homogeneous wall thickness, obvious edema of brain tissues and possible space occupying effect. The detection rate of foci by MR imaging is higher than that by CT scanning.

Case Study 1

A patient was confirmatively diagnosed as having AIDS by CDC. The patient had a history of drug abuse, with symptoms of retarded response, headache and nausea. The CD4 T cell count was 40/μl.

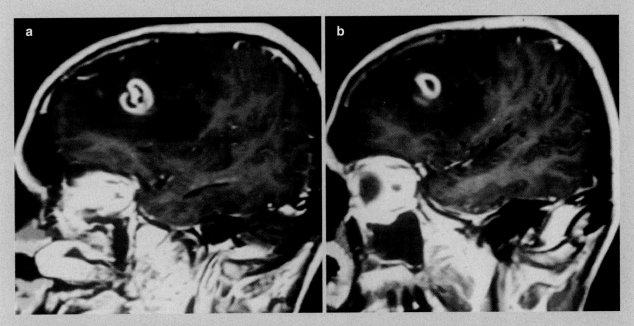

Fig. 13.28 (a, b) HIV/AIDS related intracerebral toxoplasma infection. (a) Enhanced MR imaging of IV-Gd-DTPA demonstrates spiral obvious abnormal enhancement of the left temporal lobe, obvious surrounding edema and obvious space occupying effect.

(b) Enhanced MR imaging of IV-Gd-DTPA demonstrates ring shaped obvious abnormal enhancement of the left temporal lobe, homogeneous thickness of and smooth wall, obvious surrounding edema and obvious space occupying effect

Case Study 2
AIDS patient was confirmatively diagnosed by CDC. The patient had a history of paid blood donation, with symptoms of retarded response, unconsciousness, and incontinence for 2 weeks. The CD4 T cell count was 5/μl.

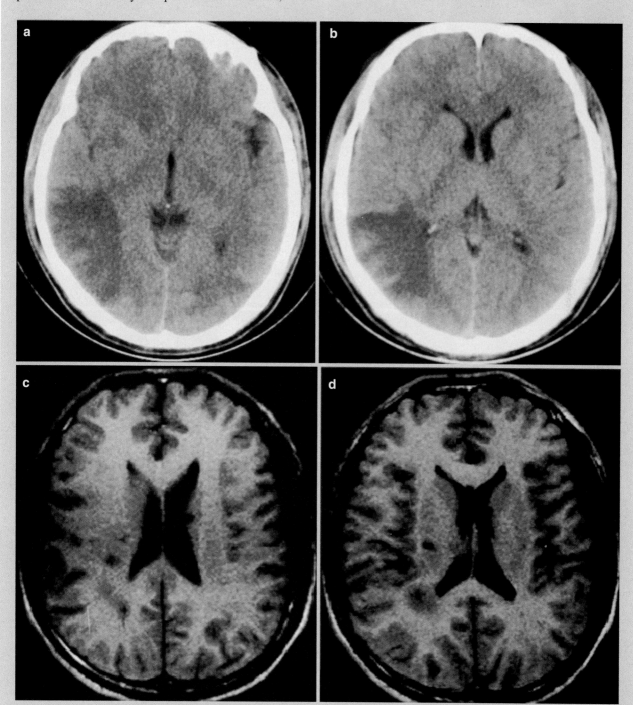

Fig. 13.29 (**a–j**) HIV/AIDS related intracerebral toxoplasma infection. (**a, b**) CT scanning demonstrates wedge shaped low density area in the right temporal and occipital lobes, obvious edema and unobvious space occupying effect. (**c–h**) MR imaging demonstrates bilateral multiple spots and flakes of long T1 long T2 signals in the brain, central short T2 signal in the focus of the right temporal and occipital lobes. (**i, j**) Enhanced imaging of IV-Gd-DTPA demonstrates ring shaped, spiral and nodular obvious abnormal enhancements and obvious edema surrounding the focus in the right temporal and occipital lobes

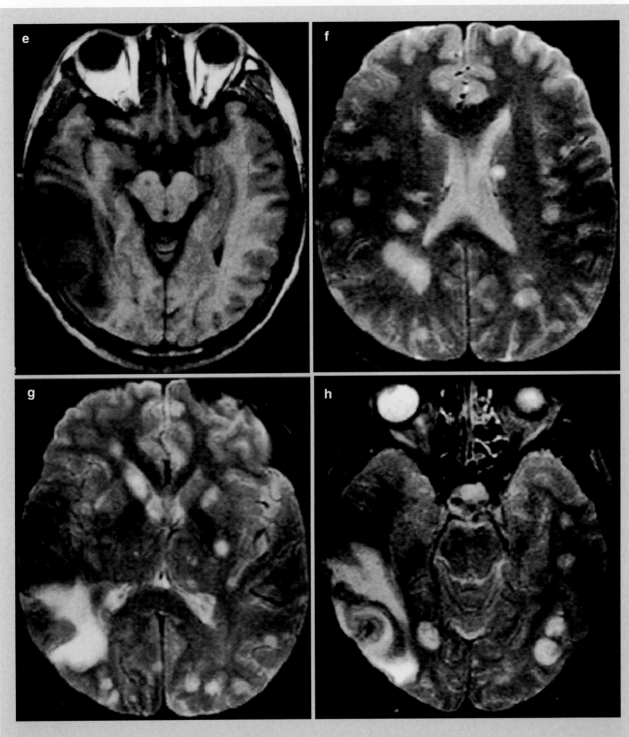

Fig. 13.29 (continued)

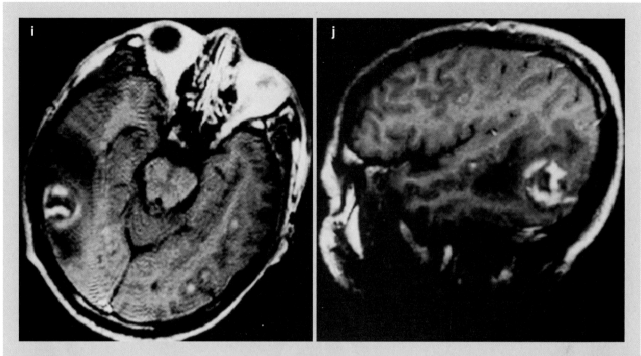

Fig. 13.29   (continued)

Case Study 3
AIDS patient was confirmatively diagnosed by the CDC. The patient had a history of drug abuse, with symptoms of headache, dizziness and nausea. The CD4 T cell count was 21/µl.

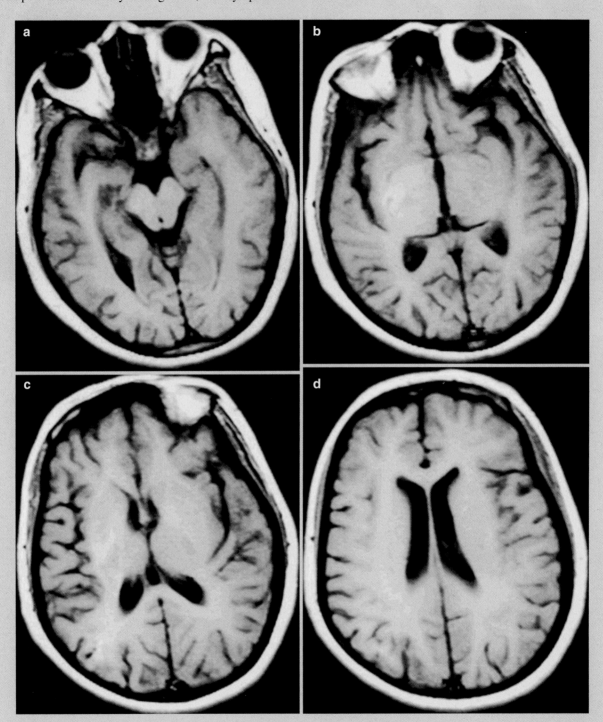

Fig. 13.30 (a–r) HIV/AIDS related intracerebral toxoplasma infection. (a–d) MR imaging demonstrates long T1 or equal T1 and stripes of short T2 signal in the right thalamus, unobvious edema and space occupying effect. (e–h) MR imaging demonstrates flame liked long T2 signal in the right thalamus and occipital lobe, obviously narrowing of the right lateral ventricle due to compression. (i–k) Enhanced MR imaging of IV-Gd-DTPA demonstrates ring shaped obvious abnormal enhancement of the right thalamus and occipital lobe, no central enhancement, homogeneous thickness of and smooth wall. (l–o) Enhanced sagittal MR imaging of IV-Gd-DTPA demonstrates multiple ring shaped obvious abnormal enhancements of the right thalamus and occipital lobe, homogeneous wall thickness and no central enhancement of the necrotic area. (p–r) Enhanced coronal MR imaging of IV-Gd-DTPA demonstrates multiple ring shaped obvious abnormal enhancements in the right thalamus and occipital lobe, homogeneous wall thickness, central nodular abnormal enhancement and no enhancement of the necrotic area

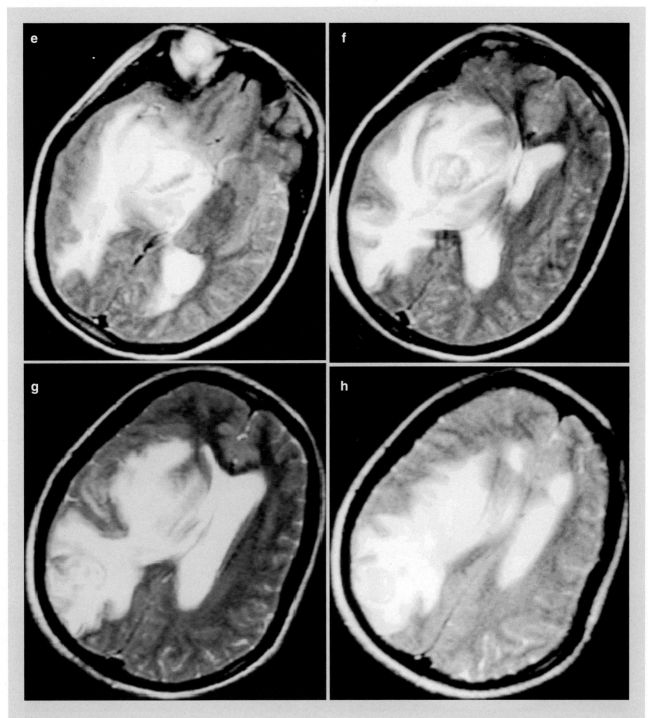

Fig. 13.30 (continued)

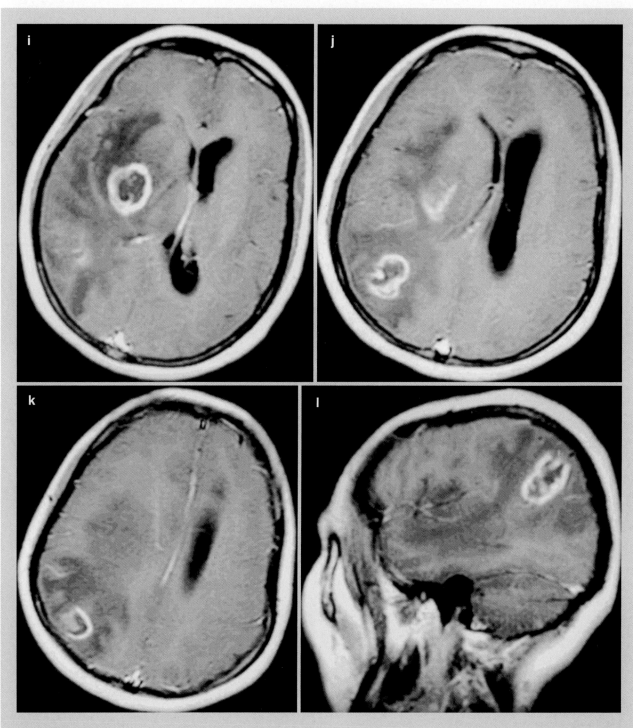

Fig. 13.30 (continued)

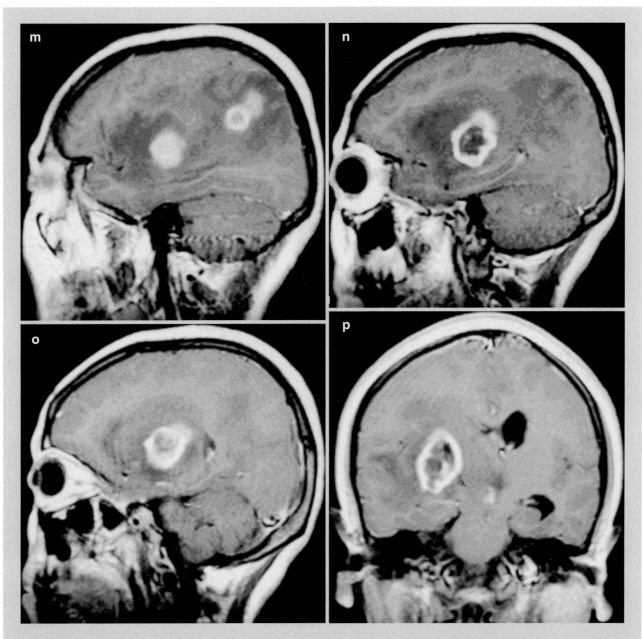

Fig. 13.30 (continued)

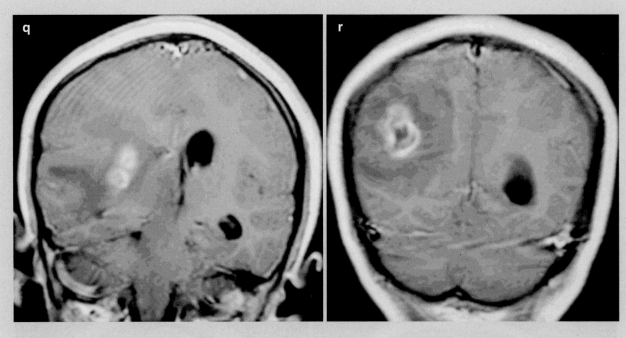

Fig. 13.30 (continued)

Case Study 4

A female patient aged 30 years was confirmatively diagnosed by the CDC as having AIDS. She had a history of paid blood donation, with symptoms of retarded response, headache, dizziness, nausea and vomiting for 1 week. Her CD4 T cell count was 31/μl.

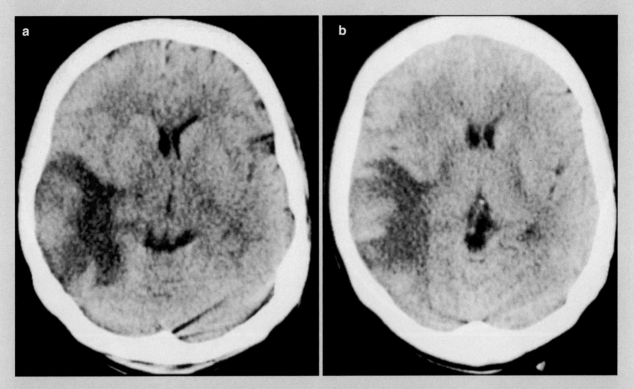

Fig. 13.31 (a–o) HIV/AIDS related intracerebral toxoplasma infection. (**a, b**) CT scanning demonstrates wedge shaped low density area in the right temporal occipital lobe, with unclearly defined borderlines; obvious edema and space occupying effect. (**c, d**) Axial MR imaging demonstrates wedge shaped long T1 signal in the right temporal occipital lobe. (**e, f**) Axial MR imaging demonstrations of large flaky long T2 signal, ring shaped short T2 signal of the focus in the right temporal occipital lobe. (**g, h**) Sagittal MR imaging demonstrates wedge shaped long T1 signal in the right temporal occipital lobe. (**i–k**) Enhanced axial MR imaging of IV-Gd-DTPA demonstrates spiral obvious abnormal enhancement in the right temporal lobe, and possible bull's eye liked abnormal enhancement. (**l, m**) Enhanced sagittal MR imaging of IV-Gd-DTPA demonstrates spiral obvious abnormal enhancement in the right temporal lobe, and bull's eye liked abnormal enhancement. (**n, o**) Enhanced coronal MR imaging of IV-Gd-DTPA demonstrates spiral obvious abnormal enhancement in the right temporal lobe, bull's eye liked obvious abnormal enhancement and nodular enhancement

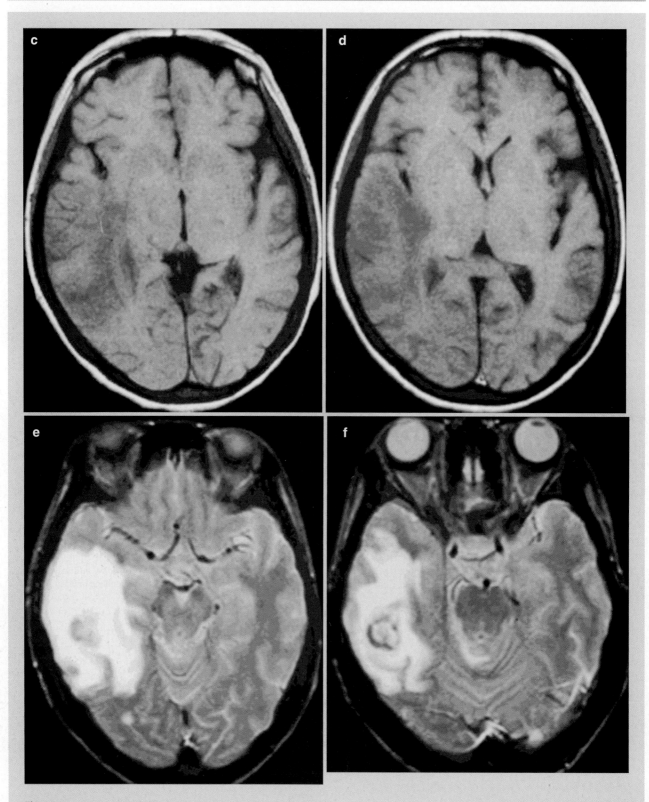

Fig. 13.31   (continued)

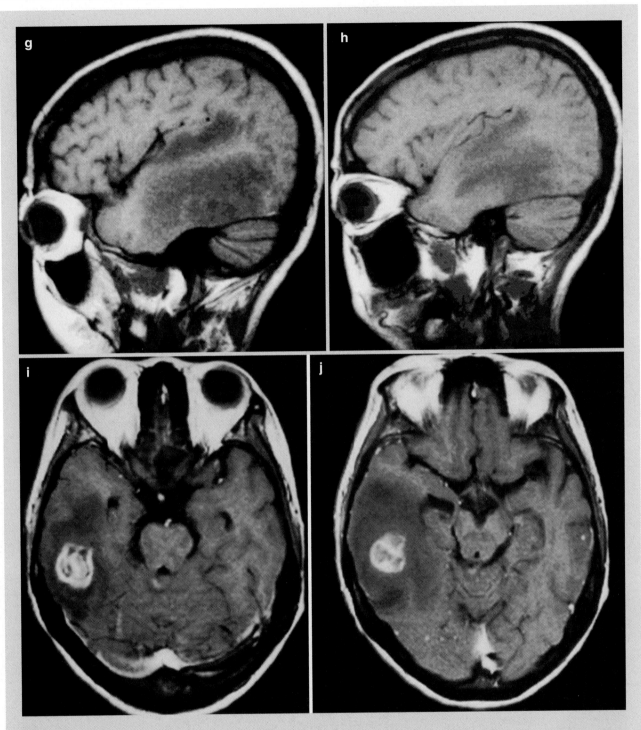

Fig. 13.31 (continued)

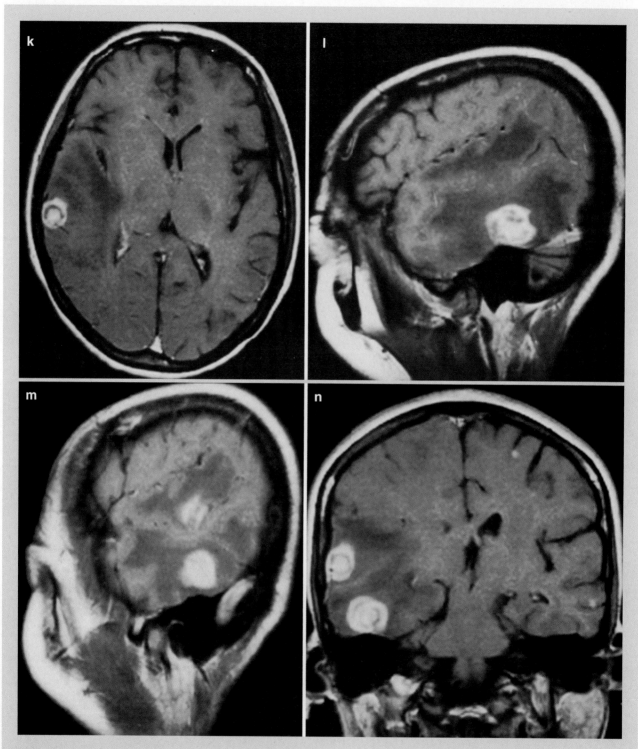

Fig. 13.31 (continued)

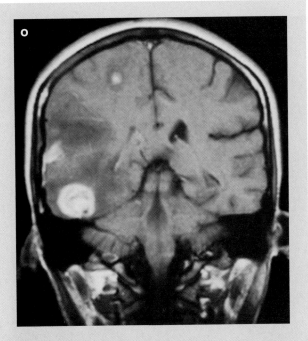

Fig. 13.31 (continued)

Case Study 5

AIDS patient was confirmatively diagnosed by the CDC. The patient had a history of paid blood donation, with symptoms of retarded response, dizziness, nausea and vomiting for 1 month. The CD4 T cell count was 11/μl.

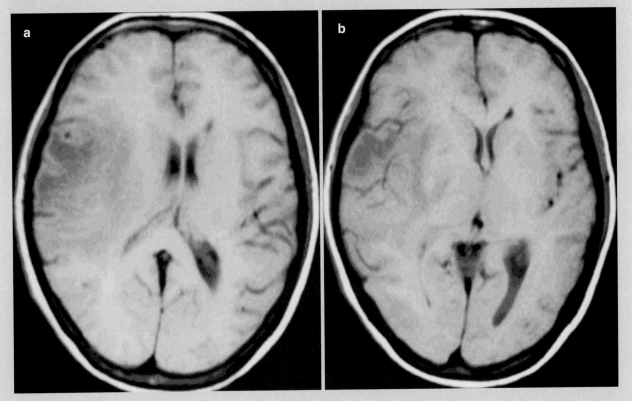

Fig. 13.32 (a–f) HIV/AIDS related intracerebral toxoplasma infection. (**a, b**) MR T1WI demonstrates large flaky low signaling area with unclearly defined borderline, slightly compressed left lateral ventricle and leftward migration of the midline. (**c, d**) MR T2WI demonstrates patchy high signaling area in the right temporal lobe and slight leftward migration of the midline. (**e, f**) Enhanced axial and sagittal MR IV-Gd-DTPA demonstrates ring shaped enhancement of the foci, with surrounding low signaling areas of edema

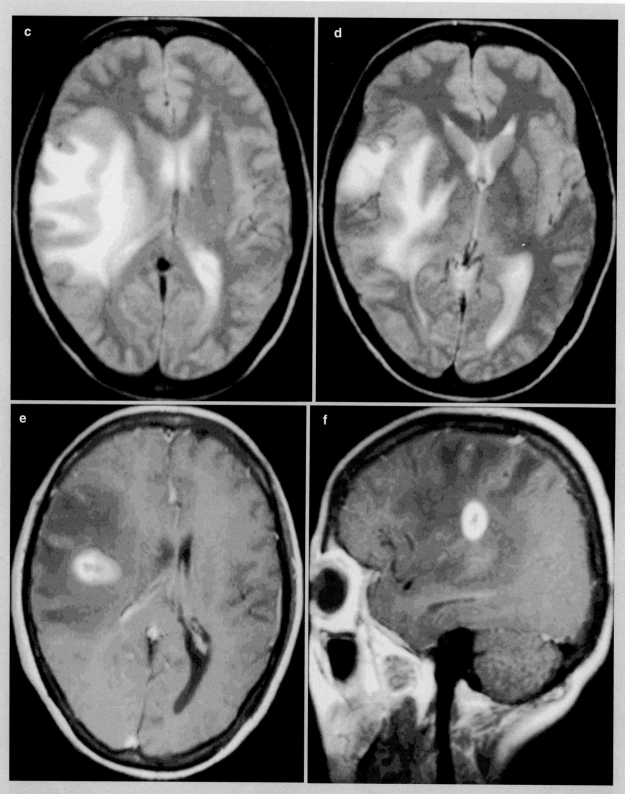

Fig. 13.32 (continued)

Case Study 6
AIDS patient was confirmatively diagnosed by the CDC. The patient had a history of paid blood donation, with symptoms of retarded response, unconsciousness and incontinence for 2 weeks. The CD4 T cell count was 51/μl.

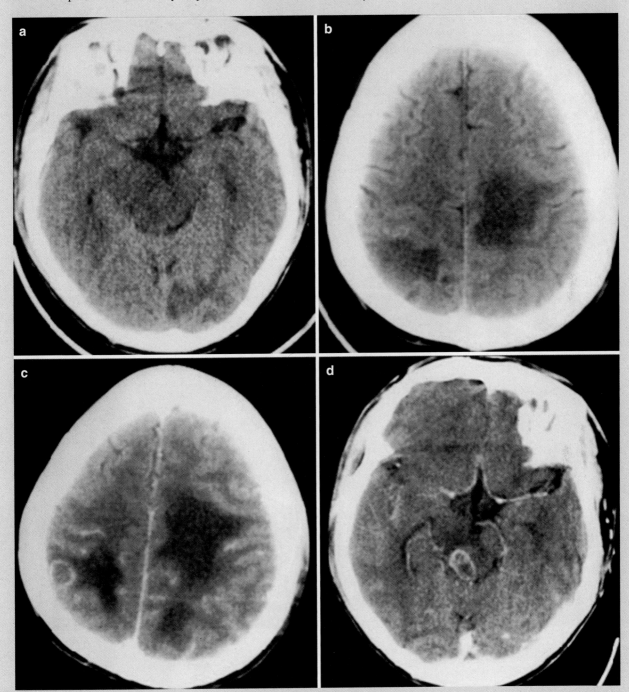

Fig. 13.33 (**a–h**) HIV/AIDS related intracerebral toxoplasma infection. (**a–c**) Plain CT scanning demonstrates patchy low density changes in the bilateral parietal occipital lobes and brainstem, with unclearly defined borderline. (**d, e**) Enhanced CT scanning demonstrates multiple ring shaped enhancement of the foci in the bilateral occipital lobes and brainstem, with surrounding low density stripes of edema. (**f**) MR imaging of IV-Gd-DTPA demonstrates multi-locular ring shaped abnormal enhancement in the brainstem. (**g**) MRI demonstrates ring shaped abnormal enhancement in the right occipital lobe, with uneven thickness of the wall. (**h**) MRI demonstrates ring shaped abnormal enhancement in bilateral parietal lobes and brainstem, obvious central enhancement and surrounding low signaling stripes of edema

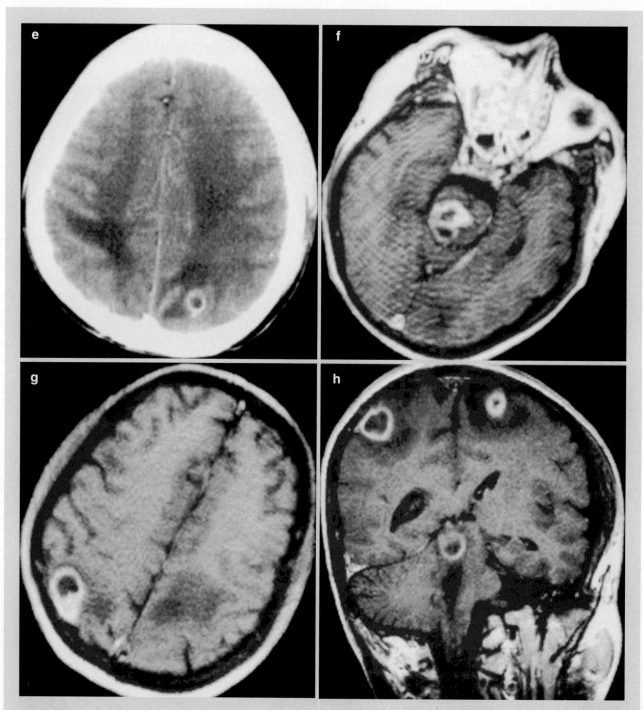

Fig. 13.33 (continued)

Case Study 7
AIDS patient was confirmatively diagnosed by the CDC. The patient had a history of paid blood donation, with symptoms of dizziness and nausea for 17 days. The CD4 T cell count was 40/μl.

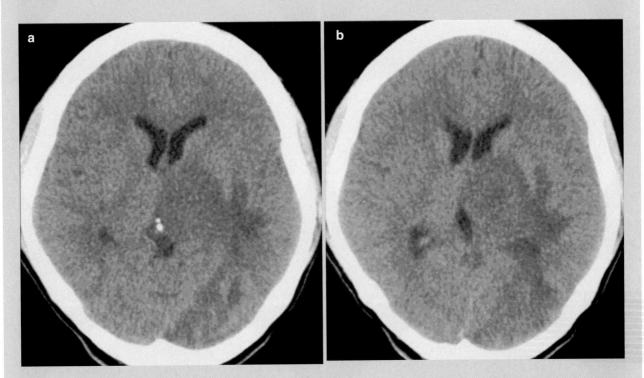

Fig. 13.34 (**a–d**) CT scanning demonstrates flaky low density area in the left basal ganglia, with obvious space occupying effect; narrowed left lateral ventricle due to compression; with significant surrounding edema and with involvements of the left temporal lobe, occipital lobe and parietal lobe. (**e**) CT scanning demonstrates flaky low density area in the right parietal lobe. (**f–j**) Enhanced CT scanning demonstrates ring shaped obvious abnormal enhancements in the left basal ganglia, occipital lobe, temporal lobe and bilateral parietal lobes in different sizes, with no central enhancement and homogeneous thickness of the wall. (**k–n**) Axial MR imaging demonstrates flaky long T1 long T2 signals in the bilateral parietal lobe and left basal ganglia, occipital lobe and temporal lobe, short T2 signal in the left basal ganglia. (**q–t**) IV-Gd-DTPA demonstrates obvious abnormal ring shaped enhancement in the left parietal lobe, with uneven central enhancement. (**a–e₁**) HIV/AIDS related intracerebral toxoplasma infection. (**u–x**) Enhanced CT scanning demonstrates small flaky low density areas in the left basal ganglia, with unclearly defined borderline; no abnormal density shadows in other parts of brain parenchyma and ventricles; shrinkage and absence of most foci compared to demonstrations before the therapy. (**a₁–b₁**) MR imaging demonstrates stripes long T2WI signal in the left parietal lobe, with ring shaped high signal and central low signal. (**c₁–e₁**) Enhanced axial imaging IV-Gd-DTPA demonstrates nodular abnormal enhancement in the left parietal lobe, and sagittal and coronal imaging demonstrations of ring shaped enhancement in the brainstem

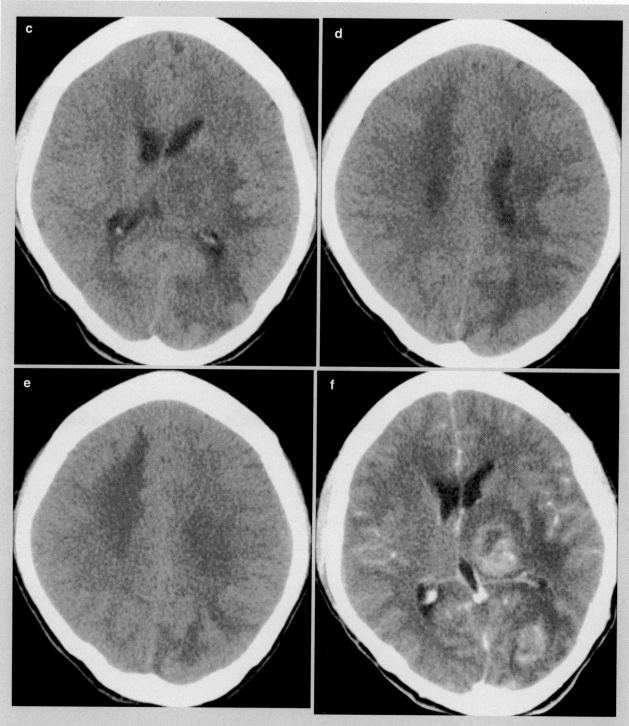

Fig. 13.34 (continued)

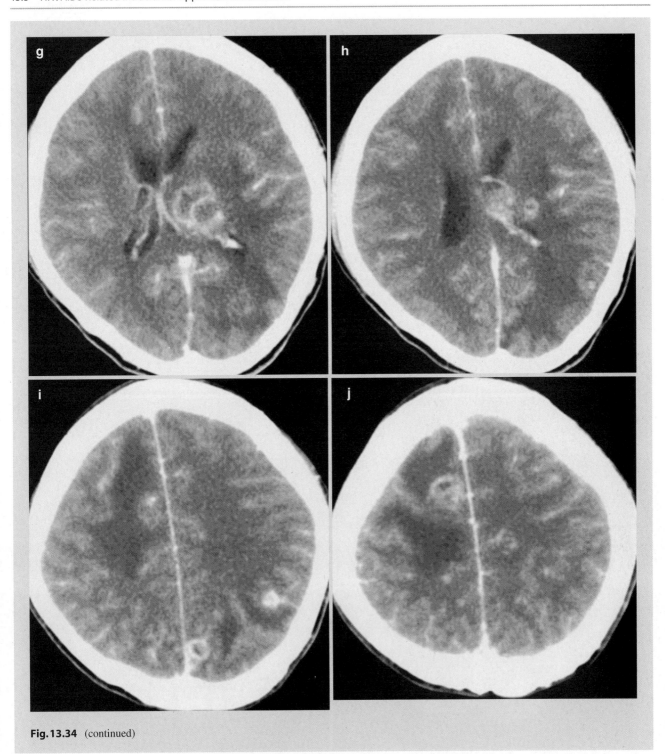

Fig. 13.34 (continued)

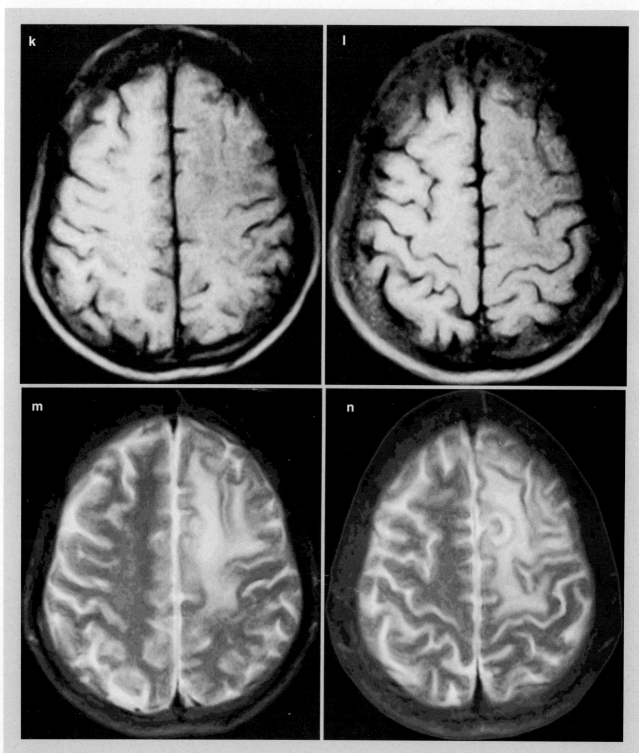

Fig. 13.34   (continued)

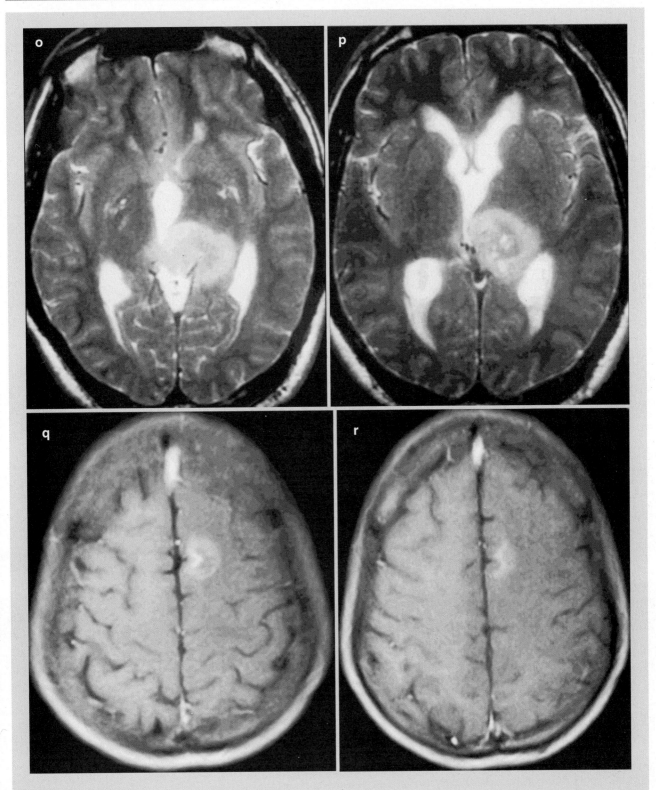

Fig. 13.34   (continued)

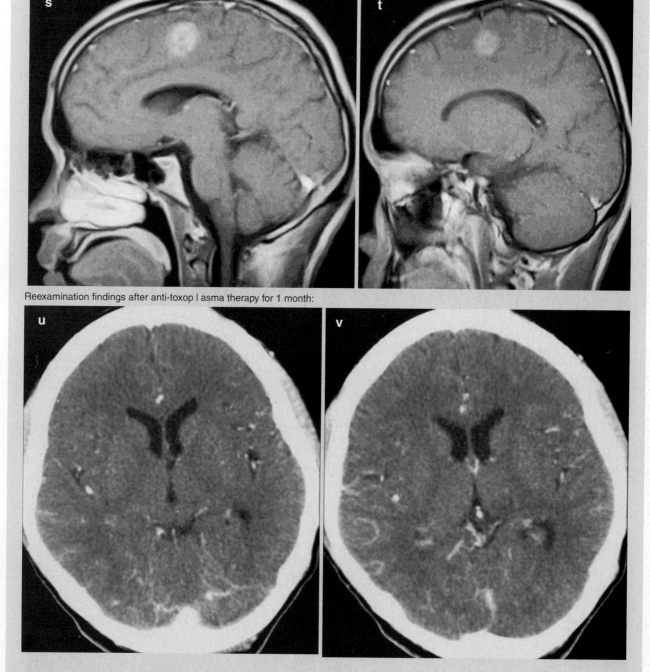

Reexamination findings after anti-toxop l asma therapy for 1 month:

Fig. 13.34   (continued)

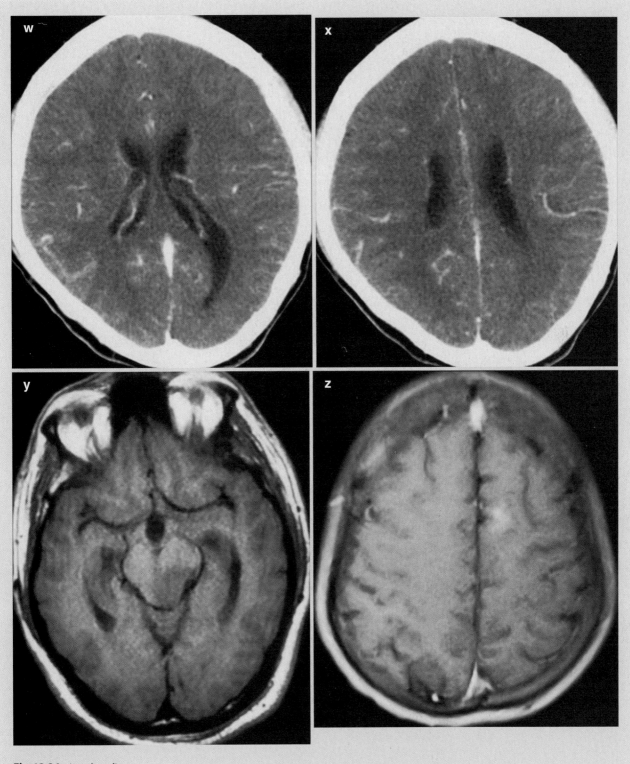

Fig. 13.34 (continued)

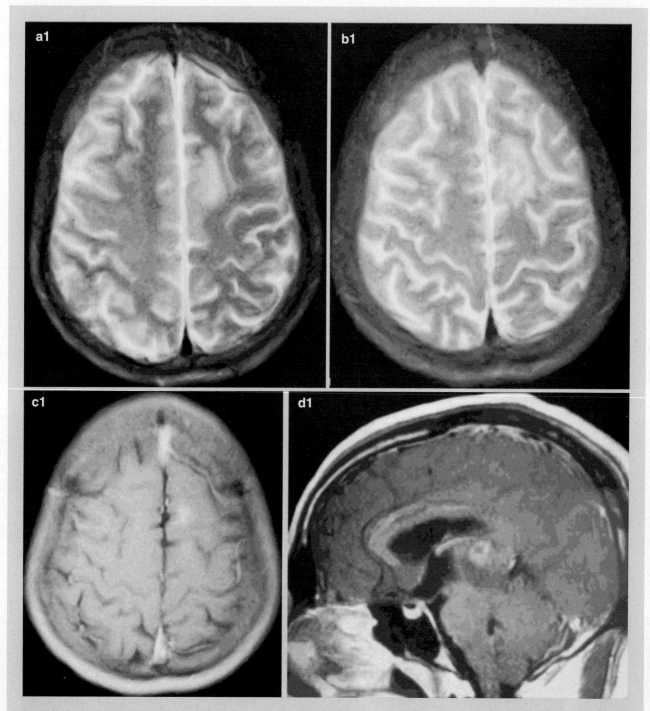

Fig. 13.34   (continued)

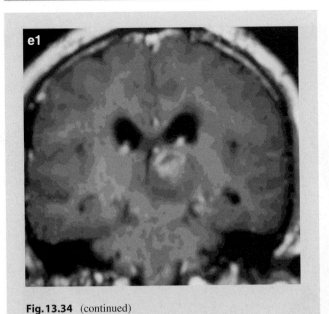

Fig. 13.34 (continued)

Case Study 8

A boy aged 5 years was confirmatively diagnosed as having AIDS by the CDC. He was vertically transmitted from his mother. When he was 6 months old, he was hospitalized due to headache and vomiting for 3 days. On March 5, 2009, he was admitted, with a CD4 T cell count of 3/μl.

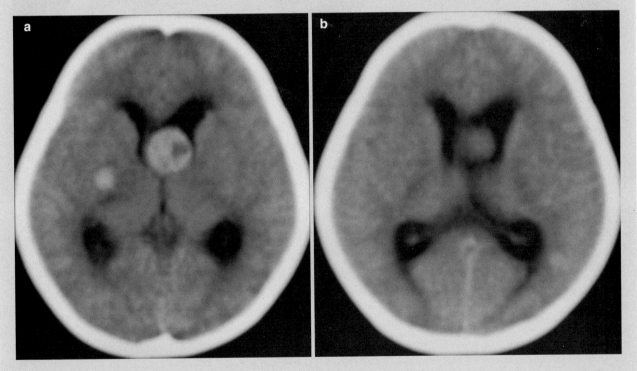

Fig. 13.35 (**a**, **b**) CT scanning demonstrates flaky high density shadow in the right basal ganglia, with clearly defined borderline, no obvious edema and space occupying effect; round liked slightly high density shadow in the frontal angle of the left lateral ventricle, with uneven central density. (**a–g**) HIV/AIDS related intracerebral toxoplasma infection. (**c–g**) CT scanning demonstrates alleviated symptoms, round liked high density focus in the frontal angle of the left lateral ventricle; slight change in size and enlarged central liquefied necrotic area compared to the imaging demonstrations before the administration of anti-toxoplasma therapy

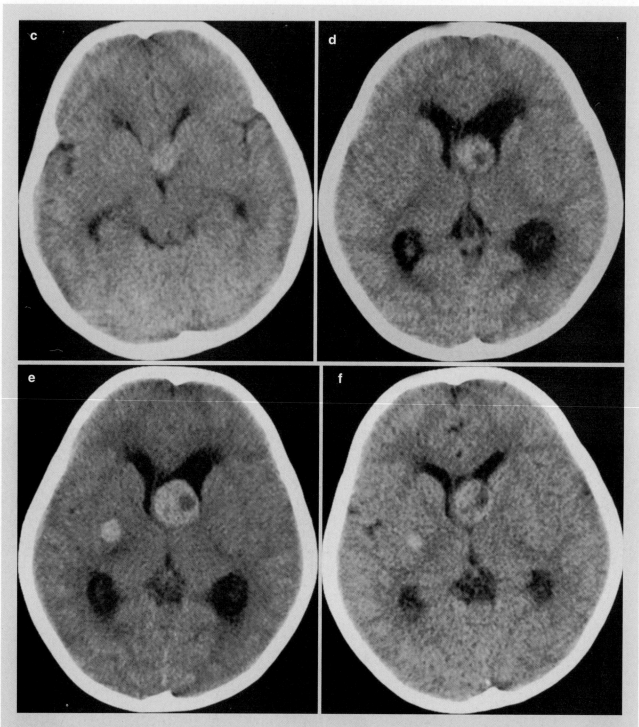

Fig. 13.35 (continued)

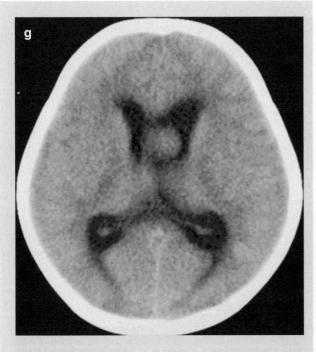

Fig. 13.35   (continued)

Case Study 9
A female patient aged 44 years was confirmatively diagnosed as having AIDS by the CDC. She had symptoms of headache, vomiting, convulsions and physical dysfunction of the right side of her body. Her CD4 T cell count was 17/µl.

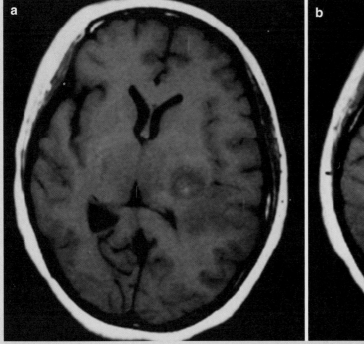
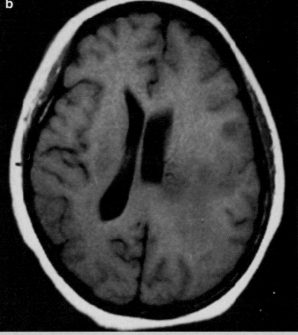

Fig 13.36 (**a–j**) HIV/AIDS related intracerebral toxoplasma infection. (**a–d**) MR imaging demonstrates large flaky long T1 and long T2 signals in the left basal ganglia and spots short T2 signal. (**e–j**) Enhanced axial, sagittal, and coronal MR imaging of IV-Gd-DTPA demonstrate spots and flakes obviously abnormal enhancement in the left basal ganglia and temporal occipital lobe, with obvious space occupying effect; narrowed left lateral ventricle due to compression and unobvious surrounding edema

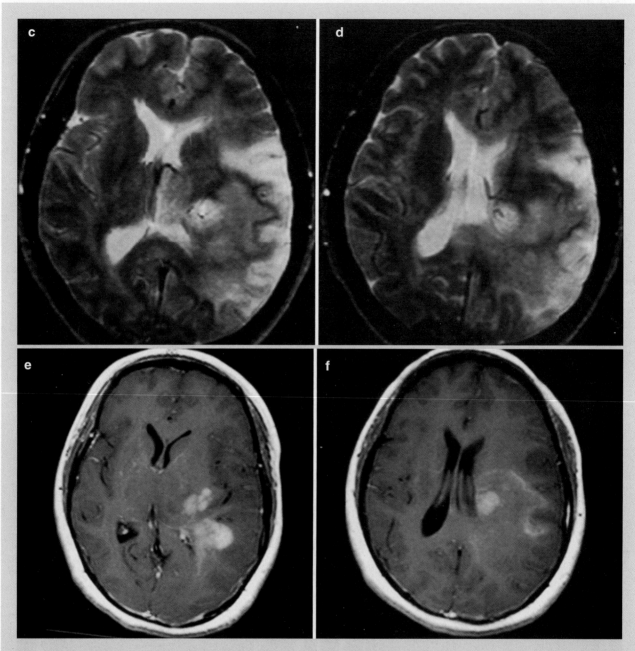

Fig 13.36   (continued)

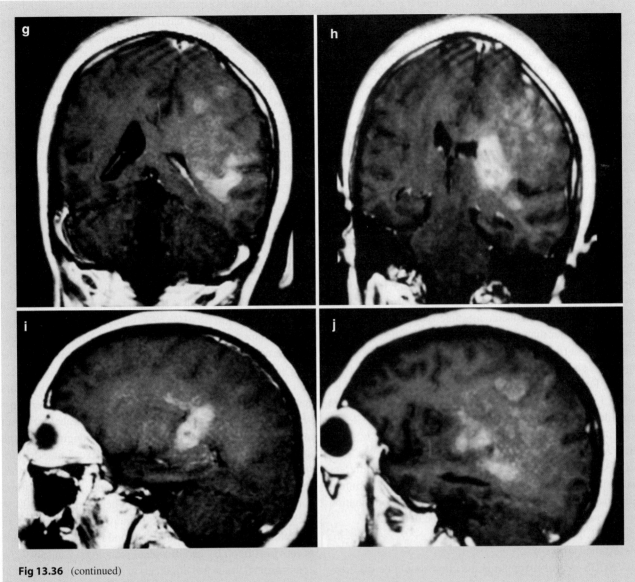

Fig 13.36 (continued)

Criteria for the Diagnosis

1. Serological tests for IgM or IgG.
2. Amniotic fluid analysis by PCR can detect the toxoplasma nucleic acid in the fetus.
3. Increased lymphocytes and protein contents in CSF.
4. Findings of toxoplasma tachyzoite by brain biopsy are specific for the diagnosis.
5. CT scanning demonstrates foci commonly at the interface between cortex and medulla and sometimes in the basal ganglia, cerebellum, brainstem and ventricles. Plain CT scanning demonstrates multiple low density areas in brain and singular low density area is rarely found. Enhanced scanning demonstrates multiple rings shaped, spiral, nodular obviously abnormal enhancement, with space occupying effect and edema effect. For the cases with occurrence of lesions in the cerebral ventricle and density difference between CSF density and space occupying density, a dense mass shadow can be demonstrated, with clearly defined borderline.

6. MR imaging demonstrates multiple or singular flaky long T1 long T2 signal, with obvious edema effect and possible space occupying effect. Enhanced imaging demonstrates multiple or singular round liked nodular, ring shaped and spiral abnormal enhancement. The resolution of MRI for soft tissues is higher than that of CT and MRI has no blind area for imaging of the brain. Therefore, the detection rate of foci by MRI is higher than that by CT.

7. PET-CT demonstrates slight and moderate increase of local metabolism.
8. Therapeutic diagnosis of toxoplasmosis: After 2–4 weeks treatment, both the size and number of intracerebral foci decrease, with alleviated brain edema and space occupying effects as well as decreased degree of enhancement.

Differential Diagnosis
Primary Brain Lymphoma
HIV/AIDS related intracerebral toxoplasma infection should be differentiated from primary brain lymphoma. Primary brain lymphoma commonly occurs in the basal ganglia and thalamus. It is usually singular, with obvious space occupying effect. Edema surrounding lymphoma is fire flame liked or finger liked. The anti-toxoplasma therapy is ineffective for it. However, intracerebral toxoplasma abscess commonly occur with multiple foci, mostly invading the interface of cortex and medulla with obvious edema around the abscess. The anti-toxoplasma treatment is obviously effective. Its diffusion coefficient by MR imaging is obviously higher than that of lymphoma. For the cases with diffusion coefficient RATIO being above 1.6, toxoplasma infection should be considered for early detection of the focus. For the cases with diffusion coefficient RATIO being less than 1.6 and above 1.0, lymphoma should be considered.

Brain Mycotic Infection
HIV/AIDS related toxoplasma infection should be differentiated from brain mycotic infections such as candida infection and cryptococcus neoformans infection. In combination with laboratory tests, the diagnosis can be defined.

Metastatic Tumors
HIV/AIDS related toxoplasma infection should be differentiated from metastatic tumors. Metastatic tumors commonly occur at the interface between cortex and medulla, with finger liked edema and primary focus. In combination with the case history, the diagnosis can be defined.

Brain Cysticercosis
HIV/AIDS related toxoplasma infection should be differentiated from brain cysticercosis. Brain cysticercosis is manifested as brain vesicle type, with cysticercosis scolex as its important indicator. Enhanced scanning demonstrates multiple thin-wall ring shaped abnormal enhancement, with findings of cysticercosis scolex.

Brain Tuberculoma
HIV/AIDS related toxoplasma infection should be differentiated from brain tuberculoma. In cases of brain tuberculoma in its early stage, edema is obvious. Edema is commonly in stripes or finger liked manifestations. The patients with brain tuberculoma are mostly having case history of tuberculosis. In combination to CSF test, the diagnosis can be defined.

Discussion
The incidence of AIDS complicated by toxoplasmic encephalitis is about 10–30 %, which is the main cause of death in AIDS patients. The clinical manifestations include fever, headache, nausea, vomiting and behavioral disorders, with a mean CD4 T cell count being lower than 50/µl. Approximately 50 % such patients have headache, memory loss, mild hemiparalysis, ataxia, half body sensory disturbance and aphasia. Serological tests can detect antibody IgA positive with high affinity, interface immune and lower antibody titer. Antibody is a relatively new biomarker for serum immunoglobulin, which are widely used in the diagnosis of chronic infection. Data indicate that 22 % AIDS patients have negative Toxoplasma antibody (IgA). In the United States, IgG positive rate in patients with AIDS complicated by toxoplasma infection is 20–30 %. The ESF blood culture is negative. Reexamination after anti-toxoplasma treatment with thiamine drugs for 2 weeks can find obvious shrinkage of the foci. The foci distribution of intracerebral toxoplasma infection in brain is the same with other infections and tumors spreading via blood flow. Cerebral hemisphere is more susceptible to involvement than brainstem and cerebellum, with most foci distributing in the bilateral basal ganglia and at the interface between cortex and medulla. CT scanning demonstrates low density for 82 % foci. Enhanced scanning demonstrates multiple nodular, ring shaped and spiral abnormal enhancement, with obvious edema. There are still 18–20 % foci with no such characteristic demonstrations. The foci in the ventricles are demonstrated as round liked or round space occupying effect. By cerebrospinal pathological autopsy, the cerebrospinal tissue has liquefaction and necrosis, with small quantity infiltration of inflammatory cells. Cystic toxoplasma tachyzoites can be found in the necrotic foci, in particles of different sizes. MRI is more favorable than CT in detecting foci and MRI is superior to CT in differentiating different tissues. The diagnosis should be in combination with clinical manifestations, pathogenic examinations and immunological assays. The final qualitative diagnosis should be confirmed by pathogenic examination findings or serological findings, sometimes even autopsy.

13.3.2.2 HIV/AIDS Related Cerebral Cysticercosis
Pathogens and Pathogenesis
Cerebral cysticercosis is a disease caused by parasitization of the cysticercus cellulosae in brain. Tapeworm eggs gain their access to the stomach via a variety of routes, which hatch in the duodenum into cysticercus cellulosae. After that, cysticercus cellulosae penetrate into the intestinal wall and into

the systemic circulation and the choroid through the mesenteric vein to invade the brain parenchyma, the subarachnoid space and the ventricular system. Therefore, a variety of lesions are caused. The pathogenesis caused by cysticercus cellulosae include: (1) The surrounding brain tissue is compressed and destructed by cysticercus cellulosae; (2) Cysticercus cellulosae as a foreign protein causes allergic responses and inflammation in brain tissue; (3) Cysticercus cellulosae obstructs cerebrospinal fluid circulation path to cause increased intracranial pressure.

Pathophysiological Basis

Cerebral cysticercosis is more common in young and middle aged adults. After cysticercus cellulosae invades into the brain, the pathological changes in different stages are as the following:

In the Early Stage

The alive cysticercus cellulosae can be found, with different sizes of the cysts, the scolex in size of millet and in color of grayish white, transparent liquid in the cyst. Inflammatory responses occur in surrounding brain tissues of the cyst, with infiltration of polymorphonuclear neutrophil granulocytes and eosinophilic granulocytes as well as collagen fibers. Vascular proliferation, edema and perivascular mononuclear cells infiltration occur around the cyst.

In the Advanced Stage

The cystic wall is thickened, with death and liquefaction of parasites and turbid cystic fluid. Chronic inflammatory changes occur around the cyst. After cystic fluid is absorbed, the cyst is decreased in size or is replaced by brain glial tissues to form fibrous nodule or calcification. The occurrence of AIDS complicated by ring shaped calcification of intracerebral foci is rare.

Clinical Symptoms and Signs

According to clinical manifestations, cerebral cysticercosis can be divided into four types: (1) epilepsic brain cysticercosis is the most common. The types of seizure include general tonic clonic seizures (major seizure) and its continuing states, partial movement episodes, complex partial seizures (psychomotor seizures). (2) Intracranial hypertensive cysticercosis has clinical manifestations of headache, vomiting, decreased vision, papilledema, and possible accompanying seizures, unconsciousness and even coma. Cysticercus parasitizes in brain ventricles with signs of ventricular involvement. (3) Meningoencephalitic cysticercosis is caused by stimulation of cysticercus to meninges and brain diffuse edema. The common clinical manifestations include headache, vomiting, meningeal irritation and fever. (4) Simple cysticercosis has no neurological symptoms.

Examinations and Their Selection

Cerebrospinal Fluid Test

CSF cytological test can find significantly increased percentage of eosinophilic granulocyte, with the maximal percentage being up to 80–90 %.

Immunological Assay

CSF cysticercus complement fixation test, indirect blood agglutination test and ELISA for cysticercus antibody are of diagnostic significance.

Diagnostic Imaging

MR imaging is the diagnostic imaging of the choice. It facilitates to define the size, morphology and localization of the focus. In addition, it can be used to assess the therapeutic efficacy. CT scanning is superior in demonstrating calcified brain cysticercus.

Imaging Demonstrations

CT Scanning

1. For the cases of brain parenchymal involvement, plain scanning demonstrates multiple diffusive small round shaped low density shadow in the hemisphere as the multiple small cysts type. Within it, there are small nodular dense shadows of cysticercus scolex. The foci are commonly found at the interface between the gray and white matters. Enhanced scanning commonly shows no enhancement or ring shaped enhancement, with slight surrounding edema. There are also cases of singular large cyst type, with growth of a singular large cysticerus cellulosae or growth of multiple cysticerus cellulosae fusion. CT scanning demonstrates intracerebral round, oval or lobulated low density shadow, with CSF density in it. The large cyst itself shows no enhancement, but with possible slight ring shaped enhancement of the surrounding tissues due to fiber tissues hyperplasia.

2. For the cases with ventricular involvement, the foci are commonly found in the fourth cerebral ventricle. CT scanning demonstrates abnormal morphology of the ventricle, restricted asymmetric dilation of the ventricle and obstructive hydrocephalus. Sometimes, the density within the cyst is higher than CSF density.

3. For the cases with meningeal involvement, there are cystic enlargement of the lateral fissure cistern and suprasellar cistern, with slight space occupying sign and symmetrically enlargement of the ventricles. Enhanced scanning demonstrates cystic wall enhancement or nodular enhancement as well as meningeal enhancement.

MR Imaging

1. For the cases with cerebral parenchymal cysticercosis, MR imaging demonstrates round shaped cystic lesions

with eccentric small spots liked cysticercus scolex shadow attaching to the cystic wall in short T1 short T2 signals. Enhanced MR imaging of IV-Gd-DTPA demonstrates cystic wall enhancement or no enhancement. In the cases of cysticercus death, scolex is unclearly defined, with aggravated surrounding edema and obvious space occupying effect. White target sign occurs, with T2WI demonstrations of high signals in the cystic fluid and peripheral

edema and low signals in the cystic wall and blurry scolex.

2. Cysticercus in the brain ventricles, cistern and groove is in long T1 long T2 signal.

3. For cases with meningeal involvement, the demonstrations are cysticercus in the brain groove adhering to the meninges. ADC value increases and MRS has fat peak, with decreased ratio of NAA/Cr.

Case Study 1

AIDS patient was confirmatively diagnosed by the CDC. The patient had one episode of epilepsy. And the CD4 T cell count was 126/μl.

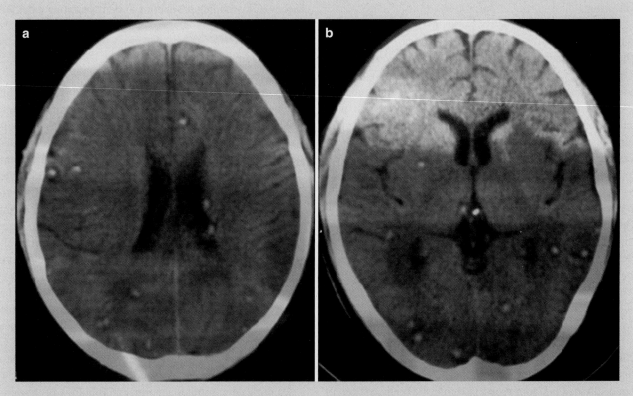

Fig. 13.37 (**a**, **b**) HIV/AIDS related cerebral cysticercosis (brain parenchymal involvement). For the cases of brain parenchymal involvement, plain CT scanning demonstrates multiple nodular high density shadow in the bilateral brain parenchyma, with surrounding ring shaped low density shadow; subependymal nodular high density shadow in the left lateral ventricle

Case Study 2

A male patient aged 34 years was confirmatively diagnosed as having AIDS by the CDC. He was admitted to hospital because of the complaints of nausea and vomiting on October 13, 2008. After symptomatic treatment, his condition improved and was discharged. He was admitted to the hospital again due to dizziness and blurry vision on October 24. His CD4 T cell count was 26/μl.

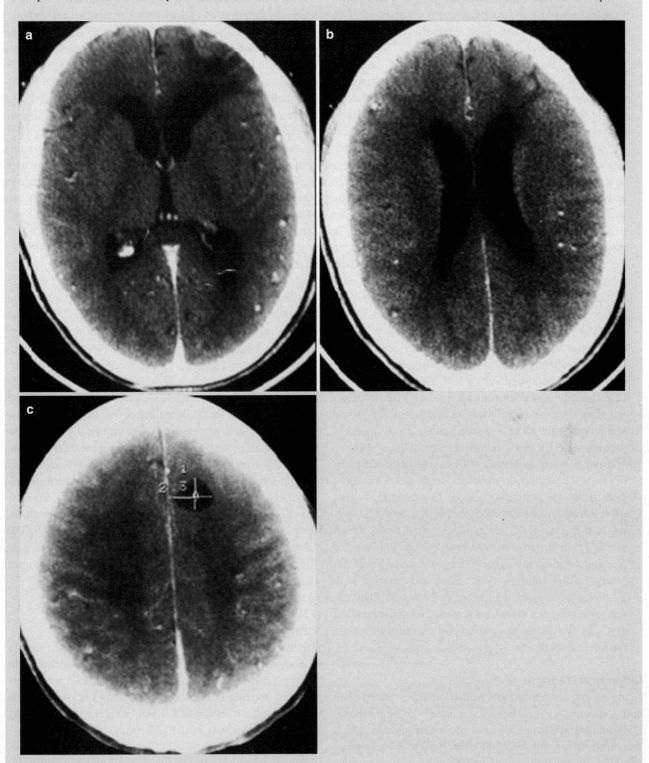

Fig. 13.38 (a–c) HIV/AIDS related cerebral cysticercosis (Multiple cerebral involvement). For cases with cerebral cysticercosis of multiple cerebral involvement (brain parenchymal and singular cystic involvements), CT scanning demonstrates multiple nodular high density shadow in the bilateral brain parenchyma and the interface between cortex and medulla; round liked cystic low density shadow in the left parietal lobe, with no cysticercus scolex

Criteria for the Diagnosis

1. The patient has a case history of defecated tapeworm and dietary measly pork.
2. The patient has neurological symptoms and signs.
3. Cystic nodules are confirmed by biopsy and pathology.
4. Immunological assay for cysticercus is positive.
5. Increased cerebrospinal fluid pressure and increased number of eosinophilic leukocytes.
6. CT scanning demonstrates foci commonly in the cortex and medulla, as well as the basal ganglia, including: (1) cystic low density focus: multiple or singular low density area in the brain parenchyma and ventricles, with clearly defined borderline, commonly in oval shape and in different sizes, central CSF density, no definitive cystic wall, commonly in the cortex and medulla as well as sometimes in the surrounding area of the midline, parasellar region and basal ganglia with balloon liked low density area, ring shaped enhancement of the cystic wall with low and even density and dull edge; (2) hydrocephalus: occurring in most patients with symmetric ventricular enlargement; in the cases of ventricular involvement with cysticercus compressing and occluding the intraventricular orifice, ventricular compression or arachnoid adhesion occurs to cause hydrocephalus; in the cases of cistern involvement, irregular small beads string liked low density shadow can be found in the basal cistern or brain fissure; (3) nodular density shadow: multiple confined low density area with obviously central abnormal enhancement; also a slightly higher density shadows in number of a few to hundreds, with surrounding stripes of edema; obvious brain edema and slight space occupying effect. (4) calcification: rarely found in patients with HIV/AIDS related cerebral cysticercosis.
7. MR imaging demonstrates: MR imaging demonstrations of cerebral cysticercosis are related to the development of cysticercus. (1) In its alive period, T1-weighted imaging demonstrates round cyst with eccentric scolex, CSF signal of the cystic fluid, scolex signal equal to the wither matter. (2) In its parenchymal edema period: T1-weighted imaging demonstrates higher intracystic signal than CSF, blurry scolex shadow and thickened cystic wall. T2-weighted imaging demonstrates intracystic high signal, lowered scolex signal, no stripes of edema around the cyst. (3) The granuloma period and calcification period are rarely found.

Differential Diagnosis

Acute encephalitis in patients with HIV/AIDS related cerebral cysticercosis should be differentiated from viral encephalitis and demyelinated disease. Demyelinated disease is demonstrated as no abnormal enhancement by enhanced scanning. In the cases with ventricular involvement, the cystic wall has spots high density shadow of the scolex or spots of calcification, which are indicative for the diagnosis. Enhanced scanning can provide more information for the diagnosis. The meningeal involvement rarely occurs.

HIV/AIDS related cerebral cysticercosis with multiple ring shaped or nodular enhancements should be differentiated from metastatic tumors and multiple tuberculoma. Cases of metastatic tumor usually have case history of primary tumor, with obvious edema around the focus. By enhanced scanning, there are different sized foci with ring shaped and nodular enhancement, different thickness of the wall and distribution at the interface between cortex and medulla. Singular large cyst should be differentiated from dermoid cyst, epidermoid cyst and arachnoid cyst. Multiple small cysts should be differentiated from brain metastatic tumor. Due to the different number of cysticercus for intracerebral invasion and different location of their invasion, as well as different developmental process and death time of cysticercus, the CT scanning demonstrations are complex and diverse. MR imaging definitely demonstrates abnormal findings in the early stage of cerebral cysticercosis. Plain and enhanced CT scanning and MR imaging can increase the detection rate of cerebral cysticercosis foci, as well as the diagnostic accuracy.

Discussion

After the intake of cysticercus larvae by human, they are hatched in the intestinal tract for general distribution and infections of muscles and brain tissues are especially common. Cerebral cysticercosis refers to the infection of the central nervous system by larvae of pork tapeworm, which is a parasitic disease. The death of larvae causes strong responses in the hosts, resulting in a wide range of brain edema. The clinical manifestations include recurrent epilepsic seizures, as well as dementia, basal cistern meningitis, increased intracranial pressure and arachnoiditis. Intraventricular cysticercus can spread along with the flow of cerebrospinal fluid, resulting in acute obstructive hydrocephalus. MR imaging demonstrates long T1 long T2 signal of cysticercus in the brain parenchyma, possible finding scolex in the cyst of cysticercus and surrounding edema. AIDS patients have no immune mediation due to their immunocompromised immunity. Therefore, HIV/AIDS related cerebral cysticercosis is commonly manifested as the vesicular period and the colloid period, with no pathological changes of granuloma and calcification.

13.3.2.3 HIV/AIDS Related Trichinosis
Pathogens and Pathogenesis

Trichinosis is a worldwide zoonotic parasitic disease. Commonly due to intake of raw or undercooked pork containing trichinella larvae cysts, it occurs in human. Larvae invasion into the brain causes lesions of central nervous system, with secondary occurrence of non-purulent meningitis and other central nervous system infections.

Pathophysiological Basis

Cerebral trichinosis is caused by invasion of trichinella into brain tissue, resulting in general strong allergic and toxic responses as well as local inflammatory responses and necrosis of local brain tissues.

Clinical Manifestations and Signs

After cerebral infection, symptoms of meningeal encephalitis occur including severe headache, unconsciousness, convulsion of the limbs, paralysis, aphasia and coma. Death may occur within 5–6 weeks after the onset of the disease.

Examinations and Their Selection

1. Cerebrospinal fluid: increased pressure and protein content, increased number of eosinophilic granulocyte and occasional findings of the larvae.
2. Diagnostic imaging: CT scanning and MR imaging are diagnostic imaging of choice. They facilitate to define the size, morphology and location of the foci. They can also be used to assess the therapeutic efficacy.

Imaging Demonstrations

CT scanning demonstrates multiple flaky low density shadow in the brain parenchyma, with unclearly defined borderline and obvious edema and space occupying effects. Enhanced scanning demonstrates nodular and flaky abnormal enhancement. MR imaging demonstrates multiple scattering nodular and flaky long T2 signal in the brain parenchyma, obviously thickened meninges, deepened and widened brain sulcis and enlarged sylvian cistern. Enhanced imaging demonstrates multiple nodular and ring shaped abnormal enhancement in the brain parenchyma, linear abnormal enhancement of the meninges, finger liked or fire flame liked obvious brain tissue edema and unobvious space occupying effect.

Case Study

A male patient aged 57 years was confirmatively diagnosed as having AIDS by the CDC. He had a history of paid blood donation in 1992, and was diagnosed as AIDS in 2002. And in 2003, he was admitted to hospital due to complaints of general soreness and pain, edema, and red rash for a week. One week before his hospitalization, he had fever, night sweats, general weakness, difficulty swallowing, coarse breathing and flustering. The history of present illness includes fever, headache, retarded response in communicating, along with right side limbs weakness and stiffness. His CD4 T cell count was 25/μl.

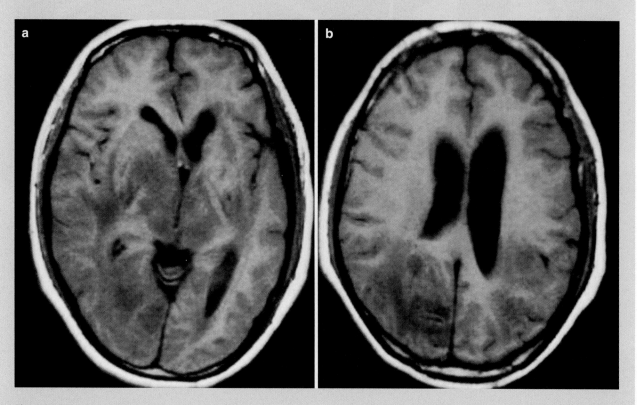

Fig. 13.39 (a–g) HIV/AIDS related cerebral trichinosis. (a–d) Enhanced axial MR imaging of IV-Gd-DTPA demonstrates multiple flaky long T1WI and long T2WI signals in the brain, obvious edema and unobvious space occupying effect. (e, f) Enhanced axial and sagittal MR imaging of IV-Gd-DTPA demonstrates multiple nodular and some ring shaped obviously abnormal enhancement in the brain, thickened meninges and abnormal enhancement in the left occipital lobe. (g) Pathological examination under an optical microscope demonstrates curled larvae of trichinella, which is surrounded by inflammatory cells to form granuloma

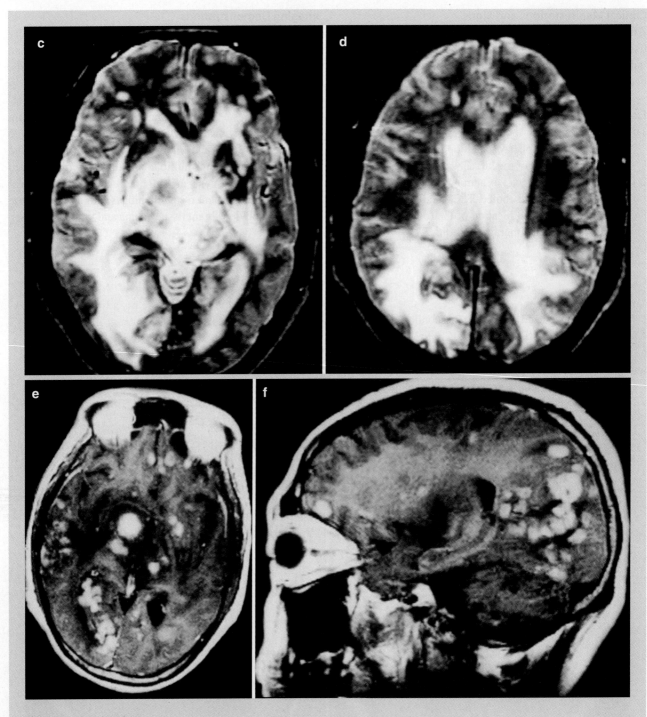

Fig. 13.39 (continued)

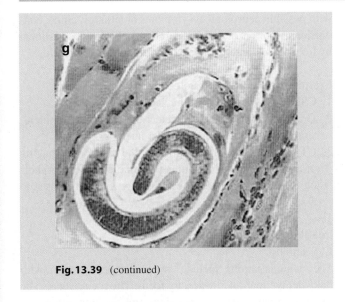

Fig. 13.39 (continued)

Criteria for the Diagnosis
1. Epidemiological data is valuable reference for the differential diagnosis. It has a history of intake raw pork 1–2 weeks (1–4 days) before the onset of the disease.
2. Clinical manifestations include fever, muscular pain, edema and skin rash. In the early stage, gastrointestinal symptoms may occur, with significantly increased total number of leukocytes and eosinophilic granulocytes.
3. Qualitative diagnosis depends on muscle biopsy to find larvae.
4. Serological tests: Trichinella antigens can be divided into the parasite antigens, parasite soluble antigen, surface antigen, and excretory-secretory antigen. Immunological test has both high specificity and sensitivity. The applicable immunological tests for the early diagnosis include indirect fluorescent antibody test (IFA), indirect hemagglutination assay (IHA), enzyme-linked immunosorbent assay (ELISA) and indirect immunoenzyme staining test (IEST).
5. CT scanning and MR imaging demonstrate foci commonly in the cortex and medulla area as well as the basal ganglia, with obvious brain tissues edema and slight space occupying effect. Enhanced CT scanning or MR imaging demonstrates irregular nodular and flaky enhancement, with occasional ring shaped enhancement.

Differential Diagnosis
1. HIV/AIDS related cerebral trichinosis should be differentiated from tuberculous brain abscess.
2. HIV/AIDS related brain trichinosis should be differentiated from toxoplasmic encephalitis.
3. HIV/AIDS related cerebral trichinosis should be differentiated from brain lymphoma.
4. HIV/AIDS related cerebral trichinosis should be differentiated from cryptococcal encephalitis.
5. HIV/AIDS related cerebral trichinosis should be differentiated from food poisoning (early stage) and diseases with increased eosinophilic granulocyte such as nodular polyarteritis, rheumatic fever, dermatomyositis, leptospirosis and epidemic hemorrhagic fever.

Discussion
Imaging demonstrations of HIV/AIDS related cerebral trichinella infection have been rarely reported. Its pathogen is trichinella, which was initially found by a British scholar James Panes Paget during an autopsy in 1835 in London, with the nomination of trichinella. Trichinosis is a zoonotic parasitic disease caused by trichinella spiralis. Its pathogenicity is related to the factors of the amount of intake larvae cysts and their vitality, and the host's immune status. The slight cases may be asymptomatic, while the severe cases may die from it. HIV/AIDS related cerebral trichinella infection occurs in patients with compromised immunity. The severe cases may have involvement of the central nervous system. The incidence of trichinella infection with involvement of the central nervous system is about 10–24 %. It was reported in the United States in 1987 that inflammatory infiltration of the central nervous system might be the brain lesions caused by antigen substances secreted by Trichinella spiralis [104]. The pathogenic processes include migration of the larvae, vascular occlusion or eosinophilic granulocytes infiltration. However, these speculations have not been scientifically proven. Trichinella infection of the central nervous system is often fatal. The patient in the case study had clinical manifestations as encephalitis and meningitis reported in literature. CT scanning and MR imaging are sensitive to intracerebral lesions. Therefore, slight lesions in brain cortex and white matter can be diagnosed by CT scanning and MR imaging. Due to the rare occurrence of HIV/AIDS related cerebral trichinella infection, our knowledge about it remains limited, which constitutes the main reason for its misdiagnosis. The key point for its differential diagnosis from lymphoma is the findings of the foci commonly at the interface between cortex and medulla, but rarely in deep brain.

13.3.3 HIV/AIDS Related Intracerebral Viral Infections

13.3.3.1 Cytomegalovirus Encephalitis
Pathogens and Pathogenesis
Cytomegalovirus (CMV) infection occurs worldwide and human is its only host. Its incidence rate is different in different countries and different regions with different economic status. The infection begins with primary detoxification,

often lasting for several weeks, months or even years, which then progresses into its latent period. The latent virus can be reactivated to cause recurrence of the infection. The clinical manifestations of CMV infection are related to immunity of the individual and his/her age. The infection of the central nervous system is commonly via placenta, occurring only in population with cellular immunodeficiency. In patients with AIDS, acquired intracerebral CMV infection causes an increased incidence of cytomegalovirus encephalitis. CMV infection in adults is closely related to the immunity, with possible occurrence of vasculitis, retinal inflammation, pneumonia and gastrointestinal infections. In most cases, the complication of Lattice-Barr syndrome can also occur.

Pathophysiological Basis

CMV infection is a sexually transmitted disease caused by cytomegalovirus. Cytomegalovirus is a DNA virus. Its characteristic lesions are enlarged infected cells, eosinophilic and basophilic inclusion bodies in the respective nuclei and cytoplasm.

Clinical Symptoms and Signs

The clinical manifestations are commonly fever, respiratory symptoms, neurological symptoms and blood symptoms. The body temperature may range from low grade fever to 40 °C,

with possible neurological symptoms of lethargy, coma, convulsions, motion disorders, cerebral palsy, and occasional hydrocephalus, intelligence decline and retinochoroiditis.

Examinations and Their Selection

1. CSF test can detect mononucleosis.
2. Urinary sediment test can detect the characteristic inclusion bodies in the magnocellular nucleus.
3. CT scanning and MR imaging are the diagnostic imaging of choice. Both can facilitate to define the size, morphology and localization of the foci. They can also be used to assess the therapeutic efficacy.

Imaging Demonstrations

CT Scanning

The demonstrations include involved basal ganglia with flaky demyelination low density focus. The focus can also be found in paraventricular area, pons and medulla oblongata, with unclearly defined borderline and unobvious space occupying effect.

MR Imaging

Demonstrations include flaky long T1 long T2 signal in the basal ganglia, with obvious edema and space occupying effect. Enhanced imaging demonstrates no enhancement.

Case Study 1

A male patient aged 26 years was confirmatively diagnosed as having AIDS by the CDC. He had a history of drug abuse, with symptoms of headache, lethargy and unconsciousness for 1 month. His CD4 T cell count was 15/μl.

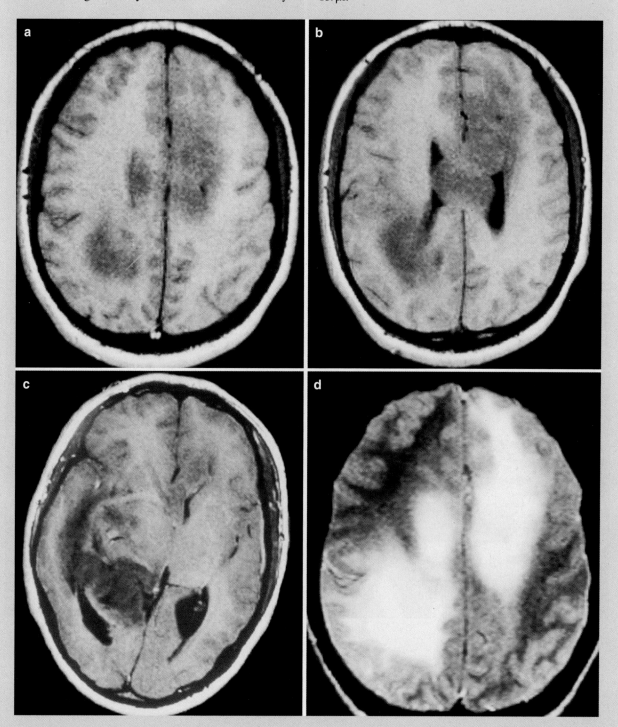

Fig. 13.40 (**a–m**) HIV/AIDS related cytomegalovirus encephalitis. (**a–c**) MR imaging demonstrates large flaky long T1 signal in bilateral parietal lobes and the right temporal lobe, with obvious surrounding edema of the brain tissue and obvious space occupying effect. (**d–f**) MR imaging demonstrates large flaky long T2 signal in bilateral parietal lobes, the right temporal lobe and the brainstem, with obvious surrounding edema of the brain tissue and obvious space occupying effect. (**g, h**) MR imaging demonstrates large flaky long T1 signal in the right temporal lobe, with obvious surrounding edema of the brain tissue and obvious space occupying effect. (**i–k**) Enhanced coronal MR imaging of IV-gd-DTPA demonstrates uneven slight enhancement of the right temporal lobe, with no central enhancement. (**l, m**) Enhanced axial MR imaging of IV-Gd-DTPA demonstrates uneven slight enhancement of the right temporal lobe, with no central enhancement; and narrowed right lateral ventricle due to compression

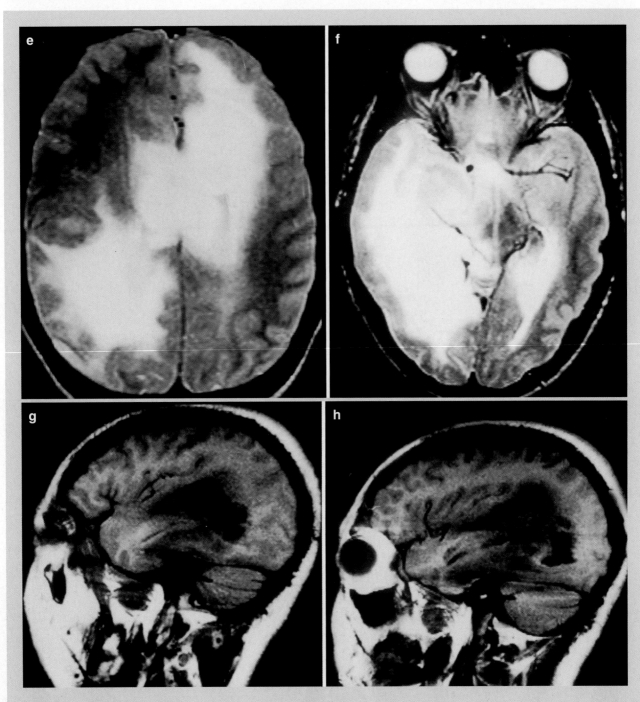

Fig.13.40   (continued)

Fig. 13.40 (continued)

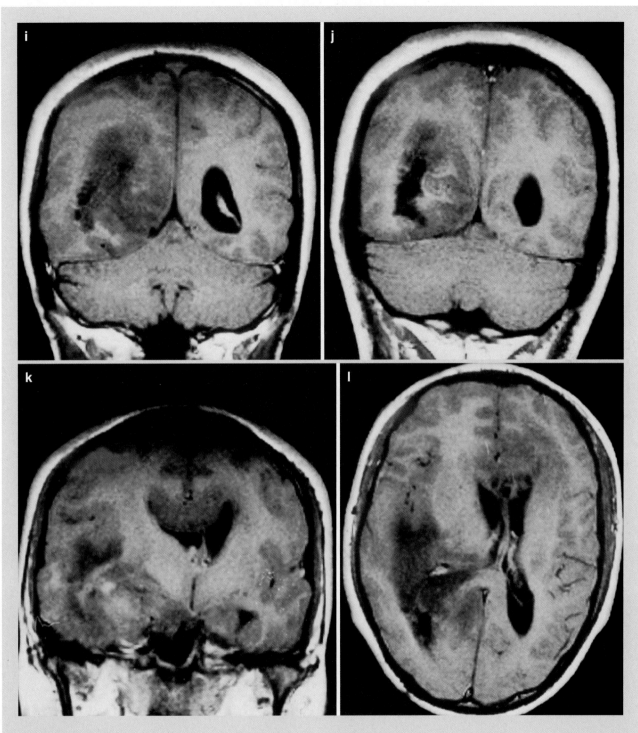

Fig. 13.40 (continued)

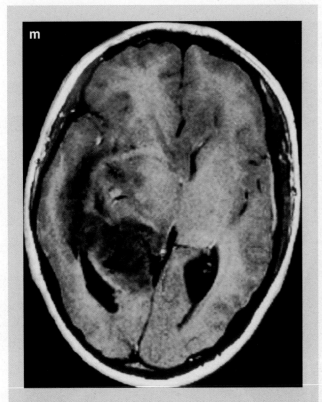

Fig. 13.40 (continued)

Case Study 2

An AIDS patient was confirmatively diagnosed by the CDC. The patient had a history of paid blood donation in 1995, and was definitively diagnosed in March 2004. The patient had symptoms of skin herpes, floaters in front of the eyes and blurry vision. In Dec. 2005, the patient complained of fever, headache, vomiting, irritation and unconsciousness. The CD4 T cell count was 10/μl.

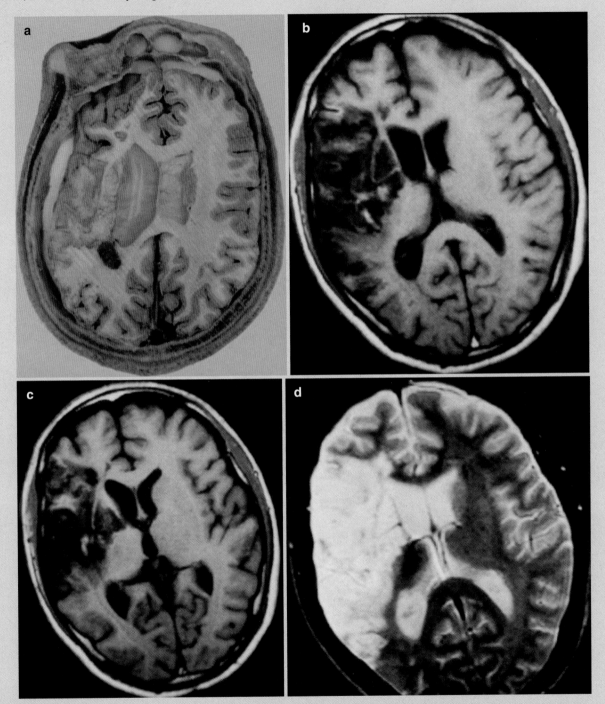

Fig. 13.41 (a–i) HIV/AIDS related cytomegalovirus encephalitis. (a) The cross sectional specimen demonstrates liquefaction, necrosis and absence of brain tissue in the right temporal parietal lobe, with purplish brown hematoma, and expansion of the right lateral ventricular top. (b–e) MR imaging demonstrates large flaky long T1 long T2 signals in the right temporal parietal lobe, with unobvious surrounding edema of the brain tissues and unobvious space occupying effect; deepened and widened brain sulci; and enlarged ventricles. (f, g) MRA demonstrates absent shadow of the right middle cerebral artery and fine anterior communicating artery. (h) It is demonstrated that cerebral CMV infection, with focal liquefaction and necrosis of the brain tissue, small quantity infiltration of chronic inflammatory cells and multiple maglocytic inclusion body. (i) It is demonstrated that cerebral liquefaction and necrosis of the brain tissue, with large quantity glial scars formation; obvious congestion of the residual tissues

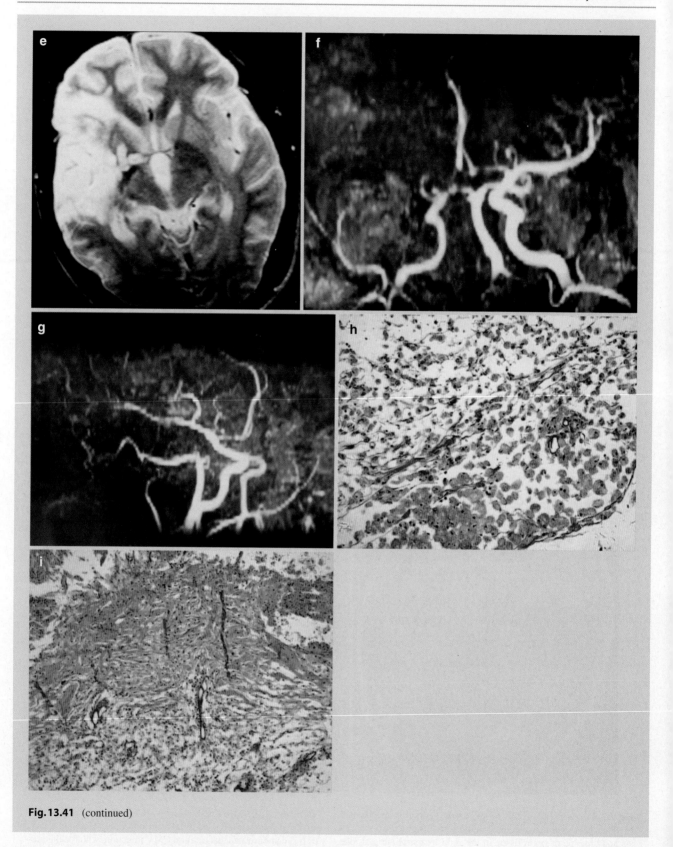

Fig. 13.41 (continued)

Case Study 3

A female patient aged 43 years was confirmatively diagnosed as having AIDS by the CDC. She had a history of extramarital affair and had symptoms of fever, headache, vomiting, irritation and unconsciousness. Her CD4 T cell count was 25/μl.

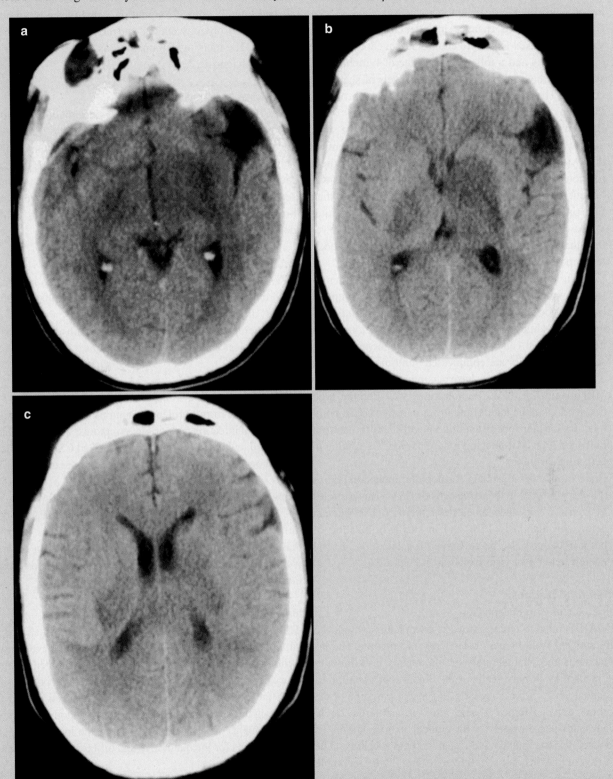

Fig. 13.42 (a–c) HIV/AIDS related cytomegalovirus encephalitis. CT scanning demonstrates symmetric low density areas in bilateral basal ganglia areas, with unclearly defined borderline and unobvious space occupying effect; communication between the left sylvian cistern and temporal horn

Criteria for the Diagnosis

1. The cases with a history of virus infection have an acute onset, with clinical manifestations of fever, headache, drowsiness, coma, convulsions, and progressive worsening of neuropsychiatric symptoms.
2. Cerebrospinal fluid changes include clear appearance, slightly increased leukocyte count with an early increase of neutrophils and a following increase of lymphocytes, slightly increased protein and normal levels of sugar and chloride. The isolation of the virus from the cerebrospinal fluid can define the diagnosis.
3. By serum neutralization test, the titers in the acute stage and that in the convalescent stage may show a difference of up to more than four times. By serum complement fixation test, the titer in the acute stage and in the convalescent stage may show a difference of up to more than four times. By hemagglutination inhibition test, the titer in the convalescent stage is four times higher or lower than that in the acute stage. Immunofluorescent antibody test is positive.
4. CT scanning demonstrates normal. In some cases, there is focal low density area in unilateral or bilateral temporal lobe, Hippocampus and its surrounding system and commonly spots high density area that indicates hemorrhagic necrosis, which can further define the diagnosis. For the severe cases, there are compressed ventricles, migration of the midline and other space occupying effects.
5. MR imaging of T2WI demonstrates well defined high density area in the middle and lower parts of the temporal lobe, the insular lobe extending upwards and the bottom of frontal lobe. MR imaging is superior to CT scanning in detecting early foci.
6. Brain biopsy demonstrates eosinophilic inclusion bodies (Cowdry A type) in the nerve cells or HSV virus particles in the nerve cells under an electron microscope, either can define the diagnosis. PCR and in situ hybridization of brain tissue can also be performed for detection of viral nucleic acid or for virus isolation and culture.

Differential Diagnosis

Herpes Zoster Virus Encephalitis

HIV/AIDS related cytomegalovirus encephalitis should be differentiated from herpes zoster virus encephalitis. Herpes zoster virus encephalitis rarely occurs, mainly invading into and incubating in nerve cells of the dorsal root ganglion of the spinal nerve or the nerve cells of sensory ganglion of the cerebral nerve. Herpes zoster virus encephalitis rarely invades the nerve system, with clinical manifestations of unconsciousness, ataxia and focal cerebral lesions. The severity of the lesions is relatively slight, with favorable prognosis. The patients commonly have a history of zoster in chest or lower back skin. By serum and cerebrospinal fluid tests, the antigens, antibodies and nucleic acid of herpes

zoster virus can be detected. Cranial CT scanning demonstrates flake or mass shaped low density area in cortex of the brain hemisphere, with obvious edema and no obvious hemorrhagic necrosis. MR imaging demonstrates flake and mass shaped long T1 long T2 signal in cortex of the brain hemisphere, with obvious edema and no obvious hemorrhagic necrosis. The imaging demonstrations can be applied for differential diagnosis.

Enterovirus Encephalitis

HIV/AIDS related cytomegalovirus encephalitis should be differentiated from enterovirus encephalitis. Enterovirus encephalitis is one of the common causes of viral meningitis and viral encephalitis. Its clinical manifestations include fever, unconsciousness, balance disorders, recurrent epilepsy seizures, and paralysis of limbs. Virus isolation from cerebrospinal fluid or PCR examination positive can help to define the diagnosis.

Acute Disseminated Encephalomyelitis (ADEM)

HIV/AIDS related cytomegalovirus encephalitis should be differentiated from acute disseminated encephalomyelitis. Acute disseminated encephalomyelitis has complex and diverse clinical symptoms and signs, with disturbance of consciousness and psychiatric symptoms.

Purulent Meningitis

HIV/AIDS related cytomegalovirus encephalitis should be differentiated from purulent meningitis. Purulent meningitis has general infection and serious symptoms, with significantly increased leukocytes in CSF, porridge liked CSF and findings of pathogenic bacteria by CSF bacteria culture or smear.

Tuberous Sclerosis

HIV/AIDS related cytomegalovirus encephalitis should be differentiated from tuberous sclerosis. Tuberous sclerosis has lesions of nodular calcification in the margin of brain ventricles and calcification in the subcortex area and cerebellum, with common findings of tumorous nodules.

Brain Tumor

HIV/AIDS related cytomegalovirus encephalitis should be differentiated from brain tumor. Both diseases have demonstrations of increased intracranial pressure. However, both primary and metastatic brain tumors have long-term progression, with increased CSF protein contents. Enhanced cranial CT scanning and MR imaging demonstrates obviously abnormal enhancement, which facilitate to define the location and size of the lesions for the qualitative and differential diagnosis.

Discussion

CMV infection is a common opportunistic infection in AIDS patients, often disseminating to involve the nervous system.

It causes encephalitis, meningoencephalitis, necrotic ependymitis, ventriculitis, choroid plexus inflammation and radiculitis. It has been internationally reported that 1–2 % AIDS patients have neurological diseases caused by CMV. CMV encephalitis is commonly subacute and diffuse, with characteristic lesions of viral inclusions and dense microglial nodules. CMV encephalitis is more frequent in advanced stage of AIDS, occurring when CD4 T cell count being lower than 50/μl. The clinical symptoms include neuropsychiatric symptoms, fever, and even nerve inhibition conditions. Diagnostic imaging demonstrates local edema, slight or no space occupying effect. Enhanced imaging demonstrates no or slight enhancement. MR imaging demonstrates flaky long T1 long T2 signal in areas surrounding brain ventricles. The findings of CMV infection of other organs can help to define the diagnosis.

13.3.3.2 HIV/AIDS Related Progressive Multifocal Leukoencephalopathy

Pathogens and Pathogenesis

Progressive multifocal leukoencephalopathy (PML) is a subacute demyelinating disease of the central nervous system due to compromised immunity. It has two predisposing factors, including a history of contacting JC virus and T cells related defense inhibition. JC virus has a worldwide distribution. Due to the compromised immunity of the host's T lymphocytes targeting JC virus, the host's immunity fails to suppress the reactivation of JC virus. Therefore, JC virus can continue its replication and dissemination. It has been proven that JC virus from papovavirus family and SV-40 (Simian virus) are the pathogens of progressive multifocal leukoencephalopathy. Onset of the disease in viruses' carriers is related to the dysfunctional immunity of the body. Studies by immunofluorescence and in situ hybridization have demonstrated that infection of papovavirus to cerebral stellate cells and oligodendrocytes in immunosuppressed patients is the cause of Progressive multifocal leukoencephalopathy.

Pathophysiological Basis

The incidence of HIV/AIDS related PML is more than 4 %. Serological studies have demonstrated that papovaviruses invade most people but with no symptoms. But for people with low level immune responses or immunodeficiency, the viruses incubating in the body are activated to cause the disease. The pathological changes include selectively destroyed oligodendrocytes by papovaviruses, multifocal lesions in the white matter to cause fusion of demyelinated foci. The cerebral hemisphere is more vulnerable than cerebellum, especially subcortex and the interface between gray and white matters. By gross observation in autopsy, multiple focal swelling plaques of demyelination can be found, yellowish diffuse asymmetric particles of fusion foci in the white matter, and the size of fused demyelination being up to several centimeters. Microscopy demonstrates demyelinated focus that is especially obvious in subcortex white matter, fusion of demyelination plaques into large demyelination area, presence of axon, absence of oligodendrocytes and medullary sheath, enlarged oligodendrocytes containing large eosinophilic nucleus inclusion bodies around the focus. There are also unclearly defined structure of eosinophilic nucleus inclusion bodies, decreased stellate neurons and slight inflammatory responses. Transmission electron microscopy demonstrates viruses in crystalline arrangement, with a size of 33–39 nm, large deformed stellate cells with pleomorphic lobulated nuclei and large quantity foamy macrophages. The virus has been isolated from the brain tissue of PML patients and the majority is papovavirus (JC virus).

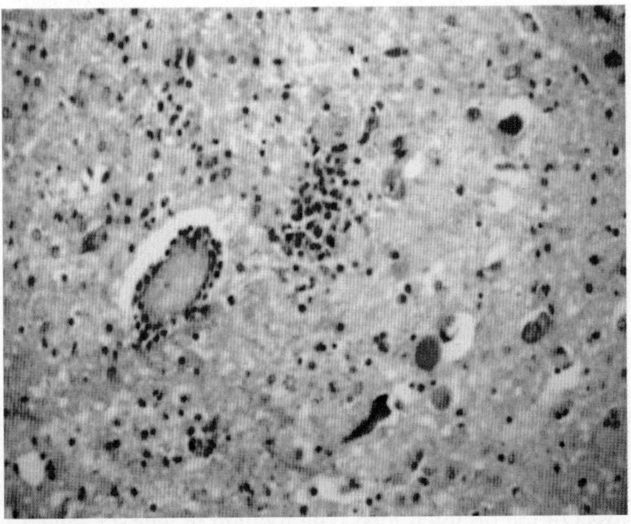

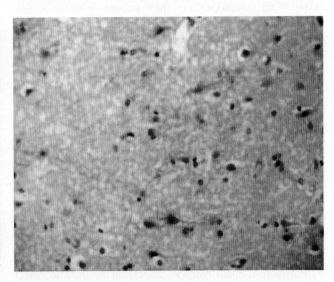

Fig. 13.43 HE staining demonstrates microglial nodules adjacent to the minor vascular vessels in the brain tissues (200×)

Fig. 13.44 HE staining demonstrates edema and demyelination in the brain tissue, especially obvious in the left brain tissue (200×)

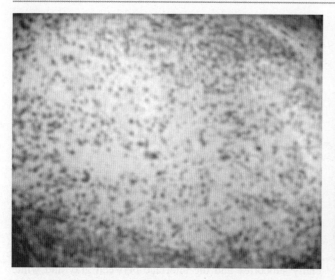

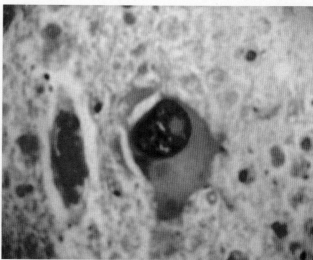

Fig. 13.45 It is demonstrated to have demyelinating lesions in the brain tissue of the patient, sparse myelin and visible multinuclear stellate cells

Fig. 13.46 It is demonstrated to have infected oligodendrocytes in the middle, with enlarged volume and large nucleus containing light red hyaloid substances (virus inclusion body)

Clinical Symptoms and Signs

HIV/AIDS related progressive multifocal leukoencephalopathy is common in male adults, with a hideous onset and diverse clinical manifestations. The disease occurs in any age group, with no definite incidence. The occurrence of PML is increasingly frequent with the wide spread of AIDS, about 2–5 % AIDS patients have the complication of PML. The early symptoms of PML include progressive mental decline, personality change and mental deterioration and characteristic neurological disorders. Its progression commonly involves the cerebral hemispheres, with occurrence of ipsilateral vision disorders, hemiplegia, hemi sensory impairments, aphasia and apraxia. Based on the scope of demyelination, the functional disorders of other cortex occur. In the advanced stage, the conscious disorder occurs. During the whole course of its progression, fever and headache rarely occur. About 10 % patients experience headaches or epilepsy seizures, with poor prognosis. Death occurs mostly in 6–12 months after the onset of the disease.

Examinations and Their Selection

1. AIDS patients or patients with compromised immunity have clinical manifestations of focal neurological disorders can be suspected diagnosed as having PML.
2. Detection of JC antigen by immunohistochemistry and detection of virus nucleic acid by molecular hybridization are valuable information for the diagnosis.
3. Brain biopsy is a reliable examination, including observation of virus particles by electron microscopy or immune electron microscopy.
4. Polymerase chain reaction (PCR) can be used to detect viral DNA in the CSF, which helps to define the diagnosis.

5. CT scanning and MR imaging are the diagnostic imaging of the choice. CT scanning is less sensitive than MR imaging in finding foci. Both have diagnostic value in finding multiple lesions as well as their qualitative diagnosis and localization. HIV/AIDS related PML commonly involves subcortical white matter of the brain. MR imaging demonstrates HIV dementia to have multi-focal abnormalities in the white matter, which seems to be PML. But HIV dementia commonly has no focal neurological symptoms and signs.

Imaging Demonstrations

CT Scanning Demonstrations

Plain CT scanning demonstrates multiple foci in the distal area surrounding ventricular system, which locate in the subcortical white matter and commonly in the parietal occipital region with an uneven distribution. Early lesions are round or oval, with following gradual fusion of the foci to enlarge. The foci are in low density, with unclearly defined borderline. Enhanced scanning demonstrates no enhancement of most foci, with rarely found enhancement. The advanced stage is demonstrated to have enlarged ventricles, deepened and widened sulci and cerebral atrophy.

MR Imaging Demonstrations

Lesions are commonly located in the frontal parietal lobe and temporal white matter, sometimes with involvement of deep gray matter. Patients with HIV/AIDS related PML have concurrent involvement of the gray matter in 50 % cases. About 1/3 patients have their lesions in the posterior cranial fossa of the occipital lobe. The foci are in long T1 long T2 signal, with clearly defined borderlines.

Case Study 1

A male patient aged 32 years was confirmatively diagnosed as having AIDS by the CDC. He had a history of drug abuse since the year of 1998. He complained of psychiatric disorder, disorder of consciousness, blurry vision and ataxia. His CD4 T cell count was 0/μl.

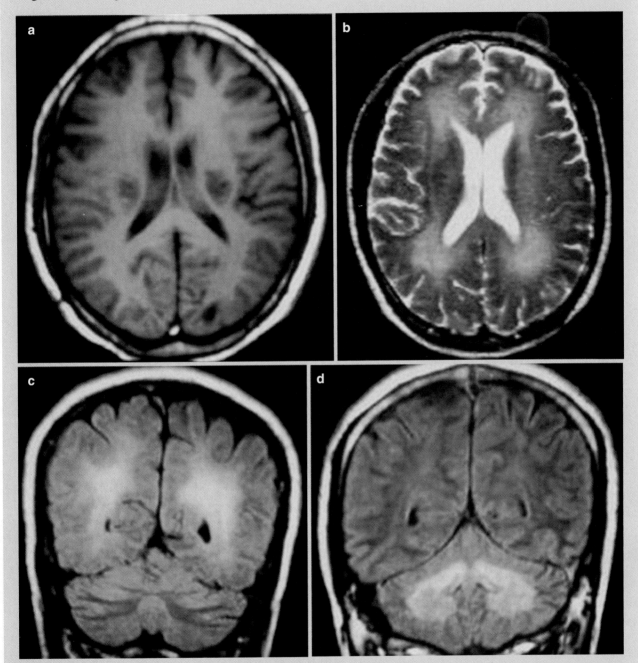

Fig. 13.47 (a–d) HIV/AIDS related PML. (a) MR imaging demonstrates symmetrical long T1 signal in bilateral basal ganglia, with quite clearly defined boundaries; no obvious edema and space occupying effect. (b) It is demonstrated to have symmetrical long T2 signal surrounding the bilateral lateral ventricles. (c, d) It is demonstrated to have symmetrical slightly short T1 signal surrounding bilateral lateral ventricles and in the cerebellar dentate nuclei, with no edema and space occupying effect

Case Study 2

An AIDS patient was confirmatively diagnosed by the CDC. She/he complained of recurrent herpes zoster, oral ulcers and facial acne for more than 3 years, with intermittent fever, malnutrition, gradual weight loss, unclear language expressions, central nervous facial palsy, shallow right nasolabial fold, being unable to stick out his/her tongue, dysphagia and weakness of the right upper limbs. MR imaging demonstrated multiple space occupying lesions in bilateral cerebral hemisphere and brainstem.

Laboratory tests demonstrated HIV antibody positive and inverse CD4/CD8 cell counts. She/he was highly suspected to have PML. PML, caused by HIV virus, is a space occupying and infiltrative disease with a rapid progression. The diagnosis mainly depends on pathological examinations, namely brain biopsy. Craniotomy was performed to collect specimens for biopsy. The following pathological examination confirmed the diagnosis of AIDS complicated by progressive multifocal leukoencephalopathy.

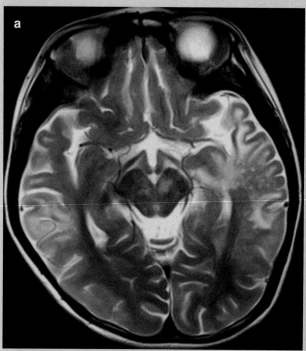 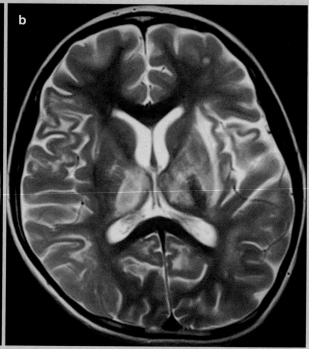

Fig. 13.48 (a–e) HIV/AIDS related PML. (a) It is demonstrated to have spots and flakes of long T2 signal in the left temporal lobe and mesocephalon, with unobvious edema and space occupying effect. (b) MR imaging demonstrates flakes of long T2 signal in bilateral basal ganglia, which is more obvious in the left basal ganglia, with quite clearly defined boundaries and with no obvious edema and space occupying effect. (c) It is demonstrated to have symmetrical flakes of long T2 signal in bilateral semioval centrum, which is more obvious in the left semioval centrum. (d) DTI demonstrates decreased blue (ascending or descending nerve fiber bundles) and green (anterior and posterior running of the nerve fiber bundles) areas in the left semioval centrum, and obvious red (horizontal running of the nerve fiber bundles) area. There are also slight elevated MRS NAA wave peak and elevated Cr wave peak

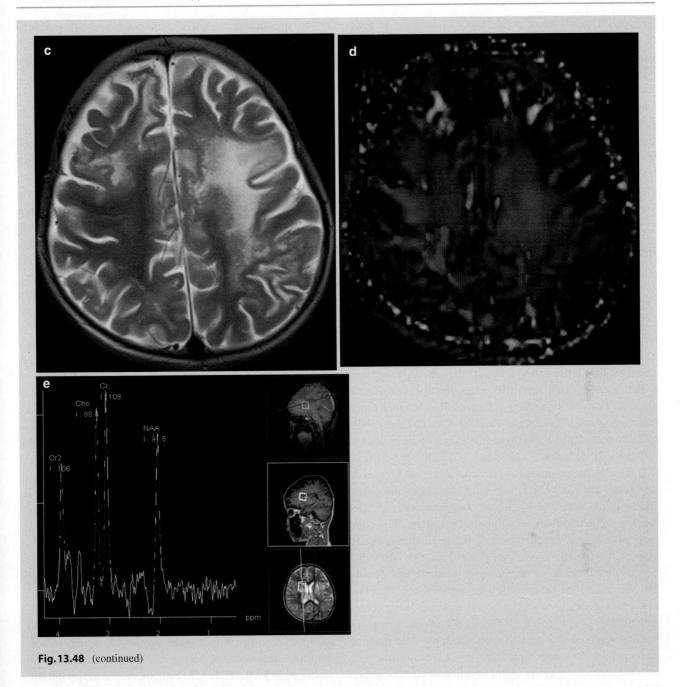

Fig. 13.48   (continued)

Criteria for the Diagnosis

1. The biopsy and pathological demonstrations are characterized by multifocal subacute demyelination of the white matter.
2. Immunocytochemistry demonstrates viral antigens. In situ hybridization and PCR can be applied to detect JC virus genes in brain tissues or CSF.
3. CT scanning demonstrates focal or diffuse white matter lesions, mostly in the white matter of distal ventricular system of the parietooccipital area with involved frontal lobe and rarely in the brainstem and cerebellum.

The foci are demonstrated as low density shadows, with unclearly defined borderlines. Enhanced scanning demonstrates no enhancement of most foci, with rarely found enhancement.

4. MR imaging demonstrates long T1 long T2 signal of the focus. Enhanced imaging demonstrates abnormal enhancement of the focus.

Differential Diagnosis

HIV/AIDS related progressive multifocal leukoencephalopathy has no specific demonstrations. Therefore, its definitive diagnosis depends on cerebral biopsy or autopsy. In terms of diagnostic imaging, it should be differentiated from other white matter diseases. The characteristic imaging findings of HIV/AIDS related PML include multiple lesions commonly distal to the surrounding tissues of the ventricular system, lesions commonly localized in the subcortical white matter of parietooccipital lobe, with gradual fusion and enlargement. However, it is difficult to be differentiated from other infectious demyelination diseases, such as (1) HIV encephalitis: HIV infectious demyelination has common manifestations of dementia and total loss of brain functions, while PML has manifestations of limited loss of brain functions. In terms of diagnostic imaging, HIV/AIDS related PML is difficult to be differentiated from demyelination diseases caused by HIV/AIDS related encephalopathy. Lesions of HIV/AIDS related infectious demyelination are more diffuse and symmetric, mostly being adjacent to the ventricles, while lesions of PML are commonly subcortical, asymmetric and multifocal. By T1WI, lesion of PML is in low signal, while HIV infectious demyelination is in equal signal by T1WI in its advanced stage. Early lesions of both diseases are in high signal by T1WI, presenting difficulty to their differentiation. It has been reported that MRI magnetization transformation (MT) can facilitate their differentiation. Magnetization transferring rates decrease in cases of both PML and HIV related encephalitis, being 26 and 38 % respectively and the difference is statistically significant. (2) Multiple sclerosis: It is the most common disease in demyelination diseases of the central nervous system, with unknown causes. Its illness course is characterized by recurrent aggravation and alleviation, with conditions being gradually worsen. The common pathological changes include scattered demyelinated plaques, destructed oligodendrocytes and vascular inflammation. Plain CT scanning demonstrates multiple low density patches around the lateral ventricles, especially in the anterior and posterior horns of the lateral ventricles, with recent and old foci mixing together. There may be concurrent low density shadows and equal density shadows. MR imaging demonstrates foci with high signal by T2WI, mostly with no space occupying effect. After injection of contrast agent, CT scanning demonstrates acute multiple sclerosis with its foci evenly enhanced. However, PML plaques are common in subcortical area, with no enhancement. Therefore, the two diseases can be differentiated. (3) Cerebrovascular disease: Cerebrovascular disease is one of the HIV/AIDS related neurological diseases. It may cause systemic vascular lesions and has clinical manifestations of brain atrophy, lacunar infarction and hemorrhagic necrosis. Brain atrophy is more commonly found in clinical practice. By CT scanning and MR imaging, there are worm bitten liked or multiple patches of foci, sometimes a large area brain infarction in unilateral brain that is asymmetric or symmetric. Enhanced scanning and imaging demonstrate varying degrees of enhancement or no enhancement. MRA demonstrates rough cerebral artery wall, stenosis of cerebral arteries, interrupted distal minor vascular vessels and weakened/absent blood flow signal. (4) Subcortical arteriosclerotic encephalopathy: It is a vasogenic demyelination disease. MR imaging demonstrates asymmetrical long T1 longT2 signal in the bilateral semi-oval centrum and paraventricular deep white matter, with no space occupying effect. There are also MR imaging demonstrations of enlarged ventricles and cisterns, widened sulci and brain atrophy, which have different locations from those demonstrations of PML. (5) Adrenal leukodystrophy: It is a rare recessive genetic disease and involves multi-system due to adipose metabolism disorder. It can be divided into four subtypes, with demyelinated areas being symmetrical distributed in the parietal, occipital and temporal white matters. Plain CT scanning demonstrates large flakes of symmetrical low density areas in the white matter around the triangle areas of the bilateral lateral ventricles, horizontal stripes of decreased density area in the corpus callosum, which across the midline to bridge the bilateral low density areas in the triangle areas. Enhanced CT scanning demonstrates stripe liked or ring shaped enhancement of the focal borders, which is active demyelinating process and perivascular mononuclear cells reaction, and manifestation of locally destructed blood–brain barrier. Adrenal leukodystrophy is significantly characterized by the progression of the lesions from the posterior to the anterior to gradually involve the occipital lobe, parietal lobe, temporal lobe and frontal lobe. Therefore, the manifestations of adrenal leukodystrophy are different from those of PML, and their differential diagnosis is less challenging.

Discussion

The imaging diagnosis of the disease should firstly define the diagnosis of AIDS or immunodeficiency caused by a variety of reasons. Its onset is generally implicit, with common manifestations of progressive psychiatric decline, personality and mental changes, memory loss, abnormal behaviors, identifying obstacles, ataxia and other symptoms, which indicate multifocal brain lesions. Mental changes are common manifestations of PML. Plain CT scanning demonstrates multiple lesions in the distal ventricular system, which is located in the subcortical white matter of the parietal occipital lobe with uneven distribution. The lesions were demonstrated as low density shadows, with unclearly defined borderlines and no space occupying effect. Enhanced scanning demonstrates no enhancement of most lesions and enhancement of the rare lesions. In the advanced stage of the disease, the manifestations are changes related to brain atrophy. MR imaging demonstrates lesions commonly located in the white matters of the frontal parietal lobe and temporal lobe, with deep gray matter involved in some cases. The foci are in long T1 long T2 signal, with clearly defined borderline. Some studies have demonstrated that lesions are commonly found in the white matter or at the interface of the gray and white matters due to the rich blood flow and staying of papovavirus infected B cells. The foci are in high signal by T2 weighted imaging and in low signal by T1 weighted imaging, which commonly have no space occupying effect but with fusion tendency. It has been reported that 23 % such patients have singular focus. It has been reported that some cases of PML may be demonstrated as intracerebral space occupying mass, which can be misdiagnosed as other diseases. Brain biopsy can define PML. In the year of 2010, the first case of HIV/AIDS related PML in China was definitively diagnosed in Peking union medical college hospital (Beijing, China). PML has a low incidence, with an average survival period of 0.5–1 year. Its treatment depends on HARRT, which can be effective with a therapeutic course of at least 3 months.

13.3.3.3 HIV/AIDS Related Herpes Simplex Virus Encephalitis

Pathogens and Pathogenesis

The pathogen of herpes simplex virus encephalitis (HSE) is the herpes simplex virus (HSV), which is a neurotropic DNA virus. The pathogenesis of HSV encephalitis is still unknown. HSV can be divided into two antigen subtypes, HSV-1 and HSV-2. HSE is commonly caused by HSV-1 and human is its unique natural host. HSV-1 infection is spread primarily via direct contacts to lesions or substances containing HSV-1 secretions, while HSV-2 infection can be transmitted via sexual contacts or to neonatals via the birth canal. HSV-2 infection can also spread via droplets. The virus invades the human body via mouth, respiratory tract and genital mucosa as well as skin defects. HSV tends to infect the sensory ganglia to cause incubated infection, which constitutes the primary reason for its recurrence. HSV is a soluble DNA virus particle, with HSV-1 incubating in the trigeminal ganglion and superior cervical ganglion, and HSV2 incubating in the sacral ganglion. When HSV-2 is attached to the peripheral nerve axis membrane, its shell is deprived, with the shell components and nucleic acid afferent to the neural nucleus. The virus replicates and proliferates, ultimately leading to death of nerve cells and tissues. The primary HSV infection has more severe clinical symptoms than the recurrent HSV infection, which may be related to the existence of antibodies and immune lymphocytes in infected patients. Studies have demonstrated that immunosuppression or immunodeficiency can reactivate HSV and lead to sensory nerve damage and neurological dysfunction. Generally, after HSV infection, humoral and cellular immune responses play important roles in preventing the spread of virus and promoting the discovery of the disease. Therefore, viremia and disseminated organ infections rarely occur in a clinical context. When cellular immunity is immaturely developed or has functional deficiency or when humoral immunity has deficiency, HSV infection commonly is disseminated and fatal. By autopsy of HSV carriers with normal immunity, HSV-DNA can be detected in the brain. However, the predictors for HSV encephalitis have been unknown. Immunosuppression is commonly not related to HSV encephalitis. HSV encephalitis occurs commonly in population with immune activity and occurs rarely in serious cases of HIV/AIDS patients. Pathological demonstrations are focal hemorrhagic and necrotic encephalitis in the temporal lobe.

Physiopathologic Basis

Regardless of primary or recurrent, HSV infection has the same pathological changes. It is generally believed that HSV usually lives in the trigeminal nerve, the olfactory nerve or spinal posterior ganglion. When the immunity is compromised, HSV may be reactivated and spread into the brain. The main pathological changes of HSV include edema, malacia and hemorrhagic necrosis of the brain tissue that are diffuse in the bilateral cerebral hemispheres, with asymmetrical distribution. The foci are the most obvious in the temporal lobe, marginal system and frontal lobe, with occasional involvements of the occipital lobe, thalamus, pons and medulla oblongata. Necrosis of the cerebral cortex is often incomplete, with intact outer layer of the cortex. The secondary sulcus herniation in the temporal lobe is fatal. Microscopically, there are extensive degeneration and necrosis of nerve cells, microglia hyperplasia, degeneration and necrosis of the vascular wall, infiltration of large quantity lymphocytes around the meninges and blood vessels to form oversleeve sign. In the nerve cells and glial cells, some infected cells are demonstrated to have balloon liked change, with accompanying concentrated intranuclear genome. There are also intranuclear inclusions and multinucleated giant cells. VZV has the same manifestations. Under an electron microscope, DNA particles and antigens of HSV can be found in the inclusion. The prominent characteristic pathological changes of the disease include hemorrhagic necrosis of the brain parenchyma and intranuclear inclusions.

Clinical Symptoms and Signs

The clinical manifestation is focal encephalitis, with acute fever, confusion, abnormal behaviors, disorders of consciousness and possible occurrence of focal neurological abnormalities. However, symptoms of HSV encephalitis are non-specific. For the cases with all symptoms indicating encephalitis, their diagnosis should be considered the possibility of HSV encephalitis. The infection of the central nervous system is a rare complication of primary/recurrent peripheral HSV infection. On the contrary, neonatal infection of the central nervous system is a common type of HSV infection, accounting for above 70 % and is commonly demonstrated as HSV encephalitis. Its clinical symptoms include acute onset, fever, headache, vomiting, unusual behaviors, olfactory hallucination, speech impairment and

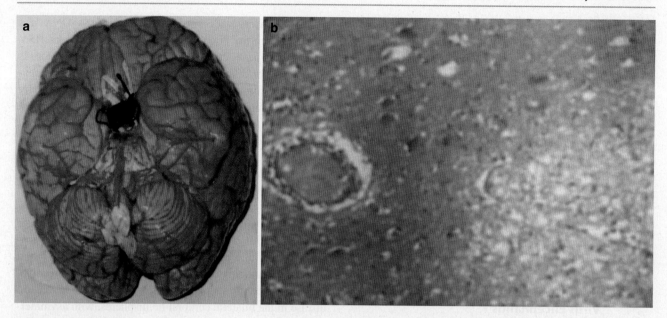

Fig. 13.49 (**a**, **b**) Herpes simplex virus encephalitis. (**a**) Gross observation of the specimen demonstrates cerebral edema, shallow sulci and widened gyri. (**b**) Histopathological analysis demonstrates liquid necrosis focus in the brain parenchyma, brain parenchymal congestion, perivascular infiltration of small quantity lymphocytes to form oversleeve sign (Provided by LANG, ZW)

focal epilepsy seizures. Some patients may suffer from disorientation, convulsion, cervical rigidity, slight paralysis and coma in a short term. The conditions are usually serious, with occurrence of death in the second week. Apart from the neonatal period, more than 95 % cases of HSV encephalitis are caused by HSV-1, which is the most common cause of acute sporadic virus encephalitis. In the prodromal stage, the clinical manifestations of HSV encephalitis include fever, headache, myalgia, drowsiness, epilepsy and other neuropsychiatric disorders, with an acute onset. The body temperature can be up to 38.4–40.0 °C. The following neurological symptoms include diffuse or focal brain lesions, with hemiopia, hemiplegia, aphasia, ophthalmoplegia, ataxia, hyperactivity and meningeal irritation.

Examinations and Their Selection

1. Blood test demonstrates increased peripheral WBC and accelerated erythrocyte sedimentation rate.
2. CSF test demonstrates increased pressure in lumbar puncture, normal or slightly/moderately increased cell account in CSF.
3. PCR examination of HSV-DNA in ESF can be performed for its early and rapid diagnosis, with high sensitivity and specificity.
4. MR imaging is the diagnostic imaging of choice, which can clearly define the location, morphology and range of the lesions. The findings are valuable in defining the diagnosis, assessing the severity and predicting the prognosis. CT scanning has less sensitivity to the lesions than MR imaging in the early diagnosis.
5. Brain biopsy, PCR of the brain tissues and in situ hybridization can also be used for detection of the virus nucleic acid in brain tissue or for virus isolation and culture.

Imaging Demonstrations

1. CT scanning demonstrates focal low density areas in unilateral/bilateral temporal lobe, hippocampus and marginal system. For the cases with high density spots, hemorrhagic necrosis is indicated, which provides evidence for the diagnosis. In serious cases, patients may have space occupying effects including ventricular compression and migration of the midline. Enhanced CT scanning demonstrates linear enhancement due to brain cells apoptosis, vascular hyperplasia and increased transparency of brain edema around the lesion.
2. MRI T2 weighted imaging demonstrates early lesions of flaky high signal area in spherical or mass like appearance in the middle and inferior temporal lobe, extending upwards to the insular lobe and frontal fundus, with clearly defined boundary from the surrounding tissues and commonly no involvement of the putamen, which is characteristic. Enhanced imaging demonstrates no abnormal enhancement. MR imaging is superior to CT scanning for early detection of the lesions.

Case Study 1

A female patient aged 40 years was confirmatively diagnosed as having AIDS by the CDC. She had a history of extramarital affair, with symptoms of mental disorders and skin herpes simplex. Her CD4 T cell count was 0/μl.

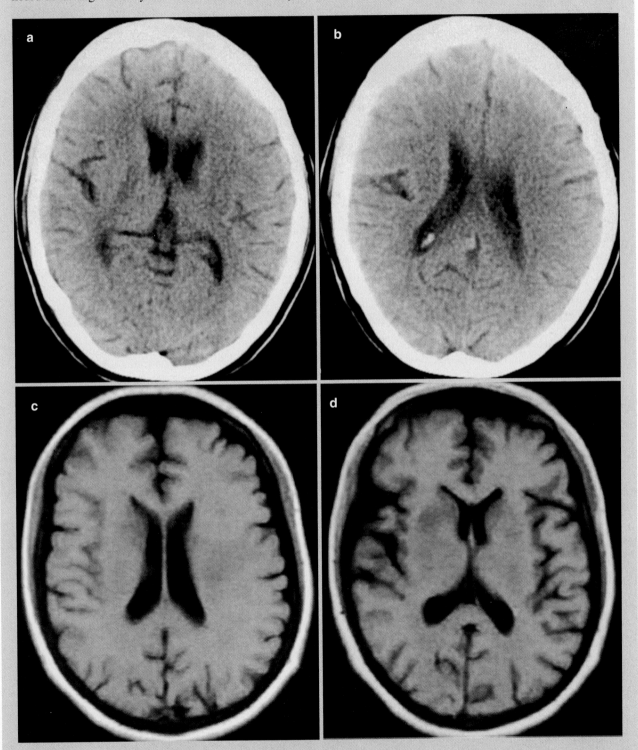

Fig. 13.50 (a–f) HIV/AIDS related herpes simplex virus encephalitis. (a, b) CT scanning demonstrates slightly low density area in bilateral basal ganglia, with unclearly defined boundary. (c, d) MR imaging demonstrates flaky long T1 signal in bilateral basal ganglia, with unclearly defined boundary. (e, f) MR imaging demonstrates flaky long T2 signal in bilateral basal ganglia, with unclearly defined boundary

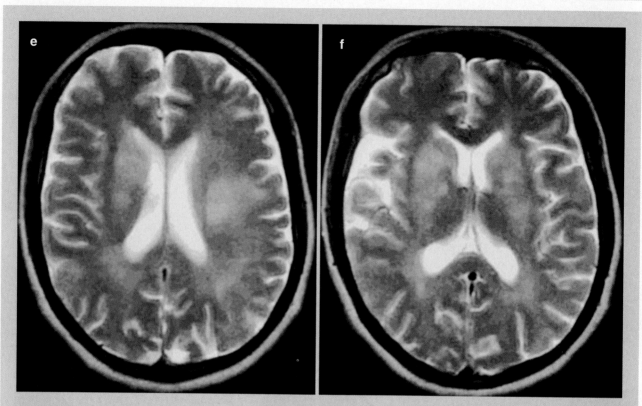

Fig. 13.50 (continued)

Case Study 2

A male patient aged 35 years was confirmatively diag-nosed as having AIDS by the CDC. He had a history of drug abuse, with symptoms of mental disorder and skin herpes simplex. His CD4 T cell count was 10/μl.

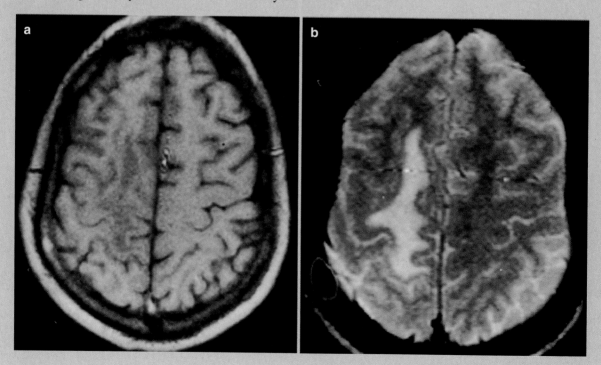

Fig. 13.51 (**a**, **b**) HIV/AIDS related herpes simplex virus encephalitis. (**a**, **b**) MR imaging demonstrates stripes long T1 and long T2 signals in the right parietal lobe, with obvious edema and no space occupying effect

Case Study 3

A female patient aged 40 years was confirmatively diagnosed as having AIDS by the CDC. She had a history of extramarital affair, with symptoms of mental disorder and skin herpes simplex. Her CD4 T cell count was 45/μl.

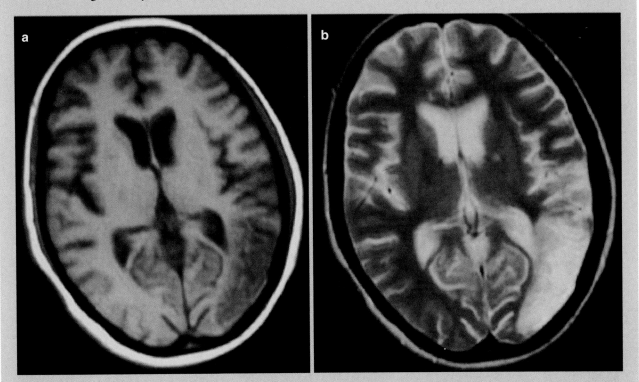

Fig. 13.52 (**a**, **b**) HIV/AIDS related herpes simplex virus encephalitis. (**a**, **b**) MR imaging demonstrates large flaky long T2 signal in the left temporal occipital lobe, and spots long T2 signal in the left basal ganglia

Case Study 4

A female patient aged 30 years was confirmatively diagnosed as having AIDS by the CDC. She had a history of extramarital affair, with symptoms of mental disorder. Her CD4 T cell count was 40/μl.

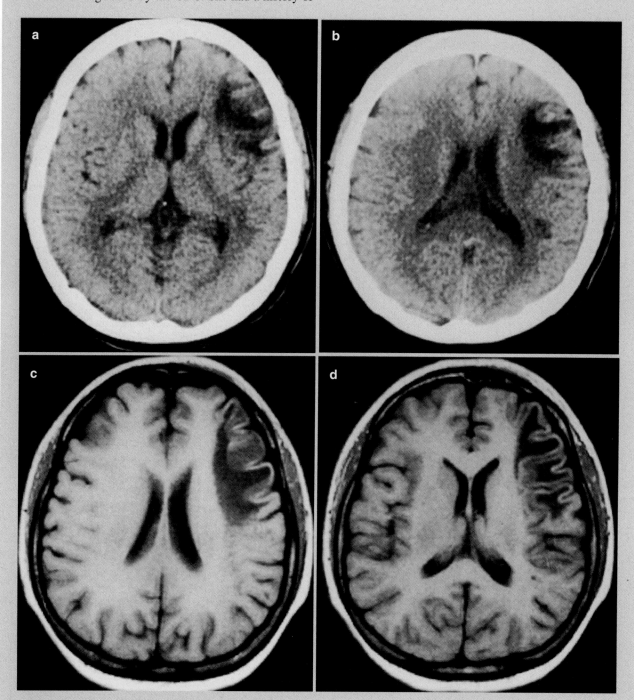

Fig. 13.53 (a–k) HIV/AIDS related herpes simplex virus encephalitis. (a, b) CT scanning demonstrates round liked low density shadow in the left frontal lobe, with swollen gyri and absent interface. (c–h) Axial MR imaging demonstrates large flaky long T1 long T2 signals in the left temporal lobe and the right occipital lobe, deepened and widened local sulci and reduced total brain volume. (i, j) Sagittal and coronal MR imaging demonstrates deepened and widened sulci in the left frontal lobe and temporal lobe and decreased total brain volume. (k) MRA demonstrates sparse distal blood vessels of the left middle cerebral artery

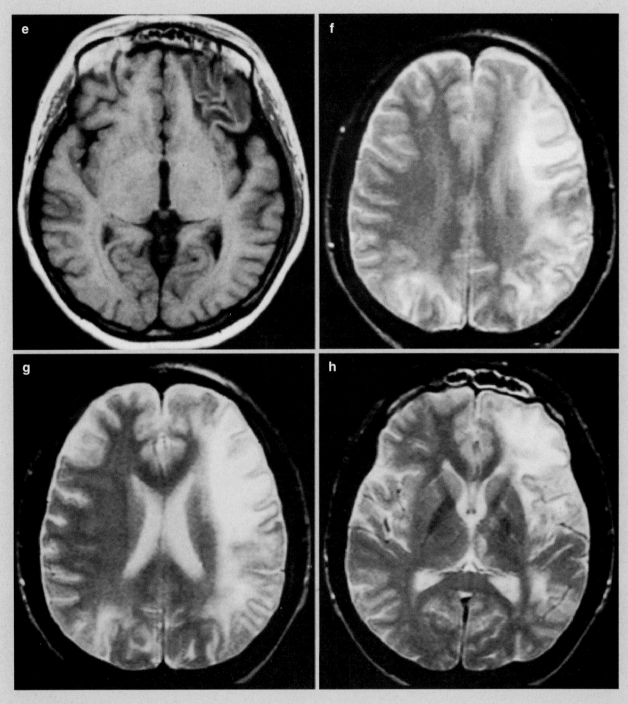

Fig. 13.53   (continued)

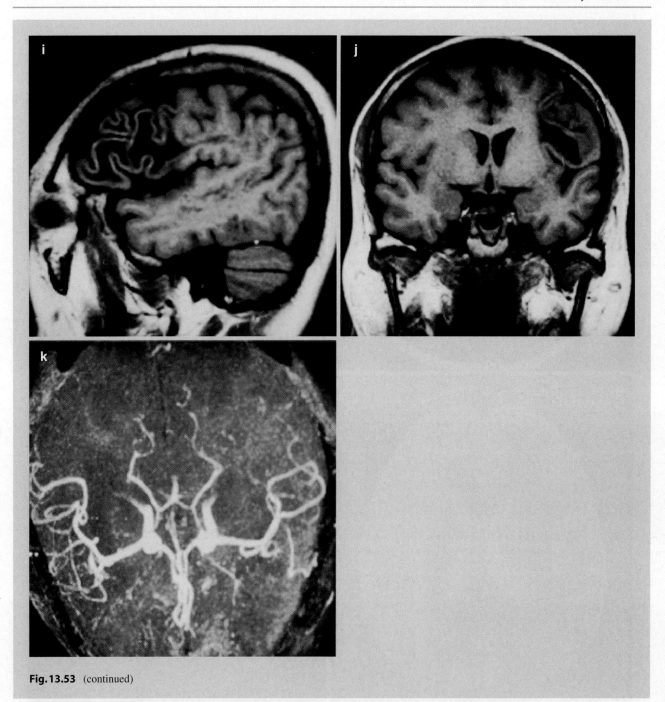

Fig. 13.53 (continued)

Case Study 5

A male patient aged 30 years was confirmatively diagnosed as having AIDS by the CDC. He had a history of drug abuse by needles, with symptoms of mental disorder. His CD4 T cell count was 70/μl.

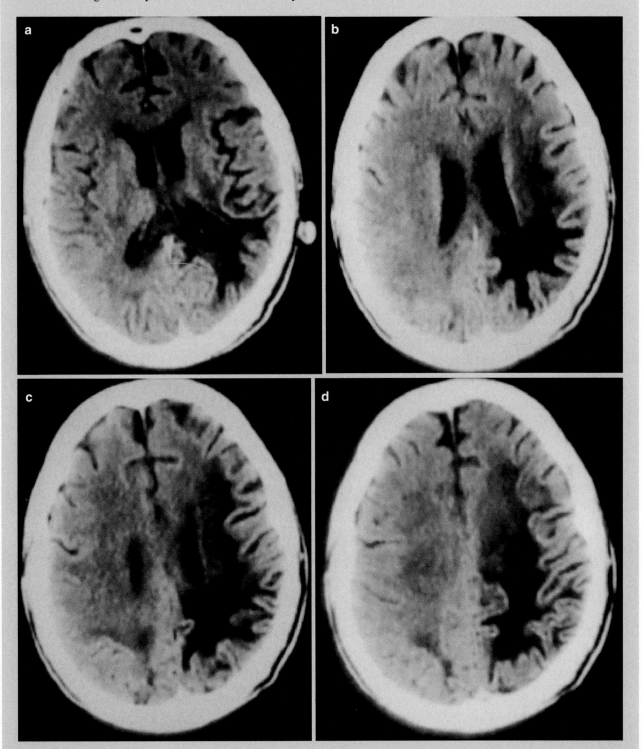

Fig. 13.54   (a–d) HIV/AIDS related herpes simplex virus encephalitis. CT scanning demonstrates large flaky low density area in the left temporal lobe and occipital lobe, deepened and widened sulci, reduced total brain volume, and enlarged left lateral ventricle

Case Study 6

A male patient aged 33 years was confirmatively diag-nosed as having AIDS by the CDC. He had a history of extramarital affair, with symptoms of headache and men-tal disorder. His CD4 T cell count was 110/µl.

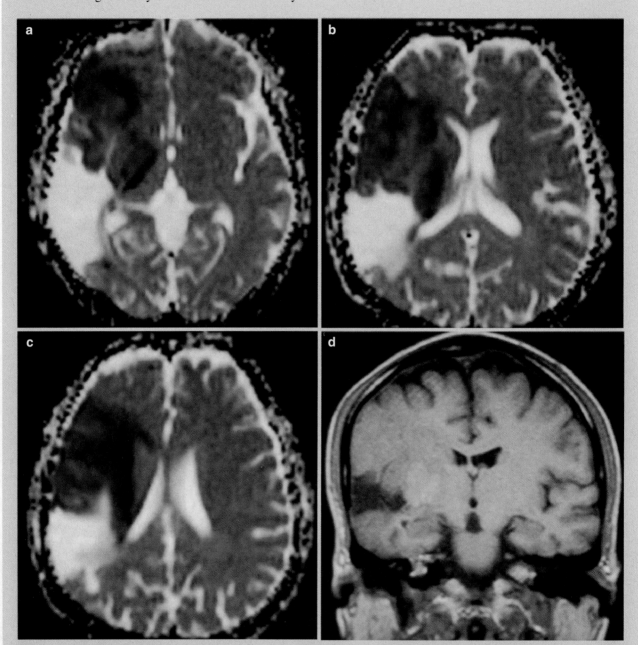

Fig. 13.55 (a–i) HIV/AIDS related herpes simplex virus enceph-alitis. (a–c) MRI FLAIR T2 imaging demonstrates large flaky long T2 signal in the right occipital lobe, and large flaky short T2 signal in the temporal lobe. (d–f) Coronal MR imaging demon-strates large flaky long T1 signal in the right temporal lobe, which is communicating with the subarachnoid space. (g–i) MRI proton density weighted imaging demonstrates high signal in the right temporal lobe, low signal in the right temporal occipital lobe and narrowed right lateral ventricle due to compression

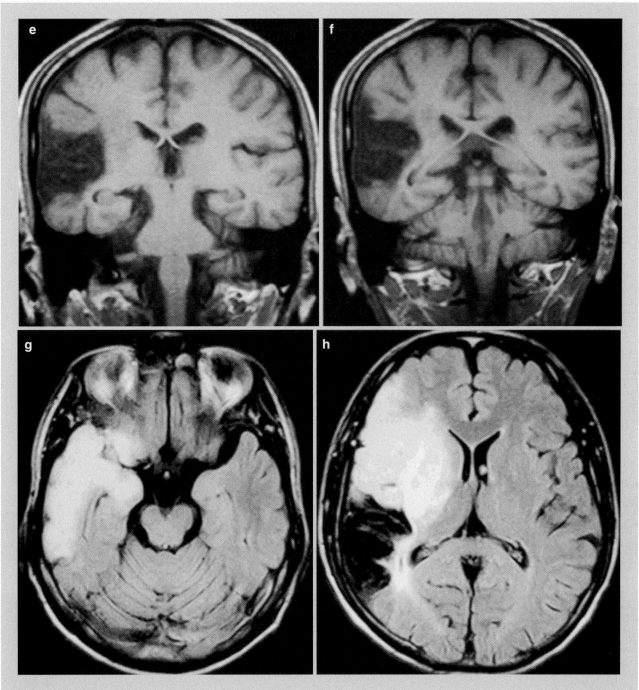

Fig. 13.55 (continued)

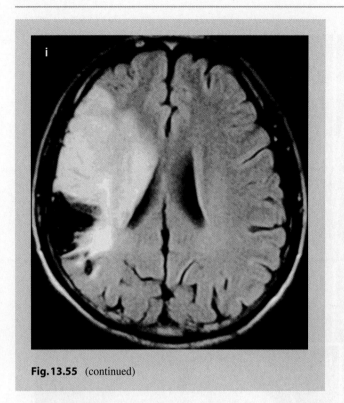

Fig. 13.55   (continued)

Case Study 7

A male patient aged 30 years was confirmatively diagnosed as having AIDS by the CDC. He had a history of sexually transmitted disease, with symptoms of headache and dizziness for 2 months. His CD4 T cell count was 40/μl.

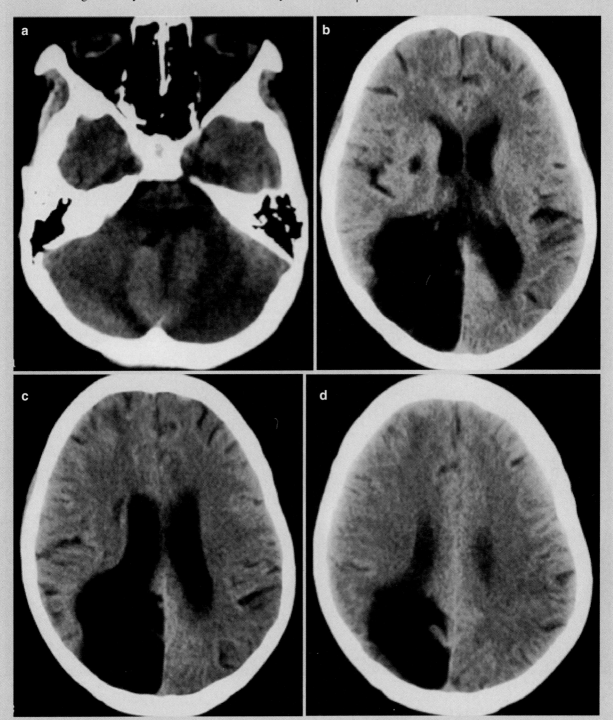

Fig. 13.56 (a–k) HIV/AIDS related herpes simplex virus encephalitis. (a) CT scanning demonstrates flaky low density shadow in the left occipital lobe, with unclearly defined interface with the gyrus. (b–d) It is demonstrated to have small flaky low density area in the right basal ganglia, with clearly defined boundary, enlarged bilateral ventricles with the right lateral ventricle communicating with the subarachnoid space to form a brain penetrating malformation. (e) Enhanced CT scanning demonstrates flaky low density shadow in the occipital lobe, widened sulci, and unclearly defined interface with the gyrus. (f–h) Enhanced CT scanning demonstrates small flaky low density area in the right basal ganglia, with clearly defined boundary, enlarged bilateral ventricles with the right ventricle communicating with the subarachnoid space to form a brain penetrating malformation. (i–k) MRI proton density weighted imaging demonstrates small flaky high signal in the right frontal lobe and in the basal ganglia, with enlarged right ventricle communicating with the subarachnoid space to form a brain penetrating malformation

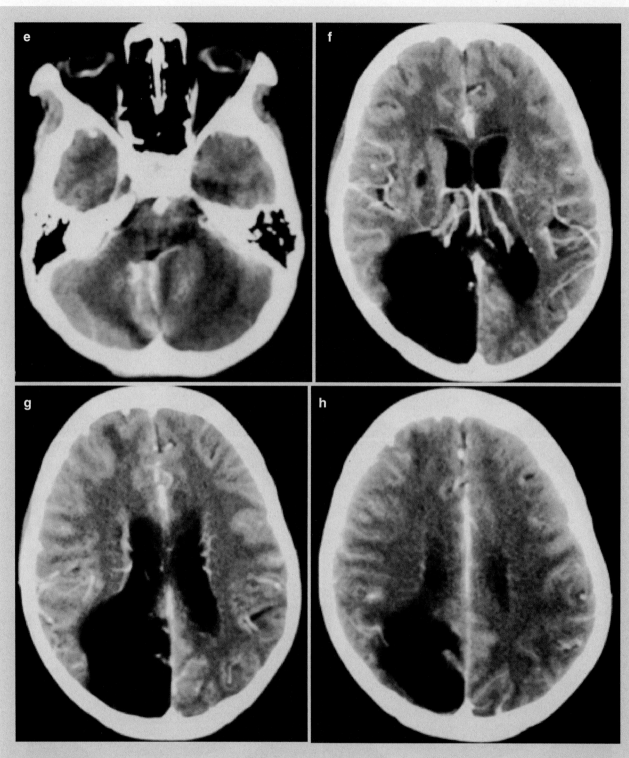

Fig. 13.56 (continued)

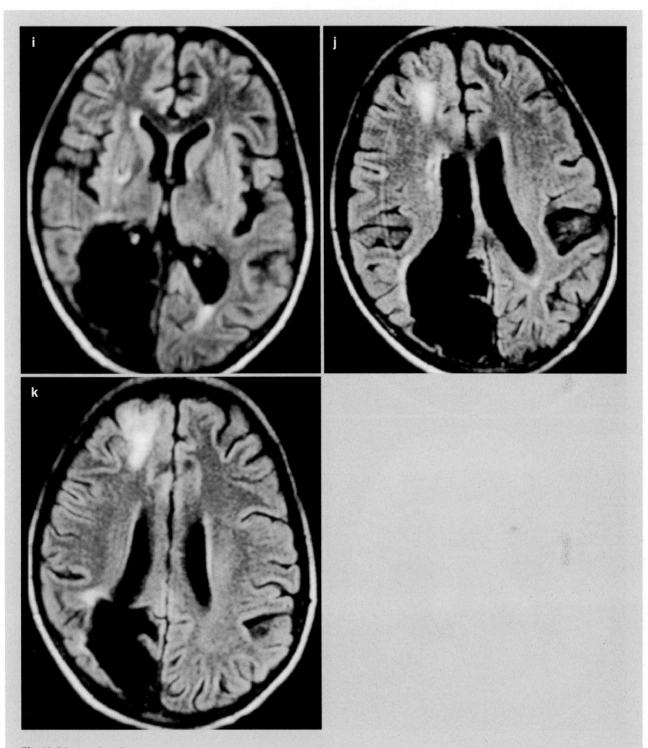

Fig. 13.56 (continued)

Case Study 8

A female patient aged 16 years was confirmatively diagnosed as having AIDS by the CDC. She had a history of surgical blood transfusion in 1994 and was definitively diagnosed in Oct. 2003. In Dec. 2004, she complained symptoms of fever, headache, dizziness, nausea, cervical stiffness and blurry consciousness. Her CD4 T cell count was 27/µl.

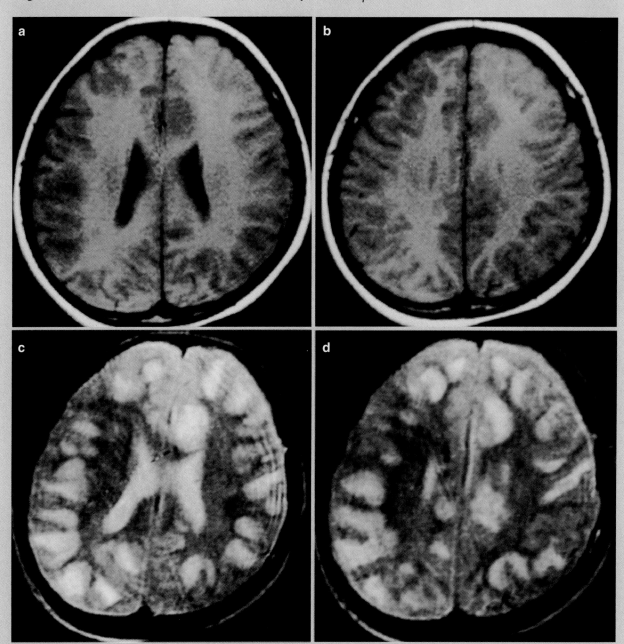

Fig. 13.57 (**a–d**) HIV/AIDS related herpes simplex virus encephalitis. (**a–d**) Axial MR imaging demonstrates swollen bilateral brain cortex in long T1 long T2 signals, absent brain interface, flaky long T1 long T2 signal of the bilateral brain white matter, with obvious edema

Case Study 9

A male patient aged 30 years was confirmatively diagnosed as having AIDS by the CDC. He had a history of paid blood donation in 1995 and was definitively diagnosed by in Feb. 2003. In Dec. 2004, he complained of symptoms of fever, headache, nausea and vomiting. His CD4 T cell count was 35/μl.

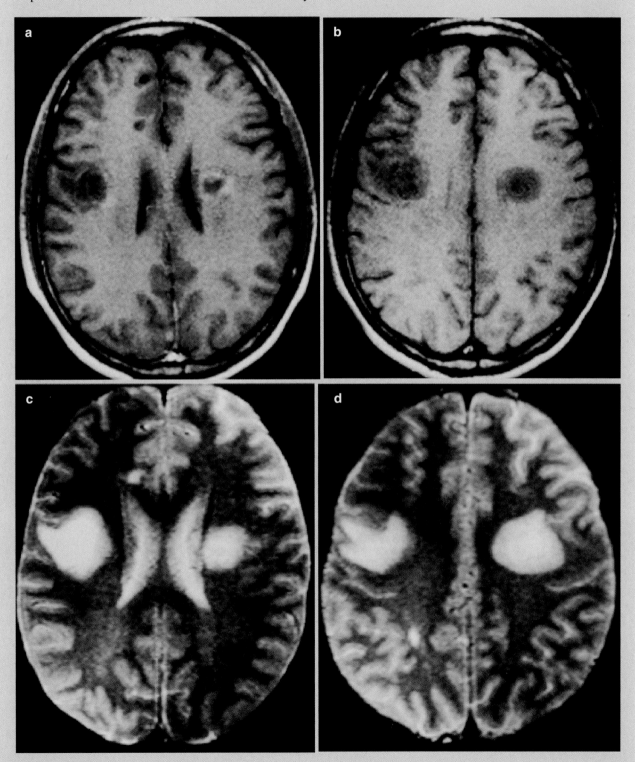

Fig. 13.58 (a–d) HIV/AIDS related herpes simplex virus encephalitis. (a, b) MR imaging demonstrates large flaky long T1 signal in right temporal parietal lobe, round liked or flaky long T1 signal in the left semioval centrum, and surrounding ring shaped short T1 signal (bleeding or gliosis). (c, d) MR imaging demonstrates large flaky long T2 signal in the right temporal parietal lobe, with finger liked edema, round liked or flaky long T2 signal in the left semioval centrum

Case Study 10

A male patient aged 40 years was confirmatively diagnosed as having AIDS by the CDC. He complained of symptoms of headache, nausea, vomiting and convulsions. His CD4 T cell count was 11/μl.

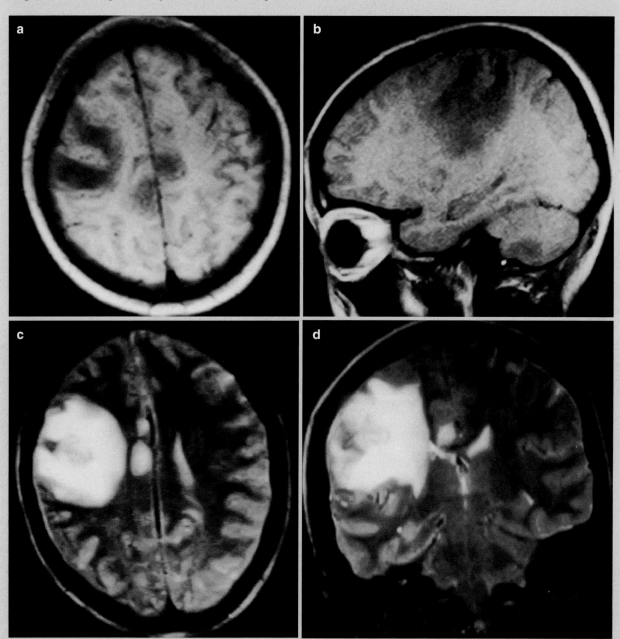

Fig. 13.59 (**a–d**) HIV/AIDS related herpes simplex virus encephalitis. (**a, b**) Axial and sagittal MR imaging demonstrates large flaky long T1 signal in the right temporal parietal lobe. (**c**) Axial imaging demonstrates round liked or flaky mass in long T2 signal in the right temporal parietal lobe. (**d**) Coronal imaging demonstrates flaky or round liked mass shadow in long T2 signal in the right temporal parietal lobe, with obvious surrounding edema effect

Criteria for the Diagnosis

1. With a case history of lips or genital herpes, or the incidence of skin and mucosal herpes with the present illness.
2. Fever, mental and behavioral disorder, convulsions, unconsciousness, and early focal neurological signs.
3. Increased leukocytes and erythrocytes in CSF (WBC $\geq 5 \times 106$/L), normal levels of sugar and chloride, PCR detection of ESF with findings of the virus DNA. HSV antibodies increased in the serum obviously.
4. HSV isolation, culture and identification are positive in the brain tissue.
5. CT scanning or MR imaging demonstrates focal hemorrhagia in the temporal lobe and round liked low density area and brain malacia focus at the interface of cortex and medulla.
6. Brain tissue biopsy or pathology demonstrates eosinophilic inclusion (Cowdry A type) in the nerve cells. Electron microscopy demonstrates HSV viral particles. Either of the above two findings can define the diagnosis. In situ hybridization demonstrates virus nucleic acid of the HSV.

Differential Diagnosis

HIV/AIDS related herpes simplex virus encephalitis should be differentiated from opportunistic infections and neoplasms of the nervous system as well as cerebrovascular diseases.

Intestinal Virus Encephalitis

HIV/AIDS related HSE should be differentiated from intestinal virus encephalitis. HIV/AIDS related intestinal virus encephalitis is relatively rare. In its early stage, there are gastrointestinal symptoms. Positive findings by virus isolation from the cerebrospinal fluid or PCR amplification can facilitate the differential diagnosis.

Cytomegalovirus Encephalitis

HIV/AIDS related HSE should be differentiated from cytomegalovirus encephalitis. Cytomegalovirus encephalitis is common in AIDS patients, with symptoms of confusion, memory loss, affective disorder, headache and focal brain damage. MR imaging demonstrates diffuse or focal abnormal signal in the white matter. Findings of typical CMV inclusion by ESF or biopsy can define the diagnosis.

Purulent Meningitis

HIV/AIDS related HSE should be differentiated from purulent meningitis. Purulent meningitis has serious systemic symptoms of infection, with significantly increased leukocytes in the cerebrospinal fluid and even porridge liked CSF. CSF bacterial culture or smear can find the pathogen, sometimes with findings of primary purulent intracerebral abscess.

Brain Neoplasms

HIV/AIDS related HSE should be differentiated from brain neoplasms. HSE sometimes has prominent focal symptoms and accompanying increase of the intracranial pressure, being similar to manifestation of brain tumor. Regardless of primary or metastatic brain tumor, its course is relatively long, with obviously increased protein in the cerebrospinal fluid. Enhanced CT scanning demonstrates enhancement. MR imaging can define the location and size of the tumor, and even its qualitative diagnosis.

Acute Demyelinating Encephalopathy

HIV/AIDS related HSE should be differentiated from acute demyelinating encephalopathy. Acute demyelinating encephalopathy commonly has an acute or subacute onset, with slight to moderate fever, psychiatric symptoms, disturbance of consciousness and focal neurological deficits, which are similar to the manifestation of HSE. CT scanning demonstrates multiple low density foci in the subcortical white matter, which is more common around ventricles with mixed new and old foci of different sizes unevenly distributed. The demyelinating plaques have enhancement effects. MR imaging demonstrates flaky slightly long T1 long T2 signal. HSE is mainly a process of necrosis and liquefaction of local brain tissues. Enhanced CT scanning and MR imaging demonstrate no enhancement.

Primary Low-Grade Glioma or Cerebral Infarction

HIV/AIDS related HSE should be differentiated from primary low-grade glioma or cerebral infarction. Involvement of the lesions to the bilateral temporal lobes with an acute onset should be considered as herpes simplex virus encephalitis rather than glioma. Cerebral cortex infarction is secondary to vascular occlusion and has the same supplying area of blood vessels. The involvement of the white matter in herpex simplex virus encephalitis occurs early, but its infarction occurs late.

Discussion

Herpes simplex virus reaches the trigeminal ganglion via the oral cavity along with sensory nerve fibers, spreading along with its branches into the temporal and frontal meninges and cerebral parenchyma innervated by the middle cranial and the anterior cranial fossa nerves. It can also reach the brainstem along the cranial IX, X nerves. And the virus can also incubate in the trigeminal ganglion and is reactivated or reinfected to cause encephalitis when the immunity of the human body decreases. The progression of HSV-1 encephalitis, the severity of its induced cerebral parenchymal changes and its prognosis are related to the virus itself and the defense mechanism of the human body. HIV/AIDS related HSV encephalitis commonly occurs in the early stage of HIV infection, especially in patients with a past history of lip and skin herpes virus infection. HIV/AIDS related HSV encephalitis occurs commonly in the frontal and temporal lobes of the cerebral hemisphere. In a short period of time, it may cause necrosis, liquefaction and abscesses of the brain tissues. The formation of brain abscesses can be divided into four stages. In the early stage of encephalitis, commonly a few days after infection, there are manifestations of absent cerebral sulci, vasogenic edema, patchy necrosis, spots bleeding and leptomeningeal enhancement. In the advanced stage of encephalitis (2 weeks after infection), the necrosis has thick cystic wall surrounding its center. There is shrinkage of the foci, surrounding glia hyperplasia, and characteristic pathological changes of paroxysmal hemorrhagic necrotizing meningitis. Virus has frequent invasion to the marginal system, including the temporal lobe, cingulate and the inferior frontal lobe. CT scanning demonstrations can be normal in the early stage of the lesions. But in the advanced stage, CT scanning demonstrates a spherical or mass liked low density shadow, with clearly defined borderline, linear abnormal enhancement of ependymitis and gyrus liked enhancement of the lesions area. There are low density lesions in the temporal lobe, with accompanying slight space occupying effect. Bleeding is the characteristic change of herpes simplex virus encephalitis. MR imaging is more sensitive than CT scanning to the early lesions of HSE. The early demonstrations include thickened gyrus with edema by T1WI in slight low or equal signal, and high signal in the cortex of the temporal lobe and cingulate gyrus by T2WI. The signal abnormalities may extend to the cortex of the insular lobe, with no involvement of the putamen. FLAIR sequence has a high detection rate of the early slight abnormal signals. In the early stage, enhanced foci and bleeding are rarely found. The characteristic spots bleeding can be favorably demonstrated by T1WI, which is more sensitive to it than CT scanning. If treated promptly, patients can have good prognosis. For the cases with lesion in the cerebrovascular watershed area, the brain tissues can be found with liquefaction and necrosis, with communication with the cerebral ventricle to form ventricular penetrating malformation.

13.3.4 HIV/AIDS Related Intracerebral Tuberculosis Infections

13.3.4.1 Pathogens and Pathogenesis

Tuberculosis is one of the most serious diseases in human history, and even today it is still a great threat to human health. TB has enormous impact on human being. For centuries, tuberculosis led to countless death of human. Due to the unique biological properties of the causative pathogen, mycobacterium tuberculosis complex strain, the incubation period lasts up to several decades. Mycobacterium

tuberculosis complex include mycobacterium tuberculosis, mycobacterium bovis and mycobacterium africanum, among which mycobacterium tuberculosis is a major pathogen. Mycobacterium tuberculosis complex has a slow growth, with reproduction of one generation usually in 20–24 h. The biological property of the pathogen brings about difficulty for its culture. And mycobacterium tuberculosis can have a long term existence in the cells or granulomas in form of dormant bacteria for up to several years. Several decades later, the dormant bacteria can be reactivated to trigger the onset of the disease. Meanwhile, its capability of replication and pathogenicity can be maintained. The epidemiological studies on TB indicated two different but interrelated possibilities. One is the possible infection of mycobacterium tuberculosis and the other is the possible progression of mycobacterium tuberculosis infection into tuberculosis. The relationship between mycobacterium tuberculosis infection and immunity can be defined by HIV infection. Although tuberculosis is related to HIV infection due to the occurrence of cellular immunity defects in HIV infected patients, in most cases the high risk groups for HIV infection are more susceptible to tuberculosis. The relative risk of tuberculosis in HIV infected populations is 200–1,000 times as high as the common populations. Like all infectious diseases, its progression into active tuberculosis depends on the amount and virulence of the pathogen as well as the resistance and sensitivity of the hosts to the pathogen. Deposition of mycobacterium tuberculosis in alveolus may lead to a series of protective reaction of the human body. Most reactions are the cellular immune response, which can prevent the progression of mycobacterium tuberculosis infection into TB. The alveolar immune response is a process of wrapping the active mycobacterium tuberculosis in the granuloma. Mycobacterium tuberculosis is usually within the macrophage and sometimes extracellular, with a large amount cells accumulating around the mycobacterium tuberculosis to form granuloma. Granulomas are composed of macrophages, CD4 T and CD8 lymphocytes, fibroblasts, giant cells and epidermal cells. HIV/AIDS related brain tuberculoma is commonly derived from pulmonary tuberculosis, which is granulomatous lesion after the infection of the central nervous system by mycobacterium tuberculosis. The incidence of cerebral tuberculoma in the general population is 1.4 % and its incidence in AIDS patients is low because granuloma rarely occurs due to immunosuppression and the loss of normal immune mediation. Cerebral tuberculoma occurs in any intracranial parts. Its occurrence in the subtentorial is more common than that in subtentorial. Intracranial TB can be divided into four categories: (1) acute meningitis (meningeal brain tuberculosis). (2) Meningitis sequelae. (3) Parenchymal brain tuberculosis. Mycobacterium tuberculosis may spread along with blood flow to cause tuberculous granuloma in the brain parenchyma and the meninges.

Tuberculous meningitis is the most common. Brain tuberculosis occurs in the cerebral parenchyma of both the supratentorial and subtentorial, mostly in temporal lobe of the cerebellum and half temporal lobe of the cerebellar hemisphere. (4) Mixed cerebral tuberculosis.

13.3.4.2 Pathophysiological Basis

Bacterial infection of the nervous system rarely occurs in AIDS patients, with main findings of mycobacterial infection by autopsy. Mycobacterium avium complex infection of the nervous system is commonly a component of disseminated infection. After the spread of primary TB along with blood is terminated, many tubercule bacilli can remain in the central nervous system. Once the cell mediated immunity changes, proliferation of the tubercule bacilli can form small nodules in diameter of less than 1 cm. These tuberculomas are in color of yellowish white or grayish yellow, with clearly defined boundaries from the surrounding brain tissue and with central caseous necrotic tissue or granulation tissue. These central foci are then liquefied to form a simple abscess. Due to the immunosuppression and the loss of immune mediated functions in AIDS patients, granulation tissue proliferation is unobvious or rarely found, and the calcification process rarely occurs. Generally speaking, the small brain tuberculosis nodules cannot break into the subarachnoid space; otherwise their invasion into the subarachnoid space can cause tuberculous meningitis. The tuberculous nodules in meninges can be in stripes of TB foci due to the thickened meninges. In the early stage of TB, there are many scattered small nodules on the meningeal surface, which mainly having infiltrations of monocytes and lymphocytes. There are meningeal congestion and edema as well as large quantity white or grayish yellow exudates depositing in the cerebral base, medulla oblongata, pons, interpeduncular cistern, sylvian fissure, the optic chiasm and ambient cistern. The exudates may compress the optic nerve, oculomotor nerve and facial nerve at the optic chiasm. Adhesion, thickening and organization of the exudates in the skull base often leads to obstruction of cerebrospinal fluid pathways and hydrocephalus. The meningeal lesions may involve superficial cerebral parenchyma to cause inflammations, and even tuberculous nodules or tuberculoma in serious cases.

13.3.4.3 Clinical Symptoms and Signs

The clinical manifestations include low grade fever, night sweats, weight loss, accelerated ESR, headache, vomiting and papilledema, hemiparalysis, aphasia, epilepsy seizures, the cerebellar symptoms, intracranial hypertension symptoms, and restricted brain lesion symptoms. The common symptoms include (1) Meningeal irritation usually occurs in the early stage, sometimes with no meningeal irritation. (2) Symptoms of increased intracranial pressure include headache, ejective vomiting, papilledema and consciousness

disorder; even cerebral herniation in the serious cases, which can lead to breathing arrest. (3) Symptoms of cranial nerves lesions include the most common symptoms related to the facial nerve, followed by the abducens nerve, the oculomotor nerve and the optic nerve. (4) Symptoms of brain parenchymal lesions include paralysis, decerebrate rigidity, hands and feet tremor and dance liked movements. The clinical manifestations are related to the location of the lesions.

13.3.4.4 Examinations and Their Selection
Epidemiological Examination

The patient has a case history of close contacts with patients of tuberculosis, with symptoms of tuberculous toxemia and accompanying intracranial hypertension, meningeal irritation, and other neurological symptoms and signs.

Acid-Fast Bacilli Staining

Mycobacterium tuberculosis can be found, with accelerated ESR.

CSF Examination

Quantitative examinations of leukocyte, protein and sugar chloride can be performed by CSF test, with demonstrations of increased protein, increased cell count predominantly monocytes and reduced sugar content.

Fundus Examination

There are round or oval pale white tuberculosis nodules with yellow ring shaped boundary adjacent to the choroidal vessels.

PPD Test

PPD test is commonly used for the diagnosis of tuberculosis, but there are some results of false positive and false negative. HIV infection is commonly demonstrated as false negative and weak positive.

Diagnostic Imaging

CT scanning and MR imaging can demonstrate the military nodules and tuberculomas in the brain parenchyma. Other indirect clinical manifestations of basal cistern and sylvian cistern exudates, cerebral edema, hydrocephalus and cerebral infarction are also reliable evidence for the diagnosis.

13.3.4.5 Imaging Demonstrations
CT Scanning

The foci can be found in any intracranial parts, including brain, ventricles and meninges. The demonstrations can be divided into:

TB Meningitis Demonstrations

Plain CT scanning fails to clearly demonstrate the lesions, while enhanced scanning can demonstrate the involved parts, with direct signs of (1) exudates in the brain basal cistern, lateral fissure, increased density with obviously abnormal enhancement; (2) miliary tuberculosis foci in small low density nodules, and obviously abnormal enhancement by enhanced scanning; and indirect signs of (1) Communicating or obstructive hydrocephalus; (2) Cerebral infarction caused by vascular stenosis or obstruction in cerebral base and the cerebral fissure, commonly found in the area supplied by the middle cerebral artery.

TB Encephalitis Demonstrations

1. In the early stage, there is equal density shadow or low density cerebral edema, funnel shaped frontal lobe and multiple fingers liked temporal parietal occipital region. Enhanced scanning demonstrates ring shaped or small nodules shaped abnormal enhancement.
2. In the middle stage of AIDS, the inflammation subsides, with proliferation of collagen tissue containing caseous substance and central sandwich low density shadow. Enhanced scanning demonstrates ring shaped obvious enhancement and surrounding low density shadows of brain edema.
3. AIDS patients finally show no calcification process.
4. TB cerebral abscess has plain CT scanning demonstrations of singular or multiple round or oval low density areas, with surrounding obvious edema and space occupying effect. Enhanced scanning demonstrates ring shaped enhancement, thick or thin wall. it can be concurrent with tuberculoma or meningitis.

MR Imaging

TB Meningitis

The direct signs include MRI T2WI findings of cerebral basal cistern occlusion, increased signals mostly in the suprasellar cistern, ambient cistern and lateral fissure cistern with long T2 signal; FLAIR sequence findings of obvious high signal, obviously thickened and enhanced meninges in the basilar cistern by enhanced imaging with involved subarachnoid space in some cases.

The indirect signs include infarction occurring in the cortex supplied by the middle cerebral artery cortex and basal ganglia in spots and flaky long T1 and T2 signals. In the early stage, hydrocephalus occurs, mostly communicating hydrocephalus and sometimes obstructive hydrocephalus.

TB Encephalitis

When intracerebral granuloma or tuberculoma occurs, plain MR imaging demonstrates singular or multiple irregular flakes of long T1 and long T2 signals. After the injection of Gd-DTPA, imaging demonstrates more tuberculoma foci than enhanced CT scanning does. Tuberculoma is commonly multiple, located in the cerebral cortex and medulla region, with nodular enhancement or ring shaped enhancement and sometimes with irregular fusion or beads string enhancement. Cases with large tuberculoma are demonstrated to have central necrosis in long T1 long T2 signal. The ring surrounding granuloma is in short T1 signal and short T2 signal. Cerebral edema is in long T2 signal.

Case Study 1

A female patient aged 34 years was confirmatively diagnosed as having AIDS by the CDC. Her CD4 T cell count was 101/μl and was pregnant for 25 weeks. After 12 weeks congestion, she began antiviral therapy for preventing mother-to-child transmission (PMTCT), with the therapeutic planning of AZT+3TC+NVP. After 2 weeks medication, she complained of nausea, vomiting, headache and general fatigue. But she continued the medication lasting for 1 month and paid her clinical visit due to the aggravated above symptoms, which was considered to be cause by adverse effects of AZT and was treated symptomatically. The symptoms were alleviated, but still with vomiting. When AZT is substituted by D4T, her conditions improved and she was discharged from the hospital. One month later, she fell at home, with symptoms of consciousness disturbance, aggravated headache, nausea, vomiting, and cervical rigidity. The body temperature was 38 °C. Physical examinations by admission revealed pulmonary tuberculosis, with no abnormalities by cranial CT scanning. But clinical analysis indicated possibility of TB meningitis due to the immune reconstitution.

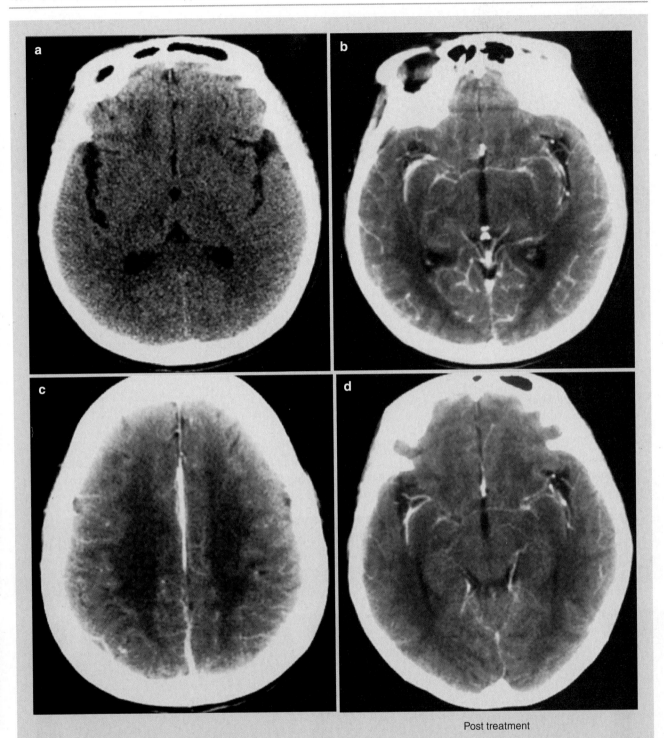

Post treatment

Fig. 13.60 (**a–e**) HIV/AIDS related intracerebral tuberculosis infection. (**a**) CT scanning demonstrates enlarged bilateral sylvian cisterns. (**b, c**) Enhanced CT scanning demonstrates thickened meninges in the bilateral sylvian cisterns and in the cerebral falx, with obviously abnormal enhancement. (**d, e**) Enhanced CT scanning after 1 month treatment demonstrates linear enhancement of meninges in the Sylvian cistern and in the cerebral falx and less thickness of the meninges compared to premedication conditions

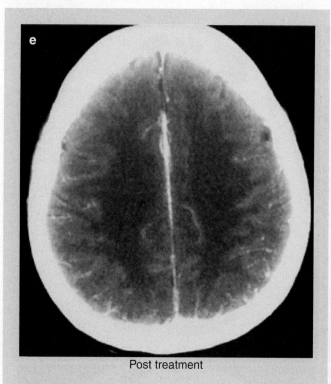

Post treatment

Fig. 13.60   (continued)

Case Study 2
A female patient aged 40 years was confirmatively diagnosed as having AIDS by the CDC. She complained

symptoms of nausea, vomiting, headache, general fatigue and left limbs weakness. Her CD4 T cell count was 80/μl.

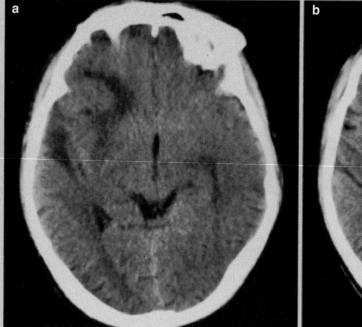

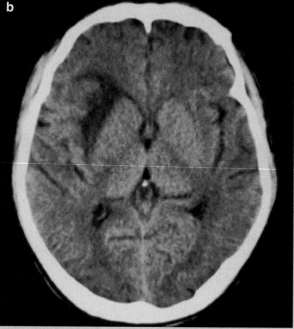

Fig. 13.61 (a–f) HIV/AIDS related intracerebral tuberculosis infection. (a–c) CT scanning demonstrates stripes and flakes of low density shadows in the right brain capsule and in the right temporal lobe, with unclearly defined boundaries. (d–f) Enhanced CT

scanning demonstrates obviously abnormal nodular, ring shaped and flaky enhancements in the bilateral sylvian cistern meninges, the capsules and the right temporal lobe

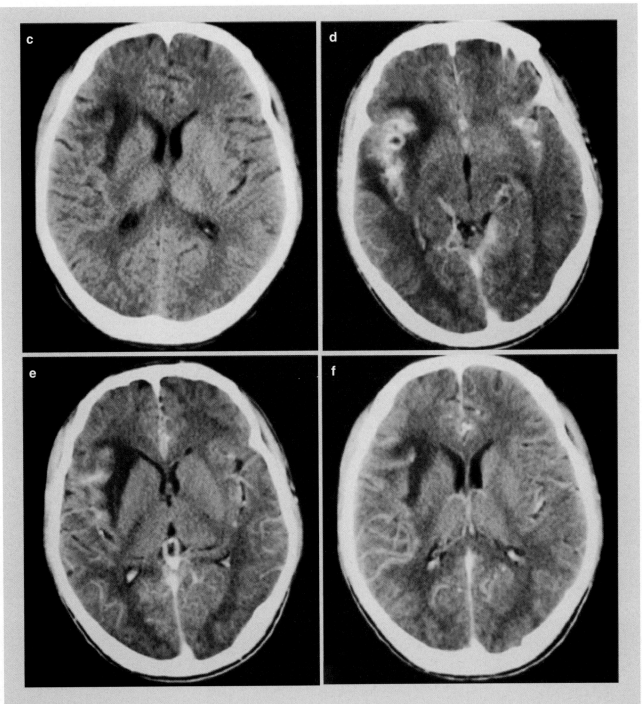

Fig. 13.61 (continued)

Case Study 3

A female patient aged 37 years was confirmatively diagnosed as having AIDS by the CDC. She had a history of paid blood donation and a history of pulmonary tuberculosis. In May. 2003, she complained symptoms of headache, nausea, vomiting, cervical rigidity and consciousness disturbance. Her CD4 T cell count was 84/μl.

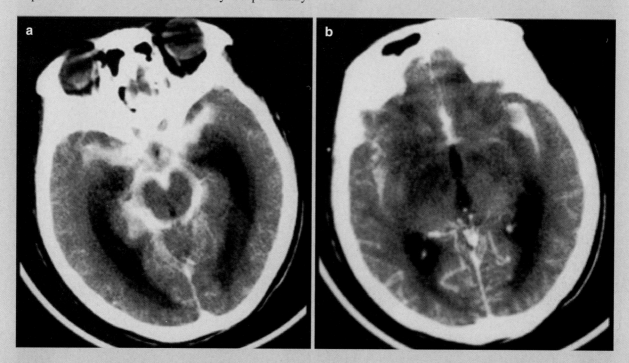

Fig. 13.62 (**a, b**) HIV/AIDS related intracerebral tuberculosis infection. (**a, b**) Axial enhanced CT scanning demonstrates obviously abnormal enhancement of the cerebral falx, lateral fissure cistern and ambient cistern, and no enhancement in bilateral basal ganglia

Case Study 4

A male patient aged 34 years was confirmatively diagnosed as having AIDS by the CDC. He had a history of intravenous drug abuse and complained symptoms of headache, nausea, vomiting, general fatigue and bilateral limbs weakness. His CD4 T cell count was 40/μl.

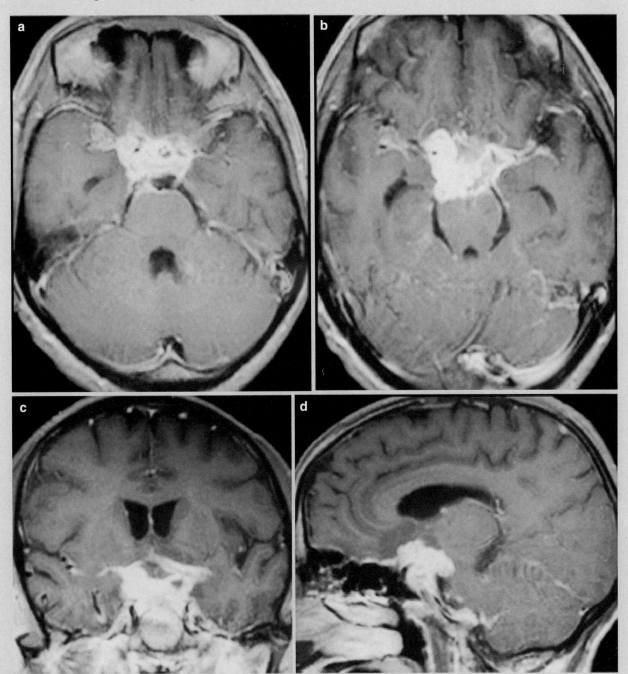

Fig. 13.63 (a–d) HIV/AIDS related intracerebral tuberculosis infection. Axial enhanced CT scanning demonstrates obvious thickened meninges in the pontine cistern and the basal temporal lobe, with obviously abnormal stripes and mass liked enhancement

Case Study 5

A female patient aged 38 years was confirmatively diagnosed as having AIDS by the CDC. She had a history of paid blood donation in 1995. In Apr. 2002, she sustained military pulmonary tuberculosis. In May, she complained symptoms of headache, dizziness, nausea, vomiting and low grade fever. Her CD4 T cell count was 68/μl.

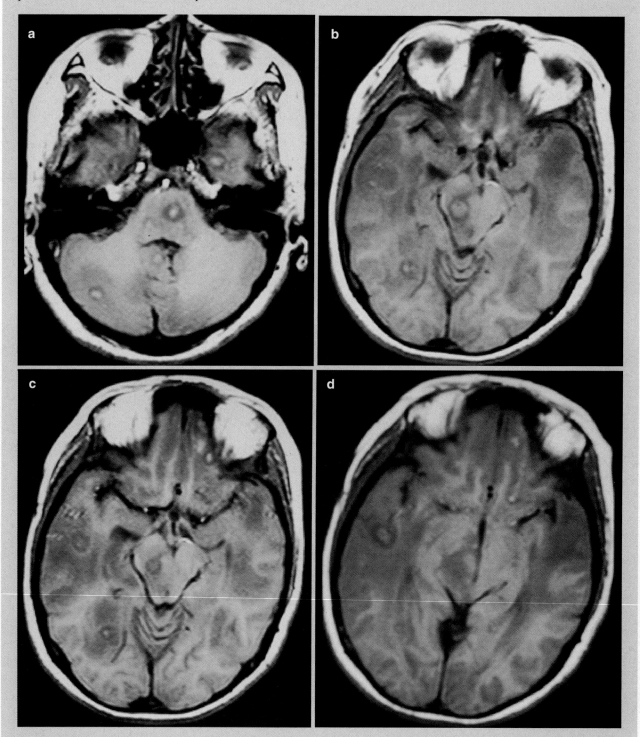

Fig. 13.64 (**a–i**) HIV/AIDS related intracerebral tuberculosis infection. (**a–d**) Axial MR imaging demonstrates multiple ring shaped long T1 signal in bilateral brain, cerebellum and brainstem, with spots slightly shorter T1 signal, peripheral edema and unclear borders. (**e, f**) Axial and sagittal MR imaging demonstrates multiple flaky long T2 signal in the brain, the cerebellum and the brain stem, with ring shaped slightly shorter T2 signal in necklace sign, obvious edema and unclear borders. (**g–i**) Axial, sagittal and frontal enhanced IV-Gd-DTPA MR imaging demonstrates multiple nodular and ring shaped abnormal enhancement in the brain, cerebellum and brainstem, with central spots of no enhancement, uniform size and regular morphology

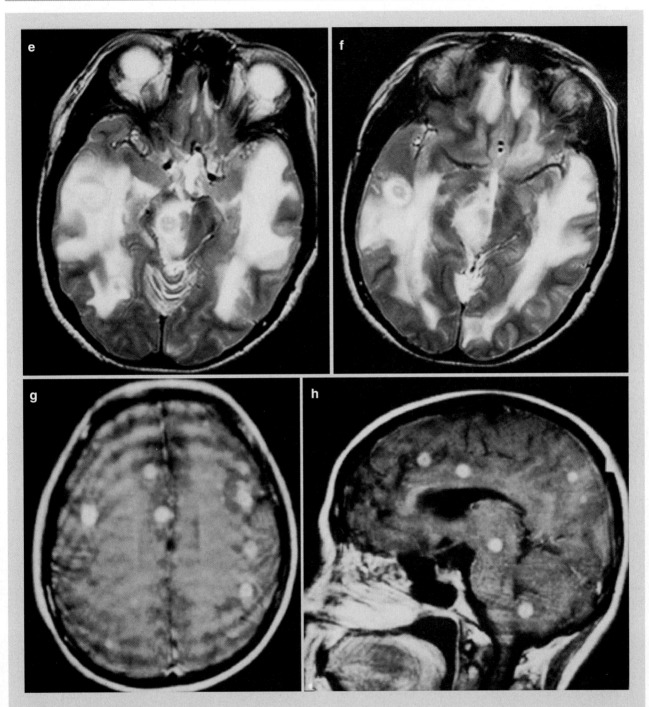

Fig. 13.64 (continued)

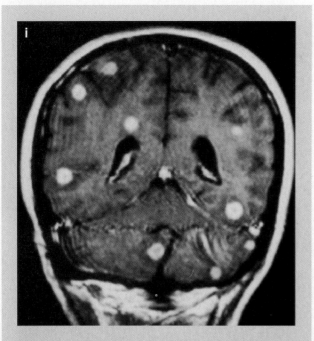

Fig. 13.64   (continued)

Case Study 6
A female patient aged 33 years was confirmatively diagnosed as having AIDS by the CDC. She had a history of extramarital affair and a history of military pulmonary tuberculosis. She complained symptoms of headache, dizziness, nausea, vomiting and low grade fever. Her CD4 T cell count was 80/μl.

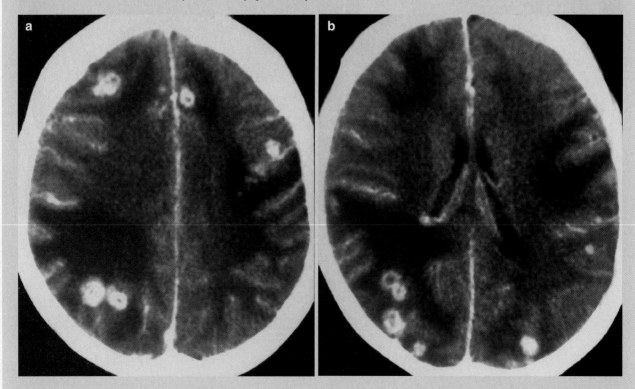

Fig. 13.65 (a–d) HIV/AIDS related intracerebral tuberculosis infection. Enhanced CT scanning demonstrates multiple round liked nodular, ring shaped abnormal enhancement in bilateral brain, with obvious brain tissue edema and mild space occupying effect, and slight leftward migration of the midline

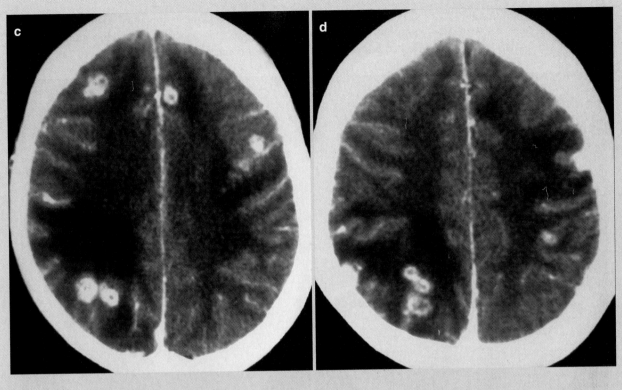

Fig. 13.65   (continued)

Case Study 7
A boy aged 4 years was confirmatively diagnosed as having AIDS by the CDC. He complained symptoms of headache, nausea and vomiting for 10 days. His CD4 T cell count was 12/μl.

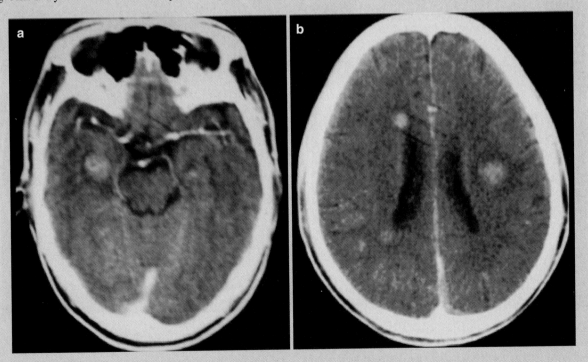

Fig. 13.66 (**a, b**) HIV/AIDS related intracerebral tuberculosis infection. Enhanced CT scanning demonstrates multiple nodular obvious abnormal enhancement in bilateral temporal horns and bilateral semioval center in various sizes, with mild edema and unobvious space occupying effect

Case Study 8

A male patient aged 38 years was confirmatively diagnosed as having AIDS by the CDC. He had a history of extramarital affair and complained symptoms of headache, dizziness, nausea, vomiting and low grade fever. His CD4 T cell count was 50/μl.

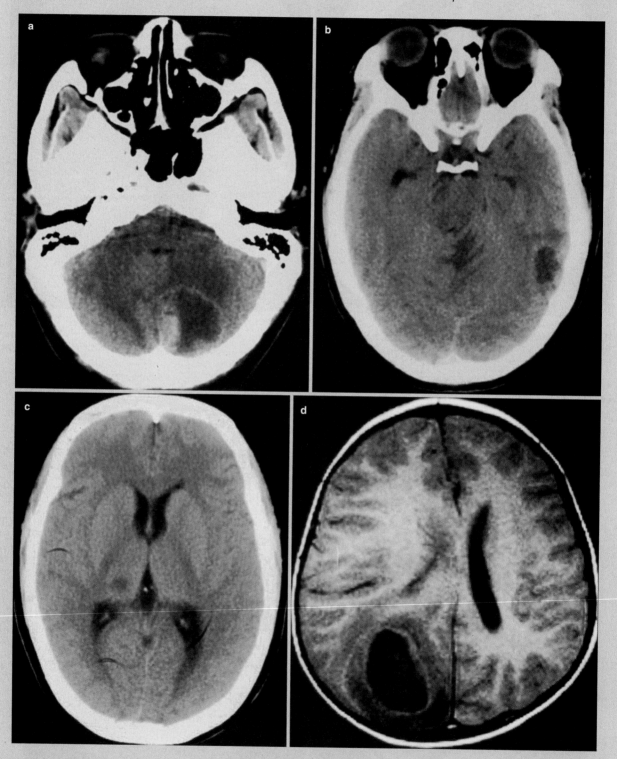

Fig. 13.67 (**a–j**) HIV/AIDS related intracerebral tuberculosis infection. (**a–c**) It is demonstrated to have cystic low density areas of different sizes in the left occipital lobe, temporal lobe, and in the right basal ganglia, with unobvious brain tissue edema and space occupying effect. (**d–j**) It is demonstrated to have large cystic long T1 long T2 signal in the right occipital parietal lobe, with surrounding slight brain tissue edema; compressed and elevated right lateral ventricular horn; Enhanced IV-Gd-DTPA imaging demonstrates ring shaped abnormal enhancements of different sizes in the left occipital lobe, temporal lobe and in the right basal ganglia, with uneven thickness and spots enhancement like buttons

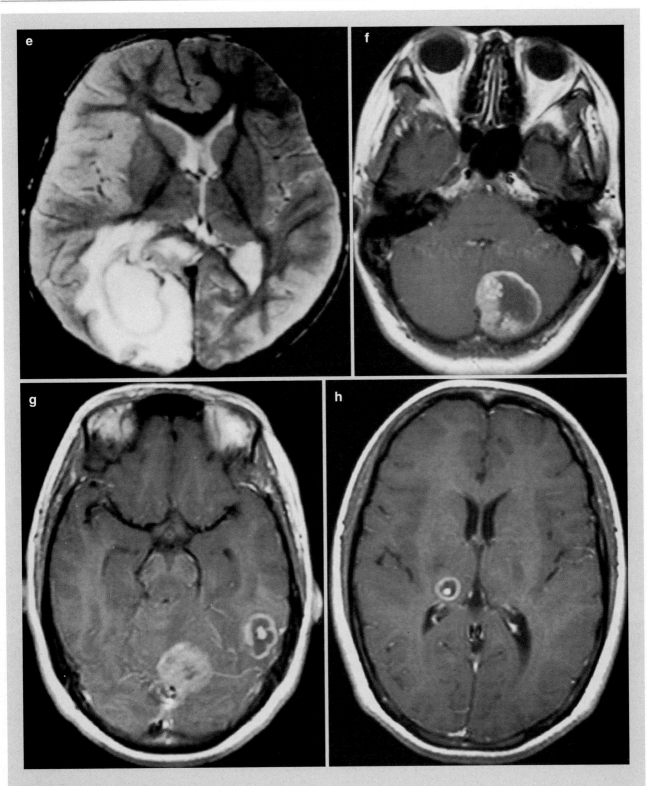

Fig. 13.67 (continued)

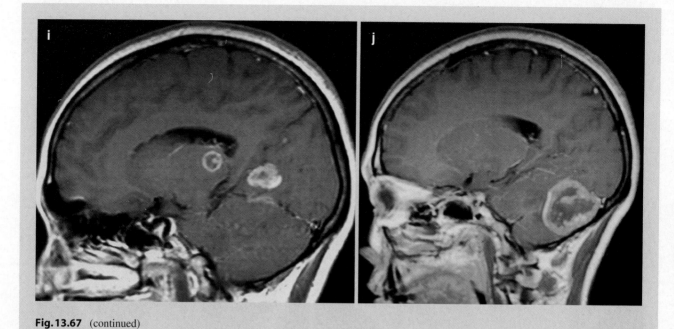

Fig. 13.67 (continued)

13.3.4.6 Criteria for the Diagnosis

1. The clinical manifestations of vision and visual field changes, fundus edema or hemiplegia, unilateral sensory disturbances, aphasia, and cerebellar signs.
2. Mycobacterium tuberculosis can be found in Acid-fast bacilli staining, with accelerated ESR.
3. CSF test for quantitative detection of leukocytes, protein and sugar chloride has the results of increased protein, increased cells counts with predominant increase of monocytes count, and reduced sugar content.
4. CT scanning demonstrates TB meningitis to have exudates occupying the cistern in the cerebral base and the lateral fissure cistern. Enhanced scanning demonstrates obvious irregular enhancement of the meninges, with occasional signs of dural matter enhancement; miliary TB nodules or large flaky low density area in the cerebral parenchyma. Enhanced scanning demonstrates nodular, ring shaped and button liked abnormal enhancement, and findings of hydrocephalus, cerebral edema, focal cerebral ischemia and cerebral infarction. Tuberculous granuloma is singular or multiple with slightly low density nodules, with perifocal edema and space occupying effect. MR imaging demonstrates stripes long/equal T1 and long T2 signals in the cistern of the cerebral base and in the lateral fissure cistern. Enhanced imaging demonstrates obviously irregular enhancement of the meninges. The foci in cerebral parenchyma are in long T1 long T2 signal, with uneven T2 signal. Granuloma is in equal T1 long T2 signal. The envelope of the foci is in equal T1 signal. Enhanced imaging demonstrates ring shaped abnormal enhancement or nodular abnormal enhancement.

13.3.4.7 Differential Diagnosis

Lymphoma

HIV/AIDS related cerebral tuberculosis infection should be differentiated from lymphoma. Lymphoma is usually singular, commonly in the basal ganglia with fire flame liked edema. The enhanced imaging demonstrates map liked abnormal enhancement, which is its characteristic demonstration. AIDS complicated by lymphoma usually shows unobvious edema lymphoma, with few cases with fire flame liked edema.

Cryptococcal Neoformans Meningoencephalitis

HIV/AIDS related cerebral tuberculosis infection should be differentiated from cryptococcal neoformans meningoencephalitis. Plain CT scanning of cryptococcal neoformans meningoencephalitis often shows no abnormalities, but enhanced scanning demonstrates linear enhancement of the meninges. The differential diagnosis should be based on the findings of cryptococcus.

Toxoplasma Encephalitis

HIV/AIDS related cerebral tuberculosis infection should be differentiated from toxoplasma encephalitis. Cerebral toxoplasma infection occurs commonly in the brain basal ganglia and the cerebral cortex and medulla. The foci are in different sizes and morphologies, commonly with spiral or ring shaped enhancement.

Abscess, Astrocytoma or Metastatic Tumors

HIV/AIDS related cerebral tuberculosis infection should be differentiated from abscess, astrocytoma or metastatic tumors. Lesions of cerebral cysticercosis have similar imaging demonstrations, being smaller than tuberculoma.

13.3.4.8 Discussion

In recent years, the incidence of TB is increasing due to the increases of intravenous drug users and HIV infected patients. The majority of patients with TB are infected by mycobacterium tuberculosis. It has been estimated that secondary tuberculosis infection of the central nervous system is due to spreading of mycobacterium tuberculosis from primary pulmonary TB along with blood flow to invade the cerebral meninges/parenchyma. Meningitis is relatively common in the central nervous system of AIDS patients, often involving the pia mater, arachnoid and its adjacent cerebrospinal fluid. The diagnosis is mainly based on the clinical data, but negative findings by the diagnostic imaging cannot exclude the possibility of meningitis. The patients often sustain pulmonary tuberculosis, with secondary intracerebral infection to cause tuberculous meningitis. Enhanced scanning demonstrates obviously abnormal enhancement of meninges. The obvious basal cistern lesions are the characteristic finding of TB meningitis. Due to the immunosuppression of the host, the capability of granuloma formation to fight against infection is impaired. Therefore, TB tends to spread, with main manifestations of intracerebral multiple space occupying edema and meningeal enhancement, even hydrocephalus. Sometimes deep brain tissue infarction is relatively common, often located in brain base supplied by the penetrating vessels. For the cases with ring shaped or nodular enhancement, it is difficult to be differentiated from intracerebral toxoplasma infection and lymphoma.

In patients with HIV/AIDS related TB infection, the incidence of TB in the central nervous system is approximately 10 %. It was speculated that TB infection of the central nervous system is due to the spreading of mycobacterium tuberculosis from primary pulmonary TB along with the blood flow to invade the cerebral meninges/parenchyma. Case studies show that the patients with intracerebral TB infection have a history of pulmonary TB, with secondary intracerebral TB infection. CT scanning demonstrates cerebral tuberculoma in its acute phase in equal or slightly high density nodules with unclear boundaries. Enhanced scanning demonstrates irregular ring shaped or nodular enhancement and mature tuberculoma in round or oval ring shaped enhancement of the foci with clear borderline. It has been reported that the incidence of TB infection is increasing in the HIV infected populations. HIV infection may promote the recessive tuberculosis to develop into clinical tuberculosis. Patients with HIV infection is found negative in PPT test due to their immunosuppression. Tuberculoma manifestations are commonly in the early stage of HIV infection, and the nodular imaging findings of tuberculoma are rarely found in the middle and advanced stages. MR imaging demonstrates scattering foci in the brain with uniform size and regular morphology, which are characteristic demonstrations.

13.3.5 HIV/AIDS Related Intracerebral Rhodococcus Equi Infections

13.3.5.1 Pathogens and Pathogenesis

Rhodococcus equi is generally considered to be the pathogens of horses, pigs and cattles. And rhodococcus equi infection rarely occurs in human. In recent years, due to increased incidence of immunodeficiency syndrome, cases of rhodococcus equi infection are increasingly reported to cause infections of brain and respiratory tract as well as sepsis. Its pathogenesis had been speculated. And recently, the findings of toxic plasmid effects on human tissues provide insightful evidence on pathogenesis of rhodococcus equi.

13.3.5.2 Pathophysiological Basis

Rhodococcus equi is the intracellular facultative parasitic bacteria, with an optimal environmental temperature for growth of 30 °C and an appropriate environmental temperature of 10–40 °C. Acid-fast staining demonstrates uncertain results of rhodococcus equi. It has various morphologies, commonly mistaken as diphtheroid bacillus, bacillus or micrococcus. The most common lesions of rhodococcus equi infection are chronic suppurative bronchopneumonia and extensive lung abscess. The diagnostic imaging demonstrates as subacute pneumonia, with formation of cavities.

13.3.5.3 Clinical Symptoms and Signs

The clinical manifestations include poor appetite, drowsiness, and fever. Other symptoms such as weight loss, diarrhea and joint pain are not representative.

13.3.5.4 Examinations and Their Selection

Bacteria Strain Identification

Various specimens are inoculated into the blood agar for 18–24 h culture at a temperature of 35 °C. The growth of 18 bacterial strains have biological properties of intransparent light yellow bacterial colony in a diameter of 0.5 mm. 48–72 h later, the bacterial colony is in size of 1–2 mm, which is prone of emulsification with mucus. Most colonies produce orange red pigment, and can grow in ordinary AGAR.

Pathological Examination

Typical histopathological changes include exudation of large quantity eosinophilic granulocytes (Von Hansemann cells). In the abscess, there are abundant polymorphonuclear leukocytes. By H&E staining, there are mainly bleeding in the alveolar cavity with large quantity epithelial cells or mainly fibroblasts with pulmonary parenchymal changes and enlarged alveolar septum intervals. By PAS staining, there are scattering or clustering rod liked Rhodococcus equi in a color of pink or purplish red.

Diagnostic Imaging

CT scanning and MR imaging are the most commonly used diagnostic imaging.

Cerebral Puncture for Biopsy

By PAS staining, the pathogen can be detected.

Case Study

A male patient aged 42 years was confirmatively diagnosed as having AIDS by the CDC. He was hospitalized due to fever, headache and inflexible movements of the left limbs for more than 20 days. His CD4 T cell count was 31/μl.

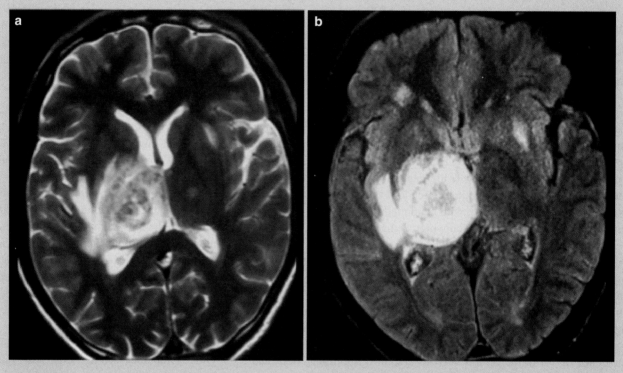

Fig. 13.68 (**a–e**) HIV/AIDS related Rhodococcus equi brain abscess. (**a**) Plain and enhanced MR imaging demonstrate flaky long T2 signal in the right basal ganglia, being uneven with unclear borderline, and obvious edema and space occupying effects. (**b**) MR diffuse imaging demonstrates high signal of the foci in the right basal ganglia and central low signal. (**c**, **d**) Enhanced imaging demonstrates ring shaped or target liked unevenly abnormal enhancement in size of 2.3×1.9 cm. (**e**) Reexamination by MR T2 imaging after anti-inflammatory therapy demonstrates small flaky short T2 signal of the space occupying lesion in the right basal ganglia, surrounding ring shaped long T2 signal, obvious decrease and shrinkage of the foci, absent edema and space occupying effects and clear borderlines

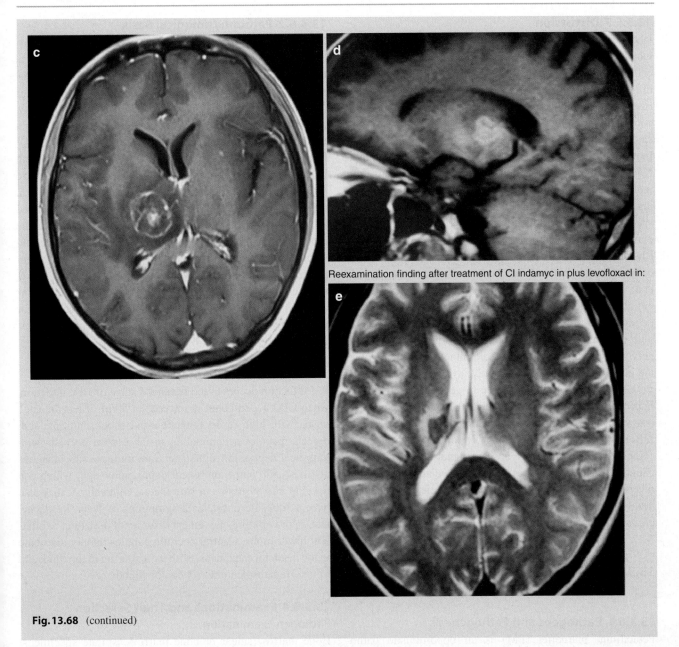

Reexamination finding after treatment of Cl indamyc in plus levofloxacl in:

Fig. 13.68 (continued)

13.3.5.5 Criteria for the Diagnosis

1. Bacterial strain identification: Strains catalase test positive.
2. Cerebral ESF culture has findings of pink or purple Rhodococcus equi.
3. Imaging demonstrations include multiple rounds or oval foci in the brain in long T1 long T2 signal, with obvious space occupying and edema effects by MR imaging. Enhanced imaging demonstrates ring shaped or target shaped obvious abnormal enhancement.
4. Therapeutic review demonstrates absence or shrinkage of the space occupying lesions by reexamination after anti-Rhodococcus equi infection therapy.

13.3.5.6 Differential Diagnosis

It should be differentiated from Toxoplasma encephalitis, Cryptococcus encephalitis, Syphilis encephalitis, TB encephalitis and Staphylococcus aureus encephalitis.

13.3.5.7 Discussion

Rhodococcus equi was firstly discovered in 1923 and nominated as Corynebacterium equi [157]. After the analysis of cellular wall structure, it was found that the bacteria are quite different from Corynebacterium. Therefore, it was categorized into Rhodococcus equi. Rhodococcus equi is generally considered to be the pathogenic bacteria of horses, pigs and cattle. Rhodococcus equi infection is rarely found in humans. In recent years, due to the increased incidence of immunodeficiency syndrome, the incidence of Rhodococcus equi induced respiratory tract infection and sepsis is also increasing. The pathogenesis of Rhodococcus equi was remained speculative in the past. Until recently, the discovery of toxic plasmid enriches our knowledge about the pathogenesis of Rhodococcus equi infection. The clinical manifestations are cough, orange sputum, high fever and other symptoms. Li et al. firstly reported a group of 13 cases HIV/AIDS related pulmonary Rhodococcus equi infection in terms of diagnostic imaging demonstrations in 2009 [86]. There was one case with the complication of Rhodococcus equi infection of the nervous system. Rhodococcus equi infection rarely involves the nervous system, but commonly involves deep brain tissues, with rapid progression, due to general dissemination. Especially the pulmonary infection of Rhodococcus equi provides chances for the secondary intracranial infections. MR imaging demonstrates long T1 long T2 signal in the cerebral parenchyma, large abscess signal in the right basal ganglia, obvious space occupying and edema effects. The imaging demonstrations are less characteristic. And it should be differentiated from toxoplasma encephalitis, Cryptococcus encephalitis, cerebral tuberculoma and lymphoma.

13.3.6 HIV/AIDS Related Intracerebral Penicillium Marneffei Infections

13.3.6.1 Pathogens and Pathogenesis

Penicillium marneffei (PM) is an opportunistic pathogen, which is the only biphasic fungus of Penicillium species. Mycelium phase colonies are grayish white in villus appearance, and the color of colonies may change in the process of differentiation. The back color is cherry red to reddish brown, like soluble red pigments penetrate into the agar medium. The surface of colony has wrinkles in gyrus liked appearance, in color of light brown to brown. Under a microscope, mycelium was singular polymorphic oval or rectangular cells. The mycelium does not split by budding. Immunodeficient individuals are susceptible to PM infection. PM can spread through rhizomyid feces contaminated soil to infect human via the respiratory tract, gastrointestinal tract, and skin defects. PM infection is one of the most common opportunistic infections in AIDS patients of the Southeast Asia, with an increasing incidence.

13.3.6.2 Pathophysiological Basis

PM invades the human body via the respiratory tract, gastrointestinal tract, and skin defects. In people with normal immunity, bacteria invade the body and form local abscess, with characteristic thick pus and mainly tissue necrosis and liquefaction. There are also less vascular reactivity, few neutrophils and body fluids exudates, and slight inflammatory signs, like cold abscess. In patients with HIV infection and decreased immunity, due to the insufficient immune factors, it is difficult for the immune cells to restrict and digest the phagocyted pathogens to form local suppurative reaction. Therefore, they have disseminated lesions. In the cases with PM spreading along with the blood flow to invade brain tissues, PM can replicate and spread to cause reactive hyperplasia of mononuclear phagocyte. Suppurative inflammation occurs in the brain, with clinical manifestations of a series of clinical syndromes induced by the involvement of mononuclear phagocytes. Generally, PM infection of the central nervous system rarely occurs.

13.3.6.3 Clinical Symptoms and Signs

PM infection occurs in the advanced stage of HIV infection, when CD4 T cell count is lower than 50/μl. It has an acute onset, with high fever, fungemia and shock, multiple skin defects, papules accumulating to the central necrosis with umbilical depression sign. There are multiple subcutaneous nodules and central umbilical depressions sign, which can develop into abscesses or skin ulcers. Clinically, it may also have a subacute onset, with symptoms of fever, headache, nausea or vomiting, movement disorder of unilateral or bilateral lower limbs. Central necrotic papules mainly distribute in the head, face and neck, with its scattering in the trunk and limbs. Hepatosplenomegaly can be found.

13.3.6.4 Examinations and Their Selection
Pathogen Examination

Bone marrow smear or bone marrow aspirate specimens/skin/lymph nodes biopsy smear is microscopically observed after Reiter staining for preliminary diagnosis. After the staining, it can be detected with a microscope to do an initial diagnosis. With staining technique, both extracellular and intracellular basophils, round, oval yeast cells can be visible. Some cells have a clear central septum, which is characteristically PM.

Pathological Examination

Biopsy of lymph nodes and defective skin should be performed with PAS staining and Wright Giemsa staining.

Laboratory Tests

Decreased leukocytes, hemachrome and platelet; increased AST; CD4 T cell count <50/μl.

Diagnostic Imaging

CT scanning and MR imaging are the diagnostic imaging examinations of the choice, which can define the size, morphology, location, amount and density of the intracerebral foci.

13.3.6.5 Imaging Demonstrations
CT Scanning

It is demonstrated multiple low density shadows in the brain. Enhanced scanning demonstrations of no enhancement or ring shaped abnormal enhancement.

MR Imaging

It is demonstrated multiple flaky long T1 long T2 signal in the brain, obvious edema and space occupying effect. Enhanced imaging demonstrations of ring shaped or target shaped obvious abnormal enhancement and multiple foci. MR imaging has a higher detection rate of the foci than CT scanning.

Case Study

A male patient aged 36 years was confirmatively diagnosed as having AIDS by the CDC. He was hospitalized due to fever for 1 month. By physical examination, he had emaciation, wartoid necrotic palpula in the face and neck, cervical resistance and movement disturbance of the right lower limb. His CD4 T cell count was 33/μl.

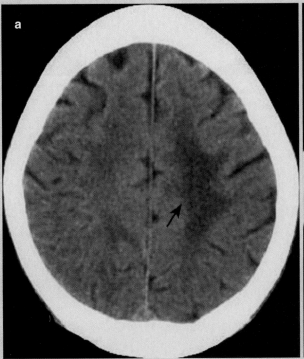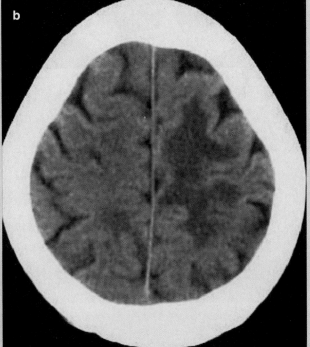

Fig. 13.69 (a–l) HIV/AIDS related Penicillium marneffei meningoencephalitis. (**a**, **b**) Brain CT scanning demonstrates irregular flaky low density shadow in the bilateral parietal lobes and obvious edema. (**c**, **d**) Enhanced scanning demonstrates surrounding gyrus liked enhancement and delayed scanning demonstrates multiple small nodular enhancement in the right parietal lobe. Both blood and CSF culture demonstrate Penicillium marneffei: (**e**, **f**) Direct microscopies by ×400 and ×100 magnification, with findings of branching, separate and broom like branching hyphae. (**g**) Microscopic observation after lactate gossypol blue staining (×1,000) demonstrates broom liked branching hyphae. (**h**) Blood culture in Sabouraud medium demonstrates red pigment. (**i**, **j**) Microscopic observation of the CSF culture demonstrates branching, separate and broom liked hyphae (×400 and ×100). (**k**) Microscopic observation after ESF lactic acid gossypol blue staining demonstrates broom liked branching hyphae (×1,000). (**l**) ESF culture in Sabouraud medium demonstrates red pigment

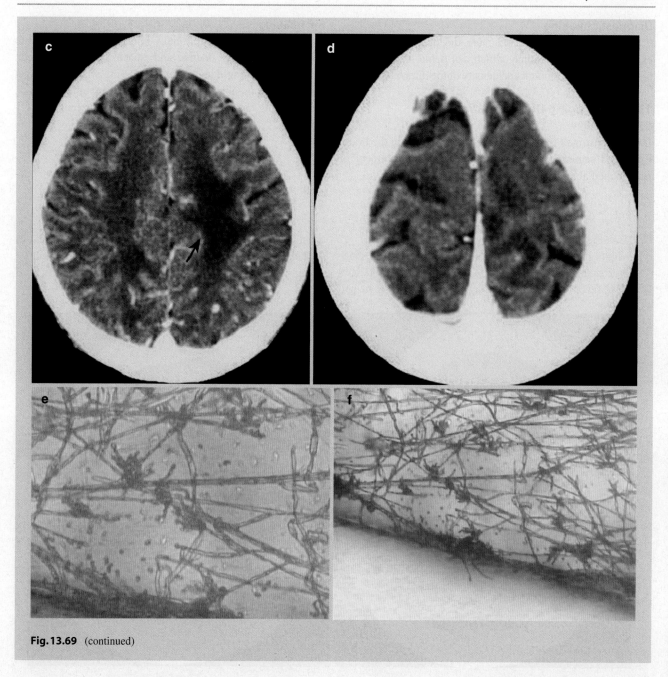

Fig. 13.69 (continued)

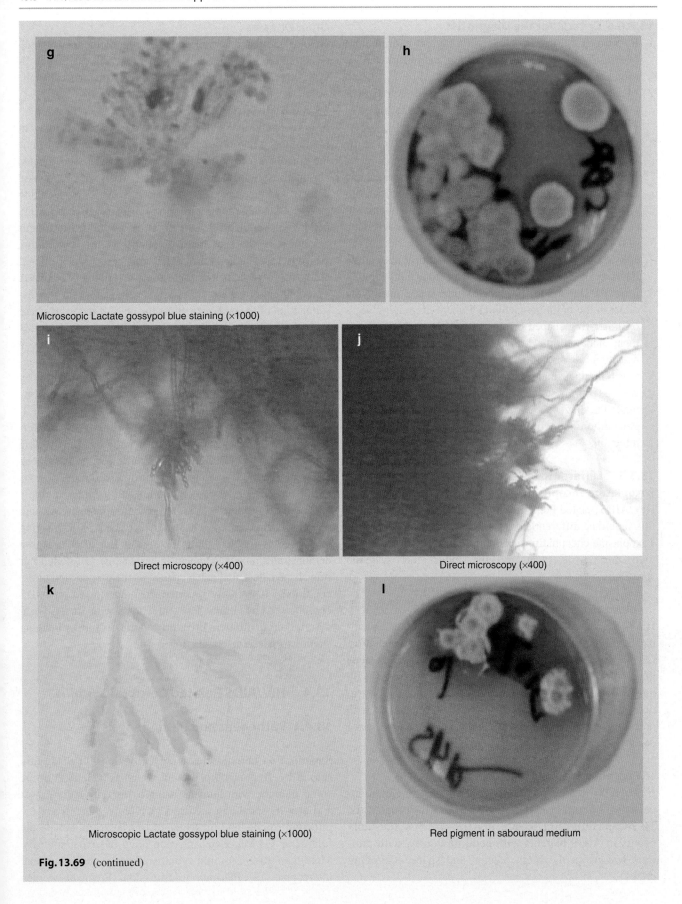

Microscopic Lactate gossypol blue staining (×1000)

Direct microscopy (×400)

Direct microscopy (×400)

Microscopic Lactate gossypol blue staining (×1000)

Red pigment in sabouraud medium

Fig. 13.69 (continued)

13.3.6.6 Criteria for the Diagnosis

1. By fungus culture and histopathological examination of the tissue sections, Penicillium marneffei can be found.
2. Metabolites of Penicillium marneffei is detected. PCR assay is performed to determine the gene sequences of Penicillium marneffei for early diagnosis.
3. CT scanning demonstrations include multiple foci at the interface of brain cortex and medulla, multiple or singular low density shadow in brain parenchyma, obvious edema and space occupying effect. Enhanced scanning demonstrates no enhancement in the early stage, with nodular or ring shaped abnormal enhancement with the progression of the infection.
4. MR imaging demonstrations include multiple foci at the interface of the cerebral cortex and medulla, flaky long T1 long T2 signal, obvious edema and space occupying effect in the brain parenchyma. Enhanced imaging demonstrates ring shaped or target liked abnormal enhancement, and multiple lesions. MR imaging has a higher detection rate of the foci than CT scanning.
5. Other findings include infections of skin and lungs as well as retroperitoneal lymphadenectasis can help to make the diagnosis because HIV/AIDS related cerebral Penicillium marneffei infection is secondary to systemic infection.

13.3.6.7 Differential Diagnosis

Toxoplasma Encephalitis

HIV/AIDS related Penicillium marneffei meningoencephalitis should be differentiated from Toxoplasma encephalitis. Toxoplasma encephalitis has multiple intracerebral lesions, with rare involvements of the lungs and systemic spreading.

Cryptococcal Encephalitis

HIV/AIDS related Penicillium marneffei meningoencephalitis should be differentiated from Cryptococcal encephalitis. Cryptococcal encephalitis has mostly gumma. Enhanced imaging demonstrates no enhancement. In the cases with gliosis or complication of other infections, the demonstrations also include multilocular and wall enhancement, with no central enhancement and generally no edema and space occupying effect.

TB Encephalitis

HIV/AIDS related Penicillium marneffei meningoencephalitis should be differentiated from TB encephalitis. TB encephalitis rarely occurs in AIDS patients. It usually occurs in AIDS patients with good immunity, with multiple lesions in the brain, edema and space occupying effect.

Other Diseases

HIV/AIDS related Penicillium marneffei meningoencephalitis should be differentiated from other diseases, such as syphiloma and intracerebral infection of Rhodococcus equi.

13.3.6.8 Discussion

PM is a conditional pathogen whose infection tends to occur in immunocompromised people. The spreading route can be the Rhizomys feces contaminated soil. People can be infected via the respiratory tract, gastrointestinal tract, and skin defects. With an increasing incidence, PSM is considered to be one of the most common opportunistic infections in AIDS patients of Southeast Asia. PM is the only biphasic fungus belonging to the species of Hyphomycetales Penicillium, which is a special Penicillium. In terms of its tissue pathogenicity, that of mold phase is inferior to that of the yeast phase. The conidium of the mold phase is responsible for the dissemiantion of the pathogen while the cells of the yeast phase are actually the pathogen. PM encephalitis is pathologically characterized by: Due to a serious failure of CD4 T cells in AIDS patients, the macrophages' phagocytic capacity is significantly weakened in the cases with AIDS complicated by PM brain infection. Central necrosis of the focus induced by inflammatory granuloma is accompanied by neutrophil infiltration containing many yeast liked PM cells. They proliferate themselves by splitting rather than budding. The imaging studies on brain Penicillium marneffei infection have been rarely reported. CT scanning demonstrates multiple lesions at the interface of the cerebral cortex and medulla, multiple or singular low density shadow in brain parenchyma, and obvious edema and space occupying effect. MR imaging demonstrates long T1 long T2 signal. Enhanced imaging demonstrates no enhancement in early stage, but nodular or ring shaped abnormal enhancement as the progression of the conditions. It is rarely reported imaging studies on AIDS complicated by brain PM infection, with inconsistent descriptions in different literature reports. Its further imaging studies still deserve conducting.

13.4   HIV/AIDS Related Cerebral Syphilis

13.4.1 Pathogens and Pathogenesis

Syphilis is a chronic classic sexually transmitted disease caused by Treponema pallidum, which is a small and fine spiral microbe with humans being as its only natural host and also its spreading media. The syphilis patients are the infection source, and its routes of transmission include the following: (1) Major transmission route of sexual contacts. More than 90 % acquired syphilis is transmitted via sexual intercourse. (2) Placenta transmission. Pregnant women with syphilis can spread the disease to the fetus via the placenta. (3) By kissing, breastfeeding and other direct contacts to the infected patients. After HIV positive patients are infected by neurosyphilis, its invasion of the central nervous system occurs in 1–3 months. After Treponema pallidum gains its access to the human body via small defects of the skin and mucous membrane, it invades the nearby lymph space and multiplies itself in a large quantity. The immune responses to its invasion cause ulceration in the invaded location, which is known as chancre. After Treponema pallidum multiplies itself in the primary lesion, they invade nearby lymph nodes and then disseminate to other tissues and organs along with blood flow, with demonstrations of mesosyphilis. If untreated, mesosyphilis in some patients may progress to tertiary syphilis, causing cardiovascular or neurological lesions as well as gummas in the skin, bone and organs. Treponema pallidum is in a large quantity with strong pathogenicity in the early stage to cause complex symptoms and signs, with main invasion of the skin and mucous membrane to cause extensive multifocal endovasculitis. Treponema pallidum is in a small quantity in the advanced stage, causing granuloma lesions with large destructive effect to local tissues. It can invade many organs in the human body, especially the invasions to the heart and the central nervous system. The clinical manifestations are related to large quantity multiplying of the pathogen and the resulted immune functional disorders.

13.4.2 Pathophysiological Basis

HIV/AIDS related neurosyphilis is more invasive, mostly involving the brain subcortical areas and spreading to the nearby brain parenchyma along blood vessels and meninges. Neurosyphilis mostly occurs in the cerebral hemispheres, occasionally in the cerebellum and brain stem, the fourth ventricle, pituitary and hypothalamus, commonly with singular lesion. The basic lesion is a dense infiltration of lymphocytes and plasma cells around the blood vessels in the brain parenchyma, which can cause meningitis, encephalitis and meningeal vascular syphilis. Cerebral syphiloma rarely occurs, and is advanced neurosyphilis of chronic granuloma. The tumor is in a shape of irregular round or oval with different diameters, rubber texture, and grayish red section. Microscopically, it can be divided into 3 regions: central region, its surrounding region and the outermost region. The central region has extensive necrosis, containing large quantity argyrophilic fibers, which is the characteristic demonstration of the disease. Its surrounding region has the peripheral cell structure with plasma cells, lymphocytes, monocytes, fibroblasts, epithelial liked cells and cytomegalovirus, with accompanying vasculitis or perivasculitis. The outermost region is an envelope composed of collagen fibers. Pathologically, the lesions of meningeal neurosyphilis can be categorized into meningitis. However, there are concurrent slight cortical lesions. By naked eyes, there are diffuse inflammatory responses in the pia matter, with increased thickness or being cloudy, and the miliary gumma in the thickened meninges resembling to miliary tuberculosis. The pathological changes is vascular neurosyphilis in the involvement of the minor and medium sized arteries in the brain and spinal cord to cause syphilitic endarteritis and brain and spinal cord tissue malacia in the corresponding area. Congenital neurosyphilis due to vertical transmission from mother to fetus commonly causes stillbirth. Fetus infected in early pregnancy sustains hydrocephalus and brain malformation, which is life threatening. In the early period after birth, the fetus may suffer meningeal vascular infection.

13.4.3 Clinical Symptoms and Signs

The clinical symptoms are atypical, including chronic headaches, memory loss or intelligence decline, history of epileptic seizure; lateral sensory or motor abnormalities, intracranial hypertension, hemiplegia, aphasia, unilateral sensory loss or cranial nerves paralysis and other local neurological signs.

13.4.4 Examinations and Their Selection

1. Pathogenic examination is the commonly used examination.
2. Syphilis immunological assay of the serum and the cerebrospinal fluid is positive.
3. Brain CT scanning or MR imaging can define the location and size of the lesions.

13.4.5 Imaging Demonstrations

13.4.5.1 CT Scanning
CT scanning demonstrates small focal low density areas with clear borders and no edema. In the cases with complicated bleeding, the demonstrations also include small spots bleeding. Syphiloma is demonstrated as granuloma, with nodular or mass liked low density shadow by CT scanning.

13.4.5.2 MR Imaging
MR imaging demonstrates intracerebral multiple spots and stripes long T1WI and long T2WI signal, and granuloma manifestations of syphiloma with long T1WI and long T2WI signal. Enhanced imaging demonstrates ring shaped enhancement and unobvious edema and space occupying effect.

Case Study 1

A female patient aged 48 years was confirmatively diagnosed as having AIDS by the CDC. She had a history of paid blood donation and a history of syphilis. She complained symptoms of headache and memory loss. Her CD4 T cell count was 43/μl.

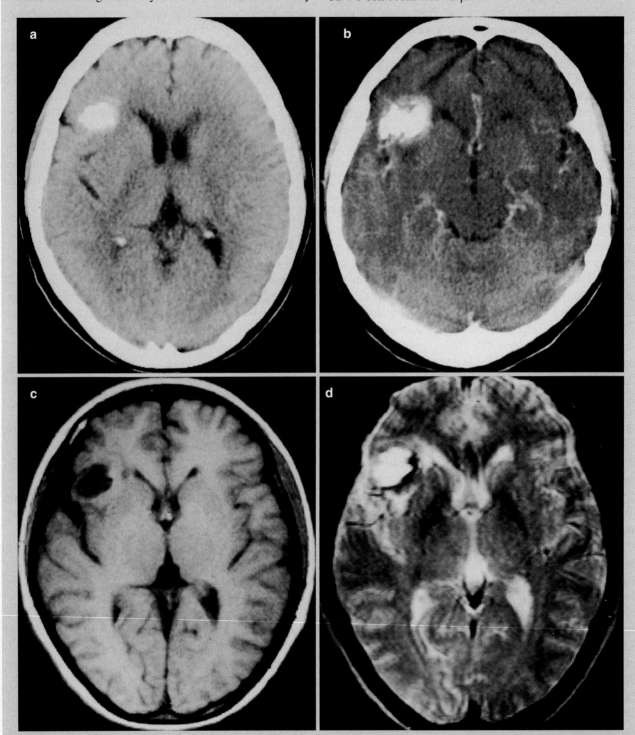

Fig. 13.70 (a–g) HIV/AIDS related brain syphiloma. (a) Axial plain CT scanning demonstrates flaky high density is in the right temporal lobe, surrounding ring shaped low density area, and unobvious edema and space occupying effect. (b) Axial enhanced CT scanning demonstrates ring halo liked abnormal enhancement in the right temporal lobe and no obvious space occupying effect. (c, d) Axial MR imaging demonstrates scanning round liked long T1 long T2 signal in the temporal lobe. (e) Axial MR imaging demonstrates round liked long T1 signal in the right temporal lobe with clear border, enlarged right lateral fissure cistern, deepened and widened local sulcus and decreased total brain volume. (f) Axial MR imaging demonstrates round liked long T2 signal in the right temporal lobe, surrounding stripes slightly short T2 signal, enlarged right lateral fissure cistern, deepened and widened local sulcus, and decreased total brain volume. (g) MRA imaging and 3-dimensional reconstruction demonstrate vascular distal occlusion of the temporal branch of the right middle cerebral artery, and no vascular network in lesions area

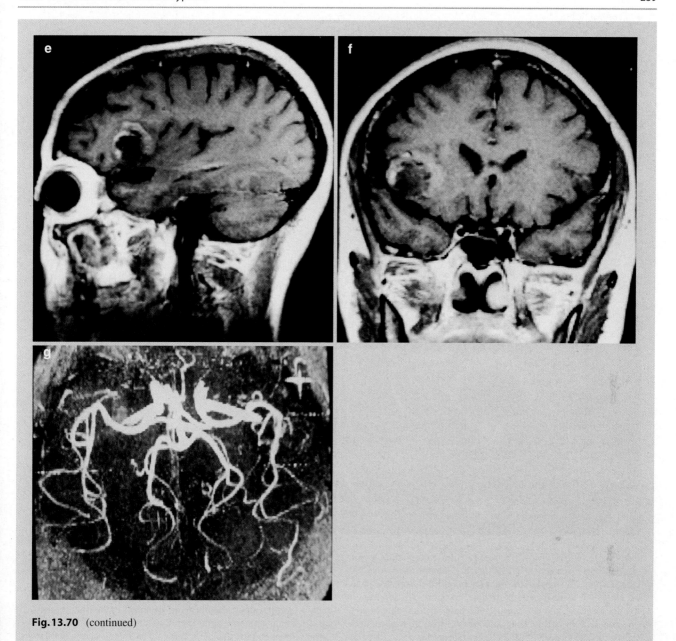

Fig. 13.70 (continued)

Case Study 2

A male patient aged 46 years was confirmatively diagnosed as having AIDS by the CDC. He complained of behavioral abnormalities and consciousness disturbance for more than 9 months and aggravated with convulsions twice. He had a history of prostitute visit and sustained sexually transmitted disease 4 years ago, without formally treated. By physical examinations on admission, his vital signs are half stable, conscious, poor calculation and orientation, increased muscular tension of lower limbs, Babinski reflex suspicious positive of lower limbs, serum syphilis antibody positive, and conditions progressively serious. Since 9 month ago, the patient had memory loss with unknown reasons, recently obvious memory loss, partial reserved long term memory, mania, anxiety, irritation, dizziness and drowsiness. His CD4 T cell count was 57/μl.

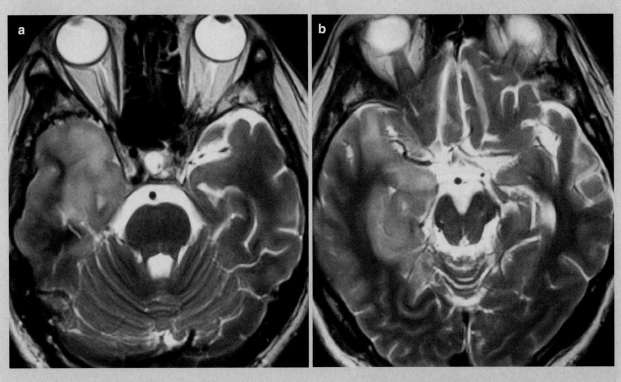

Fig. 13.71 (**a–q**) HIV/AIDS related syphilitic encephalitis, meningitis and optic neuritis. (**a–d**) MR imaging demonstrates large flaky long T1 long T2 signal in the right temporal lobe, frontal lobe and occipital lobe with unclear borderline, leftward migration of the midline structure and deformed right lateral ventricle due to compression. (**e, f**) FLAIR imaging demonstrates flaky high signal in the right temporal lobe. (**g–i**) DTI demonstrates to have decreased red area (representing horizontal course of the nerve fiber bundles) in the anterior limb of internal capsule, reduced and sparse fiber bundles. (**j**) BOLD demonstrates the left red area is the visual function area. (**k**) It is demonstrated to have a decreased MRS NAA peak and the increased creatine peak of CHO. (**l–q**) Enhanced imaging demonstrates gyrus liked abnormal enhancement in the right temporal lobe, sagittal sinus, and thickened meninges of the right cerebellar tentorium and the right lateral fissure cistern with obvious enhancement and the thickness being up to 8 mm, thickened bilateral optic nerves with enhancement

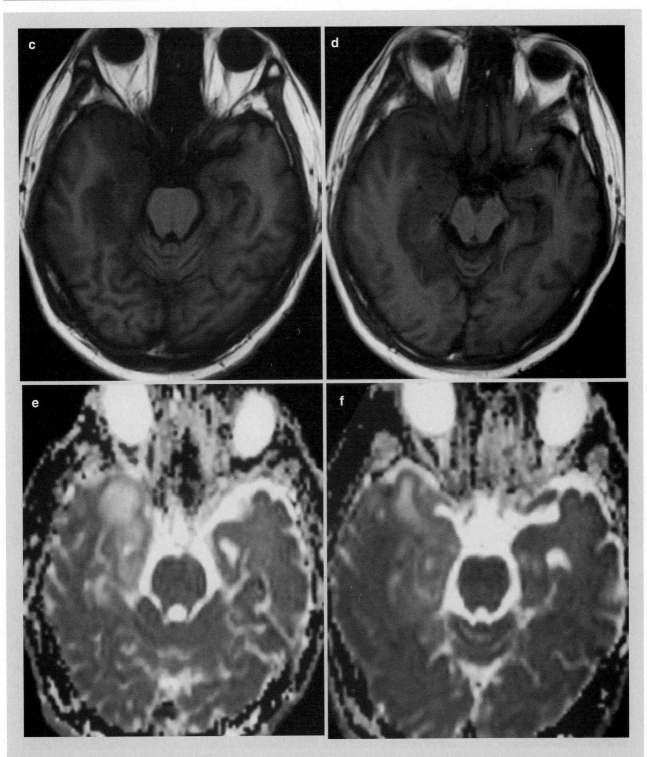

Fig. 13.71 (continued)

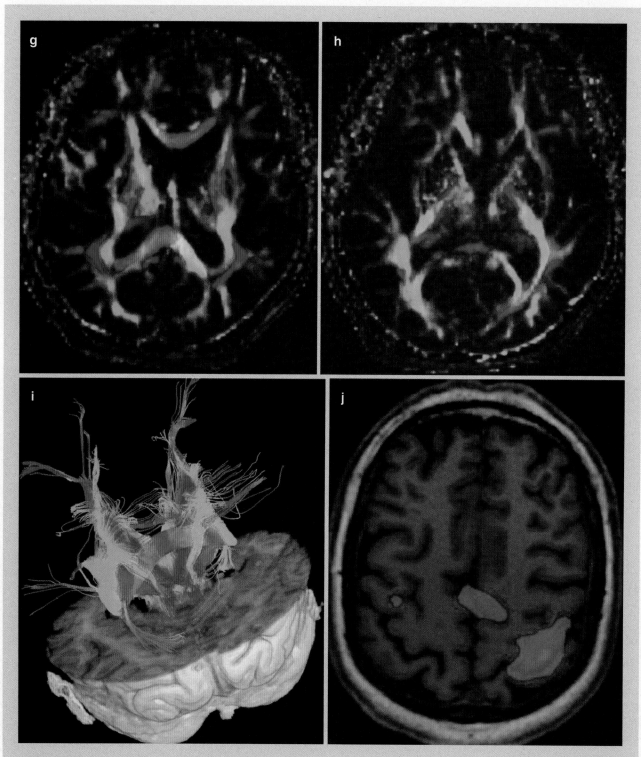

Fig. 13.71 (continued)

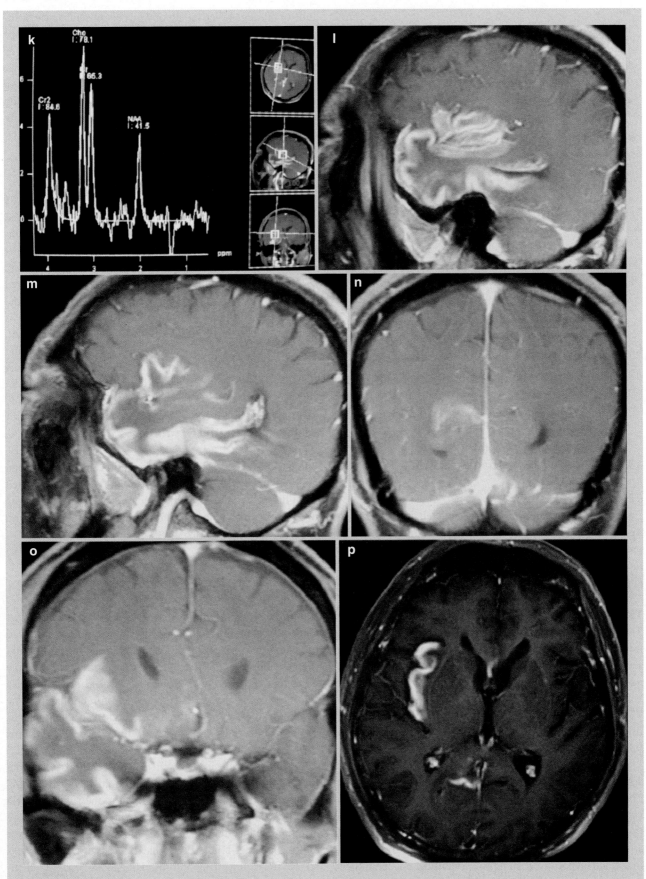

Fig. 13.71 (continued)

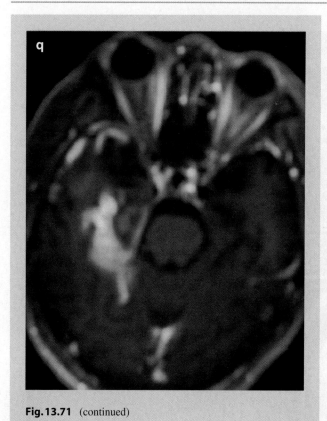

Fig. 13.71 (continued)

13.4.6 Criteria for the Diagnosis

13.4.6.1 Case History
The case history should be reported in detail, including syphilis infection, contact history with syphilitic patients, blood products transfusion, epileptic seizure, chronic headaches, memory loss, intelligent decline and lateral sensory or motor abnormalities.

13.4.6.2 Signs
The following signs should be reported, including AR pupil, intracranial hypertension, hemiplegia, aphasia, unilateral sensory decline or cranial nerves paralysis and other focal neurological signs.

13.4.6.3 Pathogenic Examination
Immunological assay of the serum and cerebrospinal fluid for syphilis is positive.

13.4.6.4 CT Scanning Demonstrations
The imaging demonstrations of AIDS complicated by brain syphilis are diverse and complex, with involvements of the brain parenchyma, spinal cord, meninges and optic nerves. It is commonly demonstrated as syphilitic vasculitis, syphiloma and syphilitic meningitis. Syphilitic encephalitis is demonstrated as flaky low density shadows in the temporal lobe or basal ganglia, and no obvious edema and space occupying effect. Enhanced CT scanning demonstrates obvious abnormal enhancement. Brain syphiloma is demonstrated as flaky low/equal density shadow in the brain. In the cases with complicated bleeding, the demonstrations can have high density shadow. In the cases with complicated liquefaction and necrosis, the demonstrations can have low density shadow, and marginal enhancement or no enhancement by enhanced scanning.

13.4.6.5 MR Imaging Demonstrations
Syphilitic encephalitis is demonstrated to have flaky long T1 and long T2 signal in the temporal lobe or basal ganglia, and obvious abnormal enhancement by enhanced imaging, common concurrent involvements of the optic nerve and spinal cord. There are also thickened optic nerve in equal T1 and slightly long T2 signal. Segmental myelitis is demonstrated to have strips long T1 and long T2 signal, obvious abnormal enhancement by enhanced imaging. Cerebral syphiloma is demonstrated to have singular long T1 and mixed T2 signal, no obvious edema and space occupying effect. Syphilitic vasculitis can result in multiple infarct and hemorrhagic foci in the cerebral cortex and the corticomedullary interface.

13.4.7 Differential Diagnosis

HIV/AIDS related syphilitic encephalitis, meningitis, optic neuritis and cerebral syphilioma should be differentiated from herpes viral encephalitis, meningioma or tuberculoma in combination with the clinical manifestations. (With detailed description in the above text).

13.4.8 Discussion

The incidence of syphilis in AIDS patients is increasing. Generally, syphilitic encephalitis is more common, followed by syphiloma. Neurosyphilis in AIDS patients can rapidly progress into the advanced stage. Due to the poor immune mediation, intracerebral syphiloma rarely occurs because syphiloma is a marker of responses from cellular immune mediation to the pathogen and facilitates to restrict the spreading of the infection. AIDS patients with intracerebral syphilis infection commonly have manifestations of cerebrovascular stenosis and occlusion, which lead to cerebral infarction, malacia and bleeding. The demonstrations in Fig. 13.69a–g include a round liked abnormal signal in the right temporal lobe, with accompanying bleeding, which is necessary to be differentiated from non-HIV/AIDS intracerebral bleeding or tumor bleeding. HIV/AIDS related cerebral syphiloma has no obvious clinical symptoms. Diagnostic imaging demonstrates no obvious edema and space occupying effect.

Cerebral bleeding in non-HIV/AIDS patient has serious clinical symptoms, commonly with inducing factors, which can be definitively diagnosed in combination with the case history. Cases with tumor bleeding commonly have obvious edema and space occupying effect, whose diagnosis can be defined in combination with the case history and laboratory tests results.

13.5   HIV/AIDS Related Intracranial Tumors

13.5.1   HIV/AIDS Related Intracerebral Non-Hodgkin's Lymphoma

13.5.1.1 Pathogens and Pathogenesis

Non-Hodgkin's lymphoma is a common malignant tumor of the nervous system in AIDS patients. As early in 80s of the twentieth century, it has been listed as the diagnostic index of AIDS. The pathogen and pathogenesis of HIV/AIDS related intracerebral non-Hodgkin's lymphoma are still unknown. Most scholars believe that since there is no lymph circulation and no lymphoid tissues accumulation in the nervous system, intracerebral non-Hodgkin's lymphoma may be derived from undifferentiated pluripotent mesenchymal cells or stem cells around the vascular vessels in the brain. Therefore, tumors and blood vessels are closely related. Currently, the virus infection theory is overwhelmingly important for immunodeficiency, which explains the pathogenesis as activation of B cells by EB virus to avoid the defense mechanism of the human body for its progression into lymphoma. Some other scholars believe that EBV contributes to the conversion of the normal growth regulatory gene into a gene that can trigger abnormal growth stimulation, whose integration into the target cells DNA causes cellular malignancy. In recent years, gene research indicated that chromosome 6q deletion and p53, bcl-6 EBER-1 are related to the occurrence of PCNSL. Montesinos-rongen et al. [106] reported the use of fluorescence in situ hybridization for analysis of lymphoma related chromosome breakage point during the interval of nuclear division in patients with PCNSL and normal immunity. They proposed that the pathogen and pathogenesis of PCNSL may be related to IGH and BCL-6 gene mutations.

13.5.1.2 Pathophysiological Basis

HIV/AIDS related intracerebral non-Hodgkin's lymphoma occurs in any age groups. Among intracranial space occupying lesions, the incidence of lymphoma is only lower than that of toxoplasmosis, with a common occurrence in the advanced stage of AIDS. Recent literature reports indicated that the incidence of extranodal lymphomas is increasing unevenly, and the most obvious increases can be found in cerebral and ocular lymphomas. The increasing incidence is possibly related to increasing infection of human immunodeficiency virus and increasing cases of transplantations as well as the increasing use of immunosuppressive therapy. Lymphoma mostly invades the cerebral hemispheres, with common involvements of the frontal lobes, parietal lobe, temporal lobe, occipital lobe, corpus striatum and lateral ventricles and with rare involvements of the brainstem, corpus callosum and cerebellum. Non-Hodgkin's lymphoma of the central nervous is commonly singular and sometimes is multiple. By gross observation, it is parenchymal masses, with irregular shapes and different sizes, in a diameter of 0.7–7 cm, no capsule. It has a clearly defined boundary from its surrounding tissue, with grayish yellow or gray red section and fish liked texture. It has a rich blood supply, commonly with hemorrhage or necrosis. Pathological changes are characterized by tumor cells around the blood vessels are central arranged and infiltrative extend outwards along the intervascular space, which is an important marker for the diagnosis of lymphoma of the nervous system. Between tumor cells, the phagocytes are in stars liked distribution. In the peritumor tissues, there are different degrees of congestion, edema, bleeding, degeneration and necrosis, with accompanying proliferation of the grid cells and glial cells. By electron microscopy, B cells are round, with a large proportion of the nuclear cytoplasm and no extracellular basement membrane or intercellular connection. There are rich ribosomes, round nuclei with nuclear fissure. The shapes of the T cells are irregular with distorted nuclei in lobulated or gyri liked appearance.

13.5.1.3 Clinical Symptoms and Signs

It commonly occurs in middle aged male AIDS patients and sometimes in young AIDS patients. Intracerebral non-Hodgkin's lymphoma, as a space occupying lesion, commonly has initial symptoms or main clinical manifestations of intracranial hypertension and localized compression symptoms, including headache, nausea, vomiting and visual disturbances. There are also cervical upset, unstable movements, drowsiness and mental disorders. For cases with intracerebral lymphoma, its complication of extracerebral lymphoma should be also considered.

13.5.1.4 Examinations and Their Selection

1. CSF examination.
2. Immunohistochemical examination.
3. Stereotactic biopsy is replacing craniotomy due to its noninvasiveness. The final definitive diagnosis of PCNSL depends on pathological examination.
4. MRI is the diagnostic imaging of the choice, which can define the size, range and amount of the tumors as well as their relationship with surrounding tissues. CT scanning is uniquely favorable in defining tumor bleeding.
5. PET-CT scanning provides valuable information for the screening and qualitative diagnosis of the disease.

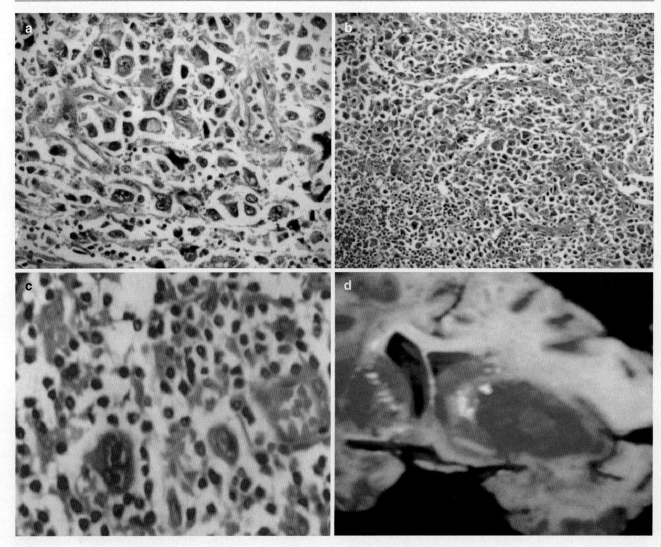

Fig. 13.72 (**a–d**) HIV/AIDS related intracerebral lymphoma. (**a**) HE staining demonstrates non-Hodgkin's lymphoma of the lymph nodes, HE ×400. (**b**) HE staining demonstrates non-Hodgkin's lymphoma of the lymph nodes, with destructed lymph nodes structure, a large volume of the tumor cells, abundant cytoplasm, and multiple mitotic count (*upper left*) HE ×200. (**c**) It is demonstrated to have large quantity lymphocytes and small quantity R-S cells, with typical mirror cells

13.5.1.5 Imaging Demonstrations
CT Scanning
Up to 90 % cases of PCNSL have singular lesions and sometimes multiple lesions. The foci are in equal/slightly low density with clear borderline. In the tumors, there are necrosis, with no/slight peritumor edema and slight space occupying effect. Enhanced scanning demonstrates many tumors in ring shaped or map liked obvious enhancement. Sometimes, the tumor margin is blurry, with irregular enhancement. In some rare cases, the lymphoma can spread downwards along ependyma to cause multiple high density foci on the brain ventricular wall. Mendenhall et al. [103] divided the CT scanning images of intracranial lymphoma into three groups: (1) multi-center group, accounting for about 50 %; (2) large lesion group (with the lesion diameter no less than 3.5 cm); (3) small lesion group (with the lesion diameter less than 3.5 cm). Ojeda divided the CT

scanning demonstrations into singular lesion group and multiple lesions group. They provided characteristic description of the CT scanning demonstrations from different perspectives.

MR Imaging
Most demonstrations by T1WI are in low or equal signal and by T2WI are slightly high signal. The MR imaging demonstrations of HIV/AIDS related lymphoma are greatly different from those of lymphoma in patients with normal immunity. Lymphomas are multiple. By enhanced imaging, there is obviously abnormal enhancement of uneven mass, ring shaped enhancements in different thicknesses and map liked enhancement, with no central enhancement due to central necrosis. It is worth noting that enhanced MR imaging demonstrates no enhancement of the tumors in patients who received hormone therapy.

PET-CT Scanning

The tumor is strongly stained with accumulated metabolites. O'Malley et al. [114] prospectively studied the diagnostic value of applied [201]T1 single-photon emission computed tomography (SPECT) for HIV/AIDS related intracranial lymphoma, with biopsy or autopsy results as the pathological control. They believed that [201]T1 single photon emission tomography (SPECT) is important in identifying space occupying lesions in the nervous system. Recently, Li et al. [90]. conducted a retrospective study to assess the diagnostic value of PET-CT for the diagnosis of HIV/AIDS related intracranial lymphoma, with autopsy results as the pathological control. They concluded that PET-CT has important value in identifying localized or diffuse lymphoma in HIV/AIDS patients as well as the benign tumor from malignancies.

Case Study 1

A female patient aged 48 years was confirmatively diagnosed as having AIDS by the CDC. She had a history of extramarital affair and complained of headache, vomiting, consciousness disturbance, irritation, incontinence and lower limbs paralysis. Her CD4 T cell count was 15/µl.

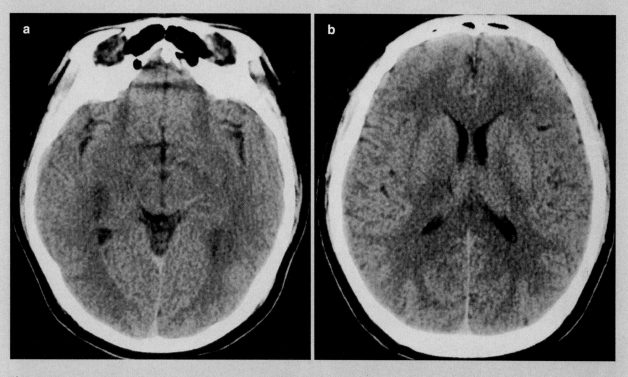

Fig. 13.73 (a–h) HIV/AIDS related intracerebral non-Hodgkin's lymphoma. (a, b) Axial CT scanning demonstrates flaky low density area in the right thalamus with blurring border, and no obvious space occupying effect and edema. (c, d) Axial MR imaging demonstrates large flaky long T1 long T2 signal in the right thalamus, obvious space occupying effect and no obvious edema. (e–h) Axial, coronal and sagittal enhanced MR imaging with IV-Gd-DTPA demonstrate ring shaped or map liked obvious abnormal enhancement of the right thalamus, no central enhancement, slight space occupying effect and narrowed right lateral ventricle due to compression; sagittal findings of oval shaped left occipital lobe, sawtooth liked abnormal enhancement, no central no enhancement, abnormal linear enhancement of the meninges in the brain falx and the right lateral ventricle

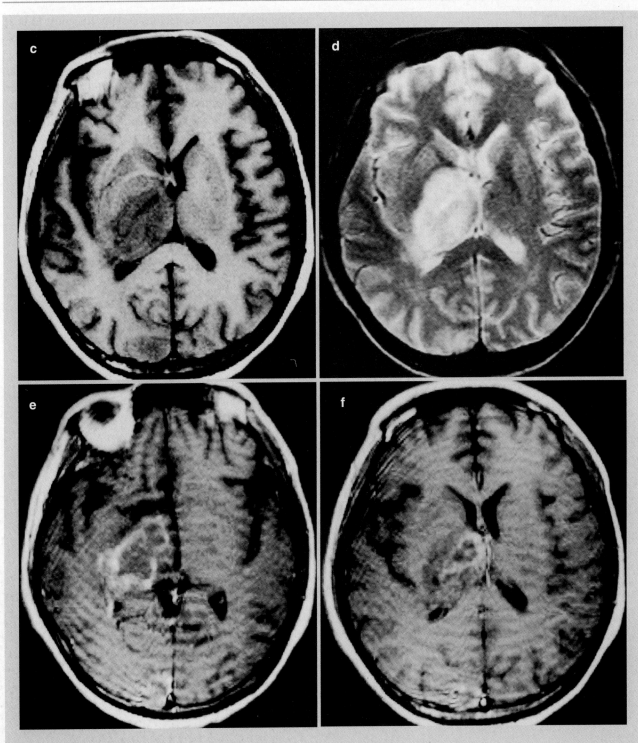

Fig. 13.73 (continued)

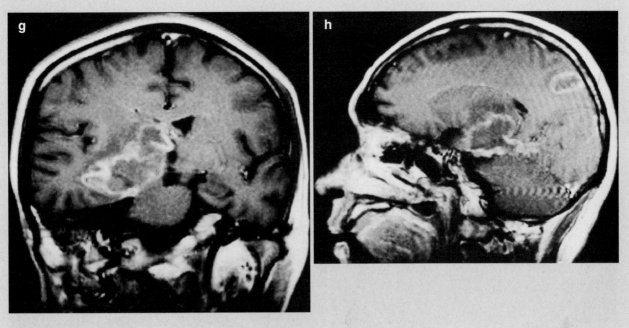

Fig. 13.73 (continued)

Case Study 2

A female patient aged 48 years was confirmatively diagnosed as having AIDS by the CDC. She had a history of extramarital affair and complained of headache, vomiting, consciousness disturbance, irritation, incontinence and lower limbs paralysis. Her CD4 T cell count was 15/µl.

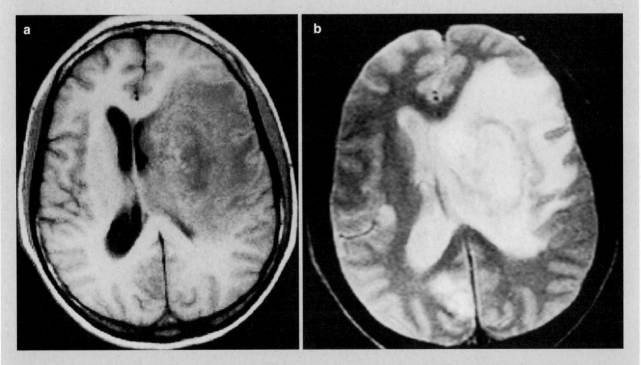

Fig. 13.74 (a–e) HIV/AIDS related brain non-Hodgkin's lymphoma. (**a**) Axial plain MR imaging demonstrates large flaky long T1 signal in deep left temporal lobe with longer T1 signal, obvious space occupying effect and obvious edema. (**b**) Axial plain MR imaging demonstrates large flaky long uneven T2 signal in deep left temporal lobe, and peripheral fire flame liked edema.

(**c–e**) Axial, sagittal and coronal enhanced MR imaging demonstrate a huge mass liked obvious abnormal enhancement in deep left temporal lobe, no central septal enhancement, obvious space occupying effect, surrounding scattered few satellite lesions in nodular abnormal enhancement

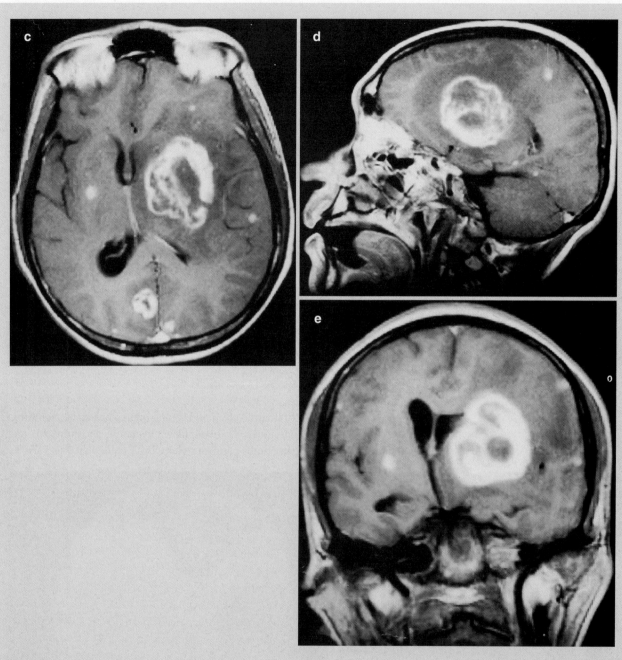

Fig. 13.74 (continued)

Case Study 3

A male patient aged 27 years was confirmatively diagnosed as having AIDS by the CDC. He had a history of extramarital affair and complained of headache, vomiting, oblique mouth and face, functional disturbance of the right limbs. His CD4 T cell count was 45/μl.

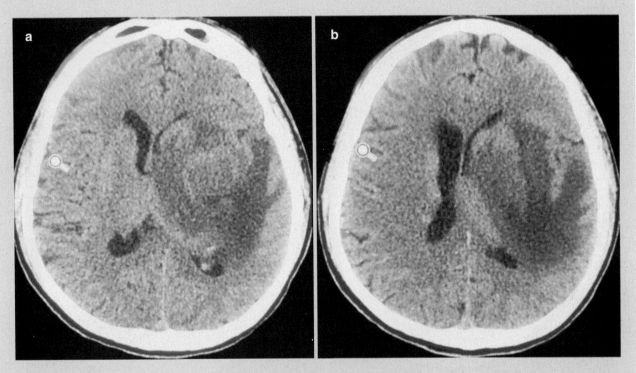

Fig. 13.75 (**a, b**) HIV/AIDS related brain non-Hodgkin's lymphoma. (**a, b**) CT scanning demonstrates Buddha's hand liked low density shadow in the left temporal lobe, rightward migration of the midline, and obvious brain tissue edema

Case Study 4

A male patient aged 77 years was confirmatively diagnosed as having AIDS by the CDC. He had a history of extramarital affair and complained of headache, vomiting, functional disorder of the limbs. His CD4 T cell count was 105/μl.

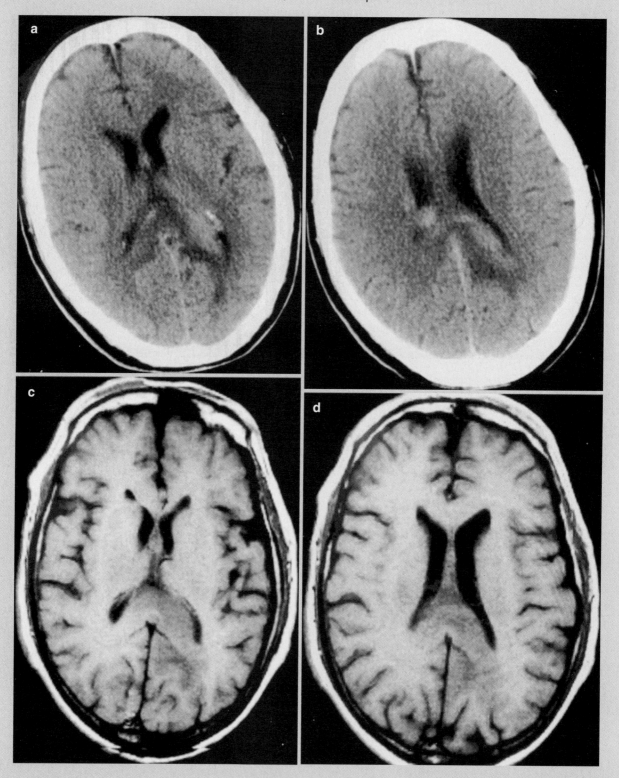

Fig. 13.76 (a–j) HIV/AIDS related brain non-Hodgkin's lymphoma. (**a**, **b**) CT scanning demonstrates stripes slightly higher density shadow in bilateral lateral ventricular occipital horns. (**c–f**) Axial MR imaging demonstrates stripes long T1 long T2 signal in ependyma of the bilateral lateral ventricular occipital horns, small flaky long T1 and T2 signal in the right basal ganglia. Enhanced MR imaging by IV-Gd-DTPA demonstrates obviously thickened ependyma in bilateral lateral ventricular occipital horns, with nodular abnormal enhancement, and involved choroid plexus

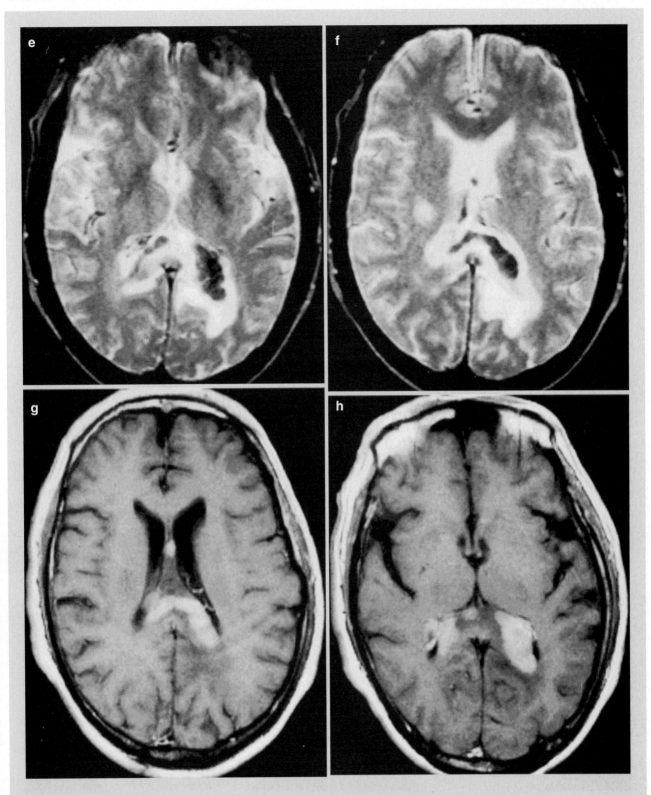

Fig. 13.76 (continued)

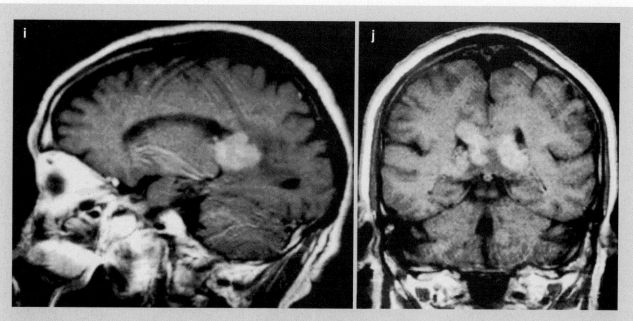

Fig. 13.76 (continued)

Case Study 5

A female patient aged 61 years was confirmatively diagnosed as having AIDS by the CDC. She was hospitalized due to numbness of the left limbs with restricted movements for 2 months, with progressive aggravation. Her CD4 T cell count was 78/µl.

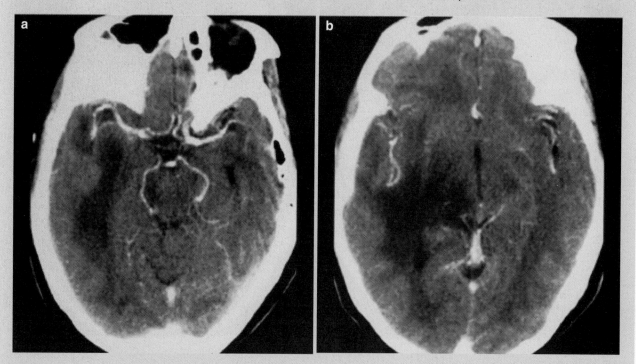

Fig. 13.77 (**a–f**) Enhanced CT scanning demonstrates horseshoe shaped obvious abnormal enhancement in the right basal ganglia, obvious edema in the surrounding brain tissue, slight space occupying effect and slight leftward migration of the midline. (**g–h**) Enhanced CT scanning demonstrates round liked mass in the left parietal lobe, with even enhancement and clear borderline, and obvious edema of the surrounding brain tissues. (**a–o**) HIV/AIDS related brain non-Hodgkin's lymphoma. (**i–k**) CT scanning demonstrates low density shadow in the right basal ganglia and the parietal lobe, finger liked edema in the surrounding brain tissue, slight space occupying effect, slight leftward migration of the midline. (**l–o**) Enhanced CT scanning demonstrates obvious abnormal horseshoe liked enhancement in the right basal ganglia, obvious edema in surrounding brain tissue, slight space occupying effect, slight leftward migration of the midline; round liked masses in bilateral parietal lobes, with even enhancement, clear borders and obvious edema of the surrounding brain tissue

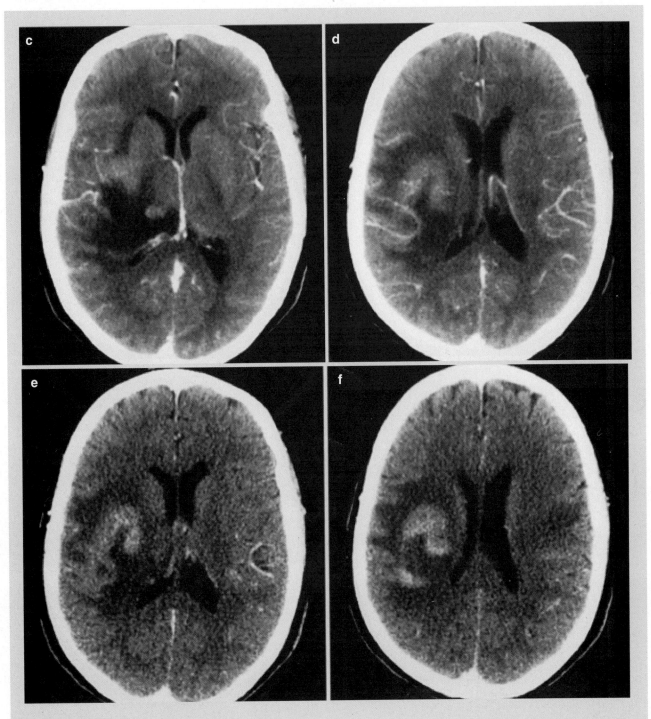

Fig. 13.77 (continued)

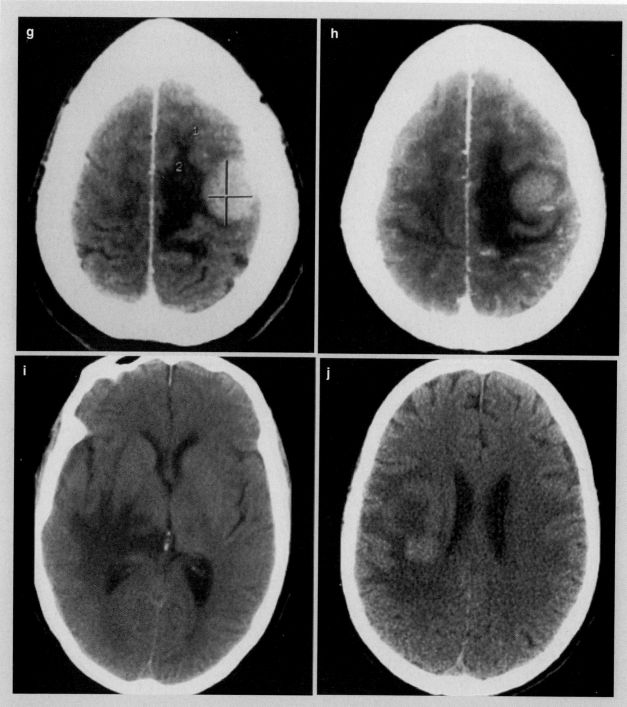

Fig. 13.77 (continued)

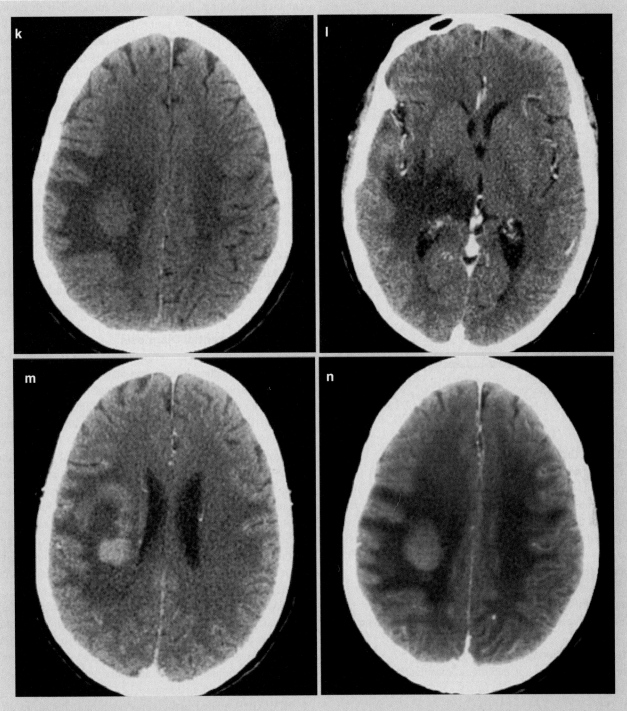

Fig. 13.77   (continued)

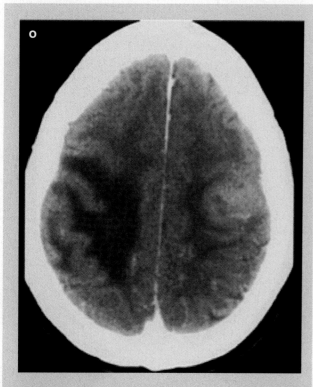

Fig. 13.77 (continued)

13.5.1.6 Criteria for the Diagnosis
CSF Examination
In patients with HIV/AIDS related PCNSL, detection of EB virus gene by PCR has a sensitivity of 100 % and a specificity of 98.5 %. sCD23 in CSF is a marker of PCNSL, with a sensitivity of 77 % and a specificity of 94 %. About 85 % patients with PCNSL have increased ESF protein and half can be detected to have tumor cells.

Immunohistochemical Assay
The tumor cells can be defined to be lymphoid or lymphoma.

Stereotactic Biopsy
Stereotactic biopsy for pathologic examination can help to find tumor cells.

CT Scanning Demonstrations
HIV/AIDS related malignant lymphoma commonly occurs in deep gray matter, periventricular area and/or the corpus callosum. It can be singular or multiple. Plain scanning generally demonstrates low density lesion with irregular border or round liked high density lesion with perifocal slight or moderate edema ring and relatively slight space occupying effect. Enhanced scanning demonstrates even enhancement of the tumor or map liked abnormal enhancement of the tumor margin, with no central necrosis enhancement. The tumor can spread along the subependymal to cause multiple high density lesions in the ventricular wall. By

enhanced scanning, the lesions are enhanced with clearer demonstrations. The key points for the diagnosis are as the following: (1) singular or multiple equal high density lesions in the deep brain; (2) relatively slight perifocal edema and space occupying effect; (3) Even enhancement of the tumor by enhanced scanning. In the cases with central necrosis, abnormal map liked enhancement can be demonstrated.

MR Imaging Demonstrations
The characteristic T2WI demonstrations of HIV/AIDS related malignant lymphoma are equal or slightly low signal. In the cases of lymphoma with more necrotic foci, high signal can be demonstrated. Most lymphomas are located in the supratentorial and communicate with ependyma and/or meninges.

PET-CT Scanning Demonstrations
HIV/AIDS related malignant lymphoma is demonstrated to be strongly stained and have accumulated metabolites. By radionuclide ^{201}T1 scanning, the lymphoma is strongly stained.

13.5.1.7 Differential Diagnosis
1. Primary lymphoma is commonly singular in about 50 % patients. It occurs in deep gray and white matters of the brain and is commonly parenchymal tumors. Enhanced scanning demonstrates even abnormal enhancement.
2. HIV/AIDS related malignant lymphoma should be differentiated from toxoplasma encephalitis. The foci of Toxoplasma encephalitis are mostly in basal ganglia and the interface of the gray-white matters. Enhanced scanning demonstrates ring or spiral shaped obvious abnormal enhancement. Radionuclide ^{201}T1 scanning demonstrates strongly stained lymphoma, while toxoplasma encephalitis shows on strong staining, which facilitates the differential diagnosis. The therapeutic diagnosis such as sensitivity of lymphoma to radiations, and sensitivity of toxoplasma to sulfa drugs also facilitates the differential diagnosis.
3. HIV/AIDS related malignant lymphoma should be differentiated from brain metastatic tumors. Brain metastatic tumors commonly occur at the interface of the gray-white matters, with multiple lesions. Enhanced scanning demonstrates nodular obvious abnormal enhancement, with obvious surrounding edema.
4. HIV/AIDS related malignant lymphoma should be differentiated from other diseases. Singular tumor should be differentiated from brain glioma and meningioma. Multiple tumors should be differentiated from multiple metastatic tumors and infectious diseases. The differential diagnosis is sometimes difficult. Experimental radiotherapy can be performed for following up observations and differential diagnosis. If necessary, biopsy can be performed to confirm the diagnosis.

13.5.1.8 Discussion
The incidence of lymphoma in immunocompetent people is relatively low, but it increases in immunocompromised

AIDS patients, being up to 2.5 %. Lymphoma in immunocompetent people commonly occurs in the age group of 60–70 years, while lymphoma in immunocompromised AIDS patients commonly occurs in the age group of 40–45 years. Pathologically, it is a large cell immune tumor, usually being monoclonal and EB positive. Tumor cells can infiltrate along the vichow-robin space to erode the vascular wall. The most common clinical symptoms of AIDS are headaches and behavioral disorders and less common symptoms of focal neurological deficits. It progresses rapidly and is sensitive to radiotherapy. Death occurs due to opportunistic infections rather than the progression of the disease.

CT scanning and MR imaging can demonstrate the lesions well. CT scanning demonstrations of the case include a huge singular lesion, nodular/ring shaped/map liked obvious abnormal enhancement by enhanced scanning. MR imaging is more sensitive to the lymphoma lesions and demonstrates characteristic lesions better. Singular lesion is more common in cases of lymphoma than in cases of toxoplasmosis. Based on statistical data, the MR imaging demonstration of singular lesion should be considered the possibility of lymphoma. In addition, primary lymphoma of the central nervous system in AIDS patients has different imaging demonstrations from primary lymphoma of the central nervous system in immunocompetent patients. Lesions of lymphoma in the central nervous system of AIDS patients are more than that in immunocompetent patients, with a higher incidence of central necrosis and less common infratentorial involvement. Due to the non-specific imaging demonstrations of lymphoma in the central nervous system of AIDS patients, CT scanning and MR imaging cannot accurately differentiate it from toxoplasmosis. The differential diagnosis only by the diagnostic imaging is subjective with less reliability.

13.5.2   HIV/AIDS Related Intracranial Hodgkin's Lymphoma

13.5.2.1   Pathogens and Pathogenesis
The pathogens and pathogenesis of this disease is not yet clear, which may be related to immunodeficiency, recurrent infections, hereditary or acquired immune disorders that lead to absent or dysfunctional T suppressor cells. The long-term overload of the immune regulatory function and the abnormal proliferative response of immune cells finally cause unlimited proliferation and onset of the disease.

13.5.2.2   Pathophysiological Basis
Young people are susceptible to it, with lesions mainly in the cervical lymph nodes and supraclavicular lymph nodes, followed by mediastinal, retroperitoneal and para-aortic lymph nodes. Lesions start from one or one group of lymph nodes, which is rarely multiple from the very beginning. It spreads gradually from the nearby lymph nodes, with involved vascular vessel, spleen, liver, bone marrow and gastrointestinal tract in the advanced stage. By naked eyes observation, the Hodgkin's lymphoma involved lymph nodes are enlarged, with no adhesion but movable in the early stage. In the cases with invasion into the adjacent tissues, the enlarged lymph nodes are unmovable. The adhesion of lymph nodes leads to formation of a nodular huge mass, with its section in fish texture and having yellow small focal necrosis. By microscopy, the normal structure of the lymph nodes is destructed and is replaced by tumor tissues. The cellular components in the tumor tissue are diverse, being composed of neoplastic components and reactive components. The neoplastic components are mainly R-S cells, while the reactive components are inflammatory cells and interstitium. The dual cores of the most typical RS cells are in an arrangement of face-to-face, both having eosinophilic nucleolus like mirror images, to form the so-called mirror cells. Such cells are of great significance in the diagnosis of the disease. Therefore, it is also known as the diagnostic RS cells. In addition to the typical R-S cells in the tumor cells of Hodgkin lymphoma, there are also tumor cells of mononuclear R-S cells or Hodgkin's cells, which may be a variant of the RS cells. Other variant RS cells are common in some special subtypes of the disease, including (1) lacunar cells, commonly in the type of nodular sclerosis; (2) popcorn cells, found in the type of predominant lymphocytes, with popcorn liked nucleus; (3) pleomorphic or undifferentiated R-S cells, found in lymphocytic depletion Hodgkin's lymphoma.

13.5.2.3   Clinical Symptoms and Signs
The clinical symptoms include fever and night sweats of unknown reasons, intermittent moderate or high fever. Pruritus is a characteristic manifestation of HLS, which can be mild and restricted but commonly progresses into generalized. In some severe cases, extensive exfoliation can be resulted in. There are also lymphadenectasis (including superficial, deep and mesenteric lymphadenectasis) and hepatosplenomegaly.

13.5.2.4   Examinations and Their Selection
1. Hemogram.
2. Bone marrow biopsy positive, with a higher positive rate than smear.
3. Serological tests for LDH and B-2 M.
4. Histological examination to detect R-S cells or atypical R-S cells or variant R-S cells with accompanying granuloma.
5. CT scanning and MR imaging are the diagnostic imaging of the choice for its diagnosis and differential diagnosis.

13.5.2.5   Imaging Demonstrations
1. CT scanning and MR imaging demonstrate superficial lymphadenectasis in the neck and supraclavicular fossa, with no fusion and fixation in the early stage but with fusion and fixation of the superficial lymph nodes in the advanced stage.

2. Enhanced CT scanning or MR imaging can demonstrate slight enhancement of mediastinal lymphadenectasis. In the cases with necrosis of lymph nodes, the demonstrations are ring shaped enhancement, with widened mediastinum, and compressed esophagus and trachea.

3. Mesenteric lymphadenectasis is demonstrated as multiple retroperitoneal lymphadenectasis, which can accumulate into a mass and fuse, with unclear structure. Enhanced CT scanning and MR imaging demonstrate network grid liked enhancement.

13.5.2.6 Criteria for the Diagnosis

1. The hemogram is normal in the early stage, occasionally with increased leukocytes. In the progressive stage, NAP slowly increases. The hemogram may show pancytopenia in the advanced stage due to chemoradiotherapy and bone marrow involvement.

2. Bone marrow biopsy positive, which has a higher positive rate than smear.

3. Serological tests demonstrate increased LDH level, indicating the loading of the tumor, and increased B-2 M, indicating low grade malignant lymphoma and predicting the possibility of relapse.

4. Histological examination demonstrates the diagnostic R-S cells or atypical R-S cells or variant R-S cells with accompanying granuloma. Most patients with typical HL have accompanying cloning cellular hereditary abnormalities.

5. CT scanning and MR imaging demonstrate multiple lymphadenectasis of different locations, fusion of lymph nodes into a mass in the advanced stage with unclear structure. Enhanced scanning and imaging demonstrate network grid liked enhancement.

13.5.2.7 Differential Diagnosis

1. Mycobacterium lymphadenectasis, which is mainly tuberculosis, non-tuberculosis mycobacterial avium infection, multiple with no fusion.
2. HIV related lymphadenectasis.
3. Idiopathic lymphadenectasis.
4. Other infectious lymphadenectasis.
5. Other malignancy metastatic lymphadenectasis.

13.5.3 HIV/AIDS Related Kaposi's Sarcoma (KS)

HIV/AIDS related Kaposi's sarcoma is commonly systemic disseminated. Brain Kaposi's sarcoma rarely occurs.

13.5.4 HIV/AIDS Related Non-Definitive Tumor

13.5.4.1 Brain Metastatic Tumor
Pathogens and Pathogenesis
The brain metastatic tumor mainly metastasizes via direct infiltration and along with blood flow.

1. Direct infiltration: The primary and secondary tumors in the peripheral cranial tissues can directly infiltrate and destruct the skull and dual mater. In some other cases, they may also gain their access to the parenchyma of the brain outermost surface via basicranial holes and spaces. After invasion of the tumor cells into the brain, they may spreading widely along with CSF in the subarachnoid space or invade into the brain parenchyma through perivascular spaces in deep brain.

2. Along with blood flow: Most tumor cells transfer into the brain along with blood flow, mostly along arterial system. In some rare cases of tumors, the tumor cells transfer into the brain along with the Batson's plexus.

3. Cerebrospinal fluid metastasis and lymph node metastasis rarely occur.

Pathophysiological Basis
Brain metastatic tumor destroys the homeostasis mechanism which is necessary to maintain the normal functions of the brain. Therefore, a variety of clinical symptoms are resulted in. Due to sudden narrowing of the cerebrovascular vessels at the interface of brain gray-white matters, the cancer cell emboli are prevented from moving forward. Therefore, most metastatic lesions are located at the interface of brain gray-white matters and commonly located in the interface area with distribution of major blood vessels, namely the watershed area. Based on the number of brain metastatic tumors, it can be divided into singular, multiple and diffuse. About 70–80 % of brain metastasis tumor are multiple, commonly with brain edema and space occupying effect.

Clinical Symptoms and Signs
Clinical manifestations are transient severe headache, intracranial hypertension, visual disturbances and psychiatric and neurological symptoms. Meanwhile there may be also sensory abnormality or weakness of unilateral limbs, olfactory hallucination, hemiplegia or faltering steps, tinnitus and deafness.

Examinations and Their Selection
1. CT scanning is the commonly applied examination recently.
2. Compared to CT scanning, MR imaging is advantageous, with more diagnostic indices, a higher detection rate of the foci, qualitative and quantitative diagnosis of the foci and their localization. In addition, it can define the pathologic changes in the craniocerebral posterior fossa, which the CT scanning is blind of.
3. PET-CT scanning can qualitatively identify the benign from malignancies. In addition, it can also be applied for the screening of the systemic tumor metastasis.
4. Stereotactic biopsy can define the qualitative diagnosis.
5. Other examinations include lumbar puncture to find increased protein and sometimes tumor cells in CSF.

Imaging Demonstrations
CT Scanning

The foci are commonly found in the cortex or subcortex of the cerebral hemispheres, multiple and in different sizes in a diameter of less than 2 cm. There are obvious peritumor edema, which constitutes a basis for the invasion and growth of the tumor cells to the normal brain tissues. The peritumor edema is commonly in palm leaf liked or Buddha's hands liked low density. By enhanced scanning, most foci are demonstrated to have obvious enhancement, in obvious even enhancement and/or ring shaped enhancement, containing an area of no enhancement. The metastatic tumor has no capsule, with rich blood supply for its rapid growth. Tumor necrosis and cystic degeneration commonly occur.

MR Imaging

Plain T1WI imaging demonstrates low signal or irregular high signal, with even or uneven signal. T2WI demonstrates equal high signal or mix signal. Because metastatic foci can be cystic parenchymal or cystic and the parenchymal foci have accompanying necrosis and bleeding, the signals are diverse and complex. T2FLAIR demonstrates foci in high signal. Due to its inhibition to the signal of the CSF, it can demonstrate the foci more clearly. DWI imaging demonstrates flaky high signal, ring shaped or mixed signal, indicating mixed multiple morphologies of the brain metastatic tumors. Enhanced imaging demonstrates obviously even enhancement of the parenchymal tumors, with the necrotic cystic metastatic tumors in ring shaped or irregular nodular enhancement and clearly defined borderlines. It can clearly define the tumor from its surrounding brain edema. The metastatic tumor has no capsule, in expansive growth with smooth and intact margin and wall nodules. There are peritumor umbilicated indentation, which limits the tumor locally from its outward expansion. And the other parts of the tumor are thin, being susceptible to the outward expansion. Multiple brain metastatic tumors have demonstrations in different sizes and with various morphologies due to the different metastatic time, location, local blood flow and anatomic structures. The peritumor edema of the metastatic brain tumors is in finger liked, with disproportional ratio of the tumor to the peritumor edema, namely a small focus but large edema sign, which is its characteristic demonstration.

PET-CT Scanning

The metastatic tumors are demonstrated to have increased glucose metabolism, with strongly stained accumulation.

Case Study

A male patient aged 43 years was confirmatively diagnosed as having AIDS by the CDC. He had a history of extramarital affair and complained of headache, nausea and vomiting for more than 1 month. His CD4 T cell count was 17/μl.

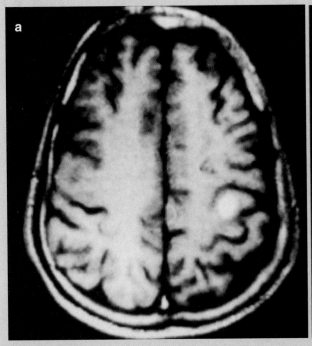 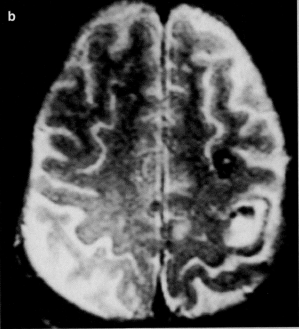

Fig. 13.78 (a–f) HIV/AIDS related brain metastatic tumor. (a) MR imaging demonstrates round liked slightly short T1WI signal in the left parietal lobe. (b, c) MR imaging demonstrates round liked uneven long T2WI signal in bilateral occipital lobes with ring shaped short T2WI signal. (d–f) Enhanced imaging by IV-Gd-DTPT demonstrates multiple nodular and mass liked obvious abnormal enhancement in bilateral occipital lobes

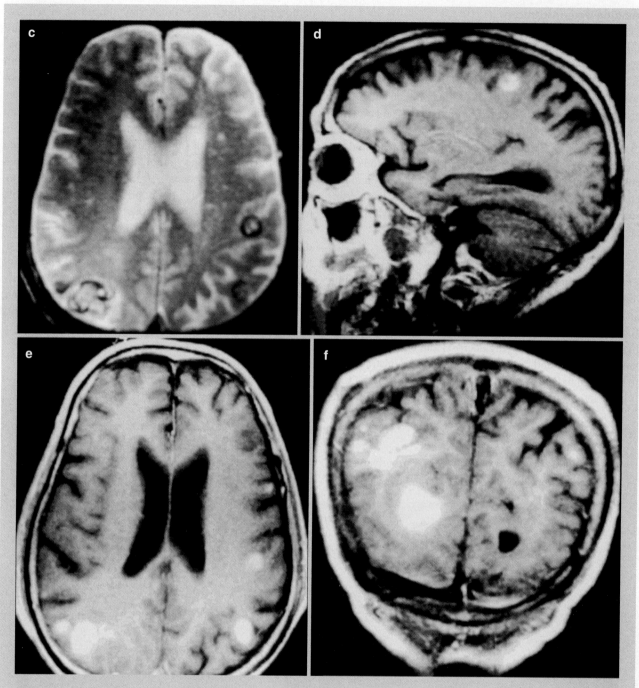

Fig. 13.78 (continued)

Criteria for the Diagnosis

1. The lesions are commonly found in the cortex of cerebral hemispheres or subcortical areas, being multiple in different sizes with a diameter of less than 2 cm. The peritumor edema is in palm leaf liked or Buddha's hand liked low density. Enhanced imaging demonstrates obvious enhancement of most lesions, with mostly even enhancement and/or ring shaped enhancement with central no enhancement. The metastatic tumor has no capsule. Tumor necrosis and cystic degeneration can occur.

2. MR imaging demonstrates cystic parenchymal or cystic metastatic tumors and the parenchymal tumors have accompanying necrosis and bleeding. Therefore, the demonstrations are diverse and complex signals, including singular or multiple round liked short T1 long T2 signal, with flaky short T2 signal, obvious edema and space occupying effect. Enhanced imaging demonstrates obvious nodular or ring shaped abnormal enhancement.

3. PET-CT scanning demonstrates multiple space occupying lesions, with increased glucose metabolites and strong staining.

4. Stereotactic pathological biopsy demonstrates tumor cells.

5. Lumbar puncture for CSF examination demonstrates increased protein content, sometimes tumor cells.

Differential Diagnosis

Primary Tumor

It is difficult to differentiate HIV/AIDS related brain singular metastatic tumor from primary tumor. The case history of primary malignancy should be combined for the diagnosis.

Meningioma

HIV/AIDS related brain metastatic tumor should be differentiated from meningioma. Brain singular metastatic tumor in the cerebral convexity or parafalx sometimes appears like meningioma. However, T2WI demonstrates meningioma as equal or slightly high signal. Enhanced imaging demonstrates obvious enhancement of the tumor for differential diagnosis.

Multiple Brain Tumors

HIV/AIDS related brain multiple metastatic tumors should be differentiated from multiple brain tumors. Brain metastatic tumors are commonly located at the interface of cortex and medulla in small lesions. Enhanced scanning demonstrates nodular or ring shaped enhancement. However, multiple malignant gliomas are commonly located in the deep brain tissues, with large sizes. Enhanced scanning demonstrates irregular ring shaped enhancement, with wall nodules. The peritumor edema is more extensive. And intratumor bleeding occurs in both diseases.

Brain Abscesses

Brain abscesses are singular/multiple ring shaped or cystic foci, with obvious enhancement by enhanced scanning. The wall is commonly thin with even thickness. In combination with clinical manifestations of infections and poisoning as well as findings of the laboratory tests, the differential diagnosis can be made.

Cerebral Cysticercosis

HIV/AIDS related brain metastatic tumor should be differentiated from cerebral cysticercosis. The cystic wall is very thin in the cases of cerebral cysticercosis, with rare enhancement by enhanced scanning. The findings of intracystic scolex or calcification facilitate the differential diagnosis.

Discussion

The common metastatic tumors in HIV infected brain parenchyma include bronchial lung cancer, breast cancer, gastrointestinal tumor, renal cell carcinoma and melanoma. Metastatic tumors often involves the interface of the cerebral cortex and medulla or the pia mater. The metastatic tumors in brain parenchyma are demonstrated to have multiple foci of different sizes, with space occupying effect. Enhanced scanning demonstrates enhancement. Enhanced MR imaging demonstrates even enhancement or marginal nodular enhancement. T2WI demonstrates extensive edema surrounding the tumors. Enhanced FLAIR sequence demonstrates the metastatic tumors in the pia mater well, with enhancement area extending from cortex surface into the sulci.

13.5.4.2 HIV/AIDS Related Leukemia

The process of ischemia in myelencephalon is chronic and progressive in AIDS patients. Due to the angiotropic and neurotropic properties of HIV, it invades myelencephalon nerves and their supplying arteries to cause apoptosis of the nerve cells, granuloma of the supplying artery intima and stenosis of the arterial lumen, resulting in myelencephalon atrophy. Infiltrative leukemia cells can directly infiltrate like other tumor cells, which can directly invade meninges, brain parenchyma, cerebrovascular vessels, spinal cord and peripheral nerves. Especially because many anti-leukemia drugs cannot or can partially pass through the blood–brain barrier, they fail to effectively kill intracerebral leukemia cells. The infiltrative lesions in the nervous system are especially common in the remission stage of leukemia. Patients with secondary infectious leukemia have dysfunctional cellular and humoral immunity, with additional decrease of the normal granulopoiesis and dysfunctional mononuclear cells and macrophages. Therefore, they are especially vulnerable to infections. The toxins produced during infection can cause nerve lesions. Leukocytosis can cause increased blood thickness and occlusion of minor vascular vessels, which lead to ischemic and anoxic changes of the nerve tissues. In addition, HARRT can also cause pathological changes of the nervous system. The increasing incidence of cerebral infarction has been reported.

Case Study

A female patient aged 32 years was confirmatively diagnosed as having AIDS by the CDC. She complained of consciousness disturbance, nausea, vomiting and incontinence. Her CD4 T cell count was 87/μl.

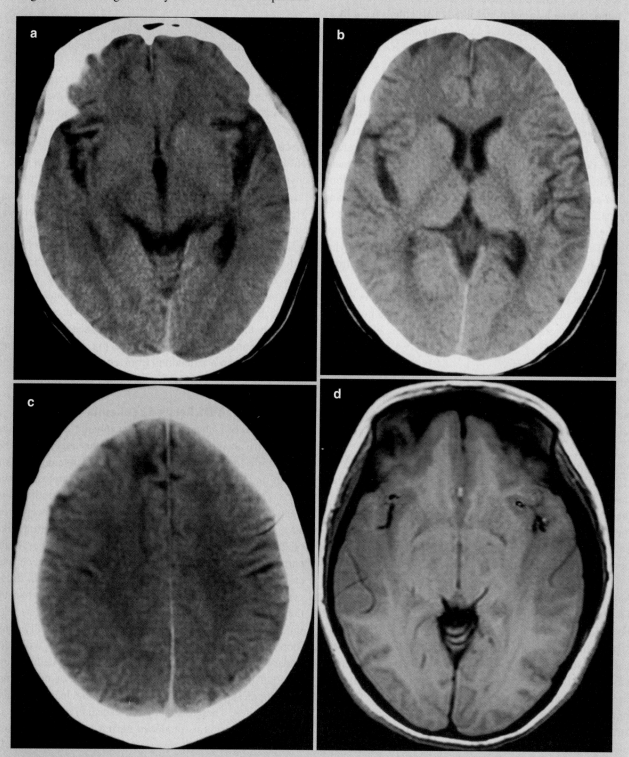

Fig. 13.79 (**a–n**) HIV/AIDS related leukemia. (**a–c**) It is demonstrated to have deepened and widened bilateral brain sulci and enlarged lateral fissure cistern. (**d–k**) Axial MR imaging demonstrates multiple flaky long T1 and long T2 signal in bilateral temporal lobes, parietal lobes and cerebellum. Reexamination of MR imaging after radiotherapy demonstrates absent intraventricular foci, deepened and widened sulcus, and enlarged lateral fissure cistern. (**l–n**) MRA demonstrates sparse and circuitous bilateral distal middle cerebral arteries

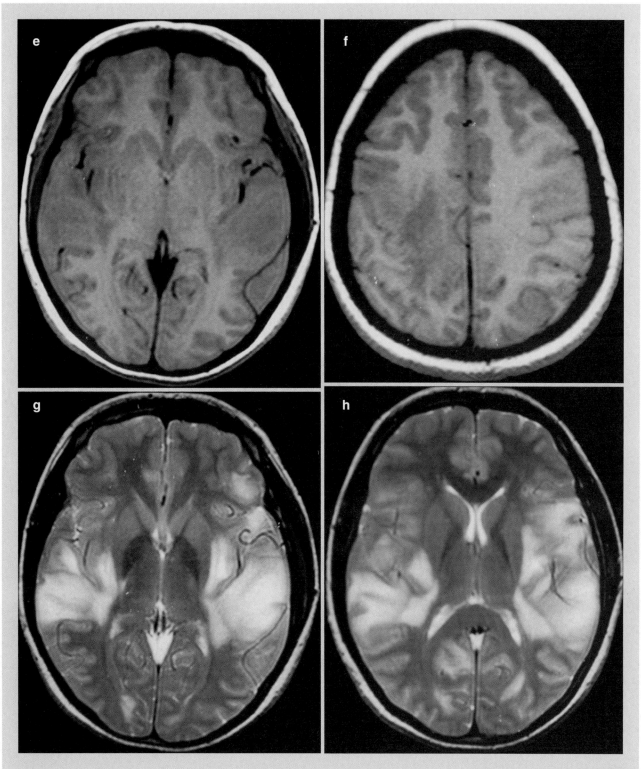

Fig. 13.79 (continued)

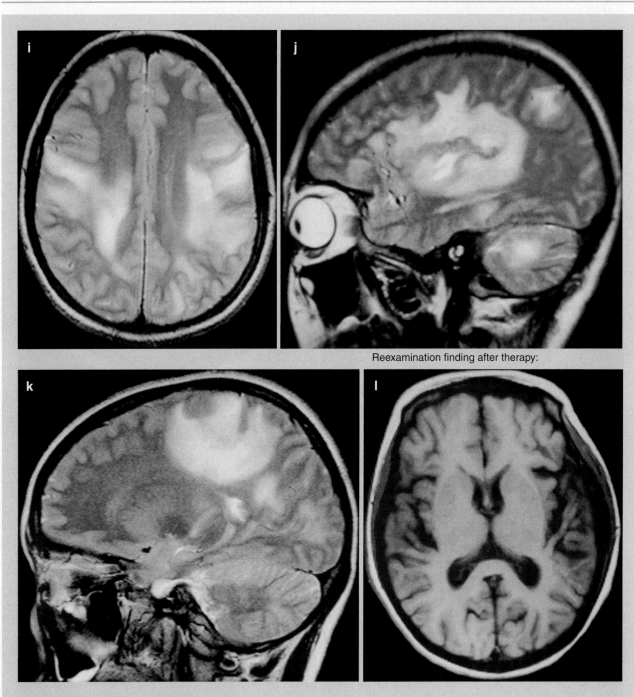

Reexamination finding after therapy:

Fig. 13.79 (continued)

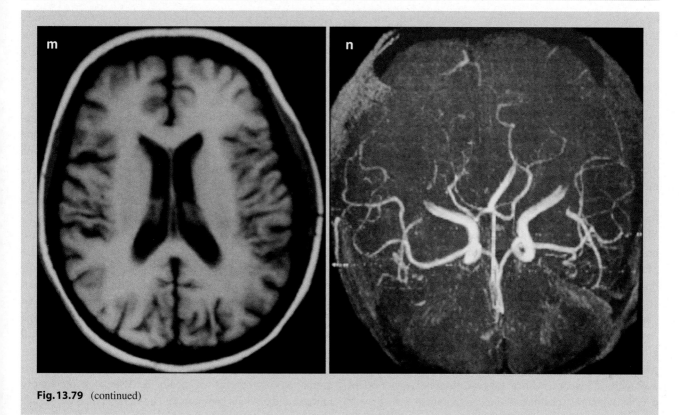

Fig. 13.79 (continued)

Key Points for the Diagnosis

1. The clinical manifestation of acute leukemia include anemia, hemorrhage, infection and infiltration (such as enlargements of the liver, spleen and lymph nodes; sternum tenderness).

2. Laboratory tests demonstrate findings or no findings of leukocytes. Myelogram has findings of leukemia cells being no less than 30 %.

3. Lesions in the nervous system include (1) symptoms and signs of the central nervous system, especially symptoms and signs of intracranial hypertension; (2) changes in the cerebrospinal fluid; (3) Leukemia cells in smear; (4) Protein being above 450 mg/L or Pandy test positive; (5) Exclusion of other reasons for similar lesions and changes of the central nervous system and cerebrospinal fluid; (6) Other lesions of the nervous system according to the clinic symptoms and signs as well as their localization.

4. Imaging demonstrations include CT findings of early low density lesions in the basal ganglia with edema effect and MRI findings of flaky long T1 and long T2 signals. In the advanced stage, imaging demonstrates brain atrophy and infection foci, and even complicated infections.

Differential Diagnosis

Brain Atrophy Induced by Other Infections

HIV/AIDS related leukemia should be differentiated from brain atrophy induced by other infections, such as herpes encephalitis and HIV encephalitis.

Brain Atrophy Induced by Other Related Factors

HIV/AIDS related leukemia should be differentiated from brain atrophy induced by other related factors.

Discussion

Due to the angiotropic and neurotropic properties of HIV, they invade the cerebral and spinal nerves and their supplying arteries to cause myelencephalon atrophy. The infiltrative leukemia cells has direct infiltrative properties as other tumor cells to directly invade the nervous system, leading to infiltrative lesions in the nervous system. Patients with HIV/AIDS related leukemia have dysfunctional cellular and humoral immunity, with additional decrease of granulopoiesis of dysfunctional mononuclear cells and macrophages. Therefore, they are especially susceptible to related intracerebral infections. In addition to the lesions directly induced by HIV infection, the occurrence of intracerebral lesions like leukemia and other related infections can aggravate the primary serious conditions of AIDS patients. The complex pathological changes and diverse imaging demonstrations require more knowledge and understanding of the diseases for the differential diagnosis. The imaging demonstrations should be in consistency with the corresponding pathology.

13.5.4.3 HIV/AIDS Related Meningioma

Pathogens and Pathogenesis

The occurrence of meningioma may be related to the changes of the internal environment and genetic variation. It is caused by multiple reasons including craniocerebral trauma, exposure to the radiation, virus infection and complicated bilateral acoustic neuroma. The etiological studies on meningioma have clarified its pathogenesis from the perspectives of the chromosome, molecular biology and receptor, which include (1) Abnormal Chromosome 22 due to its long-arm deletion or other genetic materials deletion and even total deletion. (2) Important relationship between sex hormones and meningioma. (3) Chromosome deletion caused by radiotherapy and occurrence of meningioma. (4) Occurrence of meningioma caused by trauma.

Pathophysiological Basis

Meningioma is derived from cap cells in arachnoid membrane, mostly located out of the brain parenchyma. Meningioma is in sphere shaped growth, with clearly defined borderline from the brain tissues. By naked eyes, the cross section of meningioma is found to have gray or dark red dense tissues and sometimes sand liked particles. The diameters of meningioma range from 1 to 10 cm. Benign meningioma has a slow growth and a long course of illness. The period from its origination to the early symptoms onset is averagely 2.5 years, with a longest progressive period of 6 years. General speaking, the average annual growth volume of meningioma is 3.6 %, with an expansive growth in the shapes of sphere, cone, flat or dumbbell. The common meningiomas can be divided into the following types according to their pathological features, including endothelial or fibrous type, vascular type, sand type, mixed or metastatic type, malignant type and sarcoma type. The former five types are categorized into the benign. And malignancy is commonly found in the vascular type. The cases with intratumor necrosis and multiple recurrences should also be considered as malignancy.

Microscopically, the pathological changes include typical tumor structure of some tumor tissues and malignancy manifestations of finger liked infiltration or diffuse infiltration of the brain tissues. The cells of malignant meningioma are abundant, with active growth, obvious nuclear atypia, large nuclear with strong staining, megakaryocyte and common nuclear division.

Clinical Symptoms and Signs

Females are vulnerable to meningioma, with an incidence being twice as high as that in males. It has been reported that the incidence of meningioma is high in both pregnant women and patients with breast cancer. The susceptible locations are listed as the following in the order from the most common to the least common: (1) 50 % in sagittal sinus; (2) sellar tuberculum; (3) ethmoid sinus; (4) cavernous sinus; (5) cerebellopontine horn; and (6) cerebellar tentorium. Meningioma in different locations has different clinical manifestations. For instances, the cases of cerebral convexity meningioma have

clinical manifestations of headache, psychiatric disorder, limbs movement disturbance and vision changes. About 60 % such patients may complain of symptoms caused by intracranial hypertension after 6 months. The cases of parasagittal meningioma have a slow progression of the tumor, with initial symptoms of epilepsy seizure and following psychiatric disorders such as dementia and personality change. Additionally, parasagittal meningioma in the occipital lobe may cause visual field obstacle. Sphenoid ridge meningioma is derived from anterior clinoid process, with symptoms of decreased vision and exophthalmos. Sellar tuberculum meningioma is manifested with vision and visual field obstacles, with more than 80 % patients showing visual impairment as the initial symptom. The cases of olfactory groove meningioma have early symptoms of gradual loss of olfactory sensation, vision obstacle due to intracranial hypertension, dysfunctional frontal lobe due to the tumor. Because of intracranial hypertension, there is edema in the contralateral optic nerves to form Foster-kenydy sign. Cerebellopontine horn meningioma has an incidence of 6–8 % with clinical manifestations of hearing loss, tinnitus, facial numbness, decreased sensation and other symptoms. Petroclival meningioma has symptoms of headache which is commonly ignored and obvious symptom of III-X cranial nerves lesions. Intraventricular meningioma has no obvious neurological disorders in the early stage due to its growth in the brain ventricles, with symptoms of headache, optic papilla edema, epilepsy, homonymous hemianopia and contralateral hemiparalysis. Middle cranial fossa meningioma is manifested to have trigeminal neuralgia, ocular movement disturbance, blepharoptosis, diplopia, decreased vision and homonymous hemianopia. Cerebellar tentorial meningioma has manifestations of ataxia and visual field obstacles. Paracavernous sinuses meningioma has manifestations of headache, vision and visual field change, ophthalmoplegia and pain of trigeminal nerve III innervated area. Foramen magnum meningioma has early symptoms of cervical pain, hands and upper limbs numbness, which can be misdiagnosed. Orbital and cranio-orbital meningioma has symptoms of exophthalmos, ocular movement disturbance, and decreased vision.

Examinations and Their Selection

CT Scanning

For the diagnosis of meningioma, CT scanning in high resolution can define meningiomas in size of 1 cm and even smaller meningiomas.

MR Imaging and MRA

MR imaging and MRA can directly define the size, shape, position and the blood supply of meningioma. They provide valuable information for the formulation of surgical plan and the decision making about surgical approaches and procedures.

Imaging Demonstrations

CT Scanning Demonstrations

(1) Meningioma often occurs in cerebral surface with arachnoid particles. The most common locations are cerebral convexity, cerebral parafalx and parasagittal sinus, followed by olfactory groove, sphenoid ridge, sellar tuberculum and cerebellopontine horn. The other involved locations are cerebellar tentorium, intraventricular and epiphysis. The shape of meningioma is commonly round or oval and sometimes is flat. (2) Plain CT scanning demonstrates high or equal even density lesions, and sometimes in mixed density. The size of tumor is between a few millimeters to more than 10 cm, mostly being about 5 cm. There is sometimes calcification in the tumor, in sand liked or plaque liked calcification, and even whole tumor calcification, with cystic changes and paratumor edema. (3) Because meningioma is an extracerebral tumor, its CT scanning demonstration shows a connection between the wide base and dura mater, bone hyperplasia or destruction of the adjacent internal lamina, enlarged adjacent sulcus and cistern, white matter collapse and clear boundary. (4) Enhanced CT scanning demonstrates meningioma to have obvious uniform homogenous enhancement, clearer boundary than demonstrations of plain scanning, and sometimes dural tail sign. (5) The time-density curve by enhanced CT scanning demonstrates short period of ascending time, long lasting period at the high value, and then a slow descending time. In the cases with uneven density, an uneven enhancement can be demonstrated, with possible necrosis and cystic degenerations. (6) Peritumor edema is believed to be the basis of tumor cells invasion and growth into normal brain tissue. It can separate tumor tissues from normal brain tissue which can cause tissue looseness and impair the defense mechanism of local body structure. Such characteristics of peritumor edema facilitate the malignancy of the tumor, therefore promoting invasion of the tumor cells into the host tissues. Benign meningioma usually has no obvious edema, with demonstrations of low density area and no enhancement by enhanced scanning.

MR Imaging Demonstrations

(1) Characteristic susceptible locations from the most vulnerable to the least vulnerable are parasagittal sinus, cerebral convexity, sphenoid ridge, olfactory sulcus, cerebellar tentorium, cerebellopontine horn and sellar tuberculum. (2) Plain imaging demonstrates equal or slightly lower signal comparing to the gray matter on T1WI, slightly higher or equal signal comparing to the gray matter on T2WI. The border of the tumor is smooth and intact, with internal uneven signals due to calcification, cystic degeneration, fiber septum and blood vessels. (3) Enhanced imaging demonstrates intracranial and extracerebral meningioma, with rapid and prominent enhancement of signal due to its lack of blood–brain barrier and abundant blood supply. (4) Benign meningioma usually has no obvious peritumor edema. However, in the cases with large meningioma or at a special location (to compress reflux vein or venous sinus) or malignant meningioma, peritumor edema can occur, commonly in lunar halo shape in long T1WI and long T2WI signal. (5) Enhanced imaging demonstrates thickened stripe liked adjacent meninges in about 60 % cases of meningioma, which is known as dual tail sign. It has been intensively studied, which indicates responsive hyperplasia of the meninges and hyperplasia of fibrocytes and capillaries, possibly a result of tumor infiltration into peripheral dual mater. Dural tail sign highly indicates meningioma but it is non-specific because it can also occur as a pathological change after surgery and radiotherapy, of lymphoma and brain metastatic tumor. (6) Extracerebral space occupying meningioma has pathologic changes of adjacent cranium, including hyperplasia and sclerosis, connection between the wide base and the dural mater, pseudocapsule of the tumor (linear low signal between tumor and peritumor edema) and migration of the white mater. MR imaging demonstrations of atypical meningioma include particular position, diverse signals, simultaneously involvement of multiple locations. MRS and DWI demonstrations are characterized by failed detection of NAA and Cr by MRS due to the extracerebral meningioma without neuron contents. The cases with detected NAA and Cr indicate the infiltration of the tumor into brain tissue or the interested MRS area exceeds the tumor range to include some brain tissue, which should be aware of in clinical practice. In the cases of meningioma, there are obviously increased Cho and common alanine wave (1.2–1.4 ppm), which is characteristically meningioma by MRS. These characteristics is the evidence for the differential diagnosis of hemispherical convex glioma and meningioma and is also important evidence for the diagnosis of . lateral ventricular atypical meningioma. However, these characteristics are of less significance for the differential diagnosis of sellar meningioma and pituitary tumor because of presence of alanine wave in the cases of pituitary tumor. MRS is less significant for the differentiation of benign and malignant meningiomas, but DWI can provide the useful information for their differentiation. Malignant or atypical meningioma is demonstrated as high signal by DWI, low signal by ADC with the ADC value being $0.45–0.69 \times 10^{-3}$ mm^3/s (averagely 1.03×10^{-3} mm^3/s) and being lower than that of parenchyma. However, ADC value of benign meningioma is slightly higher than that of parenchyma, being $0.62–1.8 \times 10^{-3}$ mm^3/s (averagely 1.03×10^{-3} mm^3/s). Benign meningioma is demonstrated as equal signal by DWI and ADC. The lower ADC value for malignant or atypical meningioma is possibly due to the high nucleus/cytoplasm ratio, high protein levels in the cells for restricted water molecules diffusion. It may be also due to less water content in the tumor and small extracellular space to decrease the water molecules diffusion.

Case Study

A female patient aged 56 years was confirmatively diagnosed as having AIDS by the CDC. She complained of headache and decreased vision. Her CD4 T cell count was 20/μl.

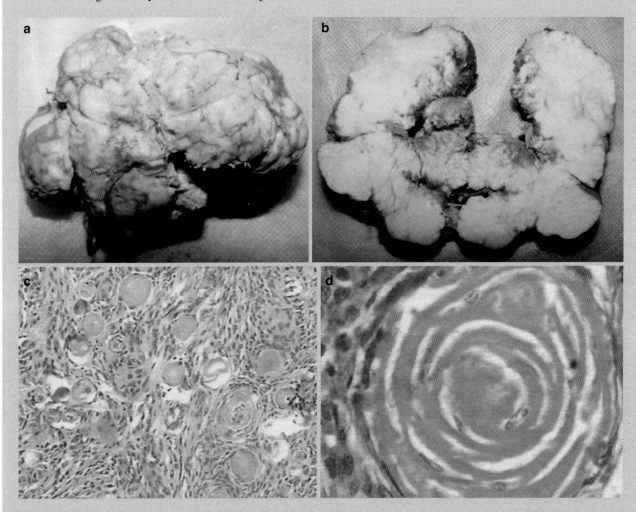

Fig. 13.80 (a–i) HIV/AIDS related meningioma. (a, b) Gross observation of the surgically removed meningioma specimen demonstrates the tumor in size of an adult's fist, in a lobulated and irregular shape, and milky white section. (c, d) Pathological analysis by autopsy demonstrates large quantity fibroblast liked tumor cells in vortex appearance and ring shaped arrangement, syncytial cells that are large in lamellar and annual ring liked arrangement. (e–i) MRI+C and MRA demonstrate equal or slightly lower T1 and slightly longer T2 signal in the brain anterior cranial fossa, occlusion of the anterior horn of lateral ventricles due to the compression, obvious space occupying effect and slight surrounding edema. Enhanced imaging by IV-Gd-DTPA demonstrates obvious point enhancement, with intact capsule and clear boundary. MRA demonstrates compressed and circuitous anterior cerebral artery in embracing ball sign

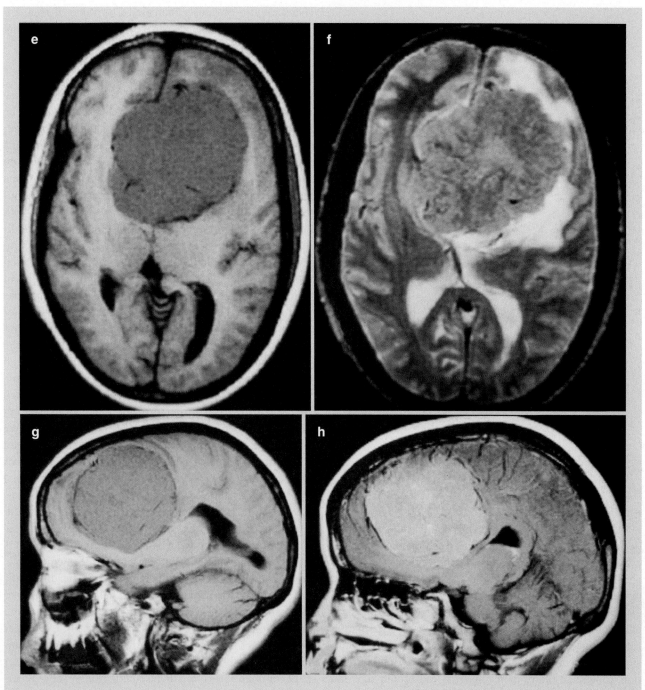

Fig. 13.80 (continued)

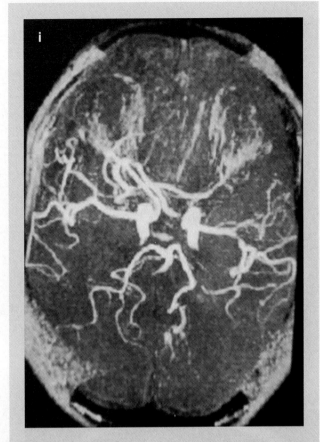

Fig. 13.80 (continued)

Key Points for the Diagnosis

(1) CT scanning and MR imaging demonstrate the space occupying lesion in parasagittal sinus, cerebral falx, cerebral convexity, olfactory sulcus and sellar tuberculum. The lesions are in equal density or slightly high density, with necrosis, cystic degeneration and sand liked calcification. There are also white matter collapse sign or gyrus compression sign; adhesion of the tumor to the dural wide base; hyperplasia, sclerosis or destruction of the local cranial lamella; occlusion of the venous sinus due to compression, brain infiltration, rough and blurry tumor margins, mushroom sign and pseudopodia sign. The tumor can be lobulated.

DSA demonstrates blood supplies around the tumors, with central blood supply by the dura mater, embracing ball sign around the tumor.

MR imaging demonstrates vascular flow void effect. Malignant or atypical meningioma is demonstrated as high signal by DWI. MRS ratio value of Cho/Cr is related to the potential of tumor hyperplasia. The failed detection of NAA and Cr has two possibilities, one is the invasion of the tumor to the brain tissue and the other is that the interested areas by MRS exceeds the range of tumor to include some brain tissue, which should be aware of in the clinical diagnosis.

There are also obviously increased Cho value of meningioma and common alanine wave (1.2–1.4 ppm), which are characteristically meningioma.

Differential Diagnosis

Meningiomas of different locations have different key points for the differential diagnosis. It usually should be differentiated from glioma, chordoma, cholesteatoma, neurilemmoma and chondrosarcoma. Large cystic meningioma often penetrates into the brain parenchyma and should be differentiated from glioma. The cysts of cystic meningioma commonly have clearly defined boundaries from the tumor parenchyma, with smooth and intact cystic wall and with similar cystic fluid signal to cerebrospinal fluid. In addition, the tumor parenchyma is demonstrated to have homogeneous and consistent enhancement, which is connected to the dural wide base or has dural tail sign. The adjacent skull may have hyperplasia. Brain glioma commonly has irregular and polycystic changes, with uneven thickness of the cystic wall and different degrees enhancement due to differently differentiated tumor tissue. In addition, the cases of meningioma commonly have slight edema and more lunar halo liked edema, while the cases of glioma commonly have serious edema and more finger liked edema. For the cases of hemorrhagic meningioma, during the subacute period of bleeding, both T1WI and T2WI demonstrate high signal, which should be differentiated from intratumor fatty tissues. At this time, the addition of STIR sequence demonstrates low signal with high signal suppressed in the cases of intratumor fatty tissues. Otherwise, it is hemorrhagic meningioma. In the later period of focus bleeding, the residual cysts are absorbed, which can be diagnosed as cystic meningioma, because it is one of the causes for occurrence of cystic meningioma. Cerebellopontine horn meningioma should be differentiated from acoustic neurinoma which belongs to tumors of VIII pair cranial nerve sheath with an origination from inner acoustic segment to cerebellopontine horn via inner acoustic canal. The common manifestations include expansion of homolateral inner acoustic canal into a loudspeaker shape, or bone absorption. Parasellar region or sellar tuberculum meningioma should be differentiated from pituitary adenoma and aneurysm. Pituitary adenoma is derived from pituitary, commonly with accompanying sellar enlargement and elevated sellar diaphragm. The downward infiltration of tumor penetrates the sellar base to the sphenoid sinus. Moreover, sagittal and coronal MR imaging fails to find the normal pituitary tissue. In the cases with sellar aneurysm and occurrence of thrombus, plain MR imaging demonstrates slightly high signal. But enhanced imaging demonstrates no enhancement or filling defects. In the cases with sellar aneurysm and no occurrence of thrombus, plain MR imaging demonstrates flow void effect. MRA or DSA can

define the diagnosis. In the cases with dual tail sign, aneurysm can be excluded. Cerebral ventricular meningioma should be differentiated from choroid plexus papilloma. The borderline of meningioma is smooth while that of choroid plexus papilloma is irregular. By T2WI, the signal of meningioma is lower than that of choroid plexus papilloma. Choroid plexus papilloma can be demonstrated to have hydrocephalus due to excessive secretion of cerebrospinal fluid. Choroid plexus papilloma occurs commonly in young adults and teenagers.

Discussion

Female is the vulnerable population to meningioma, with an incidence twice as high as that in males. It has a long progression period to the onset of symptoms, which are different according to the different locations. Meningioma mostly occurs in adults, with common symptoms of chronic headache, mental changes, epilepsy, unilateral or bilateral vision decrease and even vision loss, ataxia and local cranial mass. Especially in the cases with progressively aggravating intracranial hypertension, the possibility of meningioma should be considered. Furthermore, fundus examination commonly demonstrates chronic papilledema of the optic nerves or its secondary atrophy. Diagnostic imaging demonstration of space occupying lesion in the brain can define the diagnosis. Cystic meningioma accounts for 4–7 % of the intracranial meningioma. Due to the advantages of MR imaging in high resolution of soft tissues, its accurate diagnosis rate for cystic meningioma is obviously higher than that by CT scanning. Especially enhanced MR imaging demonstrates cystic fluid as low signal by T1WI and high or equal signal by T2WI. Enhanced imaging can define the tumor cells infiltration in the cystic wall and assess the relationship between the tumor and its surrounding tissues.

13.6   HIV/AIDS Related Cerebrovascular Diseases

13.6.1   HIV/AIDS Related Cerebral Infarction

13.6.1.1 Pathogens and Pathogenesis

HIV/AIDS related cerebral infarction is endovasculitis caused by vascular invasion of HIV, which is an opportunistic infection or complication of drug abuse. Tuberculosis, cryptococcal meningitis and meningovascular syphilis are the most common opportunistic infections with vascular involvement. The diseases with predominant vascular lesions include cerebral toxoplasmosis, mycosis and herpes virus infections. Further, various factors contribute to the aggravation of local arteriostenosis or even occlusion, leading to ischemia, hypoxia and necrosis of the brain tissues, with final occurrence of cerebrovascular diseases.

13.6.1.2 Pathophysiological Basis

HIV/AIDS Related Cerebral Infarction

In the hyperacute period of HIV/AIDS related cerebral artery occlusion, the pathological changes of brain tissues are not obvious within 6 h. However, in 8–48 h, the ischemic central tissue is demonstrated to have malacia, swelling and necrosis. There are unclearly defined interface between gray and white matters. Microscopically, the tissue structure is cloudy, with degenerations and necrosis of the neurocytes and gliacytes as well as slight dilation of capillaries. There is also surrounding fluid or erythrocytes exudation. In the acute stage of cerebral infarction, in 2–3 days after arterial occlusion, there is obvious peripheral edema. In the subacute stage of cerebral infarction, after 7–14 days of onset, the lesions are demonstrated to have malacia, absent neurocytes, liquefaction of the brain tissue, occurrence of large quantity phagocytes and stellate cells proliferation. In the chronic stage of cerebral infarction, in 21–28 days after the onset, there are proliferation of gliacytes and capillaries, formation of small foci into colloid scar and formation of large foci into malacia foci. The locations of HIV/AIDS related cerebral watershed infarction are commonly in watershed areas or marginal area of different blood supplying vessels. Generally, it is believed that cerebral watershed infarction is due to hemodynamic obstruction.

HIV/AIDS Related Cerebral Lacunar Infarction

HIV/AIDS related cerebral lacunar infarction has foci in the deep perforating arteries with a diameter of 100–400 pm. Therefore, the foci are commonly found in the putamen, caudate nucleus, internal capsule, thalamus, the basal pons and the corona radiata, in a diameter of about 0.2–15 mm. Due to the residual small cystic cavities after phagocytosis of soft and necrotic tissues, multiple cystic cavities form into lacunes. Focal cerebral atrophy and cystic degeneration are markers of chronic cerebral infarction.

13.6.1.3 Clinical Symptoms and Signs

In AIDS patients, about 12–20 % has accompanying cerebrovascular complications. The clinical manifestations are related to the location and severity of embolism and infarction. Patients may have simple sensory stroke (hemisensory obstruction), simple movement stroke, dysarthria clumsy hand syndrome, ataxic hemiparesis and blurry vision or hemianopsia. The most commonly cerebrovascular complication is singular or multiple focal cerebral infarction, with manifestations of cerebral hemorrhage and temporary ischemia.

13.6.1.4 Examinations and Their Selection

1. Lumbar puncture for brain pressure measurement can be performed. The findings of intracranial hypertension indicate large area infarction in the brain.

2. Ultrasound of carotid artery can be applied to evaluate vascular stenosis and atherosclerotic plaques, which is indicative to the diagnosis of embolism originated from the carotid artery.

3. CT scanning is the diagnostic imaging of the choice. MRI and MRA are the first choice for the diagnosis of hyperacute cerebral embolism.

13.6.1.5 Imaging Demonstrations

Routine CT scanning and MR imaging commonly demonstrate hyperacute cerebral embolism as negative. MRI diffusion-weighted imaging demonstrates high signals while CT and MRI perfusion imaging demonstrates hypoperfusion.

In the acute period, local brain tissues swelling causes decreased density and MR imaging demonstrates flaky long T1 and long T2 signals. In subacute period, routine CT scanning and MR imaging demonstrate same findings as those in the acute period. Moreover, by DWI the infarction area is in low signal and by PWI in hypoperfusion. In the chronic period, CT scanning demonstrates low density that is similar to cerebrospinal fluid and MR imaging demonstrates long T1 and long T2 signals. In addition, low signal by FLAIR with high signal of the surrounding gliosis, and low signal by DWI. CT scanning demonstrates hemorrhagic cerebral infarction as high density bleeding area in the location of primary infarction or hemorrhagic cerebral infarction in the brain cortical area.

Case Study 1

A female patient aged 40 years was confirmatively diagnosed as having AIDS by the CDC in 2003. Her husband had a history of paid blood donation and she was sexually transmitted. She complained of subjective blurry vision and nausea in Dec. 2006. Her CD4 T cell count was 50/μl.

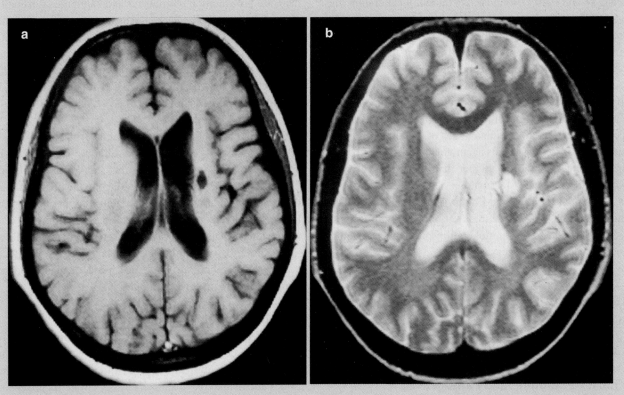

Fig. 13.81 (**a, b**) HIV/AIDS related cerebral infarction. MR imaging demonstrates small flaky long T1 and long T2 signal in the left basal ganglia with clear boundary

Case Study 2

A female patient aged 25 years was confirmatively diagnosed as having AIDS by the CDC. She was hospitalized in Mar. 16, 2009 due to dizziness for more than 2 months and accompanying blurry vision and unstable gait for more than 1 month. In early Jan. 2009, she was found HIV-Ab(+) and a CD4 T cell count of 40/μl in routine physical examinations. Later, she had symptoms of dizziness, without chills, fever, nausea, vomiting and headaches. Since Feb. 2009, she began to have blurry vision, unstable gait and left limb weakness. After being hospitalized, she received lumbar puncture with findings of intracranial pression of 130 mm H_2O and normal cerebrospinal fluid. The viruses combination in opportunistic infections is normal and all cultures for acid-fast bacillus, cryptococcus and mycobacterium tuberculosis culture were negative.

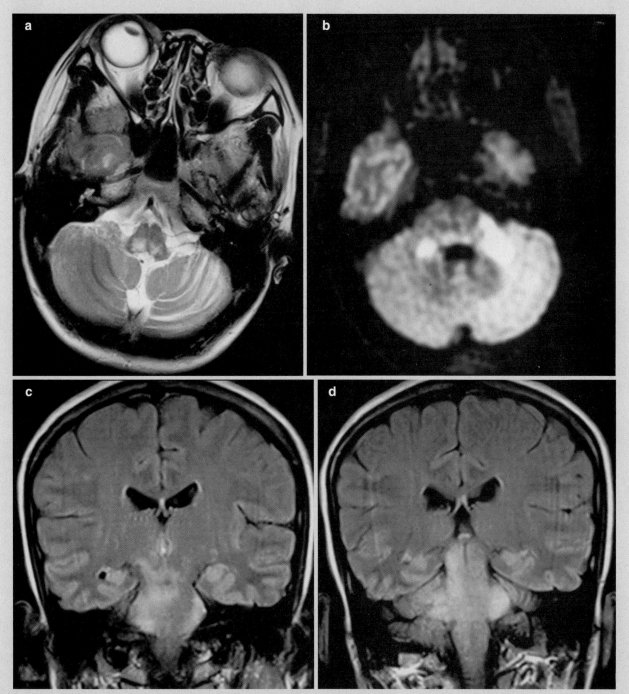

Fig. 13.82 (a–d) HIV/AIDS related cerebral infarction. (a, b) Axial MR imaging demonstrates flaky long T2 signal in the brainstem and left cerebellum. FLAIR demonstrates large flaky long and high T2 signal in the left cerebellum. (c, d) Coronal MR imaging demonstrates deepened and widened sulcus

Case Study 3
A male patient aged 28 years was confirmatively diagnosed as having AIDS by the CDC. He complained of persistent dizziness for more than 3 months, and recurrent and progressively severe headache for more than 1 month. His CD4 T cell count was 25/μl.

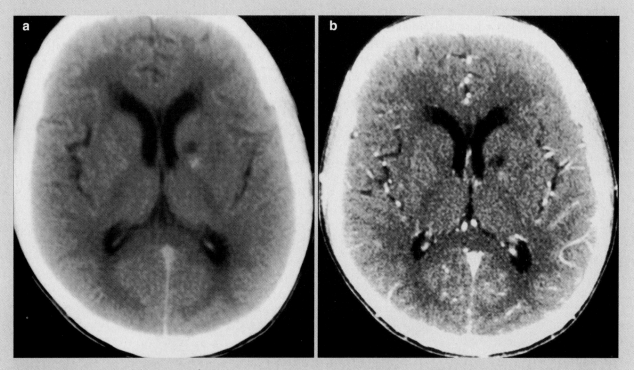

Fig. 13.83 (**a**, **b**) HIV/AIDS related cerebral infarction. (**a**) CT scanning demonstrates small flaky low density shadows in the left basal ganglia, with clear boundary. (**b**) Enhanced CT scanning demonstrates low density shadow with no enhancement in the left basal ganglia, with clear boundary

13.6.1.6 Key Points for the Diagnosis

1. The paroxysmal periods are commonly at night.
2. With a past history of hypertension or hypotension.
3. Lumbar puncture can be performed for intracranial pressure measurement. Intracranial hypertension indicates large area cerebral infarction.
4. CT scanning and MR imaging demonstrate flaky low density shadow in the brain, surrounding low density edema stripes, absent/present space occupying effect. Hemorrhagic cerebral infarction is the clinical manifestation of prior cerebral infarction. MR imaging demonstrates long T1WI and long T2WI signals. Hemorrhagic cerebral infarction is demonstrated by complex MR imaging signals. By DWI, the infarction area is in low signal. By PWI, hypoperfusion and by FLAIR, low signal.

13.6.1.7 Differential Diagnosis

It should be differentiated from cerebral hemorrhage. (1) Patients with cerebral hemorrhage commonly have a history of hypertension and cerebral arteriosclerosis, while patients with cerebral infarction commonly have a history of transient cerebral ischemia or heart attack. (2) Cerebral hemorrhage usually occurs during agitation or physical exertion while infarction often occurs in resting state. (3) Cerebral hemorrhage has an acute onset with a rapid progression. It can reach its peak within several hours, with no premonition before the onset. But cerebral infarction has a chronic progression, with gradual aggravation in 1–2 days later. The patients usually have a past history of transient cerebral ischemia. (4) Patients with cerebral hemorrhage have symptoms of intracranial hypertension, such as headache, vomiting and cervical stiffness as well as hypertension and serious consciousness disturbance. In contrast, patients with cerebral infarction usually have a normal blood pressure and are conscious. (5) By lumbar puncture, patients with cerebral hemorrhage have high CSF pressure and bloody CSF, while patients with cerebral infarction have normal CSF pressure and clear colorless CSF. (6) Patients with cerebral hemorrhage commonly have respiratory disturbance of the central nervous system, with asymmetric pupils or shrinkage of both pupils and conjugate eye deviation and floating of the eyeballs. Patients with cerebral infarction rarely have respiratory disturbance of the central nervous system, with symmetrical pupils and rarely conjugate eye deviation and floating of the eyeballs. By CT scanning and MR imaging, cerebral infarction is demonstrated to have flaky low density shadow in the brain, surrounding low density edema stripe, and absent/present space occupying effect. However, cerebral hemorrhage is demonstrated to have high density shadow. DWI of the infarction area is in low signal, with PWI hypoperfusion and FLAIR in low signal.

13.6.2 HIV/AIDS Related Cerebral Hemorrhage

13.6.2.1 Pathogens and Pathogenesis

The common causes of cerebral hemorrhage can be divided into two types, hypertensive and non-hypertensive. The pathogenesis is as the following. Due to long-term high blood pressure, vascular vessels bear great impact, with the blood flow shear stress acting on the surface of cerebral artery intima to cause damages, shedding and increased permeability of the endothelial cells. The passive blood pressure contributes to the formation of turbulent blood flow and even whirling at the arterial bifurcation and the arterial dilated part after its narrowing to cause intimal damages and atherosclerosis. In addition, it can cause occurrence of microaneurysm in the cerebral perforating artery. It has been reported that microaneurysm occurs more commonly in population aged above 50 years, with a distribution in the striate artery supplying basal ganglia, and the arteries in the pons, cerebral white matter and cerebellum. The occurrence of microaneurysm is a result of persistence high blood pressure, including pathological changes of structural changes of the vascular wall, decreased strength and elasticity of the arterial wall, and the resulted outward prominence of the thin and weak vascular wall, namely cystic microaneurysm. In the cases with sudden increase of blood pressure, rupture of the microaneurysm occurs to cause cerebral hemorrhage. Non-hypertensive cerebral hemorrhage occurs in patients with cerebrovascular malformation, cerebral artery amyloidosis, cerebroma apoplexy and brain trauma. Cerebrovascular malformation is a more common reason and is the main reason of cerebral hemorrhage in young adults, accounting for 1/4 of the non-hypertensive cerebral hemorrhage cases. Vascular malformation is commonly arteriovenous malformation. These malformed vascular vessels have segmental dilation and smooth muscle dysplasia, which make them vulnerable to rupture and hemorrhage. Cerebral artery amyloidosis is the common reason of spontaneous cerebral lobular hemorrhage, accounting for 5–10 % in cases of cerebral hemorrhage. Due to amyloidosis of the vascular wall interstitium, the vascular wall becomes fragile to cause its occurrence.

13.6.2.2 Pathophysiological Basis

The arterial system of hypertensive cerebral hemorrhage is directly from the major cerebral basal arteries. Under the impact from major arterial blood flow, due to the thin adventitia and media of cerebral arteries with less media fibers, together with pathological changes of degenerative and thickened arteriole, formation of microangioma and arteriolar wall defects, they are susceptible to rupture and bleeding. After cerebral hemorrhage, the hemorrhagic area has large quantity intact erythrocytes, with dark red hematoma and surrounding edema. The blood capillaries have congestion and rupture to form spots of bleeding. Later, the erythrocytes have rupture, with absorption of the hematoma and residual small cysts. On the cystic wall, there are tissue malacia and necrosis, spots bleeding that can be eliminated by large quantity of phagocytes, and accompanying stellate glial cells proliferation and colloid fiber formation, which can fill the cystic wall to cause local atrophy and a lacuna. In the cases with small quantity cerebral hemorrhage, the blood infiltrates between the nerve fibers to cause less damages to the brain tissue. In the cases with large quantity cerebral hemorrhage, the direct lesions can be caused, including compression, destruction, migration and malformation of the brain tissue, which further progress into hematoma, with secondary lesions of surrounding brain tissue edema and ischemia as well as CSF circulatory disturbance. Subsequently, the intracranial pressure increases gradually or rapidly to form a vicious circle. In some serious cases, cerebral herniation occurs to threaten the life.

13.6.2.3 Clinical Symptoms and Signs

Cerebral hemorrhage has an acute onset, which is life threatening with a high death rate. It commonly occurs in middle and senior aged populations, with sudden onset and symptoms of aphasia, hemiplegia, unconsciousness in serious cases, headache, vomiting, consciousness disturbance, deep and slow breathing, shrinkage/dilation of both pupils in different sizes with retarded or absent reaction to light and meningeal irritation positive. The focal location signs include (1) putamen hemorrhage of three partial syndromes (hemiplegia, hemianopsia and hemisensory obstruction), binocular gaze palsy and aphasia in the left hemisphere; (2) thalamus hemorrhage with symptoms of hemiplegia, hemisensory obstruction, binocular gaze palsy and pupils shrinkage; (3) lobular hemorrhage with symptoms of convulsion and obvious meningeal irritation and different focal signs due to differently involved lobes; (4) Pons hemorrhage with symptoms of deep coma, small pupils, fever, decerebrate rigidity or limbs paralysis; (5) cerebellum hemorrhage with symptoms of dizziness, nystagmus and ataxia (mild) as well as coma and soft loose limbs in some serious cases; (6) ventricular hemorrhage with symptoms of needle liked pupils, coma, high fever and decerebrate rigidity.

13.6.2.4 Examinations and Their Selection

1. CT scanning is the commonly used examination, especially during the hyperacute and acute periods.

2. MR imaging commonly is not used for the diagnosis of cerebral hemorrhage during the hyperacute and acute periods.

13.6.2.5 Imaging Demonstrations

1. CT scanning demonstrates the acute period as round, oval or irregular shaped high density foci in the brain, with CT values ranging from 50 to 80 HU. In the cases with penetration into the ventricles, cerebroventricular mold is formed. The atypical manifestation is equal density. In the subacute period, the density of hematoma decreases gradually to equal, with surrounding absorption and central high density ice melting sign. By enhanced scanning, there are ring shaped enhancement, decreased edema and decreased space occupying effect.

2. MR imaging demonstrates the hyperacute period as shortened T2WI signal due to the diamagnetic effect of the hemoglobin containing oxygen, and equal, uneven and high T2WI signal of the hematoma. In acute period, due to the sensitive magnetic effect which increases proton diphase, the demonstrations are shortened T2WI signal but less effect on TWI, with slightly long T1WI or equal T1WI and short T2WI signals of the hematoma. In the subacute period, due to the existence of methaemoglobin in erythrocyte, the demonstrations are shortened T1WI and T2WI signals, with central equal signals and peripheral high signals of the hematoma. In the cases with hemolysis of hematoma, methaemoglobin deposits outside the cells, in short T1WI and long T2WI signals, with long T1WI and long T2WI signal of the hematoma, decreased edema and decreased space occupying effect. Chronic hematoma is demonstrated as high signals by both T1WI and T2WI. Due to the existence of hemoglobin rings containing iron, the demonstrations are shortened T2WI signal, with equal T1WI signal and low T2WI signal of the hematoma, absent edema and space occupying effect. There are long T1WI and long T2WI signals with surrounding hemosiderin ring.

Case Study 1

A male patient aged 28 years was confirmatively diagnosed as having AIDS by the CDC. He complained of persistent dizziness for more than 3 months, and recurrent and progressively severe headache for more than 1 month. His CD4 T cell count was 25/μl.

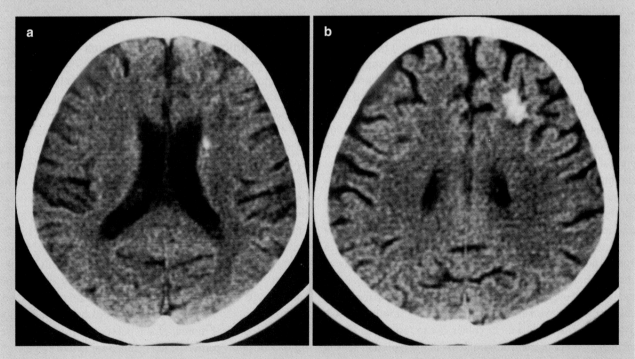

Fig. 13.84 (**a, b**) HIV/AIDS related cerebral hemorrhage. (**a, b**) CT scanning demonstrates flaky high density shadow in the left frontal parietal lobe, with no obvious edema and space occupying effect

Case Study 2

A male patient aged 31 years was confirmatively diagnosed as having AIDS by the CDC. He sustained trauma and following coma for more than 10 min and complained of headache for 6 days. His CD4 T cell count was 75/μl.

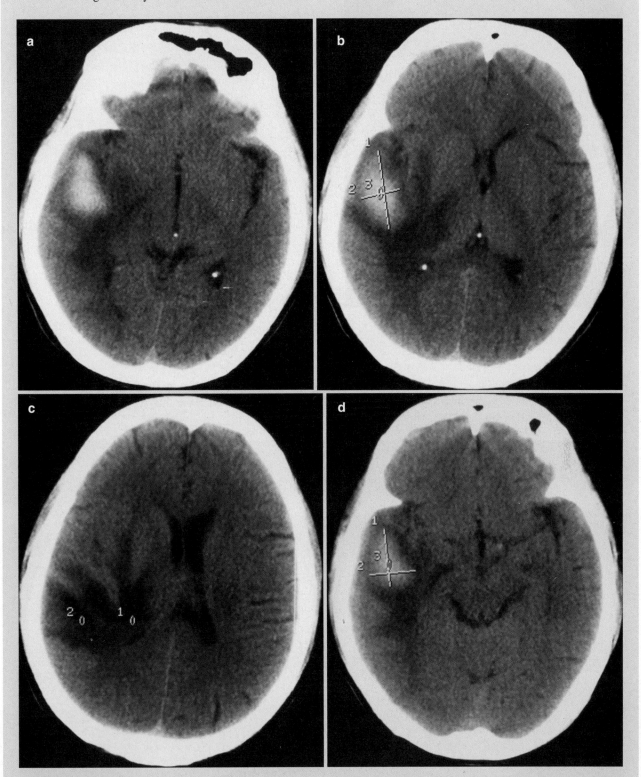

Fig. 13.85 (a–e) HIV/AIDS related cerebral hemorrhage. It is demonstrated to have large flaky high density shadow in the right temporal lobe, obvious space occupying effect, compressed and narrowed right lateral ventricle, slight leftward migration of the midline and surrounding obvious finger liked edema

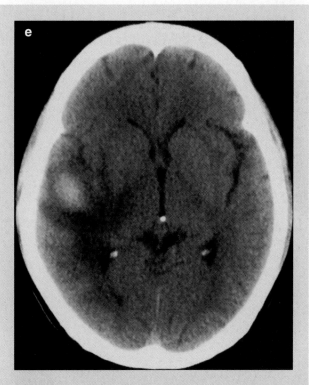

Fig. 13.85 (continued)

Case Study 3

A male patient aged 31 years was confirmatively diagnosed as having AIDS by the CDC. He complained of persistent dizziness for more than 3 months, and sudden unconsciousness for more than 10 min. His CD4 T cell count was 35/μl.

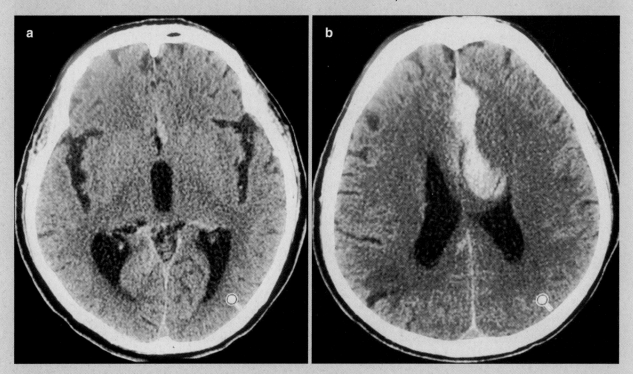

Fig. 13.86 (a–c) HIV/AIDS related cerebral hemorrhage. (a) CT scanning demonstrates enlarged bilateral lateral fissure cisterns, enlarged lateral ventricles, deepened and widened sulci. (b, c) It is demonstrated to have wide stripes of high density shadows in the left frontal parietal lobe and adjacent to cerebral falx, compressed and narrowed frontal angle of the left lateral ventricle, and rightward migration of local midline structure

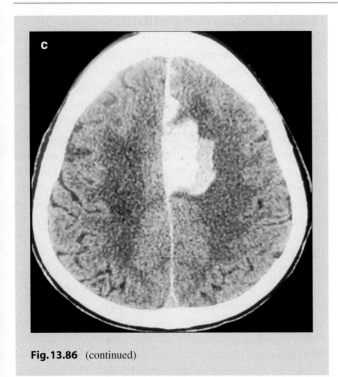

Fig. 13.86 (continued)

13.6.2.6 Key Points for the Diagnosis

1. For basal ganglia hemorrhage, there are findings of contralateral hemiplegia, aphasia caused by hemorrhage of dominant hemisphere, sensory disturbance of contralateral limbs, hemianopsia and gaze palsy. CT scanning demonstrates bilateral or unilateral flaky high density shadow, with obvious edema and space occupying effect.
2. For thalamus hemorrhage, there are clinical manifestations of thalamic sensory disturbance, thalamic aphasia and thalamic dementia. CT scanning demonstrates flaky high density shadow in the thalamus, with obvious edema and space occupying effect.
3. In the cases with brainstem hemorrhage, most have pontine hemorrhage, occasionally midbrain hemorrhage and rarely medulla oblongata hemorrhage. MR imaging can define the diagnosis.
4. For pontine hemorrhage, there are sudden headache, vomiting, dizziness, diplopia, different axis of eyeball, crossed paralysis or hemiplegia and paralysis of the limbs. MR imaging can define the diagnosis.
5. For cerebellar hemorrhage, there are sudden dizziness, vomiting posterior headache, no hemiplagia, nystagmus, unstable standing and walking, ataxia of limbs, decreased muscular tension and cervical stiffness. CT scanning demonstrates high density shadow in the cerebella hemisphere or the vermis as well as compressed four ventricles and brainstem. MR imaging can define the diagnosis, which is superior to CT scanning.

6. For lobular hemorrhage, its occurrence accounts nearly 5–10 % of cerebral hemorrhage. In the cases with frontal lobe hemorrhage, there are headache, vomiting and commonly epileptic seizure; contralateral hemiplegia, anorthopia and metal disorder; anandia in the cases of hemorrhage of dominant hemisphere. In the cases of parietal lobe hemorrhage, there are slight hemiplegia but obvious hemisensory disturbance; contralateral lower quadrantanopia; mixed aphasia in the cases with hemorrhage of dominant hemisphere. For temporal lobe hemorrhage, there are contralateral face and tongue paralysis of the central nervous system, upper limbs paralysis; contralateral upper quadrantanopia; sensory or mixed aphasia in the cases with hemorrhage of dominant hemisphere. For occipital lobe hemorrhage, there are contralateral homonymous hemianopia and sparing of macula; no limbs paralysis. CT scanning and MR imaging can define the diagnosis.
7. For ventricular hemorrhage, the clinical manifestations include sudden headache, vomiting, rapid progression into coma or gradual aggravation of coma, shrinkage of both pupils, increased muscular tension of the limbs, pathological reflex positive, early symptom of decerebrate rigidity and meningeal irritation sign positive. In addition, there are symptoms and signs of subthalamic lesions, increased CSF pressure and bloody CSF, which can be clinically misdiagnosed as subarachnoid hemorrhage. Brain CT scanning can define the diagnosis.

13.6.2.7 Differential Diagnosis
Cerebral Infarction
HIV/AIDS related cerebral hemorrhage should be differentiated from cerebral infarction. Due to the totally different therapeutic principles in clinical practice for cerebral hemorrhage and cerebral infarction, their differential diagnosis is important. Before the onset of cerebral infarction, transient brain ischemia usually occurs, with slight/absent consciousness disturbance but serious focal signs. The CSF shows no high pressure, being colorless and transparent. CT scanning demonstrates cerebral infarction as low density shadow in the brain. Enhanced CT scanning demonstrates no obvious enhancement or enhancement of the surrounding infarction area. MR imaging demonstrates cerebral infarction in long T1 long T2 signals. However, CT scanning demonstrates cerebral hemorrhage as equal or high density shadow an can define the occurrence of cerebral hemorrhage.

Intracranial Tumor Hemorrhage
Intracranial tumor, especially primary tumor, often has central ischemia and necrosis due to its rapid growth. It can be misdiagnosed as cerebral hemorrhage. Enhanced brain CT scanning and MR imaging have diagnostic value for tumor hemorrhage.

13.6.2.8 Discussion

Generally, the causes of HIV/AIDS related cerebral hemorrhage are as the follow: (1) Vascular invasion of HIV to cause vascular lesions; (2) brain tissues lesions cause by opportunistic infections; (3) cerebrovascular lesions caused by HARRT treatment; (4) syphilis or tumor hemorrhage; (5) the diseases relate to age (e.g. hypertension and diabetes). CT scanning and MR imaging can define the diagnosis. However, the diagnosis and differential diagnosis should be made based on sufficient knowledge and reasonable thinking to define the causes of hemorrhage, which is important for the following treatment and prognosis.

13.6.3   HIV/AIDS Related Encephalatrophy

13.6.3.1 Pathogens and Pathogenesis

Brain atrophy is a condition of brain metabolic abnormality and brain dysfunction with edema, degeneration and necrosis of the brain tissues caused by hypoxia, ischemia, inflammatory mediators, metabolites and oxygen derived free radicals. Any disease being capable of causing brain tissue ischemia and hypoxia disease can lead to brain atrophy.

13.6.3.2 Pathophysiological Basis

The main reasons of HIV/AIDS related brain atrophy are AIDS encephalopathy (e.g. HIV encephalopathy and encephalopathy after HARRT) and some related infections (e.g. herpes simplex virus infection). Its pathophysiological basis is changes of blood physical components that cause vascular wall malformation as well as rough vascular wall and decreased elasticity of vascular walls. The nerve fibers in the neurocytes are manifested as agglutination, curl and spiral shape, with brain cortical atrophy, narrowed gyri, widened sulci, thickened meninges and obviously enlarged ventricular system to cause brain atrophy. Brain atrophy can be focal and diffuse.

13.6.3.3 Clinical Symptoms and Signs

The early symptoms are headache, dizziness, gradual loss of memory, the decline/loss of concepts in time, place and orientation. In addition, the thought is fragmental, with major events ignored and minor events entangled. There are also intelligence decline, depression, apathia, slow response, less words and movement, bradykinesia and being indifferent to the surroundings. The personality changes are manifested as being selfish, subjective,

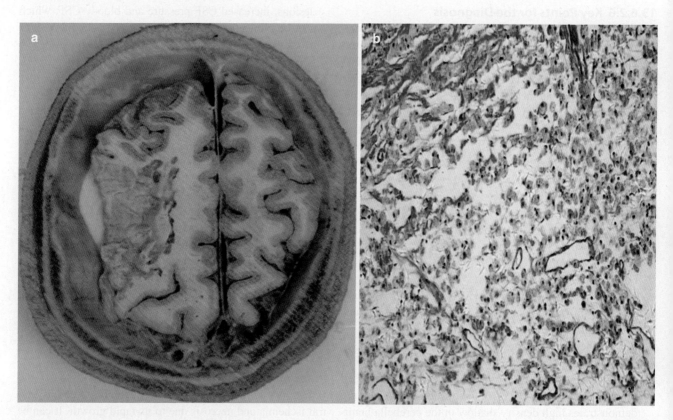

Fig. 13.87 (**a**, **b**) HIV/AIDS related cerebral infarction and brain atrophy. (**a**) Autopsy demonstrates liquefaction and necrosis after cerebral infarction in the right brain. (**b**) It is demonstrated to have no normal structures of the brain cells

stubborn, anxious, doubtful, irritation and nonsense talking. It can further progress into HIV/AIDS related vascular dementia.

13.6.3.4 Examinations and Their Selection

CT scanning and MR imaging are the diagnostic imaging of the choice. Especially MR imaging can define the abnormal change of the brain tissues for qualitative and quantitative diagnosis. MRA and brain angiography can define the morphology of brain arteries as well as the bifurcations.

13.6.3.5 Imaging Demonstrations

CT scanning and MR imaging demonstrate decreased brain parenchyma as well as enlarged brain ventricles and subarachnoid space, which are characteristic imaging demonstrations of HIV/AIDS related brain atrophy. In the cases with brain atrophy, there is enlarged subarachnoid space, symmetrically enlarged ventricular system, widened and deepened cerebral sulci, flat and narrowed gyrus, enlarged lateral ventricle and the third ventricle, decreased tissue density around anterior and posterior horns of the lateral ventricles. In the cases with local brain atrophy, the demonstrations include unilateral decrease of the local brain volume, widened cerebral sulcus and enlarged lateral fissure cistern. In the cases with cerebellar atrophy, the demonstrations are widened cerebellar sulcus, decreased volume, branch leaf liked imaging demonstrations, enlarged surrounding spaces of the cerebellum and enlarged fourth ventricle.

Case Study 1

A male patient aged 39 years was confirmatively diagnosed as having AIDS by the CDC. He had clinical manifestations of dementia and ataxia and was addicted to alcoholism and drug abuse. His CD4 T cell count was 85/μl.

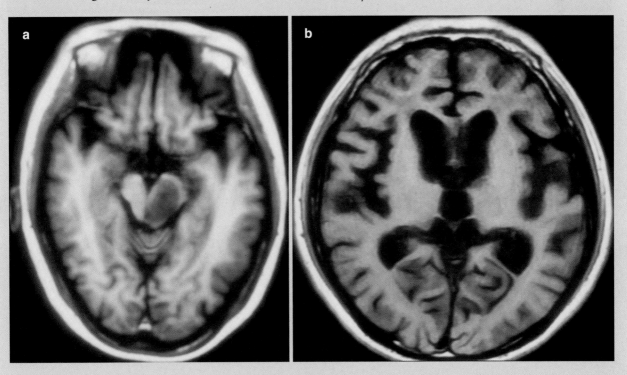

Fig. 13.88 (a–d) HIV/AIDS related brain atrophy. Axial MR imaging demonstrates long T1 and long T2 signals in the left pontibrachium, deepened and widened cerebral sulcus, enlarged lateral fissure cistern and enlarged lateral ventricle

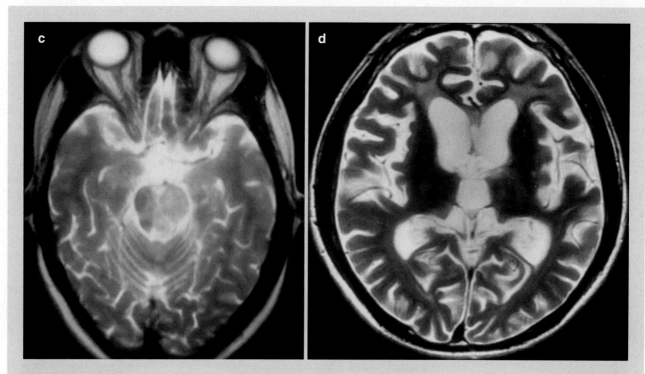

Fig. 13.88   (continued)

Case Study 2

A male patient aged 31 years was confirmatively diagnosed as having AIDS by the CDC. He had clinical manifestations of dementia and ataxia and was addicted to alcoholism and drug abuse. His CD4 T cell count was 5/μl.

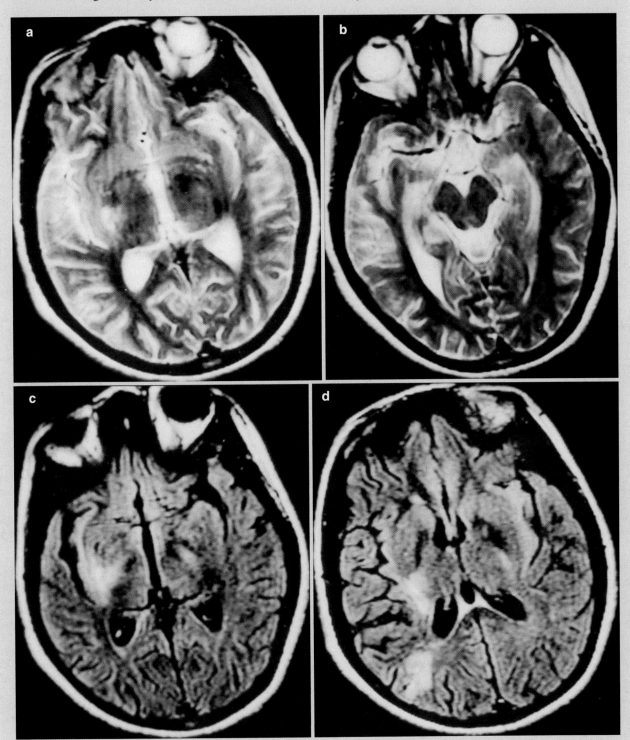

Fig. 13.89 (**a–d**) HIV/AIDS related brain atrophy. (**a–d**) Axial MR imaging demonstrates small flaky long T2WI signal in the right basal ganglia. (**c, d**) Proton density imaging demonstrates flaky high signal in the right basal ganglia, flaky high signal in the right lateral ventricular occipital horn, deepened and widened cerebral sulcus and enlarged lateral fissure cistern

13.6.3.6 Key Points for the Diagnosis

1. Symptoms of HIV encephalopathy and the history of related opportunistic infections.
2. CT scanning and MR imaging demonstrate focal or diffuse decrease of the total brain volume, deepened and widened cerebral sulcus and enlarged cistern and ventricle.

13.6.3.7 Differential Diagnosis

HIV/AIDS related brain atrophy should be differentiated from hydrocephalus, with different demonstrations of the enlarged ventricles.

	Angle between tops of both ventricles	The third Ventricle	Optic recess and infundibular recess
Brain atrophy	enlarged	Enlarged, with no obvious prominence of the anterior and posterior walls	sharp
Hydrocephalus	narrowed	In sphere shape	Blunt, shallow or absent

Extended Reading

1. Abrams EJ, Matheson PB, Thomas PA, et al. Neonatai predictors of infection status and early death among 332 infants at risk of HIV-1 infection monitored prospectively from birth, New York City perinatal HIV transmission collaborative study group. Pediatrics. 1995;96:451–8.
2. Adair JC, Beck AC, Apfelbaum RI, et al. Nocardial cerebral abscess in the acquired immunodeficiency syndrome. Arch Neurol. 1987;44:548–50.
3. American Academy of Neurology. Practice parameters for mass lesions in AIDS. Neurology. 1998;50:21–6.
4. Anders KH, Guerra WF, Tomiyasu U, et al. The neuropathology of AIDS. Am J Pathol. 1986;124:537–58.
5. Antunes F. Central nervous system AIDS —related diseases. Acta Neurochir (Wien). 2004;146(10):1071–4.
6. Anzil AP, Rao C, Wrzolek MA, et al. Amebic meningoencephalitis in a patient with AIDS caused by a newly recognized opportunistic pathogen. Arch Pathol Lab Med. 1991;115(1):21–5.
7. Ayclin F, Bartholomew PM, Vinson DG. Primary T-cell lymphoma of the brain in a patient at advanced stage of acquired immunodeficiency syndrome. Arch Pathol Lab Med. 1998;122:361–5.
8. Bale Jr JF. Human cytomegalovirus infection and disorders of the nervous system of patients with the acquired immune deficiency syndrome. Arch Neurol. 1984;41:310–20.
9. Beaman B, Burnsied J, Edwards B, et al. Nocardial infection in the United States, 1972-1974. J Infect Dis. 1976;134:286–9.
10. Berenguer J, Moreno S, Laguna F, et al. Tuberculous meningitis in patients infected with the human immunodeficiency virus. N Engl J Med. 1992;326:668–72.
11. Berger JR, Moskowitz L, Fischl M, et al. Neurological disease as the presenting manifestation of acquired immunodeficiency syndrome. South Med J. 1987;80:683–6.
12. Berkefeld J, Enzensberger W, Lanfermann H. Cryptococcus meningoencephalitis in AIDS: parenchymal and meningeal forms. Neuroradiology. 1999;41:129–33.

13. Bishburg E, Eng RH, lim J. Brain lesions in patients with acquired immunodeficiency syndrome. Arch Intern Med. 1989;149:941–3.
14. Bishburg E, Sunderama G, Reichman LB, et al. Central nervous system tuberculosis with the acquired immunodeficiency syndrome and its related complex. Ann Intern Med. 1986;105:210–3.
15. Boni J, Emmerich BS, Lein SL, et al. PCR identification of HIV-1 DNA sequences in brain tissue of patients with AIDS encephalopathy. Neurology. 1993;43(9):1813–7.
16. Bowler JV, et al. Contribution of diaschisis to the clinical deficit in human cerebral infarction. Stroke. 1995;26:1.
17. Boyd JF. Adult cytomegalic inclusion disease. Scott Med J. 1980;25:266–9.
18. Britton CB, Miller JR. Neurological complications of acquired immunodeficiency syndrome (AIDS). Neurol Clin. 1984;2:315–39.
19. Brooks BR, Walker DL. Progressive multifocal leukoencephalopathy. Neurol Clin. 1984;2:299–313.
20. Bross JE, Gordon G. Nocardial meningitis: case reports and review. Rev Infect Dis. 1991;13:160–5.
21. Bruns DK, Risser RC, White III CL. The neuropathology of human immunodeficiency virus infection. Arch Pathol Lab Med. 1991;115:1112–24.
22. Budka H, Wiley CA, Kleihues P, et al. HIV-associated disease of the nervous system: review of nomenclature and proposal for neuropathology-based terminology. Brain Pathol. 1991;1:143–52.
23. Cao ZJ, Wang W, Li LY. MRI imaging analysis of multiple sclerosis. Zhejiang Clin Med J. 2005;7(6):6561.
24. Capponi M, Sureau P. Penicillium de Rhizomys Sinensis. Bull Soc Pathol Exot. 1956;49(4):418.
25. Carbaial JR, Palacios E, Azar-kia B, et al. Radiology of cysticercosis of the central nervous system including computed tomography. Radiology. 1977;125:127–31.
26. Carne CA, Tedder RS, Smith A, et al. Acute encephalopathy coincident with seroconversion for anti-HTLV-III. Lancet. 1985;2:1206–8.
27. Centers for Disease Control. Primary resistance to anti-Tuberculous drugs – United States. MMWR Morb Mortal Wkly Rep. 1983;32:521–3.
28. Centers for Disease Control. Tuberculosis and acquired immunodeficiency syndrome – New York City. MMWR Morb Mortal Wkly Rep. 1987;36:785–95.
29. Chang L, Ernst T, Tornatore C, et al. Metabolite abnormalities in progressive multifocal leukoencephalopathy: a proton magnetic resonance spectroscopy study. Neurology. 1997;48:836–45.
30. Chen Diansen, Li Hongjun, Li li. MRI diagnosis of intracranial cryptococcus neoformans infection in AIDS patients. Radiol Pract. 2011;26(6):586–9.
31. Chrysikopoulous HS, Press GA, Grafe MR, et al. Encephalitis caused by human immunodeficiency virus: CT and MR imaging manifestations with clinical and pathological correlation. Radiology. 1990;175:185–91.
32. Cimino C, Lipton RB, Williams A, et al. The evaluation of patients with human immunodeficiency virus-related disorders and brain mass lesions. Arch Intern Med. 1991;151:1381–4.
33. Cooper Jr CR, Haycocks NG. Penicillium marneffei: an insurgent species among the penicillia. J Eukaryot Microbiol. 2000;47:24–8.
34. Cooper CR, Vanittanakom N. Insights into the pathogenicity of Penicillium marneffei. Future Microbiol. 2008;3(1):43–55.
35. Cosottini M, Tavarelli C, Del Bono L, et al. Diffusion weighted imaging in patients with progressive multifocal leukoencephalopathy. Eur Radiol. 2008;18(5):1024–30.
36. Curless RG, Mitchell CD. Central nervous system tuberculosis in children. Pediatr Neurol. 1991;7:270–4.
37. Currie BP, Casadevall A. Estimation of the prevalence of cryptococcal infection among HIV infected individuals in New York City. Clin Infect Dis. 1994;19:1029–33.

38. Amorosa JK, Nahass RG, Nosher JL, Gocke DJ. Radiologic distinction of phyogenic pulmonary infection from pneumocystis carinii pneumonia in AIDS patients. Radiology.1990;175:721–4.

39. Danner SA. Management of cytomegalovirus disease. AIDS. 1995;9 Suppl 2:S3–8.

40. Dastur DK. Neurotuberculosis. In: Minckler J, editor. Pathology of the nervous system, vol. 3. New York: McGraw-Hill; 1972. p. 2412–22.

41. de Graef M, Smadja P, Benis J, Turpin F, Liouane M, Viaud B, Ruffie P, Bourbotte G, Bonafe A. Neurotrichinosis: a case report with MRI evaluation. J Radiol. 2000;81:817–9.

42. Degirolami U, Smith TW, Henin D, et al. Neuropathology of acquired immunodeficiency syndrome. Arch Pathol Lab Med. 1990;114:643–55.

43. Deng Z, Ribas JL, Gibson DW, et al. Infections caused by Penicillium marneffei in China and Southeast Asia: review of eighteen published case and report of our mo re Chinese cases. Rev Infect Dis. 1998;10(3):640.

44. Dina TS. Primary central nervous system lymphoma versus toxoplasmosis in AIDS. Radiology. 1991;179:823–8.

45. Disalvo AF, Fickling AM, Ajello L. Infection caused by penicillium marneffei. Am J Clin Pathol. 1973;60(2):259–63.

46. Dolin PJ, Raviglione MC, Kochi A. Global tuberculosis incidence and mortality during 1990-2000. Bull World Health Organ. 1994;72(2):213–20.

47. Feydy A, Touze E, Miaux Y, Bolgert F, Martin-Duverneuil N, Laplane D, Chiras J. MRI in a case of neurotrichinosis. Neuroradiology. 1996;38 Suppl 1:S80–2.

48. Gartner S, Markovits P, Markovits DM, et al. Virus isolation from and identification of HTLV-III/LAV-producing cells in brain tissue from a patient with AIDS. JAMA. 1986;256:2365–71.

49. Gasecki AP, Steg RE. Correlation of early MRI with CT scan, EEG, and CSF: analyses in a cases of biopsy proven herpes simplex encephalitis. Eur Neurol. 1991;31:372.

50. Gelal F, Kumral E, Vidinli BD, Erdogan D, Yucel K, Erdogan N. Diffusion-weighted and conventional MR imaging in neurotrichinosis. Acta Radiol. 2005;46:196–9.

51. Gero B, Sze G, Sharif H. MR imaging of intradural inflammatory diseases of the spine. AJNR Am J Neuroradiol. 1991;12:1009–19.

52. Gonzales MF, Davis RL. Neuropathology of acquired immunodeficiency syndrome. Neuropathol Appl Neurobiol. 1988;14:345–63.

53. González RG. Imaging neuro AIDS. AJNR Am J Neuroradiol. 2004;25(2):167–82.

54. Gyure KA, Prayson RA, Estes ML, et al. Symptomatic mycobacterium avium complex infection of the central nervous system. Arch Pathol Lab Med. 1995;119:836–9.

55. Hamilton RL, Achim C, Grafe MR. Herpes simplex virus brainstem encephalitis in an AIDS patient. Clin Neuropathol. 1995;14:45–50.

56. Hanson DL, Chusy, Faizo KM, et al. Distribution of CD4+ T lymphocytes at diagnosis of acquired immunodeficiency syndrome defining and other human immunodeficiency virus-related illnesses. The Adult and Adolescent Spectrum of HIV Disease Project Group. Arch Intern Med. 1995;155(14):1537–42.

57. Harris DE, Enterline DS, Tien RD. Neurosyphilis in patients with AIDS. Neuroimaging Clin N Am. 1997;7:215–21.

58. Hassine D, Gray F, Chekroun P, et al. Early brain lesions in HIV infection post mortem radiopathology correlations in asymptomatic non-AIDS seropositive patients. J Neuroradiol. 1995;22:148–60.

59. Hassine D, Gray F, Chekroun R, et al. CMV and VZV encephalitis in AIDS. J Neuroradiol. 1995;22:184–92.

60. Ho DD, Bredesen DE, Vinters HV, et al. The acquired immunodeficiency syndrome (AIDS) dementia complex. Ann Intern Med. 1989;111:400.

61. Hurley RA, Ernst T, Khalili K, et al. Identification of HIV associated progressive multifocal leukoencephalopathy: magnetic resonance imaging and spectroscopy. J Neuropsychiatry Clin Neurosci. 2003;15(1):1261.

62. Jain K, Mittal K. Imaging features of central nervous system fungal infections. Neurol India. 2007;55(3):241–50.

63. Jiao Yan mei, Chen De xi, Li Zai cun, et al. The method of reverse establishment PCR detect HIV-1 integration sites. J Cap Med Univ. 2009;30(5):635–8.

64. Jiddane M, Nicole F, Diaz P, et al. Intracranial malignant lymphoma. Report of 30 cases and review of the literature. J Neurosurg. 1986;65:592–9.

65. Kamezawa T, Shimozuru T, M N, et al. MRI of a cerebral cryptococcal granuloma. Neuroradiology. 2000;42(6):441–3.

66. Kastrup O, Maschke M, Diener HC, et al. Progressive multifocal leukoencephalopathy limited to t he brain stem. Neuroradiology. 2002;44(3):227–9.

67. Katz DA, Berger JR. Neurosyphilis in acquired immunodeficiency syndrome. Arch Neurol. 1989;46:895–8.

68. Katz DA, Berger JR, Duncan RC. Neurosyphilis, a comparative study of the effects of infection with human immunodeficiency virus. Arch Neurol. 1993;50:243–9.

69. Kazuhiro U, Yasuo K. Brain MRI findings in cryptococcal meningoencephalitis. J Nippon Med Sch. 2000;67(4):226–7.

70. Knox JM, Musher D, Guzick ND. The pathogenesis of syphilis and related treponematoses. In: Johnson RC, editor. The biology of parasitic spirochetes. San Diego: Academic Press; 1976. p. 249–59.

71. Kovoor JM, Mahadevan A, Narayan JP, et al. Cryptococcal choroid plexitis as a mass lesion: MR imaging and histopathologic correlation. AJNR Am J Neuroradiol. 2002;23:273–6.

72. Krick JA, Remington JS. Current concepts in parasitology. Toxoplasmosis in the adult-an overview. N Engl J Med. 1978;298:550–3.

73. Kudeken N, Kawakami K, Saito A. CD4+ T cell-mediated fatal hyperinflammatory reactions in mice infected with Penicillium marneffei. Clin Exp Immunol. 1997;107(3):468–73.

74. Kuwahara S, Kawada M, Uga S. Cryptococcal meningoencephalitis presenting with an unusual magnetic resonance imaging appearance. Neurol Med Chir (Tokyo). 2001;41(10):517–21.

75. Kwee RM, Kwee TC. Virchow-Robin spaces at MR imaging. Radiographics. 2007;27(4):1071–86.

76. Lanjewar DN, Jain PP, Shetty CR. Profile of central nervous system pathology in patients with AIDS: an autopsy study from India. AIDS. 1998;12:309–13.

77. LeBlang SD, Whiteman MLH, Post MJD, et al. CNS Nocardia in AIDS patients: CT and MRI with pathologic correlation. J Comput Assist Tomogr. 1995;19:15–22.

78. Lee SC, Casadevall A, Dickson DW. Immunohistochemical localization of capsula poly saccharide antigen in the central nervous system cells in cryptococcal meningoencephalitis. Am J Pathol. 1996;148:1267–74.

79. Levy RM, Pons VG, Rosenblum ML. Intracerebral-mass lesions in the acquired immunodeficiency syndrome (AIDS). N Engl J Med. 1983;309:1454–5.

80. Levy RM, Rosenbloom S, Perrett LV. Neuroradiological findings in the acquired immunodeficiency syndrome (AIDS): a review of 200 cases. AJNR Am J Neuroradiol. 1986;7:833–9.

81. Li hongjun. Atlas of differential diagnosis in HIV/AIDS. Beijing: PMPH; 2008. First published. ISBN 978-7-117-09194-7/R.9195.

82. Li hongjun. Diagnostic imaging of AIDS in China: current status and clinical application. Chin J Magn Reson Imaging. 2010;1:5.

83. Li hongjun, Qishi. Diagnostic imaging of AIDS-related nervous system infection. Chin J Magn Reson Imaging. 2010;1:5.

84. Li hongjun, Zhao xuan. The value of image diagnosis for toxoplasma encephalitis in patients with AIDS. J Med Imaging. 2008;18:10.

85. Li hongjun, Gao yanqing, Cheng liang, et al. Diagnostic imaging, preautopsy imaging and autopsy findings of 8 AIDS cases. Chin Med J (Engl). 2009;18:2142–8.

86. Li hongjun, Meng zhihao, Huang kui, et al. Imaging finding of AIDS complicated with pulmonary Rhodococcus equi infection and correlated with pathology. Radiol Pract. 2009;24(9):943–7.

87. Li hongjun, Song Wenyan Jia cuiyu, et al. MRI in a case of neurotrichinosis. Radiol Pract. 2009;24:10.

88. Li hongjun, Zhang Yu-zhong, Cheng Jing-liang. DepaCorrelation of diagnostic imaging and autopsy findings of eight patients with acquired: immunodeficiency syndrome. Chin J Radiol. 2009;43:1196–200.

89. Li MH, Holtas S, Larsson EM. MR imaging of spinal lymphoma. Acta Radiol. 1992;33:338–42.

90. Li Yunfang, Hongjun Li. AIDS Xiangguanxing Naobing de 18F-FDG PET/CT Biaoxian. Radiol Pract. 2011;26(10):1040–2 (In Chinese).

91. Liu J, Shen JL, Zhang L. Progressive multifocal leukoencephalopathy in AIDS: case report. Chin J Med Imaging Technol. 2008;24(11):1857.

92. Lizerbram EK, Hesselink JR. Viral infections. Neuroimaging Clin N Am. 1997;7:261–80.

93. Louie E, Rice LB, Holzman RS. Tuberculosis in non-Haitian patients with acquired immunodeficiency syndrome. Chest. 1986;90:542–5.

94. Luft BJ, Remington JS. Toxoplasmmic encephalitis in encephalitis in patients with the acquired immunodeficiency syndrome. N Engl J Med. 1992;329:995–1000.

95. Lyons RW, Andriole VT. Fungal infections of the CNS. Neurol Clin. 1986;4(1):159–70.

96. Maclean H, Ironside J, Dhillon B. Acquired immunodeficiency syndrome-related primary central nervous system lymphoma. Arch Ophthalmol. 1994;112:269–72.

97. MacMahon EME, Glass JD, Hayward SD, et al. Epstein Barr virus (EBV) in acquired immune deficiency syndrome-related primary central nervous system lymphoma. Lancet. 1991;338:969–73.

98. Mathew RM, Murnane M. MRI in PML: bilateral medullary le2sions. Neurology. 2004;63(12):2380.

99. Mathews VP, Alo PL, Glass JD, et al. AIDS-related CNS cryptococcosis. Radiological-pathological correlation. AJNR Am J Neuroradiol. 1992;13:1477–86.

100. McArthur JC. Neurologic manifestations of acquired immune deficiency syndrome. Medicine. 1987;66:407–37.

101. McGee JOD, Isa-acson PG, Wright NA. Oxford of pathology. New York: Oxford University Press; 1992.

102. Mehta JB, Dutt A, Harrill L, et al. Epidemiology of extrapulmonary tuberculosis. A comparative analysis with pre-AIDS era. Chest. 1991;99:1134–8.

103. Mendenhall NP, Thar TL, Agee OF, et al. Primary lymphoma of the central nervous system, computerized tomography scan characteristics and treatment results for 12 cases. Cancer. 1983;52(11):1993–2000.

104. Miguel GM, Edward RC, Dante SZ. A probable case of human neurotrichinellosis in the United States. Am J Trop Med Hyg. 2007;77(2):347–9.

105. Miszkiel KA. The spectrum of MRI finding in CNS cryptococcosis in AIDS. Clin Radiol. 1996;51:842–50.

106. Montesions-Rongen M, Akasaka T, Zuhlke-Jenisch R, et al. Molecular characterization of BCL6 breakpoints in primary diffuse large B-cell lymphomas of the central nervous system identifies GAPD as novel translocation partner. Brain Pathol. 2003;13(4):534–8.

107. Morgello S, Soifer FM, Lin CS, et al. Central nervous system strongyloides stercoralis in acquired immunodeficiency syndrome. A report of two cases and review of the literature. Acta Neuropathol. 1993;86(3):285.

108. Moskowitz LB, Hensley GT, Chan JC, et al. Brain biopsy in patients with immune deficiency syndrome. Arch Pathol Lab Med. 1984;108:368–71.

109. Navia BA, Cho E-S, Petito CK, et al. The AIDS dementia complex: 11. Neuropathology. Ann Neurol. 1986;19:525–35.

110. Navia BA, Gonzalez RG. Functional imaging of the AIDS dementia complex and the metabolic pathology of the HIV-1 infected brain. Neuroimaging Clin N Am. 1997;7:431–45.

111. Navia BA, Jordan BD, Price RW. The AIDS dementia complex 1. Clinical features. Ann Neurol. 1986;19:517–24.

112. Navia BA, Rottenberg DS, Sidtis J, et al. Regional cerebral glucose metabolism in AIDS dementia complex. Neurology. 1985;35:226.

113. Newton HB. Common neurologic complications of HIV-1 infection and AIDS. Am Fam Physician. 1995;51:387–400.

114. O'Mally JP, Ziessman HA, Kumar PN, et al. Diagnosis of intracranial lymphoma in patients with AIDS: value of 201TI single-photon emission computed tomography. AJR Am J Roentgenol. 1994;163(2):417–21.

115. Oda M, Udaka F. Magnetic resonance imaging in multiple sclerosis. Nippon Rinsho. 2008;66(6):1098–102.

116. Offiah CE, Turnbull IW. The imaging appearances of intracranial CNS infections in adult HIV and AIDS patient s. Clin Radiol. 2006;61(5):393–401.

117. Ordan J, Enzmann DR. Encephalitis. Neuroimaging Clin N Am. 1991;1:17–38.

118. Pautler KB, Padhye AA, Ajello L. Imported penicilliosis marnefei in the United States: report of a second human infection. Sabouraudia. 1984;22(5):433–8.

119. Pitchenik AE, Cole C, Russell BW, et al. Tuberculosis, atypical mycobacteriosis, and the acquired immunodeficiency syndrome among Haitian and non-Haitian patients in South Florida. Ann Intern Med. 1984;101:641–5.

120. Pohl P, Vogl G, Fill H, et al. Single photon emission computed tomography in AIDS dementia complex. J Nucl Med. 1988;29:1382–6.

121. Porter SB, Sande MA. Toxoplasmosis of the central nervous system in the acquired immunodeficiency syndrome. N Engl J Med. 1993;2:1643–8.

122. Post MJD, Chan JC, Hensley GT, et al. Toxoplasma encephalitis in Haitian adults with acquired immunodeficiency syndrome: a clinical-pathological-CT correlation. AJR Am J Roentgenol. 1983;140:861–8.

123. Post MJD, Hensley GT, Mosowitz LB, et al. Cytomegalic inclusion virus encephalitis in patients with AIDS: CT, clinical and pathological correlation. AJR Am J Roentgenol. 1986;146:1229–34.

124. Post MJD, Sheldon JJ, Hensley CT. Central nervous system disease in acquired immunodeficiency syndrome: prospective correlation using CT, MR imaging and pathologic studies. Radiology. 1986;158:141–8.

125. Post MJD, Tate LG, Quencer RM, et al. CT, MR and pathology in HIV encephalitis and meningitis. AJNR Am J Neuroradiol. 1988;9:469–76.

126. Raez L, Cabral L, Cai JP, et al. Treatment of AIDS-related primary central nervous system lymphoma with zidovudine, ganciclovir, and interleukin 2. AIDS Res Hum Retroviruses. 1999;15:713–9.

127. Ragin AB, Storey P, Cohen BA, et al. Whole brain diffusion tensor imaging in HIV-associated cognitive impairment. AJNR Am J Neuroradiol. 2004;25(2):195–200.

128. Ramsey RG, Geremia GK. CNS complications of AIDS: CT and MR findings. AJR Am J Roentgenol. 1988;151:449–54.

129. Reichman RC. Neurological complications of varicellazoster infection. Ann Intern Med. 1978;89:375–88.

130. Remick SC, Diamond C, Migliozzi JA, et al. Primary central nervous system lymphoma in patients with and without the acquired immune deficiency syndrome. A retrospective analysis and review of the literature. Medicine. 1990;69:345–60.

131. Rhodes RH. Histopathologic features in the central nervous system of 400 acquired immunodeficiency syndrome cases: implications of rates of occurrence. Hum Pathol. 1993;24:1189–98.

132. Ribera E, Martinez-Vasquez JM, Ocana I, et al. Activity of adenosine deaminase in cerebrospinal fluid for the diagnosis and follow-up of tuberculosis meningitis in adults. J Infect Dis. 1987;155:603–7.

133. Rieder HL, Cauthen GM, Bloch AB, et al. Tuberculosis and acquired immunodeficiency syndrome – Florida. Arch Intern Med. 1989;149:1268–73.

134. Rieder HL, Cauthen GM, Kelly GD, et al. Tuberculosis in the United States. JAMA. 1989;262:385–9.

135. Rosenblum ML, Levy RM, Bredensen DE, et al. Primary central nervous system lymphomas in patients with AIS. Ann Neurol. 1988;23:S13–6.

136. Rowley AH, Whitley RJ, Lakemar FD, et al. Rapid detection of herpes simplex virus DNA in cerebrospinal fluid of patients with herpes simplex encephalitis. Lancet. 1990;335:440–1.

137. Ruzi A, Post MJD, Bundschu CC. Denate nuclei involvement in AIDS patient s with CNS crytococosis: imaging finding with pathologic correlation. J Comput Assist Tomogr. 1997;21(2):175–82.

138. Safai B, Diaz B, Schwartz J, et al. Malignant neoplasms associated with human immunodeficiency virus infection. CA Cancer J Clin. 1992;42:74–96.

139. Saigal G, Post MJ, Lolayekar S, et al. Unusual presentation of central nervous system cryptococcal infection in an immuno competent patient. AJNR Am J Neuroradiol. 2005;26(7):2522–6.

140. Satishchandra PI, Mathew TI, Gadre G, et al. Cryptococcal meningitis: clinical, diagnostic and therapeutic overviews. Neurol India. 2007;55(3):226–32.

141. Segretain G. Penicillium marneffei agent dune mycose due system reticuloendothelial. Mycopathol Mycol Appl. 1959;11(4):327–53.

142. Setinck O, Wondrusch E, Jellinger K, et al. Cytomegalovirus infection of the brain in AIDS: a clinicopathological study. Acta Neuropathol. 1995;90:511–5.

143. Shi LM, Xiao W. Epidemic status and tend of AIDS all over the world. Sci Travel Med. 2008;14(4):1241.

144. Shi DP, Yan QD, Chen SH, et al. Analysis of imaging appearances of brain lesions in AIDS patients. Pract Radiol. 2006;22(2):143–6.

145. Snider WD, Simpson DM, Nielsen S, et al. Neurologic complications of acquired immunodeficiency syndrome. Analysis of 50 cases. Ann Neurol. 1983;14:403–18.

146. Soo MS, Tien RD, Gay L, et al. MR findings in nine patiens. AJR Am J Roentgenol. 1993;160:1089.

147. Subramanian S, Mathai D. Clinical manifestations and management of cryptococcal infection. J Postgrad Med. 2005;51:S21–6.

148. Sunderam G, Mcdonald RJ, Maniatis T, et al. Tuberculosis as a manifestation of the acquired immunodeficiency syndrome (AIDS). JAMA. 1986;256:326–66.

149. Sze GK. Infection and inflammation. In: Stark DD, Bradley WG, editors. Magnetic resonance imaging. 3rd ed. St. Louis: Mosby; 1999. p. 1363–78.

150. Taratuto AL, Venturiello SM. Trichinosis. Brain Pathol. 1997;7:663–72.

151. The National Institutes of Health (NIH) the Centers for Disease Control and Prevention (CDC), and the HIV Medicine Association of the Infectious Diseases Society of America (HIVMA/IDSA). Guidelines for prevention and treatment of opportunistic infections in HIV-Infected adults and adolescents [EB/OL]. MMWR. 2009. Available from URL: http://aidsinfonih.gov/contentfiles/Adult_OI.pdf. Accessed 15 Apr 2009.

152. Tien RD, Chu PK, Hesselink JR, et al. Intracranial cryptococcosis in immunocompromised patients: CT and MR findings in 29 cases. AJNR Am J Neuroradiol. 1991;12:283–9.

153. Tien RD, Gean-Marton AD, Mark AS. Neurosyphilis in HIV carriers: MR findings in six patients. AJR Am J Roentgenol. 1992;158:1325–8.

154. Tung PP, Tchertkoff V, Win H. Fine needle aspiration biopsy of progressive multifocal leukoencephalopathy in a patient with AIDS. A case report. Acta Cytol. 1997;41:1815–8.

155. Vietzke WM, Gelderman AH, Grimley PM, et al. Toxoplasmosis complicating malignancy. Experience at the National Cancer Institute. Cancer. 1968;21:816–27.

156. Villringer K, Jager H, Dichgans M, et al. Differential diagnosis of CNS lesions in AIDS patients by FDG-PET. J Comput Assist Tomogr. 1995;19:532–6.

157. Vyslouzil L, Seidl K, Svarcova J, et al. Finding of Corynebacterium equi Magnusson 1923 in connection with focal mortality in the Eastern Bohemia. Vet Med. 1984;29(9):563–8.

158. Wang WZ. Clinical treatment and nursing of AIDS. Beijing: Peking University Press; 2003. p. 34–5.

159. Wang L, Shi DP, Li HJ. Magnetic resonance spectroscopy in the diagnosis of cognitive impairment in AIDS patients. Chin Med J (Engl). 2011;124(9):1342–5.

160. Weisberg LA, Greenberg J, Staeio A. Computed tomographic findings in acute viral encephalitis in adults with emphasis on herpes simplex encephalitis. Comput Med Imaging Graph. 1988;6:385.

161. Whiteman MLH. Neuroimaging of central nervous system tuberculosis in HIV-infected patients. Neuroimaging Clin N Am. 1997;7:199–214.

162. Wu YJ, Wu J. Medical imaging diagnosis of cerebrovascular disease. Mod J Neurol Neurosurg. 2003;3(3):187–91.

163. Yamada K, Zoarski GH, Rothman MI, et al. An intracranial aspergilloma with low signal on T2-weighted images corresponding to iron accumulation. Neuroradiology. 2001;43(7):559–61.

164. Zhang ZL, Wang H, Yin YH, et al. Value of CT and MRI features in evaluating patient s with Binswanger disease. Chin J Clin Rehabil. 2004;8(31):6950–1.

165. Zimmerman RA. Central nervous system lymphoma. Radiol Clin North Am. 1990;28:697–721.

166. Zimmerman RD, Russell EJ, Leeds NE, et al. CT in the diagnosis of herpes simplex encephalitis. AJR Am J Roentgenol. 1980;134:61.

Contents

14.1   Introduction of HIV/AIDS Related Myelopathy and Peripheral Neuropathy

Up to now, reports about HIV/AIDS related myelopathy remain rare in China. McArthur collected 186 cases of HIV/AIDS complicated by brain and peripheral nerve lesions in the year of 1987 [11]. Only 13 cases had HIV/AIDS related myelopathy, accounting for 7 %. Levy et al. [8] reported the occurrence of HIV/AIDS related myelopathy is 2–22 % based on literature analysis. In another group of 150 patients with AIDS, 42 had HIV/AIDS related myelopathy, in which 24 % with spinal degeneration, 38 % with viral infection, 5 % with toxoplasmosis, 2 % with myelitis and the other 31 % with no pathological diagnosis [2]. Surprisingly, myelopathy is commonly found by autopsy. Peter and his fellow researchers [14] found 50 % of the total 178 patients with AIDS have myelopathy, with 29 % spinal degeneration, 5 % HIV myelitis, 8 % viral infection, 7 % other infections and 2 % lymphoma. Budka [3] retrospectively reviewed autopsies of 475 death cases from AIDS in 1997 and found that 22.5 % had spinal degeneration, 6 % myelitis, 58 % viral infection and 4.1 % fungal, bacterial and protozoal infections as well as 2.3 % lymphoma. Since the year of 1997, knowledge about the clinical treatment for HIV/AIDS complicated by myelopathy has been greatly improved.

HIV/AIDS related myelopathy had been rarely reported probably due to the difficulty in its differential diagnosis from encephalopathy based on the clinical manifestations and the difficulty in its diagnosis resulted from its complex lesions.

H. Li (ed.), *Radiology of HIV/AIDS*,
DOI 10.1007/978-94-007-7823-8_14, © Springer Science+Business Media Dordrecht and People's Medical Publishing House 2014

HIV infected patients commonly have complicated peripheral neuropathy, which is clinically manifested as neuropathic pain. Its incidence rate is much higher than myelopathy and the diagnosis rarely depends on the diagnostic imaging. In cases complicated by central nervous disorders, the clinical manifestations are complex. The diagnosis of cerebral and spinal lesions can be greatly facilitated by the diagnostic imaging.

In the year of 1985, Petito et al. [15] confirmed by pathological examinations that HIV/AIDS related spinal lesions are commonly accompanied by spinal degeneration, peripheral neuropathy and dementia and about 20 % have ataxia and sphincter impairments. Nevertheless, there still have no explicit diagnostic criteria. Due to the high degree of immunodeficiency in patients with AIDS, spinal lesions are commonly secondary rather than primary. Abnormal findings of myelopathy by the diagnostic imaging are usually demonstrated in the advanced stage of AIDS. The commonly seen HIV/AIDS complicated by myelopathy include viral myelitis, spinal bacterial infection and myeloma.

14.1.1 HIV/AIDS Related Spinal Toxoplasma Infection

Patients with AIDS are highly susceptible to toxoplasma infection, especially recurrence of latent infection. In such cases with acquired toxoplasmosis, lymphadenopathy may be less evident but acute fetal infections with extensive dissemination may occur. The clinical manifestations include high fever, pneumonia, skin rash, hepatosplenomegaly and myocarditis. Sometimes, spinal toxoplasmosis occurs as a complication of HIV/AIDS.

14.1.2 HIV/AIDS Related Viral Myelitis

Patients with AIDS can develop myelitic lesions induced by multiple viruses, such as cytomegalovirus (CMV), varicella zoster virus (VZV) and herpes simplex virus (HSV). It is commonly believed that the lesion is resulted from demyelination secondary to infection and is related to the autoimmunity. The foci can be found at any part of spinal white matter, with characteristic demonstrations of concurrent lesions around the veins and under the soft pia mater in the diseased white matter area. The lesion may involve the gray matter, with a diffusive distribution.

Viral myelitis has an acute onset, with initial clinical manifestations of fever, headache, nausea and vomiting 1–2 weeks prior to the onset. The following manifestations are anxiety, deliration, lethargy, stiffness and coma.

The imaging demonstrations are not characteristic, making it difficult to be differentiated from acute multiple sclerosis. CT scanning demonstrates diffusive low-density area in the spinal white matter. MR imaging demonstrates swollen spinal cord, with equal or low signal of T1WI and high signal of T2WI. The focus is prone to be complicated by hemorrhage and swollen and enlarged spinal cords show no enhancement by enhanced imaging. In the chronic stage, the spinal cord may be shrunk and thin, with dilated central duct. However, the manifestations are not specific, making it difficult to be differentiated from lymphoma.

14.1.3 HIV/AIDS Related Spinal Bacterial Infection

HIV/AIDS complicated by spinal tuberculosis [4] and syphilis [12] have been reported. Tuberculosis mycobacterium can cause meningoradiculitis or intramedullary tuberculoma. Syphilis may cause syphiloma within the spinal canal. In patients with frequent intravenous drug abusers, bacteremia commonly occurs, with possible occurrence of epidural abscess that may extend to paravertebral. The most common pathogen of epidural abscess is staphylococcus; tuberculosis mycobacterium, Nocardia and Aspergillus [13] are also reported to cause high fever with progression to paralysis within 24–72 h. The lesion may be sub-acute, with nerve symptoms in 1 week or several months. Intramedullary infection is resulted from venous occlusion by bacteria colonies, leading to spinal venous occlusion. CT and MRI scanning can definitively demonstrate the location and range of the abscesses. Plain CT scanning demonstrates local spinal thickening, irregular morphology, and clearly defined boundary of intraspinal foci. The enhanced scanning shows ring shaped enhancement of the capsule. MRI demonstrates low signal of T1WI and T2WI of the capsule, low signal of T1WI and high signal of T2WI of the abscess fluid. The enhanced MR imaging demonstrates ring shaped enhancement of abscess wall by T1WI. Both CT and MRI demonstrate flaky or nodular enhancement before the formation of large abscess cavity at the inflammation phase.

14.1.4 HIV/AIDS Related Myeloma

Due to dependence on the immune response, patients with AIDS rarely have myeloma. The rarely found reports also include cases of spinal lymphoma and plasmocytoma. Lytic enzyme in the extraspinal Kaposi's tumor (KS) can also impair the spinal cord. In HIV/AIDS related neoplasms, the accompanying spinal metastasis tumor may occur.

14.1.5 Other HIV/AIDS Related Diseases

HIV/AIDS related multiple sclerosis is related to HIV-induced immunodeficiency, with acute or sub-acute onset. Its initial symptoms include bilateral or unilateral visual impairment. Spinal cord lesions commonly occur in the dorsal horn, with clinical manifestations of limbs pain, paresthesia, weakness and paralysis of limbs or hemiplegia. Some patients may develop sensory disturbance, specifically sensing the plane as incomplete. Plain CT scanning demonstrations are negative; uneven ring shaped enhancement of the spinal cord in the acute phase can be found by enhanced scanning, with low sensitivity. Sagittal MR imaging demonstrates clearly the range of the lesions by T1WI and T2WI. In the acute phase, T1WI only demonstrates thickened spinal cord, with normal intraspinal signal; T2WI demonstrates intraspinal singular or multiple high signal foci, with space occupying effects of different degrees. By enhanced imaging, some foci are in ring shaped enhancement. Increased dosage of the contrast reagent can increase the detection rate of the foci.

Diagnostic examinations for HIV/AIDS related myelopathy include: For patients with spastic paralysis or paraplegia of the lower extremities, CSF test should be firstly performed to find the common pathogenic microorganisms and PCR can be performed to detect myelitis related viruses. For patients with large epidural abscess, lumbar puncture is of tremendous risk. CT scanning can effectively detect epidural lesions, but with poor demonstration of intraspinal lesions. MR imaging is ideal for clinical diagnosis of HIV/AIDS related myelopathy to distinguish epidural and subdural structures, demonstrate spinal degeneration, extensive necrosis and hemorrhage. When MR imaging is not available or feasible, enhanced CT scanning can facilitate the preliminary diagnosis.

14.2 HIV/AIDS Related Spinal Toxoplasma Infection

14.2.1 Pathogen and Pathogenesis

Toxoplasma invades the human body via the digestive tract. Firstly, sporozoites or trophozoites invade intestinal mucosal cells and reproduce there to cause the rupture of the intestinal mucosal cells. The released trophozoites are disseminated along with blood or lymph flow throughout the body to cause parasitemia. The further involvement of the spinal tissues renders toxoplasma rapidly divide and proliferate in tissue cells to cause damages to the host cells and invasion of their adjacent cells. The repeated pathogenic processes cause necrosis of local tissue cells to form necrotic foci and to induce acute inflammatory responses predominantly with monocytes infiltration.

14.2.2 Pathophysiological Basis

By autopsy, the spinal cord is found to have tissue liquification and necrosis, with few inflammatory cells infiltration. Within the necrotic foci, there are cystic toxoplasma trophozoites, as granules of different sizes.

14.2.3 Clinical Symptoms and Signs

Typical spinal toxoplasmosis has a sub-acute onset, with clinical manifestations of headache, hemiplegia, seizure, visual disturbance, unconsciousness and even coma. The symptoms of fever and meningeal irritation are rarely found.

14.2.4 Examinations and the Selection of Examinations

14.2.4.1 Examinations for Pathogens
Cerebrospinal fluid, sputum, pleural effusion, ascites and marrow are collected for smears. Alternatively, lymphnode-imprintslide and tissue sections may also be prepared. Subsequently routine staining or immunocytochemistry can be performed to detect toxoplasm trophozoites or cysts. Moreover, the toxoplasm can be isolated by inoculating the above specimens in mice or by tissue culture. In recent years, nucleic acid hybridization in situ or PCR has been used to examine toxoplasma DNA, which might facilitate diagnosis of toxoplasma infection. Especially, PCR examination of toxoplasma DNA in cerebrospinal fluid and amniotic fluid is of great significance for diagnosis of spinal toxoplasmosis and congenital spinal toxoplasmosis.

14.2.4.2 Immunological Assays
A widely used technology in recent years is to examine toxoplasma circulating antigen (CAg) in the serum or body fluid with specific antibody to toxoplasma. Toxoplasma CAg positive is an indicator of pathogen, facilitating the diagnosis of acute toxoplasma infection.

14.2.4.3 CSF Test
Cerebrospinal fluid (CSF) pressure is commonly normal, with yellowish appearance, positive globulin test and a slight increase in cell count, which is commonly $(100–300) \times 10^6$/L and monocytes. The glucose level remains normal or decreased, with increased level of protein and normal level of chloride.

14.2.4.4 Diagnostic Imaging

MR imaging can clearly define the size, shape, location of the foci as well as their relationship with the adjacent tissues, which is of great importance to the diagnosis of cerebral toxoplasmosis and its outcomes.

14.2.5 Imaging Demonstrations

14.2.5.1 CT Scanning

The brain and spinal cord commonly have multiple foci. The plain CT scanning demonstrates thickened spinal cord, foci in equal or low signal, foci complicated by calcification in high signal, surrounding edema in strip liked low density foci, and ring liked and target shaped enhancement of foci by enhanced scanning.

14.2.5.2 MR Imaging

Plain MR imaging demonstrates thickened and swollen spinal cord, foci in short T1 and T2 signals, surrounding edema in long strip liked high T1 and T2 signals. By enhanced imaging, the foci are in ring shaped or target liked enhancement, highly indicative of spinal cord infection.

Case Study 1

A patient aged 36 years was confirmatively diagnosed as having AIDS by CDC, with positive toxoplasma IgG and a CD4 T cell count of 45/μl.

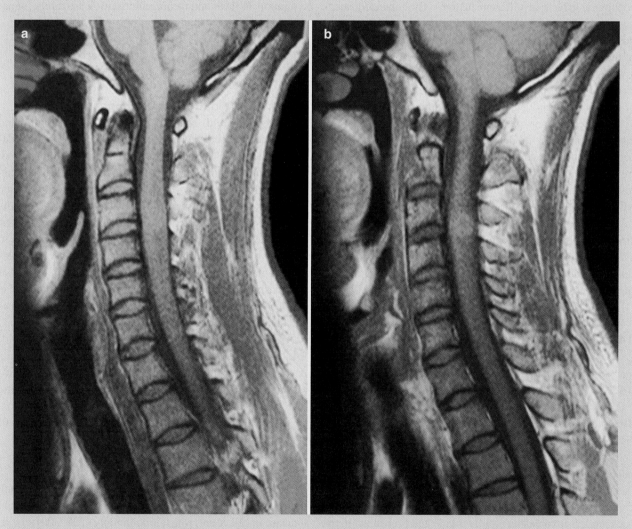

Fig. 14.1 (a–j) HIV/AIDS related spinal toxoplasma infection. (a–g) Pre-treatment. (h, j) Post-treatment. (a, b) Sagittal T1WI demonstrates round liked and slightly short T1 signal at C3–C4 level, equal T1 signal within it, swollen and thickened cervical spinal cord in the focal site. (c, d) Sagittal T2WI demonstrates long T2 signal of the focal margin with central even and short T2 signals, surrounded by spindle shaped edema. (e, f) Coronal and sagittal enhanced T1WI demonstrate obvious ring shaped enhancement of the foci. (g) Coronal enhanced T1WI demonstrates evident homogeneous enhancement of the foci. (h) Sagittal T1WI demonstrates shrunk foci. (i) Sagittal T2WI demonstrates ring shaped high signal of the foci with unobvious peripheral edema. (j) Saggital enhanced T1WI demonstrates shrunk foci with ring shaped enhancement

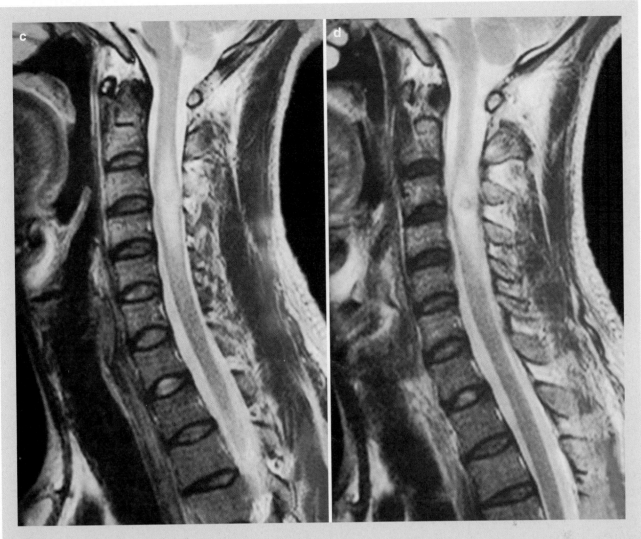

Fig. 14.1 (continued)

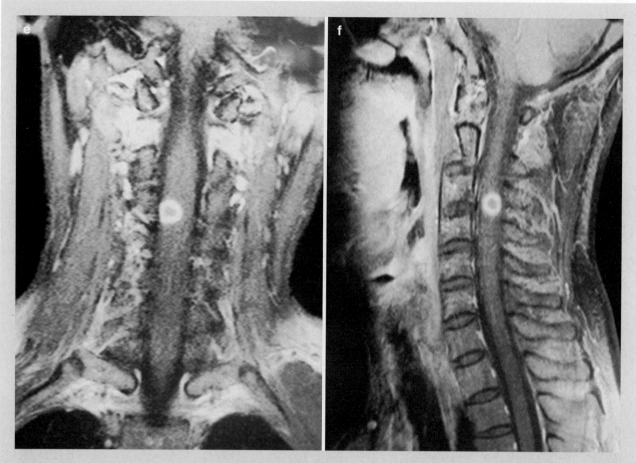

Fig. 14.1   (continued)

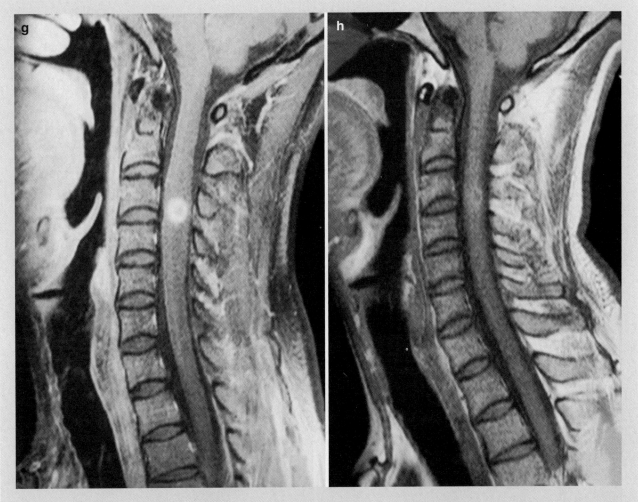

Fig. 14.1 (continued)

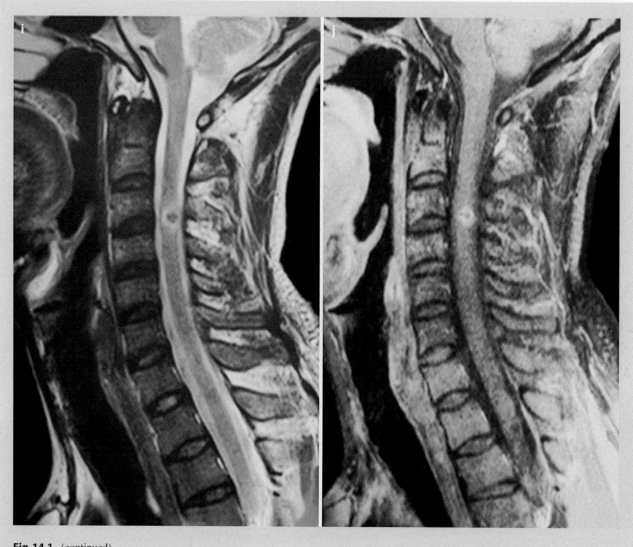

Fig. 14.1 (continued)

Case Study 2

A male patient aged 51 years was confirmatively diagnosed as having AIDS by CDC. His CD4 T cell count was 45/µl.

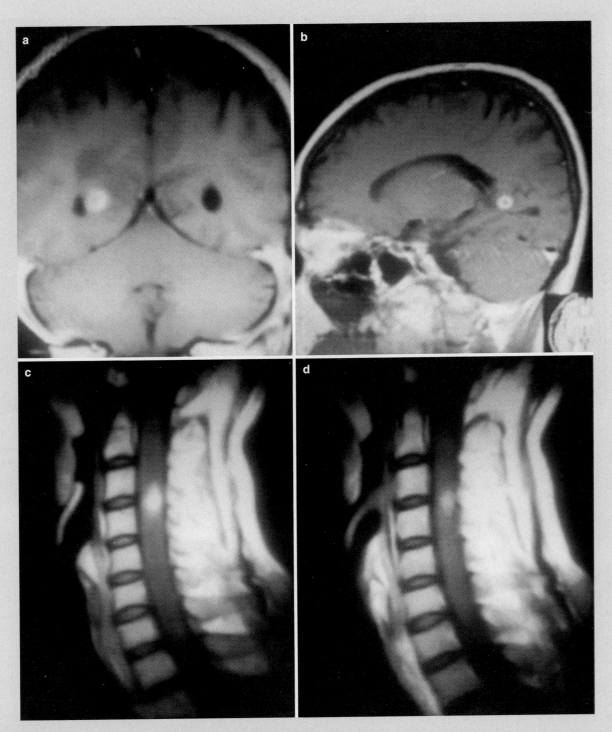

Fig. 14.2 (a–d) HIV/AIDS related cerebral and spinal toxoplasma infection. (a) Coronal enhanced T1WI demonstrates ring shaped enhancement of the foci adjacent to the right ventricle, with slightly compressed and deformed right ventricle. (b) Sagittal enhanced T1WI demonstrates ring shaped enhancement of the foci posterior to the body of lateral ventricle. (c, d) Sagittal enhanced T1WI demonstrates irregular foci at C3–C4 level, with homogeneous enhancement and blurry borderline

Case Study 3

The male patient aged 41 years was confirmatively diagnosed as having AIDS by CDC. His CT4 T count was 55/μl.

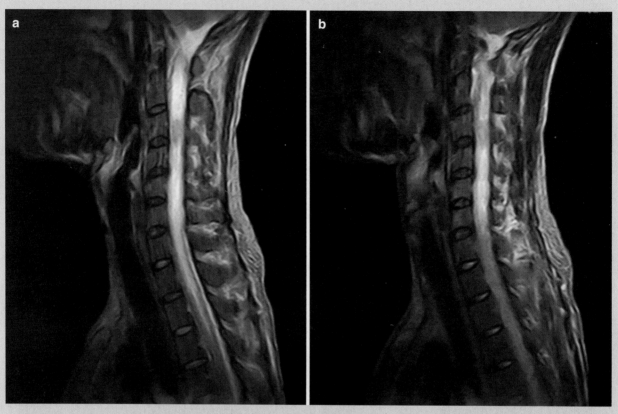

Fig. 14.3 (a–g) HIV/AIDS related spinal toxoplasma infection. (**a, b**) Sagittal T2WI demonstrates slightly swollen and enlarged cervical spinal cord, irregular short T2 signal of the foci at C3 level and peripheral long strips of edema with long T2 signal. (**c**) Sagittal enhanced T1WI demonstrates annular ring shaped enhancement of the spinal foci. (**d**) Coronal enhanced T1WI demonstrates inhomogeneous enhancement of the focuses. (**e, f**) Sagittal T2WI demonstrates no foci after treatment. (**g**) Coronal T1WI demonstrates no detectable foci

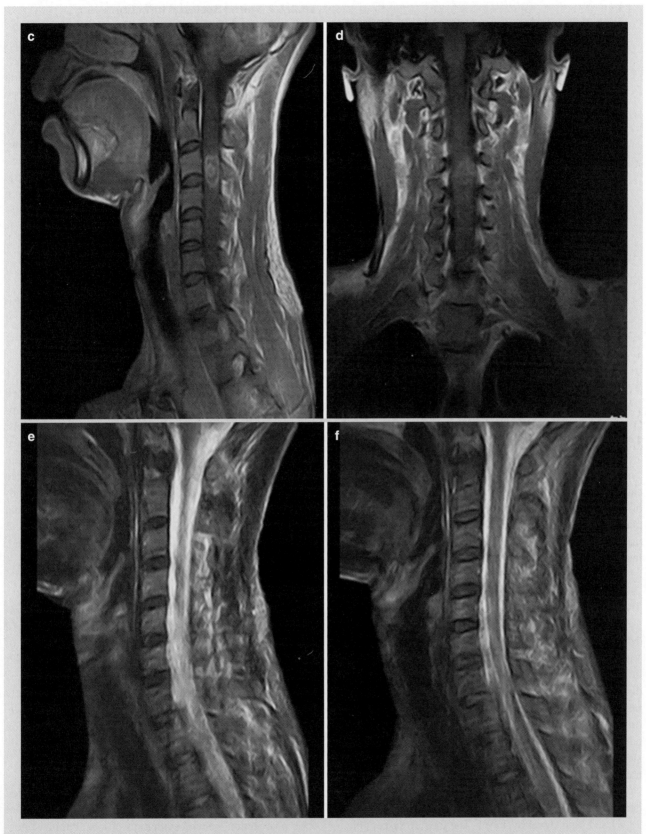

Fig. 14.3 (continued)

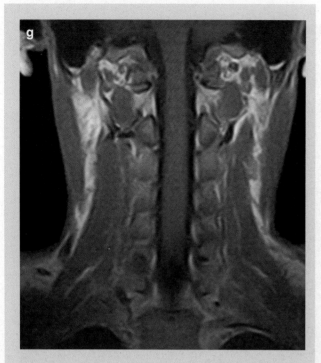

Fig. 14.3 (continued)

14.2.6 Criteria for the Diagnosis

The definitive diagnosis is based on the corresponding clinical manifestations. CSF test demonstrates a slight increase of white cells, increased proteins and positive serum toxoplasma antibodies IgA and IgG. The diagnosis can also be made based on biopsy of cerebrospinal fluid and histopathological examination.

14.2.7 Differential Diagnosis

14.2.7.1 Viral Myelitis

Viral myelitis has typical manifestations of concurrence of lesions around the veins and under the soft pia mater in the diseased white matter, with possible involvement of the gray matter, in a diffusive distribution. The disease has an acute onset, with initial clinical symptoms of fever, headache and nausea and the following symptoms of irritation, delirium, sleepiness and coma. The imaging demonstrations are not characteristic. CT scanning demonstrates diffusive low density areas in the white matter of the spinal cord. MR imaging demonstrates swollen spinal cord, equal or low signal by T1WI and high signal by T2WI. The foci are susceptible to bleeding. Enhanced scanning demonstrates no enhancement of the foci. The differential diagnosis depends on the test for serum anti-toxoplasma antibody, CSF biopsy and histopathological examination.

14.2.7.2 Spinal Bacterial Infection

Plain CT scanning demonstrates locally thickened spinal cord with irregular morphology, clearly defined border of intraspinal foci, and ring shaped enhancement of envelope membrane by enhanced scanning. Plain MR imaging demonstrates long T1 and short T2 signals of the envelope membrane, long T1 and T2 signals of the inner abscess fluids; and ring shaped enhancement of the abscess wall by enhanced imaging. CT and MRI demonstrate flaky or nodular enhancement before the formation of larger abscess cavity in the inflammation phase. By the diagnostic imaging, it is difficult to differentiate spinal bacterial infection from spinal toxoplasma infection. Laboratory tests and histopathological examinations should be performed for their differential diagnosis.

14.3 HIV/AIDS Related Viral Myelitis

14.3.1 HIV/AIDS Related Herpes Simplex Virus Myelitis

14.3.1.1 Pathogen and Pathogenesis

Herpes simplex virus (HSV) consists of double-stranded DNA genome and is transmitted via intimate or sexual contacts to patients and healthy virus carriers or via droplets. Virus in latency can be activated in immunocompromised AIDS patients to cause more severe symptoms and organ damages. HSV latent in the neural ganglia is activated when cellular immunodeficiency occurs, followed by its descending course along the sensory nerve fiber axon to its terminal to infect the neighboring skin or mucosa epithelium and to proliferate there. Therefore, recurrent local herpes is caused. This is known as the neuron triggering theory.

14.3.1.2 Pathophysiological Basis

The pathological changes include inflammation and degeneration, with manifestations of edema and degeneration of soft pia mater and spinal cord, infiltration and effusion of monocytes and lymphocytes, swollen neural cells and detectable intranuclear inclusions in the infected cells. The infected cells commonly fuse into multinuclear giant cells. In severely ill patients, myelomalacia, spinal necrosis and hemorrhage, nerve cells atrophy in the chronic phase, loss of myelin, axon degeneration and gliocyte hyperplasia may occur.

14.3.1.3 Clinical Symptoms and Signs

For patients of the initial occurrence, due to no produced antibody in the acute phase, they usually show symptoms of fever or irritation, general symptoms of local lymphadenectasis, muscular pain, and disseminative infections. The spinal cord is often invaded, including transverse injury, with initial symptoms of lower extremities weakness, sensory disturbance and urine retention. Brown-Sequard syndrome has manifestations of unilateral extremities weakness, diminished deep sensation and involved contralateral algesia and thermesthesia.

14.3.1.4 Examinations and Their Selection
Laboratory Test

HSV-DNA-PCR antibody in the CSF and serum specific IgM is one of the laboratory tests for accurate and rapid diagnosis.

Diagnostic Imaging

CT scanning has a limited diagnostic value. MRI can clearly define the size, shape, location of the foci as well as their relationship with the surrounding tissues, facilitating the clinical diagnosis.

14.3.1.5 Imaging Demonstrations
CT Demonstrations

CT scanning usually is applied together with myelography, with demonstrations of slightly thickened spinal cord with uneven density.

MRI Demonstrations

MRI provides evidence for understanding of HSV myelitis, whose demonstrations include one or several thickened spinal segments with irregular long T1 and T2 signals, bleeding foci, swollen and thickened spinal cord and no enhancement by enhanced imaging. In the chronic phase, the demonstrations are shrunk and thinner spinal cord, accompanying enlargement of the central canal, but no MRI demonstrations characteristic of HSV myelitis.

Case Study

A male patient aged 38 years was confirmatively diagnosed as having AIDS by CDC. His CD4 T cell count was 55/μl.

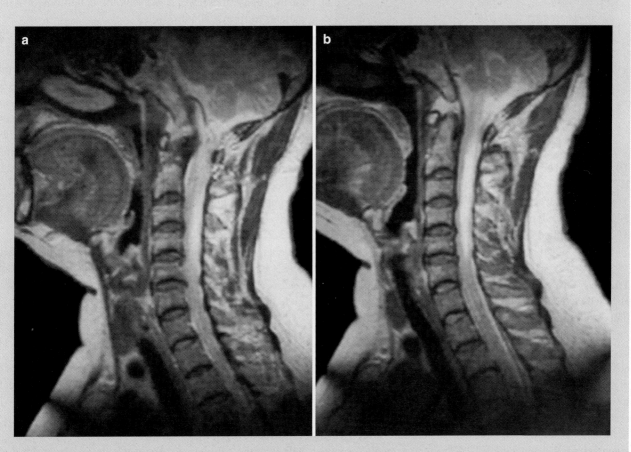

Fig. 14.4 (**a–c**) HIV/AIDS related herpes simplex virus myelitis. (**a–c**) Sagittal T1WI demonstrates strip liked short T1 signals at C2–C5 level and slightly swollen and enlarged cervical spinal cord at the lesion

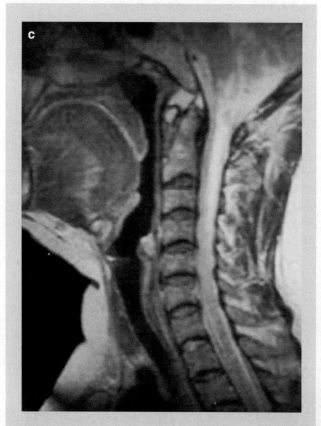

Fig. 14.4 (continued)

14.3.1.6 Criteria for Diagnosis
1. Typical clinical manifestations of limbs dysfunction as well as urinary and fecal incontinence.
2. Increased CSF proteins
3. Swollen spinal cord by MR imaging, with equal T1 and long T2 signals.

14.3.1.7 Differential Diagnosis
HIV/AIDS related multiple scleroses are related with HIV-induced immunodeficiency, with an acute or sub-acute onset. Its initial symptoms include bilateral or unilateral visual disturbance. Plain CT scanning demonstrations are commonly negative, but demonstrations of uneven ring shaped enhancement of spinal cord in the acute phase by enhanced scanning, with a low sensitivity. Sagittal MRI of T1WI and T2WI clearly demonstrate the range of the lesions. By T1WI, the demonstration of the acute phase includes thickened spinal cord, with normal signal within the spinal cord. T2WI suggests singular or multiple high signal foci, with accompanying space occupying effects of various degrees. By enhanced imaging, some foci are demonstrated in ring shaped enhancement. Appropriate increase of the contrast reagent dosage can improve the detection rate of the foci. Acute multiple sclerosis has similar manifestations to the disease and their differential diagnosis should incorporate clinical and other examinations.

14.3.2 HIV/AIDS Related Cytomegalovirus Myelitis

14.3.2.1 Pathogen and Pathogenesis
Cytomegalovirus (CMV) infection is the most common viral opportunistic infection in AIDS patients, with an occurrence of 40 % in terminal patients with AIDS. By autopsy, the occurrence of HIV/AIDS related cytomegalovirus infection is up to 62 %. CMV can remain latent within the human body over a long period, reactivated and triggering onset of CMV infection due to compromised or deficient immunity. The virus can spread to impair other organs via viremia or carried by lymphocytes and monocytes. As a typically active infection, over 90 % patients are CMV antibody positive and over 50 % develop viremia. CMV is suppressive to cellular immunity; therefore, it worsens the conditions of AIDS patients to form a vicious cycle.

14.3.2.2 Pathophysiological Basis
The pathophysiological findings include hypermyelohemia, edema and demyelination. The lesions are initially in the perivascular area, followed by fusion into flakes with adjacent lesions to cause myelomalacia or even necrosis-induced cavities. Blood vessels in the lesion area enlarge, with infiltration of peripheral granular cells, inflammatory cells and gliocytes. The vascular endothelium is swollen to occlude some vessels. In the advanced stage, the spinal cord obviously shrinks, with accompanying gliosis and scars following myelomalcia.

14.3.2.3 Clinical Symptoms and Signs
Patients with CMV infection have symptoms of fever, headache, general upset, skin rash and involvement of some organs. The impaired spinal cord commonly causes incomplete flaccid paralysis or paraplegia.

14.3.2.4 Examinations and Their Selection
Laboratory Tests
CSF cytological changes should be observed and culture of CSF after its isolation should be performed. And PCR technology facilitates the diagnosis.

Diagnostic Imaging
MR imaging can define the size, shape and location of the foci as well as their relationship with the surrounding tissues. But the MRI demonstrations are not characteristic of CMV infection. The diagnosis should based on incorporation of the case history.

14.3.2.5 Imaging Demonstrations
CT Scanning Demonstrations

Lesions in the cervical and lumbar spinal cord is common, non-AIDS patients with cervical thoracic is common. CT scan shows mildly thickened spinal cord and uneven density spinal cord.

MR Imaging Demonstrations

MRI demonstrations are not specific, commonly thickened singular or multiple segments of the spinal cord, irregular long T1 and T2 signals in the spinal cord. Enhanced imaging commonly demonstrates no enhancement of the foci.

Case Study

A male patient aged 50 years was confirmatively diagnosed as having AIDS by CDC. The onset of the illness is acute and sudden. Viral retinitis occurred suddenly 2 weeks ago, causing rapidly decreased vision that progresses into blindness, with companying lower extremities numbness and weakness, unsmooth urine and dry stool. Three days ago, he suddenly developed paralysis, with urinary and fecal incontinence. His CD4 T cell count was 50/µl.

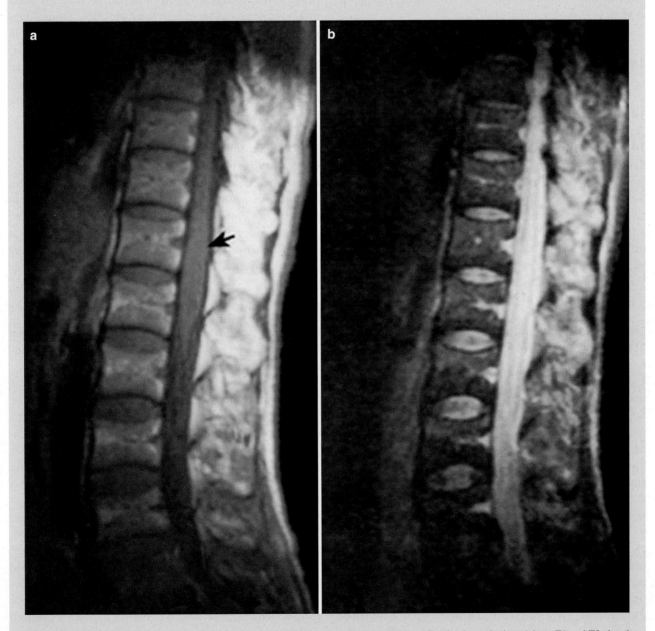

Fig. 14.5 (**a, b**) HIV/AIDS related CMV myelitis. (**a, b**) MR imaging demonstrations swollen lumbar spinal cord, long T1 and T2 signal in the spinal cord (*arrow*)

14.3.2.6 Criteria for Diagnosis

1. Clinical manifestations include lower extremities numbness and weakness, sudden attack of paralysis as well as urinary and fecal incontinence.
2. After CSF cytological test, isolation and culture of CSF and PCR, only half of the clinically typical cases have positive findings in cell culture.

14.3.2.7 Differential Diagnosis

HIV/AIDS related CMV myelitis should be differentiated from neoplasms of the spinal cord. The neoplasms commonly have slow progressions, with accompanying hemorrhage and necrosis of the neoplasms in uneven enhancement. CMV myelitis has sudden and acute onset, with no enhancement or even enhancement of the foci.

14.4   HIV/AIDS Related Spinal Bacterial Infection

14.4.1   Staphylococcus Aureus Infection

14.4.1.1 Pathogen and Pathogenesis

Spinal staphylococcus aureus infection is commonly caused by infections secondary to acute epidural or subdural abscess. It may also be caused by direct bacterial infection of the spinal cord. No matter of the primary or secondary infection, primary foci or primary history of infection commonly occur before the symptoms of the spinal cord, including septicemia, abscess of adjacent tissues and pyogenic infection of lungs. They are usually caused by attack of bacteria into the spinal cord and pia matter along with blood flow.

14.4.1.2 Pathophysiological Basis

The pathological changes vary with the routes of bacterial invasion. For those with local invasion by the bacteria, the lesions of spinal cord are confined within several spinal segments. For those with invasion by contaminated blood, multiple or disseminated foci commonly occur, mostly in the thoracic and lumbar area. By anatomy, it may be found to have swollen spinal cord, congestion and edema of the involved blood vessels, purulent secretions in the involved area, obviously thickened meninges, inflammatory effusion and granuloma formation. In addition, congestion and effusion of adjacent and supplying blood vessels occurs with thickened vascular walls to cause vascular occlusion. In the early stage of the inflammation, the spinal cord is congested with edema, followed by purplish gray and soft spinal cord, necrosis in the advanced stage. Its incision indicates scattered small foci of myelomalacia in the spinal tissues. Under a microscope, congestion of meningeal blood vessels can be found, with degeneration or obliteration of spinal neurons, dissolution of neuron axons, degeneration and loss of myelin.

In addition, there is infiltration of disseminated inflammatory cells as well as proliferation of phagocytes and gliocytes. Multiple small abscesses in the spinal cord may integrate themselves into larger abscesses and massive necrosis of neural tissues. Purulent myelitis secondary to epidural or subdural abscess mainly demonstrates thickened and adhesion of meninges as well as vascular occlusion. The involved spinal cord is characterized by infiltration of inflammatory cells and ischemic necrosis. Upwards and downwards conductive bundles in the spinal cord can degenerate due to insufficient supply of nutrients by neuron axons.

14.4.1.3 Clinical Symptoms and Signs

Prior to onset of myelitis symptoms, patients usually exhibit toxic symptoms including high fever and chills. Several days later, complete or incomplete paraplegia may occur, with dysfunction urination and defecation. The location of lesions is commonly thoracic segment of the spinal cord, followed by the lumbar segment. The location of the lesions usually has the sensations of pain and girdling, with general muscular soreness.

14.4.1.4 Examinations and Their Selection
Laboratory Tests

Early blood culture is commonly positive. CSF is transparent or yellowish, with increased cells that are mainly neutrophils. It is commonly found to have increased protein, decreased glucose and chlorides and unobstructed vertebral canal. CSF smears or culture can detect the pathogens and the results of drug sensitivity test can provide basis for its treatment.

Diagnostic Imaging

CT scanning and MR imaging can define the size, shape and location of the foci as well as their relationship with the surrounding tissues.

14.4.1.5 Imaging Demonstrations

Imaging demonstrations of staphylococcus aureus myelitis is not characteristic, similar to other non-infective inflammations and demyelination. Plain CT scanning demonstrates locally thickened spine cord with irregular shapes, clearly defined borderline of the focus. For cases with abscess, enhanced CT scanning reveals ring shaped enhancement of the abscess wall. T2WI of MR imaging demonstrates confined or disseminated high signals within the spinal cord, with or with no space occupying effects. Enhanced MR imaging demonstrates diffusive, flaky and ring shaped enhancement. After the formation of abscess, the abscess wall demonstrates long T1 and short T2 signals and its inside abscess demonstrates long T1 and T2 signals. Enhanced T1W1 demonstrates ring shaped enhancement of the abscess wall and compressed thinner spinal cord.

Case Study

A male patient aged 48 years was confirmatively diagnosed as having AIDS by CDC. The illness was progressively severe, with lower extremities weakness as well as urinary and fecal incontinence for over 1 month. The sensory level of T10–T12 decreased, with grade III right muscle strength, grade II left muscle strength and positive muscular reflex. By bacteria culture, staphylococcus aureus infection was indicated.

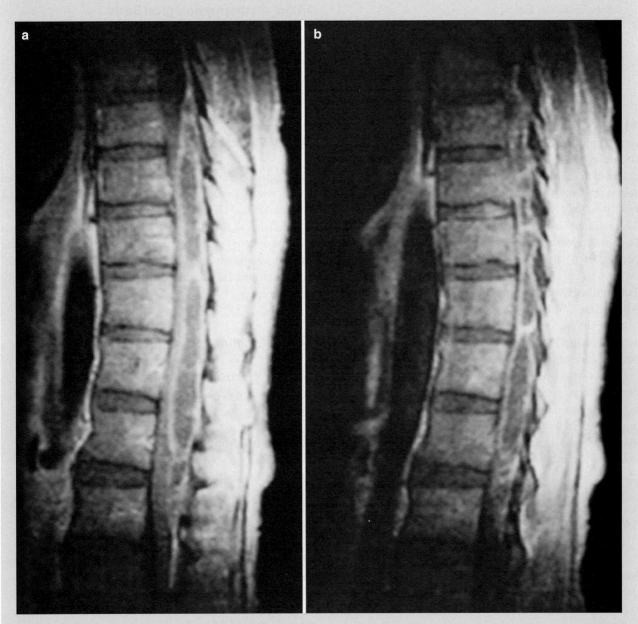

Fig. 14.6 (**a, b**) HIV/AIDS related spinal bacterial infection. (**a, b**) MR imaging demonstrates abnormal strip liked long T1 and T2 signal in the vertebral canal of thoracic and lumbar segments. Enhanced imaging demonstrations of grid liked enhancement of the paraspinal abscess wall, and obviously compressed spinal cord

14.4.1.6 Criteria for the Diagnostic

1. Clinical manifestations include a history of general or local infection, with sudden onsets of paralysis, urination and defecation dysfunction as well as high fever.
2. Increased cell count and protein in CSF, decreased glucose and chloride and unobstructed spinal canal, which can facilitate the diagnosis
3. MR imaging demonstrates strip liked abnormal long T1 and T2 signals within thoracic and lumbar spinal canal; enhanced imaging demonstrates ring shaped or grid shaped enhancement of paravertebral abscess wall and obviously compressed spinal cord.

14.4.1.7 Differential Diagnosis
Acute Epidural Abscess

It develops 3–4 weeks after acute bacterial infection, with companying evident and severe nerve root pain and obvious spinal tenderness. Lumbar puncture suggests Queckenstedt test positive, yellowish CSF and increased proteins. Myelography indicates canal blockage, which should be further differentiated. If necessary, MRI examination can be performed to define the location and size of the abscess.

Tuberculosis Myelitis and Tuberculosis Paravertebral Abscesses

It has a chronic onset, with no accompanying fever or with accompanying low grade fever after noon. For cases with complication of tuberculosis abscess, the illness has an acute onset. However, the spinal cord commonly has kyphosis and obvious local tenderness. Plain chest X-ray demonstrates vertebral bone destruction, narrowed intervertebral space in angular deformity. Lumbar spinal puncture indicates obstructed spinal canal. The CSF test shows decreased glucose and chloride and increased protein. These findings are characteristic for differential diagnosis.

14.5 HIV/AIDS Related Vacuolar Myelopathy

Vacuolar myelopathy (VM) or chronic progressive myelopathy (CPM) is the most common primary infections of the nerve system in patients with AIDS. About 1/3 patients with AIDS suffer from vacuolation of the spinal white matter. By autopsy, 20–30 % cases have such an illness. However, its symptoms show up in cases with vacuolation and evident demyelination.

14.5.1 Pathogen and Pathogenesis

The pathogen and pathogenesis of vacuolar myelopathy (VM) is still unknown. Although findings of HIV by culture

of the spinal cord have been reported [1], it has not been clarified whether HIV is the direct pathogen of VM. It is speculated that abnormal transmethylation induced by HIV or cytokine is the possible cause of VM.

14.5.2 Pathophysiological Basis

VM is pathologically typical of vacuoles in the spinal white matter, with invasion to the lateral and posterior columns, especially the thoracic spinal cord. It is commonly companied with spinal swelling or demyelination.

14.5.3 Clinical Symptoms and Signs

The clinical manifestations include progressive spastic paraplegia with accompanying deep sensation disturbance and sensory ataxia. The majority of such patients are bound to wheelchairs in weeks or months and minorities of such patients undergo painless progression in several years. Some patients also have vacuolar changes in the brain, with clinical manifestations of progressive dementia. Spinal spasticity rarely occurs.

14.5.4 Examinations and Their Selection

14.5.4.1 Electrophysiological Examination
Asymptomatic sub-acute spinal diseases can be detected in the early stage.

14.5.4.2 MR Imaging
MR imaging has no specific demonstrations, but can accurately locate the lesions.

14.5.5 Imaging Demonstrations

MR imaging commonly demonstrates long T1 and T2 signals of the lesions as well as myelatrophy.

14.5.6 Criteria for the Diagnosis

1. Clinical manifestations are progressive spastic paraplegia, wit accompanying deep sensation disturbance and sensory ataxia.
2. The diagnosis should exclude the possibility of compressive myelopathy, sub-acute combined degeneration and secondary infection.
3. MR imaging demonstration is commonly myelatrophy.

14.5.7 Differential Diagnosis

14.5.7.1 Differential Diagnosis from Toxoplasmosis

As an opportunistic infection, toxoplasmosis is commonly found in patients with compromised immunity. But simple toxoplasmosis is rarely seen. Most patients have motion disorder, especially the dismal lower extremities, which progresses into paraplegia. The sensory disturbance is commonly bilateral, with detectable sensory level in physical examinations. The common symptoms also include local pain, urinary disturbance and fever. Moreover, protein in CSF significantly increases with positive findings of serum toxoplasma antibody. Spinal MR imaging demonstrates intraspinal confined foci, which demonstrate enhancement by enhanced imaging. Most patients are sensitive to antibiotics therapies, with improved conditions.

14.5.7.2 Differential Diagnosis from Subacute Combined Myelopathy

Subacute combined myelopathy is commonly found in the thoracic spine. Plain CT scanning and enhanced scanning demonstrate no positive findings. MR imaging is the unique method for its detection. The imaging demonstrations include long strip liked equal T1 and long T2 signals of the posterior and lateral cords of the spine. Generally, there is no enhancement as well as thickened and swollen spinal cord, presenting difficulty in its differential diagnosis. For cases with anemia and decreased level of B12, diagnosis can be established.

14.5.7.3 Differential Diagnosis from Syringomyelia

Syringomyelia is congenital, with other complicated congenital abnormalities, such as spina bifida, spinal fusion and Arnold-Chiari malformation, which make it easy to be differentiated from VM. For cases with syringomyelia secondary to spinal neoplasms, spinal trauma, spinal hemorrhage or arachnoiditis, the case history, clinical manifestations and laboratory tests should be combined for its differential diagnosis from VM.

14.6 HIV/AIDS Related Myelatrophy

14.6.1 Pathogen and Pathogenesis

Ischemia of AIDS patients is a chronic progressive course. Due to angiotropic nature of HIV, its invasion to supplying arteries of spinal cord leads to endothelial granuloma of the supplying arteries and vascular lumen stenosis. Thereby, ischemia of spinal cord is caused to finally develop into myelatrophy.

14.6.2 Pathophysiological Basis

The pathological changes of myelatrophy are thinner spinal cord, dilated central canal of several segments and of the whole spinal cord in rare cases.

14.6.3 Clinical Symptoms and Signs

Clinical manifestation is motor and sensory disturbance of the corresponding spinal levels.

14.6.4 Examinations and Their Selection

Both CT scanning and MR imaging are important ways for the diagnosis of myelatrophy, with MR imaging being more accurate and convenient. Sagittal T1WI can directly demonstrate the range and severity of myelatrophy.

14.6.5 Imaging Demonstrations

MRI examination is the imaging of choice. Sagittal T1WI can directly demonstrate the range and severity of myelatrophy, which is commonly limited to several segments and rarely involves the whole spinal cord. There are intact appearance, possible dilation of central canal, widened subarachnoid space and often normal signals in the spinal cord.

Case Study 1

A male patient aged 34 years was confirmatively diagnosed as having AIDS by CDC. His CD4 T cell count was 10/μl.

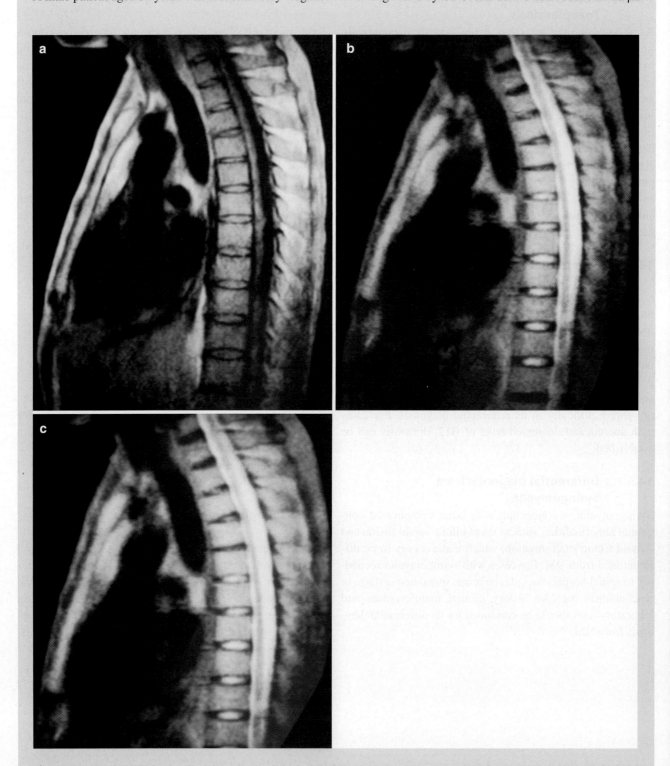

Fig. 14.7 (**a–c**) HIV/AIDS related myelatrophy. (**a–c**) Sagittal T1WI and T2WI demonstrate the thinner spinal cord and widened subarachnoid space

Case Study 2

A male patient aged 30 years was confirmatively diagnosed as having AIDS by CDC. His CD4 T cell count was 35/μl.

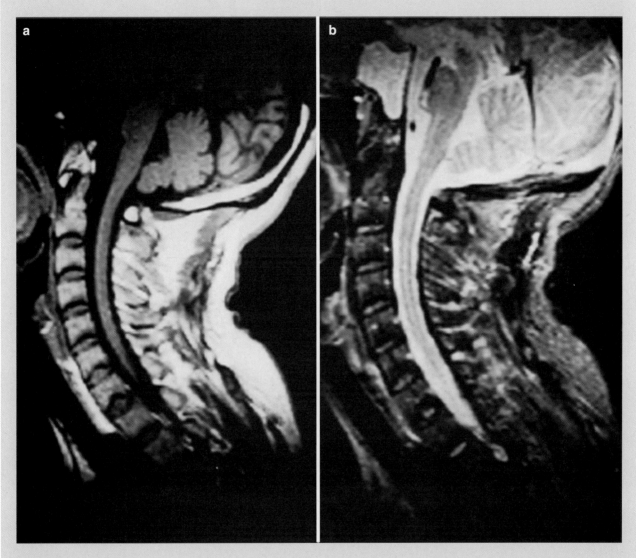

Fig. 14.8 (**a–h**) HIV/AIDS related myelatrophy. (**a–d**) Sagittal T1WI and T2WI demonstrate thinner cervical spinal cord and widened subarachnoid space. (**e, f**) Sagittal T1WI and T2WI demonstrate thinner thoracic spinal cord and widened subarachnoid space. (**g, h**) Sagittal T1WI and T2WI demonstrate the thinner lumbar spinal cord and widened subarachnoid space

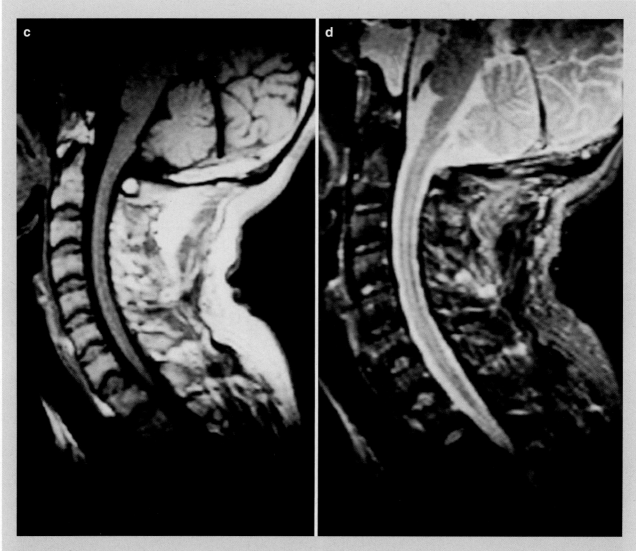

Fig. 14.8 (continued)

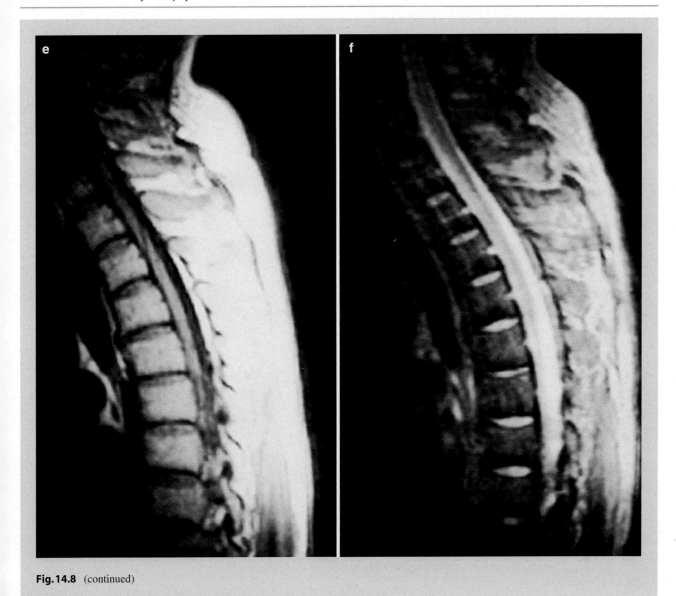

Fig. 14.8 (continued)

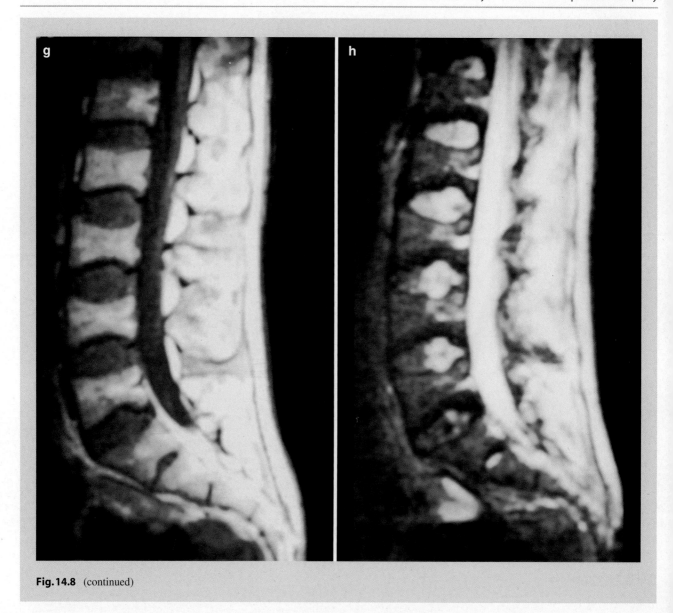

Fig. 14.8 (continued)

14.6.6 Criteria for the Diagnosis

1. It is clinically manifested as motor and sensory disturbance of the corresponding spinal levels.
2. MR imaging suggests myelatrophy.

14.6.7 Differential Diagnosis

HIV/AIDS related myelatrophy should be differentiated
from myelatrophy caused by trauma, vascular malformation
and myelitis. The diagnosis can be clarified in combination
of the case history and imaging demonstrations.

14.7   HIV/AIDS Related Peripheral Neuropathy

14.7.1 HIV/AIDS Related Sensory Neuropathy

HIV/AIDS related sensory neuropathy is the most important HIV/AIDS related neuropathy, characteristic of the
advanced stage of AIDS. About 45 % patients with AIDS
have such an illness, but children with it are rarely found.
Its pathogenesis remains unclear, which might be related
with HIV or CMV infections. Pathological changes are
macrophage infiltration in the peripheral nerves of the
patients.

In the early stage of the infection, the temperature of both lower extremities slightly decreases, with no ankle reflex or decreased ankle reflex. The patients have no symptoms or slight symptoms. With the progression of the illness, tingling or numbness of the feet occurs, with the sensation extending to the knees. Both hands are rarely involved, but with occasionally obvious weakness of the extremities. In some patients, painful distal sensory neuropathy may occur, with its progression into the condition of difficulty walking. Electrophysiology, electromyography and sural nerve biopsy can facilitate its diagnosis.

14.7.2   HIV/AIDS Related Autonomic Neuropathy

A minority of patients may develop autonomic neuropathy in the advanced stage of HIV infection, with clinical manifestations of postural hypotension, diarrhea and sudden attack of arrhythmia. The sub-clinical autonomic neuropathy has an occurrence of 50 % in patients with advanced HIV infection. Autonomic neuropathy is usually accompanied by sensory neuropathy. Electrophysiology, electromyography and sural nerve biopsy can facilitate its diagnosis.

14.7.3   Human Cytomegalovirus Myelopathy (HCMV)

14.7.3.1   Pathogen and Pathogenesis
HCMV usually occurs in patients with CD4 T cell count being less than 0.1×10^9/L. In patients with their CD4 T cell counts being less than 0.05×10^9/L, the occurrence of HCMW is 30–40 %. Once the virus gains their access to the cells, the envelope of the virus adheres to the cell membrane and the viral genome integrates with the host cell nucleus. In cases with immature or compromised immunity, primary HCMV, reactivation of the latent virus or the newly emerging HCMV virus strain can cause massive duplication of the virus. Therefore, damages and diseases are resulted in. Most cases of HCMV are caused by reactivation of latent viruses.

14.7.3.2   Pathophysiological Basis
HCMV is pathologically characterized by arachnoid thickening, minor vessel dilation, a few lymphocytes infiltration, loosen and swollen spinal cord with disseminated small necrotic foci. Within the foci, 1–10 cytomegalic inclusions can be found, with no inflammatory responses in the surrounding tissues of the foci. Nervous system infected by cytomegalic inclusions demonstrates disseminated and nodular infiltration, with involvement of the nerve cells, especially obvious in the medullary olivary nucleus.

14.7.3.3   Clinical Signs and Symptoms
HCMV mainly invades the lower extremities, with accompanying myelopathies. Patients usually complain of ascending numbness of lower extremities, with companying weakness of both lower extremities and backache. Sometimes, sensory loss of sellar region occurs, with its progression into urination dysfunction. With the symptoms develop for days or weeks; the loss of deep tendon reflex occurs, with loss of distal sensation and accompanying weakness of the lower extremities and occasional occurrence of hand lesions.

14.7.3.4   Examinations and Their Selection
Laboratory Tests
CSF test has findings of increased cell count, mainly multinuclear leukocytes. Virus culture is negative, but positive in antibody or DNA assays.

Imaging Examinations
Imaging examinations are used to exclude the space occupying lesions of the lower spinal cord or the nerve root.

14.7.3.5   Imaging Demonstrations
Thoracic and lumbar MR imaging demonstrates swelling and aggregative changes of the cauda equine.

14.7.3.6   Criteria for the Diagnosis
1. CSF tests of CMV culture, antibody staining or DNA assay are positive.
2. Clinical manifestations are ascending numbness of lower extremities with weakness of both legs and urinary dysfunction. The loss of deep tendon reflex of legs occurs, with distal sensation loss and weakness of both legs.
3. MR imaging demonstrates swelling and agglutinative cauda equine.

14.7.3.7   Differential Diagnosis
The condition should be differentiated from varicella zoster virus (VZV) myelitis, which has a sub-acute onset. Patients with VZV myelitis commonly have a case history of VZV infection. By CSF test, there are increased protein, motor/sensory disturbance, sphincter dysfunction and lesions of the skin innervated by corresponding nerve system. Myelitis generally occurs 2–3 weeks after skin rash, with nerve lesions of the thoracic segment. The differential diagnosis should be based on the combination of case history and skin lesions.

Case Study

The female patient aged 31 years was confirmatively diagnosed as having AIDS by CDC. Her CD4 T cell count was 25/μl.

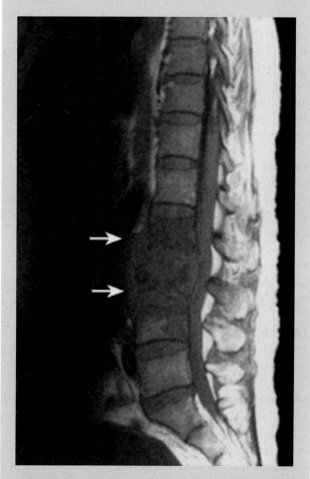

Fig. 14.9 HIV/AIDS related CMV myelitis. Sagittal T2WI demonstrates L2–L4 spinal cord lesions, paravetebral mass shadows with heterogeneous signals and enlarged masses with its extra-epidural part (*arrow*)

14.7.3.8 Compound Mononeuritis

Compound mononeuritis occurs in a minority of AIDS patients in its advanced stage. The illness occurs when CD4 T cell count is no less than 0.25×10^9/L (250/mm³). Compound mononeuritis can also be caused by CMV when CD4 T cell count is below 0.05×10^9/L (50/mm³). For cases with CD4 T cell count above 200/μl, neural biopsy demonstrates axon degeneration and peripheral inflammatory infiltration of blood vessels. For patients in the advanced stage, neural biopsy demonstrates compound demyelination and axon degeneration, with accompanying macrophage infiltration characteristic of CMV infection. The diagnosis of compound mononeuritis usually depends on the clinical manifestations.

Electromyelography suggests multiple local axon neuropathies. By CSF, the findings are non-specific, only with an increase of protein and a slight increase of monocytes. The imaging demonstrations are also non-specific.

14.7.4 Distal Symmetrical Polyneuropathy (DSPN)

DPSN is also known as progressive peripheral neuropathy, characterized by delayed sensation of pain. Such patients have moderate loss of symmetrical distal sensation or numbness, burning sensation and itches. These symptoms initially occur in hands and feet with a stock liked or glove liked distribution. Physical examination demonstrates loss of warm and painful sensation of hands and feet, loss or decreased ankle reflex, weakness and shrinkage of distal muscles. CSF test indicates normal or an increase of proteins. Electromyelography and nerve conduction velocity usually indicate distal sensory and motor evidence of neuropathy characteristic of demyelination and mild nerve conduction deceleration. This disease is predominant of delayed and decreased painful sensation, occasional with mild distal weakness and decreased or loss of ankle reflex. Neural pathological examination demonstrates axon degeneration, occasional segmental demyelination, which is closely related with AIDS.

The diagnosis of HIV/AIDS related DPSN is based on detailed case history in neurology and physical examinations. Laboratory tests can be used to exclude the potential causes of neuropathy, including diabetes, vitamin deficiency, hereditary factors and other infections. Electromyelography, CSF test and biopsy can facilitate the diagnosis.

14.7.5 Multiple Mononeuropathy

Multiple mononeuropathy demonstrates cerebral nerve involvement, distal symmetrical or asymmetrical neuropathy. The involved areas innervated by nerves have motor or sensory deficiency. The pathological findings include segmental demyelination of the peripheral nerves and/or axon degeneration. CSF test indicates normal or a mild increase of protein and an increase of IgG potency. Electromyelography suggests axonal multi-neuropathy. Neural biopsy can provide accurate evidence for the determination of the nature and degree of neural injuries.

14.7.6 Chronic Infectious Demyelinating Polyneuropathy (CIDP)

CIDP occurs with an acute onset when serum HIV antibody inverts positive or with a chronic onset in the advanced stage of AIDS with mild immunodeficiency. Local lesions are loss or thinner myelin sheath, decreased myelinated nerve fibers, distribution of proliferated Schwan cells in concentric circles like onions and lymphocytes infiltration. Lesions can be found in spinal nerves and proximal nerve trunk. Demyelination and regeneration of nerves roots and trunks as well as lymphocytes infiltration can cause painful extremities, exercise fatigue, decreased tendon reflex and sensory disturbance. CSF test shows increased protein and lymphocytes and an increase of globulin potency. The diagnosis of CIDP can be made based on the symptoms and signs, CSF and electrophysiology. The definitive diagnosis sometimes needs nerves biopsy.

Case Study 1
A male patient aged 51 years was confirmatively diagnosed as having AIDS by CDC. His CD4 T cell count was 45/μl.

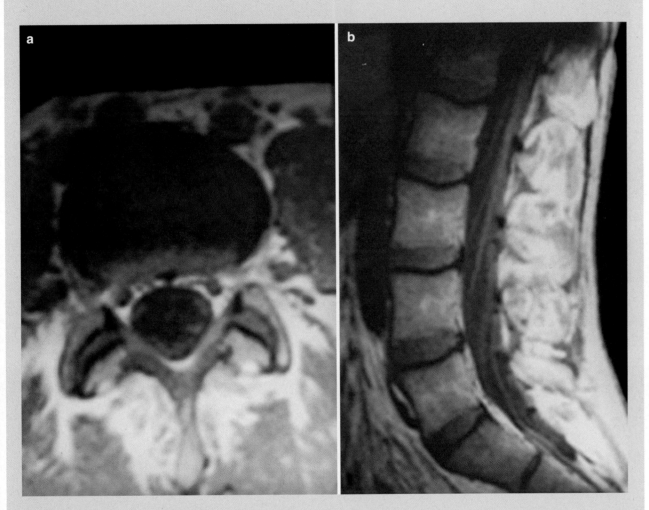

Fig. 14.10 (a–d) HIV/AIDS related CIDP. (a, b) Plain T1WI imaging of HIV/AIDS related CIDP. (c, d) Enhanced T1WI imaging demonstrates enhancement of intrathecal nerve roots

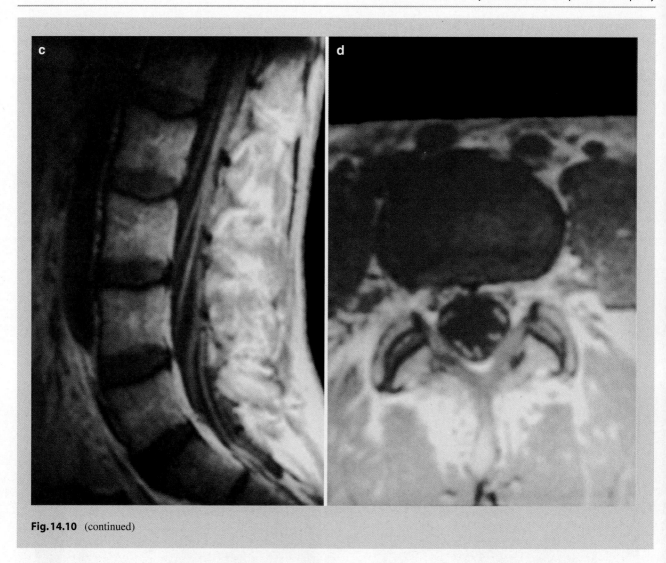

Fig. 14.10 (continued)

Case Study 2

A male patient aged 42 years was confirmatively diagnosed as having AIDS by CDC. His CD4 T cell count was 65/µl.

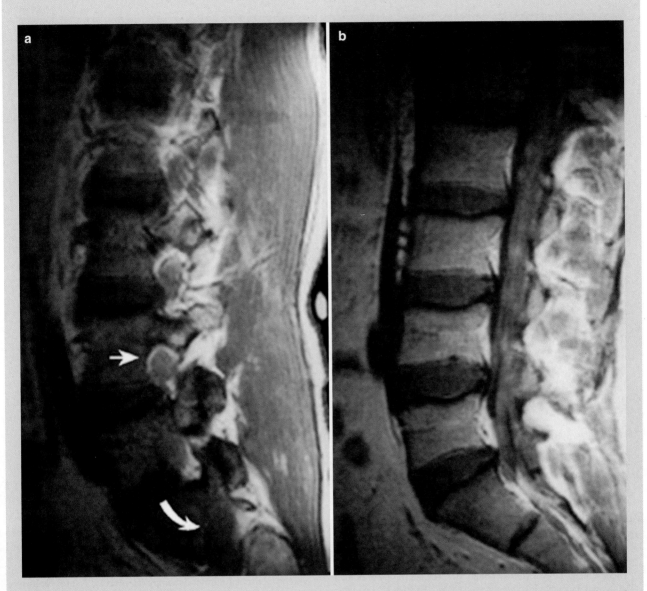

Fig. 14.11 (**a, b**) HIV/AIDS related CIDP. (**a, b**) Enhanced sagittal T1WI imaging demonstrates agglutinative nerves of cauda equian and their nodular enhancement (*arrow*)

Case Study 3

A male patient aged 34 years was confirmatively diagnosed as having AIDS by CDC. His CD4 T cell count was 25/μl.

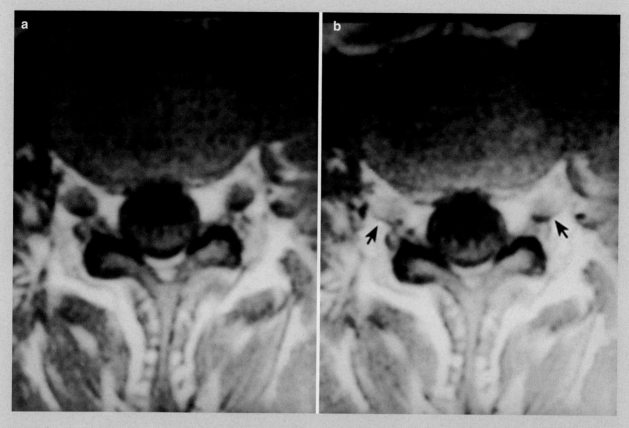

Fig. 14.12 (**a**, **b**) HIV/AIDS related CIDP. (**a**) T1WI scanning. (**b**) Enhanced T1WI imaging demonstrates enhanced swollen nerve roots (*arrow*)

Extended Reading

1. Anneken K, Fischera M, Evers S, et al. Recurrent vacuolar myelopathy in HIV infection. J Infect. 2006;52(6):e181–3.
2. Bredesen DE, Levy RM, Rosenblum ML. The neurology of human immunodeficiency virus infection. Q J Med. 1988;68(25):665–77.
3. Budka H. Neuropathology of myelitis, myelopathy, and spinal infections in AIDS. Neuroimaging Clin N Am. 1997;7(3):639–50.
4. Claeke TR, Barrow G, Glibert DT, et al. A possible case of spinal tuberculosis in a HIV-positive male. West Indian Med J. 2010;59(4):453–4.
5. England JD, Gronseth GS, Franklin G, et al. Practice parameter: the evaluation of distal symmetric polyneuropathy: the role of laboratory and genetic testing (an evidence-based review): report of the American Academy of Neurology, the American Association of Neuromuscular and Electrodiagnostic Medicine, and the American Academy of Physical Medicine and Rehabilitation. PM&R. 2009;1:5–13.
6. Fuller GN. Cytomegalovirus and the peripheral nervous system in AIDS. J Acquir Immune Defic Syndr. 1992;5(Suppl):33–6.
7. Husstedt IW, Evers S, Reichelt D, et al. Screening for HIV-associated distal-symmetric polyneuropathy in CDC-classification stages 1, 2 and 3. Acta Neurol Scand. 2000;101:183–7.
8. Levy RM, Bredesen DE, Rosenblum ML. Neurological manifestations of the acquired immunodeficiency syndrome(AIDS):experience at UCSF and review of the literature. J Neurosurg. 1985;62(4):475–95.
9. Marra CM, Boutin P, Collier AC. Screening for distal sensory peripheral neuropathy in HIV-infected persons in research and clinical settings. Neurology. 1998;51:1678–81.
10. Maschke M, Kastrup O, Esser S. Incidence and prevalence of neurological disorders associated with HIV since the introduction of highly active antiretroviral therapy (HAART). J Neurol Neurosurg Psychiatry. 2000;69:376–80.
11. McArthur JCN, Hoover DR, Bacellar H, Miller EN, et al. Dementia in AIDS patients : incidence and risk factors. Multicenter AIDS Cohort Study. Neurology. 1993;43(11):2245–52.
12. Molina-Olier O, Tunon-Pitalua M, Alcala-Cerra G, et al. Spinal cord compression due to intraspinal gumma in one patient. Clinical case. Acta Ortop Mex. 2012;26(3):197–201.
13. Nakamura M, Fujishima S, Hori S, et al. An adult case of cervico-mediastinal tuberculous lymphadenitis. Nihon Kokyuki Gakkai Zasshi. 2000;38(3):223–8.
14. Peter SA, Brignol YF, Razavi MH, et al. Diffuse hyperpigmentation associated with acquired immunodeficiency syndrome. J Natl Med Assoc. 1992;84(11):977–9.
15. Petito CK, Navia BA, Cho ES, et al. Vacuolar myelopathy pathologically resembling subacute combined degeneration in patients with the acquired immunodeficiency syndrome. N Engl J Med. 1985;312(14):874–9.
16. Wulff EA, Wang AK, Simpson DM. HIV-associated peripheral neuropathy epidemiology. Pathophysiology and treatment. Drugs. 2000;59(6):1251–60.

HIV/AIDS Related Eye Diseases

Contents

15.1   Introduction to HIV/AIDS Related Oculopathy

In patients with AIDS, over 90 % have ocular manifestations of opportunistic infections and over 70 % have accompanying signs of oculopathy. CMV infection is the most common HIV/AIDS related oculopathy and PCP, tuberculosis, HSV infection, fungus infection, toxoplasmic infections and Kaposi's sarcoma rarely occur. Oculopathy is commonly opportunistic infections, with involvement of both intraocular and extraocular tissues. Concurrent infections may be found, such as concurrence of fungal infection and CMV infection. Some oculopathies occur in the early stage of AIDS, being an indicator of HIV infection. With the prolonged course of the illness, the occurrence of complications increases.

15.1.1   HIV/AIDS Related Retinitis

HIV/AIDS related fundus microvascular lesions is also known as HIV/AIDS related retinitis, which may result in retinal capillary occlusion, retinal nerve fiber necrosis, microaneurysms and flaky retinal hemorrhage, with cotton-wool liked exudating plaques or round/oval Roth plaques with white centers. Ophthalmoscopy demonstrates white cotton wool liked effusions at the posterior end of the retina, with unclearly defined boundary. The old lesions are in lightened color in whitish gray with clearly defined boundary. The absorbed white plaques have remained slight retinal pigment disorder. The pathological changes of retinal microvascular lesions include: (1) vascular endothelial cells swelling; (2) globulin sedimentation or increased immune complexes; (3) increased blood viscosity; (4) cellular necrosis surrounding blood vessels and thickened basal membrane of endothelia cells. Pathological examination suggests immune complexes sedimentation, followed by microvascular occlusion and local ischemia. In addition, edema, degeneration, necrosis and rupture of the nerve fiber can be found, with swelling of neural terminals.

H. Li (ed.), *Radiology of HIV/AIDS*,
DOI 10.1007/978-94-007-7823-8_15, © Springer Science+Business Media Dordrecht and People's Medical Publishing House 2014

15.1.2 Cytomegalovirus (CMV) Infection

In patients with AIDS, disseminative CMV infection is common, with a death rate of 30 % directly from CMV infection. In the advanced stage of AIDS, CMV may involve eyes. The incidence rate of HIV/AIDS related CMV retinitis is about 10–15 %, and about 30 % by autopsy. With the prolonging of the survival period, its incidence is increasing. Retinitis is a local manifestation of disseminative CMV infection, with characteristics of chronic and progressive necrosis of the whole retina (necrotic retinitis) with following blindness after several months' progression. Its clinical manifestations include unilateral visual field defect or decreased vision, sense of floating materials or dark spots in front of eyes. By oph-thalmoscopy, typically large yellowish white opaque foci scatter along the vascular vessels. Sometimes, the accompanying inflammatory effusion or bleeding surrounding vascular vessels may occur, with necrosis at the focal center. The necrotic retina and normal retina are clearly defined, with yellowish white particles at the margin of the foci. At the early stage, the lesions are found at the peripheral area of the fundus, with light gray cotton wool liked exudates of blurry borderline, which extends later to the macula and the optic papilla. Macular edema can lead to decreased vision, with retinal congestion and edema or even hemorrhage and necrosis in the active phase in tomato sauce liked appearance of the fundus. The active lesions are grayish white at the edges with a rapid progression while lightened color at the edges of foci. The small granules are relatively static. Meanwhile, the foci can gradually enlarge, possibly with newly occurring foci. It has been reported that the foci may enlarge 1–2 times within 1 month. CMVR is a complication in terminal AIDS patients, which usually occur in cases with CD4$^+$ T count being less than 0.05×10^9/L. At this level of CD4 T count, the incidence of CMVR is about 24.6 %. It can be manifested as a sudden outbreak or regional granular. The pathological basis is that retinal microvascular lesions cause local insufficiently of blood supply and formation of cotton wool liked plaques. The foci of the infection distribute along vascular vessels. Commonly, CMV invades blood vessels to cause toxemia, leading to multi-focal infection. Invasion of CMV into retinal gliocytes and pigment epithelial cells renders CMV to duplicate actively in them to cause irreversible damages to the infected cells. Therefore, necrosis of large areas of retina occurs. For cases of AIDS have blurry vision or sense of floating materials in front of eyes, fundus examination should be performed under dilated pupil. CMV retinitis typically occurs at the retinal peripheral area or at the posterior pole, commonly with hemorrhage and vascular inflammatory changes. Thereby, in the year of 1987, CDC of the United States listed CMV retinitis as an indicator of AIDS in the diagnosis, with following diagnostic criteria: specific changes by ophthalmoscopy such as scattered retinal white effusions with blurry boundaries disseminating along the blood vessels centrifugally. Its progression lasts for several months, with occurrence of accompanying retinal vasculitis, hemorrhage and necrosis. After acute lesions subside, the retinal scars and atrophy remain with accompanying retinal pigment epithelial spots. CMV retinitis is irreversible. Isolation of CMV from the patient's aqueous humour and tear is of diagnostic value. PCR technology has high specificity and sensitivity, facilitating the diagnosis of pathogen.

15.1.3 Herpes Virus Induced Lesions

Herpes virus induced lesions are commonly caused by Herpes simplex virus(HSV) and varicella-zoster virus (VZV) infections, both of which can lead to acute retinal necrosis with a rapid progression. Within 2–4 days, the whole retina can be completely destroyed. The foci are grayish white, with clearly defined borderline. Such patients usually have a recent history of herpes zoster or herpes simplex infection.

15.1.4 Toxoplasma Retinitis

Toxoplasma retinitis is usually congenital or can be found in patients with AIDS. Retinochoroiditis initially occurs, with lesions in the peripheral area of the fundus in the early stage. In the following stages, the foci may involve macula and optic papilla. Fundus examination indicates singular or multiple light yellow retinal lesions at the fundus at the acute phase, being irregular in shape. It may develop into necrotic retinochoroiditis, chronic choroiditis or optic neuritis, with accompanying vitreitis.

15.1.5 Other Infections

Other infections include tuberculosis, pneumocystosis, cryptococcal and bacterial infections, which may result in conjunctivitis, cornea ulcer and meibomian gland cyst. Viral infections usually lead to molluscum contagiosum and in children lead to a typical viral skin infection, which can involve eyelid and conjunctiva. Molluscum contagiosum is clinically manifested as grayish white nodules at the eyelids, 2–3 mm in diameter with a central hilar depression. Herpes zoster is also common.

15.1.6 Eye Neoplasms

Kaposi's sarcoma commonly occurs at the eyelids and conjunctivas of AIDS patients, with an incidence rate of about 20–24 %. It can be found in the tissues of eyelids, tarsal gland, lacrimal gland and conjunctiva. The diseased eyelids may have light purple colored lesion or bright/dark red flat plaques and nodules, with involvement of both upper and lower eyelids. The lesions are confined painless nodules, with local lumps which gradually enlarge. The conjunctival lesions are relatively flat, being prone to be confused with subconjunctival hemorrhage and nodules. Orbital involvement causes exophthalmos, blepharoedema, and ptosis of the upper eyelid.

15.2 HIV/AIDS Related Orbitopathy

15.2.1 HIV/AIDS Related Intraorbital Mucormycosis

15.2.1.1 Pathogen and Pathogenesis
Mucor spores are commonly found in soil and air, which can be inhaled into nasal sinus and lung. It seldom causes disease in healthy populations and mucormycosis occurs commonly in immunocompromised people and is generally secondary. The pathogen invades the body through nasal mucosa where black necrotic foci are formed. Then they spread around and extend to the orbit of the same side to involve eyeballs, intraorbital soft tissues, blood vessels and nerves. Mucor invasion into ophthalmic artery can cause thrombosis that further leads to facial, orbital content and eyelid infarction as well as local skin gangrene.

15.2.1.2 Pathophysiological Basis
HIV/AIDS related orbital mucormycosis is not the same as other mycoses which have a chronic progression. It is an acute inflammation with a rapid progression to trigger extensive dissemination. It spreads to the surrounding tissues rapidly, commonly invading blood vessels to cause thrombosis and infarction. Sometimes the illness is chronic, with multitude macrophages and foreign giant cells, infiltration of massive neutrophils and eosinophils, interstitial fiber hyperplasia and thickened capillary walls. The necrotic area, vascular wall, vascular lumen and thrombosis contain quantities of mucor hyphas. HIV/AIDS related orbital mucormycosis is manifested as acute suppurative inflammation, which has a more severe invasion to the blood vessels than aspergillus to cause a higher occurrence of vascular thrombosis and infarction. Therefore, severe necrosis and purulence of the tissues might be the results of concurrence direct action of mucor and vascular blockage by mold embolus.

15.2.1.3 Clinical Symptoms and Signs
Clinically the ocular symptoms include orbital pain, eyelid ptosis, exophthalmos, fixation and loss of sight, orbital infection (cellulitis) companied with exophthalmos, pus discharge from the nasal cavity, possible damage of nasal septum, roof of the mouth (palate), orbital bones or sinus tract. The pathogens may also invade major blood vessels to cause thrombosis and necrosis. Death may rapidly occur in such patients.

15.2.1.4 Examinations and Their Selection
1. Direct microscopic examination and culture of fungus: The specimens are collected from superior turbinate scrapings or biopsy.
2. Histopathological examination facilitates the qualitative diagnosis.
3. CT scanning and MR imaging facilitate the shape of the occupied space and its surrounding tissues.

15.2.1.5 Imaging Demonstrations
CT scanning demonstrates an increase in orbital density, loss of posterior fat space of eyeballs and exophthalmos, diffuse shadows of increased density at the orbital conical area, effusion in nasal cavity and maxillary sinus, mucosal hypertrophy of maxillary sinus and ethmoidal sinus, curved nasal septum. The severely ill patients may develop orbital cellulitis, suggesting of pathogenic invasion into eyes and the central nervous system to cause paralysis of multiple cranial nerves such as V and VII.

Case Study

A male patient aged 43 years was confirmatively diagnosed as having AIDS by CDC. He had a history of paid blood donation and his CD4 T cell count was 55/μl.

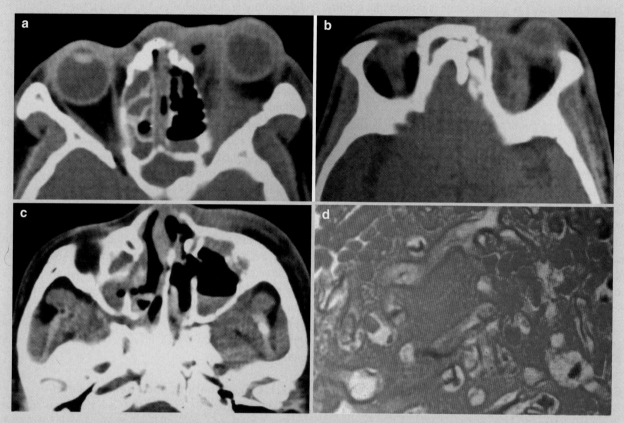

Fig. 15.1 (a–d) HIV/AIDS related mucormycosis. (a–b) CT scanning demonstrates increased tissues density in the left eye, deformed eyeball and diffuse shadows of increased density at the orbital conical area. (c) CT scanning demonstrates liquid level of the left maxillary sinus, mucosa hypertrophy of the right maxillary sinus and ethmoidal sinus, and curved nasal septum. (d) Pathological analysis of perforated tissues indicates light staining of hyphas with varied diameters

15.2.1.6 Criteria for the Diagnosis

1. Etiological examinations
2. Histopathological examinations

   It usually demonstrates suppurative inflammation companied with abscess formation and suppurative necrosis. The necrotic tissue may contain broad hyphas, with peripheral narrow band of neutrophils. Chronic infection rarely occurs, with common manifestations of simplex granuloma or concurrent purulent inflammation and granuloma inflammation. Invasion of blood vessels by pathogens may be found, with vascular wall necrosis, fungal embolism and tissue infarction.
3. CT scanning and MRI imaging

   CT scanning and MR imaging demonstrate intraorbital space occupying effects, loss of orbital posterior fat space and protruding eyeball due to compression.

15.2.1.7 Differential Diagnosis

Patients with normal immunity usually have chronic nasal mucormycosis with local nasal granuloma containing hyphae. In some patients, only cranial or cerebral granuloma occurs, with demonstrations of intracranial space occupying effects. The immunocompromised patients with AIDS rarely have granuloma, making it difficult to be identified from other fungal infections and bacterial infections. Therefore, the diagnosis should be based on the etiological examinations.

15.2.2 HIV/AIDS Related Intraorbital Lymphoma

15.2.2.1 Pathogen and Pathogenesis

Compromised immunities caused by AIDS, some hereditary diseases, acquired immunodeficiency diseases or autoimmune diseases such as ataxia telangiectasia, combined immunodeficiency syndrome, rheumatoid arthritis, systemic lupus erythematosus, hypogammaglobulinemia and patients receiving long-term immunosuppressing medication (such as medication after organ transplantation) are high risks for occurrence of non-Hodgkin's lymphoma.

15.2.2.2 Pathophysiological Basis

According to the latest classification, orbital lymphoma is categorized into non-Hodgkin's lymphoma, accounting for about 0.01 % in patients with lymphoma and 3 % in patients with extraglandular malignancies. It can occur in conjunctiva and lacrimal gland or posterior to eyeballs, complicating central nervous system lymphoma. It occurs in patients aged above 30 years, with homogeneously yellowish or pinkish masses. Its inside lobule is obvious, with clearly defined borderline. The neoplasms have a uniform shape, composed of immature lymphocytes or evidently deformed lymphocytes. The tumor cells are in diffusive infiltration, with various morphologies. The tumor cells may be atypical T lymphocytes in different sizes, concurrently exist with possible involvement of the blood vessels.

15.2.2.3 Clinical Symptoms and Signs

It is clinically manifested as unilateral or bilateral swelling and ptosis of the eyelids, with palpable painless hardened lumps. The eye ball bulges, migrating laterally. Chemosis occurs, with infiltrative hyperplasia to involve optic nerves and extraocular muscles. In the cases with invasion to subconjunctiva, lumps like pink fish can be observed through conjunctiva.

Non-Hodgkin's lymphoma is a definitive illness of AIDS. Orbital lymphoma is commonly non-Hodgkin's lymphoma (originating from B lymphocytes). It has a unilateral occurrence (more common) or bilateral concurrence (rarely found). Clinically, it can be divided into acute and chronic. The chronic type has a hideous onset, with slow progression and mild symptoms, while the acute type has clinical manifestations of eyelid swelling, palpable painless hardened nodular intraorbital lumps; propelled eyeballs out of the orbits, eyeballs motion disorders and decreased eyesight.

15.2.2.4 Examinations and Their Selection

1. Ultrasonography.
2. CT scanning
3. MR imaging
4. Pathological examinations provide essential evidence for the diagnosis of MHL and its category.

15.2.2.5 Imaging Demonstrations

B Ultrasound

The B mode ultrasonography demonstrates irregular lesions in flat or oval pattern with clearly defined borderline, less echoes, and decreased ultrasound attenuation. Generally, CDI can detect the relatively rich blood flow within the lesions.

CT Scanning

Lymphoma usually occurs in the extraconal space, with concurrent involvement of orbit and extraconal space. It has unclearly defined borderline with peripheral extraocular muscle and eye ring, with even density of orbital foci by CT scanning. Lymphoma shows a diffuse growth inside and outside of muscular cone, and grows encompassing eyeballs with a cast liked condition, whereas the eye ring is complete without confined thickening. The intraorbital fat space cannot be found. Enhanced scanning suggests mildly or moderately even enhancement. Based on the range of the involvement, lymphoma is divided into local and diffuse. (1) Most lesions are located anterior to the extraconal space, immediately posterior to orbital septum and anterior area of the orbital septum, with a growth tendency of encompassing eyeballs. (2) Unilateral lesions are common with rare occurrence of bilateral involvements. The lesions grow backward along extraconal space with a sharp posterior margin of the lump in a cast liked change. (3) Due to no envelope surrounding the tumors, the tumors have infiltrative growths, with no obvious mechanical space occupying effects. Therefore, it commonly involves extraconal space, with unclearly defined borderline with eye ring, extraocular muscle and optic nerve. The interface between the wall of eyeball and the tumor has no depression, with no obvious thickened eye ring. (4) Plain CT scanning demonstrates homogeneous density, similar to the density of the extraocular muscle. By enhanced scanning, moderately homogeneous enhancement of the tumors can be found. (5) Orbital bone injury is rarely found, but can be found in cases with lesions resulted from orbital lymphoma invasion. (6) In some cases, the lymphoma can spread to intracranial and extracranial areas via superior or inferior orbital fissure.

MR Imaging

Lymphoma commonly occurs in the extraconal space, with concurrent involvements of the orbit and extraconal space. It is unclearly defined from peripheral extraocular muscle and eye ring. Moreover, MRI shows equal T1 and long T2 signals and a moderate enhancement by enhanced imaging. Lymphoma often involves eyelid and the peripheral tissues of the orbit, with rare involvement of the orbit itself.

Case Study

A female patient aged 54 years was confirmatively diagnosed as having AIDS by CDC. She had a history of paid blood donation and her CD4 T cell count was 15/µl.

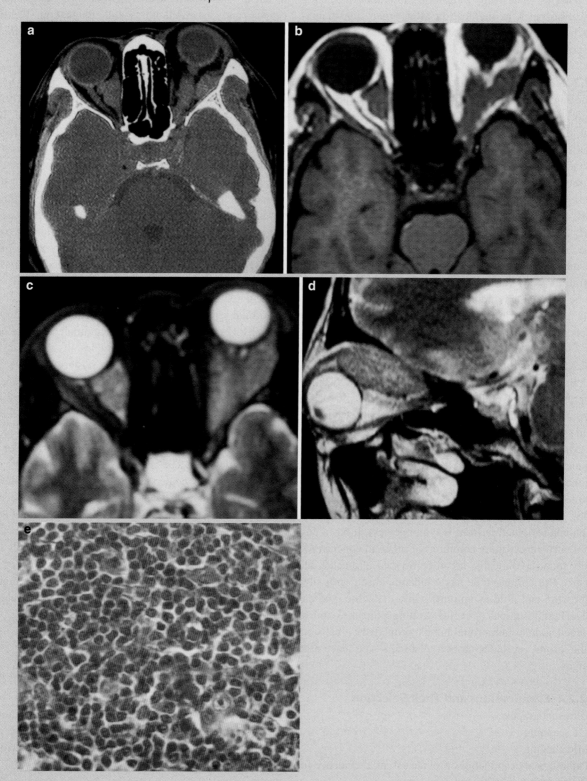

Fig. 15.2 (a–e) HIV/AIDS related orbital lymphoma. (a) The bilateral orbits demonstrates irregular shaped mass shadows of soft tissues. (b, c) Axial MRI demonstrates equal T1 and long T2 signals of intraorbital soft tissues. (d) Sagittal MRI demonstrates spindle shaped soft tissue signals above optic nerves. (e) Pathological analysis of perforated tissues demonstrates mirror cells as a main type of lymphocytes

15.2.2.6 Criteria for the Diagnosis

1. CT scanning demonstrates lump shadows of soft tissue density superior to the orbit and surrounding eyeballs have an unclearly defined borderline with their neighboring eyelid, extraocular muscle and lacrimal gland. The lumps are of homogeneous density with moderately even enhancement. The orbits are rarely involved.
2. MR imaging indicates frequent occurrence of lymphoma in the extraconal space, with equal T1 and long T2 signals. Enhanced imaging demonstrates a moderate enhancement. The orbits are rarely involved.
3. Biopsy of pathological tissues suggests mirror cells as a main type of lymphocyte.

15.2.2.7 Differential Diagnosis

Diffuse Inflammatory Pseudotumor

It commonly has an uneven density with extraocular hypermyotrophy. Its typical manifestations include simultaneous thickening of the muscular belly and tendon, companied by thickened eye ring and enlarged lacrimal gland. Hormone therapy is effective but it commonly recurs.

Orbital Cellulitis

The symptoms include swollen eyelid soft tissues with unclear borderline, swollen and thickened extraocular muscles. Enhanced scanning suggests inhomogeneous but evident enhancement of the foci. Thereby, diagnosis can be made in combination of its inflammatory manifestations. Its clinical medical history and blood biochemical examination has specific indicators.

Diffuse Lymphangioma

It generally has a long-term progression, with manifestations of large lumps, irregular shapes, uneven density, obvious enlargement and no damages to bones.

15.2.3 HIV/AIDS Related Fungal Suppurative Panophthalmitis

15.2.3.1 Pathogen and Pathogenesis

The vitreum is a tissue with no blood supplying, only containing water and protein. The invasion of pathogens and their duplication may cause inflammation and abscess. The pathogens are usually from eyelid and conjunctival sac, fungus accounting for 26 %. The invasion of pathogens into eyes and duplication there produces endotoxins and exotoxins which triggers violent inflammatory reactions of the ocular tissues. Thereby, a series of clinical symptoms show up.

15.2.3.2 Pathophysiological Basis

The common pathological changes include extensive suppurative inflammation, large quantities of neutrophils infiltration. Separated small abscesses adjacent to foci may be found. At the terminal phase, polymorphonuclear white cells encompass the fungus to trigger granuloma reactions.

15.2.3.3 Clinical Symptoms and Signs

According to the severity of clinical manifestations, endophthalmitis falls into three categories.

1. Acute endophthalmitis The incubation period is about 3 days or just hours. The symptoms are severe, with a rapid progression, which is usually caused by staphylococcus aureus, pseudomonas aeruginosa and bacillus cereus with strong virulence.
2. Sub-acute endophthalmitis The incubation period is about 1 week. The symptoms are evident, caused by streptococcus and diplococcus pneumonia.
3. Chronic endophthalmitis The incubation period is over 1–2 weeks. The symptoms are slight, with a slow progression or recurrence. The pathogens include staphylococcus epidermidis, staphylococcus albus, fungus and propionibacterium acnes with weak virulence.

Suppurative endophthalmitis and endophthalmitis induced by bacillus cereus commonly have a sudden outbreak, which should be given focused attention.

15.2.3.4 Examinations and Their Selection

1. Bacterial culture and smear staining of aqueous humour and the vitreum is of critical value for the definitive diagnosis.
2. Ultrasound can identify the severity of vitreous opacity, retinal detachment and presence of bulbar wall or retrobulbar abscess, which is key for the diagnosis and treatment.
3. CT scanning demonstrates heterogeneously moderate density, with the eye rings bulging inward and deformed.
4. MR imaging is of high resolution for soft tissues, which can provide more information about the tissue structure for the diagnosis.

15.2.3.5 Imaging Demonstrations

B Ultrasound

B ultrasound demonstrates spot or strip liked echo of the vitreum and posterior high intensity echo band connected to the optic disc, which indicates retinal detachment.

CT Scanning

CT scanning demonstrates enlarged eyeballs with uneven density and unclear borderline with peripheral tissues. The eye ball bulges inward with obvious deformity.

MR Imaging

MR imaging demonstrates equal T1 and long T2 signals of eyeballs, deformed eyeball, thickened eye ring and enhanced signaling from the vitreum. IV-GD-DT-PA demonstrates obviously ring shaped abnormal enhancement of retrobulbar lumps.

Case Study

A male patient aged 31 years was confirmatively diagnosed as having AIDS by CDC. He had a history of paid blood donation, with a progressive loss of right eyesight and bulging eye ball with pain for 1 month. His CD4 T cell count was 75/μl.

Diagnosis: AIDS complicated by fungal suppurative panophthalmitis and interior staphyloma.

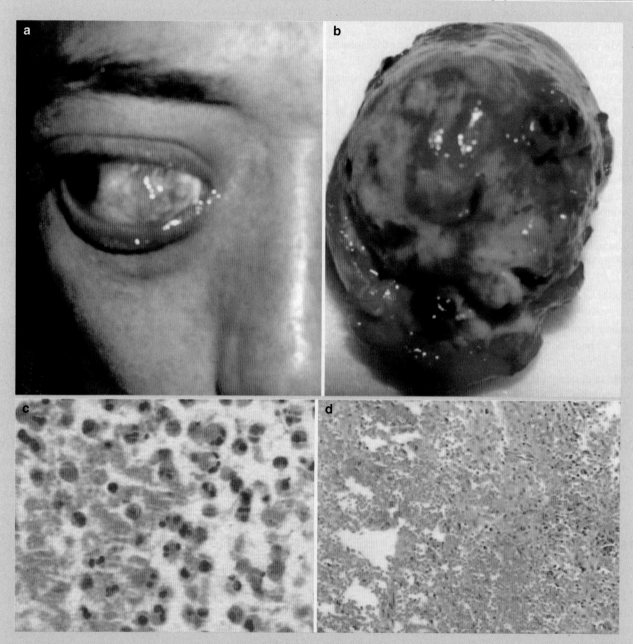

Fig. 15.3 (a–j) HIV/AIDS related fungal suppurative panophthalmitis and interior staphyloma. (**a**) Right eyeball protruding outward with exterior rotation as well as ocular medial masses. (**b**) Manifestations before and after enucleation of the right eyeball, with abscesses and protrusion of the medial sclera to cover the surface of the eyeball. (**c**) Pathological analysis demonstrates inflammatory necrotic tissues in the ocular infected area, with congestion and small vessel hyperplasia; chronic suppurative necrosis in the ocular abscess area with abundant neutrophils and local acidophils; blood clots in the ocular necrotic tissues and melanin deposit in the cavity wall with obvious congestion. (**d**) Massive inflammatory necrotic tissues and fungal hyphae with slight staining. (**e**) B ultrasound demonstrates spot and strip liked echo in the vitreum and posterior light bands with strong echo connected to the optic disc, indicating retinal detachment. (**f**) CT scanning demonstrates heterogeneously moderate density area in size of 2×2 cm in the right eye, with the eye ring protruding inward and deformed eyeball. (**g, h**) MR imaging demonstrates equal T1 and long T2 signal posterior to the eyeball. (**i**) Coronal MR imaging demonstrates enlarged and deformed right eyeball, with heterogeneous signaling from the vitreum. (**j**) MRI IV-GD-DTPA demonstrates retrobulbar masses with obviously ring shaped enhancement but no central enhancement

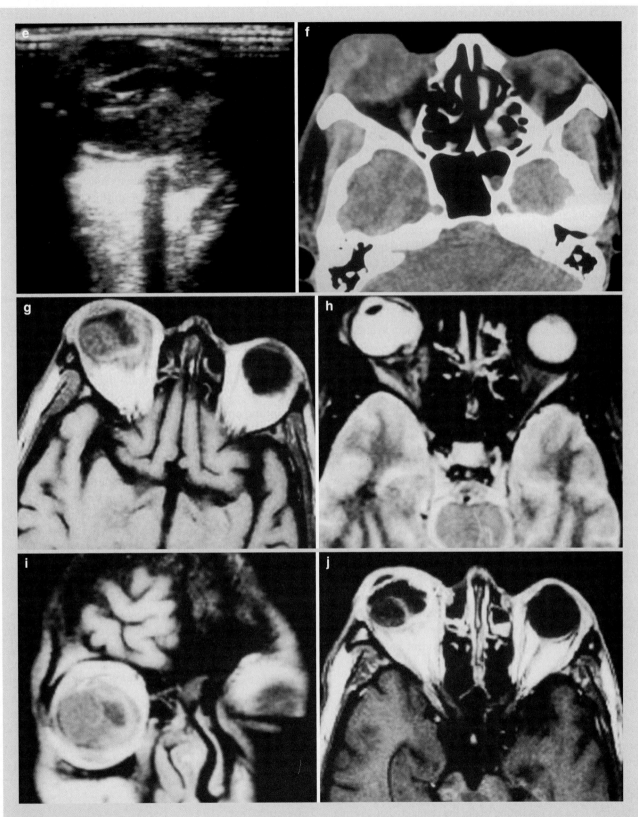

Fig. 15.3 (continued)

15.2.3.6 Criteria for the Diagnosis
B Ultrasound
B ultrasound demonstrates spot and strip liked echo in the vitreum, with posterior light band of high intensity connected to the optic disc, indicating retinal detachment.

CT Scanning
CT scanning demonstrates enlarged eyeballs with uneven density and vague borderline with peripheral tissues, inward bulging eye ring and obviously deformed eyeball.

MR Imaging
MR imaging demonstrates equal T1 and long T2 signals of eyeballs, deformed eyeball, thickened eye ring and enhanced signaling from the vitreum. IV-GD-DT-PA demonstrates abnormal ring shaped enhancement of retrobulbar lumps but no central enhancement.

15.2.3.7 Differential Diagnosis
It should be differentiated from traumatic hemorrhage and ocular neoplasms.

15.2.4 HIV/AIDS Related Choroidal Tuberculosis

15.2.4.1 Pathogen and Pathogenesis
Choroidal tuberculosis falls into two categories according to the lesions nature. One is caused by direct invasion of tissues by mycobacterium tuberculosis. Due to the rich choroidal blood vessels and slow blood flow, bacteria are likely to remain there to cause choroidal tuberculosis. Therefore, choroidal tuberculosis is common in ocular tuberculosis. This type of choroidal tuberculosis is characterized by chronic proliferative lesions, with no severe inflammatory reactions. The other category is caused by direction invasion of other bacteria than mycobacteria, namely allergic responsive inflammation of tissues to tuberculoplasmin which is characterized by acute progression with evident inflammatory effusion.

15.2.4.2 Pathophysiological Basis
In the acute stage, the fundus usually presents yellowish white or grayish white exudative foci in round or oval shapes or circumscribed by satellite spots. It can be found across the fundus, but commonly in the peripheral area. For cases with prolonged course or renal pigment degeneration caused by other factors, retina-choroid barrier may be damaged with choroidal fluid accumulating under the retina to cause retinal detachment. Thereby it should be differentiated from primary retinal detachment. After inflammation subsides after treatment, shrinkage foci may be remained at the fundus, with

pigment sedimentation. It may recur in the peripheral area of the foci or in the areas adjacent to the inflammatory lesions.

15.2.4.3 Clinical Symptoms and Signs
Clinical manifestations of tuberculous chorioretinitis can be divided into four types, namely exudative, chronic miliary tuberculosis, acute miliary tuberculosis and choroidal tuberculoma. Their clinical manifestations include: (1) concurrence of retinal tubercles with choroidal tuberculosis, (2) tuberculous retinitis with yellowish white exudative foci, hemorrhage and venectasia, (3) tuberculous retinal periphlebitis and (4) tuberculous retinal arteritis that has a rare occurrence, with white effusions and tuberculous choroiditis in the retinal arteries.

15.2.4.4 Examinations and Their Selection
Ultrasonography
B ultrasound demonstrates retrobulbar thickened sclera that protrudes towards vitreous space and retrobulbar abscess. Retina-choroid detachment occurs due to retrobulbar scleritis. Retrobulbar abscess surrounds the optic nerve in a T shaped sign. A ultrasound demonstrates thickened posterior eyeball wall showing a massive spike liked echo.

CT Scanning and MR Imaging
CT scanning demonstrates thickened posterior eye ring, thickened junction between the optic nerve and eyeball, concurrent exophthalmos and retrobulbar edema. Injection of contrast reagent can more clearly demonstrate the findings. MR imaging demonstrates thickened posterior eyeball wall with long T1 and T2 signals and enhanced imaging demonstrates enhancement. Signal intensity of weighted imaging can distinguish choroid and retina, which is of great value for the diagnosis of retrobulbar scleritis.

Fundus Fluorescein Angiography (FFA)
FFA demonstrates retinal pigment epithelial detachment, exudative retinal detachment, optic disc edema and macular cystoid edema. In the early stage of exudative retinal detachment, the manifestations include mottling background fluorescence of the choroid. In the middle stage, diffuse multiple highlighted areas in the size of needle points are demonstrated, and subretinal fluid staining in the advanced stage. Choroidal folds are demonstrated as striped hypofluorescence and hyperfluorescence, while retinal folds show no fluorescence. FFA demonstrations are non-specific to posterior scleritis.

Tuberculin Test
Tuberculin test positive indicates a history of tuberculosis, while ocular tuberculosis cannot be excluded even in cases with negative results.

15.2.4.5 Imaging Demonstrations
CT Scanning

CT scanning demonstrates flaky high density areas peripheral to the eyeball, deformed eyeball and thickened eye ring protruding into vitreous cavity.

MR Imaging

MR imaging demonstrates strip liked equal T1 and long T2 signals surrounding the eye ring, thickened and bulging eye ring below the right temple, increased signal of the vitreous cavity and diffuse increased signals in the eyeball.

Case Study

A male patient aged 38 years with AIDS was confirmatively diagnosed. He had a history of paid blood donation, progressive decrease of the right eyesight, ocular pain and fever for 2 weeks. He also had pulmonary miliary tuberculosis, with positive staining for sputum acid-fast bacilli and weakly positive for tuberculosis antibody. His CD4 T cell count was 55/ μl.

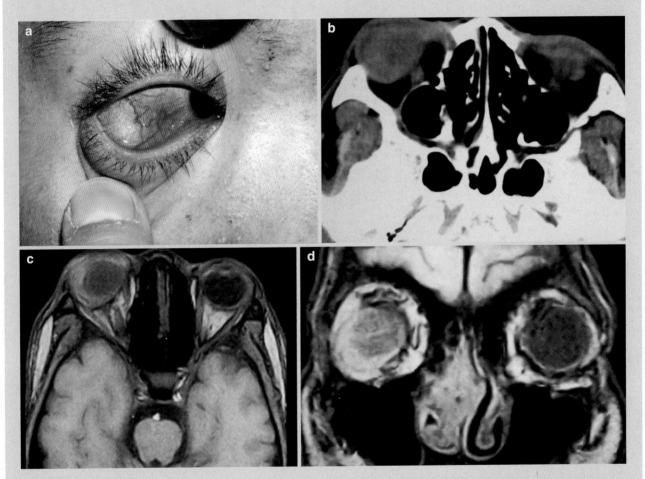

Fig. 15.4 (a–g) HIV/AIDS related choroidal tuberculosis. (a) It is demonstrated to have masses below the temple of the right eye, conjunctival congestion, and superficial large blood vessels. (b) CT scanning demonstrates flaky high density areas lateral to the right eyeball, deformed eyeball, thickened right eye ring protruding toward the vitreous cavity. (c, d) Coronal and sagittal MR imaging demonstrates strip liked slightly long T1 and long T2 signals lateral to the right eye ring, thickened and protruding right eye ring below the right temple, increased signaling of the vitreous cavity and increased diffuse signals within the eyeball. (e) There is flaky long T2 signal at the right parietal lobe, with peripheral finger liked findings. (f, g) After surgical removal of the eyeball, pathological analysis demonstrates caseous necrosis of the choroid with abundant inflammatory effusions and visible tuberculous nodules

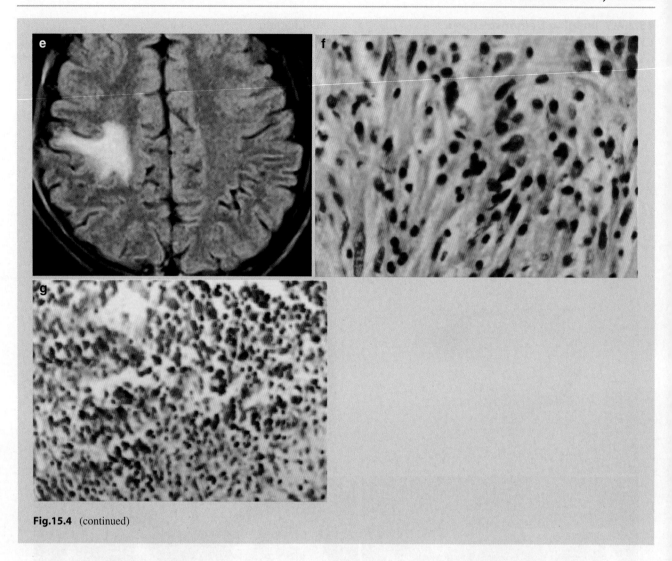

Fig.15.4 (continued)

15.2.4.6 Criteria for the Diagnosis

1. By ELISA (enzyme-linked immunosorbent assay), tuberculosis antibody is positive, especially the ratio of titers in serum and aqueous.
2. Biopsy of the peripheral retinal lesions.
3. DNA probe produced with ribosomal nucleotide of the mycobacterium as the template.
4. CT scanning demonstrates lumps peripheral to the right eye, flaky high density areas lateral to the eyeball, deformed eyeball, thickened temporal eye ring protruding into the vitreous cavity.
5. MR imaging demonstrates thickened eye ring with equal T1 and long T2 signals, tuberculosis of other areas, such as pulmonary tuberculosis.
6. Pathological analysis indicates caseous necrosis of the choroid, with abundant inflammatory effusions and visible tuberculous nodules.

15.2.4.7 Differential Diagnosis

It should be differentiated from intraorbital neoplasms.

15.3   HIV/AIDS Related Fundus Diseases

15.3.1 HIV/AIDS Related Microangiopathy

15.3.1.1 Pathogen and Pathogenesis

HIV/AIDS related microangiopathy is also known as HIV/AIDS retinopathy, which is the most frequent oculopathy after HIV infection, with an incidence of 40–60 % in HIV positive patients and 89 % in autopsy samples. The incidence of its complications increases as CD4 T count decreases. It may be caused by HIV direct infection of vascular epithelium or immune complex deposits at the retinal arterioles, suggestive of blood-retina barrier damage. In addition, hemodynamic changes may also contribute to its pathogenesis, leading to retinal capillary occlusion, retinal neural fiber necrosis, microaneurysms, flaky retinal hemorrhage, cotton-wool liked effusions and round/oval shaped Roth spots with white centers.

15.3.1.2 Pathophysiological Basis

The pathological process of retinal microangiopathy includes: (1) swollen vascular epithelia; (2) globulins sedimentation or increased immune complex; (3) increased blood viscosity; (4) perivascular cells necrosis and thickened epithelial basal membrane. The pathological examination reveals microvascular occlusion and ischemia caused by immune complex deposits, and the resulted swelling, degeneration, necrosis, rupture of the neural fiber layer and swelling of the nerve terminals.

15.3.1.3 Clinical Symptoms and Signs

Its clinical manifestations include blurry vision, progressively decreased eyesight and evident floaters in front of eyes.

15.3.1.4 Examinations and Their Selection

1. Ophthalmoscopy
2. Fundus fluorescein angiography (FFA)

15.3.1.5 Imaging Demonstrations

It is initially demonstrated as optic papilla swelling and unclearly defined optic disc borderline. With the development of the conditions, the demonstrations include abundant cotton wool liked spots and stellate effusions in the superficial retina around the optic disc, occasionally with superficial hemorrhagic spots along the course of the blood vessels. White segmental sheath of the venous wall can be found, with uneven diameters of the arteries and veins. In the advanced stage, the diameter of the veins are varying, with cotton wool liked plaques, yellowish white effusions and superficial bleeding. FFA demonstrates retinal fluorescein staining corresponding to the optic disc and cotton wool liked plaques, vascular fluorescein effusions in the lesion areas, coverage of fluorescence by bleeding.

Case Study 1

A male patient aged 37 years with AIDS was confirmatively diagnosed by CDC. He had binocular retinal arteriosclerosis of II degree, with a CD4 T count of 25/μl.

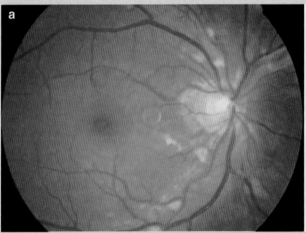
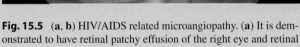
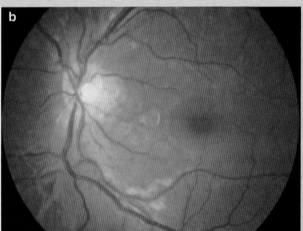

Fig. 15.5 (**a, b**) HIV/AIDS related microangiopathy. (**a**) It is demonstrated to have retinal patchy effusion of the right eye and retinal small patchy bleeding. (**b**) It is demonstrated that retinal arteriosclerosis of II degree of the left eye

---

Case Study 2

A female patient aged 36 years with AIDS was confirmatively diagnosed by CDC. She experienced decreased eyesight and blurry vision. Ophthalmological examination indicates 4.7 of the right eyesight and 0.06 of the left eyesight, binocular absence of ciliary congestion, transparent cornea, KP negative, normal depth of the anterior chamber, aqueous flaring negative and transparent lens.

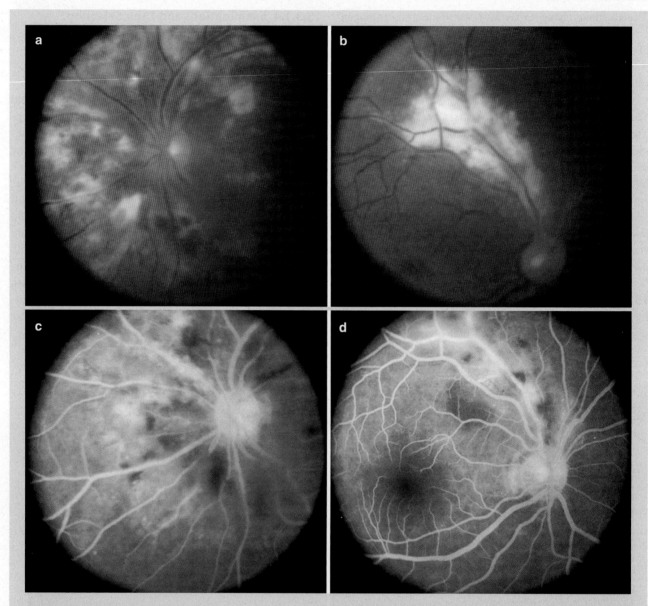

Fig. 15.6 (**a–d**) HIV/AIDS related microangiopathy. (**a**) There is an unclearly defined borderline of the left optic disc, massive cotton wool liked and star liked effusions in the retina peripheral to the optic disc, sporadic superficial patchy bleeding along the course of the blood vessels, segmental white sheath of the venous wall and varying diameters of the arteries and veins. (**b**) There is a cotton wool liked plaques along the direction of the right superior temporal vein, yellowish white effusions and superficial hemorrhage, different diameters of the superior temporal vein. (**c**) FFA demonstrates the left eye in the terminal stage, enhanced cotton wool liked plaques corresponding to retinal fluorescence, diffuse fluorescein staining of the lesions in the retina, coverage of the fluorescence by hemorrhage, the optic disc staining with unclearly defined borderline, segmental staining of the vascular wall. (**d**) FFA demonstrates the right optic disc staining, cotton wool plaques corresponding to retinal fluorescein staining; vascular fluorescein leakage in the lesions and coverage of fluorescence by hemorrhage

15.3.1.6 Criteria for the Diagnosis

1. HIV infection confirmed by CDC
2. Progressively decreasing eyesight, blurry vision.
3. Ophthalmoscopy shows congestion and edema of arteries and brush liked hemorrhage along the blood vessels. Fundus Fluorescein Angiography (FFA) manifests fluorescein effusions peripheral to blood vessels.

15.3.1.7 Differential Diagnosis

It should be differentiated from CMV retinitis/diabetes, hypertension and fundus arteriosclerosis and hemorrhage.

15.3.2 HIV/AIDS Related Cytomegalovirus Retinitis (CMVR)

15.3.2.1 Pathogen and Pathogenesis

In patients with AIDS, over 90 % have ocular lesions from opportunistic infections and over 70 % have accompanying oculopathy, 60–75 % have fundus complications and 30–40 % have complicated CMV retinitis among which 30–50 % have binocular involvement. Cytomegalovirus is a kind of herpes simplex viruses, and most patients with AIDS are serum CMV positive, with findings of CMV after blood culture. Clinically, CMVR infection is one of the manifestations of terminal HIV infection. When CD4 T count is less than 50/µl, the incidence of cytomegalovirus retinitis in patients with HIV/AIDS is 40 %.

15.3.2.2 Pathophysiological Basis

CMV infection can result in necrosis of the whole retina layer and loss of intact retinal structure. Most cases with CMV retinitis have initial cotton wool liked lesions. And the destructed blood-retina barrier can be caused by invasion of CMV into the retina. Because arteriole occlusion may lead to swelling of local retinal nerve fibers and axoplasmic flow stagnation, with subsequent occurrence of cotton wool liked plaques. The cotton wool plaque may be simple or compound with other microvascular abnormalities.

15.3.2.3 Clinical Symptoms and Signs

The clinical manifestations of CMVR include red eye, blurry vision, defective lesion and floaters in front of eyes.

Typical CMVR presents cream liked yellowish white retinal opacity with varied retinal hemorrhage. Lesions show different degrees of vascular stenosis and occlusion as well as white sheathing. The condition can usually involve posterior polar area, initially optic papilla and macula leading to irreversible vision loss. About 50 % cases of CMVR have retinal detachment which is another essential cause of vision loss resulted from CMV retinopathy, with a common occurrence in the advanced stage after retinal infection.

15.3.2.4 Examinations and Their Selection

1. Ophthalmoscopy
2. FFA
3. PCR
4. Pathological biopsy

15.3.2.5 Imaging Demonstrations
Ophthalmoscopy

Ophthalmoscopy demonstrates white cotton wool liked effusions in the posterior pole of the fundus, initially white with unclearly defined borderline as well as lightened and grayish color with well-defined borderline.

FFA

FFA demonstrates abnormal microcirculation and capillaries blocked region.

Case Study 1

A male patient aged 30 years with AIDS was confirmatively diagnosed by CDC. Six months ago, he developed local itchy papules, with orbital pain, itchy and sore throat, decreased eyesight and binocular blurry vision. Ophthalmology demonstrated 4.4 of the right eyesight and 0.06 of the left eyesight as well as binocular anterior segments negative.

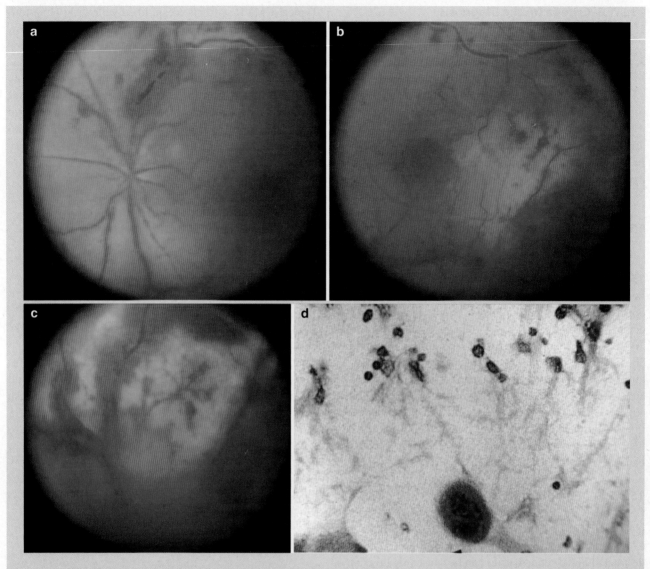

Fig. 15.7 (**a**–**d**) HIV/AIDS related cytomegalovirus retinitis. (**a**, **b**) There is an unclearly defined left optic disc, segmental stenosis of the retinal arteries with white sheathing of arteriovenous walls, hemorrhage along the retinal central veins in brush liked morphology, hemorrhage of the peripheral retina like wintersweet flower and large flaky yellowish white effusions as well as hematocele in the inferior peripheral vitreum. (**c**) There is a brush liked hemorrhage beside the retinal blood vessels of the right eye, yellowish white effusions of the deep retina and large flaky yellowish white effusions along the blood vessels in the paranasal retina. (**d**) Pathological analysis demonstrates retinal macrophages into "eagle eye" sign containing inclusion bodies

Case Study 2

A female patient aged 35 years with AIDS was confirmatively diagnosed by CDC. She had a history of paid blood donation in 1995 and the symptoms occurred in 2002 with general itchy skin papules. Currently, she had head-ache, faintness, numbness of hands and feet. Her left eyesight decreased with blurry vision for 5 days. Ophthalmological examinations indicates 5.0 of the right eyesight and 4.2 of the left eyesight. Binocular anterior segments are normal. And her CD4 T count was 1/μl.

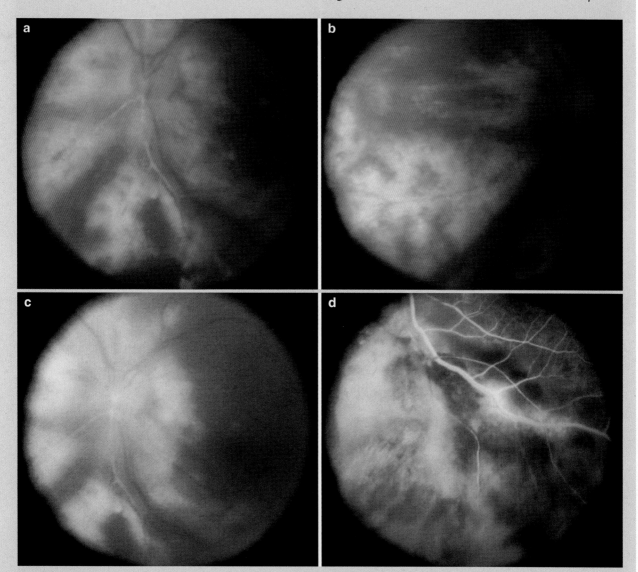

Fig. 15.8 (**a, b**) There is an unclearly defined left optic disc, slightly dilated veins, inferior retinal arterial stenosis into a white line, yellowish white foci and flaky hemorrhage along the venous wall in the superior, inferior nasal and inferior temporal retina. Little spots of irregular yellowish white particles scattered in the macula, a flaky yellowish white effusion with a bleeding cap in the retina surrounding temporal macula. (**c, d**) FFA demonstrates early superficial capillary dilation of the left optic disc, delayed filling time of the inferior artery and vein, weakened background fluorescence of the yellowish white lesion areas, with visible retinal atrophy and flaky penetrating fluorescence, incomplete filling of inferior temporal arteries, large flakes of no filling areas surrounding the optic disk and inferior to the retina. Flaky hemorrhage of the retina to cover the fluorescence, low fluorescence of the retina corresponding to the yellowish white particles of the macula, unclearly defined structures of the macular arch. In the advanced stage, fluorescein effusions from the left optic disk in locally strengthened fluorescence, fluorescein staining of the borderlines of non-filling areas in the inferior retina and in peripheral areas of the optic disc, segmental staining of the arteries and veins in the lesion areas with fluorescein effusions and strong fluorescence of the retina in the lesion areas. (**a–f**) HIV/AIDS related cytomegalovirus retinitis. (**e**) It is demonstrated to have retinal atrophy in the original foci, with scattering spot liked and flaky pigment deposit and thinner blood vessels. (**f**) FFA demonstrates weakened fluorescence of the retinal blood vessels, fluorescein staining of the lesions in the advanced stage and staining of some blood vessels

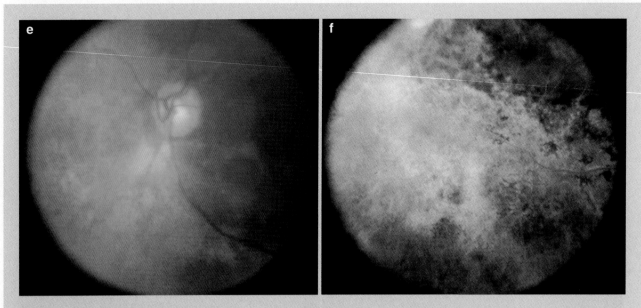

Fig.15.8 (continued)

Case Study 3

A female patient aged 52 years with AIDS was confirmatively diagnosed by CDC. She had no history of hypertension and arteriosclerosis but had symptoms of general weakness and pain, binocular blurry eyesight, cough, fever, gastric upset and poor appetite. Her BP was 12/8 kPa and CD4 T cell count was 13/μl. Ophthalmological examinations indicated right eyesight 4.3 and left eyesight 4.7, binocular ciliary congestion, transparent cornea, KP negative, aqueous flaring negative, floaters negative and transparent lens.

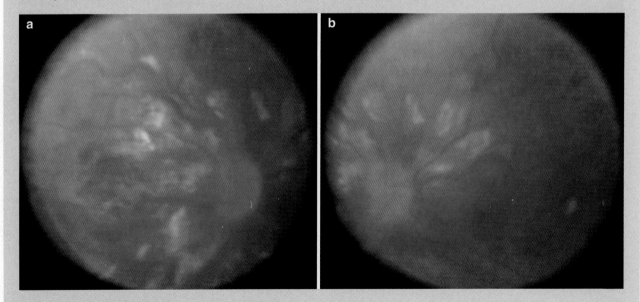

Fig. 15.9 (a–d) HIV/AIDS related cytomegalovirus retinitis and central retinal vein occlusion of the left eye. (**a**, **b**) There is an unclearly defined right optic disc, abundant cotton wool plaques and scattering strips and flakes of hemorrhage surrounding the optic disc, diffuse hemorrhage of the retinal veins with circuitous venules with some minor branches like white lines, mostly lateral to the nose. (**c**) FFA demonstrates delayed reflux time of the right ocular vein, arteries with different diameters, circuitous veins, fluorescein effusions of the optic disc to cover fluorescence, retinal minor vessel occlusion and unclearly defined structure of macular arch. In the advanced stage, stained retinal arterial and venous walls, leakage of different severities, hemorrhage to cover the fluorescence. (**d**) FFA demonstrates fluorescein effusions of the optic disc with peripheral fluorescence covered, retinal minor vessel occlusion

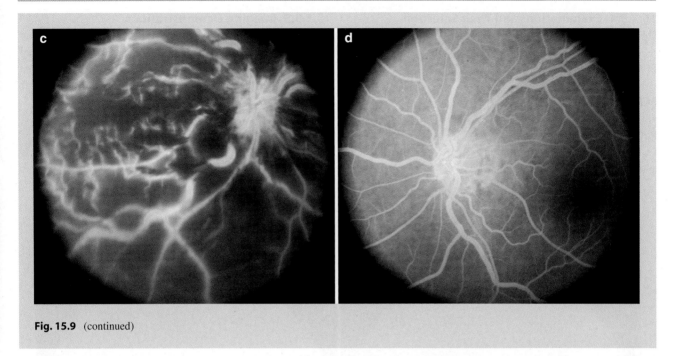

Fig. 15.9 (continued)

15.3.2.6 Criteria for the Diagnosis

1. HIV infection confirmed by CDC.
2. Progressive decrease of the eyesight, blurry vision and floaters in front of the eyes.
3. Ophthalmoscopy demonstrations of fundus artery congestion and edema with brush-liked hemorrhage along the vessels as well as cotton wool liked plaques.
4. FFA demonstrations of fluorescein effusions peripheral to blood vessels.
5. Giant cells inclusions by biopsy.
6. Detectable CMV by PCR.

15.3.2.7 Differential Diagnosis

1. It should be principally differentiated from atypical CMV retinitis. Such patients usually have vitreous infiltration with involvements of peripheral retina. For cases with severe vision loss, acute retina necrosis is most likely to occur.
2. In patients with HIV infection, when no other general diseases occur they may develop uveitis, retinal vasculitis and optic neuritis, with manifestations of vitreous humour infiltration as well as retinal and choroidal infiltrations.
3. It is generally difficult to be differentiated from other infectious retinitis. However, CMV retinitis can be complicated by typical changes of vascular infiltration and hemorrhage along vessels. Therefore, it can be differentiated from other infectious retinitis by laboratory tests. Most importantly, it should be differentiated from toxoplasma retinitis, for which about 15 % patients have poor outcomes after treatments, with unclearly defined lesions and a chronic

progression. Acute retinal necrosis is common in herpes retinitis of AIDS patients, mostly caused by VZV.

15.3.3 HIV/AIDS Related Varicella-Zoster Virus Retinitis

15.3.3.1 Pathogen and Pathogenesis

VZV infection in AIDS patients can result in necrotic herpes retinopathy (NHR), whose incidence is less than 1 %.

15.3.3.2 Pathophysiological Basis

VZV infection can cause necrosis of the whole retina and loss of retinal structure. When blood-retina barrier is invaded, VZV invades the retina. The minor arterial occlusion causes swelling of the local retinal nerve fibers and stagnation of axoplasmic flow, which further leads to cotton-wool which liked plaques in the fundus.

15.3.3.3 Clinical Symptoms and Signs

NHR is clinically divided into acute retina necrosis syndrome and progressive retina necrosis syndrome. The acute type commonly occurs in the healthy populations or AIDS patients with slightly compromised immunity. The progressive type occurs in AIDS patients with severely compromised immunity. Both have fast progression clinically, with poor prognosis. The acute type has three combined clinical manifestations, namely peripheral retinitis, vitritis and retinal arteritis. About 59–70 % cases of NHR show involvement of both eyes, sometimes with retrobulbar optic neuritis and vision loss that is irresponsible to macular degeneration.

15.3.3.4 Examinations and Their Selection
Ophthalmoscopy

FFA

PCR

Pathological Examinations
Pathological examinations demonstrate inclusion bodies and antigens in VZV cells.

15.3.3.5 Imaging Demonstrations
The diagnostic imaging demonstrates swollen, blurry and effusion of the optic papilla, with flakes and spots liked retinal hemorrhage. FFA demonstrates thinner and circuitous retinal blood vessels and hidden fluorescence by hemorrhage.

Case Study 1
A boy aged 2 years was confirmatively diagnosed as having AIDS by CDC. He was infected by vertical transmission. His CD4 cell count was 8/μl.

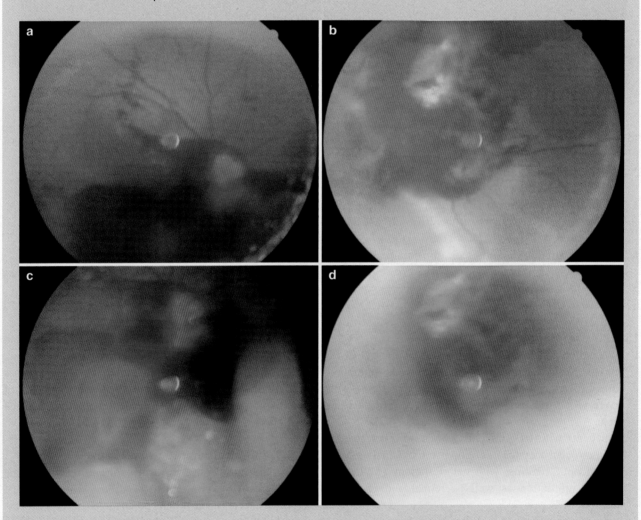

Fig. 15.10 (**a–d**) Ophthalmoscopic demonstrates flakes and spots liked hemorrhage and old effusions of the binocular retina. (**a–f**) HIV/AIDS related VZV retinitis. (**e, f**) Ophthalmoscopic demon- strates spot liked and flakes of yellowish effusions and organized plaques in the binocular retina

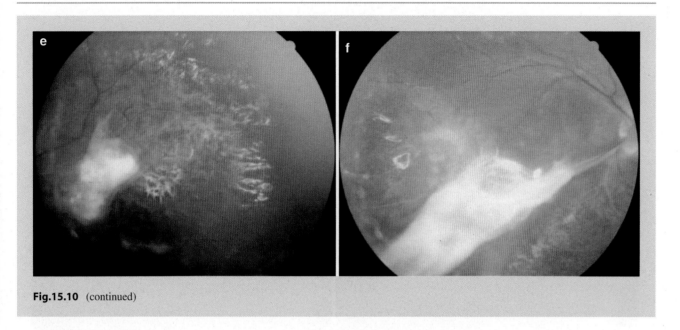

Fig.15.10   (continued)

Case Study 2

A male patient aged 30 years with AIDS was confirmatively diagnosed by CDC. He had a history of paid blood donation and now developed high fever, lung infection, progressively severe vision decrease and evident floaters in front of the right eye. And his CD4 T cell count was 4/μl.

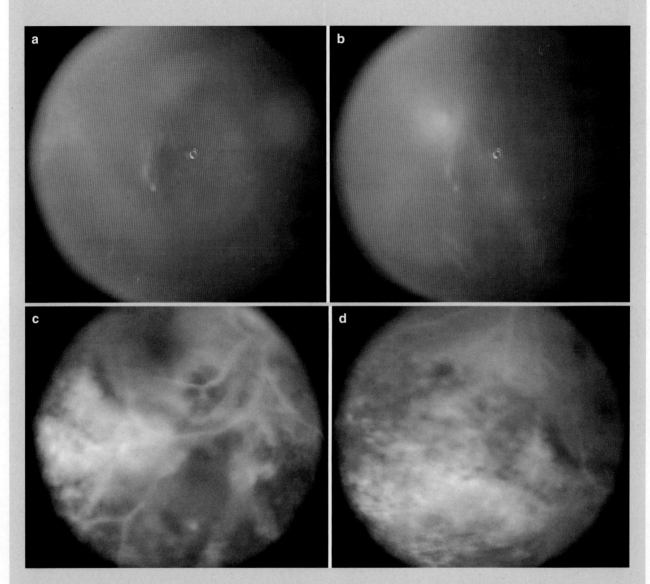

Fig. 15.11 (**a–d**) HIV/AIDS related VZV retinitis, retrobulbar scleral staphyloma and retinal detachment. (**a, b**) It is demonstrated to have opaque binocular vitreous humor, flush optic papilla with unclearly defined boundaries, scattering flakes and strips of hemorrhage with yellowish white effusions at the posterior pole of the right eye, scattering small flakes of hemorrhage along the inferior or superior temporal blood vessels, yellowish white effusions and hemorrhage in the peripheral retina. (**c, d**) FFA demonstrates fluorescein staining of the right optic disc with fluorescence covered by hemorrhage, diffuse fluorescein effusions in the inferior retina, segmental staining of the retinal vessels in the lesion areas, and involvement of the macular region

15.3.3.6 Criteria for the Diagnosis

1. HIV infection confirmed by CDC.
2. Progressive decrease of vision, blurry vision and floaters in front of the eyes.
3. Ophthalmoscopic demonstrations of fundus arteriectasis from congestion and exudative changes of fundus vessels.
4. FFA demonstrations of fluorescein effusions surrounding the vessels.
5. Detectable VZV by PCR.

15.3.3.7 Differential Diagnosis

1. Generally, CMV retinitis occurs based on VZV infection.
2. HIV-infected patients can develop uveitis, retinal vasculitis and optic neuritis, with manifestations of vitreous infiltration as well as retinal and choroidal infiltration.
3. Its differentiation from other infectious retinitis should depend on laboratory tests for the definitive diagnosis.

15.3.4 HIV/AIDS Related Toxoplasma Retinitis with Accompanying Retinal Detachment

15.3.4.1 Pathogen and Pathogenesis

In patients with AIDS, the incidence rate of toxoplasma retinitis is 1–2 %. About 56 % patients with ocular toxoplasmosis have concurrent cerebral toxoplasma infection.

Toxoplasma gondii can be found in the retina, optic nerve and uvea of the affected eye.

15.3.4.2 Pathophysiological Basis

HIV/AIDS related toxoplasma retinitis has more evident intraocular inflammatory responses, with common manifestations of retinal necrosis but less obvious hemorrhage.

15.3.4.3 Clinical Symptoms and Signs

Clinical manifestations of HIV/AIDS related toxoplasma retinitis are similar to CMV infection, including blurry vision, defected vision fields and floaters in front of the eyes.

15.3.4.4 Examinations and Their Selection

1. Ophthalmoscopy.
2. FFA.
3. PCR is facilitative to its etiological diagnosis.
4. Pathological examination can detect inclusion bodies and antigens in VZV cells.

15.3.4.5 Imaging Demonstrations

Ophthalmoscopic demonstrations include large flakes of dense yellowish white effusions with patches of hemorrhage, the involvement of macula region, varied severities of artery stenosis, circuitous and dilated veins, white sheathing of arteriovenous walls; FFA demonstrations of artery stenosis and circuitous arteries as well as fluorescein effusions of the lesion areas.

Case Study

A female patient aged 30 years was confirmatively diagnosed as having AIDS by CDC. She had symptoms of headache and nausea for 1 week. Head MR imaging demonstrated cerebral toxoplasma infection. After therapies against toxoplasma gondii for 1 month, she had blurry vision and floaters in front of the eyes. Her CD4 T cell count was 17/μl. Toxoplasma antibody was positive.

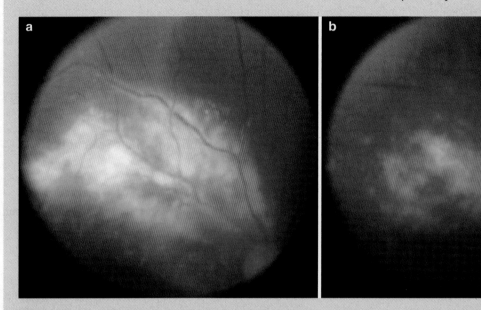

Fig. 15.12 (**a**, **b**) HIV/AIDS related orbital toxoplasma retinitis accompanied with retinal detachment. (**a**, **b**) There is a large flakes of dense yellowish white effusions with patches of hemorrhage in the superior temporal retina of the right eye, involvement of the macular region, stenosis of arteries with varied severity, circuitous and dilated veins as well as accompanying white sheathing in arteriovenous walls

15.3.4.6 Criteria for the Diagnosis

1. HIV infection confirmed by CDC.
2. Progressive decrease of vision and blurry vision
3. Ophthalmoscopy indicates fundus arteriectasis from congestion with brush-liked hemorrhage, large flakes of dense yellowish white effusions in the retina companied with patches of hemorrhage.
4. FFA shows fluorescein effusions around blood vessels.
5. Immunological examination indicates positive for IgG and IgE antibodies.
6. Biopsy can detect toxoplasma tachyzoite.

15.3.4.7 Differential Diagnosis

1. CMV retinitis
2. VZV retinitis
3. PCP retinitis

15.3.5 HIV/AIDS Related Pneumocystis Carinii Retinitis

15.3.5.1 Pathogen and Pathogenesis

HIV/AIDS related pneumocystis carinii infection is a clinically common general infection, mostly involving lungs. Ocular pneumocysis carinii infection has an occurrence of less than 1 %. Occurrence of pneumocystis carinii choroiditis indicates general spreading of pneumocysis carinii.

15.3.5.2 Pathophysiological Basis

HIV/AIDS related histopathological examinations can detect cystic or crescent shaped pneumocystis carinii enveloped by foam liked substances.

15.3.5.3 Clinical Symptoms and Signs

HIV/AIDS related pneumocysis carinii choroiditis has a chronic progression, with unobvious decrease of the vision; fundus demonstrations of multiple yellowish choroidal foci with clearly defined borderlines at the posterior pole and mild inflammatory responses.

15.3.5.4 Examinations and Their Selections

1. Ophthalmoscopy
2. FFA
3. Pathological biopsy

15.3.5.5 Imaging Demonstrations

Ophthalmoscopy indicates light-colored optic papilla, massive yellowish white effusions in its surrounding retina, bleeding at the surfaces of the effusions, stenosis and thinner retinal arteries and veins, white sheathing of some retinal veins and arteries, white line liked arteries; FFA demonstrates fluorescein effusions and retinal artery stenosis.

Case Study

A male patient aged 43 years was confirmatively diagnosed as having AIDS by CDC. He had symptoms of severe decrease of vision and his CD4 T cell count was 26/μl.

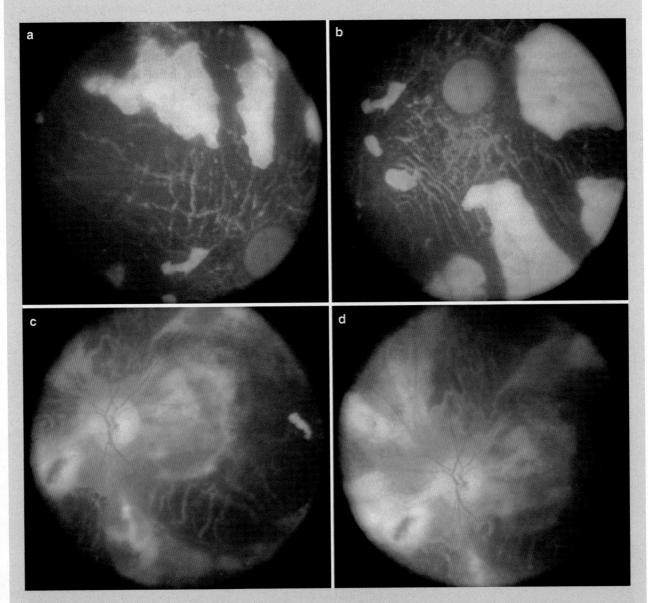

Fig. 15.13 (a–d) HIV/AIDS related pneumocystis carinii retinitis and optic nerve atrophy. (a) It is demonstrated to have right optic papilla in color of wax yellow, abundant yellowish white effusions in the papillary peripheral retina and stenosis of retinal blood vessels. (b–d) It is demonstrated to have light-colored left optic papilla, abundant yellowish white effusions in the papillary peripheral retina with hemorrhage at the surface of the effusions, stenosis of retinal arteries and veins sometimes with white sheathing, and inferior nasal artery shown in white line

15.3.5.6 Differential Diagnosis
It should be differentiated from CMV retinitis and VZV retinitis.

15.3.6 HIV/AIDS Related Tuberculous Retinitis

15.3.6.1 Pathogen and Pathogenesis
Dissemination of M. tuberculosis via blood causes tuberculous retinitis, which hyperplastic inflammation with large quantity of infections and weak allergic responses of tissues. In HIV-infected patients, Gram-positive bacteria infections commonly occur, with involvement of mycobacterium infection such as MTB and MAC to eyes. For instance, Shafran et al. [36]. reported in 1994 the symptoms of uveitis caused by MAC.

15.3.6.2 Pathophysiological Basis
It is rarely found, characterized by formation of atypical granulomas, absence of caseous necrosis and presence of numerous giant cells. In these giant cells, acid-fast bacilli tuberculosis can be detected. Choroidal granuloma can involve peripheral retina to cause edema and inflammatory effusions.

15.3.6.3 Clinical Symptoms and Signs
Tuberculous disseminated chorioretinitis is transient bacteremia secondary to general inactive primary foci. It is commonly found in the young or the middle-aged populations, with onset in both eyes. MAC infection can also result in choroidal granuloma which is a local manifestation of disseminated MAC infection and is usually concurrent with CMV retinitis. In the early stage, the patients only experience photopsia or floaters in front of the eyes.

15.3.6.4 Examinations and Their Selections
1. Ophthalmoscopy
2. FFA
3. Pathological biopsy

15.3.6.5 Imaging Demonstrations
Ophthalmoscopy shows unclear refractive media, blurry large flakes of hemorrhage and yellowish white effusions along the blood vessels in nasal lateral optic disk and superior retina, varying degrees of vascular stenosis and white sheathing in the lesions, clear refractive media of the left eye and slight varicose of fundus veins.

Case Study
A male patient aged 30 years was confirmatively diagnosed as having AIDS by CDC. He had a history of cervical lymphoid tuberculosis and miliary pulmonary tuberculosis. Currently, his eyesight had decreased for 2 weeks, with the right eye being more severe and blurry eyesight of the left eye. His CD4 T cell count was 3/μl.

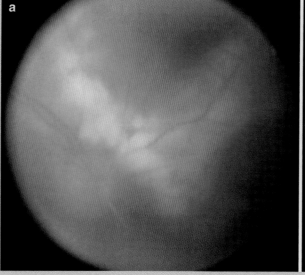
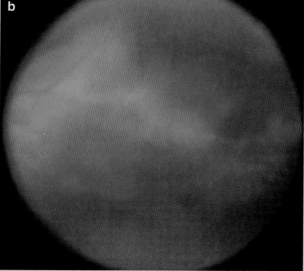
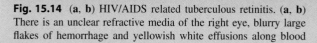

Fig. 15.14 (**a, b**) HIV/AIDS related tuberculous retinitis. (**a, b**) There is an unclear refractive media of the right eye, blurry large flakes of hemorrhage and yellowish white effusions along blood vessels in the nasal lateral optic disc and superior retina; varying degrees of vascular stenosis and white sheathing; clear refractive media of the left eye; slight varicose of the fundus veins

15.3.6.6 Criteria for the Diagnosis

1. HIV infection confirmed by CDC
2. Progressive decrease of eyesight and blurry vision
3. Ophthalmoscopy indicates light-colored optic papilla surrounded by large quantity of yellowish white effusions topped by hemorrhage, stenosis and thinner retinal arteries and veins sometimes with white sheathing, white line liked subnasal artery.
4. FFA indicates fluorescein effusions around blood vessels.
5. Acid-fast bacilli staining of the biopsy can detect acid-fast bacilli.

15.3.6.7 Differential Diagnosis

It should be differentiated from CMV retinitis and VZV retinitis.

15.3.7 HIV/AIDS Related Cryptococcal Retinitis

HIV/AIDS related cryptococcus infection rarely occurs singularly, usually as local manifestations of general cryptococcosis that may be caused by dissemination of meningeal, pulmonary foci or foci of other areas. The common manifestations are circuitous retinal artery, swollen optic papilla, hemorrhage, necrosis, and occasional granuloma in AIDS patients. Subjective symptoms are not severe but with a long duration.

Case Study 1

A female patient aged 34 years was confirmatively diagnosed as having AIDS by CDC. She had a history of drug abuse and complained of headache, hands and feet numbness and severe decrease of eyesight. Her CD4 T cell count was 10/μl.

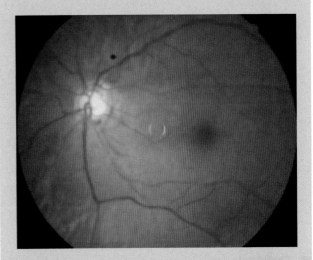

Fig. 15.15 HIV/AIDS related cryptococcus retinitis. Ophthalmoscopic demonstrates swollen right optic papilla with unclearly defined borderline, and circuitous binocular retinal arteries

Case Study 2

A male patient aged 44 years was confirmatively diagnosed as having AIDS by CDC. He complained of decreased binocular eyesight and blurry vision. His CD4 T cell count was 44/μl.

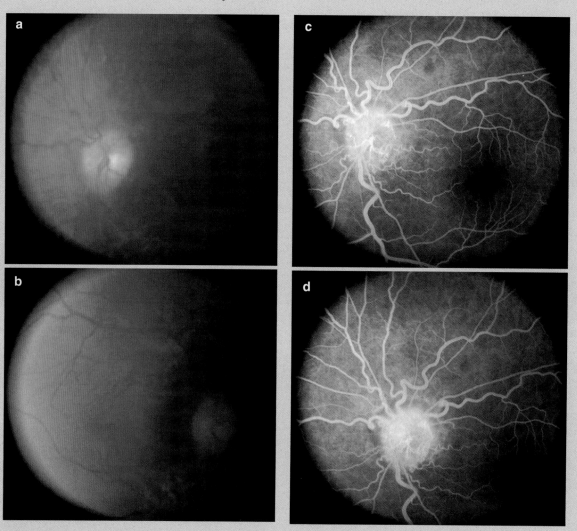

Fig. 15.16 (**a–d**) HIV/AIDS related cryptococcal retinitis and binocular optic nerve injuries. (**a, b**) It is demonstrated to have flushing binocular optic discs with blurry borderlines, circuitous and dilated veins as well as straightened and thinner arteries. (**c, d**) FFA demonstrates lesions of the advanced stage, high fluorescence of the binocular optic discs

15.3.8   HIV/AIDS Related Optic Neuropathy

In HIV infected patients, autoimmune diseases can be readily found, especially in the latent period with favorable immune functions but dysfunctional immunity control mechanism. Optic nerve papilla edema, papillitis and retrobulbar neuritis may occur, for which HARRT therapy could be tried for their treatment. Sometimes, clinical symptoms are not in consistency with the findings by fundus examination. In cases of photopsia and progressive defects of vision field, the fundus examination may show normal findings. HIV/AIDS related optic neuropathy is related to the decrease of the CD4 T cell count. About 50 % AIDS patients suffer from immunosuppressive oculopathy without opportunistic infections. Such oculopathy has no impact on the vision, with a stable duration for 3–4 weeks and automatic subsiding.

Case Study

A female patient aged 54 years was confirmatively diagnosed as having AIDS by CDC. She had a history of paid blood donation and currently experienced blurry vision of the right eye, feet and hands numbness, headache, and tremendous decrease of eyesight. Her CD4 T cell count was 10/ μl

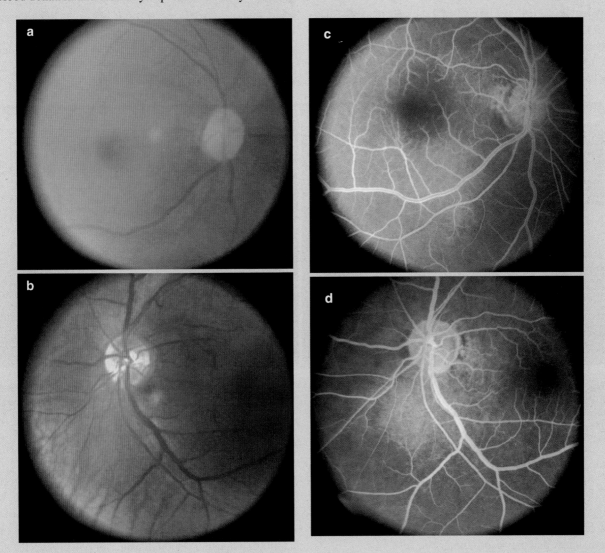

Fig. 15.17 (**a–d**) HIV/AIDS related optic nerve injuries. (**a, b**) It is demonstrated to have flushing right optic disc with unclear borderline as well as circuitous retinal veins. (**c**) There is a circuitous of left retinal veins. (**c, d**) FFA demonstrates primary stage of right optic nerve injuries, dilated capillaries of the optic disc, and slight staining of the optic disc; advanced stage of right optic nerve injuries, fluorescein staining of the optic disc with blurry borderline, normal fluorescence of the optic disc, circuitous and dilated retinal blood vessels

15.3.9   HIV/AIDS Related Retinal Detachment

The retinal pigment epithelium and the retinal inner nine layers are closely connected at the optic papilla and the ora serrata. The other parts of the retinal pigment epithelium and the retinal inner nine layers are loosely bound by pigment epithelium processes and mucopolysaccharide with potential spaces between them. The basilar membrane of the pigment epithelium, the coating of hyaline membrane of the choroid, is formed by small enclosed bands between pigment cells to prevent choroidal fluid effusion into the inner layer of the retina. It also sustains the metabolisms of optic rods and cones cells to form the exterior barrier of the retina to maintain its dryness. The endothelial cells of the retinal blood vessels are closely connected with presence of pericytes in the vascular walls to serve as the interior barrier of the retina that prevents plasma or other tangible substances from permeating out. Therefore, barrier dysfunction of any cause can lead to retinal detachment which is a relatively severe and common oculopathy in young and middle aged patients with AIDS that may cause blindness.

Case Study

A female patient aged 51 years was confirmatively diagnosed as having AIDS by CDC. She had onset of symptoms in 2006. About 3 months ago, she suddenly had blurry vision of the right eye that was progressively severe, swelling and pain of the left eye, right side headache and absent contents of vision. Ophthalmological examination indicates normal left eyesight, light sensation of inferior right eye within 0.5 m, transparent cornea, clear lens, and no obvious opacity of the vitreum. Fundus examination shows retinal detachment with dark grey in color. Her CD4 T cell count was 30/ μl.

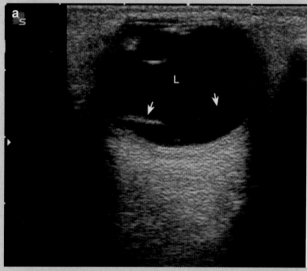 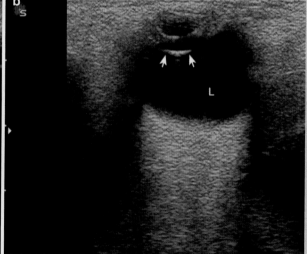

Fig. 15.18 (**a, b**) HIV/AIDS related Retinal Detachment. (**a, b**) Color Doppler ultrasound demonstrates strong echo light band in the left optic vitreum in a shape of V with the depression forwards and posterior motion negative (*arrow*). CDFI demonstrations of visible blood flow signals continuing to the retinal central arteries and veins; its frequencies spectrum being identical to the retinal central arteries and veins (*arrow*)

Oculopathy is a sign of AIDS. Because the autoimmune defects in AIDS patients, above 75 % AIDS patients have ocular involvement. About 25 % AIDS patients have retinal detachment of varying severities, which is a common and severe illness that may cause blindness.

15.3.10   HIV/AIDS Related Posterior Vitreous Detachment

The vitreum is a clear gel structure filling 4/5 retrobulbar space, which is composed of collagen fibers, mucopolysaccharide or matrix and soluble proteins. Its cortex is relatively compact, known as the boundary membrane. The normal vitreum is immediately posterior to the lens with touch, with an interface of its other part to the internal coating of the eyeball, and is immediately anterior to the peripheral optic papilla and macular region. Its anterior part crosses the anterior part of the retinal ora serrata to reach the ciliary pars plana. Anterior or posterior to the retinal ora serrata of about 6 mm, the ring shaped area is the basilar vitreum, with the closest interconnection of tissues. Vitreous degeneration necessarily causes posterior vitreous detachment with the vitreum detached from the retina. With the increased range of detachment, the closely bound optic disc and the vitreous basement is remained. At this time, the rapid movement of eyes could induce the vitreous movement, which leads to separation of the vitreum from the retina at the optic disc with final occurrence of complete vitreous detachment. The

detached vitreum exerts traction on the retina, which may lead to retinal rupture that contributes to retinal detachment.

Case Study

A female patient aged 45 years was confirmatively diagnosed as having AIDS by CDC. Her onset of symptoms was in 2005. She complained of evident eyesight decrease for several months. Her CD4 T cell count was 55/µl.

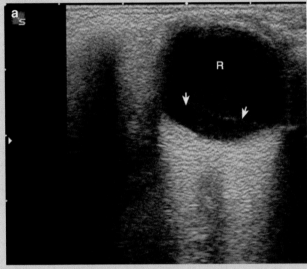

Fig. 15.19 (a, b) HIV/AIDS related posterior vitreous detachment. (a, b) Color Doppler ultrasound demonstrates continuous light strip band in the right vitreum (*arrow*), disconnected to the fundus; obvious mobility and posterior motion; CDFI demonstrates no obvious blood flow signals

---

Color Doppler flow imaging (CDFI) has been an important examination for the diagnosis of oculopathy. Ultrasound can provide reliable diagnostic information as a clinical and specialized examination. With aging, severe myopia and degeneration of collagen fibers and hyaluronic acid, namely the liquefaction and fusion of the gel, can reach the posterior vitreous boundary membrane anterior to the macula to cause rupture of the posterior boundary membrane. Therefore, the liquid flows into the retinal-vitreous space to cause posterior vitreous detachment. With the increased flow of the liquid into the space, the condition is progressively severe. The high liquefaction of the vitreum causes high incidence of posterior vitreous detachment. The complete posterior vitreous detachment, separation of the vitreous posterior boundary membrane from the retinal inner boundary membrane, ranges from the posterior pole to ora serratta (the vitreous base). The ultrasound demonstrations include retrobulbar continuous arc-shaped light strips disconnected to the fundus, evident motion degree and backward movement, no blood flow signal from the strip liked echo band. Partial posterior vitreous detachment is referred to as the vitreous posterior boundary membrane is connected to the fundus by its partial adherence to the optic disc, peripheral macula, peripheral major blood vessels or inner boundary membrane of the

degenerative retina, with obvious motions along with the motions of the eyeball. In addition, the static eyeball is along with motions of the lesions, namely posterior motion test positive. The demonstrations include the continuous light strips to the retina being smooth, arch shaped, large range of motion, obvious posterior motion and no blood flow signal from the light strips of vitreum. The ultrasound can be applied for the differential diagnosis of posterior vitreous detachment to other light strips of intraocular organized membrane, such as retinal detachment, choroid detachment and vitreous organized membrane. In cases of retinal detachment, the light strip of strong echo in the vitreum is in shape of V with its depression facing the front, with posterior motion negative. CDFI demonstrates continuous blood flow signal to the retinal central arteries and veins in the light strips, identical frequencies spectrum to the retinal central arteries and veins. In the vitreum with choroid detached, there are multiple arch shaped light strips connecting to the eyeball wall, with convex toward the vitreum. The eyeball rotates toward the lateral nose, with intravitreous multiple continuous light strips, namely rose sign positive. The complete choroid detachment demonstrates a shape of X, with central anastomosis. There is blood flow signal in the light strips with blood flow frequencies spectrum of arterial type, being close to posterior ciliary artery. The light strip of the vitreous organized membrane is irregular in shape, being curved with branches in different sizes. The intensity of echoes is heterogenous, with unclearly defined borderline, contact to the eyeball wall and obvious motions. For cases with multiple adhesion points, the posterior motions is not obvious. CDFI demonstrates no blood flow signal in the organized membrane. Posterior vitreous detachment has typical demonstrations by ultrasound. Based on the findings in static images, in combination of dynamic observation and 3 dimensional reasoning, the currently applied high frequency probe equipped with Color Doppler ultrasonograph can accurately diagnosed posterior vitreous detachment.

Extended Reading

1. Barnes PF, Bloch AB, Davidson PT, et al. Tuberculosis in patients with human immunodeficiency virus infection. N Engl J Med. 1991;324:1644–50.
2. Barre-Sinoussi F, Chermann J, Rey P, et al. Isolation of a T-lymphotrophic retrovirus from a patient at risk for AIDS. Science. 1983;220:868–71.
3. Baxter J, Mayers D, Wentworth D, et al. A pilot study of the short term effects of antiretroviral management based on plasma genotypic antiretroviral resistance testing (GART) in patients failing antiretroviral therapy. In: Sixth conference on retroviruses and opportunistic infections, Chicago, Feb 1999. Abstract LB8.
4. Behrens G, Schmidt H, Meyer D, et al. Vascular complications associated with the use of HIV protease inhibitors. Lancet. 1998;351:1958.
5. Biggar RJ, Rabkin CS. The epidemiology of acquired immunodeficiency syndrome-related lymphomas. Curr Opin Oncol. 1992;4:883–93.
6. Brau N, Leaf HL, Wieczorek RL, et al. Severe hepatitis in three AIDS patients treated with indinavir. Lancet. 1997;349:924–5.
7. Brennal R, Durack D. Gay compromise syndrome. Lancet. 1981;2:1338–9.
8. Budka H. Human immunodeficiency virus (HIV)-in-duced disease of the central nervous system: pathology and implications for pathogenesis. Acta Neuropathol. 1989;77:225–36.
9. Buv'e A. HIV/AIDS in Africa: why so severe, why so heterogeneous?. In: 7th conference on retroviruses and opportunistic infections, San Francisco, 30 Jan–2 Feb 2000. Abstract S28.
10. Caccamo D, Pervez NK, Marchevsky A. Primary lymphoma of the liver in the acquired immunodeficiency syndrome. Arch Pathol Lab Med. 1986;110:553–5.
11. Centers for Disease Control and Prevention U.S. HIV and AIDS cases reported through December 1999. Year-End Edition. vol 11, No. 2.
12. Deeks SG, Smith M, Holodniy M, Kahn J. HIV-1 protease inhibitors. A review for clinicians. JAMA. 1997;277:145–53.
13. DHHS Panel on Clinical Practices for Treatment of HIV Infections Guidelines for use of antiretroviral agents in HIV-infected adults and adolescents. 28 Jan 2000 revision. Available at: http://havatis.org.
14. Di Barbaro G, Lorenzo G, Grisorio B, Barbarini G. Incidence of dilated cardiomyopathy and detection of HIV in myocardial cells of HIV-infected patients. N Engl J Med. 1999;399:1093–9.
15. Gal AA, Klatt EC, Koss MN, et al. The effectiveness of bronchoscopy in the diagnosis of pneumocystis carinii and cytomegalovirus pulmonary infections in acquired immunodeficiency syndrome. Arch Pathol Lab Med. 1987;111:238–41.
16. Gallo R, Salahuddin S, Popovic M, et al. Frequent detection and isolation of cytopathic retroviruses (HTLVIII) from patients with AIDS and at risk for AIDS. Science. 1984;224:500–3.
17. Garcia PM, Kalish LA, Pitt J, et al. Maternal levels of plasma human immunodeficiency virus type 1 RNA and the risk of perinatal transmission. Women and Infants Transmission Study Group. N Engl J Med. 1999;341:394–402.
18. Gold JE, Altarac D, Ree HJ. HIV associated Hodgkin disease: a clinical study of 18 cases and review. Am J Hematol. 1991;39:93–9.
19. Goldman GD, Milstone LM, Shapiro PE. Histologic findings in acute HIV exanthem. J Cutan Pathol. 1995;22:371–3.
20. Grody WW, Cheng L, Lewis W. Infection of the heart by the human immunodeficiency virus. Am J Cardiol. 1990;66:203–6.
21. Hammer SM, Squires K, Hughes M, et al. A controlled trial of two nucleoside analogues plus indinavir in persons with human immunodeficiency virus infection and CD4 cell counts of 200 per cubic millimeter or less. AIDS Clinical Trials Group 320 Study Team [see comments]. N Engl J Med. 1997;337:725–33.
22. Janssen RS. Epidemiology and neuroepidemiology of human immunodeficiency virus infection. In: Berger JR, Levy RM, editors. AIDS and the nervous system. 2nd ed. Philadelphia: Lippincott-Raven; 1996. p. 13–37.
23. Levine AM. Epidemiology, clinical characteristics, and management of AIDS-related lymphoma. Hematol Oncol Clin North Am. 1991;5:331–42.
24. Li HJ. The complicated by CMV infection of the eyes with HIV/AIDS. Chin J AIDS STD. 13, 2007–6, No. 3.
25. Lucas SB. Tropical pathology of the female genital tract and ovaries. In: Fox H, editor. Haines and Taylor obstetrical and gynaecological pathology. Edinburgh: Churchill Livingstone; 1995. p. 1209–31.
26. Lucas SB, Hounnou A, Paecock CS, et al. The mortality and pathology of HIV disease in a West African city. AIDS. 1993;7:1569–79.
27. Mehta JB, Dutt A, Harrill L, et al. Epidemiology of extrapulmonary tuberculosis. A comparative analysis with pre-AIDS era. Chest. 1991;99:1134–8.
28. Mellors J, Munoz A, Giorgi J, et al. Plasma viral load and CD4+ lymphocytes as prognostic markers of HIV1 infection. Ann Intern Med. 1997;126:946–54.
29. Oettle AG. Geographical and racial differences in the frequency of Kaposi's sarcoma as evidence of environmental or genetic causes. Acta Unio Int Contra Cancrum. 1962;18:330–63.
30. Paxton LA, Janssen RS. The epidemiology of HIV infection in the era of HAART. J HIV Ther. 2000;5:2–4.
31. Perrients J. AIDS- a global overview. In: Program and abstracts of the 7th European conference on clinical aspects and treatment of HIV-infection, Lisbon, 23–27 Sep 1999.
32. Piot P, O' Rourke M. AIDS in the developing world: an interview with Peter Piot. AIDS Clin Care. 2000;12:1–5.
33. Race EM, Adelson-Mitty J, Barlm TF, et al. Focal mycobacterial lymphadenitis following initiation of pro-tease-inhibitor therapy in patients with advanced HIV-1 disease. Lancet. 1998;351:252–5.
34. Radin DR, Baker EL, Klatt EC, et al. Visceral and nodal calcification in patients with AIDS-related Pneumocystis carinii infection. AJR Am J Roentgenol. 1990;154:27–31.
35. Schwartz DA, Sobottka I, Leitch GJ, et al. Pathology of microsporidiosis. Arch Pathol Lab Med. 1996;20:173–88.
36. Shafran SD, Deschenes J, Miller M, et al. Uveitis and pseudojaundice during a regimen of clarithromycin, rifabutin, and ethabutol. MAC study group of the Canadian HIV trials network. N Engl J Med. 1994;330(6):438–9.

37. Tappero JW, Conant MA, Wolfe SF, et al. Kaposi's sarcoma. Epidemiololgy, pathogenesis, histology, clinical spectrum, staging criteria and therapy. J Am Acad Dermatol. 1993;72:254–61.

38. Thomas D, Astemborski J, Rai R, et al. The natural history of hepatitis C virus infection. JAMA. 2000;284:450–6.

39. Thomsen H, Jacobsen M. Kaposi sarcoma among homosexual men in Europe. Lancet. 1981;2:688.

40. Tschirhart DL, Klatt EC. Disseminated toxoplasmosis in the acquired immunodeficiency syndrome. Arch Pathol Lab Med. 1998;112:1237–41.

41. Vella S, Giuliano M, Pezzotti P, et al. Survival of zidovudine-treated patients with AIDS compared with what of contemporary untreated patients. JAMA. 1992;267:1232–6.

42. Volberding PA, Lagakos S, Kocth M, et al. Zidovudine in asymptomatic human immunodeficiency virus infection: a controlled trial in persons with fewer than 500 CD4-posi-tive cells per cubic millimeter. N Engl J Med. 1990;322:941–9.

Contents

16.1   An Overview of HIV/AIDS Related Neck Diseases

AIDS patients often develop otorhinolaryngological diseases as Marcuser and Sooy [9] reported in 1985 that 165 cases among 399 AIDS patients (41 %) have cranial and cervical symptoms, including oral and pharyngeal KS, candida infection and the most commonly found nasal sinusitis.

HIV/AIDS related lymphoid tuberculosis results in cervical lymphadenectasis. The swollen lymph-node cells are exhausted to necrosis and liquefaction.

HIV/AIDS related otorhinolaryngological diseases include suppurative otitis externa, otitis media, tonsillitis, chronic pharyngitis and sinusitis caused by pathogens of anaerobes, candida, cryptococcus and herpesvirus. All these opportunistic infections are manifestations of compromised immunity.

In terms of HIV/AIDS related thyroid and parathyroid diseases, it is reported that patients with HIV infection have thyroid infections by pathogens of pneumocystis carinii, cryptococcus, CMV and toxoplasma. Thyroiditis can cause functional morphological changes and it has been reported that patients with advanced stage of HIV infection complicated by lymphoma have accompanying hypercalcemia and serum PTH inhibition yet no reports about thyroid lesions in the cases of hypercalcemia.

16.2   HIV/AIDS Related Thyromegaly

16.2.1   Pathogens and Pathogenesis

AIDS can indirectly or directly involve all the systems in the human body and endocrine system is not an exception. HIV/AIDS induced infections, non-specific inflammations, hemorrhage and cancer all wreck damages to the endocrine tissues. Antibodies and cytokines produced by acute and chronic complications such as tumor necrosis factor (TNF), IF-1 and IF-N may interfere functions of the endocrine

H. Li (ed.), *Radiology of HIV/AIDS*,
DOI 10.1007/978-94-007-7823-8_16, © Springer Science+Business Media Dordrecht and People's Medical Publishing House 2014

glands. Medications for their treatment may also impose adverse effects on the endocrine tissues. For instance, Ketoconazole for fungal infections can inhibit synthesis of cortisol and testosterone; Rifampicin against tuberculosis can promote cortisol catabolism; Pentamidine for PCP can result in damages to the islet beta cell. Endocrine dysfunction of AIDS patients vary with severities of the particular conditions and its occurrence may be due to conditions ranging from slightly abnormal hormonal secretions and metabolism to complete failure of an endocrine gland.

It has consistently been reported that changes of thyroid functions and morphology occur in patients with AIDS and the related research has been attracted increasingly focused attention. Asymptomatic patients with AIDS predominantly have normal thyroid function, and increased levels of T3 and T4 are rarely found due to increases of TBG concentration of unknown reasons. However, with progression of AIDS and decrease of TBG level, serum levels of T3 and T4 decline gradually as T4 transforms into T3 in the peripheral tissues and TSH secretion decreases. In advanced stage of AIDS, the patients may sustain slight decrease of HSH level. The changes of thyroid hormone level in patients with AIDS are similar to those with other general chronic diseases. However, the decrease of T3 level in AIDS patients is not as obvious as patients with other general chronic diseases in frequency and severity. There have also been reports about diffuse thyroid enlargement and hyperthyroidism in a few cases of AIDS and it has been speculated in these reports that the compromised immunity of AIDS patients causes immune damages to the thyroid and further causes hyperthyroidism/hypothyroidism and its morphological enlargement. The morphological and structural changes of enlarged thyroid can be detected by the diagnostic imaging.

The causes of HIV/AIDS related thyromegaly remains unclear. It is generally believed that the clinically defined causes of thyromegaly are also applicable to HIV/AIDS related thyromegaly. However, the underlying relations between these causes and AIDS remain elusive.

16.2.1.1 Iodine Deficiency and Thyromegaly Caused by Excessive Iodine

Iodine deficiency is the main cause of endemic thyromegaly, mostly found in inlands and mountain areas with a high altitude far away from oceans. Increased demand for thyroxin in periods of puberty, pregnancy, lactation and menopause as well as a result of mental stimulation and traumas can lead to relative iodine deficiency. In cases of environmental iodine deficiency or decreased serum inorganic iodine concentration, hyperplasia of the thyroid tissues occurs to boost its function of iodine intake. Therefore, the thyroid can take in enough iodine from blood under low iodine condition to ensure synthesis of enough thyroid hormones for physiological demand of the body tissues. However, in cases of severe deficiency of

iodine, this compensation mechanism can not maintain normal thyroid functions so the thyroid preferably synthesizes and secretes T3 which needs less iodine but has stronger activity and T4 synthesis decreases. Moreover, as T4 concentration is an essential cause for pituitary stimulation to produce TSH, decreased T4 concentration increases the pituitary stimulation to produce more TSH which further aggravates thyroid hyperplasia and enlargement. Contrarily, for cases with long-term excessive intake of iodine, excessive inorganic iodine ions in the thyroid tissues can impede iodine organizing process, resulting in decreased synthesis of thyroxin. Additionally, thyroxin release inhibition by abundant iodine contributes to further deficiency of blood thyroxin, which increases TSH synthesis and secretion and causes thyromegaly.

Clinical observation reveals that blood T3 and T4 levels decrease significantly with accompanying decrease of sex hormones. According to the above-mentioned mechanism, decreases of T3 and T4 levels can likewise lead to thyromegaly. Moreover, T3 and T4 level are associated with the survival rate of AIDS patients. The decreases of T3 and T4 levels are the accurate predictor for occurrence of death in AIDS patients.

16.2.1.2 Substances Causing Thyromegaly

It has been demonstrated that some food and drugs may be of certain relations with thyromegaly. For instances, long-term intake of cabbages in a large quantity can result in thyromegaly. It has been found by researchers that organic cyanides in cabbages can interfere in iodide oxidation to affect the synthesis of the thyroid hormones, therefore leading to compensatory thyroid enlargement. Prolonged oral administration of some medicines as potassium cyanide, potassium perchlorate, Aminosalicylic acid, phenyl-butazone, Sulfanilamide and Thioureas can hinder the synthesis of thyroid hormones and inhibit their releases. Consequently, thyroxin in blood decreases and TSH level increases, lead to thyromegaly. AIDS patients are commonly treated with various combinations of drugs. It cannot be excluded that some medicines have impacts on synthesis and release of thyroxin, leading to thyromegaly.

16.2.1.3 Congenital Defects in Thyroid Hormone Synthesis

Synthesis of thyroid hormones cannot be completed without the catalyses of various specialized enzymes. AIDS patients probably have congenital defects in thyroid hormone synthesis. The related symptoms are prone to be clinically manifested in the stage of AIDS.

16.2.1.4 Thyroid Immune Damage due to the Compromised Immunity

It has been reported that AIDS patients may be complicated by hyperthyroidism or hypothyroidism. Observation of thyroid hormone level and immunity suggests that immunological damages to the thyroid tissues may occur but its underlying mechanism has not be definitively reported.

16.2.2 Pathophysiological Basis

The lesion of HIV/AIDS related thyromegaly is diffuse and soft, with no nodules and with diffuse enlargement of the volume including the both lateral lobes and isthmus. Cases with persistent long-term thyromegaly may have multiple nodules, with various sizes, heterogeneous density and possibly formation into cysts, sometimes with accompanying hemorrhage.

16.2.3 Clinical Symptoms and Signs

Thyromegaly complicating HIV/AIDS has principal demonstrations of diffuse enlargement of the thyroid, being soft and with no nodules by palpitation. Thyromegaly can be graded into 3° according to the findings by palpitation: degree I—invisible but palpable enlargement of the thyroid; degree II—visible and palpable enlargement of the thyroid but the thyroid being within sternocleidomastoid; degree III—the enlarged thyroid exceeding the lateral margin of sternocleidomastoid. Diffuse thyroid enlargement rarely results in symptoms of local compression. In the nodular stage, nodules of different sizes occur to compress the trachea, resulting in dyspnea. Or the nodules compress the recurrent laryngeal nerve, resulting in coarse sound. Changes of thyroid functions occur in the advanced stage of AIDS, commonly decreased thyroid functions but with rare reports of hyperthyroidism. The corresponding symptoms of hypothyroidism/hyperthyroidism are concurrent with the clinical symptoms of HIV/AIDS, presenting great difficulty for the differential diagnosis. Therefore, diagnosis of thyroid functions should be based on the blood T3 and T4 levels.

16.2.4 Examinations and Their Selection

Nuclear imaging and ultrasound are important examination methods for thyroid diseases. ECT of thyroid mainly demonstrates iodine intake rate by the thyroid, based on which the differential diagnosis of nodular lesions can be made. Ultrasound can provide a detailed assessment on the shapes and sizes of the thyroid and can sensitively detect the thyroid nodules, calcification and cysts as well as the blood supply of the lesions. CT scanning is commonly applied for the assessment of the thyroid, demonstrating the size, shape and density of the thyroid as well as the nodules, cysts, bleeding and calcification in it. Concerning the invasion and extension of the lesions to the surrounding tissues, CT scanning plays an important role. For instance, in cases of giant thyromegaly compressing the trachea, CT scanning can show the mass extension posterior to the trachea or superior to the mediastinum as well as the compressed changes of the trachea.

16.2.5 Imaging Demonstrations

16.2.5.1 Nuclear Imaging Demonstrations

Nuclear imaging demonstrates homogeneous radioactive distribution of the bilateral lobes that are similar to the normal thyroid or homogeneous increase of radioactive concentration. For cases with nodules, the demonstrations include local defects of radioactive distribution in the thyroid parenchyma, being worm-eaten liked.

16.2.5.2 Ultrasound Demonstrations

Ultrasound demonstrates homogeneous enlargement of thyroid parenchyma, with its severity being related to the course and severity of the illness. The interior echo is normal, moderate and homogeneous, with occasionally scattering cystic nodules in homogeneous non-echo areas with smooth borderlines. CDFI generally demonstrates no obvious abnormalities.

16.2.5.3 CT Scanning Demonstrations

CT scanning demonstrates diffuse enlargement of the thyroid with symmetric enlargement of the bilateral lobes and isthmus. The tissues density may be normal but commonly decreases. It is likely to be diffuse scattering spot liked lower density shadows in the thyroid. By enhanced scanning, there is obvious homogeneous enhancement with clearly defined borderlines. The highly enlarged thyroid can compress its surrounding tissues for their morphological changes. The compressed trachea can be narrowed and prolonged. For cases with nodular thyromegaly, there are multiple round shaped low density areas in the thyroid parenchyma, with different sizes and clearly defined borderlines. Enhanced scanning demonstrates the lower enhancement of the thyroid than its surrounding parenchyma. No obvious enhancement of the foci indicates formation of cysts.

16.2.5.4 MR Imaging Demonstrations

MR imaging demonstrates the same morphological changes. Enlarged thyroid parenchyma shows homogeneous moderate high signal by T2WI and homogenous equal or slightly high signal by T1WI based on the varying protein concentrations in the parenchyma. The cysts show regional higher signal by T2WI and relatively lower signal by T1WI with smooth borderlines. The enlarged nodules are demonstrated as moderate high signal that is slightly lower than the peripheral parenchyma by T2WI, and regional high signal by T1WI with smooth borderlines.

Case Study 1

A female patient aged 49 years with AIDS was confirmatively diagnosed by CDC. The onset of symptoms was accidentally found in 2001. The mass was located in the right anterior cervical thyroid which could move upward and downward along with swallowing. Her CD4 T cell count was 37/μl.

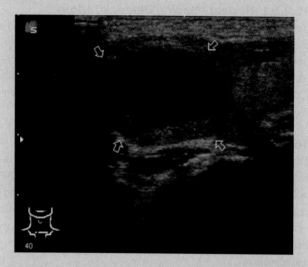

Fig. 16.1 HIV/AIDS related thyroid adenoma (follicular adenoma). Color ultrasonography demonstrates cystic parenchymal mass in size of 45×35 mm in the right thyroid lobe (*arrows*), with clearly defined borderline, predominant liquid low echo inside with intervals of strip liked slightly high echo. CDFI demonstrates unobvious blood flow signal in and surrounding the mass

Case Study 2

A female patient aged 53 years with AIDS was confirmatively diagnosed by CDC. The onset of symptoms was in 2003. She had fever and was detected with nodules in the left thyroid lobe by cervical examinations. Her CD4 T cell count was 37/μl.

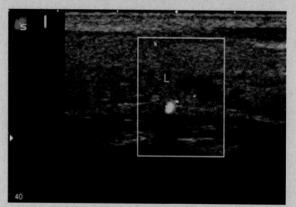

Fig. 16.2 HIV/AIDS related thyroid adenoma (papillary adenoma). Color ultrasonography demonstrates a cystic parenchymal low echo nodule in the left thyroid lobe. The nodule is clearly defined in size of 12×6 mm with liquid low density inside and a papillary adhesive wall with slightly high echo. CDFI demonstrates papillary blood flow signals with slightly high echo

16.2.6   Discussions

Occurrence of thyroid diseases in AIDS patients is increasingly high in recent years, and thyroid adenoma is the most commonly seen disease. Clinically, thyroid adenoma is common, with a high occurrence, which mostly has benign lesions and rarely malignancies. The pathogenesis remains unclear and pathological changes include thyroid follicular hyperplasia and enlargement of thyroid tissues. The begin lesions are soft in texture while the malignant ones are hard. The benign cervical mass is commonly singular, with slow growth. The large one may compress its surrounding tissues. The mass may move upward and downward along with swallowing and is smooth, soft, round or oval in shape, which may cause hyperthyroidism. Conclusively, the principal pathogenic causes include excessive estrogen induced by endocrine disorder, excessive iodine intake and mental conditions.

Pathological classification of thyroid adenoma

1. Follicular adenoma

   The most commonly benign thyroid tumors which can further divided into the following five types: (1) Embryonal adenoma; (2) Fetal adenoma; (3) Colloidal adenoma, also known as Giant follicular adenoma; (4) Simple adenoma; (5) Acidophilic adenoma.

2. Papillary adenoma

   Papillary adenomas are rarely benign and mostly cystic, therefore they are also known as papillary cystadenoma. Thyroid adenoma with papillary structures is most likely to develop into malignancy.

3. Atypical adenoma

   It is relatively rare with complete capsule of the tumor and being hard in texture

4. Thyroid cyst

   It can be classified into colloid cyst, serous cyst, necrotic cyst and hemorrhagic cyst according to its contents.

5. Autonomous hyperfunctioning thyroid adenoma

   In the neoplasm parenchyma, foci of old hemorrhage necrosis, cystic changes, hyaline change, fibrosis and calcification can be found. The tumor tissues are clearly defined, commonly with atrophy of its surrounding thyroid tissues.

6. Toxic thyroid adenoma

   Toxic thyroid adenoma shows enhanced function of thyroid to synthesize and secrete large amount of thyroid hormones resulting in hyperthyroidism. Toxic thyroid adenoma is mostly found in females aged 30–40 years. The adenoma is usually singular and multiple in rare cases. The patients have symptoms of hyperthyroidism and by physical examinations thyroid nodules are commonly found, generally being large in size of several centimeters. Serum T3 and T4 levels increase, especially significant T3 level increase. Thyroid scanning demonstrates that the nodules are hot nodules but radioactive isotopes usually are deficient or decreased in the peripheral thyroid tissues.

16.2.7   Criteria for the Diagnosis

The relationship between HIV infection and thyromegaly remains unclear; hence the diagnosis of HIV/AIDS related thyromegaly basically depends on diagnosis of HIV infection in combination with diagnosis of thyromegaly. In addition to the understanding of pathological and morphological changes of the tissues, a basic illness history of HIV infection should also be taken into account as well as the blood test results, such as CD4 T count and its ratio to CD8 T count as well as serum HIV antibody positive. Meanwhile, thyromegaly caused by other factors should be differentially diagnosed, especially autoimmune induced thyromegaly (Hashimoto thyroiditis).

16.2.8   Differential Diagnosis

HIV/AIDS related thyromegaly should be differentially diagnosed from following diseases:

16.2.8.1   Diffuse Thyromegaly

Hyperplasia may be caused by dietary iodine deficiency or hyperthyroidism or inflammation. The diffusely enlarged thyroid commonly extends to retrosternal or other areas. CT scanning demonstrates CT values of the thyroid tissues mostly above 70 Hu due to abundant contents of iodine. Tracheas and brachiocephalic blood vessels are compressed for migration and deformation and the superior vena cava is compressed for secondary venectasia. For cases with degeneration, it may demonstrate flaky calcification and cystic changes. By enhanced scanning, the thyroid tissues show enhancement, with no enhancement of cysts and rare enhancement of the degenerating lesions. Differential diagnosis of HIV/AIDS related thyromegaly from simple thyromegaly is difficult. For cases with diffuse thyromegaly complicating HIV/AIDS, the common causes of simple thyromegaly should be firstly excluded for the diagnosis of HIV/AIDS related thyromegaly.

16.2.8.2   Hashimoto Thyroiditis

It has manifestations of diffuse enlargement of the thyroid with infiltration toward the peripheral area. The enlargement is lobulated with unclearly defined borderlines and a density generally lower than normal thyroid tissues but close to the peripheral muscular tissues. It can be complicated by calcification and cystic changes. After intravenous injection of reagent, there is heterogeneous enhancement. Generally, the illness course is long. Based on the clinical manifestations and case history, its diagnosis can be made. Only by CT scanning, the differential diagnosis from neoplasms is difficult.

16.2.8.3   Thyroid Carcinoma

Differential diagnosis of obvious thyroid carcinoma is not necessary. Thyroid carcinoma initially shows local nodules in thyroid parenchyma, which should be differentiated from nodules manifested in cases of HIV/AIDS related thyromegaly.

Thyroid carcinoma can be divided into five types: papillary, follicular, encephaloid, giant cell and Hürthle cell. CT scanning can define the range of the lesions as well as lymphoid metastases. In terms of thyroid masses, there are no reliable signs to differentiate the benign from the malignant. For cases with regional lymphadenectasis, recurrent laryngeal nerve paralysis and injuries of thyroid cartilage or other laryngeal cartilages, it is facilitative for the diagnosis of malignancy. Calcification is not the evidence for the differentiation of the benign from the malignant because calcification occurs in cases of benign tumors. Nuclear imaging can roughly evaluate the biological activity of thyroid nodules, which facilitates the differential diagnosis. Thyroid carcinoma commonly shows cold nodules, mostly common with adenoma hyperplasia which can be cystic or parenchymal. Only 20 % nodules are malignant.

16.3   HIV/AIDS Related Cervical Lymphoid Tuberculosis

16.3.1   Pathogen and Pathogenesis

HIV/AIDS related cervical lymphoid tuberculosis can be classified into primary and secondary.

16.3.1.1   Primary Lymphoid Tuberculosis

Cervical lymphoid tuberculosis is a part of primary tuberculosis infection. Primary infection foci can be caused by invasion of M. Tuberculosis via upper respiratory tract or the oral cavity and nasopharynx. The most common location of the primary infection is the tonsil. The infection further spreads to the cervical superficial or deep lymph nodes or submandibular lymph nodes along lymph vessels, with possible involvement of preauricular and retroauricular lymph nodes. At this time of infection, the primary foci may have been absorbed gradually. But lymphoid tuberculosis may progress into cold abscess or ulcer.

16.3.1.2   Secondary Lymphoid Tuberculosis

After the primary tuberculosis or during the progression of secondary tuberculosis, tuberculosis invades the cervical lymph nodes via blood-borne transmission. The involved cervical lymph nodes are extensive, with bilateral involvements. Alternatively, deep cervical lymph nodes may be infected by tuberculosis that primarily invades the thoracic or abdominal lymph nodes and spreads via lymph vessels.

In the above two types of HIV/AIDS related cervical lymphoid tuberculosis, the secondary type is more common. Compromised immunity is an important factor for its onset. Secondary oral suppurative infection contributes to its occurrence and progression.

16.3.2 Pathophysiological Basis

Commonly found in the middle and advanced stages of AIDS, HIV/AIDS related cervical lymphoid tuberculosis shows multiple enlarged lymph nodes in unilateral or bilateral neck, with varying sizes and being at the anterior or posterior margin of the sternocleidomastoid muscle (SCM). Initially, the enlarged lymph nodes are relatively hard, painless and movable. With its progression, perilymphadenitis occurs, with lymph nodes adhering to skin or peripheral tissues or with lymph nodes adhering to each other to fuse into unmovable nodular masses. In its advanced stage, caseous necrosis and liquefaction of lymph nodes occurs to form cold abscesses. The rupture of the abscess releases pus to result in long-term unhealed sinus or chronic ulcer. The skin margin of ulcer is in dark red color and sinking in the skin, with pale granulation and edema. Different lymph nodes in patients may have different manifestations of above three stages.

16.3.3 Clinical Symptoms and Signs

The symptoms include bilateral cervical lymph nodes enlargement, showing multiple nodules and being painless at palpitation. Initially, the nodule is singular, smooth and movable. After that, the nodules fuse into irregular masses, with poor mobility. The mass may have abscesses with a sense of fluctuation and its rupture may result in formation of sinus canal to sink into skin in a long-term unhealing state. The secretion is commonly loose, containing caseous materials and unhealthy granulation of the wound surface. The general toxic symptoms of tuberculosis may show up including low grade fever, night sweating, fatigue and emaciation.

16.3.4 Examinations and Their Selection

Chest X-ray is of limited diagnostic value for cervical tuberculosis. Ultrasound clearly demonstrates the location, shape, size, amount and interior echo of the diseased cervical lymph nodes. Especially, ultrasound can probe the involvement of deep cervical lymph nodes that are difficult to be palpitated. CDFI can further demonstrate the blood supply of the lymph nodes, which provides abundant diagnostic information for the diagnosis and differential diagnosis of cervical tuberculosis. Compared to other imaging examinations, ultrasound is of the first choice due to its non-invasiveness, low cost and dynamic demonstration. Cervical CT scanning can identify the location, distribution

and size of the enlarged lymph nodes in neck and their relationship with their adjacent structures. Enhanced scanning demonstrates obvious enhancement of the lymph nodes, which facilitates the differential diagnosis. The cervical MRI functions similarly to cervical CT scanning in its diagnosis, whereas MRI can demonstrate the relationship between lesions and their adjacent structures from multiple perspectives, and is more sensitive to the necrosis of lymph nodes.

Indirect laryngoscopy and nasopharynx endoscopy can occasionally detect laryngeal tuberculosis and nasopharyngeal tuberculosis. Clinically, tuberculin test and ESR (erythrocyte sedimentation rate) are facilitative for the diagnosis.

16.3.5 Imaging Demonstrations

16.3.5.1 Ultrasound

Unilateral cervical lymphoid tuberculosis is as common as bilateral cervical lymphoid tuberculosis, predominantly middle and root cervical multiple lymphoid tuberculosis and occasional involvement of the superficial cervical lymph nodes. Based on the pathological manifestations in different stages, cervical lymphoid tuberculosis can be divided into three types, namely lymphadenitis, low-echo mass and liquefaction. Lymphadenitis type of cervical lymphoid tuberculosis is corresponding to the pathological stage of proliferative granuloma, with intact envelope, no obvious damage to its inner structures, clear boundary between cortex and medulla, relatively thickened cortex and decreased homogeneity of echoes. Due to uncompleted damages to the lymph nodes, dots and strips of blood flow can be found. The type of low-echo mass corresponds to the pathological stage of caseous lesions, characterized by formation of abundant tubercles due to lymphoid proliferation to cause medulla disappearance or medulla being pushed to the border showing eccentric narrow band or twig liked high echo while heterogeneous distribution of coarse echo in the cortex. In this stage, the lymph nodes commonly have abundant blood supply. The liquefaction type shows fused flakes of caseous changes and liquefaction necrosis, typical of large light spots, patches and masses in the liquefied foci. In cases of necrotic lymph nodes, absence of any blood flow signal can be demonstrated.

16.3.5.2 CT Scanning

CT scanning demonstrates the same involved range of lesions as ultrasound. CT scanning demonstrates obviously enlarged lymph nodes, with diameters exceeding 10 mm. The lymph nodes being less than 10 mm may also be lymphoid tuberculosis. The involved lymph nodes are in round, oval or irregular shapes, commonly with intact and smooth margins. For cases with effusion or fusion of lymph nodes, the margins are blurry. The ruptured envelope of lymph nodes results in the thickened neighboring superficial fascia. Plain CT scanning demonstrates homogeneous soft tissue density of the lymph nodes, with lower central density in the cases of liquefaction and necrosis. Enhanced scanning demonstrates different findings according to the different pathological stages of lymph nodes. During the stage of lymphadenitis, the enhanced scanning demonstrates homogeneous enhancement, with no lower central density area. During the stage of caseous necrosis, enhanced CT scanning demonstrates heterogeneous enhancement, with no central enhancement of different degrees. The typical findings include ring shaped enhancement of the thin wall and no central enhancement. In some cases, the demonstrations include irregular ring shaped enhancement of the thick wall, with central septal enhancement. In addition, some lymph nodes show enhancement of incomplete ring, with no surrounding fat space.

16.3.5.3 MR Imaging

The range and size of lymph nodes are as the above mentioned. By T1WI, the enlarged lymph nodes are in low signals, with lower signals in the cases with central necrosis. By T2WI, the enlarged lymph nodes are demonstrated by slightly higher signals, with increased signals in cases with central necrosis. In the predominant lymphadenitis stage, T2WI with additional fat suppression imaging demonstrates increased signal of the peripheral tissues, groups of aggregated lymph nodes with some fused. Sagittal or coronal MR imaging demonstrates lymph nodes in arrangement like a string of beads. Enhanced imaging demonstrates similar enhancement of enlarged lymph nodes to that by enhanced CT scanning.

Case Study 1

A female patient aged 43 years was confirmatively diagnosed as having AIDS by CDC. She complaint of intermittent fever, no local tenderness as well as swollen and cystic changes of the left retroauricular lymph nodes. Her CD4 T cell count was 107/μl.

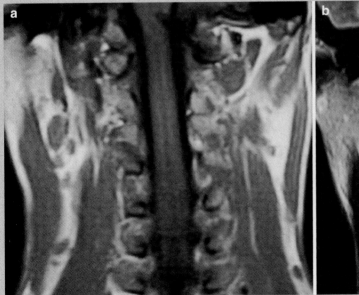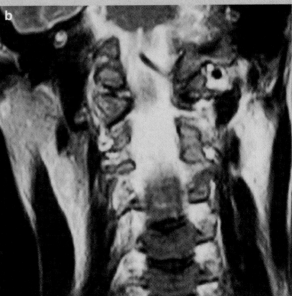

Fig. 16.3 (a, b) HIV/AIDS related cervical lymphoid tuberculosis. (a, b) MR T1WI demonstrates multiple oval signals of soft tissue density with varying sizes and clearly defined borderlines under the right cervical mastoid muscle

Case Study 2

A female patient aged 43 years was confirmatively diagnosed as having AIDS by CDC. She complained of intermittent fever, local distending pain and swelling and cystic changes of the left periotic lymph nodes.

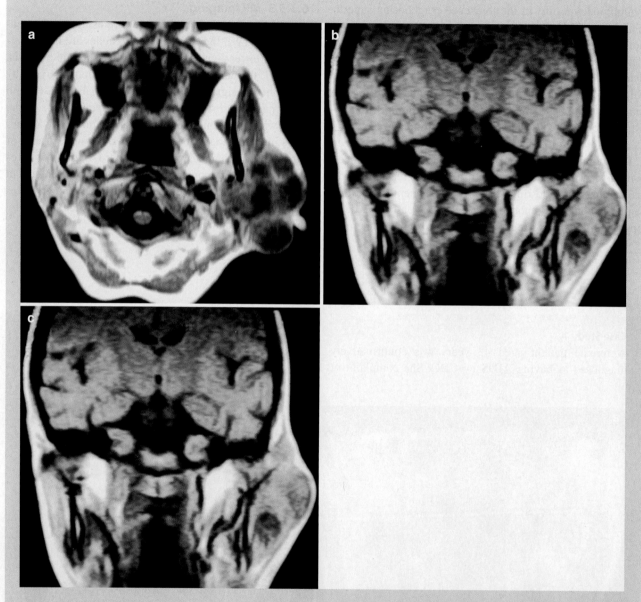

Fig. 16.4 (**a–c**) HIV/AIDS related cervical lymphoid tuberculosis. (**a, b**) Axial T1WI demonstrates left periotic multiple oval shaped low signals that fuse into masses, some being eccentric with low signals, thick wall and clearly defined borderlines. (**c**) Coronal T1WI demonstrates left periotic multiple oval shaped low signals that fuse into masses with clearly defined borderlines, thinner subcutaneous fat tissue behind ears due to compression

Case Study 3

A patient was confirmatively diagnosed as having AIDS by CDC, with cervical lymphoid tuberculosis.

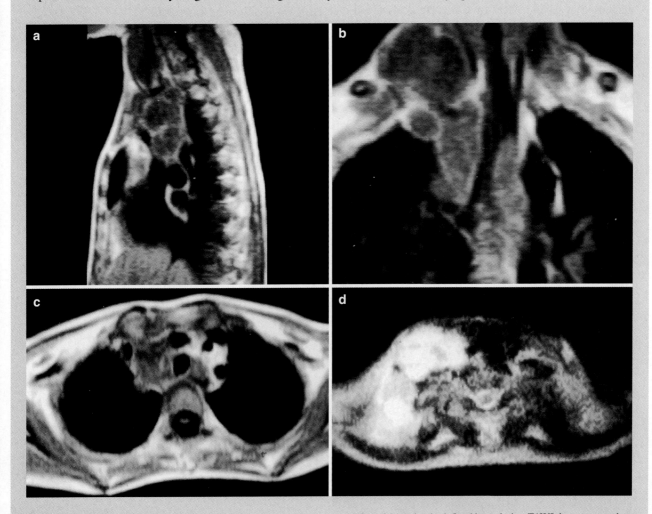

Fig. 16.5 (**a–d**) HIV/AIDS related cervical lymphoid tuberculosis. (**a–c**) MR imaging demonstrates multiple nodules with soft tissue signal in bilateral cervical roots and superior mediastinum, the lesions dominantly distributed in the right neck root, fusion of nodules with unclearly defined boundaries. T1WI demonstrates heterogeneous low signals and lower signals inside. (**d**) Flat trachea due to compression, T2WI demonstrates heterogeneous high signals and higher central signals

Case Study 4

A male patient aged 28 years was confirmatively diagnosed as having AIDS by CDC. He complained of intermittent fever, local distending pain as well as swelling and cystic changes of the right cervical lymph nodes. His CD4 T cell count was 107/μl.

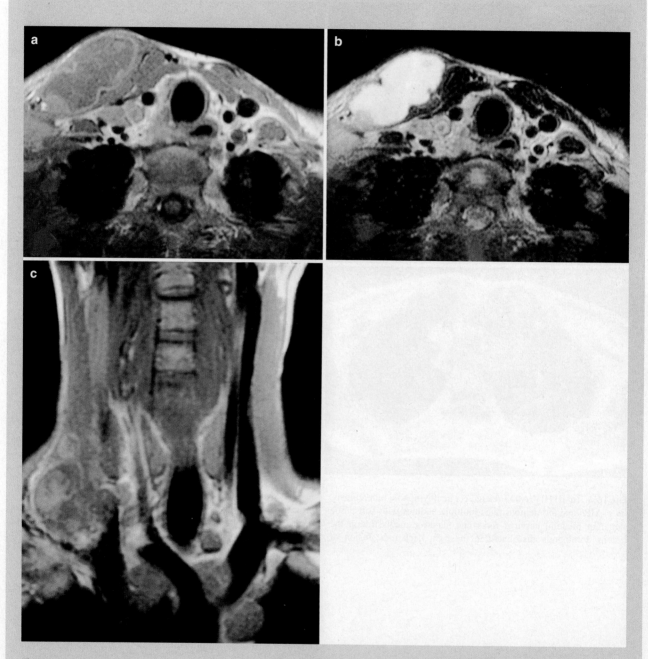

Fig. 16.6 (**a–c**) HIV/AIDS related cervical lymphoid tuberculosis. (**a, b**) MR imaging demonstrates dumbbell liked space occupying effect in the right supraclavicular fossa; T1WI demonstrates slightly low signals, thin but homogeneous slightly high signals of the borders, with clearly defined boundary. (**b**) T2WI demonstrates obviously homogenous high signals, thin but homogeneous moderate signals of borders, several small nodules superior and posterior to the lesions with similar demonstrations to the lesions

Case Study 5

A female patient aged 50 years was confirmatively diagnosed as having AIDS by CDC. She had a history of paid blood donation in the year of 1993 and symptoms onset in the year of 2006. She now complained of fever and numerous palpable bean liked lumps in the neck. Her CD4 T cell count was 30/μl.

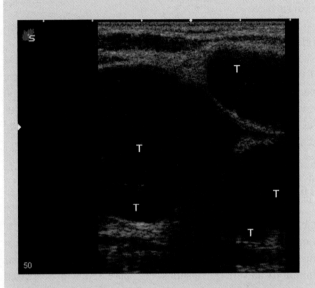

Fig. 16.7 HIV/AIDS related cervical lymphadenectasis. Ultrasound demonstrates multiple parenchymal low echo nodules of various sizes surrounding the bilateral cervical major blood vessels (*T*), with clearly defined boundaries and heterogeneous inner echo; CDFI demonstrates unobvious interior blood flow in the nodules, the larger nodules being in size of 30×20 mm

Case Study 6

A male patient aged 47 years was confirmatively diagnosed as having AIDS by CDC. He had a history of paid blood donation in 1995. The onset of symptoms was in the year of 2006. She complained of fever and emaciation. And her CD4 T cell count was 39/μl.

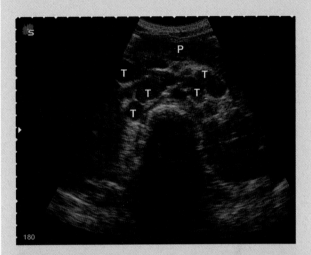

Fig. 16.8 HIV/AIDS related epigastric lymphadenectasis. Color ultrasound demonstrates multiple parenchymal low-echo nodules surrounding the bilateral cervical major blood vessels (*T*, *P*), with clearly defined boundaries, fusion of some nodules and relatively heterogenous echo in the nodules; CDFI demonstrates spots or strips liked blood flow signals in the nodules, the larger one being in size of 25×17 mm

Case Study 7

A male patient aged 39 years was confirmatively diagnosed as having AIDS by CDC. He had a history of paid blood donation in 1993. The onset of symptoms was in 2004, with complaints of fever, emaciation and abdominal upset. His CD4 T cell count was 29/μl.

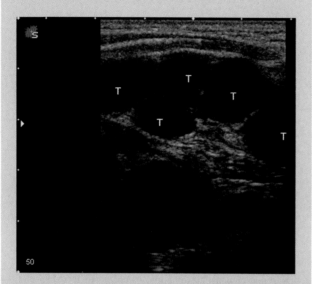

Fig. 16.9 HIV/AIDS related mesenteric lymphadenectasis. Color ultrasound demonstrates multiple parenchymal low echo nodules of various sizes in the mesentery of the lower abdomen (*T*), with clearly defined boundaries and relatively heterogeneous echo within nodules; CDFI demonstrates spots and strips liked blood flow signals in the nodules, with the larger one being in size of 21 × 17 mm

16.3.6   Discussions

Lymph nodes are important immune organs in the human body, with about 500–600 lymph nodes in a healthy person. According to their location, lymph nodes can be divided into superficial lymph nodes and deep lymph nodes. A normal lymph node is commonly 0.2–0.5 cm in diameter, with distribution in groups and smooth surface. Lymph nodes are soft in texture, with no tenderness and no adhesion to the peripheral tissues. Except for 1–2 occasionally palpable lymph nodes in submandibular area, groin and armpit, the lymph nodes are generally unpalpable. However, enlarged lymph nodes are palpable due to occurrence of inflammations or tumors. Each group of lymph nodes collects lymph fluid of the corresponding drainage area, and understanding of the relationship facilitates the localization of the primary foci and its properties.

Among the AIDS patients in our hospital, the epigastric (portal hepatis) lymphadenectasis is the most common. In the early stage of AIDS, the incidence of lymphadenectasis

is about 55–100 %. A patient from high risk populations and sustaining general lymphadenectasis of unknown reasons is possibly an HIV infected patient.

Lymphadenectasis can be general, but commonly in the posterior neck, supraclavicular and submandibular areas and armpit. The enlarged lymph nodes do not fuse and are hard in texture. Occasionally, the tenderness of enlarged lymph nodes can be found. And no change can be found across the skin surface.

In the advanced stage of AIDS, lymphadenectasis is complicated by bacterial infection, with symptoms of redness, swelling, fever and pain. Especially in cases with their CD4 T cell count being lower than 200/μl, patients usually have persistent fever, cervical singular or multiple enlarged lymph nodes. Even for cases with no focus of pulmonary tuberculosis, lymphoid tuberculosis should 3,000 be suspected for the diagnosis.

16.3.7   Criteria for the Diagnosis

Generally, the positive rate of PPD test in common populations with TB is above 90 %. However, due to the compromised immunity of HIV infected patients, their cellular immunity and allergic response are depressed, with decreased response or negative response in PPD test. The positive rate of PPD test in patients with HIV/AIDS complicated by TB is less than 10 %. The diagnosis of cervical lymphoid tuberculosis in AIDS patients principally depends on imaging demonstrations and puncture for biopsy.

Imaging demonstrations provide important information for the diagnosis of lymphoid tuberculosis. The typical findings include multiple enlarged lymph nodes of different sizes in unilateral or bilateral neck, generally at the anterior or posterior margins of sternocleidomastoid muscle (SCM), numerous swollen nodule shadows in soft tissues density that fuse into flakes with central lower density. Meanwhile, multiple swollen lymph nodes may fuse into petal or polycyclic masses to form multi-room sign. Enhanced imaging demonstrates ring liked enhancement of central lower density in the nodules, homogeneous thickness of the ring wall and smooth interior and exterior walls. These are characteristic findings of HIV related lymphoid tuberculosis.

16.3.8   Differential Diagnosis

16.3.8.1 Cervical Lymphoid Metastatic Neoplasms

The most common demonstrations are multiple mass shadows in soft tissue density in the areas of sub-mastoid, submandibular and carotid sheath, with clearly defined borderlines. They may fuse into flakes or lobules. Enhanced scanning demonstrates slight or medium enhancement of the foci, being clearly defined from blood vessels, and ring liked enhancement in cases with companying liquefaction necrosis, heterogeneous and irregular thickness of the ring wall. These are the most important imaging demonstrations for the differential diagnosis of lymphoid tuberculosis. Cervical lymphoid metastasis can invade jugular veins to cause venous thrombosis, and it can invade other cervical structures.

16.3.8.2 Cervical Lymphoma

Cervical lymphomas include Hodgkin's and Non-Hodgkin's lymphoma, more common in the young. Multiple enlarged lymph nodes are commonly found in the neck, which fuse into larger masses to embed the cervical major vessels, forming vascular embedding sign. CT scanning demonstrates homogeneous low density. Enhanced scanning demonstrates homogeneous enhancement, with rare occurrence of liquefaction necrosis.

16.3.8.3 Cervical Schwannoma

CT scanning demonstrates round or oval mass shadows in soft tissue density in the carotid sheath, with clearly defined borderlines. The long axis has a tendency to travel along the nerve; the internal and external carotid arteries migrate forward while the temporal styloid process migrates backward. Cystic necrosis in the masses is common. Enhanced scanning demonstrates heterogeneously obvious enhancement, with no enhancement in the area of cystic necrosis.

16.4 HIV/AIDS Related Neoplasms

In the stages of acute HIV infection, AIDS associated syndrome and typical AIDS, lymphoid system is involved. Lymph node is one of the earliest and the most susceptible tissues. Therefore, the disease of lymph node is the most common or sometimes the earliest manifestations of HIV infection. Lymph nodes are important immune organs distributed all through the body and play an essential role in defense mechanism. Lymphadenopathy is a generalization of numerous diseases or lesions manifested as lymphadenectasis of various causes, including reactive hyperplasia, acute or chronic inflammation, primary or metastatic neoplasms of lymph nodes as well as persistent general lymphadenopathy (PGL). HIV/AIDS related lymphadenectasis includes infectious lymphadenectasis such as lymphoid tuberculosis, neoplastic lymphadenectasis such as lymphoma and metastatic neoplasm of lymph nodes, and lymphadenectasis resulted from concurrent contributing factors. Therefore, the clinical diagnosis of HIV/AIDS related lymphadenopathy depends on further examinations to find the pathogens for its differential diagnosis. Biopsy of lymph node is an important method for clinical diagnosis.

16.4.1 Pathogen and Pathogenesis

HIV infection can directly cause changes of tissue structures of lymph nodes and the corresponding pathological changes. On the basis of the illness course, the pathogenesis can be divided into four stages, namely follicular hyperplasia, follicular degeneration, follicular absence and lymphocytic failure. During the initial illness course of AIDS, reactive hyperplasia of lymph nodes occurs due to HIV stimulation, which causes B lymphocytic proliferation and phagocyte accumulation and consequent lymphadenectasis. Thereafter T lymphocytic failure in the lymph nodes occurs to cause lymphocytic shrinkage but formation of nodules due to histiocytic hyperplasia. In the advanced stage of illness course, liquefaction necrosis or disappearance of lymph nodes may occur. During different illness courses, the structural and cellular changes of lymph nodes are different, but all demonstrate reactive hyperplasia of lymph nodes. In the later two stages, multiple infections may complicate AIDS due to the compromised immunity of the patients to aggravate the severity of lymphadenectasis. In the enlarged lymph nodes, the pathogens of complicating infections can be found.

16.4.2 Clinical Symptoms and Signs

HIV/AIDS related cervical lymphadenectasis has manifestations of bilateral cervical deep and superficial lymph nodes enlargement of different degrees. The symptoms and signs vary with pathogenic factors. Cervical lymphadenectasis caused by HIV infection is manifested as painless nodules with a persistent progression, which fuse with each other to cause poor mobility in the advanced stage. In cases complicated by lymph node infection, it manifests inflammatory responses of lymph nodes of different degrees, pain and swelling. Lymphoid tuberculosis can form cervical cold abscess or sinus canal.

For cases of malignant neoplastic lymphadenectasis, tumor cells proliferate and multiply in the lymph nodes to cause enlarged, dense and hard lymph nodes, with smooth surface or with processes from the surface. The lymph nodes adhere to their surrounding tissues, with poor mobility and no tenderness.

16.4.3 Examinations and Their Selection

16.4.3.1 Hemogram

Leukocyte count and differential blood counts in the peripheral blood is of certain reference value for identifying causes of lymphadenectasis. Lymphadenectasis and companying increased leukocyte count and neutrophil count is commonly found in bacterial infections but for some cases with Gram-negative bacilli infections, leukocyte count may not increase yet neutrophil count usually increases. Lymphadenectasis with normal or decreased leukocyte count but increased lymphocyte count often suggests viral infection but for patients with infectious mononucleosis due to EB virus infection, leukocyte count usually increases in the second week after infection. In addition, in the third week after infection abnormal lymphocytes (at least 10–20 %) can be found, with increased eosinophil count, which are suggestive of parasitic infection or eosinophilic granular cell granuloma. Lymphadenectasis with accompanying immature cells in the peripheral blood indicates leukemia or carcinoma. Malignant histiocytosis usually manifests fever, hepatic and splenic lymphadenectasis and pancytopenia.

16.4.3.2 Bone Marrow Examination

Bone marrow smear for cell morphological examination can confirm the diagnosis of leukemia, plasmacytoma, malignant histiocytosis, Gaucher disease and Niemann-Pick disease. If necessary, pathological examination of bone marrow should be performed. It is difficult to identify the primary location of metastatic carcinoma, but of decisive significance in identifying metastatic cancer cells.

16.4.3.3 Diagnostic Imaging

Ultrasonography can demonstrate the location, amount, size of lymph nodes and their relationship with the surrounding structures. CT scanning and MR imaging can also define the location, amount, size of lymph nodes and their relationship with the surrounding structures. In addition, CT scanning and MR imaging are more favorable in defining the relationship between lymph nodes and their peripheral structures as well as the degrees of involvement. Especially T2WI fat suppression sequence of MR imaging can further demonstrate peripheral reactions to lymph node lesions. Enhanced CT scanning or MR imaging is facilitative for finding the causes of lymphadenectasis based on the degrees and types of enhancement of lymph nodes. For instance, ring shaped enhancement of lymph nodes is commonly suggestive of lymphoid tuberculosis.

16.4.3.4 Puncture of Lymph Nodes for Needle Suction and Smear

For patients with evident superficial lymphadenectasis, a comparatively large sized injection needle could be used for puncture of lymph nodes, followed by needle suction of a few contents via a large negative pressure for smear. The method is simple and convenient to apply and the findings have a high positive rate.

16.4.3.5 Pathological Examination of Lymph Nodes

Patients with evident lymphadenectasis of unknown reasons, if without surgical contraindications, generally undergo routine histopathological biopsy of lymph nodes. Meanwhile lymph node imprinting can be performed for morphological examination of the diseased cells.

16.4.4   Imaging Demonstrations

16.4.4.1 Ultrasonography

Cervical lymphadenectasis is commonly bilateral, with involvement of both the superficial and the deep lymph nodes. The enlarged lymph nodes are different in size, oval or round in shape with clearly defined borderline and homogeneous inner echo. For cases complicated by lymph node infection, manifestations vary with pathogenic factors (for details, check relevant chapters). The lymph nodes in cases of lymphoma and metastatic lymphoid neoplasms have the common manifestations as those in other body parts.

16.4.4.2 CT Scanning

CT scanning demonstrates the same involved range of lymph nodes as by ultrasound. The involved lymph nodes are different in size, mostly being obviously enlarged ones in diameters of above 10 mm. The lymph nodes are oval or round in shape, predominantly with clear and smooth boundaries. Plain scanning demonstrates homogeneous soft tissue density of the lymph nodes. Enhanced scanning demonstrates homogeneous slight enhancement of lymph nodes. For cases complicated by opportunistic infections of lymph nodes, the manifestations are different for various infections. Generally, the boundaries of lymph nodes from peripheral tissues are blurry, increased peripheral fat density and thus opaque, as well as peripheral lymph nodes enhancement by enhanced scanning. For cases of tuberculous lymphadenitis, the lymph nodes are demonstrated as typical ring shaped enhancement with no central enhancement in lower density.

16.4.4.3 MR Imaging

MRI imaging demonstrates the same range and size of lymph nodes as the above mentioned. The enlarged lymph nodes are in slightly low homogeneous signal by T1WI and are in slightly high homogeneous signal by T2WI. For cases complicated by lymphoid infection, the lymph node boundary is blurry with an increased signal, which is more obvious by T2WI fat suppression imaging of the peripheral tissues. The typical manifestations of lymphoid tuberculosis include central caseous necrosis signals of lower signal by T1WI and higher signal by T2WI. By enhanced imaging, typically ring shaped enhancement can be found.

Case Study 1

A male patient aged 32 years was confirmatively diagnosed as having AIDS by CDC. He had a history of drug abuse and symptoms of fever and cough with phlegm. By acid-fast staining of the sputum, acid-fast bacilli negative. And he was tested as HIV positive. CT scanning indicated pulmonary tuberculosis and his CD4 T cell count was 600/μl.

Immunohistochemistry indicated CD3 weak positive, CD20 negative, CD30 negative and CD45R0 weak positive. Stereological examination demonstrated large nasal ala with ulceration and black scab, communication between palate and nasal cavity, pus discharge with a stench smelling. Reexamination after 3 months found loss of right nasal ala, expanded ulceration, fever and paranasal pain.

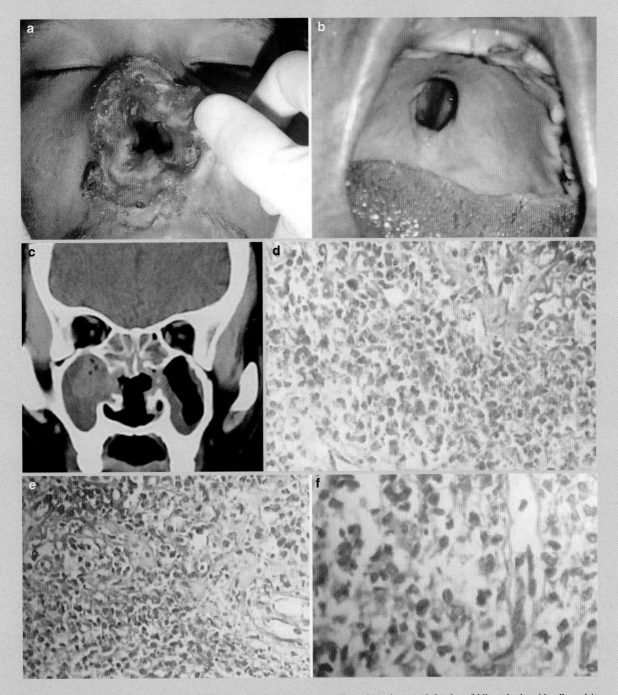

Fig. 16.10 (**a–h**) HIV/AIDS related lymphoma. (**a**) It is demonstrated that defection of most nasal ala, red granulation of the surface, partially with scab. (**b**) It is demonstrated that Perforation of palate to render communication between nasal and oral cavities. (**c**) Coronal plain CT scanning demonstrates absent bilateral middle nasal concha, thinner and irregular soft tissues of bilateral inferior nasal concha, thickened mucosa of bilateral maxillary sinus, filling of tissues with soft tissue density within the right maxillary sinus, increased density of bilateral ethmoid cells and intact bone of the sinal wall. (**d–f**) Nasal histopathology demonstrates a few atypical proliferative lymphoid cells, immunohistochemical labeling being in line with manifestations of lymphoma. (**g**, **h**) Chest X-ray and plain chest CT scanning demonstrate infiltrative pulmonary tuberculosis in superior lobes of both lungs and in middle lobe of the right lung

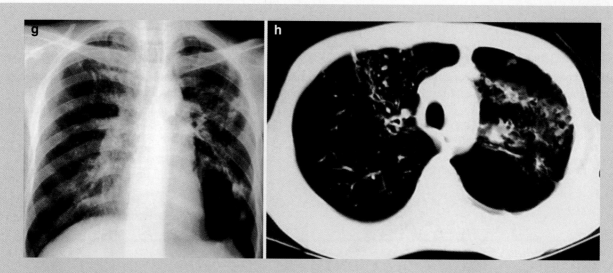

Fig. 16.10 (continued)

Case Study 2

A female patient aged 34 years was confirmatively diagnosed as having AIDS by CDC. The cervical lump was punctured for pathological examination. Microscopic examination found a few fibrins, lymphocytes but no tumor cells. Gram staining of specimens collected by puncture indicated Gram-positive bacteria. By acid-fast staining, there was no growth of acid-fast bacilli. And bacteria culture of the specimens suggested no growth of bacteria. Her CD4 T cell count was 17/μl.

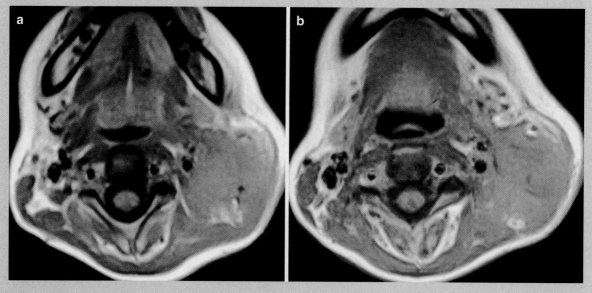

Fig. 16.11 (a–d) Cervical lymphoma. (a, b) Cervical plain CT scanning demonstrates mass with homogeneous density inferior to the left mandible angle and lateral to carotid sheath, with even interior density but unclearly defined boundary. (c, d) Enhanced scanning demonstrates obvious enhancement of its most part, irregular septal enhancement of its interior tissues, unsmooth inner wall, inward migration of the carotid sheath due to compression, outward migration of sternocleidomastoid muscle is press

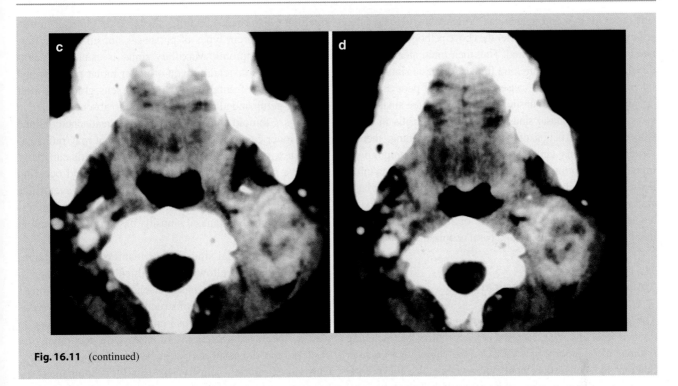

Fig. 16.11 (continued)

16.4.5   Criteria for the Diagnosis

Diagnosis of HIV induced lymphadenopathy should be made in combination with the laboratory blood test results, such as serum HIV antibody positive, CD4 T cell count and its ratio to CD8 T cell count. Based on the clinical evidence of HIV infection, diagnosis for cases with cervical diffuse multiple lymphadenectasis can be defined. In addition, imaging demonstrations and, if necessary, biopsy of lymph nodes should be combined for further differentiation of neoplastic lymphadenectasis and inflammatory lymphadenectasis.

16.4.6   Differential Diagnosis

16.4.6.1   Reactive Follicular Hyperplasia

It may be caused by various factors. Hyperplastic lymphoid follicles are mostly located in the cortex, with uniform structure and shape but with no fused and strangely shaped ones. The ratio of CD4 T cell count to CD8 T cell count in the terminal blood shows no conversion.

16.4.6.2   Vascular Immunoblast Lymphadenopathy

It commonly occurs in senior population aged above 60 years, with atypical lymphoid follicular hyperplasia, increased immunoblast with diffuse infiltration, and companying venular hyperplasia after capillaries. The inner structures of lymph nodes are not very clearly defined, with sediment of PAS staining positive substances. Morphologically, there is no obvious malignant evidence. But recently, TCR clonal rearrangement has been reported. The recent classification by WHO has listed vascular immunoblast lymphadenopathy as T cell lymphoma.

16.5   HIV/AIDS Related Paranasal Sinusitis

16.5.1   Pathogen and Pathogenesis

In a healthy condition, various species of pathogenic bacteria can be found in the nasal cavity, including bacteria and a few fungi. Detoxification of the nasal cavity ensures the above bacteria/fungi within the amount that the human body can resist. The factors such as cold, rain and fatigue can decrease the detoxification ability of the nasal cavity to defer the above pathogens within the nasal cavity for a longer period. Thus their multiplication during this time may cause rhinitis, and further paranasal sinusitis. The inflammatory stimulation causes obstruction of paranasal sinus opening, which leads to unsmooth discharge of the sinal mucus to exacerbate paranasal sinusitis. Paranasal sinusitis in return worsens the obstruction of paranasal sinus opening, thereby forming a vicious circle. For AIDS patients, compromised immunity is the primary cause of paranasal sinusitis due to infections of nasal cavity and paranasal sinus. Some diseases of nasal cavity are fundamental causes of paranasal sinusitis, including deviated nasal septum, hypertrophy of middle nasal concha, nasal polyps, allergic rhinitis and nasal neoplasms.

16.5.2 Pathophysiological Basis

The principal pathology of acute paranasal sinusitis can be divided into following stages: (1) Catarrhal stage, including findings of temporary mucosa ischemia, subsequent vascular dilation and congestion, epithelial swelling, lamina propria edema, polymorphonuclear leukocytes and lymphocytes infiltration, slowed ciliary movement and serous/mucus hypersecretion; (2) suppurative stage, including findings of epithelial necrosis, cilia shedding, minor vascular hemorrhage and purulent secretions; (3) complication stage, including inflammatory invasion of bone or inflammatory spreading via blood flow to cause myelitis or intraorbital/intracranial complications.

For cases of chronic paranasal sinusitis, the pathological findings include thickened mucosa, lamina propria edema, thickened vascular wall with stenosis or even occlusion of vascular lumen, abundant interstitial round cells infiltration. After acute suppurative paranasal sinusitis progresses into chronic period, the pathological findings include partially damaged mucosa with companying squamous metaplasia and granulation, evidently thickened lamina propria with infiltration of large amount of lymphocytes and plasmacytes, as well as local polyps. In cases of fungal paranasal sinusitis, calcified foci can be found in the sinal cavity.

16.5.3 Clinical Symptoms and Signs

The clinical manifestations of acute paranasal sinusitis include nasal obstruction, thick nasal discharge, temporary smelling disturbance, chill, fever and general upset. Moreover, different types of paranasal sinusitis have different typical symptoms. Maxillary sinusitis usually is manifested as facial distending pain or upper molar pain. Frontal sinusitis shows frontal pain which worsens gradually after morning getup and alleviates after noon to absence of pain in evenings. Ethmoid sinusitis causes slight headache confined within inner canthus or nasal root region that may radiate to the vertex, or top of the head. Sphenoid sinusitis can cause deep eye pain that may radiate to the vertex, and occipital pain slight in mornings but severe after noon. However, since most patients have symptoms in different body parts and it is difficult to locate paranasal sinusitis based on the symptom of headache.

Chronic paranasal sinusitis has manifestations of abundant yellowish or yellowish green thick nasal discharge in uncertain quantity. The nasal discharge commonly flows towards the throat. Nasal obstruction has different severities, caused by nasal mucosa congestion and swelling as well as increased secretions. In cases with accompanying nasal polyps, the nasal cavity can be completely obstructed. Chronic paranasal sinusitis is usually accompanied by headache, which is dull pain or heaviness sensation of the head being severe in the day and slight in the evening. Anterior paranasal sinusitis principally has manifestations of distending pain or dull pain in frontal and nasal root regions, while posterior paranasal sinusitis shows vertex, temporal or occipital pain.

16.5.4 Examinations and Their Selection

The traditional plain X-ray of the paranasal sinus cannot demonstrate paranasal sinus lesions in details and its application is limited. CT scanning is an important method for the diagnosis of paranasal sinusitis, which is also a compulsory examination before surgeries for paranasal sinusitis. It can clearly demonstrate the subtle structures of the paranasal sinus and its neighboring area, thereby providing essential information for the diagnosis and treatment of paranasal sinusitis. CT scanning is sensitive and accurate in demonstrating bones of paranasal sinus, which provides information for the differential diagnosis of paranasal sinusitis. MR imaging is of high resolution for soft tissues of paranasal sinus and could reveal the spatial structures from multiple dimensions, which renders it more favorable to differential diagnosis of paranasal sinus lesions. MR imaging can be applied when lesions are complex or failed defining of lesions by CT scanning.

16.5.5   Imaging Demonstrations

16.5.5.1   Acute Paranasal Sinusitis

Plain X-ray demonstrates increased density and opacity of the sinus cavity, which is more obvious in cases of maxillary sinusitis. In cases with gas in sinal cavity, gas-fluid level can be found. There are evenly thickened mucosa, clearly defined bony white line in submucosal sinus wall and thickened mucosa of nasal cavity. Plain CT scanning suggests thickened mucosa in nasal cavity and sinus, effusion and gas-fluid level in the sinus cavity and no damage to the bone of the sinus wall. MR imaging indicates diffuse homogeneous thickening of the mucosa in nasal cavity and sinus, and more sensitive demonstrations to sinus effusions. T1WI demonstrates slightly low signal and T2WI demonstrates bright high signal.

16.5.5.2   Chronic Paranasal Sinusitis

Plain X-ray demonstrates increased density of sinus cavity and more obviously thickened mucosa which is uneven like polyps, blurry white line of submucous bone of sinus wall, whitening and hardening of bone, as well as bone absorption in some cases. CT scanning indicates unevenly thickened mucosa of sinus cavity that even fills the whole cavity, necrotic tissues accumulating in the sinus cavity to relatively increase the density, no obvious changes of the bone of sinus wall but some cases possibly with bone absorption or hyperplasia, thickened mucosa of nasal cavity, asymmetric thickening of turbinate, and obstruction of the opening of maxillary sinus due to prominent thickening. MR imaging shows unevenly thickened mucosa in a slight low signal by T1WI and high signal by T2WI, extremely high signal of the cysts and no obvious signal changes of the bone of sinus wall.

16.5.5.3   Fungal Paranasal Sinusitis

As a type of chronic sinusitis, it has its typical characteristics. In addition to the common manifestations of chronic sinusitis, it has demonstrations of increased density of the sinus cavity with higher density shadows in it.

CT scanning demonstrates calcification of different degrees, with their surrounding mucus fluid of slightly lower density, which is characteristically fungal paranasal sinusitis. In some cases, fungal paranasal sinusitis can cause distended sinus cavity and even damage and absorption of bone of sinus wall, which may be misdiagnosed as tumors. MR imaging demonstrates heterogeneous signals in the sinus cavity, especially obvious in the maxillary sinus. It demonstrates heterogeneous signals by T1WI and flakes of low signals in the high signals by T2WI. The sinus cavity usually enlarges, with increased signal of the sinus wall by T2WI.

Case Study 1

A male patient aged 39 years was confirmatively diagnosed as having AIDS by CDC. He had cysts in the maxillary sinus.

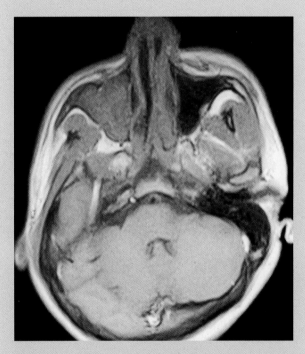

Fig. 16.12   HIV/AIDS related cyst in the right maxillary sinus. Axial T1WI demonstrates slightly lower homogeneous signals filling in the right maxillary sinus, clearly defined and continuous bone of the sinus wall, thickened left inferior concha compared to the right side and narrowed nasal cavity

Case Study 2

A male patient aged 14 years was confirmatively diagnosed as having AIDS by CDC. His CD4 T cell count was 87/μl.

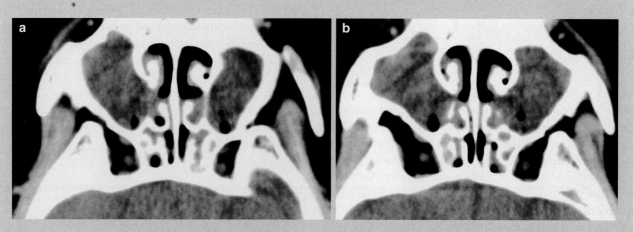

Fig. 16.13 (**a, b**) HIV/AIDS related bilateral maxillary sinusitis. Coronal CT scanning demonstrates heterogeneous low density shadows filling in the bilateral maxillary sinuses with gas in the superior section, thickened soft tissues at the opening of the bilateral sinuses, no damages to the bone of the sinus wall and increased density of the bilateral ethmoid cells

Case Study 3

A male patient aged 32 years was confirmatively diagnosed as having AIDS by CDC. He had maxillary sinusitis. And his CD4 T cell count was 69/μl.

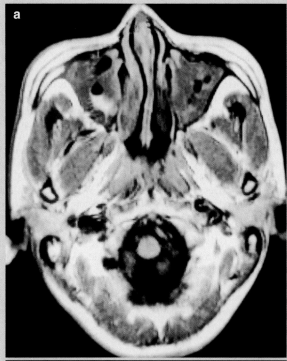

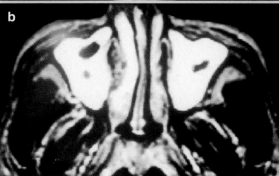

Fig. 16.14 (**a, b**) HIV/AIDS related bilateral maxillary sinusitis. Axial MR imaging demonstrates heterogeneously thickened mucosa of bilateral maxillary sinuses, with low T1 signal and bright high T2 signal; obviously shrunk sinus cavities with only a little air; a few different signals area posterior to the right sinus cavity, with mucous retention of high T1 and T2 signal

16.5.6   Diagnostic Criteria

Paranasal sinusitis can be definitely diagnosed based on clinical symptoms and imaging demonstrations. But further diagnosis of HIV related paranasal sinusitis should combine the laboratory blood test results, including CD4 T cell count, its ratio to CD8 T cell count and serum HIV antibody positive.

Clinical symptoms are as mentioned above. Imaging demonstrations are important information for definitive diagnosis. CT scanning demonstrates turbinate hypertrophy, thickened paranasal sinus mucosa that generally parallel to the sinus wall. Cases with obvious mucosa edema have lobulated polyp liked hypertrophy. There are also CT scanning demonstrations of secretion retention in the sinus, air-fluid level changing with the posture. Plain scanning demonstrates low density secretions or a density similar to that of the mucosa, occasionally with flakes of high density that may be mould mass or necrotic tissue. Enhanced scanning demonstrates obvious enhancement of the mucosa. In the chronic stage, the bone of sinus wall is hardened and thickened, possibly with distention and damage. MR imaging demonstrates thickened paranasal sinus mucosa having equal T1 and long T2 signals. In the acute stage, effusion from the sinus cavity is serous fluids with a few visible component such as proteins, in long T1 and long T2 signals which are higher than mucosa signals. Cases with more proteins content demonstrate equal/short T1 signals and long T2 signals.

16.5.7   Differential Diagnosis

16.5.7.1 Chronic Rhinitis

The nasal discharge in patients with chronic rhinitis is not green and purulent yet without odors, which is the key for differential diagnosis. Plain X-ray can accurately diagnose the condition. Lesions of chronic rhinitis are limited in the nasal cavity while chronic paranasal sinusitis has changes like thickened paranasal sinus mucosa.

16.5.7.2 Nervous Headache

Some patients with nervous headache sustain long-term headache that frequently recurs, which is commonly misdiagnosed as having paranasal sinusitis. However, these patients have no nasal symptoms and the differential diagnosis can be made based on clinical manifestations and plain X-ray findings.

16.5.7.3 Paranasal Sinus Cyst

MR imaging is of great value for differential diagnosis of paranasal sinus cystic or parenchymal lesions. Retention cyst shows homogeneous low signals by T1WI and homogeneous high signals by T2WI, while mucous cyst shows homogenous slightly higher signals.

16.5.7.4 Paranasal Sinus Neoplasms

Neoplasms are masses of soft tissue signals or densities. MR imaging demonstrates long T1 and long T2 soft tissue signals with space occupying effects or mixed signals. Enhanced imaging demonstrates obvious enhancement of the lumps. CT scanning can demonstrate the damages of the bone of paranasal sinus wall.

Extended Reading

1. Chen WL, Lin YF, Tsai WC, et al. Unveiling tuberculous pyomyositis: an emerging role of immune reconstitution inflammatory syndrome. Am J Emerg Med. 2009;27(2):251.El-2.
2. Chong WK, Hall-Craggs MA, Wilkinson ID, et al. The prevalence of paranasal sinus disease in HIV infection and AIDS on cranial MR imaging. Clin Radiol. 1993;47(3):166–9.
3. De Backer AI, Mortele KJ, De Keulenaer BL, et al. Tuberculosis: epidemiology, manifestations, and the value of medical imaging in diagnosis. JBR-BTR. 2006;89(5):243–50.
4. Del Borgo C, Del Forno A, Ottaviani F, et al. Sinusitis in HIV-infected patients. J Chemother. 1997;9(2):83–8.
5. Greaves WO, Wang SA, et al. Selected topics on lymphoid lesions in the head and neck regions. Head Neck Pathol. 2011;5(1):41–50.
6. Hoffmann CJ, Brown TT. Thyroid function abnormalities in HIV-infected patients. Clin Infect Dis. 2007;45(4):488–94.
7. Madedde G, Spanu A, Chessa F, et al. Thyroid function in human immunodeficiency virus patients treated with highly active antiretroviral therapy (HAART): a longitudinal study. Clin Endocrinol (Oxf). 2006;64(4):375–83.
8. Madge S, Smith CJ, Lampe FC, et al. No association between HIV disease and its treatment and thyroid function. HIV Med. 2007; 8(1):22–7.
9. Marcuser DC, Sooy CD. Otolaryngologic & head & neck manifestation of AIDS. Laryngoscope. 1985;95:401.
10. Masgala A, Christopoulos C, Giannakou N, et al. Plasmablastic lymphoma of visceral cranium, cervix and thorax in an HIV-negative woman. Ann Hematol. 2007;86(8):615–8.
11. Robinson MR, Salit RB, Bryand-Greenwook PK, et al. Burkitt's/Burkitt's-like lymphoma presenting as bacterial sinusitis in two HIV-infected children. AIDS Patient Care STDS. 2001;15(9):453–8.
12. Sathekge M, Maes A, AI-Nahhas A, et al. What impact can fluorine-18 fluorodeoxyglucose PET/computed tomography have on HIV/AIDS and tuberculosis pandemic. Nucl Med Commun. 2009;30(4):255–7.
13. Sathekge M, Maes A, Kgomo M, et al. Use of 28F-FDG PET to predict response to first –linetuberculostatics in HIV –associated tuberculosis. J Nucl Med. 2012;52(6):880–5.
14. Steinfort DP, Smallwood D, Antippa P, et al. Endobronchial extension of granulomatous lymphadenitis in an HIV-positive man with immune reconstitution syndrome. Respirology. 2009;14(7):1064–6.

HIV/AIDS Related Respiratory Diseases

17

Contents

17.1 General Overview of HIV/AIDS Related Respiratory Diseases

Lungs are the most commonly involved organ by HIV/AIDS related diseases, and pulmonary infections are the main reasons for the increasing death rate from AIDS. Pathogens of HIV related pulmonary infections include parasites, fungi, mycobacteria, viruses, bacteria and toxoplasma gondii. According to international reports, pathogens have different geographical distribution, which is also closely related to the socioeconomic status of the region to produce varied AIDS related diseases spectra. For instance, in the United States, pneumocystis carnii pneumonia (PCP), tuberculosis and recurrent bacterial pneumonia (at least twice within 1 year) occur frequently in HIV infected patients. An international report published 10 years ago indicated that PCP is the most common and serious pulmonary opportunistic infections in HIV infected patients. Now its incidence has dropped with the application of antiretroviral treatment and preventive measures. PCP will continue to occur initially in patients who are aware of their HIV infection. In addition, HIV related viral and parasitic infections have been reported both domestically and internationally. In this section, the clinical manifestations and imaging findings of HIV related pulmonary infections are analyzed and discussed, which provide effective diagnosis basis, so as to reduce the incidence of HIV-related pulmonary infections.

17.1.1 AIDS Related Pulmonary Infections

17.1.1.1 Pneumocystis Carnii Pneumonia

Pneumocystis has been believed to be a kind of protozoon. Recently, based on its ultrastructure and ribosomal RNA phylogenetic analysis, pneumocystis is now believed to be a kind of fungus, with high affinity to the lung tissues. Due to the compromised immunity, 95 % AIDS patients sustain different types of pulmonary infections, of which PCP is the most common life-threatening opportunistic infection with an incidence rate of about 60–85 %. About 90–95 % patients suffering from AIDS complicated by PCP are adolescents and adults with their CD4 T cell counts being less than 200/μl. Clinical manifestations of typical PCP are fever, cough (dry cough without phlegm), dyspnea, chest distress and shortness of breath. Dyspnea is shown as progressive difficulty in breathing, which initially occurs after physical activities and develops into difficulty breathing even in resting state. PCP is commonly accompanied by weight loss, fatigue, anemia, general upset and lymphadenectasis. All these symptoms are non-specific, but patients often report subjective feelings of severe symptoms while physical signs are mild. By auscultation, the lungs are normal or with slightly dry, moist rales. These are the clinical findings characteristic to AIDS complicated by PCP. In most patients with PCP, the serum LDH level increases but it is non-specific. In cases of AIDS complicated by PCP, the blood PO2 reduces, commonly being lower than 70 mmHg in patients in the middle and advanced stages. The diagnostic imaging for PCP includes chest X-ray and CT scanning. Due to the low resolution of chest X-ray, its demonstrations are negative for PCP patients in the early stage or only include thickened pulmonary markings and decreased pulmonary transparency. However, CT scanning demonstrates tiny lesions or more detailed changes in lungs. Especially with the application of HRCT, the detection rate of PCP lesions has been greatly improved. It has been internationally reported that nearly 10 % of PCP patients show negative findings by the chest X-ray but with abnormal findings by HRCT. Due to the rapid progression of PCP as well as its complex pathological changes, CT scanning demonstrations are diverse with specificity. According to different pulmonary CT scanning demonstrations in different stages of the illness, PCP is divided into early stage (exudative and infiltrative stage), middle stage (fusion and parenchymal stage) and advanced stage (absorption or fibrosis stage). The early typical manifestations include intrapulmonary multiple miliary nodules, mainly distributed in both middle and lower lung fields.

It may be accompanied by enlarged hilar shadow, which should be differentiated from acute miliary tuberculosis.

The middle stage is a period of infiltration. As the disease progresses, miliary and patchy shadows fuse and expand into a dense infiltrative shadow with even density, showing a diffuse ground glass liked change. The typical manifestations include bilaterally symmetric foci with the hilus as the center. The foci infiltrates from the hilus to bilateral pulmonary interstitium, progressing from the both middle lungs to both lower lungs. HRCT can more clearly demonstrate the foci, showing a map liked or gravel road liked appearance, with clearly demonstration of gas containing bronchus penetrating the foci. The pulmonary apex is involved later. The exterior stripe of the lung field has increased transparency, showing typical willow leaf sign or moon bow sign which is the manifestation of compensatory pulmonary emphysema.

During the late compensatory repair period, the intrapulmonary lesions are mainly parenchymal changes and fibrosis, with large flaky high density shadows as well as cords liked and reticular changes. Pneumothorax, mediastinal emphysema, pneumatocele, pleural effusion and other complications may occur, with an incidence of pneumatocele in about 10–20 % patients. The autopsy grossly demonstrates swelling of the lung tissue, and the alveoli are filled with large quantity foamy liquid. The pathological changes mainly manifested as interstitial pneumonia, with early manifestations of increased permeability of the capillary wall basement membrane in the alveolar walls, which leads to fluid exudation. The Pneumocystis carinii proliferate in large quantity and adhere to cause degeneration of the type I alveolar epithelial cells and shedding of the basement membrane. Vascular congestion, edema as well as infiltration of lymphocytes, plasma cells and mononuclear cells can be found in the pulmonary interstitium.

17.1.1.2 Fungal Infections

Due to the extensive existence of aspergillus in natural world, sputum smear positive often fails to define its invasive infection. In the cases with aspergillus infection, hyphae can be found in the sputum. Fungal infections often occur in patients with CD4 T cell count below 100/μl, of which the most common pulmonary infection is aspergillus infection, followed by penicillium marneffei infection. Pulmonary infections caused by Candida albicans and histoplasma are rarely found. The incidence of cryptococcal pulmonary infection is still in a disagreement, which is increasing recently. There are also some common endemic fungal infections, such as the most commonly found fungal infections of AIDS complicated by penicillium infections in Guangxi Zhuang Autonomous Region and Hong Kong, China. Aspergillus has an extensive existence in the natural world. AIDS complicated by aspergillus infection is related to the application of corticosteroid hormone or broad-spectrum antibiotics, which occurs commonly in the advanced/critical stage of AIDS. The cases of pulmonary fungal infections, with findings of hyphae (aspergillus or candida) or yeast in cytoplasm (Histoplasma capsulatum) in tissue sections and simultaneous findings of histiocytic reactions including the infiltration of neutrophilic granulocyte and the necrosis of histocytes, can be diagnosed as having invasive fungal infection.

Cryptococcal Pneumonia

Cryptococcal infection occurs when CD4 count is below 200/µl. Especially when CD4 count is below 50/µl, the incidence is increasing. Cryptococcal infection often manifests as meningitis or meningoencephalitis. Its pulmonary infection is simple or with accompanying meningitis. The clinical manifestations are the fever, cough, shortness of breath and rarely accompanying chest pain. About 10 % patients with cryptococcal infection have respiratory failure. Cryptococcal pneumonia can occur in any part of the lungs, commonly with multiple foci in both lower lungs. Its imaging demonstrations commonly include increased pulmonary markings, singular or multiple nodules and the fusion of multiple nodules into mass. In 1992, Jones et al. [103] divided the pulmonary lesions into four groups: (1) Primary syndrome composed of subpleural lesions and the involved lymph nodes; (2) Granuloma, which is larger parenchymal granuloma; the granuloma contains large quantity inactive yeast and surrounded by fibrous granulation tissues, which contains large quantity macrophages. (3) Intrapulmonary miliary lesions, the lesions being in miliary size and diffusively distributing; (4) Formation of cavities, with central necrosis of the foci to form cavity; 10–16 % patients may have thin wall cavities. The manifestations of bilateral diffuse interstitial infiltration, patchy fusion, nodules, pleurisy, and hilar lymphadenectasis have also been reported. There are also some individual reports of cryptococcal pneumonia with pulmonary mass, singular pleural effusion and pneumothorax. In addition, some cases of cryptococcal infection may show negative pulmonary manifestations. The pathological changes include mainly exudative or granulomatous reaction, infiltrations of macrophages, lymphocytes and multinuclear macrophages in the foci, and rarely found purulent lesions. Chronic granuloma may be accompanied with extensive fibrosis.

Aspergillus Pneumonia

Aspergillus is a conditional pathogenic fungus. In AIDS patients, aspergillus invades the bronchial wall and the lung tissues after inhaled to cause exudative and necrotic lesions as well as secondary suppurative pneumonia and lung abscess. After the pus fluids and necrotic substances expelled, cavity forms. Sometimes a fungus ball occurs in the cavity. Due to the different types of aspergillus as well as their different targets of invasion and different defense mechanism of the human body, the demonstrations of aspergillus pneumonia are also varying, which can be divided into four types. The first type includes bronchial pneumonia, disseminated aspergillus sepsis, aspergillus ball, and allergic reaction, with clinical manifestations of chills, fever, wheezing, cough, mucous sputum, hemoptysis and chest pain. Hemoptysis is a serious symptom of pulmonary aspergillosis, which can be the main reason of death. By chest X-ray, there are pulmonary infiltration and cavity lesion that is a round shadow with clear boundary, movable with posture. In the cases with bronchial occlusion, the fluid in the cavity shows liquid level, and sometimes in air crescent sign, based on which neoplasm can be excluded. Aspergillus infection secondary to the cavity is the specific demonstration for the imaging diagnosis of aspergillosis.

Penicillium Marneffei Pneumonia

Penicillium marneffei is a new species of penicillium genus, which was discovered in 1956 [104], with a distribution in Southeast Asia and southern China. Rhizomys is its natural host. As an conditional pathogen, people with compromised immunity are susceptible to Penicilliosis marneffei (PSM). Penicillium marneffei can spread through the contaminated soil by faeces of Rhizomys, and infect people via the respiratory tract, gastrointestinal tract and skin defects. PSM is believed to be one of the most common opportunistic infections in AIDS patients of Southeast Asia, and its incidence is still increasing. The clinical manifestations include long-term fever, progressive weight loss, cough and expectoration, skin rash, anemia, and lymphadenectasis. The pathological process of PM pneumonia is that PM yeast phase pigment with a strong hydrophobicity promotes the conidium of the mould phase and the cells of the yeast phase to adhere to the alveolar macrophages and macrophages in other parts, which enlarge the organs with abundant mononuclear macrophages, such as lymphadenectasis. Macrophagic granuloma may occur, with multinucleated cytomegalic responses. Kudeken et al. [13] conducted a study on PM infected but immunocompetent rats, which demonstrated that PM can cause fatal high inflammatory responses after complex CD4 T cells mediation. But in AIDS patients with PM pulmonary infections, due to the serious insufficiency of the CD4 T cells, the phagocytosis of macrophages is obviously weakened, with less exudative changes but commonly proliferative changes to cause only non-reactive necrotic inflammation with cavity formation. Zhang et al. [105] studies a group of cases, with imaging characteristic demonstrations of clustering cavities in the irregularly thick wall, reflecting its pathological features of mainly proliferation and necrotic cavities. The clustering may be related to the spreading of PM along the bronchi. The pulmonary puncture for biopsy demonstrates that microscopically tissue culture at a temperature of 25 °C may find mycelium branches and septa as well as the string of microspores or growth of hyphae in broom liked appearance.

Candida Pneumonia

Candida albicans is yeast liked fungus, which is widespread in the natural world. It can parasitize in the mocous of skin, oral cavity, intestinal tract and vagina of the human being. Candida albicans cannot cause disease in immunocompetent people but is pathogenic in immunocompromised population. After its invasion into the tissues, it turns into mycelia and multiplies in large quantity with great toxicity. It also has the ability to fight against phagocytosis. Clinically, its infection is characterized by a chronic onset and clinical symptoms of low and moderate grade fever but rarely high fever, cough, shortness of breath, cyanosis, irritation or dysphoria. The pulmonary signs include weakened breathing sounds by auscultation and obvious moist rales of lungs. The serious cases may have symptoms of systemic poisoning. The illness is prolonged and repeated during its whole progression. By diagnostic imaging demonstrations, it can be divided into the following types: (1) Bronchitis type, with chest X-ray demonstrations of increased pulmonary markings in lower fields of both lungs; (2) Pneumonia type, commonly with accompanying extrapulmonary lesions. The lesions are mainly located in the middle and lower lung fields and lesions in the lower lung field are more common. The apex is generally not involved. The lesions are recurring one after another. A small number of patients may sustain complications of exudative pleurisy. (3) Disseminated type, with miliary shadows, diffuse nodular shadows or multiple small abscesses. The lesions often involve the middle and lower lungs. Chest X-ray demonstrates thickened pulmonary markings and accompanying spots, small flakes and large flakes of parenchyma shadows, in manifestations of bronchial pneumonia. In some serious cases, the foci may fuse together and enlarge to involve the entire lobe. CT scanning demonstrates pulmonary nodules and few have ground glass liked changes of the lungs. Pathological changes include acute inflammatory lesions in the lungs, alveolar exudation and infiltration of monocytes, lymphocytes and neutrophils. Acute disseminated lesions often cause multiple small abscesses, central caseous necrosis, spores and hyphae in and around the lesions.

Histoplasma Capsulatum Pneumonia

Histoplasma capsulatum belongs to moniliales family, deuteromycetes class and fungal kingdom, whose growth requires organic nitrogen. It is often isolated from the soil with abundant contents of birds or bats faeces and spreads along with chickens, birds, dogs, cats, and mice. When the conidia and mycelial fragments of histoplasmosis are inhaled, most can be expelled by the defense mechanism of the human body. Granulomas may form, but in immunocompromised patients, it may cause disseminated histoplasmosis. When the CD4 T cell count in AIDS patients is less than 150/µl, histoplasma capsulatum infection of lungs may

occur. Histoplasma capsulatum pneumonia has a higher incidence in South America, Africa and India. In the slight cases, the clinical manifestations are similar to symptoms of the cold, with low-grade fever, cough, and general upset. In the serious cases, there are symptoms of influenza, including chills, high fever, cough, chest pain, dyspnea, fatigue and poor appetite. In the cases of acute cavity, thin-walled cavity may form within a month. Complications may be pericarditis, arthritis, skin nodules, rash fibrous mediastinitis and mediastinal granuloma. Diagnostic imaging demonstrations are non-specific, with scattering pulmonary acinus exudation, multiple nodules in a diameter of about 3 mm with accompanying thickened septa, and formation of granulomas with accompanying calcification. It should be differentiated from bacterial pneumonia, tuberculosis and other pulmonary fungal infections by laboratory tests to define the diagnosis. The specificity of the glycogen antigen detection of histoplasma capsulatum is up to 98 %.

Mucor Pneumonia

Mucor spreads through the respiratory tract. It commonly invades the blood vessels, especially arteries. It reproduces locally or causes thrombosis and embolism. Clinical manifestations are high fever, cough, sputum, shortness of breath, chest distress, chest pain and hemoptysis (pulmonary artery involvement). The diagnostic imaging demonstrates flakes inflammatory foci, with manifestations of pulmonary cavity and pulmonary infarction. The pathological changes are hemorrhagic infarction of local tissue, pneumonia and exudation of neutrophils. Hemorrhagic infarction of local tissue may be related to hyphae induced minor arteries lesions.

17.1.1.3 Pulmonary Tuberculosis

It is estimated that one third of the world population was/is infected with tubercle bacillus and 9 % of them are AIDS patients. The WHO reported that there are 88,000 newly infected patients of TB each year and 8.4 % of them arc caused by AIDS. It is estimated that each year in 1,000 HIV infected patients, 35–162 sustain active TB, and there is a great risk of active TB progressed from the latent tuberculosis infection. HIV infected patients with tuberculosis are commonly young and middle aged adults, with more male patients than female patients. Tuberculosis can occur at any stage of AIDS and at any level of CD4 T cell counts. It has been internationally reported that HIV infection complicated by TB has no specific imaging demonstrations. It has an acute onset, with an incidence of acute onset 2.5 times as high as that in non-HIV infected patients. The lesions are morphologically diverse, which are different from non-HIV infected patients with TB. HIV infection complicated by TB has commonly an acute onset, while TB in non-HIV infected patients is commonly secondary to other lesions, with cavities, fibrosis, pleural thickening and calcification. A study conducted in China has demonstrated that for AIDS complicated by TB, the acute cases mainly have military and exudative lesions, with an incidence of 33 and 49 % respectively; while the incidence of chronic cases including cavity, fibrosis and calcification is declining, being 11, 11 and 2 respectively. A later occurrence of tuberculosis in HIV infected patients indicates a more seriously immunocompromised immunity, with less typical clinical manifestations and imaging demonstrations. When the CD4 T cell count level is above 350–400/μl, the systemic symptoms are fever, chills, night sweating, fatigue, poor appetite and weight loss. Respiratory symptoms are cough, expectoration, hemoptysis, chest pain and dyspnea. It manifests as primary tuberculosis, with its foci distributing in the middle and lower lungs, involving multiple lobes and segments. When the CD4 T cell count decrease, the impact of TB increase including the occurrence of extrapulmonary tuberculosis and disseminated disease. When the CD4 T cell count drops below 200/μl, pulmonary tuberculosis manifests as acute onset (such as miliary tuberculosis) or extrapulmonary tuberculosis (such as ileocecal tuberculosis) and peripheral lymph nodes tuberculosis. Its difference from the clinical manifestations of non-HIV infected patients is as the following: (1) More common pulmonary infiltration with multiple involvements and rare cavities; (2) Higher incidence of dissemination (87–96 %) commonly along with blood flow and higher incidence of extrapulmonary tuberculosis (60–70 %); (3) More common lymph node tuberculosis, such as hilar, mediastinal and extrapleural lymphadenectasis; (4) Lower positive rate of tuberculin test (PPD); (5) More patients with no expectoration, with sputum smear for acid-fast bacilli staining is negative; (6) Higher incidence of resistant strains, high recurrence rate, and higher mortality (Table 17.1).

Foci in the cases with AIDS complicated by pulmonary tuberculosis are change quickly. After anti-TB treatment, the lesions are absorbed quickly. Those receiving no anti-TB therapy, the foci tend to fuse together to form a mass or diffusely distribute.

17.1.1.4 Bacterial Pneumonia

Bacterial septicemia often occurs in AIDS patients. Many opportunistic pathogens can cause respiratory infections, including bacterial bronchitis, pneumonia and pleuritis. The incidence rate of bacterial pneumonia (BP) is 3–5 %. BP has a larger range of impact on HIV infected patients than on non-HIV infected groups. Repeated episode of BP is considered to be the first manifestations of latent HIV infection. Therefore, for those individuals who have recurrent pneumonia without other risk factors, they should be alert to HIV infection. The common pathogenic bacteria include Streptococcus pneumoniae, Staphylococcus aureus, Rhodococcus equi, Haemophilus and pseudomonas aeruginosa. As non-HIV infected patients, the most common pathogens of pneumonia

Table 17.1 Clinical manifestations of HIV/AIDS related tuberculosis and Non-HIV/AID related tuberculosis

	HIV/AID tuberculosis	Non-HIV/AID tuberculosis
Tuberculin test	Early positive	Accumulation of somatic cells
	Advanced conversion into negative	Generation of lymphokine (ThI type)
Chest X-ray	Atypical	Infiltration
	More common in the lower lung	More commonly cavity
	Rare cavity	Common occurrence in the apex and posterior segment, with downwards spreading
Extrapulmonary TB	More common	Mainly intrapulmonary, rarely extrapulmonary
	Spreading to extrapulmonary tissues	
Detection rate of MTB	Low (19 %)	High (30–73 %)
Anti-TB therapies	Poor efficacy and more side effects	Favorable efficacy and less side effects

are Streptococcus pneumoniae and Haemophilus influenzae. Legionella and Klebsiella are also common. Many factors, such as the reduced T lymphocytes in HIV infected patients, manufacturing disorders of neutrophils, mononuclear cells and cytokines, and dysfunctional B lymphocytes, provide chances for opportunistic bacterial infections. In addition, the application of broad-spectrum antibiotics also increases the chance of opportunistic infections. BP can occur in any stage of HIV and at any level of CD4 T cell count. When the CD4 T cell count decreases, the incidence of BP also increases. The clinical manifestations of HIV infected patients are the same as non-HIV infected patients, with acute onset (3–5 days), high fever (39–40 °C), chills, chest pain, dyspnea, cough, purulent sputum (bloody or rusty). Being different from non-HIV infection, pulmonary infection in HIV-infected patients is often recurrent.

The imaging demonstrations of HIV/AIDS related bacterial pneumonia are similar to those in non-HIV infected patients. Most cases of streptococcal pneumonia and haemophilus pneumonia have unilateral, confined and partially fused foci with accompanying pleural effusion. The imaging demonstrations include thickened and deranged pulmonary markings, alveolar filling of inflammatory exudates with the progression of the illness, large flaks inflammatory infiltration shadows or parenchymal shadows, bronchial gas filling phase in the parenchymal shadows. The lesions distribute along the pulmonary segments or lobes, rarely with accompanying pleural effusion. During the absorption period, the density of the parenchymal shadows gradually reduces and the scope narrows down. There may be cavities in some individual cases. But in most cases it is completely absent after

3–4 weeks. Lesions absorption are slow in elderly patients and recurrent patients, which is difficult to be completely absorbed and often develop into organic pneumonia.

Rhodococcus equi was initially discovered in 1923 and nominated as corynebacterium equi. After structure analysis of the cell wall, it was found to be different from Corynebacterium, and therefore it is classified into Rhodococcus. Rhodococcus equi is generally considered as the pathogens of horses, pigs and cattle. Human rhodococcus equi infection is rare. But in recent years, due to an increase in patients with immunodeficiency syndrome, reports of rhodococcus equi induced human respiratory infection and sepsis are increasing. Rhodococcus equi is an intracellular facultative parasitic bacterium. Its optimum temperature for growth is 30 °C, and suitable temperature for its growth is 10–40 °C. The acid-fast staining for rhodococcus equi shows uncertain results. Due to its various morphology, it is commonly mistaken as diphtheroids bacilli, Bacillus or Micrococcus. On sheep blood agar plate, the bacterium can have synergistic hemolysis with staphylococcus aureus, mononuclear Listeria and Corynebacterium pseudotuberculosis. Toxicity mechanisms of Rhodococcus equi has been recently discovered the existence of toxic plasmid, which provides a new idea for the full understanding of its pathogenesis. Clinical symptoms are usually cough, orange red sputum, high fever and other symptoms. E Marchiori et al. in 2005 studied five cases of AIDS complicated by Rhodococcus equi pulmonary infection. All the patients had a case history of cough and fever history for 1–2 months with accompanying shortness of breath and chest pain. Li et al. in 2009 [106] studied a group of 13 cases. All patients had fever, with a body temperature being 38–40 °C, cough, orange red sputum. The typical clinical manifestations of the disease are fever, dyspnea and chest pain. Other symptoms such as weight loss, diarrhea and joint pain are not representative. Based on the course of the disease, the diagnostic imaging demonstrations of Rhodococcus equi pulmonary infection can be divided into early stage, showing round liked flaky blurry shadows surrounding unilateral hilum that has blurry boundary; middle stage (parenchymal change), showing central sphere liked high density shadow surrounding unilateral hilum, in parenchymal changes and with clear boundary; advanced stage (necrosis) showing secondary cavity of the pulmonary mass, possibly with hydropneumothorax and pleurisy. The imaging demonstrations are characteristic, but lack of specificity. And it should be differentiated from pulmonary tumors. The pathological changes include the most commonly chronic suppurative bronchopneumonia and extensive pulmonary abscesses. The histopathology demonstrates massive bleeding in alveolar space, large quantity erythrocytes, intact cellular wall and large quantity epithelial cells. The predominant pathological changes may also be fibroblasts, with parenchymal changes of lung tissue and thickened alveolar septa. Accumulating piles of strip liked purple Rhodococcus equi can be found by PAS staining.

17.1.1.5 Viral Pneumonia

Common pathogenic viruses of the opportunistic pulmonary infections in HIV infected patients are cytomegalovirus (CMV) and influenza virus. CMV is the most common pathogen of HIV/AIDS related pulmonary infection. By autopsy, 49–82 % patients with HIV/AIDS have CMV infection, only second to Pneumocystis carinii pneumonia. Moskowitz et al. [32] reported that among the direct causes of death in AIDS patients, 19 % is due to pulmonary cytomegalovirus infection. Because of the lack of typical clinical manifestations and sensitive examinations for its early diagnosis, the definitive diagnosis rate of cytomegalovirus pneumonia is only 13–24 % before autopsy. The clinical manifestations of CMV infection are non-specific. The systemic symptoms are fever, soreness of joints and muscles. Respiratory symptoms are paroxysmal dry cough, progressive shortness of breath, difficulty in breathing during activities. Pulmonary CMV infection may develop secondary fungal infection or be complicated by bacterial, fungal, and Pneumocystis carinii infections. The cytomegalovirus can widely spread in the organs and tissues of the infected patients, and the infections can directly lead to the damage of infected host cells. In addition, the virus can also cause pathogenic effects via immune pathological mechanism. Some scholars classified CMV pneumonia into diffuse, miliary necrosis and cytomegalic. Diffuse and cytomegalic CMV pneumonia are often accompanied by diffuse alveolar damage (DAD), which is more common in the diffuse type of CMV pneumonia but less common in cytomegalic type of CMV pneumonia. The pathological basis of diffuse small nodules in lungs is hemorrhagic necrosis. Sometimes CMV infection is concurrent with other infections in the lungs, and even co-infects one cell. Pulmonary parenchymal changes indicate bacterial and fungal infections, such as findings of inclusion bodies in the cells, commonly known as Eagle's Eye sign. The imaging demonstrations of cytomegalovirus pneumonia are diverse. Some studies summarize that the lungs commonly have manifestations of diffuse interstitial infiltration or alveolar infiltration, with ground glass liked changes, pulmonary parenchymal changes, grid liked changes, thickend bronchial wall, bronchiectasis, pulmonary nodules or masses. The principal changes include the early lesions of ground glass liked changes and advanced lesions of pulmonary masses.

17.1.1.6 Lymphoid Interstitial Pneumonia

Lymphoid interstitial pneumonia is the abnormal hyperplasia of the pulmonary lymphoid tissue. Its occurrence is related to autoimmune diseases, and is believed to be a direct response of the lungs to HIV. The clinical manifestations are recurrent infections, poor appetite, hepatomegaly and splenomegaly, and arrested development. The diagnostic imaging demonstrates no characteristic changes by CT scanning, with thickened bronchial wall, diffuse central lobular nodules or bronchiectasis, grid liked and cords liked shadows in uneven thickness. The pathological changes include accumulating lymphocytes and plasma cells that are mixed to infiltrate the pulmonary interstitium and expand to surrounding areas of the bronchi.

17.1.1.7 Toxoplasma Pneumonia

Toxoplasma pneumonia is caused by the infection of the intracellular parasite, Toxoplasma gondii. Ludlam et al. in 1963 firstly proposed the concept of pulmonary toxoplasmosis, which was believed to cause atypical pneumonia [107]. The clinical manifestations are cough and expectoration. In the serious cases, dyspnea and cyanosis can occur. In the chronic cases, there are long term low grade fever, cough, weight loss and enlarged lymph nodes. The diagnostic imaging demonstrates bronchopneumonia, interstitial pneumonia and pleurisy. (1) Bronchial pneumonia is also known as lobular pneumonia, with scattered patchy and blurry density shadows. (2) Interstitial pneumonia has typical manifestations of reticular and nodular shadows. (3) Pleurisy is rare, showing pleural effusion, limited diaphragmatic activity. The imaging demonstrations are non-specific, which can be defined in combination with the etiologic examinations. The pathological changes are congestion and edema of the surrounding connective tissue of the alveolar wall and bronchial walls, widened pulmonary interstitium, small quantity serous fibrin exudation from alveoli and pulmonary interstitium, and infiltration of macrophages and lymphocytes. Toxoplasma cysts and tachyzoites may be found in pulmonary interstitium and macrophages as well as alveolar epithelium.

17.1.2 HIV/AIDS Related Pulmonary Tumors

17.1.2.1 Kaposi's Sarcoma

Kaposi's sarcoma, a vascular tumor, was discovered in 1872, and is also known as multiple hemorrhagic sarcomas, multiple vascular sarcomas, or multiple pigmented sarcomas. Kaposi's sarcoma is believed to be the defining tumor of AIDS. Outbreak of KS occurred in male homosexuals in Europe and the United States. Data show that in about 30 % Caucasian homosexuals, Kaposi's sarcoma is a major complication of in HIV/AIDS patients. It has been confirmed that, though Kaposi's sarcoma has strong invasion, the disease itself has little impact on the mortality of AIDS. The cause of death in majority of the patients is still opportunistic infections. The clinical manifestations include face and neck lesions in dark red to purple red plaques. The plaques do not fade away when pressed, with surrounding brown ecchymosis. It commonly involves multiple organs including lungs, spleen, oral cavity, lymph nodes, gastrointestinal tract and liver. The lungs are the major target of invasion. The diagnostic imaging demonstrates hilar lymphadenectasis and its surrounding nodular infiltration, bilateral interstitial changes, and pleural effusion that are its typical X-ray demonstration. Early pathological changes are similar to those of common angioma; with gathering of capillaries into groups containing histocytes engulfed hemosiderin and orderly arranged vascular endothelial cells. It further progression see active proliferation of endothelial cells and fibroblasts, increased nuclear mitosis with anaplasia, and scattered lymphocytes and histocytes between blood vessels. In the advanced stage, occlusion and necrosis of the vascular lumen can be found. Irregular lumen and fissures of the new capillaries can be commonly found in the tumor, filled with blood and common hemorrhage. In China, KS is relatively rare. Its definitive diagnosis can be made by pathological examination.

17.1.2.2 Other HIV/AIDS Related Malignancies

Other HIV/AIDS related malignancies include Burkitt's lymphoma, non-Hodgkin's lymphoma, Hodgkin's lymphoma and lung cancer. In summary, HIV/AIDS related pulmonary infections are important diseases in the disease spectrum of HIV/AIDS imaging. The diagnostic imaging is irreplaceable examinations for pulmonary infections. Early prevention and correct diagnosis are the keys to improve the quality of life and prolong the lives of patients. The complexity and multiplicity of HIV/AIDS related pulmonary diseases present challenges for the clinicians. Firstly, HIV/AIDS related diseases should be optimally classified. Each type should has a disease spectrum, which can be used for exclusion in combination with immunological indices to make the diagnosis and differential diagnosis. The diagnosis of HIV/AIDS related pulmonary infections should be made in combination with case history and laboratory tests for targeting individualized diagnosis to serve clinical practice.

17.2 HIV/AIDS Related Pneumocystis Carnii Pneumonia (PCP)

Pneumocystis carinii (PC) pneumonia is caused by the opportunistic fungus, Pneumocystis carinii. The disease occurs in immunocompromised patients, mostly are HIV infected persons. In these patients, PCP is one of the manifestations of AIDS. The risk factors of PCP include HIV infection, primary immunodeficiency, premature birth, neoplasms, the use of immunosuppressant after organ transplantation and long-term use of high dose corticosteroids. Currently, HIV infection is the cause of the vast majority cases of PCP. The Pneumocystis carinii is re-classified as a fungus by genome, which is a widespread micro-organism. Immunocompromised people are susceptible to its infection. In the early 1980s, due to the limited knowledge about HIV/AIDS complicated by opportunistic infections, Pneumocystis carinii infection is rarely diagnosed. In the recent 15 years, since the worldwide prevalence of AIDS, Pneumocystis carinii infection is the most common and serious opportunistic infection in HIV infected patients. In North America, Pneumocystis carinii infection is listed as the defining disease of AIDS, with more than 85 % HIV infected patients can be infected by Pneumocystis carinii and their CD4 T cell count is usually lower than 100/μl. When PCP is diagnosed, the average CD4 T cell count is approximately 50/μl. The mortality rate of Pneumocystis carinii infection induced acute respiratory failure is higher than 80 %, which can be reduced to 50 % after systematic treatment. Pneumocystis carinii infection has a high recurrence rate, being more than 65 % within 18 months. Therefore, when the CD4 T cell count of HIV infected patients is lower than 100/μl, preventive treatment against Pneumocystis carinii infection should be administered.

17.2.1 Pathogens and Pathogenesis

The pathogen is the trophozoites and cysts produced by Pneumocystis carinii, principally living in the lungs. Pneumocystis carinii was used to being categorized as as protozoon, but recently, it is believed to be belonged to fungus according to its ultrastructure and Pneumocystis ribosomal RNA phylogenetic analysis. The main infection route of PCP is airborne transmission and reactivation of in vivo latent Pneumocystis carinii. Inflammatory and immune responses of the host include phagocytosis of Pneumocystis carinii by the alveolar macrophages, infiltration of lymphocytes in peribronchial and vascular area, proliferation of type II alveolar cells, local and systemic increase of antibody.

17.2.2 Pathophysiological Basis

By naked eyes observation, there are extensive and diffuse invasion of lungs, which is soft like waterlogged sponge and in milky white with black spots. The filled foamy substance in the alveoli and bronchioles is a mixture of necrotic fungus and immunoglobulin. The alveolar septum has infiltration of plasma cells and lymphocytes, resulting in thickened alveolar septa up to 5–20 times as the normal thickness that occupy 3/4 of the entire lung volume. The cysts are firstly located in the macrophage cytoplasm of the alveolar septa. Subsequently, the alveolar cells containing cysts sheds off into the alveolar space. After the rupture of the cystic wall, sporozoite is discharged to turn into free trophozoites, which

gains its access into the alveolar space. The alveolar exudates include plasma cells, lymphocytes and histocytes (Fig. 17.1a–c).

17.2.3 Clinical Symptoms and Signs

The clinical symptoms include dry cough, shortness of breath and an indoor hypoxia. About 95 % AIDS patients have multi-pathogens induced pulmonary infections. The most significant laboratory abnormality in most PCP patients is hypoxemia. Based on correlation between PCP and arterial oxygen partial difference, hypoxemia is divided into three degrees. The slight cases at indoor conditions have their PaO_2 being above 70 mmHg, or alveolar-arterial oxygen pressure difference being less than 35 mmHg, or both. The moderate and severe cases have their PaO_2 being usually less than 70 mmHg, or alveolar-arterial oxygen pressure difference being above 35 mmHg, or both. The most common manifestations of AIDS complicated by PCP are progressive subacute onset of dyspnea, fever, dry cough and chest distress, the symptoms aggravating in a few days or weeks. Pulmonary examination is usually negative in slight cases. As the disease aggravates, the cases show shortness of breath, cyanosis, tachycardia, and diffuse dry rales. Pneumocystis carinii infection accounts for 60–85 % of AIDS patients, which is one of the major causes of death in AIDS patients.

17.2.4 Examination Methods and Selections

17.2.4.1 Diagnostic Imaging
The diagnostic imaging examinations include chest X-ray, CT scanning and nuclear medicine examination. (1) Chest X-ray is the conventional examination for screening. Early lesions tend to be missed for the diagnosis due to the limited resolution or atypical lung lesions. (2) CT scanning with high resolution is superior to chest X-ray. (3) Nuclear medicine examination demonstrates increased uptake of the isotope-labeled monoclonal antibodies in the lung tissues of the PCP patients.

17.2.4.2 Etiological Examination
(1) By tracheal suction or lung tissue biopsy, the detection rate of Pneumocystis carinii is up to 90 %. By tissue section staining, abundant protozoa can be found in intra-alveolar foamy eosinophil substance mass (By methenamine silver nitrate staining, the dark brown round or oval shaped cysts can be found in a diameter of 6–8 μm out of the cells). (2) By ELISA, Pneumocystis IgG antibody can be detected and by latex particle agglutination test, the protozoa antigen can be detected. (3) Molecular biology techniques, such as PCR can be applied for early diagnosis.

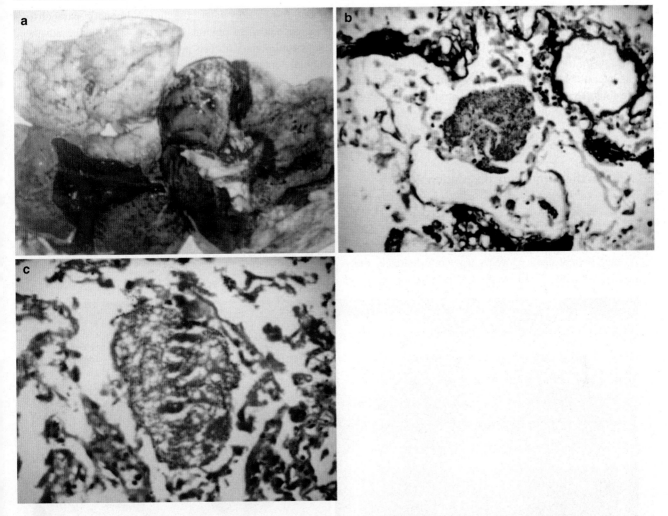

Fig. 17.1 (**a**) Gross specimens' observation demonstrates foamy liquid filling in the lung tissues. (**b**) HE demonstrates pneumocystis in the alveolar exudates, which can be stained black by silver methenamine staining, ×400. (**c**) HE demonstrates the foamy substance in the alveolar space, ×400

17.2.4.3 Other Examinations

The following examinations are non-specific, but can be used to assess the severity of PCP and its progression. (1) By arterial blood gas analysis, the patients may show reduced blood oxygen saturation and respiratory alkalosis. (2) By serum enzyme spectrum analysis, the patients may show increased LDH. (3) It can be detected to have increased alveolar-arterial oxygen partial pressure difference.

17.2.5 Imaging Demonstrations

17.2.5.1 Chest X-ray

In the early stage (exudation period), alveolar fluids exudate, with diffuse granular shadows in the bilateral lung fields extend from the hilum to the surrounding. In the middle stage (infiltration and fusion period), the intrapulmonary lesions fuse, with ground glass liked or cloudy shadows that are bilaterally symmetric like butterfly wings. In the middle and advanced stages (parenchymal changes period), the lung tissues show parenchymal changes, with high density shadows and accompanying air bronchogram. The lung periphery shows stripes of transparent shadows. In the advanced stage (pulmonary fibrosis period), the pulmonary interstitium is thickened in dense cords liked appearance, with interval irregular patchy shadows. The pulmonary ventilation improves and the lung periphery shows dense parenchymal shadows with emphysema, pneumomediastinum and pneumothorax.

17.2.5.2 CT Scanning

In the early stage (exudation period), the lesions radiatus develop from the hilum to lung field. In the early stage, the diffuse exudative lesions distribute as pulmonary acinus, with changes similar to pulmonary interstitial changes. It was believed to be interstitial pneumonia. However, acute PCP is actually exudation of alveoli and spaces containing gas. The parenchymal changes are accompanied by infiltration of small quantity plasma cells, with demonstrations of spots and granular shadows with clear boundaries. In the middle stage (infiltration and fusion period), about 3–4 weeks later, the lesions fuse to show typical alveolar exudative lesions. The fused foci are demonstrated as non-specific infiltration shadows in ground glass liked appearance. In the middle and advanced stages (parenchymal changes period),

about 5–6 weeks later, the intrapulmonary parenchymal changes show an obvious bronchus sign. In the advanced stage (pulmonary fibrosis period), about 7–8 weeks later, the lobular septa of both lungs are significantly thickened, with cords liked pulmonary fields, grid liked changes and decreased transparency. It can be complicated by pulmonary psuedocysts, with thin and clear cystic wall and with no liquid gas level.

17.2.5.3 In the Early Stage (Exudation Period)

Case Study 1

A male patient aged 34 years was confirmatively diagnosed as having AIDS by the CDC. He complained of dyspnea and wheezing for 3 days and his CD4 T cell count was 85/µl.

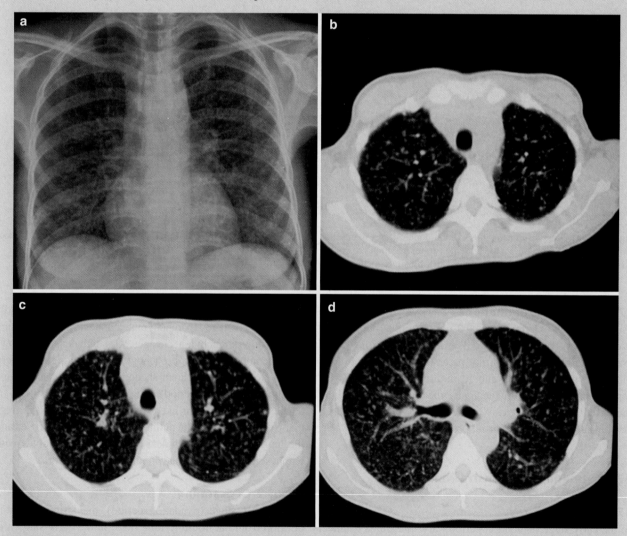

Fig. 17.2 (**a–f**) HIV/AIDS related Pneumocystis carinii pneumonia. (**a**) DR demonstrates scattered miliary increased density shadows in both lungs, with even size, density and distribution. The shadows of both hila are dense, with sharp both costophrenic angles. (**b–f**) CT scanning demonstrates scattered miliary nodular shadows in both lungs, which is more obviously in the middle pulmonary strip and with quite even size and density. Trachea and bronchi are unblocked

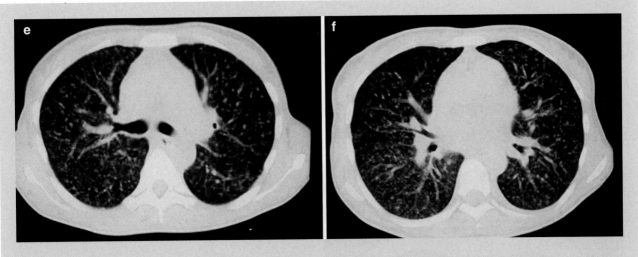

Fig. 17.2   (continued)

Case Study 2

A male patient aged 31 years was confirmatively diagnosed as having AIDS by the CDC. He complained of dyspnea and wheezing for 1 week and his CD4 T cell count was 115/μl.

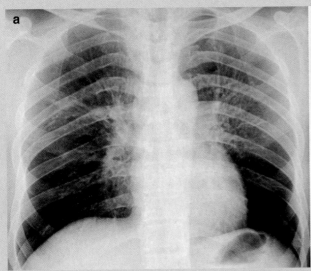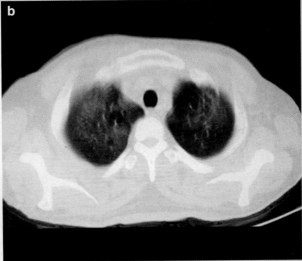

Fig. 17.3   (**a–e**) HIV/AIDS related Pneumocystis carinii pneumonia. (**a**) DR demonstrates cloudy and scattered miliary increased density shadows in both lungs, with enlarged and thickened hilum of both lungs. (**b–e**) CT scanning demonstrates even miliary increased density shadows in the middle and upper lungs as well as the dorsal segment of the lower lung field, with some fused in thin cloudy shadows

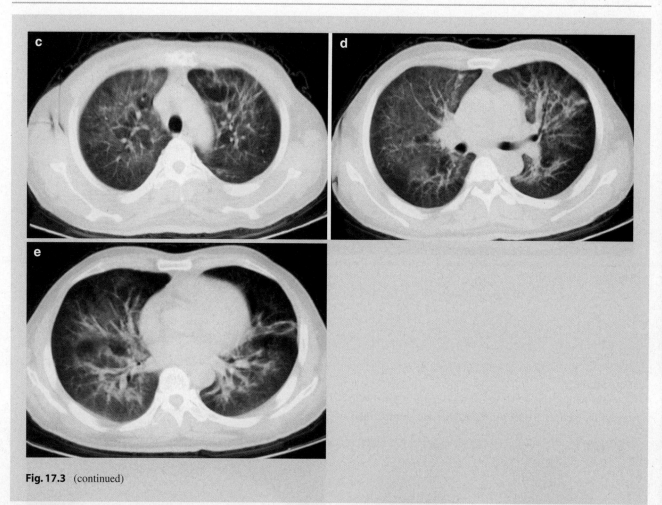

Fig. 17.3 (continued)

17.2.5.4 In the Middle Stage (Infiltration and Fusion Period)

Case Study 3

A male patient aged 38 years was confirmatively diagnosed as having AIDS by the CDC. He complained of dyspnea and wheezing for 20 days and his CD4 T cell count was 105/μl.

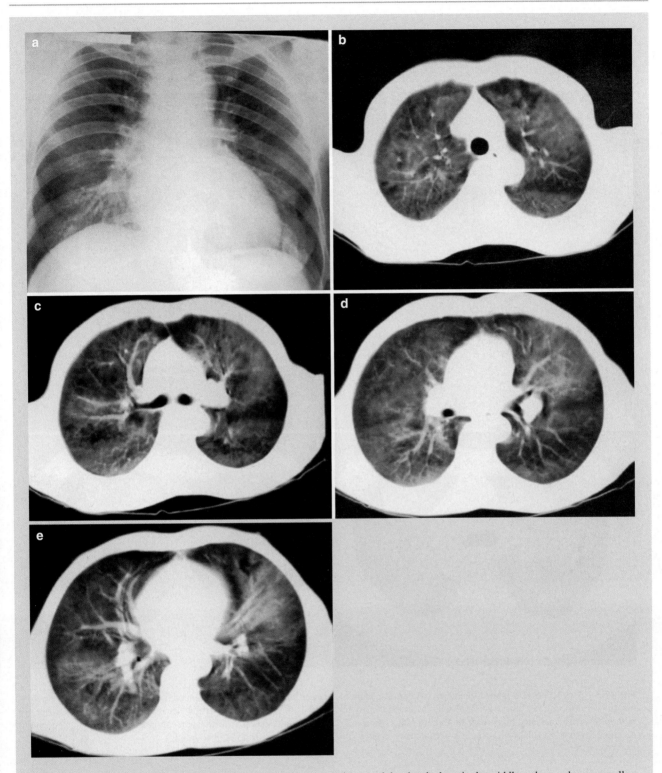

Fig. 17.4 (a–e) HIV/AIDS related Pneumocystis carinii pneumonia. (a) DR demonstrates cloudy or ground glass liked increased density shadows in both lungs, with enlarged and thickened hilum of both lungs. (b–e) CT scanning demonstrates even miliary increased density shadows in the middle and upper lungs as well as the dorsal segment of lower lungs, with some fused into thin cloudy ground glass liked shadows with increased density, with decreased transparency of both lungs and enlarged hilar shadows in both lungs

Case Study 4

A male patient aged 41 years was confirmatively diagnosed as having AIDS by the CDC. He complained of chest distress, dyspnea and wheezing for 1 month and his CD4 T cell count was 104/μl.

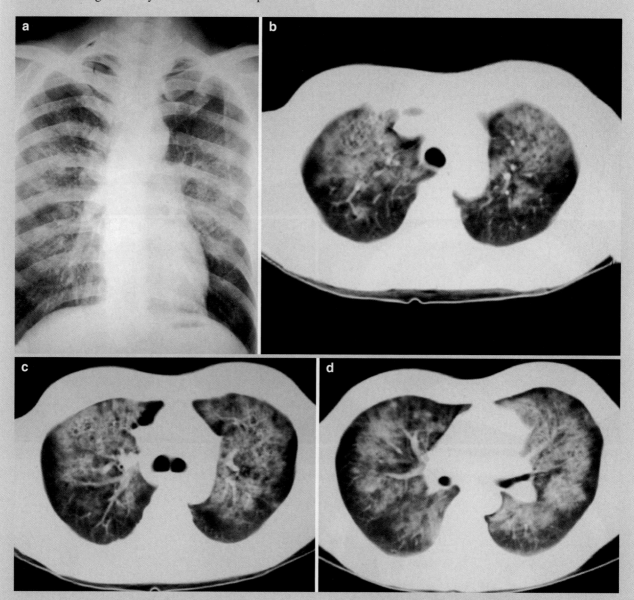

Fig. 17.5 (a–g) HIV/AIDS related Pneumocystis carinii pneumonia. (a) DR demonstrates patchy shadows with increased density in both lungs, with thickened hilar shadows in both lungs. (b–g) CT scanning demonstrates flaky ground glass liked density shadows in upper lungs and dorsal segment of both lungs, which is more obvious in the middle inner strips. There are extrapulmonary stripes transparent shadows, with some bronchial walls thickened and enlarged hilar shadows in both lungs

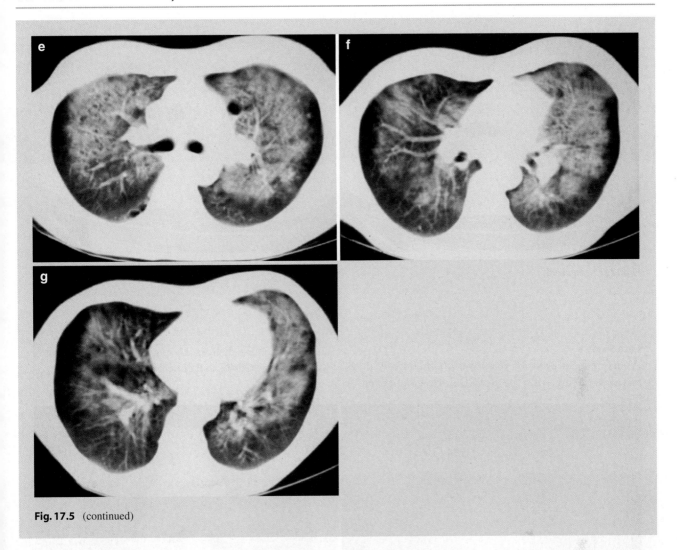

Fig. 17.5 (continued)

Case Study 5

A female patient aged 31 years was confirmatively diagnosed as having AIDS by the CDC. She complained of chest distress, dyspnea and wheezing for 1 week and her CD4 T cell count was 115/μl.

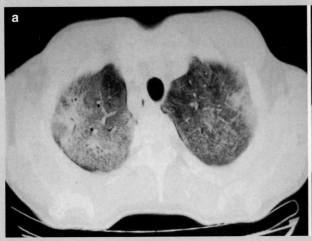

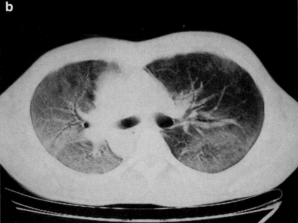

Fig. 17.6 (**a-d**) HIV/AIDS related Pneumocystis carinii pneumonia. (**a–d**) CT scanning demonstrates flaky ground glass liked density shadows in upper lobes of both lungs, with bronchial shadows in them; flaky parenchymal shadows in the subpleural apical segment; and thickened bronchial walls in the anterior and posterior segments of the right upper lobe

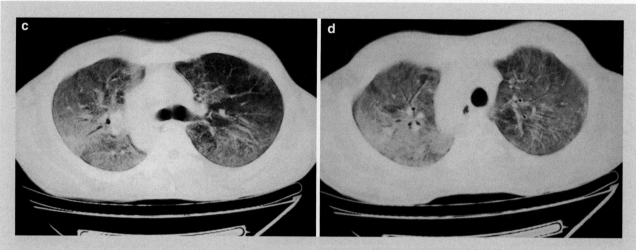

Fig. 17.6 (continued)

Case Study 6

A male patient aged 31 years was confirmatively diagnosed as having AIDS by the CDC. He complained of chest pain, chest distress, dyspnea and wheezing for 2 weeks and his CD4 T cell count was 85/μl.

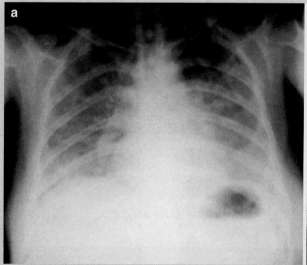

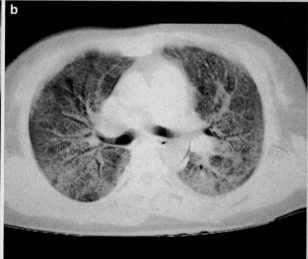

Fig. 17.7 (a–d) HIV/AIDS related Pneumocystis carinii pneumonia. (**a**) DR demonstrates diffusely distributed shadows with increased density in both lungs that is more obvious in the middle and lower lungs. The hilar shadows in both lungs are enlarged. Both diaphragmatic surfaces and phrenic angles are blurry. (**b–d**) CT scanning demonstrates flaky shadows with increased density in both lungs, with parenchymal shadows in the lingular segment of left upper lobe and in the dorsal segments of both lower lobes and bronchial shadows in them. There are also thickened bronchial walls and enlarged hilar shadows in both lungs

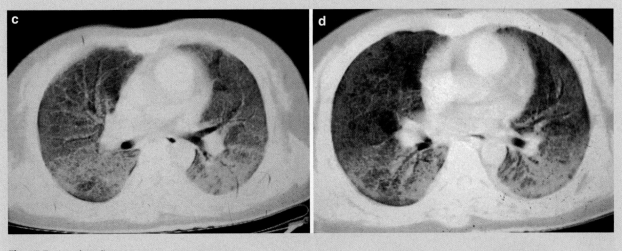

Fig. 17.7   (continued)

17.2.5.5 In the Middle-Advanced Stage (Parenchymal Changes Period)

Case Study 7

A male patient aged 31 years was confirmatively diagnosed as having AIDS by the CDC. He complained of dyspnea, cyanosis and wheezing for 3 weeks, with obviously decreased oxygen saturation. His CD4 T cell count was 45/µl.

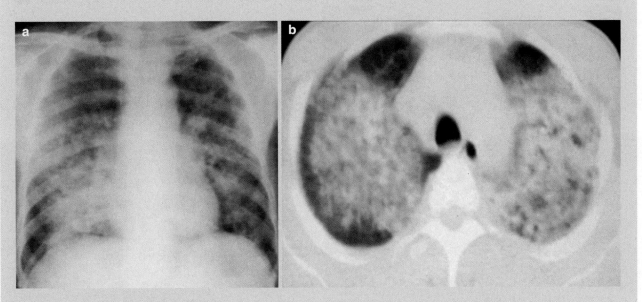

Fig. 17.8   (a–g) HIV/AIDS related Pneumocystis carinii pneumonia. (**a**) DR demonstrates large flaky parenchyma shadows in both lungs which is more obvious in the middle and lower lobes of both lungs. There are also enlarged hilar shadows in both lungs and sharp both costophrenic angles. (**b–g**) CT scanning demonstrates large flaky parenchyma shadows in concentric and symmetrical distribution, bronchial shadows in them and thickened bronchial walls

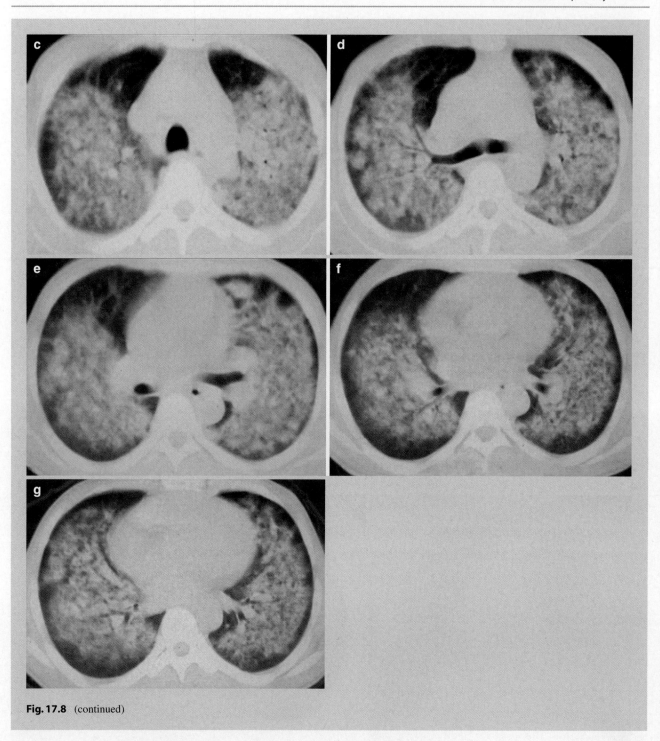

Fig. 17.8 (continued)

Case Study 8

A male patient aged 31 years was confirmatively diagnosed as having AIDS by the CDC. He complained of dyspnea, cyanosis and wheezing for 4 weeks, with obviously decreased oxygen saturation. His CD4 T cell count was 45/μl.

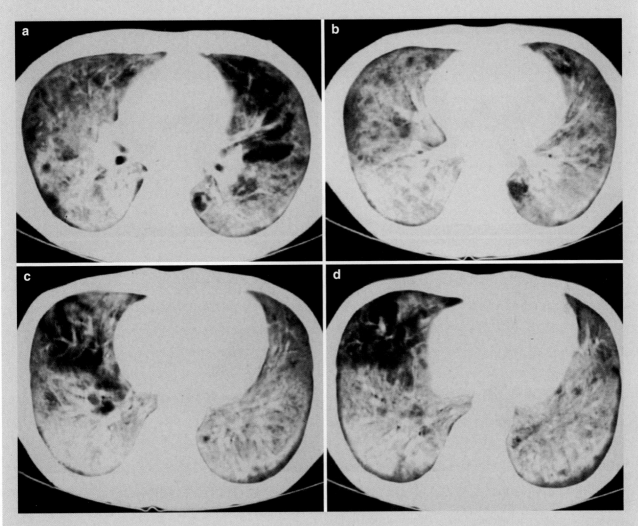

Fig. 17.9 (**a–d**) HIV/AIDS related Pneumocystis carinii pneumonia. (**a–d**) CT scanning demonstrates large flaky parenchyma shadows in both lungs, with transparent areas in some foci. The trachea and bronchi are unblocked, with thickened bronchial walls in the middle and lower lobes

Case Study 9

A male patient aged 43 years was confirmatively diagnosed as having AIDS by the CDC. He complained of dyspnea, cyanosis and wheezing for 4 weeks, with obviously decreased oxygen saturation. His CD4 T cell count was 45/μl.

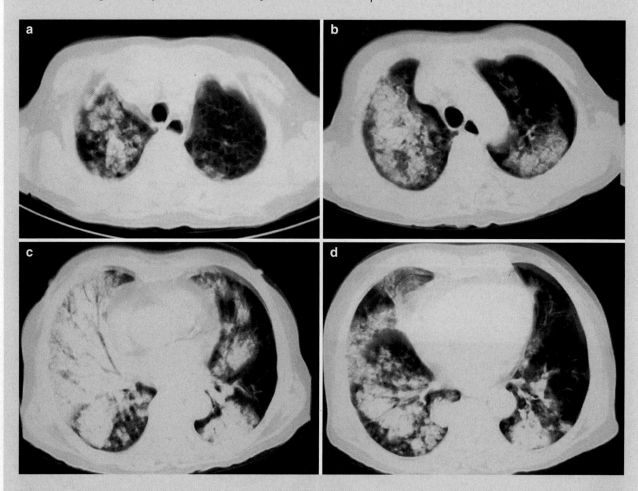

Fig. 17.10 (a–d) HIV/AIDS related Pneumocystis carinii pneumonia. (a–d) CT scanning demonstrates large flaky and mass liked parenchyma shadows in both lungs which is more obvious in the right lung, bronchial shadows in them, and thickened bronchial walls in the middle lobe of the right lung

17.2.5.6 In the Absorption Period

Case Study 10

A male patient aged 31 years was confirmatively diagnosed as having AIDS by the CDC. He complained of dyspnea, cyanosis and wheezing for 7 weeks, with obviously decreased oxygen saturation. His CD4 T cell count was 75/μl.

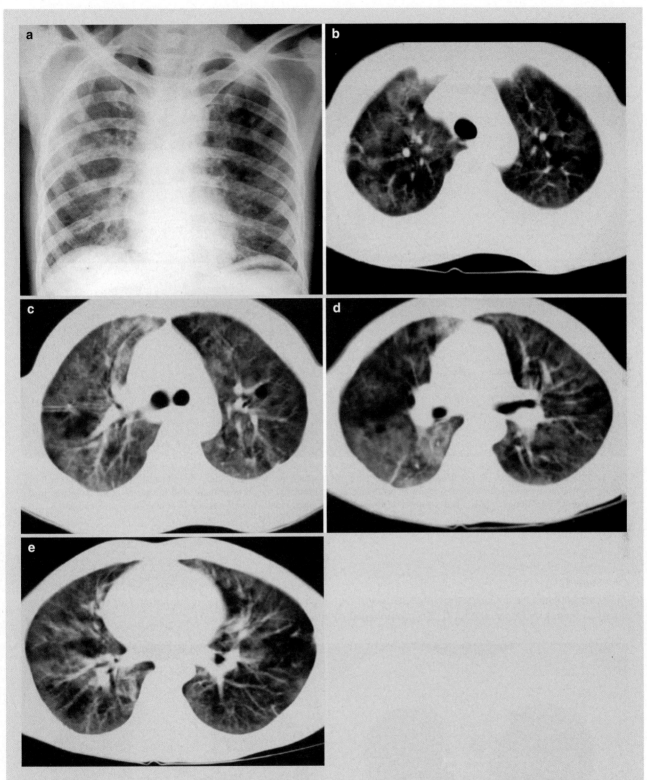

Fig. 17.11 (a–e) HIV/AIDS related Pneumocystis carinii pneumonia. (a) DR demonstrates scattered patchy shadows with increased density in both lungs and a few cords liked shadows which are more obvious in the right lung. There are thickened both hilar shadows and sharp both costophrenic angles. (b–e) CT scanning demonstrates flaky and mass liked ground glass density shadows in both lungs and a few cords liked shadows which are more obvious in the right lung. The trachea and bronchi are unblocked

Case Study 11

A female patient aged 51 years was confirmatively diagnosed as having AIDS by the CDC. She complained of dyspnea, cyanosis and wheezing for 8 weeks, with obviously decreased oxygen saturation. Her CD4 T cell count was 65/ μl.

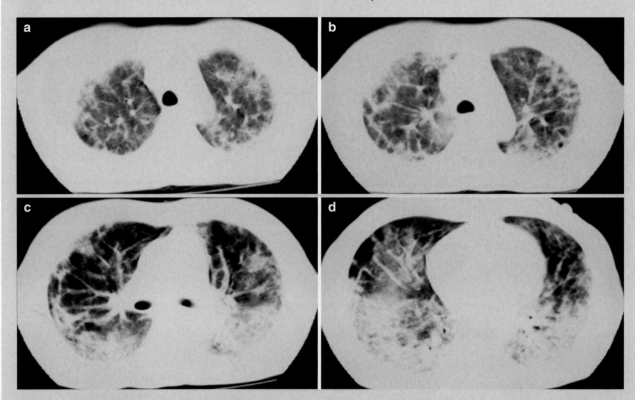

Fig. 17.12 (**a–d**) HIV/AIDS related Pneumocystis carinii pneumonia. (**a–d**) CT scanning demonstrates multiple patchy parenchyma shadows and fibrous cords liked shadows in both lungs which are more obvious in the dorsal segment of both lower lungs, bronchial shadows in them, and thickened bronchial walls in the middle lobe. The hilar shadows in both lungs are enlarged

Case Study 12

A female patient aged 37 years was confirmatively diagnosed as having AIDS by the CDC. She complained of dyspnea, cyanosis and wheezing for 8 weeks, with obviously decreased oxygen saturation. Her CD4 T cell count was 45/ μl.

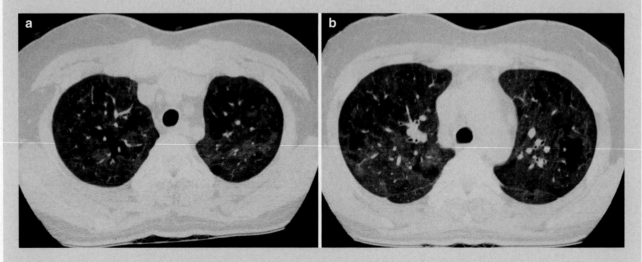

Fig. 17.13 (**a–c**) HIV/AIDS related Pneumocystis carinii pneumonia. (**a–c**) CT scanning demonstrates multiple ground glass liked density shadows in both lungs, transparent areas in them and unblocked trachea and bronchi

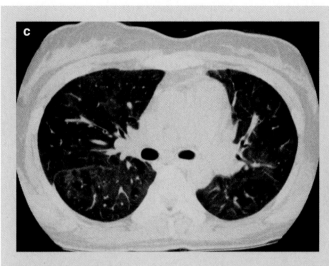

Fig. 17.13   (continued)

Case Study 13

A male patient aged 41 years was confirmatively diagnosed as having AIDS by the CDC. He complained of dyspnea, cyanosis and wheezing for 8 weeks. His CD4 T cell count was 45/μl.

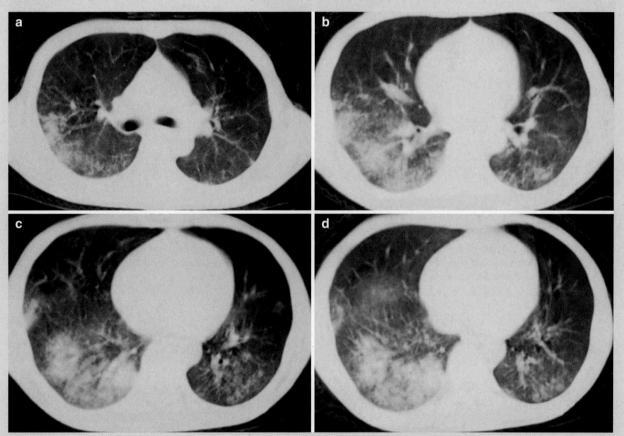

Fig. 17.14   (a–d) HIV/AIDS related Pneumocystis carinii pneumonia. (a–d) CT scanning demonstrates multiple ground glass liked density shadows in both lungs, mass and flakes of parenchymal shadows in the posterior segment of the right upper lobe and in the dorsal segment of both lower lobes which is more obvious in the right lung, and bronchial shadows in them

17.2.5.7 In the Advanced Stage (Pulmonary Fibrosis Period)

Case Study 14

A female patient aged 31 years was confirmatively diagnosed as having AIDS by the CDC. She complained of dyspnea, cyanosis and wheezing for 5 weeks, with obviously decreased oxygen saturation. Her CD4 T cell count was 45/ μl.

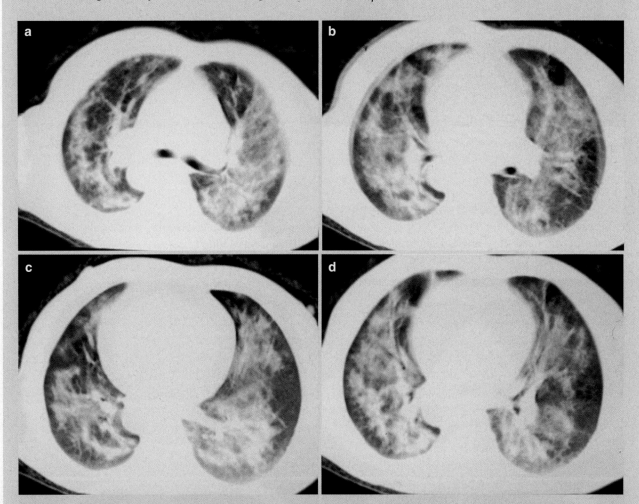

Fig. 17.15 (a–d) HIV/AIDS related Pneumocystis carinii pneumonia. (a–d) CT scanning demonstrates multiple patchy blurry shadows and fibrous cords liked shadows in both lungs which are more obvious in the middle inner parts of both lungs, with transparent areas in them. The bronchial walls are thickened

Case Study 15

An AIDS patient was confirmatively diagnosed by the CDC. He sustained Pneumocystis carinii pneumonia.

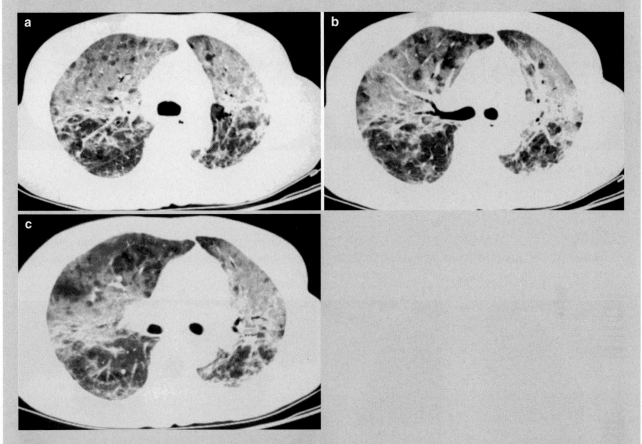

Fig. 17.16 (a–c) HIV/AIDS related Pneumocystis carinii pneumonia. (a–c) CT scanning demonstrates multiple fibrous cords liked shadows in lungs, multiple patchy parenchyma shadows and ground glass liked density shadows in both upper lobes, with multiple transparent areas in them. The bronchial walls are thickened in the anterior and posterior segments of the right upper lobe as well as in the lingual segment of the left lung

Case Study 16

A female patient aged 30 years was confirmatively diagnosed as having AIDS by the CDC. She complained of dyspnea, cyanosis and wheezing, with obviously decreased oxygen saturation. Her CD4 T cell count was 3/μl.

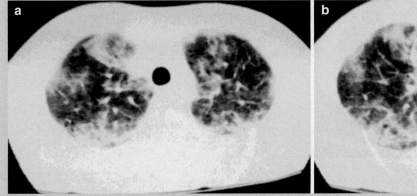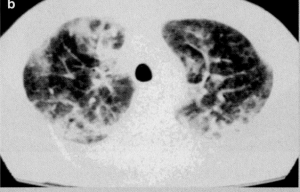

Fig. 17.17 (a–d) HIV/AIDS related Pneumocystis carinii pneumonia. (a–d) CT scanning demonstrates multiple patchy parenchymal shadows and fibrous cords liked shadows in both lungs which are more obvious in both lower lungs. The trachea and bronchi are unblocked, with enlarged hilar shadows in both lungs

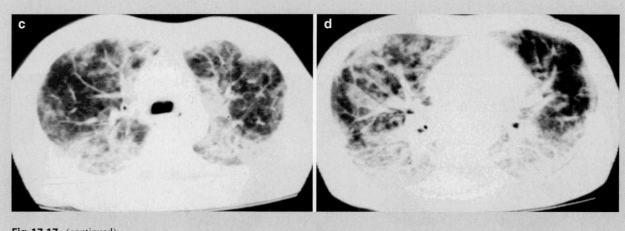

Fig. 17.17 (continued)

Case Study 17

A female patient aged 38 years was confirmatively diagnosed as having AIDS by the CDC. She complained of dyspnea, cyanosis and wheezing, with obviously decreased oxygen saturation. Her CD4 T cell count was 5/μl.

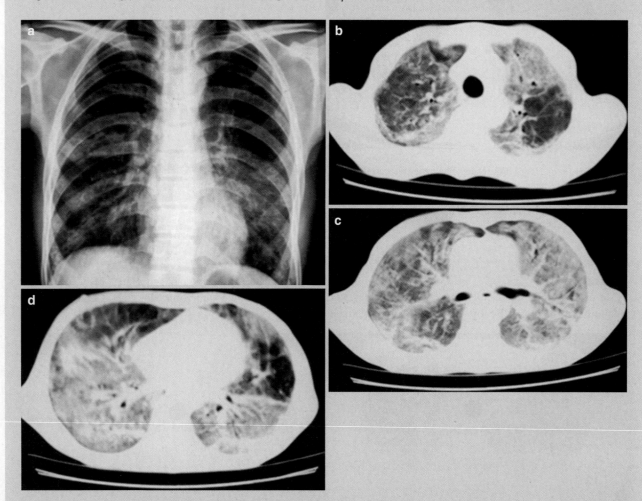

Fig. 17.18 (a–d) HIV/AIDS related Pneumocystis carinii pneumonia. (a) DR demonstrates multiple patchy shadows with increased density in both lungs which are more obvious in both middle and lower lungs. The hilar shadows in both lungs are enlarged, with sharp both costophrenic angles. (b–d) CT scanning demonstrates multiple patchy and mass liked parenchyma shadows in both lungs, ground glass density shadows in the apical segment of both upper lobes, transparent areas in the medial segment of the right middle lobe as well as in the lingual segment of the left upper lobe, and unobstructed trachea and bronchi

17.2.6 Diagnostic Basis

17.2.6.1 Case History
Patients with acquired immunodeficiency.

17.2.6.2 Clinical Symptoms
The early symptoms include fever, dry cough and shortness of breath. The advanced symptoms are serious dyspnea, cyanosis, progressive hypoxemia and respiratory failure. By pulmonary examinations, scattered dry and moist rales can be heard.

17.2.6.3 Bronchoalveolar Lavage (BAL)
Trophozoites of Pneumocystis cysts can be found by liquid Giemsa staining.

17.2.6.4 Biopsy or Autopsy for Pathological Examination
Slight and moderate interstitial inflammation responses mainly involve lymphocytes and alveolar macrophages. The detection of cysts containing sporozoites is the basis to define the diagnosis.

17.2.6.5 Imaging Demonstrations
Chest X-ray
Chest X-ray demonstrations of PCP can be classified into four types. (1) Early pulmonary interstitial infiltration and diffuse miliary alveolar exudation; (2) In the middle stage, there are alveolar exudates, with fusion and parenchymal changes; (3) In the middle-advanced stage, diffuse parenchymal changes; (4) Pulmonary interstitial fibrosis and lung cavity or lung bulla, as well as pneumothorax and emphysema.

CT Scanning with High Resolution
For the cases with negative or atypical findings by chest X-ray, CT scanning with high resolution should be performed. CT scanning demonstrates early lesions of multiple symmetric diffuse miliary nodal shadows, which have clear boundaries. In the middle stage, there are thin cloudy shadows or ground glass liked density shadows. In the middle-advanced stage, the lung tissues show parenchymal shadows, with trachea-bronchial sign. In the outer strip of the lung, a transparent area in shape of willow leaf can be demonstrated. In the advanced stage, fibrous cords liked shadows are demonstrated some lung tissues with compensatory emphysema and even pulmonary pseudocysts.

Nuclear Medicine Examinations
The intake of the isotope-labeled monoclonal antibody by lung tissues of PCP patients increases.

17.2.7 Differential Diagnosis

HIV/AIDS related PCP should be differentiated from bacterial pneumonia, pulmonary tuberculosis, viral pneumonia, fungal pneumonia, ARDS, and lymphocytic interstitial pneumonia (LIP).

17.2.7.1 Bacterial Pneumonia
Bacterial pneumonia has more focal lesions but less diffuse lesions.

17.2.7.2 Pulmonary Mycobacterium Tuberculosis Infection
Pulmonary mycobacterium tuberculosis infection has manifestations of military pulmonary tuberculosis by chest X-ray, which is difficult to be differentiated from early PCP. HIV/AIDS related PCP shows miliary nodules, which further fuse into cloudy or ground glass liked shadows or parenchymal changes. The lesions are commonly symmetrical, with the hilus as the center. The clinical manifestations include fever, dry cough or accompanying difficulty breathing, and even cyanosis. But in the cases of pulmonary Mycobacterium tuberculosis infections, most show miliary nodules, which further fuse into large nodules or mass. After about 2 weeks treatment in the early stage, the military nodules in both lungs can be absent, with common clinical symptom of high fever. Correlation studies of miliary tuberculosis and peripheral blood CD4 T cell count have demonstrated that the general incidence of miliary tuberculosis is low, only 6–9 %, but it is the main manifestation of HIV/AIDS related pulmonary miliary tuberculosis. Generally, when CD4 T cell count is below 200/μl, the incidence of cavity lesions is 29 %, non-cavity lesions 58 %, complicated by pleural effusion 11 % and lymphadenectasis 20 %. When CD4 T cell count is between 200 and 390/μl, the incidence of cavity lesions and non-cavity lesions each accounts for 44 %, complicated pleural effusion 11 % and lymphadenectasis 14 %. When CD4 T cell count above 400/μl, the manifestation is commonly pneumonia type, in flaky shadows or parenchymal shadows in just one pulmonary segment. The incidence of cavity lesions is 63 %, non-cavity lesions 33 %, complicated by pleural effusion 3 % and no lymphadenectasis.

17.2.7.3 Cytomegalovirus Pneumonia
Chest X-ray demonstrates cytomegalovirus pneumonia negative in 1/3 patients. The foci are commonly bilateral, with reticular particles in 33 % patients, alveolar foci in 22 % patients, nodular foci in 11 % patients, complicated by cavity in 11 % patients, cysts in 6 % patients, pleural effusion in 33 % patients and lymphadenectasis in 11 % patients.

17.2.7.4 Cryptococcus Neoformans Pneumonia
The incidence of diffuse foci in the cases of cryptococcus neoformans pneumonia is 76 %, interstitial foci or mixed foci 76 %, alveolar foci 19 %, nodular foci 5 %, lymphadenectasis 11 % and pleural effusion 5 %.

17.2.7.5 Lymphoid Interstitial Pneumonia
HIV/AIDS related PCP is more likely to occur in children with AIDS, which presents difficulty for its differentiation

form lymphoid interstitial pneumonia. However, lymphoid interstitial pneumonia commonly has a chronic onset, with commonly manifestations of cough and dry rales. Systemic lymphadenectasis and enlargement of salivary glands can also be found. By lung tissues biopsy, EBV-DNA1 can be detected, which provides basis for their differentiation.

17.2.8 Discussion

Pneumocystis, a unicellular organism, is the pathogen of Pneumocystis carinii pneumonia. Pneumocystis carinii pneumonia is one of common opportunistic infections in AIDS patients, which is also the leading cause of death in AIDS patients. In the initial episode of PCP, most patients have a CD4 T cell count of less than 100/μl. Diagnostic imaging demonstrates bilaterally symmetrical ground glass liked shadows, which can be diffusely distributed and tend to mainly involve the periphery of the hilus or the middle and lower lung fields. HRCT scanning is commonly applied to assess early PCP that is demonstrated negative by chest X-ray. HRCT scanning demonstrates bilaterally symmetric patchy or fused ground glass liked shadows. The pathological basis of ground glass liked shadows and parenchymal areas reflect that the acinus is filled by the foamy exudates, which are composed of surface active substances, cellulose and cell debris. All of the ground glass liked shadows, overlapping septa and the intralobular linear shadows are in gravel road liked manifestation. The septa and intralobular linear shadows demonstrate pulmonary interstitial edema or cellular infiltration.

In the middle-advanced stage of PCP, there are manifestations of small pulmonary nodules, pulmonary parenchymal changes, thickened interlobular septa, intralobular linear shadows, mass like lesions, pleural effusion, and lymphadenectasis. The cysts tend to mainly involve the upper lobes, which can be unilateral or bilateral pulmonary cysts, pneumothorax, mild or severe interstitial fibrosis and traction bronchiectasis. HRCT scanning demonstrations of PCP are non-specific. Its diagnosis should be in combination with HIVPH13 and etiological examinations.

17.3   HIV/AIDS Related Pulmonary Bacterial Infections

17.3.1 HIV/AIDS Related Tuberculosis

17.3.1.1 Pathogen and Pathogenesis

Mycobacterium tuberculosis is still an important pathogen for pulmonary infection in HIV positive patients. Since the mid-1980s, the main cause of the increasing incidence of tuberculosis is the prevalence of HIV infection. The incidence

of tuberculosis in AIDS patients is 200–500 times higher than the general population. HIV infection is the most dangerous factor for progression of latent tuberculosis into active tuberculosis. Tubercle bacillus belongs to Mycobacterium family of Mycobacterium genus, which is divided into types of human, bovine and murine. The main cause of human tuberculosis is human Mycobacterium tuberculosis, which is known as acid-fast bacilli. Tubercle bacillus wall is the complex containing high molecular weight fatty acids, lipids, proteins and polysaccharides, which are related to its pathogenicity and immune responses. Lipid can cause the infiltration of human monocytes, epithelial cells and lymphocytes to form tuberculous nodules. Its protein contents can cause allergic reactions, and infiltration of neutrophils and mononuclear cells. Polysaccharides participate in certain immune responses (such as agglutination). These pathogenic factors lay the foundation for the occurrence of tuberculosis in AIDS patients.

17.3.1.2 Pathophysiological Basis
Human immunity, allergic responses as well as the number and pathogenicity of tubercle bacilli are closely related to the quality, range, spreading rate and the progression of tuberculosis. Its pathological changes are characterized by exudation, infiltration, proliferation and hyperplasia, degenerative necrosis (caseous necrosis) and cavity formation.

Exudation Based Lesions
The manifestations include congestion, edema and infiltration of leukocytes. The exudative lesions occur in early stage of tuberculosis inflammation or when the lesions deteriorate. It can also be found in the serosa tuberculosis. There is neutrophilic granulocytes in the exudative lesions, which are gradually substituted by monocytes (phagocytes). The engulfed tubercle bacilli can be found in the large mononuclear cells. The exudative lesions are absorbed and dissipated through the phagocytosis of the mononuclear-phagocyte system, even with no scar.

Proliferation Based Lesions
When large mononuclear cells engulf and digest tubercle bacilli, the phospholipid of the bacteria render the large mononuclear cells to enlarge and be flat, similar to epithelial cells, which is known as epithelioid cells. These epithelioid cells gather into groups, with central Langhans giant cells that pass the messages of the bacteria antigens to lymphocytes. Surrounding the Langhans giant cells, there are often many lymphocytes to form typical tuberculous nodules, which are characteristic lesions of tuberculosis. This is why it is called Tuberculosis. In the tuberculous nodules, tubercule bacilli are usually undetectable. Proliferation based lesions often occur in the cases with less bacteria invasion and when human cells mediated immunity is predominant.

Degeneration Based Lesions (Caseous Necrosis)

Degeneration often occurs on the basis of the exudative or proliferative lesions. Tubercle bacilli overcome macrophages and then continually proliferate in large quantity. After the cells become cloudy and swelling, the foci show fatty degeneration, dissolved into fragments, until the occurrence of necrosis. After the death of inflammatory cells, proteolytic enzymes are released to dissolve the tissues that results in necrosis, which is coagulative necrosis. By naked eyes observation, they are yellowish gray, with loose and brittle quality like caseous. Therefore it is known as caseous necrosis. Microscopic examination demonstrates an area of solid and Eosin staining red necrotic tissues with no tuberculosis.

Results of Tuberculosis

Tubercle bacilli in the foci of caseous necrosis proliferate in large quantity to cause liquefaction, which is related to infiltration of neutrophile granulocytes and large monocytes. Part of

liquefied caseous necrotic substances can be absorbed and part can be discharged by the bronchus to form cavities. Otherwise, it may cause intrapulmonary spreading along with bronchi. The small caseous necrosis or proliferative lesions can be shrunk and absorbed after treatment, with only residues of slight fibrous scars. Due to the compromised immunity in AIDS patients, the lesions rarely show fiber tissues proliferation, but form cords liked scar. Calcification rarely occurs.

Spread and Deterioration of Tuberculosis Lesions

If the necrotic lesions erode the blood vessels, tubercle bacilli can cause systemic miliary tuberculosis along with blood flow, including brain, bones and kidneys. Large quantity sputum containing tubercle bacilli gains its access into the gastrointestinal tract. It can also cause intestinal tuberculosis and peritoneal tuberculosis. Pulmonary tuberculosis can cause tuberculosis pleurisy via direct spreading to the pleura (Fig. 17.19a–c).

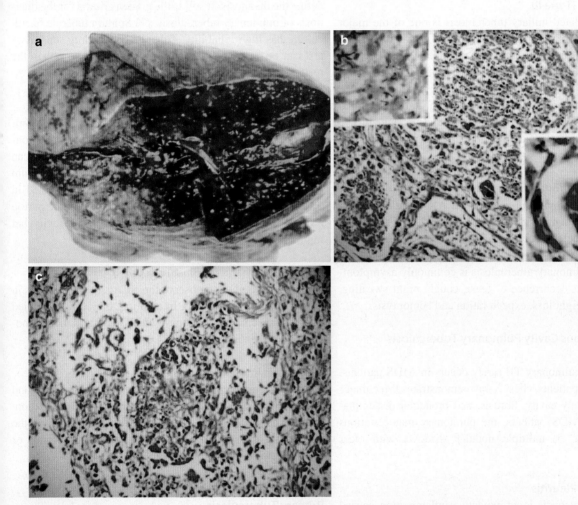

Fig. 17.19 (a) Gross observation in autopsy demonstrates disseminated pulmonary tuberculosis, with grayish white military nodules in diffuse distribution in the lung tissues section. (b) It is demonstrated that mycobacteriumavium-intracellularcomplex infection in the lung tissue, with atypical tuberculosis nodules and acid-fast staining

positive (*left top*). There are a subnodular giant cell, eosinophilic inclusion bodies in the nucleus and bradyzoites in cytoplasm of T. gondii. HE × 100. (c) HE demonstrates mycobacteriumavium-intracellularcomplex infection, with atypical tuberculosis nodular changes, HE × 200

17.3.1.3 Clinical Symptoms and Signs

Clinically, it is a chronic progression, with rare acute onset. The clinical symptoms are commonly systemic, with fever and fatigue. The respiratory symptoms include cough and hemoptysis. Pulmonary TB can be divided into primary and secondary, with the initial episode commonly being primary (type I). The residual bacteria after primary infection can cause secondary infection (type II-IV) when the immunity is compromised via spreading along blood flow or direct spreading.

Primary Tuberculosis (Type I)

It is common in HIV positive children. Most cases are asymptomatic, sometimes with symptoms of low grade fever, mild cough, sweating, rapid heartbeat, and poor appetite.

Hematogenous Disseminated Pulmonary Tuberculosis (Type II)

HIV/AIDS related miliary tuberculosis is one of the major manifestations of pulmonary tuberculosis, which is more common. The onset of acute miliary tuberculosis is rapid, with symptoms of chills and high fever with a body temperature up to 40 °C, mostly remittent fever or continuous fever. There may be decreased leukocytes count and accelerated sedimentation rate. The progression of subacute and chronic hematogenous disseminated pulmonary tuberculosis is relatively slow.

Infiltrative Pulmonary Tuberculosis (Type III)

Infiltrative pulmonary tuberculosis in AIDS patients commonly occurs in both middle and lower lung fields, with flaky and flocculent foci or parenchymal changes in lobes or segments. Caseous lesions are rare. The early stage of infiltrative pulmonary tuberculosis is commonly asymptomatic, with later occurrence of fever, cough, night sweating, chest pain, weight loss, expectoration and hemoptysis.

Chronic Fibrous Cavity Pulmonary Tuberculosis (Type IV)

This type of pulmonary TB rarely occurs in AIDS patients. In non-AIDS patients, chest X-ray demonstrates three major changes, namely cavity, fibrosis, and bronchial dissemination. In the AIDS patients, the pulmonary manifestations include single or multiple nodular shadows with clear boundaries.

Tuberculous Pleuritis

Tuberculous pleuritis is an exudative inflammation caused by the direct invasion of tubercle bacillus from the primary lesion near the pleura into the pleura, or hematogenous dissemination via the lymphatic vessels to the pleura. The routes for occurrence of tuberculous pleurisy include: (1) The bacteria in the hilar lymph tuberculosis counterflow to the pleura along lymph vessels. (2) TB lesions adjacent to pleura rupture to cause direct access of the tubercle bacilli or products of tuberculosis infection into the pleural cavity. (3) Acute or subacute hematogenous disseminated tuberculosis causes pleuritis. (4) Due to the increased allergic responses, the pleura highly respond to tuberculosis toxins to cause exudation. (5) Thoracic tuberculosis and rib tuberculosis rupture into the pleural cavity. Clinically, pleuritis can be divided into three types, dry pleuritis, exudative pleuritis and tuberculous empyema (rare). The common clinical manifestations are fever, cough with accompanying chest pain of the affected side and shortness of breath.

17.3.1.4 Examinations and Their Selection
Sputum Tuberculin Test

(1) Sputum smear examination is simple to manipulate, with high accuracy rate. The findings of the tubercle bacilli can define the diagnosis. It still is the golden criteria for the diagnosis of pulmonary tuberculosis. (2) Sputum tubercle bacilli culture has high reliability. Tubercle bacilli drug sensitivity test can be performed but requires 6–8 weeks to obtain the results. Therefore, its application is limited.

Immunological Diagnosis of Pulmonary TB

(1) Tuberculin purified protein derivative (PPD) test is commonly used. Its positive result is one of the evidence confirming a past history of TB infection. (2) BACTEC test can be performed to detect the metabolites of mycobacterium tuberculosis. Generally, mycobacterium can be detected in 2 weeks. The quantity of mycobacteria can affect the period required for test results. (3) PCR has poor specificity but high sensitivity of up to 98–100 %.

Thoracoscopy and Mediastinoscopy

Both can be applied to observe the enlarged lymph nodes in the chest and mediastinum. In addition, they can be applied to obtain specimens for biopsy, which facilitates the diagnosis and differential diagnosis.

Diagnostic Imaging

Diagnostic imaging examinations include chest X-ray and CT scanning. Chest X-ray can demonstrate the location, quality and range of the lesions. It can also help to assess the therapeutic efficacy. CT scanning can demonstrate small or hidden lesions, with a high resolution.

17.3.1.5 Imaging Demonstrations
Primary Tuberculosis

Primary pulmonary tuberculosis, also known as primary syndrome, is rare in adult AIDS patients. Chest X-ray demonstrates intrapulmonary patchy or large flaky parenchymal changes, hilar and mediastinal lymphadenectasis in connection to irregular cords liked shadows (located between intrapulmonary lesion and the hilum). Lymph node tuberculosis is demonstrated to have mediastinal lymphadenectasis that sometimes fuse into mass. In AIDS patients, simple mediastinal lymph node tuberculosis is more common than primary syndrome.

Hematogenous Disseminated Pulmonary Tuberculosis

(1) The acute cases are demonstrated to have diffused miliary nodules in both lungs with even distribution, even size and even density. (2) The subacute and chronic cases are demonstrated to have nodules in both lungs, with uneven distribution, uneven size and uneven density. Sometimes calcification occurs in the nodules, with fibrous cords and thickened pleura.

Secondary Pulmonary Tuberculosis

Infiltrative pulmonary tuberculosis are demonstrated to have patchy parenchymal changes in the middle and lower lung fields as well as parenchymal changes, cavities and fibrous cords liked foci in the segments and lobes. It can also occur in the upper lung fields, commonly with accompanying mediastinal and hilar lymph node tuberculosis.

Chronic Fibrous Cavity Pulmonary Tuberculosis

It commonly occurs in the advanced stage of AIDS,, with manifestations of pulmonary interstitial fibrosis and formation of cavities. This type of pulmonary tuberculosis is less common.

Tuberculous Pleuritis

It rarely occurs, mostly in the early stage of AIDS. It is rare in the middle and advanced stages of AIDS. Dry pleuritis has manifestations of blunt costophrenic angle and limited diaphragm mobility. Exudative pleuritis is manifested as small quantity pleural effusion and thickened pleura, commonly with encapsulated effusion of the lateral pleura. Calcification is rare.

HIV/AIDS Related Lymph Node Tuberculosis

Case Study 1

A male patient aged 28 years was confirmatively diagnosed as having AIDS by the CDC. He complained of dull chest pain, dyspnea, fever, night sweating, fatigue and anorexia. His CD4 T cell count was 65/μl.

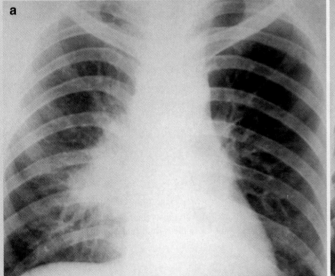
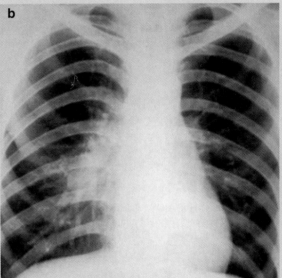
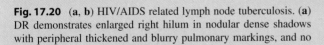

Fig. 17.20 (a, b) HIV/AIDS related lymph node tuberculosis. (a) DR demonstrates enlarged right hilum in nodular dense shadows with peripheral thickened and blurry pulmonary markings, and no obvious abnormalities of the left hilum. (b) DR demonstrates smaller right hilum after treatment for 1 month

Case Study 2

A male patient aged 37 years was confirmatively diagnosed as having AIDS by the CDC. He complained of dull chest pain, dyspnea, fever, night sweating and fatigue. His CD4 T cell count was 65/μl.

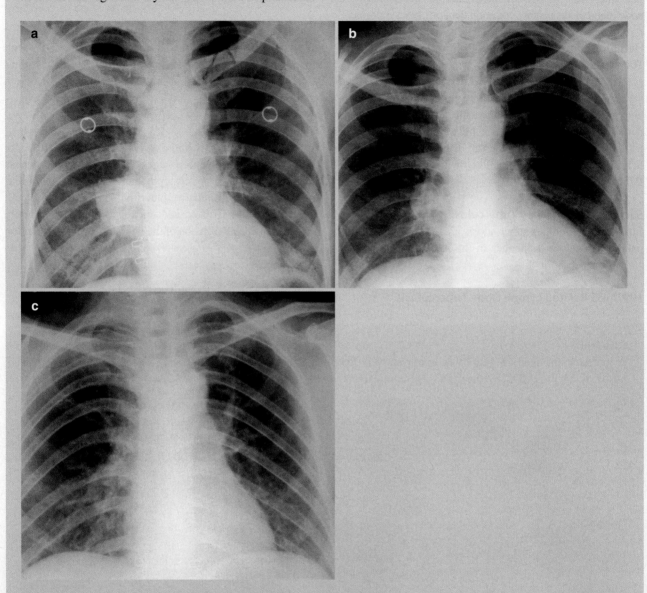

Fig. 17.21 (a–c) HIV/AIDS related lymph node tuberculosis. (**a**) DR demonstrates enlarged right hilum in mass liked dense shadow, with peripheral thickened and blurry pulmonary markings, and no obvious abnormalities of the left hilum. (**b**) DR demonstrates smaller right hilum after anti-tuberculosis therapy for 1 month. (**c**) DR demonstrates absent tumor in the right hilum and normal left hilum

Case Study 3

A male patient aged 48 years was confirmatively diagnosed as having AIDS by the CDC. He complained of dull chest pain, dyspnea, fever, night sweating, fatigue and anorexia. His CD4 T cell count was 45/μl.

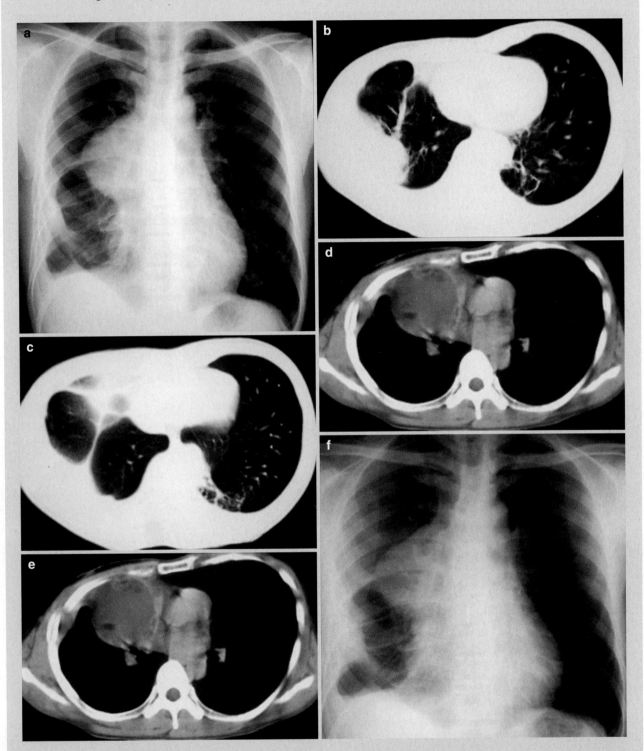

Fig. 17.22 (a–f) HIV/AIDS related lymph node tuberculosis. (a) DR demonstrates semicircular mass liked dense shadow in the right hilum that protrudes to the lung field with peripheral thickened and blurry pulmonary markings, thickened pleura of lateral chest wall, and blunt costophrenic angle in Jan. 2008. (b–e) CT scanning demonstrates narrowed right thorax, thickend pleura of lateral chest wall with encapsulated effusion, uneven density mass in the right hilum, thinner right bronchus due to compression and no obvious abnormalities in the left hilum. (f) DR in Aug. 2008 demonstrates no obvious changes of the lesions after anti-tuberculosis treatment for 1 month

Case Study 4

A female patient aged 36 years was confirmatively diagnosed as having AIDS by the CDC. She complained of dull chest pain, dyspnea, fever, night sweating, fatigue and anorexia. Her CD4 T cell count was 55/µl.

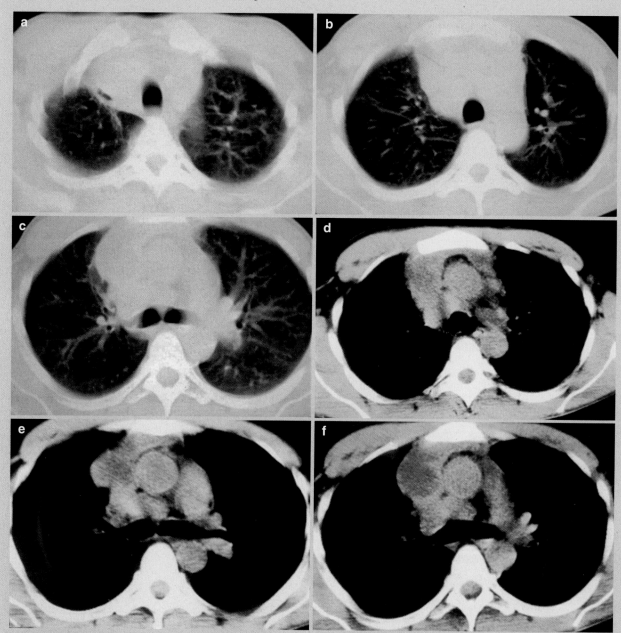

Fig. 17.23 (**a–f**) HIV/AIDS related lymph node tuberculosis. (**a–c**) CT scanning of the pulmonary window demonstrates dense mass shadow beside the right aortic arch, and thinner right bronchus due to compression. (**d–f**) CT scanning of the mediastinal window demonstrates low density mass shadow besied the right aortic arch with clear boundary

Case Study 5

A female patient aged 46 years was confirmatively diagnosed as having AIDS by the CDC. She complained of dull chest pain, dyspnea, fever and fatigue. Her CD4 T cell count was 35/µl.

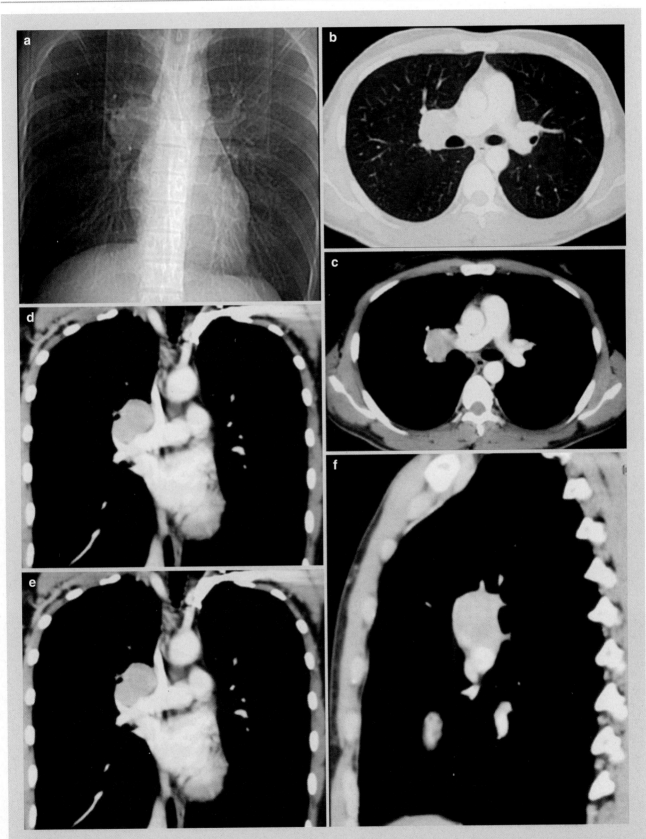

Fig. 17.24 (a–g) HIV/AIDS related lymph node tuberculosis. (a) DR demonstrates circular mass dense shadow in the right hilum that protrudes to the lung field with peripheral thickened and blurry pulmonary markings, thickened pleura in the lateral chest cavity and blunt costophrenic angle in Jan. 2008. (b–e) CT scanning demonstrates multiple uneven mass density shadows in right hilum in a size of about 3×3.5×3.8 cm. (f–g) Enhanced CT scanning demonstrates slight uneven enhancement of the lesion and no obvious abnormalties in the left hilum

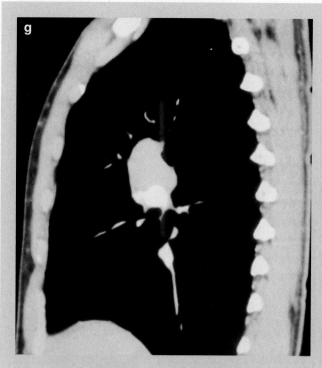

Fig. 17.24 (continued)

Case Study 6

A female patient aged 36 years was confirmatively diagnosed as having AIDS by the CDC. She complained of dull chest pain, dyspnea, fever, night sweating and fatigue. Her CD4 T cell count was 85/μl.

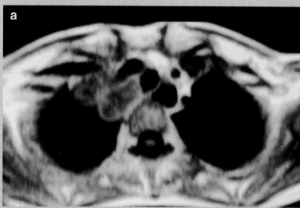
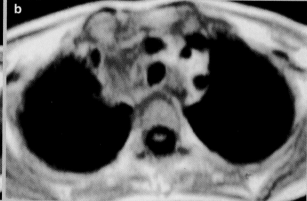

Fig. 17.25 (**a–m**) HIV/AIDS related lymph node tuberculosis. (**a–f**) MR imaging demonstrates multiple round liked long T1WI long T2WI signal adjacent to the right sternocleidomastoid as well as in the supraclavicular fossa and the right upper mediastinum. (**g–j**) Sagittal MR imaging demonstrates multiple round liked sugar-coated haws liked masses in the entrance of the thorax and right upper mediastinum, with central long T1WI signal and unclear boundary. (**k, l**) Axial MR imaging demonstrates round liked long T1WI long T2WI signal in the right cardiophrenic angle (*arrow*). (**m**) Coronal MR imaging demonstrates round liked equal signal shadow

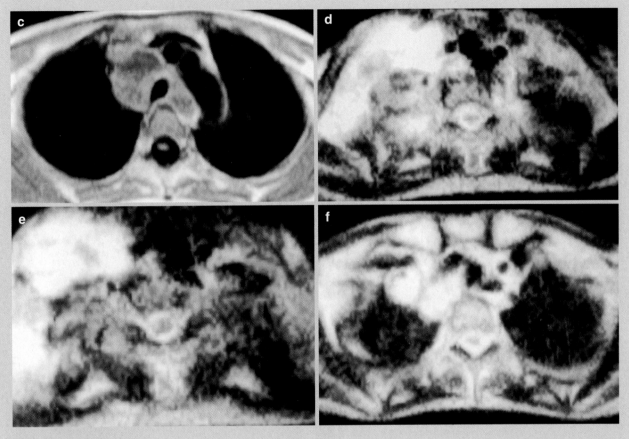

Fig. 17.25   (continued)

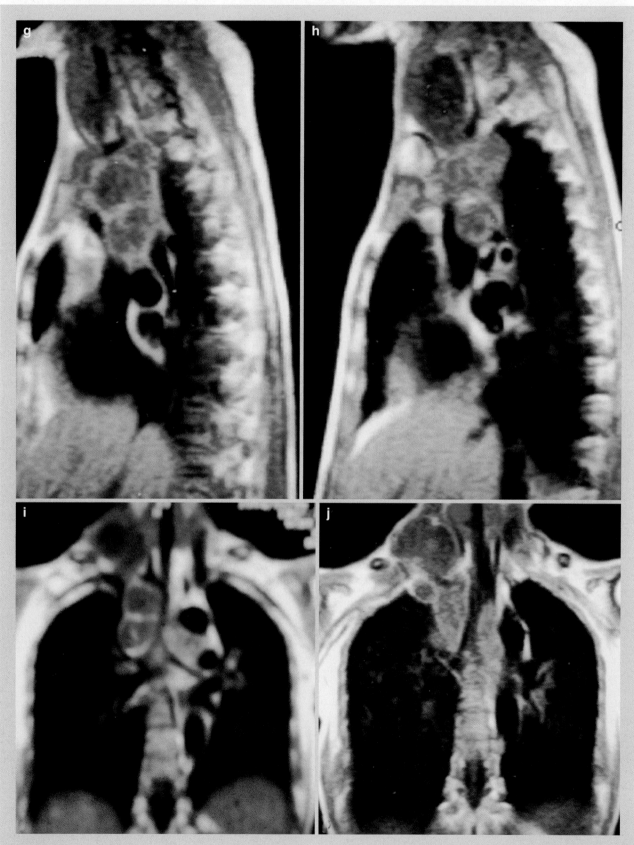

Fig. 17.25 (continued)

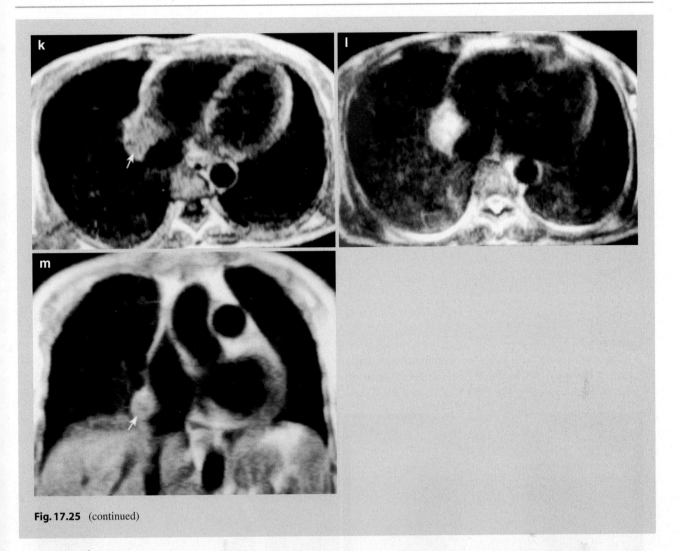

Fig. 17.25 (continued)

Miliary Tuberculosis

Case Study 1

A male patient aged 41 years was confirmatively diagnosed as having AIDS by the CDC. He was infected HIV via blood transfusion, with complaints of cervical lymph node tuberculosis, ascites and abdominal infection, fungal stomatitis, biliary stones with infection and severe anemia. His CD4 T cell count was 33/μl.

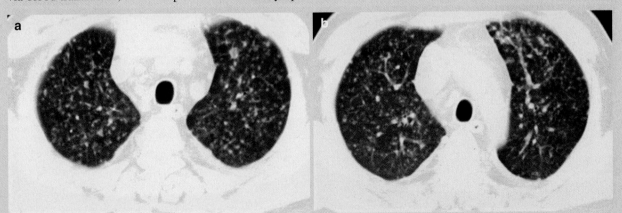

Fig. 17.26 (a–d) HIV/AIDS related miliary tuberculosis. (a–d) CT demonstrates diffuse scattering miliary shadows with increased density in both lungs, which are bilaterally symmetric as well as in even size and distribution

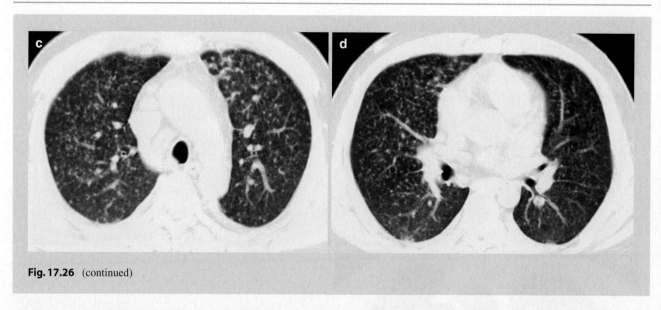

Fig. 17.26 (continued)

Case Study 2

A female patient aged 39 years was confirmatively diagnosed as having AIDS by the CDC. She complained of fever and night sweating. Her CD4 T cell count was 73/μl.

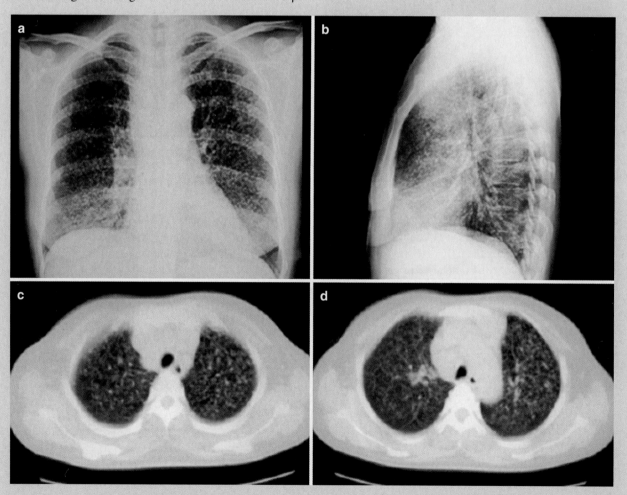

Fig. 17.27 (a–f) HIV/AIDS related miliary tuberculosis. (a–b) Anteroposterior and lateral DR demonstrates diffuse miliary shadows in both lungs, which are bilaterally symmetric and in even size and distribution. (c–f) CT demonstrates diffuse scattering miliary shadows with increased density in both lungs, which are bilaterally symmetric as well as in even size and distribution

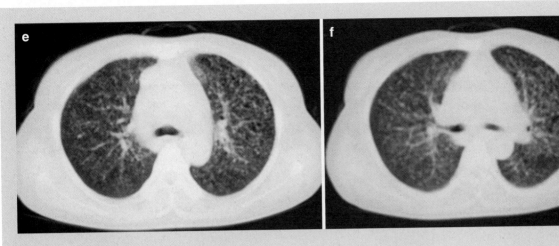

Fig. 17.27 (continued)

Case Study 3

A female patient aged 42 years was confirmatively diagnosed as having AIDS by the CDC. In the recent 1 month, she sustained chills, fever, aggravating night sweating and diarrhea with watery stools for five to six times daily and no bloody mucopurulent stool as well as obvious weight loss. By physical examinations on admission, T 35.6 °C, P 80/min, R 20/min, BP 90/60 mmHg; by laboratory tests, AST 83 u/l, ALB 26.7 g/L, GLO 36.4 g/L, GGT 233u/L, ALP 438 u/L; electrolytes normal; WBC 1.4/L, LYM% 12.1 %, NEuT% 84.4 %; blood sedimentation 20 mm/h; RPR-Ab Weak positive. Her CD4 T cell count was 53/μl.

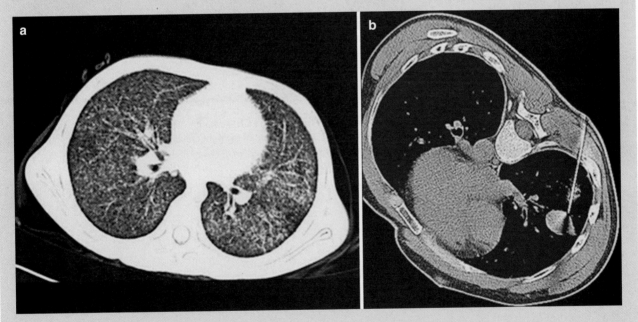

Fig. 17.28 (a–b) HIV/AIDS related miliary tuberculosis. (a) CT scanning demonstrates diffuse scattering miliary shadows with increased density in both lungs, which are bilaterally symmetric and in even size and distribution. (b) CT scanning of the mediastinal window demonstrates round liked nodular shadows in the right lower lung. CT guided puncture for biopsy is performed to define the diagnosis

Case Study 4

A female patient aged 46 years was confirmatively diagnosed as having AIDS by the CDC. She complained of chills, fever and night sweating for 1 week. Her CD4 T cell count was 23/μl.

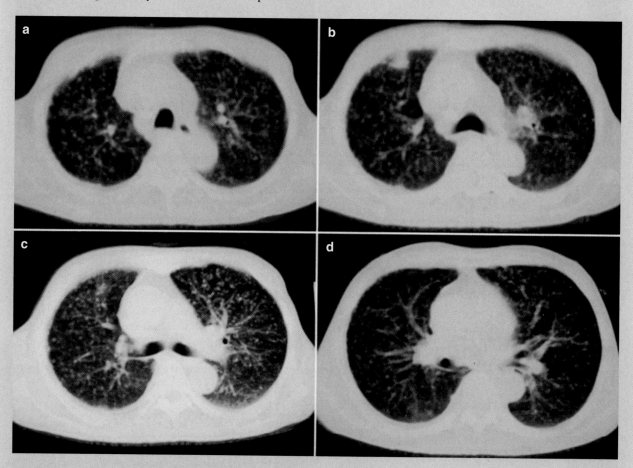

Fig. 17.29 (a–d) HIV/AIDS related miliary tuberculosis. (a–d) CT scanning demonstrates diffuse scattering miliary shadows with increased density in both lungs, which are bilaterally symmetric and in even size and distribution. There are nodular shadows in the anterior segment of the right middle lung lobe with clear boundary

Case Study 5

A female patient aged 32 years was confirmatively diagnosed as having AIDS by the CDC. She complained of chill and fever for 2 weeks. Her CD4 T cell count was 63/μl.

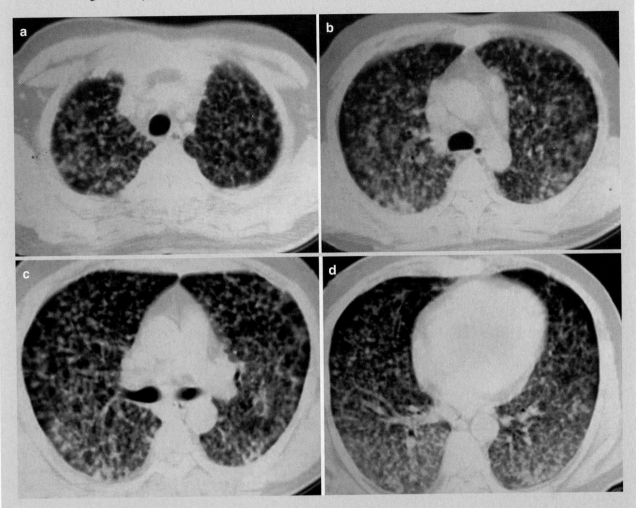

Fig. 17.30 (**a–d**) HIV/AIDS related miliary tuberculosis. (**a–d**) CT scanning demonstrates diffuse scattering miliary shadows with increased density in both lungs and fusion of some military shadows, which are bilaterally symmetric and in even size and distribution

Case Study 6

A male patient aged 37 years was confirmatively diagnosed as having AIDS by the CDC. He had a history of blood transfusion, with complaints of finding HIV infected for 4 years, intermittent cough and fever for 6 months. His CD4 T cell count was 50/μl.

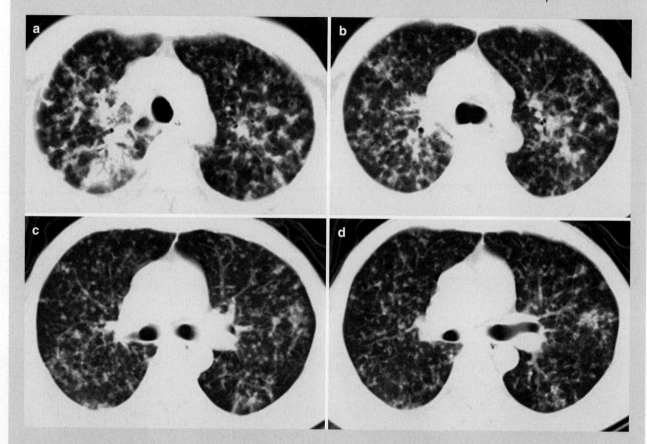

Fig. 17.31 (a–d) HIV/AIDS related miliary tuberculosis. (a–d) CT scanning demonstrates diffuse scattering miliary shadows with increased density in both lungs, fusion of some military shadows into patchy or mass liked shadow, diffusely distributed lung lesions

Fusion Period of Miliary Pulmonary TB

Case Study 7

A male patient aged 47 years was confirmatively diagnosed as having AIDS by the CDC. He had a history of blood transfusion, with complaints of finding HIV infected for 6 years, intermittent cough and fever for 6 months. His CD4 T cell count was 10/μl.

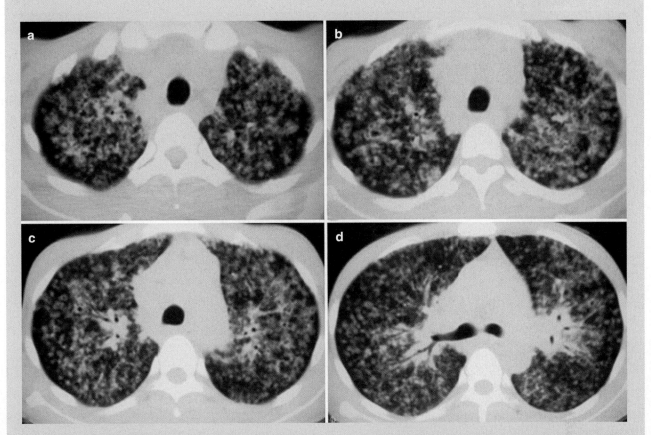

Fig. 17.32 (**a–d**) HIV/AIDS related miliary tuberculosis. (**a–d**) CT demonstrates diffuse scattering miliary shadows with increased density in both lungs, fusion of some military shadows into patchy or mass liked shadows and diffusely distributed lung lesions

Infiltrative Pulmonary Tuberculosis

Case Study 1

A male patient aged 41 years was confirmatively diagnosed as having AIDS by the CDC. He sustained HIV infection for 7 years, with chief complaints of cough and dyspnea. His CD4 T cell count was 14/μl.

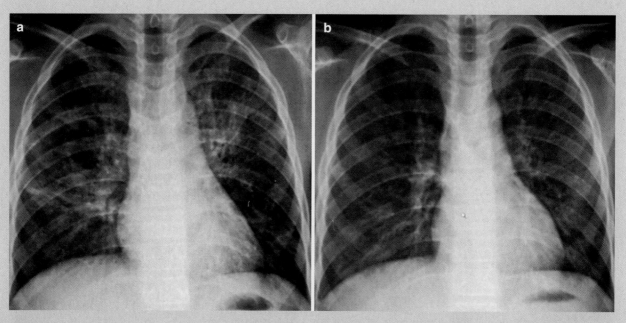

Fig. 17.33 (**a, b**) HIV/AIDS related infiltrative pulmonary tuberculosis. (**a**) DR demonstrates scattering patchy and cords liked blurry density shadows in the right middle and upper lung fields as well as enlarged and thickened hilum. (**b**) DR demonstrates that the lungs lesions are almost absent compared to (**a**), after anti-TB treatment for 5 months

Case Study 2

A female patient aged 31 years was confirmatively diagnosed as having AIDS by the CDC. She sustained HIV infection for 8 years, with chief complaints of cough and dyspnea. Her CD4 T cell count was 34/μl.

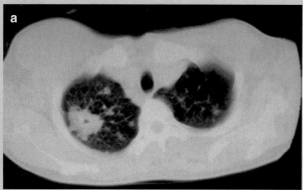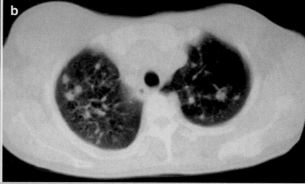

Fig. 17.34 (**a–c**) HIV/AIDS related infiltrative pulmonary tuberculosis. (**a, b**) CT scanning of the pulmonary window demonstrates patchy shadows with increased density in the right upper lung and multiple satellite lesions scattering around. (**c**) CT scanning of the mediastinal window demonstrates lymphadenectasis of aortic window, subcutaneous soft tissue mass shadow in the left anterior chest wall with central low density shadow as well as right axilliary lymphadenectasis

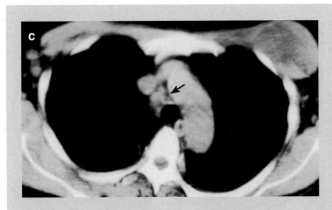

Fig. 17.34 (continued)

Case Study 3

A male patient aged 41 years was confirmatively diagnosed as having AIDS by the CDC. He sustained HIV infection for 7 years, with chief complaints of cough and dyspnea. His CD4 T cell count was 14/μl.

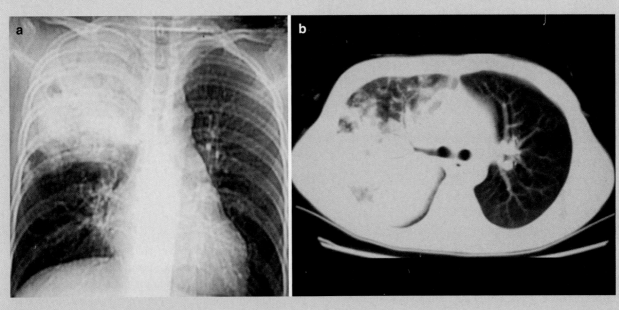

Fig. 17.35 (**a–e**) HIV/AIDS related infiltrative pulmonary tuberculosis. (**a**) DR demonstrates diffuse large flaky dense shadows in the right upper lung with transparent areas in them. (**b–c**) CT scanning of the pulmonary window demonstrates large flaky shadows with increased density in the right upper lung, with multiple satellite lesions scattering around. (**d, e**) CT scanning of the mediastinal window demonstrates large flaky parenchymal shadows in the right upper lung with air bronchogram sign as well as mediastinal lymphadenectasis

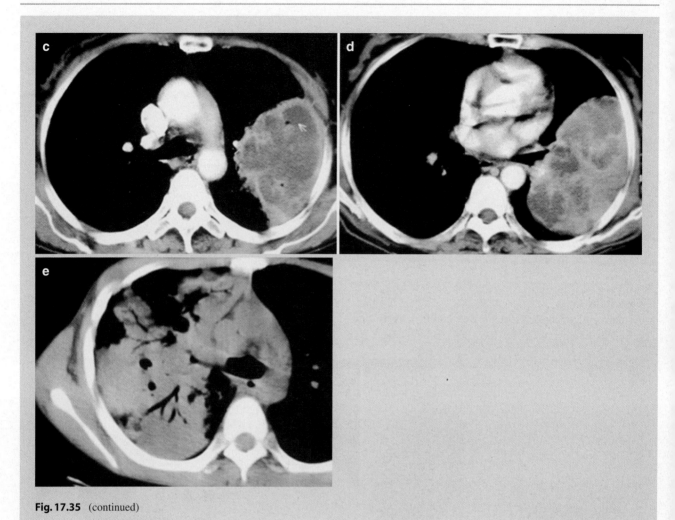

Fig. 17.35 (continued)

Case Study 4

A male patient aged 36 years was confirmatively diagnosed as having AIDS by the CDC. He sustained HIV infection for 6 years, with chief complaints of fever and left chest pain for more than 1 month. Examinations demonstrated HIV positive, acid-fast bacilli positive in sputum culture, PPD strong positive; CD4 T cell count 168/μl, CD4/CD8 0.27. Pathology demonstrated caseous and granulation tissue. The clinical diagnosis was type III tuberculosis with accompanying left pleurisitis.

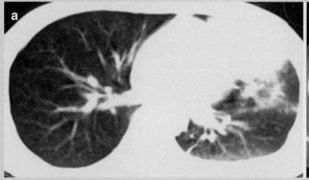
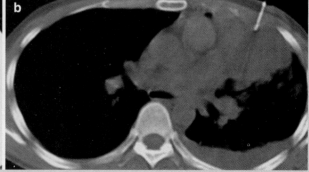

Fig. 17.36 (a–c) HIV/AIDS related infiltrative pulmonary tuberculosis. (a) Pulmonary CT scanning of the pulmonary window demonstrates parenchymal shadows in the left lingual lobe with surrounding pulmonary acinar nodular shadows. (b) CT guided pucture biopsy of left lingula. (c) The pathology demonstrates granulation tissue and caseous necrosis, being in consistency with tuberculosis changes. HE×100

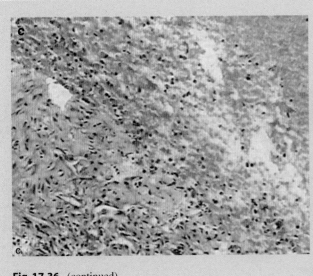

Fig. 17.36   (continued)

Chronic Fibrous Cavity Pulmonary Tuberculosis (with Rare Occurrence)

Case Study 1

A male patient aged 38 years was confirmatively diagnosed as having AIDS by the CDC. He complained of fever and left chest pain for 1 month. By examinations, HIV positive, acid-fast bacilli positive in the sputum culture and a CD4 T cell count 201/µl.

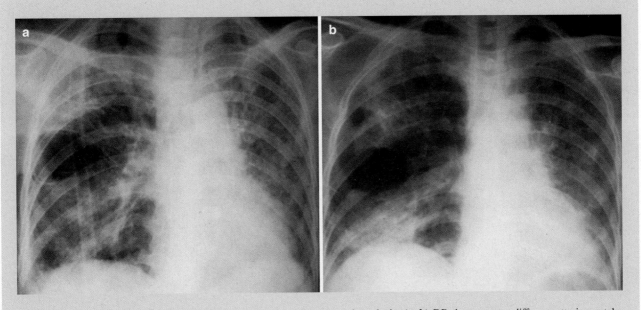

Fig. 17.37   (**a, b**) HIV/AIDS related chronic fibrous cavity pulmonary tuberculosis. (**a, b**) DR demonstrates diffuse scattering patchy shadows with increased density, and oval thin wall cavity shadows in the right middle lung field

Case Study 2

A male patient aged 43 years was confirmatively diagnosed as having AIDS by the CDC. He complained of finding HIV positive for 6 years, as well as fever, cough and left chest pain for 1 month. The acid-fast bacillus was positive in sputum culture and his CD4 T cell count was 261/μl.

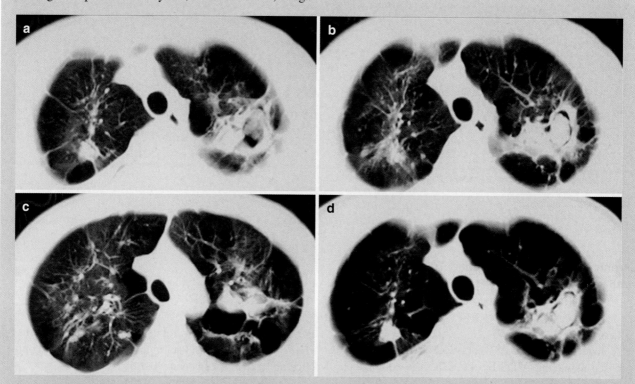

Fig. 17.38 (**a–d**) HIV/AIDS related chronic fibrous cavity pulmonary tuberculosis. (**a**) CT scanning of the pulmonary window demonstrates patchy shadows with increased density in both upper lungs, peripheral crab feet liked or cords liked shadows due to pleural traction with cavity shadows in them and periperal satellite lesions. (**b–d**) CT scanning of the mediastinal window demonstrates round liked mass shadows with high density in the cavities of the left upper lung, surrounding transparent shadows, no nodules in the walls and surrounding nodular satellite lesions. By pathological examination, the diagnosis is defined as chronic fibrous cavity pulmonary tuberculosis complicated by Aspergillus infection

Case Study 3

A female patient aged 41 years was confirmatively diagnosed as having AIDS by the CDC. She had a case history of cavity pulmonary tuberculosis for several years, with complaints of fever, cough and chest pain for 2 months. Acid-fast bacilli were positive in the sputum culture. Her CD4 T cell count was 151/μl.

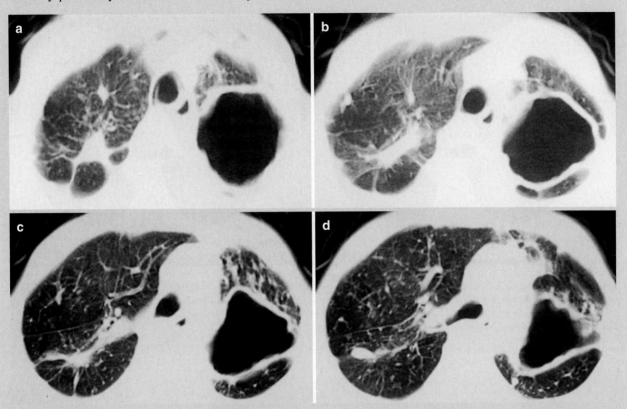

Fig. 17.39 (a–d) HIV/AIDS related chronic fibrous cavity pulmonary tuberculosis. (a, b) CT scanning of the pulmonary window demonstrates patchy shadows with increased density in the right upper lung, periphery crab feet liked or cords liked shadows due to pleural traction and satellite lesions. (c, d) CT scanning of the mediastinal window demonstrates round liked or triangle shaped thick wall cavities in the left upper lung, no nodules in the wall and peripheral nodular satellite lesions

Case Study 4

A female patient aged 35 years was confirmatively diagnosed as having AIDS by the CDC. She was hospitalized due to complaints of chest distress, cough and expectoration for 2 months, with after noon low grade fever and weight loss. On admission, she was confirmed HIV positive and a CD4 T cell count of 120/μl.

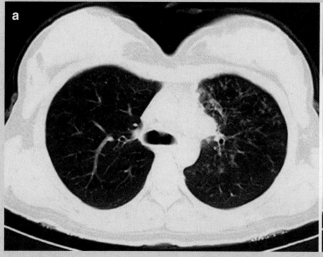 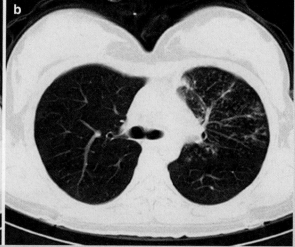

Fig. 17.40 (**a**, **b**) HIV/AIDS related endobronchial tuberculosis. (**a**, **b**) Chest CT scanning demonstrates narrowed left major bronchus, irregular thickening of the brounchial wall, multiple irregular flaky, patchy and military shadows in the posterior apical, anterior and lingual segments of the left upper lung. Bronchobierscopy demonstrates narrowed left major bronchus, which is possibly caused by endobronchial tuberculosis

Tuberculous Pleuritis

Case Study 1

A female patient aged 37 years was confirmatively diagnosed as having AIDS by the CDC. She complained of fever and chest pain for 2 months, with acid-fast bacilli positive in the pleural fluid culture. Her CD4 T cell count was 71/μl.

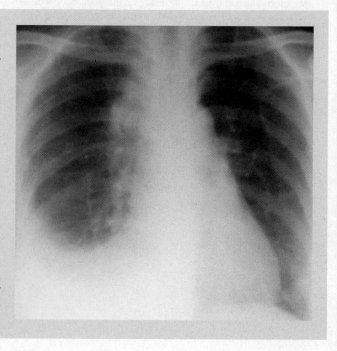

Fig. 17.41 HIV/AIDS related tuberculous pleuritis. DR demonstrates arch shaped dense shadows with higher exterior density and lower interior density in the right lower lung field and covered right edge of the heart

Case Study 2

A female patient aged 40 years was confirmatively diagnosed as having AIDS by the CDC. She complained of fever and chest pain for 2 months, with acid-fast bacilli positive in the pleural fluid culture. Her CD4 T cell count was 891/μl.

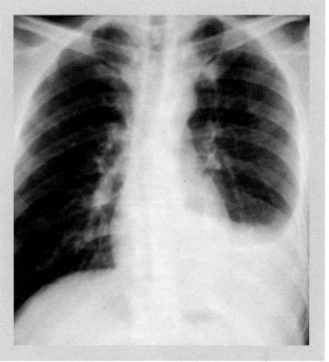

Fig. 17.42 HIV/AIDS related tuberculous pleuritis. DR demonstrates arch shaped dense shadows with higher exterior density and lower interior density in the left lower lung field and covered right edge of the heart

Case Study 3

A female patient aged 34 years was confirmatively diagnosed as having AIDS by the CDC. She complained of fever and chest pain for 2 months, with acid-fast bacilli positive in the pleural fluid culture. Her CD4 T cell count was 51/μl.

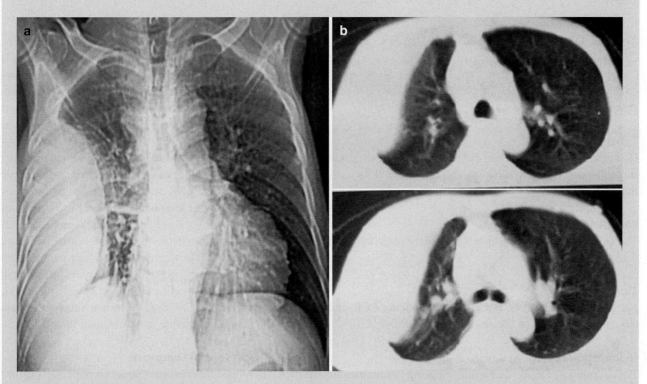

Fig. 17.43 (a–c) HIV/AIDS related tuberculous pleuritis. (a) DR demonstrates thickened pleura in the right lateral chest wall in spindle liked dense shadows. (b) CT scanning of the pulmonary window demonstrates thickened pleura in the right lateral chest wall in spindle liked dense shadows. (c) CT scanning of the mediastinal window demonstrates encapsulated fluid density shadow in the pleura of the right lateral chest wall

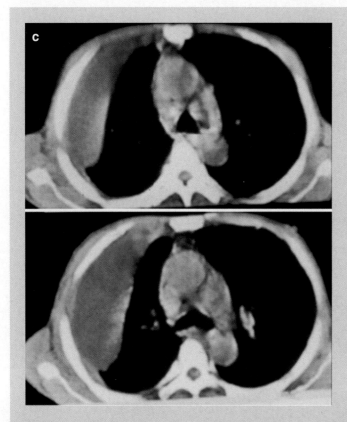

Fig. 17.43 (continued)

17.3.1.6 Diagnostic Basis
Clinical Symptoms and Signs
Cough expectoration, chest pain, dyspnea, fever, night sweating, fatigue, anorexia, lymphadenectasis and rapid progression of the conditions.

Tuberculin Test
PPD skin test with a resulted diameter of more than 5 mm should be considered as tuberculosis infection. But its positive rate remains low.

Bacterial Culture
The culture of sputum and bronchoalveolar lavage fluid can detect the pathogens.

Molecular Biology Examination
Nucleic acid analysis or DNA probe technique, PCR and chromatography can be applied to detect tubercle bacilli.

Diagnostic Imaging
The commonly used diagnostic imaging examinations include chest X-ray and CT scanning. The main demonstrations include (1) intrapulmonary and extrapulmonary lymphadenectasis; (2) miliary tuberculosis manifestations; (3) infiltrative (pneumonia type) pulmonary tuberculosis; (4) Pulmonary interstitial fibrosis, cavity, pulmonary emphysema, nodules, emphysema, and bronchiectasis with accompanying infections. In the cases with their CD4 T cell count being above 400/µl, the imaging demonstrations are similar to those of non-HIV/AIDS patients with pulmonary tuberculosis. In the cases with their CD4 T cell count being above 400/µl, the manifestations are intrapulmonary large flaky parenchymal changes, surrounding satellite lesions as well as mediastinal and hilar lymphadenectasis. Sometimes the manifestations may be only mediastinal lymphadenectasis and their fusion into mass. In the cases with CD4 T cell count being above 200/µl, there may be accompanying extrapulmonary tuberculosis, such as tuberculous peritonitis, bone tuberculosis, brain tuberculosis and splenic tuberculosis. In the cases with their CD4 T cell count being lower than 100/µl, the manifestations are mostly miliary tuberculosis.

17.3.1.7 Differential Diagnosis
HIV/AIDS related tuberculosis should be principally differentiated from pneumocystis carinii pneumonia, fungal infections, other pneumonia and lung cancer.

Pneumocystis Carinii Pneumonia

HIV/AIDS related tuberculosis should be differentiated from PCP. PCP is mainly manifested as multiple lesions with hilum as the center to extending symmetrically to outside of the lungs. In the advanced stage, PCP has main lesions of pulmonary interstitial fibrosis, with less accompanying mediastinal and hilar lymphadenectasis. The laboratory tests can facilitate to define the diagnose.

Fungal Infections

HIV/AIDS related tuberculosis should be differentiated from fungal infections. Fungal infections are relatively less common than tuberculosis. The imaging findings of HIV/AIDS related pulmonary fungal infections are diverse, with manifestations of miliary, flaky flocculent liked, parenchymal, mass, and interstitial changes. In general, the diffuse lesions are mainly interstitial changes, while confirmed lesions, compared to TB lesions, are more likely to have thick walled cavities. Satellite lesions of fungal infections are less than those of tuberculosis, with less accompanying mediastinal and hilar lymphadenectasis. Sometimes laboratory tests are necessary to define the diagnosis.

Non-tuberculosis Mycobacteria Pneumonia

HIV/AIDS related tuberculosis should be differentiated from non-tuberculosis mycobacteria pneumonia. Their imaging findings are similar to each other, which presents challenges for their differential diagnosis. Molecular biology examinations play an important role in the differentiation.

Other Pneumonia

HIV/AIDS related tuberculosis should be differentiated from other pneumonia. Non-bacterial pneumonia (mycoplasma, viral and allergic) often shows patchy shadows, which are similar to the manifestations of early infiltrative pulmonary tuberculosis. When bacterial pneumonia shows lobar lesions, it may be confused with tuberculous caseous pneumonia, which should also be differentiated for the diagnosis. Symptoms of mycoplasma pneumonia are mild, with imaging findings being always inconsistency with the clinical symptoms, which usually subside within 2–3 weeks. In the cases of allergic pneumonia, eosinophils in the blood increase, with intrapulmonary mobile shadows, which are the basis for their differentiation. Bacterial pneumonia can have acute onset, with chills, high fever, rust colored sputum, and streptococcus pneumoniae positive. Recovery is rapid after antibiotic treatment and all these symptoms can subside within 1 month.

Pulmonary Abscesses

HIV/AIDS related tuberculosis should be differentiated from pulmonary abscesses. In the cases of infiltrative pulmonary tuberculosis with cavities, it should be differentiated from pulmonary abscess. Especially, tuberculosis with cavities in the apical segment of inferior lobe should be differentiated from acute pulmonary abscess. Chronic fibrous cavity tuberculosis should be differentiated from chronic pulmonary abscess. The key points for the differentiation are tubercle bacilli positive by sputum culture in the cases of TB, while tubercle bacilli negative by sputum culture in the cases of abscesses. Pulmonary abscess has an acute onset, with increased leukocytes and neutrophils as well as favorable therapeutic efficacy of antibiotics. But sometimes tuberculosis with cavity may develop into bacterial infection, with undetectable tubercle bacillus by sputum culture.

Lung Cancer

HIV/AIDS related tuberculosis should be differentiated from lung cancer. The central type of lung cancer has nodular shadow in the hilum or hilar and mediastinal lymph node metastasis, which should be differentiated from lymphatic tuberculosis. The peripheral type of lung cancer has small flaky infiltration and nodules in the periphery of the lungs, which should be differentiated from tuberculoma or tuberculosis infiltrative lesions. Lung cancers occur commonly in people aged above 40 years. The central type mainly is squamous carcinoma and the cases often have a history of long term smoking, with symptoms of no fever but difficulty breathing or chest distress as well as gradually increasing chest pain. There are also symptoms of irritated cough with blood phlegm and progressive weight loss. The cases with supraclavicular metastasis have palpable harden lymph nodes. The intrapulmonary nodules can lobulated with fine spikes, no satellite lesions, generally no calcification and possible vacuole sign. The peripheral type of lung cancer shows pleura invagination sign. Tuberculin test often shows negative in the cases of lung, positive or weakly positive in the cases with TB, and negative or weak positive in AIDS patients.

17.3.1.8 Discussions

HIV infection is known to be the main factor for the development of latent tuberculosis into active tuberculosis. It has been estimated that there are globally about 42 million HIV infected patients, of which more than 25 % sustains active tuberculosis. Most of these patients are in Africa and some developing countries of Asia, with insufficient health care resources. The clinical manifestations of tuberculosis in AIDS patients are affected by the degree of immunosuppression. The imaging findings in the cases with slight immunosuppression are similar to those of secondary tuberculosis in healthy hosts. The disease mainly involves the posterior apical segment of the upper lobe to show focal parenchymal areas and nodular shadows. About 20 % patients may have cavities and 10 % patients may have lymphadenectasis. The imaging demonstrations in the cases with serious immunosuppression are similar to those in the cases with primary tuberculosis, with characteristic abnormal manifestations of hilar and/or mediastinal lymphadenectasis and parenchymal changes of the air chambers. CT scanning demonstrates enlarged nodules with low density. Enhanced scanning demonstrates marginal enhancement of the lymph nodes. The incidence of military tuberculosis in AIDS patients is increasing due to reduced thymic T lymphocytes in AIDS patients and the defects of delayed allergic responses, which result in the formation of granulomas and impaired functions to kill bacilli and confine the lesions.

17.3.2 HIV/AIDS Related Pulmonary Nontuberculous Mycobacterial Infections

Nontuberculous mycobacteria (NTM) refer to the mycobacteria except for mycobacterium tuberculosis complex (human, cattle, African and vole) and mycobacterium leprae. The most commonly known nomination is nontuberculous mycobacteria (NTM). More than 100 kinds of NTM have been found so far. According to Berger Manual of Systematic Bacteriology, NTM is divided into two categories, rapid growth type and slow growth type.

17.3.2.1 Pathogens and Pathogenesis

NTM are widely spread in nature, such as soil, dust, flowing water and raw milk. Under a microscope, NTM is morphologically similar to tubercle bacilli, with red stained findings by acid-fast staining. According to the growth of NTM in solid medium, the Runyon classification divides NTM into the following four groups, light chromogenic bacteria; dark chromogenic bacteria that can cause cervical lymphnoditis in children, intrapulmonary or extrapulmonary infections and abrasive abscess; non-chromogenic bacteria including mycobacterium avium complex, intracellular mycobacteria that can cause pulmonary infections, lymphnoditis, arthritis and meningitis; rapid growth bacteria including mycobacterium fortuitum, mycobacterium, mycobacterium abscessus that can cause pulmonary diseases and skin infections.

17.3.2.2 Pathophysiological Basis

Immunocompromised populations, such as HIV infected patients, patients with neoplasms, patients with long-term use adrenocortical hormone or immunosuppressive agents, are more susceptible to disseminated NTM infection. Immunocompetent people may have mycobacterium kansasii and mycobacterium avium infections. It was reported in the United States that the occurrence of mycobacterium avium complex infection in HIV positive patients is up to more than 95 %. The pathological changes of NTM infections are similar to those of tuberculosis. NTM lymphnoditis is pathologically characterized by granulomatous inflammation.

Tuberculous nodules formed by epithelioid cells and Langhans giant cells are rare, with no accompanying central caseous necrosis. Due to the weak pathogenicity of NTM, the pathological changes are slight, but there is difference in the pathological changes of NTM infections in terms of location, type and host. Cavities are common in the cases with pulmonary NTM infection, commonly being multiple or multilocular thin wall cavities. The pleuron is rarely involved, with non-specific pathological changes of inflammation but with large quantity pathogens of NTM.

17.3.2.3 Clinical Symptoms and Signs

Patients often have a history of chronic obstructive pulmonary disease, tuberculosis, silicosis, pulmonary abscess, bronchiectasis, cystic fibrosis, diabetes, ulcer as well as use of hormone or immunosuppressive agents. Its occurrence is more common in males than in females. The symptoms include cough, expectoration, hemoptysis, chest pain, difficulty breathing, low grade fever, weight loss and fatigue. The symptoms are non-specific and the conditions progress slowly.

17.3.2.4 Examinations and Their Selection
Bacteriologic Examinations

For patients with suspected diagnosis of pulmonary NTM infection, sputum smear for acid-fast staining, sputum culture and bronchial lavage specimen culture can be performed. The positive findings should be identified with two to three times repeated culture. The same finding of NTM can define the diagnosis.

Pathological Examinations

Pathological biopsy can be performed for the diagnosis of NTM lymphnoditis.

Molecular Biological Examinations

Using 16S-23 SrDNA gene spacer sequence (IGS) of NTM for PCR-restriction fragment length polymorphism analysis (PCR-RFLP), NTM species can be identified, which is more accurate, faster and simpler than the conventional morphological and biochemical examinations.

Mantoux Skin Test

Mycobacterium tuberculosis and NTM have common antigen. PPD skin test produces cross-reaction, but there are still differences between mycobacterium tuberculosis and NTM. PPD-T of the mycobacterium tuberculosis and PPD-NTM of NTM are simultaneously obtained for Mantoux skin tests. The induration diameter of PPD-T in NTM patients is generally within 15 mm. For the cases with the induration diameter of PPD-NTM skin test being 5 mm larger or over 25 % larger than that of PPD-T skin test, NTM infection can be confirmed.

Chest X-ray and CT Scanning

Both are the most commonly used imaging examinations.

17.3.2.5 Imaging Demonstrations

Imaging demonstrations include various lesions such as infiltration, cavity, nodules, fibrous caseation and extensive fiber contraction in unilateral or bilateral lungs. The incidence of cavity is up to 80 %, being singular or multiple. Cavities caused by intracellular Mycobacterium are mostly found in the pleura, with thin wall and less surrounding exudates.

Case Study

A female patient aged 26 years was confirmatively diagnosed as having AIDS by the CDC. She complained of cough and chest distress for half a month, fever for 10 days, 1 day after cesarean section and finding of HIV positive for 1 day. Her CD4 T cell count was 54/μl, with Treponema pallidum antibody negative and PPD test negative.

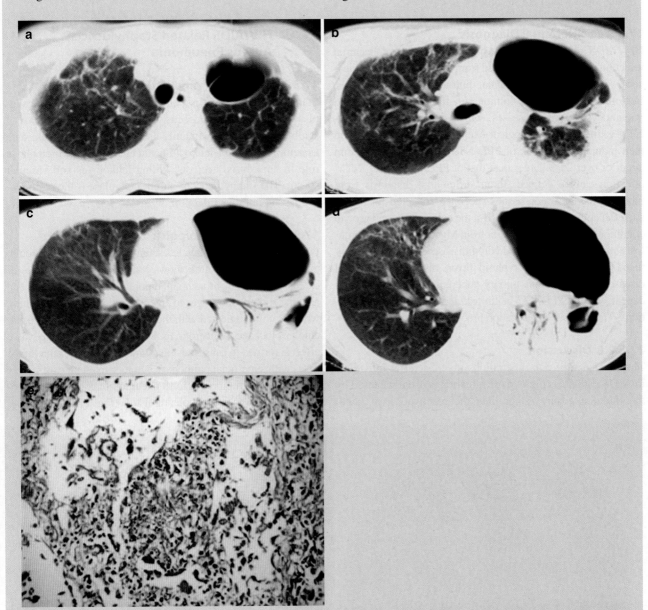

Fig.17.44 (a–e) HIV/AIDS related pulmonary nontuberculous mycobacterial infection. (a–d) CT scanning demonstrates multiple cavities in the left lung field, bilateral multiple lobular central nodules and extensive branches liked linear shadows in tree buds sign. There are also large flaky parenchymal changes of the lung tissues in the left lower lung field in high density shadows, with accompanying air bronchogram sign. (e) HE staining demonstrates avium intracellular complex mycobacteria infection of lung tissues in atypical tuberculous nodular changes. (HE×200)

17.3.2.6 Diagnostic Basis

1. Respiratory symptoms or accompanying systemic symptoms.
2. Sputum culture find the same kind of NTM three times.
3. Bronchial biopsy for NTM culture is positive and lung tissue biopsy demonstrates similar granuloma to NTM lesions.
4. Chest X-ray demonstrates a variety of lesions, such as infiltration, cavity, nodules, fibrous caseation and extensive fiber contraction in the right upper lung. CT scanning demonstrates multiple lobular central nodules and tree buds sign, which are susceptible to cavities.

17.3.2.7 Differential Diagnosis

HIV/AIDS related pulmonary nontuberculous mycobacterial infection should be differentiated from tuberculosis, bronchiectasis, mycoplasmal pneumonia, pulmonary cystic fibrosis, Legionnaires disease, pulmonary fungal diseases and Pneumocystis carinii diseases, which depends on the PPD-NTM skin test and etiological examinations. The cases with their induration diameter of PPD-NTM skin test being 5 mm larger or over 25 % larger than that of PPD-T skin test, NTM infection can be defined. In its differential diagnosis from tuberculosis, the lesion tissues specimen collected for mycobacterial culture is all positive. But the colony state and growth conditions of NTM are different from Mycobacterium tuberculosis complex. Disseminated NTM disease should be differentiated from septicemia, typhoid fever, disseminated fungal diseases, and systemic miliary tuberculosis, which mainly depends on the PPD-NTM skin test and etiological examinations. The specific identification procedures are as above.

17.3.2.8 Discussion

The incidence of non-tuberculous mycobacterial infections in AIDS patients is high. MAC infection is usually caused by the initial exposure rather than the reactivation of latent pathogens. In patients with complications of MAC related lung diseases, most of the imaging findings are normal. The most common manifestation is mediastinal or hilar lymphadenectasis. And the pulmonary symptoms are similar to those of tuberculosis. In the cases with multiple patchy parenchymal changes, cavities can be found, as well as nodules with blurry boundaries, pleural effusion and rarely found miliary nodules. Sputum or bronchoalveolar lavage fluid culture positive, clinical symptoms, imaging findings, and response to treatment can define the diagnosis.

17.3.3 HIV/AIDS Related Staphylococcus Aureus Pneumonia

17.3.3.1 Pathogens and Pathogenesis

Staphylococcus aureus is a Gram positive coccus and is coagulase positive staphylococcus. The pathogenic substances of staphylococcus aureus mainly are toxins and enzymes, such as hemolytic toxins, leukocidin and enterotoxin, which play a role in hemolysis, necrosis, killing leukocytes and vascular spasm. The staphylococcus aureus coagulase is the main reason for suppurative infection.

17.3.3.2 Pathophysiological Basis

Pneumonia caused by inhaled staphylococcus aureus through the respiratory tract often shows lesions in the large lobes or extensive fusion of bronchopneumonia lesions. Bronchial and alveolar rupture allows gas to enter the pulmonary interstitium, which is communicated with the bronchi. In the cases of bronchiolar blockage by necrotic tissues or pus, the one-way valve effect is formed to cause tension pulmonary emphysema. In the cases with superficial pulmonary emphysema with excessively high tension, it ruptures to form pneumothorax or pyopneumothorax, as well as bronchooleural fistula (Fig. 17.45a, b).

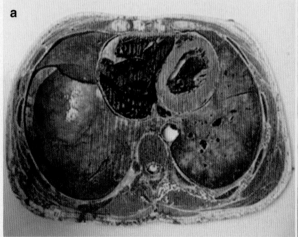
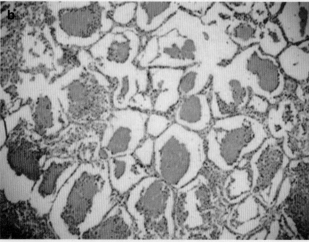
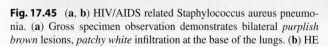

Fig. 17.45 (a, b) HIV/AIDS related Staphylococcus aureus pneumonia. (a) Gross specimen observation demonstrates bilateral *purplish brown* lesions, *patchy white* infiltration at the base of the lungs. (b) HE staining demonstrates alveolar diffuse lesions, exudation of the serous fluid and inflammatory cells in the alveolar cavity, and alveolar wall congestion

17.3.3.3 Clinical Symptoms and Signs

The symptoms include chills, persistent high fever, cough, expectoration, chest pain and other symptoms. There is no sign in the early period. Symptoms are scattered moist rales in both lungs, being in consistency to severe toxic symptoms and respiratory symptoms. Yellow purulent sputum is the typical characteristics of staphylococcus aureus pneumonia. In the cases with larger lesions or fusion of lesions, signs of parenchymal changes, pneumothorax or pyopneumothorax can be found.

17.3.3.4 Examinations and Their Selection

Bacteriological Examinations

In the sputum or pleural fluid smears examinations, the bacteria with a concentration being no less than 107 cfa/ml is the pathogen, the bacteria with a concentration being 105–107 cfa/ml is the suspected pathogen, and the bacteria with a concentration being less than 105 cfa/ml is the contaminated bacteria.

Blood Tests

There are increased WBC count and neutrophils, leftward migration of the nucleus and possibly no increase of WBC count in AIDS patients.

Immunological Examinations

Immunofluorescence, enzyme-linked immunosorbent assay and counter immunoelectrophoresis can be performed to detect serum antigen or antibody of the pathogenic bacteria, which can define the diagnosis. Polymerase chain reaction has certain significance in pathogen detection.

Bronchofiberoscopy

The protected bronchoscopic specimen (PBS) and bronchoalveolar lavage (BAL) can be applied to collect the specimen, which has reduced chances of specimens contamination by oral bacteria.

Percutaneous Puncture Biopsy

Biphasic TV monitors guided pulmonary puncture and suction for pulmonary tissues examinations can be performed to detect the real pathogenic bacteria.

Chest X-ray and CT Scanning

Both are the most commonly used imaging examinations.

17.3.3.5 Imaging Demonstrations

The diagnostic imaging demonstrates staphylococcus aureus pneumonia as lesions in the inner zone of both middle lower lungs. There are singular or multiple parenchymal changes in patchy or lobar distribution that may fuse into large flakes. It may be complicated by cavity and pulmonary emphysema, with surrounding compensatory emphysema.

Case Study 1

A male patient aged 37 years was confirmatively diagnosed as having AIDS by the CDC. He complained of high fever with a body temperature of about 39 °C and chest pain for 2 months. His CD4 T cell count was 31/μl.

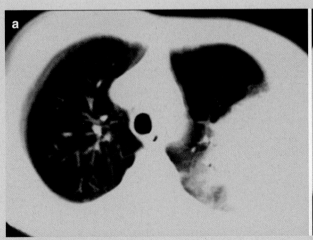 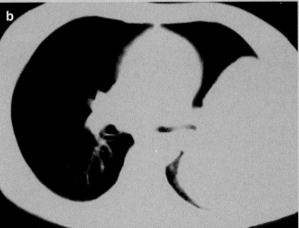

Fig. 17.46 (**a–f**) HIV/AIDS related staphylococcus aureus pneumonia. (**a–c**) CT scanning demonstrates large flaky dense shadows in the middle-outer zone of the left middle lung field, and narrowed left bronchus. (**d–f**) CT scanning demonstrates large flaky shadows with uneven density in the left lateral chest wall and even lower density shadow in them

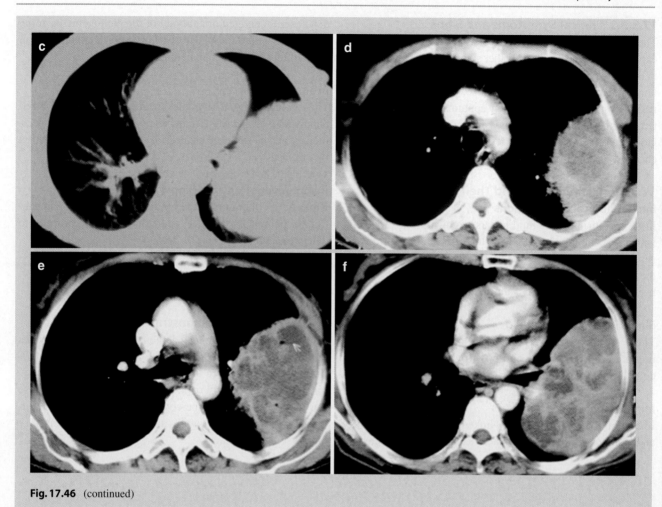

Fig. 17.46 (continued)

Case Study 2

A male patient aged 40 years was confirmatively diagnosed as having AIDS by the CDC. He complained of high fever with a body temperature of about 40 °C and chest pain for 2 months. His CD4 T cell count was 85/μl.

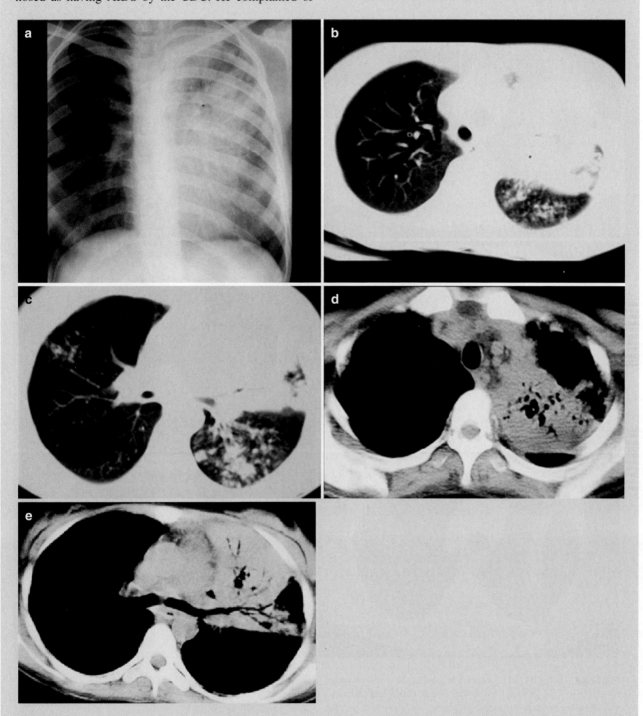

Fig. 17.47 (a–e) HIV/AIDS related staphylococcus aureus pneumonia. (a) DR demonstrates large flaky dense shadows with increased density in the middle-inner zone of the left upper lung field, with blurry boundaries. The lung tissue are atelectatic and the mediastinum migrates leftwards. (b, c) CT scanning demonstrates large flaky dense shadows with increased density in the middle-inner zone of the left upper lung field, with blurry boundaries, with surrounding acinar or particle liked shadows that fuse into flaky shadows. (d, e) CT scanning demonstrates large flaky shadow of parenchymal changes in the middle-inner zone of the left upper lung field, with cyst liked transparent shadows and air bronchogram sign in them, as well as mediastinal lymphadenectasis

Case Study 3

A male patient aged 40 years was confirmatively diagnosed as having AIDS by the CDC. He complained of general fatigue and dizziness for more than 2 months as well as cough and expectoration for 1 month. His CD4 T cell count was 46/μl.

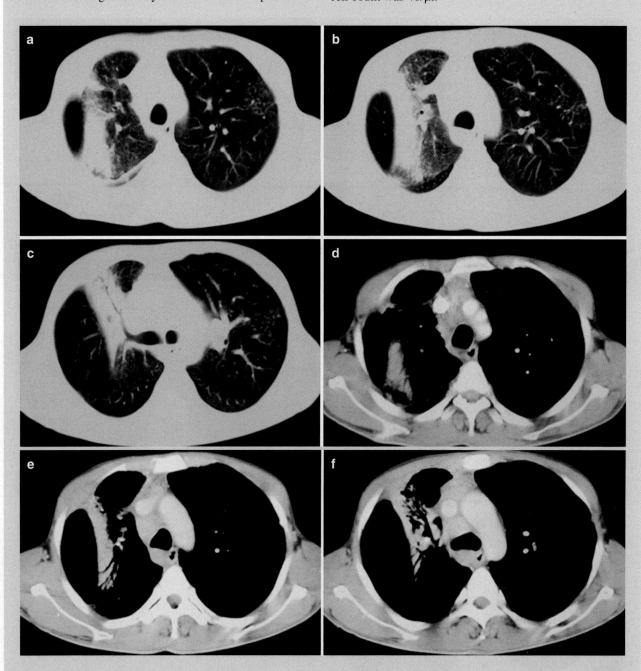

Fig.17.48 (a–f) HIV/AIDS related Staphylococcus aureus pneumonia. (a–c) CT scanning demonstrates broad band liked high density shadows in the right middle lung field, with air bronchogram sign in them. (d–f) CT scanning of the mediastinal window demonstrates broad band liked uneven parenchymal shadows in the right middle lung field, with uneven thickness of air bronchogram sign

Case Study 4

A male patient aged 40 years was confirmatively diagnosed as having AIDS by the CDC. He complained of general fatigue and dizziness for more than 2 months as well as cough and sore throat for 1 month. His CD4 T cell count was 76/μl and was clinically diagnosed as bacterial pneumonia of the right lung.

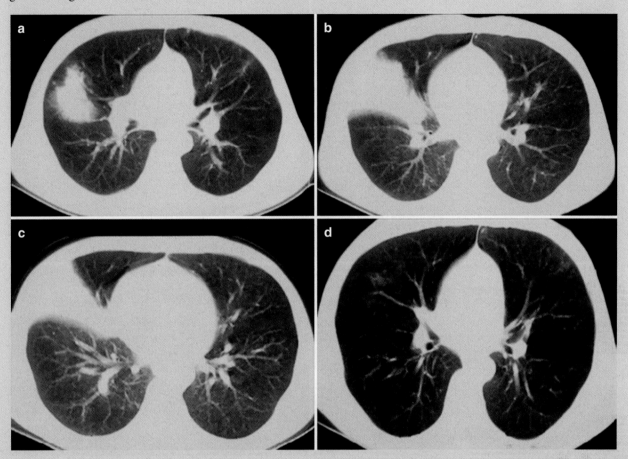

Fig.17.49 (**a–d**) HIV/AIDS related staphylococcus aureus pneumonia. (**a–c**) CT scanning demonstrates fan shaped shadow in the right middle lung field with its apex pointing to the hilar dense shadow, with clear boundaries. (**d**) CT scanning reexamination demonstrates absence of the lesions in the right lung after anti-bacteria treatment for 2 weeks

Case Study 5

A male patient aged 44 years was confirmatively diagnosed as having AIDS by the CDC. He complained of high fever, cough and expectoration for 1 week. His CD4 T cell count was 116/μl.

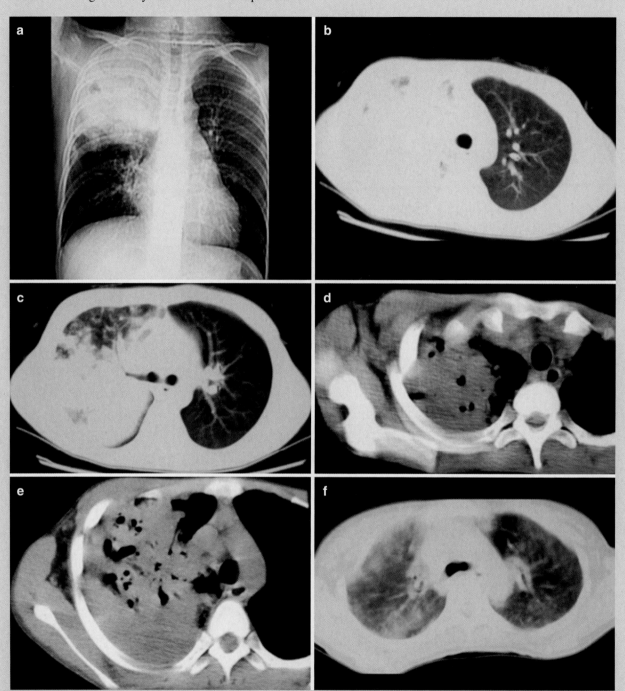

Fig.17.50 (a–f) HIV/AIDS related Staphylococcus aureus pneumonia. (a) DR demonstrates large flaky dense shadow in the right middle-upper lung field, with blurry boundary. (b, c) CT scanning demonstrates large flaky dense shadow in the right middle upper lung field, with blurry boundary. (d, e) CT scanning demonstrates large flaky dense shadow in the right middle upper lung field, with cystic transparent area in it. (f) Reexamination demonstrates obviously improved pulmonary lesions in the right lung after anti-bacteria treatment for 3 weeks

Case Study 6

A male patient aged 29 years was confirmatively diagnosed as having AIDS by the CDC. He had a history of multiple sexual partners. He was definitively diagnosed in Otc. 2004 and showed symptoms in Dec. 2005. He complained of high fever with the highest body temperature of 39 °C, cough and expectoration of thick sputum, weight loss and fatigue. His CD4 T cell count was 20/μl.

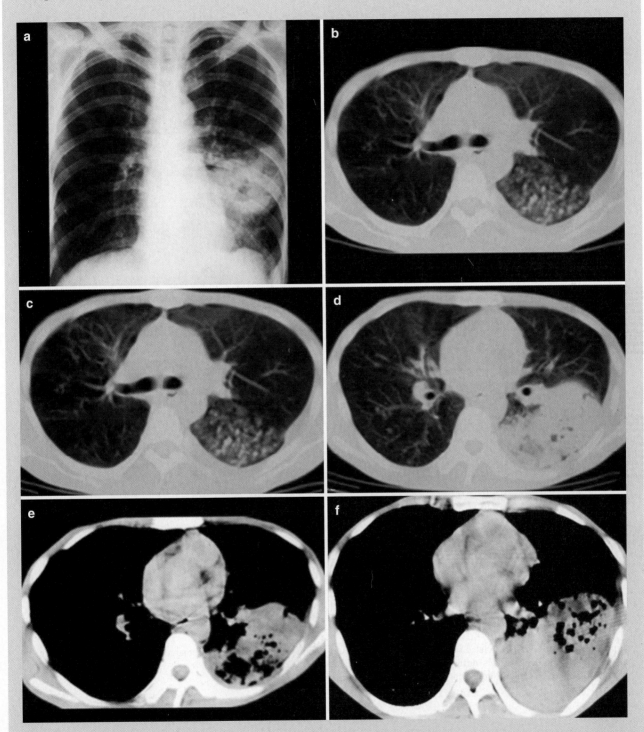

Fig. 17.51 (**a–h**) HIV/AIDS related staphylococcus aureus pneumonia. (**a**) Chest X-ray demonstrates large flaky high density shadow in the left middle-lower lung field, with central transparent areas in different sizes and blurry boundaries; parenchyma changes of the left lower lung, predominantly in the posterior and exterior basal segments; unobstructed brounchus and thickened adjacent pleura. (**b–d**) CT scanning demonstrates large flaky shadows in fan shaped distribution along the bronchus in the left middle-lower lung, with gas containing cavities and high density shadows; and thickened adjacent pleura of the lateral chest wall. (**e, f**) CT scanning of the mediastinal window demonstrates large flaky fan shaped parenchymal shadows in the left middle-lower lung field, with ventilation shadows in them; and thickened pleura of the lateral chest wall. (**g, h**) Pathological examination showed staphylococcus aureus

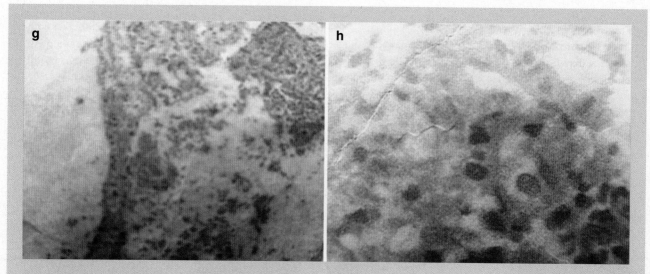

Fig. 17.51   (continued)

Case Study 7

A male patient aged 38 years was confirmatively diagnosed as having AIDS by the CDC. He had a history of multiple sexual partners. He complained of fever with the highest body temperature of 39 °C, cough and expectoration of thick sputum for 1 week. His CD4 T cell count was 30/μl.

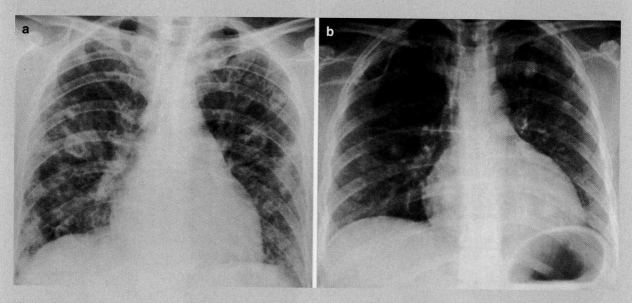

Fig. 17.52   (**a, b**) HIV/AIDS related staphylococcus aureus pneumonia. (**a, b**) DR demonstrates diffuse scattered multiple thin-walled transparent areas in both lungs, increased and blurry pulmonary markings, and enlarged heart shadow in flask shape (pericardial effusion)

17.3.3.6 Diagnostic Basis
Clinical Symptoms
Chills, fever, cough, expectoration, chest pain and other symptoms commonly; hemoptysis and dyspnea rarely

Clinical Signs
The patients may be found with fever appearance, rarely shortness of breath and cyanosis. In the serious cases, the body temperature can be as high as 39–40 °C and blood pressure decreases, with signs of shock. By chest examinations, decreased ipsilateral respiratory motion; increased or decreased fremitus, dull sound in percussion; bronchial breathing sounds or moist rales by auscultation; rarely pleural friction and weakened breathing sounds.

Blood Tests
Increased WBC count and neutrophils, possible the nucleus left shift; no increase or even decrease of WBC count in AIDS patients; Staphylococcus aureus positive by blood culture.

Bacteriological Examinations
Sputum or pleural fluid smears examinations for pathogenic bacteria culture is positive, and antibiotic sensitivity test is positive.

Chest X-ray and CT Scanning
By chest X-ray and CT scanning, the most common demonstrations are lesions of bronchial pneumonia. The findings of pulmonary emphysema and cavities can facilitate the diagnose.

17.3.3.7 Differential Diagnosis
The lesions should be differentiated from infiltrative parenchymal bronchioloalveolar carcinoma. The smaller lesions should be differentiated from pulmonary infarction. The large lesions should be differentiated from obstructive pneumonia. It is difficult to identify the types of common bacterial pneumonia simply by chest X-ray and CT scanning. In combination to the laboratory tests, the diagnosis can be defined.

17.3.3.8 Discussion
The incidence of pyogenic bacterial infection is increasing in AIDS patients, which is caused by their weakened cellular and humoral immunity. The manifestations of these most common bacterial infections are similar to those of non-HIV infected patients by chest X-ray. Bacterial pneumonia and purulent bronchitis are the most common causes of pulmonary infections in AIDS patients. Particularly, they are frequently found in patients with a history of intravenous drug abuse and smokers. They are histologically characterized by inflammations of the bronchi and bronchioles as well as inflammatory exudates and mucus in the airway lumens. CT scans facilitates the diagnosis of bronchiolitis and early bronchial pneumonia. The demonstrations are characterized by (1) small centrilobular nodular shadows, which is the cross sectional demonstration of bronchioles filled with inflammatory substances and its surrounding inflammations; (2) Branched linear shadows, which is the long axis demonstration of abnormal bronchioles; (3) Focal parenchymal areas caused by bronchial pneumonia. Bacterial infection usually is the unilateral segmental alveolar infiltration, with manifestations of lobar segmental pneumonia in the exudation period. Early lesions show exudative inflammation in lobar and segmental distribution. The pathological changes are mainly alveolar exudates in a small quantity. The lesions progress into parenchymal changes. According to the case history and the clinical manifestations, the lesions are in lobar and segmental distribution by chest X-ray and CT scanning, with the bronchi in railway track sign for the diagnosis. CT scanning demonstrates fan-shaped or broad band liked distributions of infiltration and parenchymal changes in the lungs.

17.3.4 HIV/AIDS Related Rhodococcus Equi Pneumonia

17.3.4.1 Pathogens and Pathogenesis
Rhodococcus equi infection is one of the zoonotic diseases, which commonly occurs in the grazing areas. Patients with T lymphocyte immunodeficiency caused by AIDS and other factors are especially susceptible to the infection. Rhodococcus equi was firstly discovered in 1923 and was nominated as corynebacterium equi. After structure analysis of the cell wall, it was found that the bacterium is quite different from Corynebacterium, and therefore classified as Rhodococcus. Rhodococcus equi infection in human is rare. But in recent years, due to an increase of patients with immunodeficiency syndrome, reports on rhodococcus equi caused human respiratory infections and sepsis are increasing. In the past, the toxicity mechanism of Rhodococcus equi was mostly speculated. Until recently, the damage process of toxic plasmid to human tissue is discovered, which presents a new way for the study of the pathogenesis of Rhodococcus equi infections.

17.3.4.2 Pathophysiological Basis
Rhodococcus equi is one of the facultative parasites in the cells and its optimum growth temperature is 30 °C, with a suitable growth temperature of 10–40 °C. Acid-fast staining of Rhodococcus equi shows uncertain results. Due to its morphological diversity, it is often mistaken as diphtheroid bacillus, bacillus or micrococcus. In sheep blood agar, rhodococcus equi can have synergistic hemolysis with

staphylococcus aureus, Listeria monocytogenes and coryne-bacterium pseudotuberculosis, which is a characteristic manifestation of Rhodococcus equi. The most common pathological changes in Rhodococcus equi infection are chronic purulent bronchitis and extensive lung abscess. Imaging often demonstrates subacute pneumonia, commonly with cavities.

17.3.4.3 Clinical Symptoms and Signs

The clinical manifestations are poor appetite, drowsiness, fever and shortness of breath. Studies by E Marchiori et al. [30] in 2005 revealed that all the 5 cases of AIDS complicated by rhodococcus equi pulmonary infection have cough and fever lasting for 1–2 months, with accompanying shortness of breath and chest pain. All the 13 cases, studied by Li et al. in 2011 [106], have fever with a body temperature up to 38–40 °C and cough. In addition, there are also expectoration with orange red sputum in 10 cases, hemoptysis in 4 cases, dyspnea in 11 cases, moist rales of lungs in 13 cases, emaciation in 6 cases, poor appetite in 6 cases, diarrhea in 2 cases, joint pain in 1 case, oral candidiasis infections in 13 cases, oral herpes in 4 cases, chest pain in 4 cases, no obvious symptoms in 1 case and hepatitis B in 3 cases. Typical clinical manifestations of this disease are fever, cough, dyspnea and chest pain, while others such as emaciation, diarrhea and joint pain are not representative symptoms.

17.3.4.4 Examinations and Their Selection

Identification of the Bacteria

Various specimens were inoculated on blood plates at a temperature of 35 °C for 18–24 culture, with bacteria growth of 18 strains. They are biologically characterized by a diameter of about 0.5 mm, non-transparent and slight yellowish colonies. After 48–72 h, the colonies expand to 1–2 mm, which can be emulsified in mucous fluid liked state. Most of the colonies produce orange and orange red pigments, which can be cultured in ordinary agar.

Pathological Examinations

Histopathological findings are typical for Rhodococcus equi infection. H&E staining demonstrates mainly bleeding in the alveolar space, large quantity epithelial cells, possibly predominant fibroblasts, parenchymal changes of lung tissue and thickened alveolar septa. PAS staining demonstrates scattered or clustered rhodococcus equi in pink or purplish red.

Chest X-ray and CT Scanning

Both are the most commonly used imaging examinations.

Percutaneous Lung Puncture for Biopsy

Biphasic TV monitor guided lung puncture can be performed to suck lung tissues for biopsy, based on which the real pathogenic bacteria can be detected.

17.3.4.5 Imaging Demonstrations

The typical demonstrations include central hilar sphere liked shadow with increased density in unilateral lung, accounted for 70 %. There are also manifestations of exudative infiltration and large flaky or spherical mass shadows in the right or left hilar area. The lesions are in patchy or flaky appearance, radiating from the hilum to the lung field with blurry boundaries.

Case Study 1

A male patient aged 30 years was confirmatively diagnosed as having AIDS by the CDC. He complained of recurrent fever, cough and chest pain for 13 days; and was found HIV positive for 8 days. He was also a carrier of hepatitis C virus, with symptoms of fever with no known causes, cough, chest distress and weak limbs. By examinations, he was found to have complexion of chronic conditions; many moist and dry rales by cardiopulmonary auscultation. He had a past history of HIV positive for 8 years, with drug abuse and extramarital affairs. The history of present illness includes fever, paroxysmal cough with a little whitish yellow thick sputum since May 8, 2008. He also had subjective paroxysmal dull pain in the left chest, and hemoptysis once which was bright red with blood clot in a volume of about 80 ml. His CD4 T cell count was 10/µl. By sputum culture, Rhodococcus equi was found positive. After receiving antibiotic treatment, his conditions improved and he was discharged from the hospital.

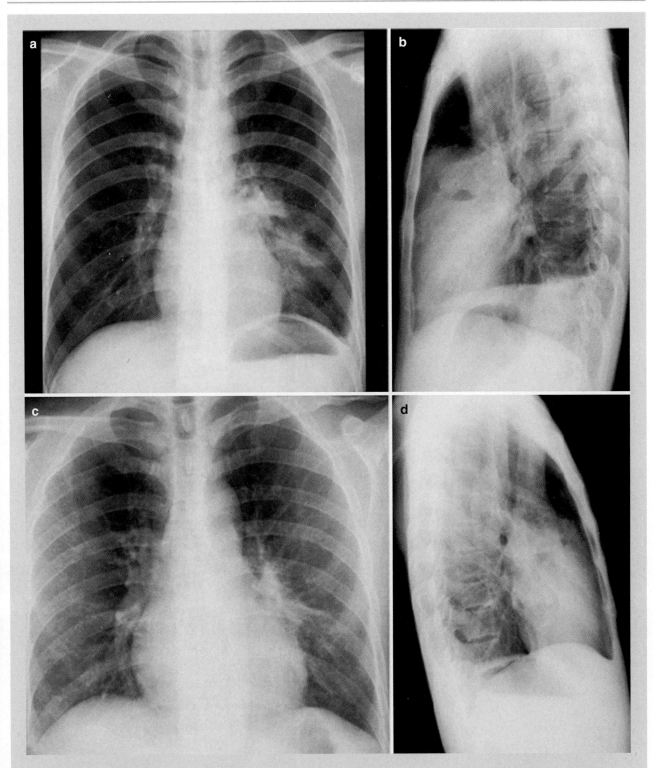

Fig.17.53 (a–d) HIV/AIDS related Rhodococcus equi pneumonia. (**a**, **b**) Anteroposterior and lateral DR demonstrates enlarged and thickened left hilum, and large flaky blurry shadows with increased density in the left lower lung. (**c**, **d**) Reexamination demonstrates normal lungs after antibiotic treatment

Case Study 2

A male patient aged 43 years was confirmatively diagnosed as having AIDS by the CDC. He complained of fever with the highest body temperature of 39 °C with no known causes for more than 3 months, with accompanying paroxymal cough and expectoration of small quantity white thick sputum. By blood culture, Rhodococcus equi was found positive. He was confirmatively diagnosed as HIV positive 3 months ago and his CD4 T cell count was 15/µl. By examinations, he had a complexion of chronic illness and many moist and dry rales by cardiopulmonary auscultation.

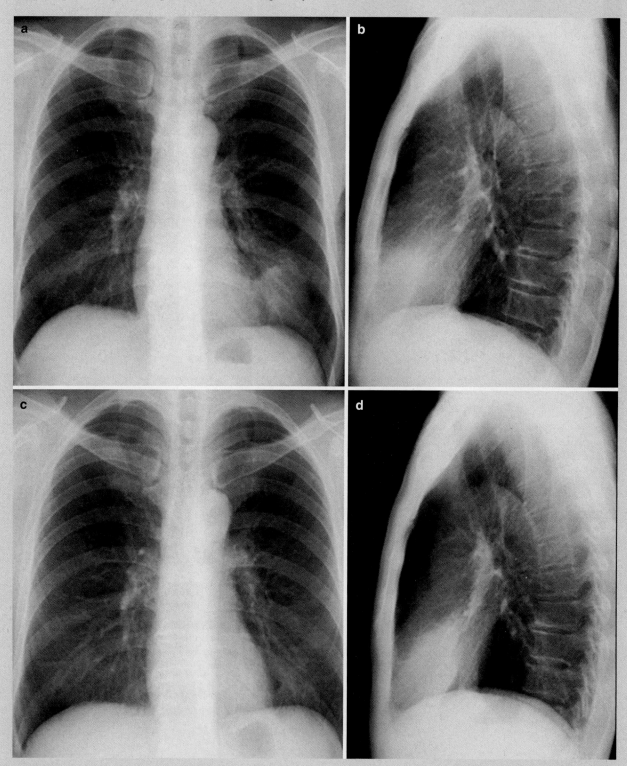

Fig. 17.54 (a–d) HIV/AIDS related Rhodococcus equi pneumonia. (a, b) DR demonstrates round liked large flaky shadows with increased density in the left lower lung, enlarged and thickened hilus. (c, d) DR reexamination after treatment demonstrates flocculent shadows in the left lower lung, with improved conditions than previous findings before treatment (a, b)

Case Study 3

A male patient aged 49 years was confirmatively diagnosed as having AIDS by the CDC. He complained of paroxymal cough and expectoration of white diluted bubble sputum with no known causes since Dec. 2007, as well as other symptoms of after noons fever with the highest body temperature of 40 °C and obvious night sweating. He also complained of chest distress and weak limbs for 5 months, finding of HIV positive for 14 days. By examinations, he had a complexion of chronic illness and his CD4 T cell count was 53/μl. After anti-infection treatment, his conditions were not improved, but deteriorated to cause death.

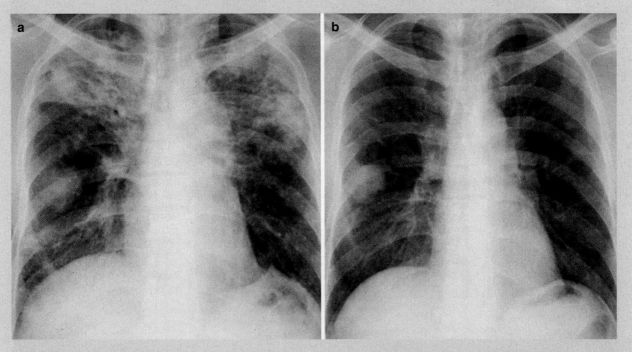

Fig. 17.55 (**a**, **b**) HIV/AIDS related Rhodococcus equi pneumonia. (**a**, **b**) DR demonstrates round liked large flaky shadows with increased density in the right lower lung, cords liked and flocculent liked blurry shadows in both middle-upper lung fields and in the right lower lung field, and enlarged and thickened hilus

Case Study 4

A male patient aged 38 years was confirmatively diagnosed as having AIDS by the CDC. He complained of fever, cough, expectoration, chest distress and weak limbs for 5 months. His CD4 T cell count was 63/μl.

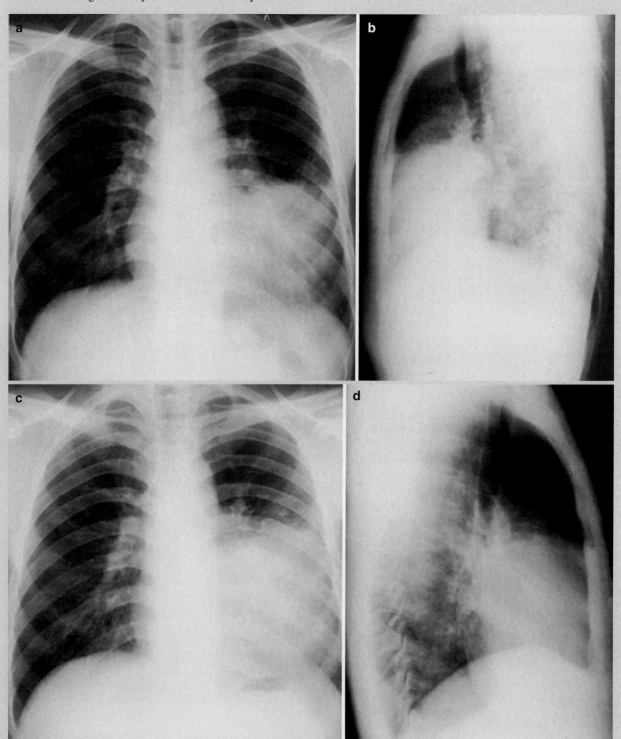

Fig.17.56 (**a–e**) HIV/AIDS related Rhodococcus equi pneumonia. (**a, b**) DR demonstrates huge round large flaky shadows with increased density in the left lower lung, enlarged and thickened hilum and covered right heart edge. (**c, d**) DR reexamination after treatment for 1 week demonstrates flocculent shadow in the left lower lung, improved than those before the treatment (**a, b**). (**e**) DR reexamination after treatment demonstrates flocculent liked shadows in the left lower lung, obviously improved than before the treatment (**c, d**)

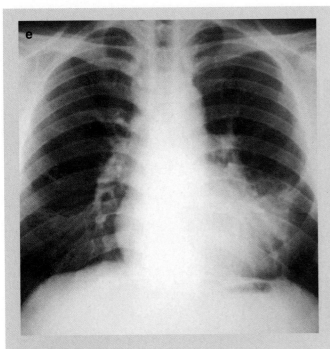

Fig. 17.56 (continued)

Case Study 5

A male patient aged 39 years was confirmatively diagnosed as having AIDS by the CDC. He complained recurrent cough and fever for 3 days. His CD4 T cell count was 50/μl. Multiple times sputum smears demonstrated Gram positive bacilli, Rhodococcus equi, and yeast liked fungus. Multiple times sputum culture demonstrated smooth ball liked Candida glabrata, Rhodococcus equi and fungi. By lung tissues culture, Rhodococcus equi was detected.

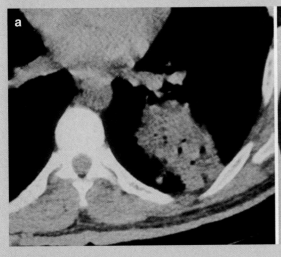

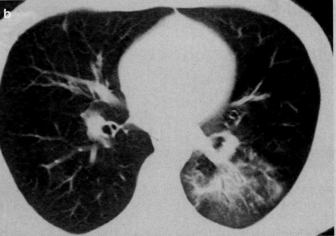

Fig. 17.57 (a, b) HIV/AIDS related Rhodococcus equi pneumonia. (a) CT scanning of the mediastinal window demonstrates soft tissue mass shadows in the dorsal segment of the left lower lung, with ventilation shadows in them. (b) CT scanning of the pulmonary window after the treatment demonstrates absence of the soft tissue mass shadows, and flocculent liked shadow in the left lower lung, obviously improved than previous findings (a)

Case Study 6

A male patient aged 39 years was confirmatively diagnosed as having AIDS by the CDC. He complained of

recurrent cough and chest distress for 2 months. His CD4
T cell count was 50/μl.

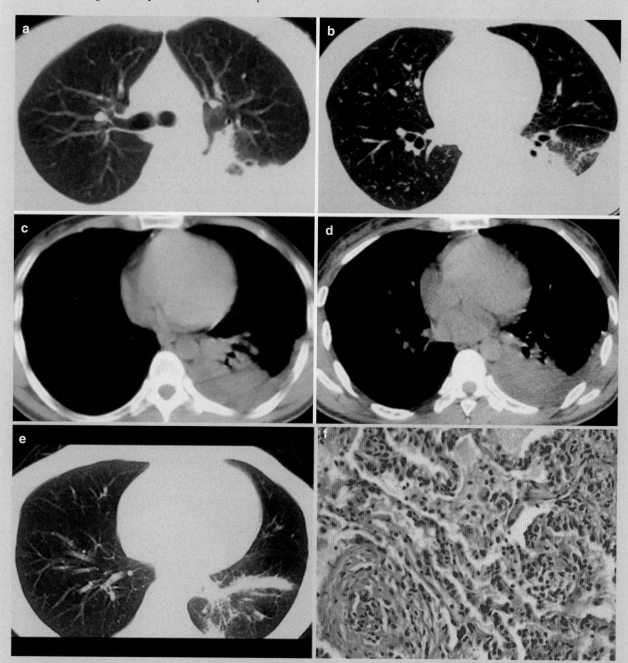

Fig.17.58 (a–i) HIV/AIDS related Rhodococcus equi pneumonia.
(a, b) CT scanning of the pulmonary window before the treatment
demonstrates flaky dense shadows in the dorsal segment of the left
lower lung, with ventilation shadows in them. (c, d) CT scanning of
the mediastinal window before the treatment demonstrates flaky dense
shadows in the dorsal segment of the left lower lung, pulmonary atelectasis and pleural effusion, with ventilation shadows in them. (e) CT
scanning of the pulmonary window after the treatment demonstrates

absence of the mass shadows in the left lower lung with transverse
stripes shadows, obviously improved than previous findings (a, b). (f)
HE staining demonstrates thickened alveolar septa and exudates from
the alveolar cavity. (g) HE staining demonstrates massive bleeding in
the alveolar cavity, large quantity erythrocytes and intact cell walls. (h)
HE staining demonstrates phagocytized basophilic granules in the leukocytes. (i) HP staining demonstrates *purplish red* Rhodococcus equi
in a shape of crescent in orange red sputum

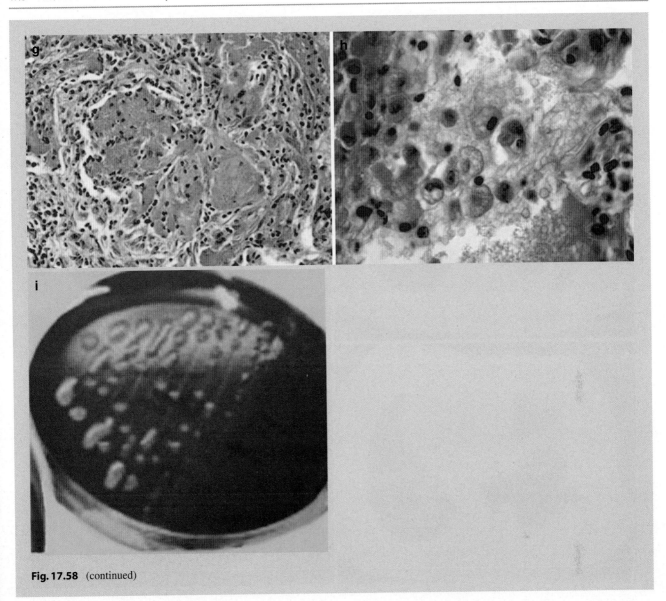

Fig. 17.58   (continued)

Case Study 7

A male patient aged 48 years was confirmatively diagnosed as having AIDS by the CDC. He complained of fever, cough, expectoration, chest distress and weak limbs for 3 months. His CD4 T cell count was 53/μl.

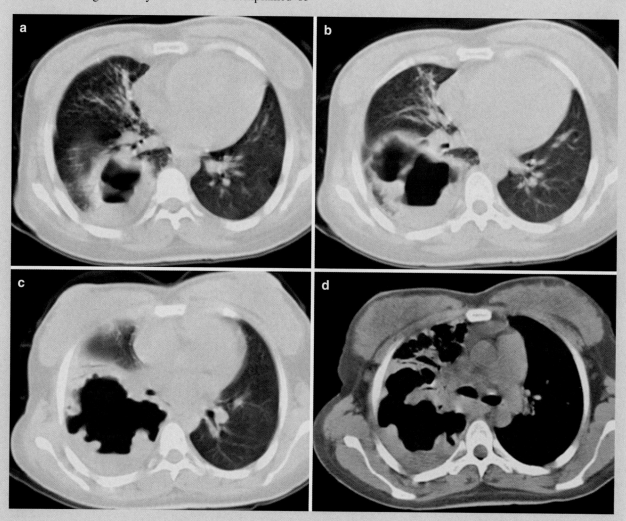

Fig. 17.59 (a–d) HIV/AIDS related Rhodococcus equi pneumonia. (a–c) CT scanning of the pulmonary window demonstrates thick walled cavities shadows in the dorsal segment of the right lower lung, with irregular wall thickness and liquid gas level in them. (d) CT scanning of the mediastinal window demonstrates thick walled cavities shadows in the dorsal segment of the left lower lung, with irregular wall thickness and liquid gas level in them

Case Study 8

A male patient aged 40 years was confirmatively diagnosed as having AIDS by the CDC. He complained of fever, cough, expectoration and chest distress for 1 month. His CD4 T cell count was 70/μl.

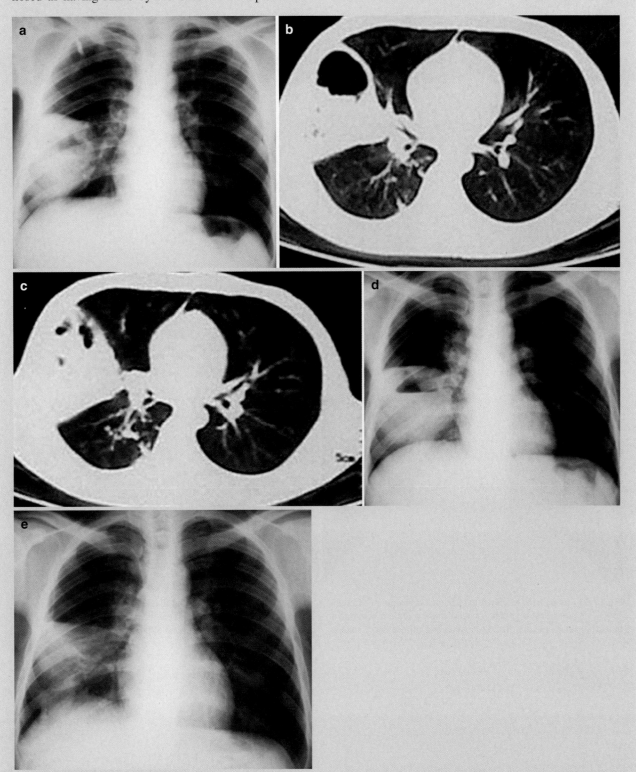

Fig. 17.60 (**a–e**) HIV/AIDS related Rhodococcus equi pneumonia. (**a**) DR demonstrates huge sphere liked mass shadow in the middle-outer zone of the right lower lung field, with cavities shdows in them. (**b–d**) CT scanning demonstrates triangular dense shadow in the middle-outer zone of the right lower lung field, with its apex pointing to the hilum and round liked cavities shadows in them. (**e**) Reexamination after the treatment demonstrates shrinkage of the huge sphere liked mass shadow in the middle-outer zone of the right lower lung field, with closure of the cavities

Case Study 9

A male patient aged 30 years was confirmatively diagnosed as having AIDS by the CDC. He complained of fever, cough, expectoration and chest distress for 1 week. His CD4 T cell count was 90/μl.

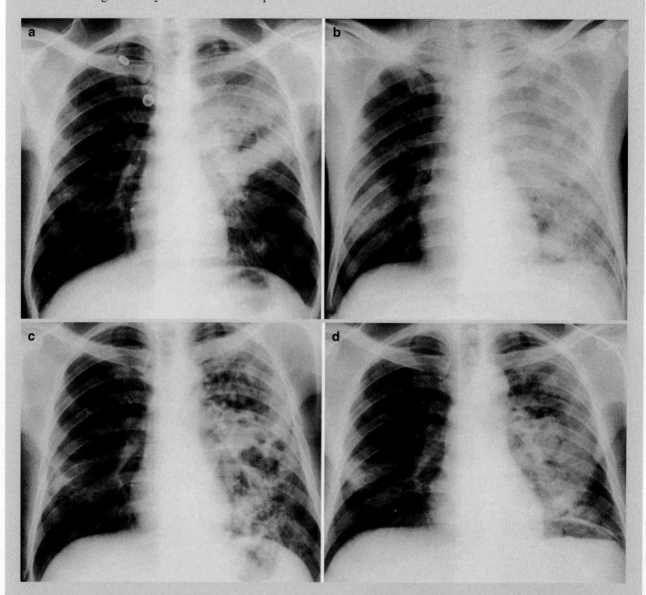

Fig.17.61 (**a–d**) HIV/AIDS related Rhodococcus equi pneumonia. (**a**) DR demonstrates large flaky shadow in the middle-outer zone of the left upper lung field. (**b**) DR demonstrates diffuse dense shadow in the left lung field, with round liked cavities shadows in them. (**c–d**) Reexamination after treatment demonstrates multiple cavities shadows in the middle-outer zone of the left upper lung field

Case Study 10

A male patient aged 35 years was confirmatively diagnosed as having AIDS by the CDC. He complained of paroxymal cough, expectoration of white diluted bubble sputum and fever with the highest body temperature of 40 °C. His CD4 T cell count was 93/μl.

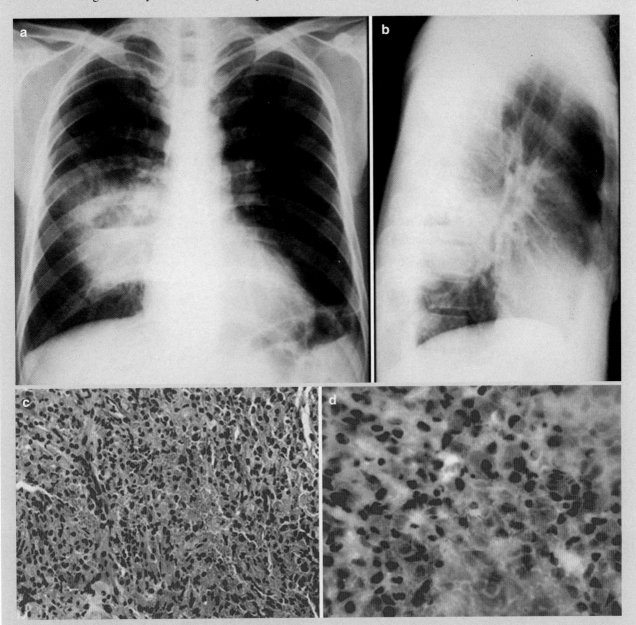

Fig. 17.62 (a–d) HIV/AIDS related Rhodococcus equi pneumonia. (**a**, **b**) Anteroposterior and lateral DR demonstrates huge sphere liked mass shadow in the right hilum, with cavities shadows and liq-uid gas level in it. (**c**) HE staining demonstrates bleeding in the lung tissues and aggregation of large quantity lymphocytes. (**d**) Masson staining demonstrates branches liked *purplish red* Rhodococcus equi

Case Study 11

A male patient aged 34 years was confirmatively diagnosed as having AIDS by the CDC. He complained of right chest pain and hemoptysis for 5 months for admission and was confirmed as HIV positive. His CD4 T cell count was 11/μl.

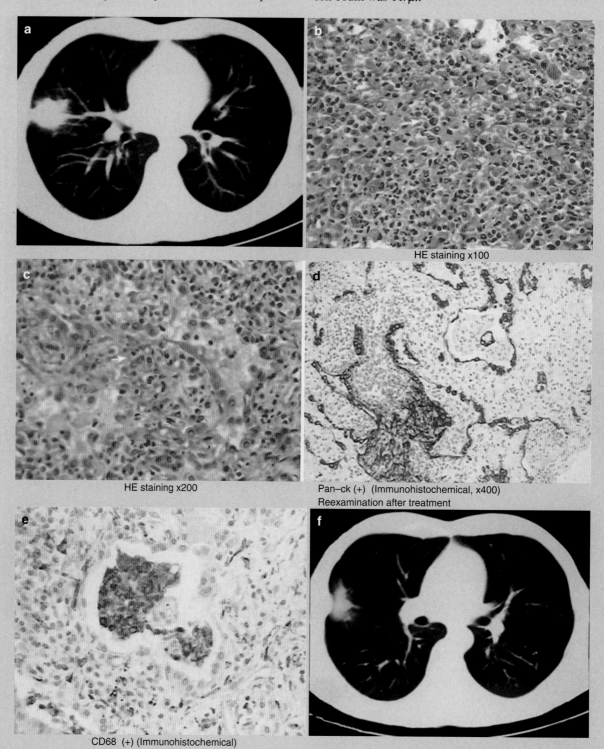

HE staining x100

HE staining x200

Pan–ck (+) (Immunohistochemical, x400)
Reexamination after treatment

CD68 (+) (Immunohistochemical)

Fig.17.63 (**a–f**) HIV/AIDS related Rhodococcus equi pneumonia. (**a**) Pulmonary CT scanning demonstrates a mass shadow in the lateral segment of the right middle lobe in size of 4.7×3.7×3.2 cm with uneven density and lace liked boundary, and small bubbles shadows in it. By both sputum culture and lung tissue culture, Rhodococcus equi can be detected. (**b, c**) Pathological biopsy and HE staining demonstrate inflammatory pseudotumor. (**d, e**) Immunohistochemistry demonstrates Rhodococcus equi antibody positive. (**f**) Reexamination after treatment demonstrates obvious shrinkage of the original lung lesions

17.3.4.6 Diagnostic Basis

Strain Identification

Catalase test of the strain is positive, which is confirmed as Rhodococcus equi by API CORYNE system.

Pulmonary Puncture for Biopsy and Pathological Examinations

H&E staining demonstrates mainly bleeding in the alveolar space, large quantity epithelial cells or mainly fibroblasts, parenchymal changes of lung tissue and thickened alveolar septa. PAS staining and Masson staining demonstrate scattered or clustered distribution of rod rhodococcus equi in pink or purplish red.

Imaging Demonstrations

AIDS complicated by pulmonary rhodococcus equi infection shows subacute inflammation. Firstly, there are exudates in the surrounding area of unilateral hilum as well as sphere shaped mass shadows which is centrally dense and peripherally blurry, with its apex pointing to the hilum. The lesions can be complicated by cavities and fluid level, with thick wall of the cavities. As the disease progresses, the abscess cavities have increased tension, with gradually thinner abscesss cavity walls and uneven wall thickness, even showing pleural effusion. These are its characteristic imaging findings.

Differential Diagnosis

It often needs to be differentiated from Pneumocystis carinii pneumonia, tuberculosis, staphylococcus aureus pneumonia, central type lung cancer and other diseases. Imaging findings of Pneumocystis carinii pneumonia usually are ground glass liked changes in the lung field, with parenchymal changes and centrilobular nodules. Tuberculosis often shows miliary tuberculosis, with lymphadenectasis, large tubercles and parenchymal changes. These characteristic pathological and imaging findings of staphylococcus aureus pneumonia are similar to those of bronchial pneumonia (lobular pneumonia). The lesions are nodules with blurry boundaries in a diameter of 4–10 mm. The disease progresses rapidly, while pulmonary rhodococcus equi infection has a chronic progression. HRCT scanning demonstrates staphylococcus aureus pneumonia as centrilobular nodules and branch linear shadows (tree buds sign), which can be found in 40 % patients, with 15–30 % will develop into commonly singular pulmonary abscess. Chest CT scanning demonstrates round liked abscess cavity with thick wall and liquid level in it. The inner wall of the abscess cavity is often irregular, with various changes within short period. The central type of lung cancer is commonly demonstrated as round liked shadow of unilateral hilum with rough boundary. Lobulation or bronchial stenosis sometimes occurs. However, AIDS complicated by Rhodococcus equi pneumonia is demonstrated as sphere liked mass in the hilum; mostly sphere liked increased density shadow with hilum as the center. The shadow is centrally dense and peripherally blurry, with no bronchial stenosis.

17.3.4.7 Discussion

Rhodococcus equi was firstly discovered in 1923 and was nominated as corynebacterium equi. After structure analysis of the cell wall, it was found that the bacterium is quite different from Corynebacterium, and therefore classified as Rhodococcus. Rhodococcus equi is generally believed to be the pathogen for horses, pigs and cattle. Human Rhodococcus equi infection is rare. But in recent years, due to an increase of patients with immunodeficiency syndrome, reports on human respiratory tract infection and sepsis caused by Rhodococcus equi are increasing. In sheep blood agar, Rhodococcus equi may have synergistic hemolysis with staphylococcus aureus, Listeria monocytogenes and corynebacterium pseudotuberculosis, which is characteristically rhodococcus equi. Studies by E Marchiori et al. [30] in 2005 revealed that all the 5 cases of AIDS complicated by Rhodococcus equi pulmonary infection have cough and fever lasting for 1–2 months, with accompanying shortness of breath and chest pain. All the 13 cases, studied by Li et al. in 2009 [106], have fever with a body temperature of 38–40 °C and cough. There are symptoms or signs of orange red sputum in 10 cases, hemoptysis in 4 cases, dyspnea in 11 cases, lung moist rales in 13 cases, emaciation in 6 cases, poor appetite in 6 cases, diarrhea in 2 cases, joint pain in 1 case, oral candidal infections in 13 cases, oral herpes in 4 cases, chest pain in 4 cases, no obvious symptoms in 1 case and hepatitis B in 3 cases. In the studies of the horse infected with Rhodococcus equi, Professor CHEN [108] found that it is characterized by chest X-ray demonstrations of abscesses in different sizes in the lungs and significant alveolar fusion in the lesion site. Its basic pathological changes are chronic suppurative bronchopneumonia and extensive pulmonary abscesses. The imaging demonstrations are commonly subacute pneumonia, often with cavities. Among the 13 cases of AIDS patients, studied by Li et al. in 2009 [106], 9 cases have central type sphere liked shadows with increased density distributed in the unilateral hilar region, accounting for 70 %. The largest shadow is in size of 5×6 cm, which is centrally dense and peripherally blurry, in a halo sign. The imaging findings are similar to those of lung tumor; with exudative infiltration and large flaky or sphere shaped mass shadow in the right hilar region in 4 cases, infiltration and large patchy or sphere shaped mass shadow in the outer zone of the right lung in 1 case, exudative infiltration and large flaky or sphere shaped mass shadow in left hilar region in 4 cases, diffuse atelectasis in the left lung in 1 cases, partial atelectasis in 5 cases, singular pulmonary abscess cavity in 9 cases, multiple honeycomb liked cavity in 1 case, cavity shadow in the right lung in 6 cases, complicated by fluid level in 4 cases, cavity in the left lung in 3 cases, complicated by fluid level in 1 case, flakey shadows in bilateral hilar regions in 1 case, left pleural effusion in 3 cases and mediastinal lymphadenectasis in 2 cases. Exudative inflammation often occurs around the abscess cavity, possibly with small quantity pleural effusion and/or thickened and adhesive pleura. In the study of 5 cases AIDS complicated by pulmonary Rhodococcus equi infection, conducted by E Marchiori et al. [30] in 2005, CT scanning demonstrates 3 cases with fusion of centrilobular nodules and tree buds sign around the parenchymal changes, among which one case has the lesions in the both lower lobes. Donisi investigated 12 patients with HIV positive complicated by Rhodococcus equi infection and found its mortality rate is 58 % [37]. Harvey reported 11 cases of HIV positive complicated by Rhodococcus equi infection, with 6 cases of death, accounting for 54.5 % [38]. The study of 13 cases of AIDS complicated by Rhodococcus equi infection, conducted by Li et al. [106] found its mortality rate of 7 %. The very different mortality of the two groups may be closely related to the regional economic and medical conditions as well as the administration of antibacterial and HAART therapies. In the study of the AIDS complicated by Rhodococcus equi pulmonary infection, conducted by E Marchiori et al. in 2005 [30], the CD4 T cell count is below 50/µl. In the study of AIDS complicated by Rhodococcus equi pulmonary infection conducted by Donisi et al. in 1996 [37], CD4 T cell count is 47.7/µl. The 13 cases of AIDS complicated by Rhodococcus equi infection studied by Li et al. in 2009 [106] showed a CT4 T cell count of lower than 49/µl. All the results are in consistency. In conclusion, AIDS complicated by pulmonary Rhodococcus equi infection is mainly subacute inflammation. There are exudation around the unilateral hilum as well as centrally dense and peripherally blurry sphere shaped mass shadows, with secondary cavities and parenchyma changes and even pleural effusion. All of these are characteristic imaging demonstrations.

17.4   HIV/AIDS Related Pulmonary Fungal Infections

17.4.1   HIV/AIDS Related Pulmonary Aspergillus Infection

17.4.1.1 Pathogens and Pathogenesis

Most cases of HIV positive complicated by respiratory or pulmonary diseases are caused by Aspergillus fumigatus. Aspergillus fumigatus belongs to filamentous fungi, which is a common opportunistic fungus and has a wide distribution in the nature. As conditional pathogenic bacteria, it can parasitize in the human skin and upper respiratory tract. Human has certain resistance to Aspergillus so it commonly fails to cause diseases. In immunocompromised AIDS patients, the pathogenic bacteria can pass through the defects in the skin and mucous membrane into the blood flow to infect the tissues and organs.

17.4.1.2 Pathophysiological Basis

Aspergillus commonly violates bronchus and lung, with involvements of rhinal sinuses, external auditory canal, eye and skin. Otherwise, it disseminates to organs of the body along with blood flow. The early lesions are diffuse infiltrative and exudative changes. And advanced lesions are necrosis, pyogenesis or granuloma. Large quantity hyphae can be found in the lesions. The hyphae penetrate the blood vessels to cause vasculitis, perivascular inflammation and thrombosis. And thrombosis can cause ischemia and necrosis of the tissue. According to the pathological changes and imaging findings, it can be divided into three major types: vascular invasion type, bronchopneumonia type and allergic bronchopulmonary aspergillosis type. (1) The vascular invasion type is the result caused by toxins released in the process of aspergillus spreading extensively from the primary focus to the lungs. Vascular infiltration of the pulmonary parenchyma and coagulative necrosis are believed to be the cause of vascular occlusion and pulmonary infarction. (2) Bronchopneumonia type is acute bronchitis caused by inhalation of Aspergillus spores. In the cases of hyphae invasion into the lung tissues, extensive infiltrative pneumonia or focal granuloma are resulted in. It can also cause necrosis, pyogenesis and multiple small abscesses. Spherical pulmonary aspergillosis is often secondary to bronchiectasis, tuberculosis, carcinous cavity and other lung diseases. Mycelia multiply and gather in the cavities of the lungs to form a spherical mass with fibrin and mucosal cells, which are called aspergillar glomera, which do not invade the lung tissue. (3) Allergic bronchopulmonary aspergillosis type is the proliferation and germination of inhaled Aspergillus spore in the airway, often showing obvious related mucosal lesions and eventually resulting in bronchiectasis (Fig. 17.64a–c).

17.4.1.3 Clinical Symptoms and Signs
HIV/AIDS Related Aspergillus Bronchopneumonia

The cases with acute onset have symptoms of high fever or irregular fever, cough, shortness of breath and green purulent sputum. The cases with a chronic onset have symptoms of repeated cough and hemoptysis, which are similar to those of tuberculosis. The pulmonary signs are not obvious, with occasional findings of moist rales.

HIV/AIDS Related Spherical Pulmonary Aspergillosis

Most cases are asymptomatic and sometimes there are fever, cough, shortness of breath, and mucous purulent sputum.

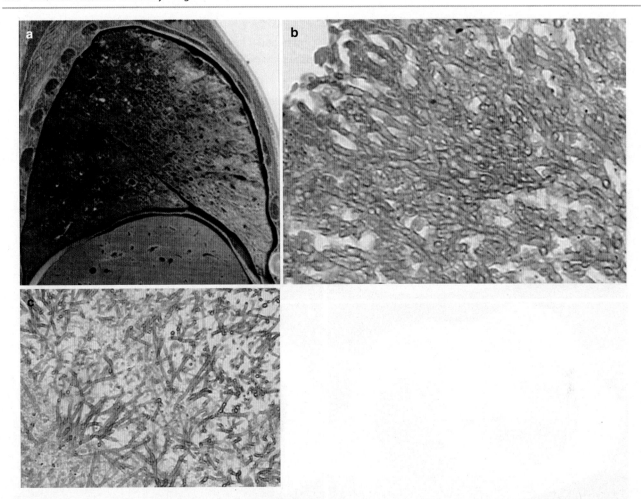

Fig. 17.64 (**a**) Gross observation demonstrates *dark brown* lungs in appearance. (**b, c**) Thology demonstrates hemorrhage and edema of the lung tissue and focal necrosis, with large quantity Aspergillus hyphae and spores in the surrounding area of the necrosis (Combined with pulmonary CMV infection)

Invasive Pulmonary Aspergillosis
The main symptoms are persistent fever, cough and chest pain. In the serious cases, there is dyspnea.

17.4.1.4 Examinations and Their Selection
Microscopic Examination of Sputum
By microscopic examination of sputum, Aspergillus hyphae can be found. The culture for aspergillus fumigatus is positive.

Immunologic Assays
Serum IgE is commonly above 2,500 µg/L. Skin test for aspergillus antigen is positive. Serum anti-Aspergillus antigen IgG antibody precipitin is positive.

Fiberobronchoscopy Lavage and Biopsy
Puncture of lungs and pleura for biopsy facilitates the diagnosis of pulmonary fungal infections.

Chest X-rays and CT Scanning
Both are the most commonly used imaging examinations.

17.4.1.5 Imaging Demonstrations
HIV/AIDS related aspergillus bronchopneumonia is commonly demonstrated to have increased pulmonary markings, diffuse patchy blurry shadows and mass shadows in both lungs. Spherical pulmonary aspergillosis is commonly demonstrated to have sphere liked aspergillar glomera suspending in the cavities to form a crescent shaped transparent area, in characteristic meniscus sign, rolling ball sign and fingertip sign. Meniscus sign is nominated due to a meniscus liked space between the aspergillar glomera growing in the cavity and the cavity wall. Rolling ball sign means that the aspergillar glomera moves along with the changes of posture. Fingertip sign indicates that the substance formed by aspergillar glomera in dilated bronchi is in a finger shape, sometimes in V shape sign and Y shape sign. Invasive lesions refer to lesions invading or destroying lung structures, such as pneumonia, parenchymal changes and necrosis.

Case Study 1

A female patient aged 28 years was confirmatively diagnosed as having AIDS by the CDC. She complained of cough and chest distress, with increased eosinophilic granulocytes. Her CD4 T cell count was 45/µl.

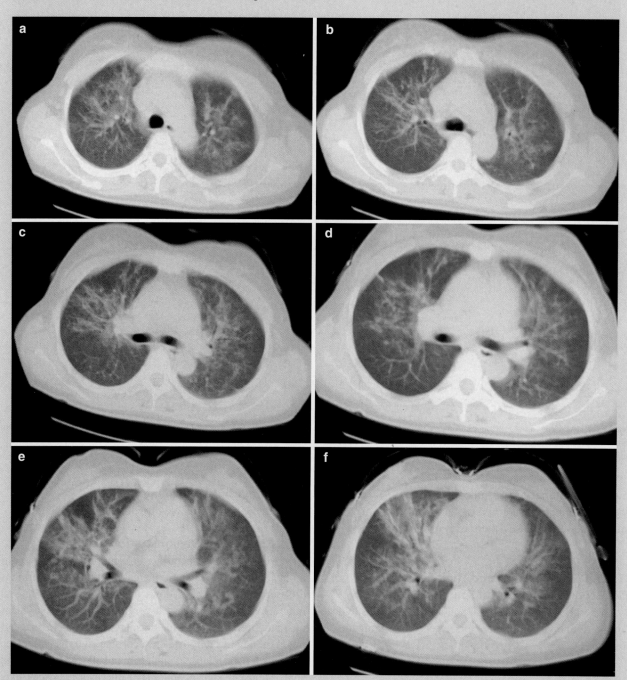

Fig. 17.65 (a–g) HIV/AIDS related allergic pulmonary Aspergillus infection. (a–f) CT scanning of the pulmonary window demonstrates thickened central pulmonary markings in both lungs, which is turtuous and deranged with fingertip infiltration shadows. (g) DR demonstrates hyperinflation of the right lung, increased and thickened pulmonary markings and ground glass liked shadows with increased density in the right lower lung and left lung lobe

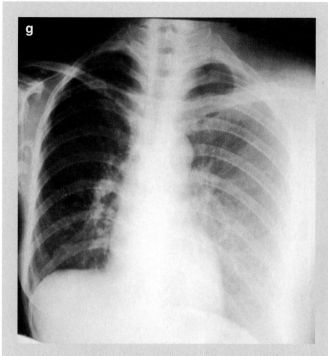

Fig. 17.65 (continued)

Case Study 2

A female patient aged 30 years was confirmatively diagnosed as having AIDS by the CDC. She complained of high fever or irregular fever, cough and shortness of breath. Her CD4 T cell count was 56/μl.

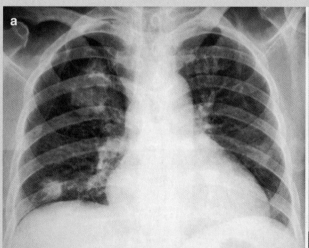

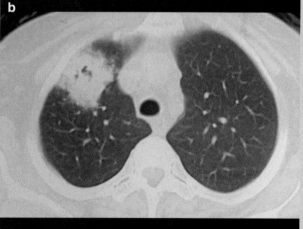

Fig. 17.66 (a–g) HIV/AIDS related pulmonary aspergillosis infection. (**a**) DR demonstrates large flaky shadows with increased density in the right upper lung, with blurry boundaries; round liked or sphere shaped mass shadows in the right lower lung, with uneven density. (**b–e**) CT scanning of the pulmonary window demonstrates multiple round liked thick-wall cavities in the dorsal segment of the right lower lung, with small nodular shadow adhering on the cavity wall; and surrounding small nodular shadows and infiltration shadows. (**f, g**) Coronal CT scanning reconstruction demonstrates a huge thick-wall cavity in the right upper lung, with irregular thickness of the wall; round liked cavity shadows in the right lower lung, with thick and multilocular walls; and flaky shadows with increased density in the outer zone of the left lower lung

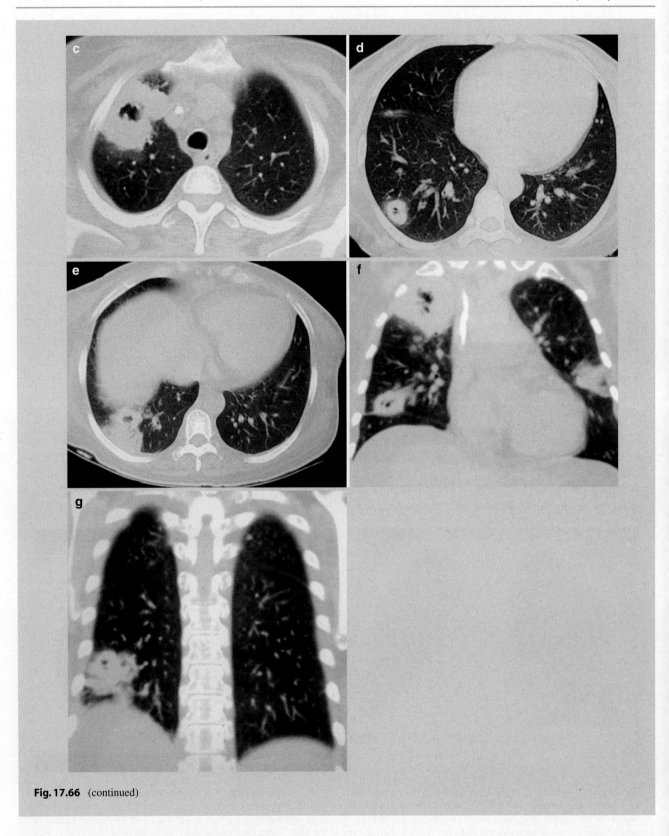

Fig. 17.66 (continued)

Case Study 3

A male patient aged 36 years was confirmatively diagnosed as having AIDS by the CDC. He complained of high fever or irregular fever, cough and shortness of breath. His CD4 T cell count was 96/μl.

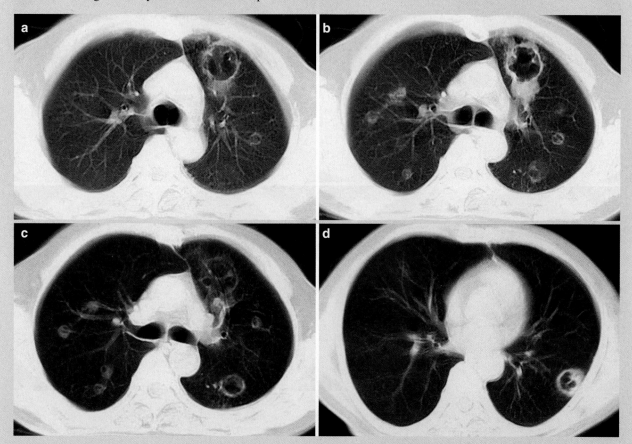

Fig. 17.67 (**a–h**) HIV/AIDS related pulmonary aspergillosis infection. (**a–d**) CT scanning of the pulmonary window demonstrates multiple scattered round liked nodular shadows and thick-wall cavity shadows in both lungs, with small nodular shadows in the cavity shadows. (**e–h**) Reexamination of the pulmonary window after 3 months treatment demonstrates multiple scattered round liked nodular shadows and thick wall cavity shadows in both lungs, with small nodular shadows in the cavity shadows which obviously increase and enlarge compared to previous lesions, with accompanying infiltration shadows around the lesions

Images demonstrations after 3 months treatment:

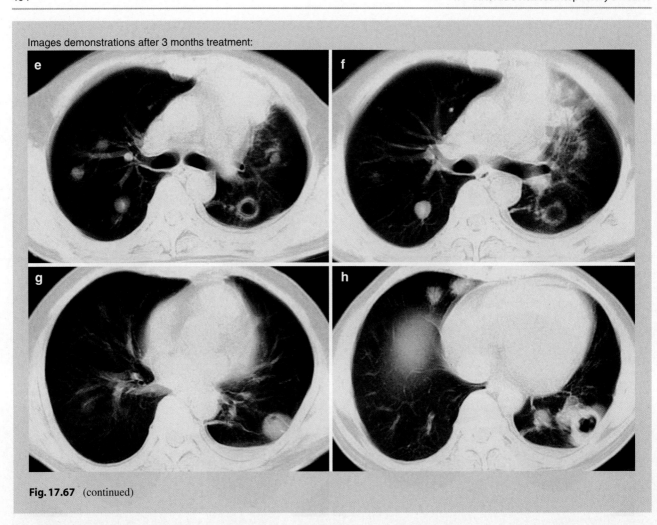

Fig. 17.67   (continued)

Case Study 4

A male patient aged 38 years was confirmatively diagnosed as having AIDS by the CDC. He complained of high fever or irregular fever, cough and shortness of breath. His CD4 T cell count was 76/µl.

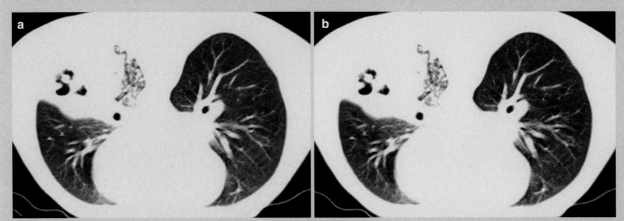

Fig. 17.68 (**a–d**) HIV/AIDS related pulmonary aspergillosis infection. (**a, b**) CT scanning of the pulmonary window in prone posture demonstrates mass shadow and thick wall cavity in the dorsal segment of the right lower lung, small nodular shadows in the cavities, surrounding fused miliary infiltration shadows. (**c, d**) CT scanning of the mediastinal window in the prone posture demonstrates mass shadow and thick wall cavity shadows in the dorsal segment of the right lower lung, small nodular shadows in the cavities, and involved pleura of partial lateral chest wall

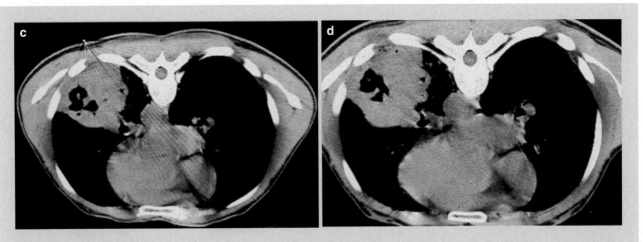

Fig. 17.68 (continued)

Case Study 5

A female patient aged 35 years was confirmatively diagnosed as having AIDS by the CDC. She complained of irregular fever, cough and chest distress. Her CD4 T cell count was 16/μl.

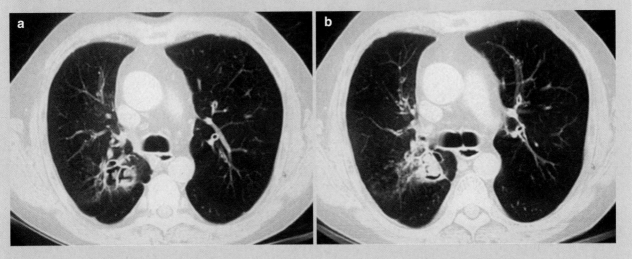

Fig. 17.69 (**a**, **b**) HIV/AIDS related pulmonary aspergillosis infection. (**a**, **b**) CT scanning of the pulmonary window in the prone posture demonstrates mass shadow and thick wall cavity shadows in the medial basal segment of the right lower lung, irregular nodular shadows in the cavities, and surrounding fused miliary infiltration shadows

Case Study 6

A female patient aged 40 years was confirmatively diagnosed as having AIDS by the CDC. She complained of irregular fever, cough and shortness of breath. Her CD4 T cell count was 36/μl.

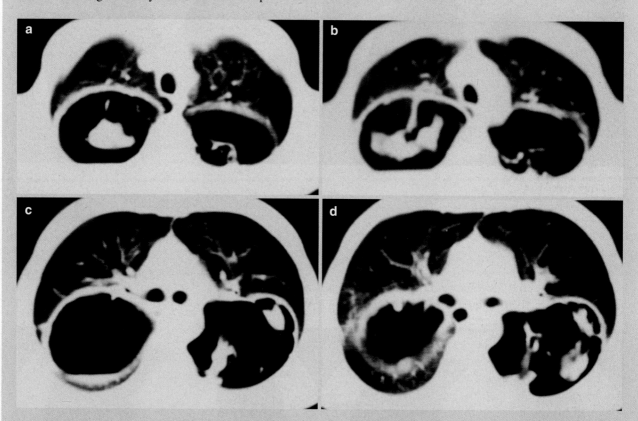

Fig. 17.70 (**a–d**) HIV/AIDS related pulmonary aspergillosis infection. (**a**, **b**) CT scanning of the pulmonary window demonstrates a huge cavity shadow in the dorsal segment of the right lower lung, large nodular shadows in it, liquid gas level in the basal cavity, and the evenly thick wall. (**c**, **d**) CT scanning of the mediastinal window in the prone posture demonstrates a huge cavity shadow in the dorsal segment of the left lung, multiple large nodular shadows in it, and involved pleura of the lateral chest wall

Case Study 7

A male patient aged 38 years was confirmatively diagnosed as having AIDS by the CDC. He complained of high fever, cough and chest distress. His CD4 T cell count was 76/μl.

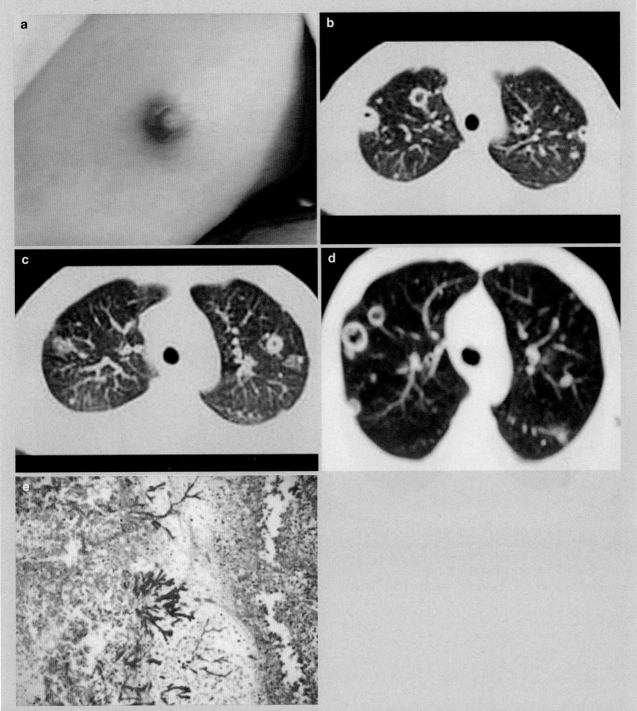

Fig. 17.71 (a–e) HIV/AIDS related pulmonary aspergillosis infection. (a) The gross specimen demonstratesAspergillus abscess in the skin of the forearm. (b–d) CT scanning of the pulmonary window demonstrates multiple round liked nodular shadows and cavity shadows in both lungs, even thickness of cavity wall, and small nodular shadows in some cavities. (e) Pulmonary Aspergillus infection, demonstration purplish blue branches liked or grasses liked growth of hyphae, HE×400

Case Study 8

A male patient aged 26 years was confirmatively diagnosed as having AIDS by the CDC. He had history of drug abuse and complained of nausea, vomiting gastric contents after meals, abdominal distension, abdominal pain and shortness of breath. By physical examinations, cardiopulmonary auscultation positive, edema of lower limbs. By laboratory tests on admission, WBC 15.8×10^9/L, NEuT 0.534 %, RBC 3.08×10^{12}/L, HGB 77 g/L, LYM 0.334 %, GLu 1.1 mmol/L, APTT 64.4 s; liver functions: TBIL 24.6 μmol/L, ALT 88.0 u/L, AST 528 u/L; electrolyte K 5.8 mmol/L; renal functions: HCO_3^- 10.1 mmol/L, blood tuberculosis antibody positive, Ascites protein positive, karyocyte 900×10^6/L. Oxygen inhalation was prescribed, with anti-PCP, anti-infection, anti-virus, intravenous dripping, therapies for electrolytes and acid-base balance, diuresis therapies are administered after hospitalized. After 6 o'clock pm, he showed exacerbated shortness of breath, which was diagnosed as episode of PCP. The emergency rescuing was ineffective and death occurred. By B ultrasound, there were hepatosplenomegaly, diffuse lesions in both kidneys, and large quantity ascites.

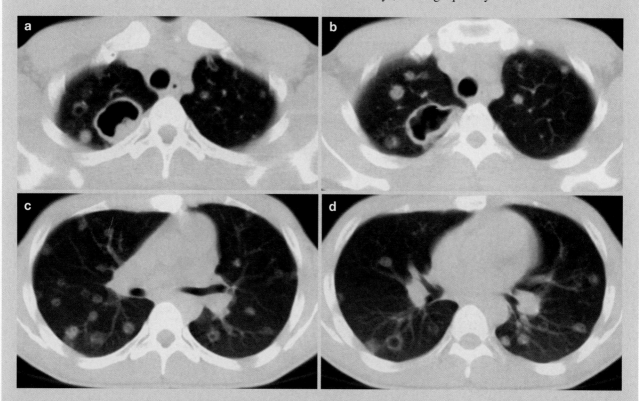

Fig. 17.72 (**a–d**) HIV/AIDS related pulmonary aspergillosis infection. (**a–d**) CT scanning of the pulmonary window demonstrates multiple scattered round liked nodular shadows and cavity shadows in both lungs, with even wall thickness and small nodular shadows in some cavities

Case Study 9

A male patient aged 48 years was confirmatively diagnosed as having AIDS by the CDC. He complained of high fever, cough and shortness of breath. His CD4 T cell count was 19/ μl.

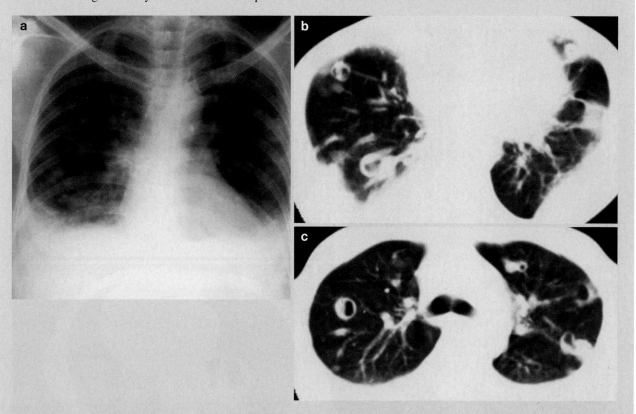

Fig. 17.73 (**a–c**) HIV/AIDS related pulmonary aspergillosis infection. (**a**) DR demonstrates diffuse dense shadows in both lower lung fields which is in a arcuate surface with exterior high and interior low (pleural effusion). (**b, c**) CT scanning of the mediastinal window demonstrates multiple scattered round liked nodular shadows and thick-wall cavity shadows in both lungs, with small nodular shadows in the cavities; thickened pleura of the lateral chest wall, with accompanying encapsulated effusion

Case Study 10

A male patient aged 39 years was confirmatively diagnosed as having AIDS by the CDC. He complained of high fever, cough and chest distress for 1 month. His CD4 T cell count was 29/μl.

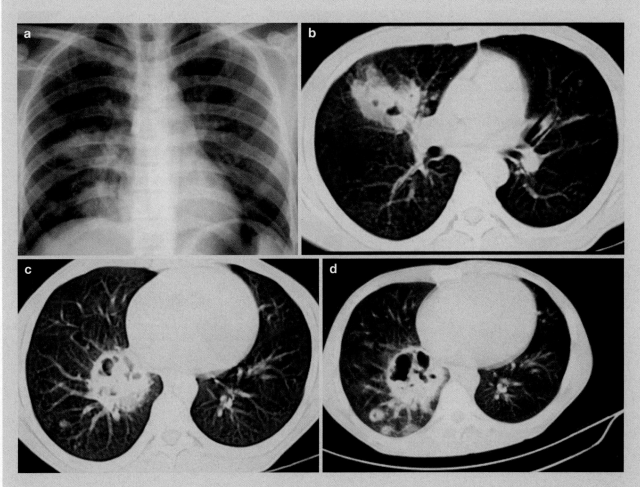

Fig. 17.74 (**a–d**) HIV/AIDS related pulmonary aspergillosis infection. (**a**) DR demonstrates round liked uneven density shadows in the medial segments of both middle and lower lungs, multilocular hollow holes in the cavities, surrounding multiple round liked thick-wall small cavity shadows and ground grass liked infiltration shadows. (**b–d**) CT scanning of the pulmonary window demonstrates scattered round liked uneven density shadows in the right hilum and lower lung, multilocular hollow holes in the cavities; and surrounding multiple round liked thick-wall small cavity shadows and ground grass liked infiltration shadows

Case Study 11

A male patient aged 34 years was confirmatively diagnosed as having AIDS by the CDC. He complained of high fever, cough and chest distress for 3 months. His CD4 T cell count was 49/μl.

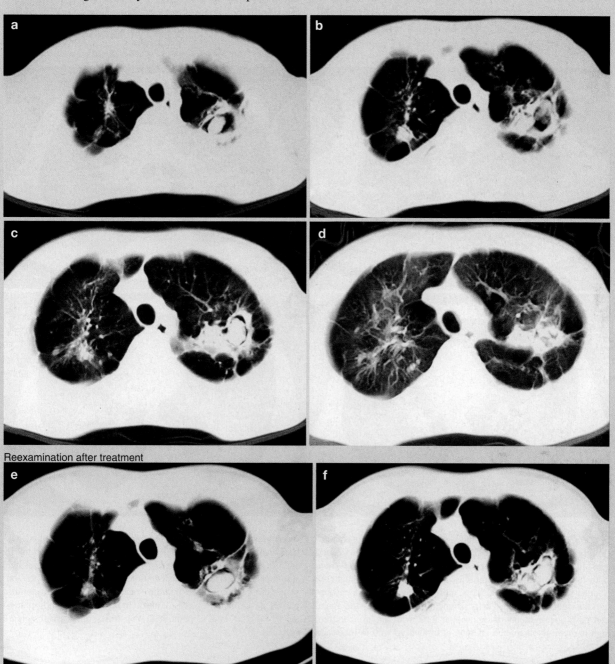

Reexamination after treatment

Fig. 17.75 (**a–f**) HIV/AIDS related pulmonary aspergillosis infection. (**a–d**) CT scanning of the pulmonary window demonstrates multiple scattered round liked nodular shadows and irregular thickwall cavity shadows in both lungs, oval or sphere shaped nodular shadows in the cavities with smooth boundaries. (**e, f**) Reexamination after treatment demonstrates multiple scattered round liked nodular shadows and irregular thick-wall cavity shadows in both lungs, oval nodular shadows in the cavity with smooth boundaries. Compared to the previous imaging findings, the lesions are shrunk, with improved surrounding infiltration

Case Study 12

A male patient aged 35 years was confirmatively diagnosed as having AIDS by the CDC. He was hospitalized due to complaints of fever for 1 week, chest distress and shortness of breath for 1 day. On admission, he was confirmed as HIV positive, with a CD4 T cell count of 9/μl.

By physical examinations, he was in poor physical conditions, respiratory rate 27/min, lips cyanotic, coarse breathing sounds of both lungs with small quantity dry rales. His conditions progressed rapidly and death occurred due to respiratory failure after 3 days.

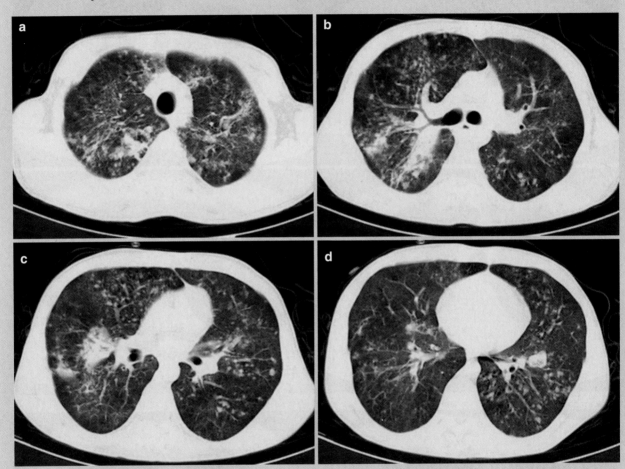

Fig. 17.76 (a–g) HIV/AIDS related pulmonary aspergillosis infection. (a–d) CT scanning demonstrates diffuse scattered thin ground glass liked, patchy, flaky blurry shadows and cords liked shadows in both lungs, with blurry boundaries and uneven density; scattered nodular shadows in different sizes; more lesions in both upper lobes and the right middle lobe; flaky parenchyma shadows in the apical and posterior segments of right upper lobe, with air bronchogram sign in them; unobstructed opening of bronchi as well as lobar and segmental bronchi without stenosis and obstruction; lymphadenectasis in the right hilar region; detected Aspergillus fumigatus by sputum culture. (e, f) Culture for 72 h, lactic acid gossypol blue staining and microscopic observation at ×200 and ×400 demonstrate short column liked conidial head, smooth wall of conidiophores, flask-shaped top capsule and monolayer microconidiophores. (g) Culture in Paul's medium demonstrates dark green colored colonies

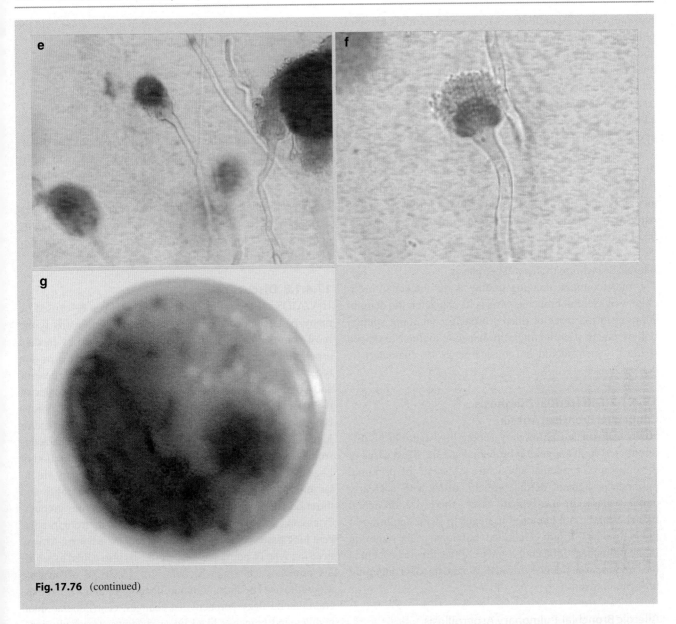

Fig. 17.76 (continued)

17.4.1.6 Diagnostic Basis
Fiberobronchoscopy Lavage and Biopsy
Lung and pleura puncture for biopsy can detect the growth of Aspergillus hyphae.

Sputum Culture
Sputum culture can detect Aspergillus hyphae, with findings of Aspergillus fumigatus positive.

Immunologic Assays
In the cases with allergic bronchopulmonary aspergillosis, the serum IgE is above 2,500 μg/L. Skin test of aspergillus antigen is positive. The serum anti-Aspergillus antigen IgG antibody precipitin is positive.

Diagnostic Imaging
Characteristic CT scanning demonstrations of HIV/AIDS related parasitic aspergillar glomera include pulmonary cavities or cavity lesions with spherical contents, smooth boundaries of the spherical contents with even density, lunate shaped or ring shaped transparent shadows between cavity or cavity walls and the contents, migration of the contents with the body postures. According to the pathological and imaging demonstrations, it can be divided into three major types:

Vascular Invasion Type of Pulmonary Aspergillosis
In the early stage, CT scanning demonstrates soft tissue density nodules or light ground glass liked halo sign around the mass, which is the evidence for the diagnosis of the invasion

type pulmonary aspergillosis. Air cresent sign refers to round pulmonary infiltration with accompanying central necrosis and surrounding lunate or ring shaped cavity. Other non-characteristic CT scanning demonstrations include multiple lobular parenchyma lesion shadows or lobular fusion shadows, parenchyma lesion shadows in the lobes, segments and subsegments, nodular or mass shadows and thin/thick wall cavities or low density areas in the mass shadows.

Airway Invasion Type of Pulmonary Aspergillosis
It is demonstrated to have parenchymal lesions around the airway or/and central small nodules in the lower lobes. The parenchymal lesions prove the occurrence of mycotic bronchopneumonia.

Allergic Bronchopulmonary Aspergillosis
The most common imaging finding is the thickened bronchial wall. Central bronchiectasis is its characteristic demonstration. In the cases of dilated bronchi containing sputum bolt or mucus, it shows fingertip shaped or toothpaste shaped shadow, which should be considered as its characteristic demonstration.

17.4.1.7 Differential Diagnosis
Congenital Bronchial Atresia
HIV/AIDS related pulmonary aspergillosis should be differentiated from congenital bronchial atresia. Most cases of the congenital bronchial atresia are atresia at the proximal pulmonary segment of the bronchi, often with a clearly defined mass. In the typical cases, there are bronchial branches and more branches in fingertip shape, pointing to the pulmonary hilum. Confined pulmonary air retention in the pulmonary lobe and segment of the atresic bronchi is the important evidence for the diagnosis of congenital bronchial atresia.

Allergic Bronchial-Pulmonary Aspergillosis
HIV/AIDS related pulmonary aspergillosis should be differentiated from allergic bronchial-pulmonary aspergillosis. In the cases of allergic bronchial-pulmonary aspergillosis have no clearly defined mass, with demonstrations of V shaped, Y shaped, grapes shaped or fingertip shaped shadows with clearly defined boundaries, which are characteristic in those patients with bronchial asthma or a case history of exposure to dusts containing fungi. There is also increased proportion of eosinophilic granulocytes in the peripheral blood. Detection of aspergillus in phlegm can define the diagnosis.

Central Lung Cancer
HIV/AIDS related pulmonary aspergillosis should be differentiated from central lung cancer. Central lung cancer also can cause mucus impaction of the distal bronchi, with manifestations of bronchial arctia and/or truncation, and the surrounding soft tissue mass shadows.

Pulmonary Cavities and Abscesses Induced by Tuberculoma Dissolved, Secondary Pulmonary TB, Chronic Lung Abscess and Peripheral Lung Cancer as Well as Cystic Bronchiectasis
HIV/AIDS related pulmonary aspergillosis should be differentiated from pulmonary cavities and abscesses induced by dissolved tuberculoma, secondary pulmonary TB, chronic lung abscess and peripheral lung cancer as well as cystic bronchiectasis. Except aspergilloma, spheric morphology caused by other causes is commonly irregular. The cavity contents cannot migrate with body postures, which is the key point for the differential diagnosis.

17.4.1.8 Discussion
HIV/AIDS related pulmonary aspergillosis can be caused by many pathogenic bacteria and aspergillus fumigatus is the most common one. The infection is often caused by inhaled aspergillus fumigatus in the environment. Vascular invasion type of pulmonary aspergillosis usually has multiple lesions and nodular changes. Generally in pathology, the center of nodule presents typical pale color; commonly with fibrous ring surrounding the nodules resulted from hemorrhage and/or lung parenchymal changes. Histologically, they are characterized by coagulative necrosis of the lung tissues, infiltration of large quantity hyphae in the necrotic tissue, pulmonary vascular infiltration, but usually without responses of vasculitis and thrombosis. The enzymes released by neutrophile granulocytes can cause the separation of necrotic tissue from its adjacent lung tissues to form necrotic mass in the cavities. Airway invasion type of pulmonary aspergillosis, also called aspergillus bronchopneumonia, accounts for 15–30 % of invasive aspergillosis. The most common imaging findings are unilateral/bilateral flaky parenchymal changes, centrilobular small nodules and branches liked linear shadows (tree buds sign). Histologically, it is characterized by necrosis and infiltration of neutrophil granulocytes. The lesions surround the bronchiole and the bronchiole. The invasion of the pulmonary artery can cause bleeding of the adjacent pulmonary parenchyma. Allergic bronchopulmonary aspergillosis rarely has lesions, with no unknown pathogenesis, which is generally believed to be related to type I and type II allergic reactions. It usually shows obvious asthma related mucosal lesions. Hyphae generated by aspergillus fumigatus can induce the production of mucus and additional mucosal lesions, eventually leading to bronchiectasis. Dilatate bronchial lumen is filled with mucus or with absence of epithelium, which is replaced by a granulomatous inflammatory infiltration. The most common imaging manifestations are migratory flocculent, branched Y shaped and V shaped (fingertip sign) shadows in the pulmonary parenchyma, which are related to the infiltration of eosinophils.

Pathologically, bronchial cystic dilatation in the pulmonary segment and sub-segment occurs, with large quantity eosinophils in the bronchial mucus and scattered broken aspergillus hyphae. In combination with the case history, the diagnosis can be defined.

17.4.2 HIV/AIDS Related Pulmonary Cryptococcus Infection

17.4.2.1 Pathogens and Pathogenesis

Compromised immunity is an important cause of cryptococcosis, especially in patients with AIDS or abnormal lymphoproliferative diseases. Cryptococcus neoformans, a single phase mould, exists widely in the natural world. The cryptococcus has a diameter of less than 10 μm, which can be inhaled into the human body via respiratory tract. Under the impact of a high concentration carbon dioxide, it forms a clearly defined protective layer composed of polysaccharide capsule to antagonize the defense mechanisms of the host. Thus, lung infection occurs after its inhalation in immunocompetent people, which is commonly asymptomatic. of cryptococcus, Inhalation of cryptococcus by AIDS patients can lead to hilar lymphadenopathy, as well as singular or multiple subpleural small nodules, being similar to those in the cases of Mycobacterium tuberculosis infection.

17.4.2.2 Pathophysiological Basis

In the early stage of cryptococcal infection, only a mild inflammatory reaction or diffuse infiltrative exudative changes occur. But in the advanced stage, necrosis, suppuration or granuloma is formed. Large quantity hyphae can be found in the focus. In the cases with hyphae penetrating the blood vessels, vasculitis, perivascular inflammation and thrombosis occur. And thrombosis leads to ischemia and necrosis of the tissue (Fig. 17.77).

17.4.2.3 Clinical Symptoms and Signs

Pulmonary cryptococcus infection in AIDS patients often is extensively disseminating, with symptoms of fever, cough, difficulty breathing, expectoration, chest pain caused by pleuritis, and even acute respiratory distress syndrome (ARDS).

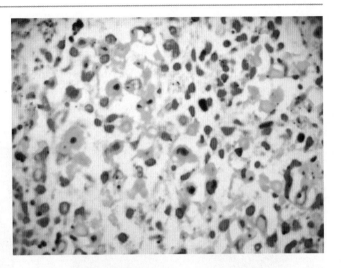

Fig. 17.77 HE staining demonstrates isseminated cryptococci, the Cryptococcus is stained red after mucin carmine staining of cryptococcus neoformans spores in lungs, (HE × 200)

17.4.2.4 Examinations and Their Selection

1. Chest X-ray and CT scanning are the most commonly used diagnostic imaging examinations.
2. Laboratory tests include India ink smear or culture of phlegm, chest liquid and CSF; and complement binding reaction test.
3. Routine blood test can detect slightly and moderately increased WBC count and neutrophils.

17.4.2.5 Imaging Demonstrations

HIV/AIDS related pulmonary cryptococcus infection has no characteristic imaging demonstrations. Chest X-ray and CT scanning show multiple morphology of the lesions. In the slight cases, there are thickened pulmonary markings in both lower lungs or isolated nodular shadows, and occasionally cavities. In the cases of acute interstitial inflammation, there are diffuse infiltrative or miliary foci, with infiltration, nodules or exudation in any lobe which is more common in bilateral middle and lower lungs, in unilateral lung or confined to one lobe. The foci may be isolated huge spherical or multiple nodular, without obvious surrounding inflammatory responses, similar to those of tubercles or tumors. Otherwise, they are diffuse miliary shadows or flaky infiltrative shadows.

Case Study 1

A male patient aged 38 years was confirmatively diagnosed as having AIDS by the CDC. He had history of paid blood donation for more than 100 times from the year of 1990 to 1994 and was detected HIV positive on Jan. 18, 2004. His CD4 T cell count was 246/μl in the year of 2004, 212/μl in 2005, 120/μl in 2006, 166/μl in 2007, and 27/μl in 2008. He complained of intermittent diarrhea, fever and chest distress for more than 4 months, with alternate occurrence of intermittent diarrhea and fever by watery stool.

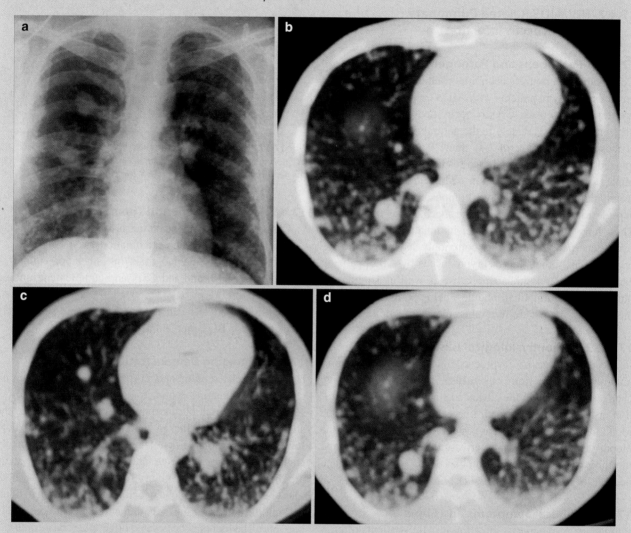

Fig. 17.78 (a–d) HIV/AIDS related pulmonary cryptococcus infection. (a) DR demonstrates multiple scattered nodular and miliary shadows in both lungs. (b–d) Chest CT scanning demonstrates multiple dense nodular shadows with different sizes in both lungs, with clear boundaries. They are intensively distributed in the dorsal segment and the largest one has a diameter of about 2 cm

Case Study 2

An AIDS patient was confirmatively diagnosed by the CDC. He sustained pulmonary Cryptococcus infection.

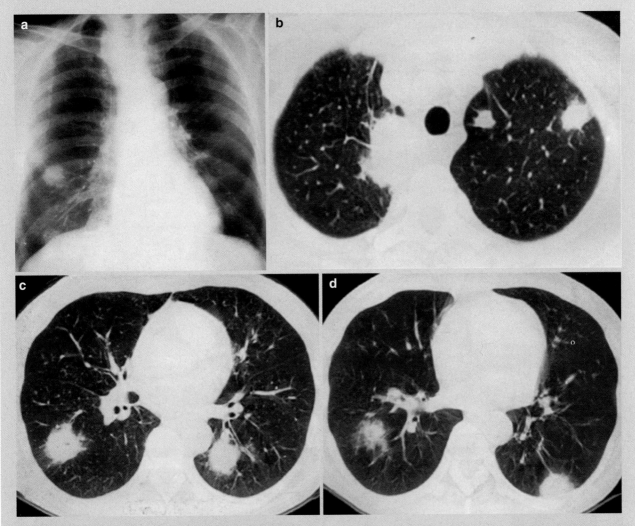

Fig. 17.79 (**a–d**) HIV/AIDS related pulmonary cryptococcus infection. (**a**) DR demonstrates multiple scattered nodular shadows in both lower lungs. (**b–d**) Chest CT scanning demonstrates multiple dense nodular shadows with different sizes and mass shadows in both middle and lower lung fields, with clear boundaries. They are more common in the dorsal segments

Case Study 3

A female patient aged 54 years was confirmatively diagnosed as having AIDS by the CDC. She complained of repeated fever, headache and vomiting for more than 10 days. More than 10 days ago, she was confirmatively diagnosed as having cryptococcus infection by lumbar puncture for the second time. On May 25, 2009, pressure at lumbar puncture 100 mmH$_2$O; Biochemistry findings: mononuclear cells 74 %, lobulated neutrocytes 26 %, WBC 0.1×10^9/L, PanDi's test ++, ALT 20 u/L and AST 24 u/L. On Jun. 6, 2009, pressure at lumbar puncture 330 mmH$_2$O; Biochemistry findings: mononuclear cells 74 %, lobulated neutrocytes 26 %, WBC 0.1×10^9/L, PanDi's test +, cryptococcus (+). Her CD4 T cell count was 153/µl.

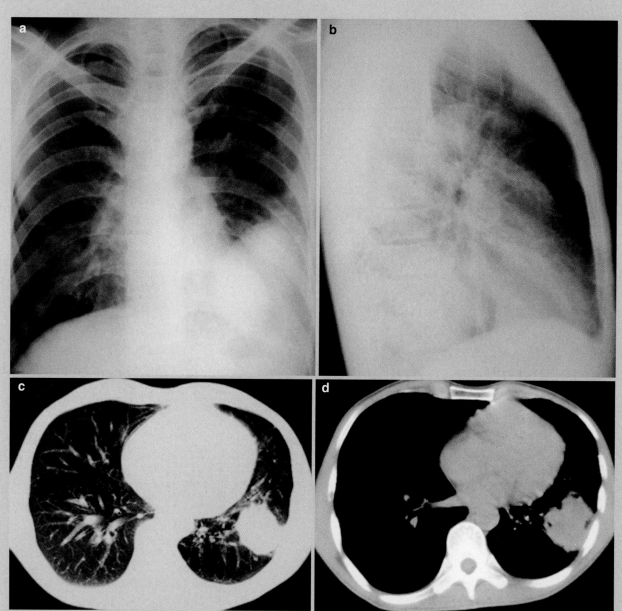

Fig. 17.80 (**a–d**) HIV/AIDS related pulmonary cryptococcus infection. (**a, b**) Anteroposterior and lateral DR demonstrate a huge dense mass shadow in the left lower lung, with clear boundary. (**c**) CT scanning of the pulmonary window demonstrates round liked high density shadow in the left lower lung near left chest wall, with even density. (**d**) CT scanning of the mediastinal window demonstrates round liked soft tissue density shadows in the left lower lung near left chest wall, with even density, lobulation, and surrounding thick spikes

Case Study 4

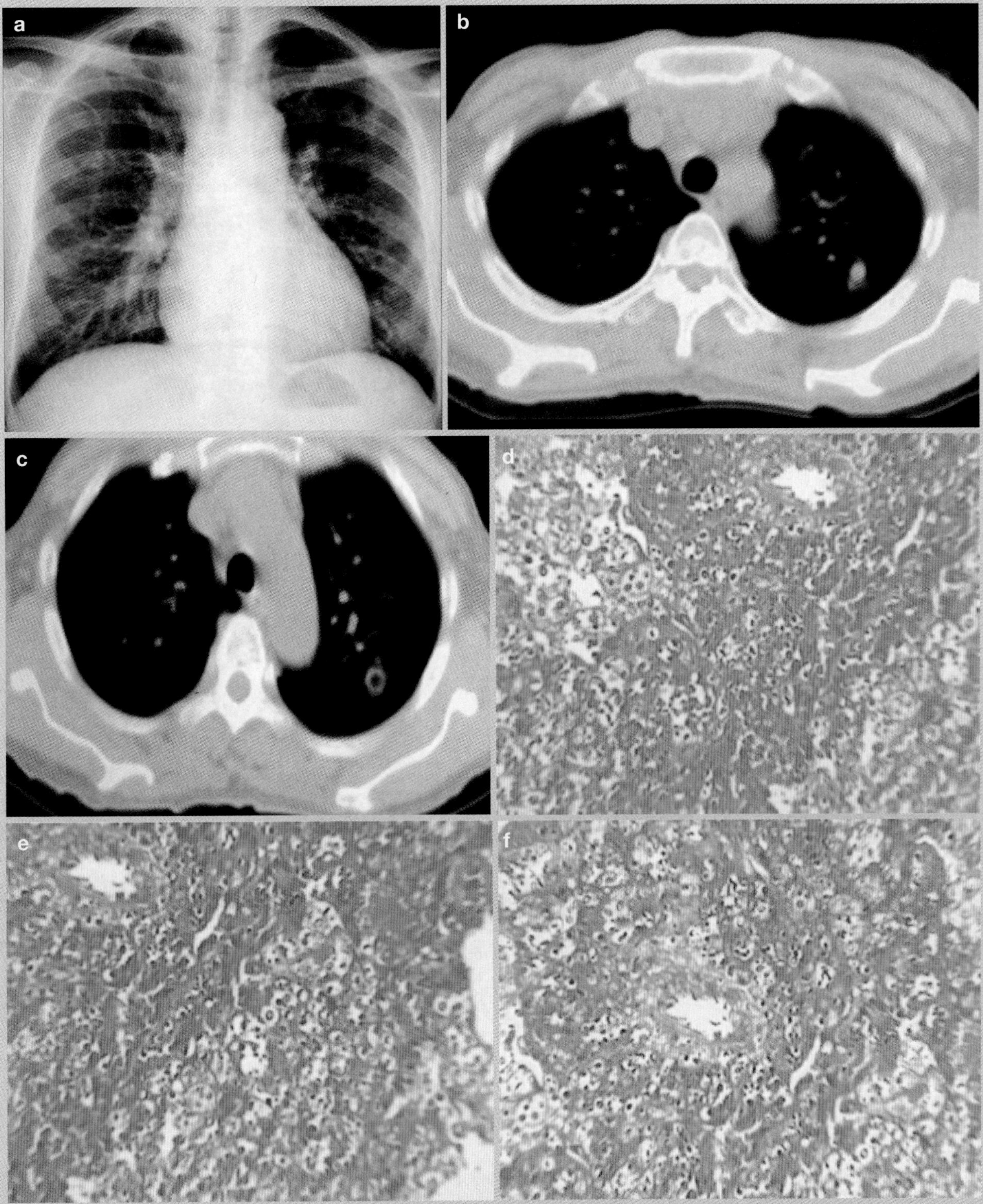

Fig. 17.81 (**a–f**) HIV/AIDS related pulmonary cryptococcus infection. (**a**) DR demonstrates thickened lung markings in both lungs and flaky blurry shadows in the left lower lung. (**b, c**) CT scanning demonstrates round liked nodular and small cavity shadows in the left upper and lower lung, with clear boundaries. (**d–f**) Pathology demonstrates transparent substrate in lung tissues and many bi-capsular cryptococci in cytoplasm

Case Study 5

An AIDS patient was confirmatively diagnosed by the CDC. He/She was diagnosed as having pulmonary Cryptococcus infection.

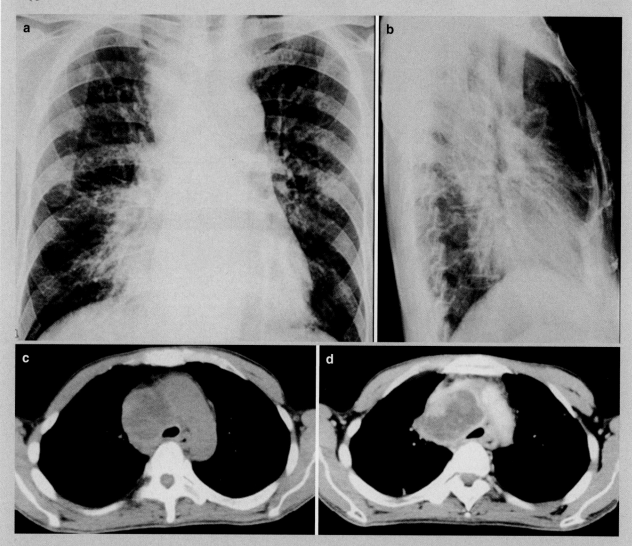

Fig. 17.82 (a–d) HIV/AIDS related pulmonary cryptococcus infection. (a, b) DR demonstrates enlarged blurry hilum in both lungs and thickened pulmonary markings. (c, d) CT scanning demonstrates mediastinal lymphadenectasis, narrowed trachea due to compression with liquefactive necrosis. Enhanced scanning demonstrates marginal enhancement and no central enhancement

Case Study 6

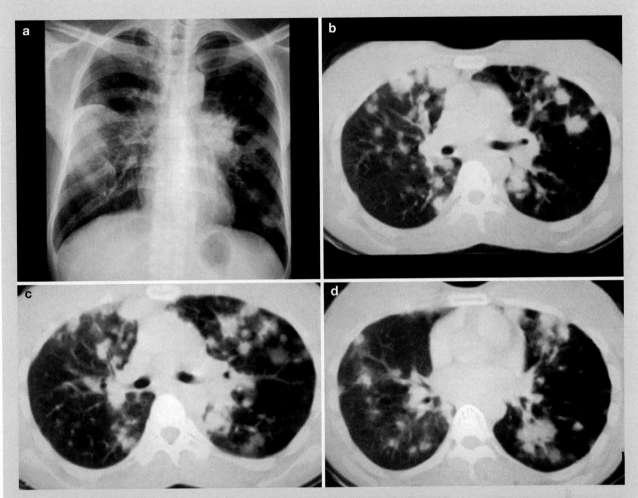

Fig. 17.83 (**a–d**) HIV/AIDS related pulmonary cryptococcus infection. (**a**) DR demonstrates enlarged blurry hilum in both lungs and thickened lung markings. (**b–d**) CT scanning demonstrates multiple scattered nodular or mass dense shadows in both lungs, with lobulation, rough spikes around and fusion of some shadows into mass; surrounding small flaky infiltrative shadows; and mediastinal lymphadenectasis

Case Study 7

A male patient aged 60 years was confirmatively diagnosed as having AIDS by the CDC. He was hospitalized on 2009-2-19 due to headache and vomiting for more than 10 days. In the CSF, Cryptococcus was found. By blood and sputum culture, cryptoccocus was detected. The diagnosis was cryptococcal meningitis, cryptococcal pneumonia and cryptococcal sepsis. After receiving amphotericin

B antifungal treatment and dehydration, headache and vomitting were relieved. But chest CT scanning reexamination demonstrated increased pulmonary lesions, which was considered as tuberculosis. On 2009-4-1, he was given HERV anti-tuberculosis treatment. Twenty days ago he sustained weakened lower limbs, which gradually aggravated and completely paralyzed in the recent 1 week, His CD4 T cell count was 34/μl.

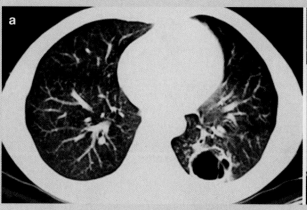

Fig. 17.84 (**a**, **b**) HIV/AIDS related pulmonary cryptococcus infection. (**a**) CT scanning demonstrates round liked cavity shadows in the left upper and lower lung, with uneven thickness of the cavity wall and surrounding infiltrative shadows. (**b**) CT scanning demonstrates round liked dense mass shadows in the right upper lung, with clear boundaries and bulky drainage vessel shadows

Case Study 8

A male patient aged 50 years was confirmatively diagnosed as having AIDS by the CDC.He complained of cough and chest distress for 3 months. His CD4 T cell count was 35/μl.

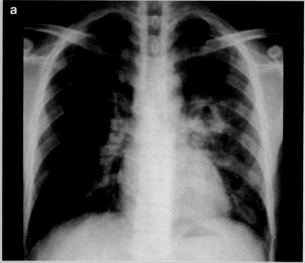
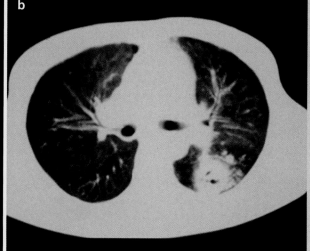

Fig. 17.85 (**a–f**) HIV/AIDS related pulmonary cryptococcus infection. (**a**) DR demonstrates round liked thick-wall cavity in the left hilum, with blurred boundary; ground-glass liked shadows with increased density in the left middle and lower lung. (**b–d**) CT scanning of the pulmonary window demonstrates thick-wall cavity in the dorsal segment of the left lower lung, with uneven thickness of cavity wall. (**e**, **f**) CT scanning of the mediastinal window demonstrates thick-wall cavity in the dorsal segment of the left lower lung, with uneven thickness of the cavity wall and surrounding thick spikes

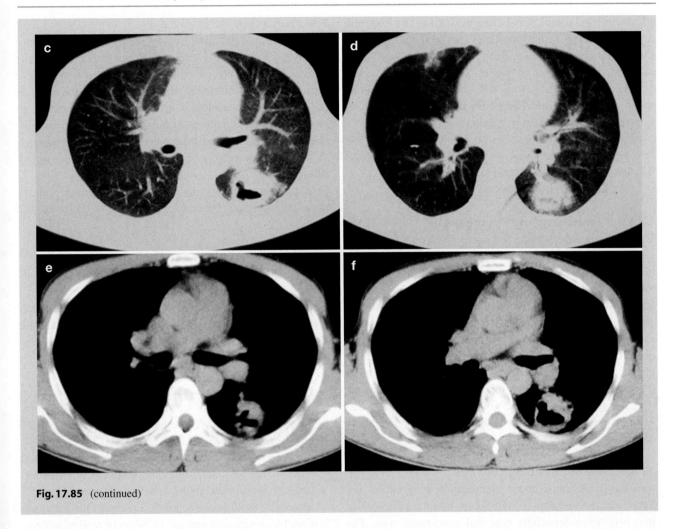

Fig. 17.85 (continued)

17.4.2.6 Diagnosis Basis

1. Most AIDS patients are asymptomatic, but they may have low-grade fever and slight cough, usually without positive signs.
2. Findings of cryptococcus by sputum smear and India ink staining or culture can define the diagnosis.
3. Blood related antibodies positive by indirect immunofluorescence test can assist the diagnosis.
4. Findings of Cryptococcus by percutaneous lung biopsy, PAS staining or Alcian blue staining.
5. Imaging demonstrations of thickened lung markings, scattered nodular or isolated spherical mass under the pleura and surrounding infiltrative lesions commonly in the dorsal segment of the lower lungs, and rarely cavities and mediastinal lymphadenectasis.

17.4.2.7 Differential Diagnosis

HIV/AIDS related pulmonary cryptococcus infections should be differentiated from tuberculosis, primary or metastatic lung cancer. Tuberculosis mostly is secondary tuberculosis, which is caused by repeated infections of tubercule bacillus. Lesions show flaky or flocculent shadows in the two upper lungs, with blurry boundaries. The wrapped necrotic foci by fibers develop into nodules. It can also show miliary shadows, mostly with mediastinal lymphadenectasis. It should also be differentiated from primary or metastatic lung cancer.

17.4.2.8 Discussion

Cryptococcus is a relatively common pathogen of pulmonary fungal infection, and mostly develops in AIDS patients. Usually, it is a disseminated disease, with common involvement of the central nervous system and the lungs. In immunocompetent patients, the nodular granuloma caused by the pathogen is similar to those of other pulmonary fungal infections. In patients with serious immunosuppression, wide tissue infiltration of the pathogens may occur in the lungs. A series of imaging demonstrations of pulmonary cryptococcus infection includes reticular or reticulated nodular interstitium. Other less common demonstrations are ground-glass liked shadows, parenchymal changes of air cavity and miliary nodules. The pathogenic fungi can be found mainly in the pulmonary interstitium. Imaging findings include singular or multiple nodules or masses, parenchymal changes of lung lobes and lung segments with clear or unclear boundaries in size of 1–10 cm. There may be also miliary lesions, lymphadenectasis and cavity shadows.

17.4.3 HIV/AIDS Related Pulmonary Candida Infection

17.4.3.1 Pathogens and Pathogenesis

Candida is an opportunistic pathogen, which widely exists in nature. Candida albicans parasitize in the oral cavity, laryngopharynx, upper respiratory tracts, vaginal and intestinal mucosa of human being. Pulmonary and bronchial moniliasis is commonly caused by candida albicans which has the strongest pathogenicity. After its invasion into the tissues, candida transforms into hyphae and multiplies in a large quantity, with strong toxicity and ability to fight against phagocytosis. AIDS patients may have disseminated pathological changes. Only when the immunity is compromised, the pathogen invades into the bronchus or lungs to cause diseases. Therefore, pulmonary candida infection is commonly secondary.

17.4.3.2 Pathophysiological Basis

Candidosis can cause acute inflammation in bronchus and lungs, mainly exudation of neutrophils, which can be divided into two types: bronchitis type and pneumonia type. The pathological changes in the early stage are acute suppurative inflammation, accompanied with the formation of abscesses. By the naked eyes observation, they are large flaky parenchymal changes, with central grayish white coagulative necrosis. Under a microscope, the lesions are large flaky caseous necrosis, accompanied with the formation of abscesses, and surrounding infiltration of hyphae and phagocytes. In the advanced, there are caseous necrosis, formation of cavities, fibrosis and granuloma.

17.4.3.3 Clinical symptoms and signs
Bronchitis Type

Symptoms in AIDS patients are mild, with frequent cough, with a small amount of white mucous phlegm or thick phlegm, no fever or low grade fever; scattered spots of white membranes in the mucosa of oral cavity, throat and bronchus. Dry rales can be heard occasionally in both lungs.

Pneumonia Type

In AIDS patients, the manifestations are mostly acute pneumonia or sepsis, with chills, fever, cough, expectoration of white mucous jelly liked phlegm or thick phlegm often with blood or necrotic tissue. The thick sputum, candidal hyphae and shedding cell debris can be condensed into small colloid clumps, with yeast smell. Other symptoms include even haemoptysis and difficulty breathing. Dry and moist rales can be heard in lungs.

Allergy Type

Symptoms may be difficulty breathing, rhinocnesmus, runny nose and sneezing. Wheezing rales can be heard in both lungs.

17.4.3.4 Examinations and Their Selection

1. Chest X-ray and CT scanning are the most commonly used diagnostic imaging examinations.
2. Sputum smear for direct microscopy can show candida. By fungus culture, the fungus strain can be identified based on colonies growth and microscopy.
3. Histopathologically, fiberobronchoscopy lavage for smear and biopsy can be performed.
4. By fungus skin test, candida skin test can provide information for the diagnosis of candida infection. Generally, the results are positive. In the serious cases, the results may be negative.
5. Fluorescent antibody test for direct smear specimens, colonies by fungus culture and pathohistological tissue section has certain value in the detection of the pathogens.
6. Molecular biology can be applied to detect the pathogen.
7. Candida metabolites test and PCR can be applied to determine the gene sequence of candida for the early diagnosis.

17.4.3.5 Imaging Demonstrations
Chest X-ray

Chest X-ray demonstrates nodular shadows and flaky parenchyma changes in unilateral or bilateral lungs. Sometimes there is miliary infection.

CT Scanning

CT scanning demonstrates most lesions in the middle and lower lung fields, with rare involvement of the apex. There are thickened lung markings or diffuse small flaky/patchy shadows, some of which can fuse into large flaky dense shadows, with blurry boundaries. Nodules, due to bleeding around it, may be surrounded by ground glass liked shadows, which is necrotic bronchopneumonia, usually accompanied with a large quantity neutrophils.

Case Study
A male patient aged 40 years was confirmatively diagnosed as having AIDS by the CDC. He complained of high fever, cough, expectoration, chest pain and shortness of breath, with pulmonary parenchymal changes sign and moist rales. His CD4 T cell count was 18/μl.

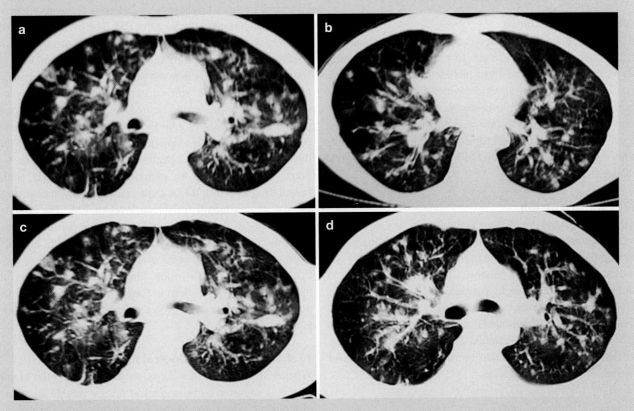

Fig. 17.86 (a–d) HIV/AIDS related pulmonary candida infection. (a–d) CT scanning demonstrates thickened and deranged lung markings in both lungs, diffuse small flaky or patchy shadows, fusion of some small shadows into large flaky dense shadows, with blurry boundaries, enlarged hilum and blurry structures

17.4.3.6 Diagnostic Basis
Clinical Symptoms
Cough expectoration with white mucous phlegm or thick phlegm, hemoptysis and shortness of breath.

Signs
Examinations of the oral cavity and the throat demonstrate spots liked white membrane covering the surface, and dry and moist rales in the lungs.

Cultures
Successive cultures of phlegm, lung tissue, pleural fluid or cerebrospinal fluid repeatedly demonstrate the same strain of candida, or direct microscopic findings of large quantity pseudohyphae or hyphae and groups of spores can define the diagnosis.

Chest X-ray and CT Scanning
It is demonstrated to have thickened and deranged lung markings in double lung, diffuse small flaky/patchy shadows, fusion of some small shadows into large flaky dense shadows, with blurry boundaries, enlarged hilum and blurry structures. The conditions progress rapidly, with repeated lesions occurrence.

17.4.3.7 Differential Diagnosis
Bacterial Pneumonia
HIV/AIDS related pulmonary candida infection should be differentiated from bacterial pneumonia. Bacterial pneumonia often has symptoms such as high fever, cough, expectoration, chest pain and shortness of breath. CT scanning demonstrates flocculent infiltrative shadows or parenchyma changes and cavities. The pathogen can be detected in the sputum or chest liquid.

Virus Pneumonia
HIV/AIDS related pulmonary candida infection should be differentiated from virus pneumonia. Viral pneumonia firstly causes upper respiratory tract infection, which spread downward to cause pulmonary inflammation. The demonstrations

include ground glass liked changes in the lung fields or mass shadows. The definitive diagnosis should be based on throat swabs, virus isolation from the sputum and serum specific antibodies test.

Pulmonary Tuberculosis

HIV/AIDS related pulmonary candida infection should be differentiated from pulmonary tuberculosis. In the early stage, the symptoms and signs include irritative dry cough, expectoration, hemoptysis and cavities in lungs. (Detailed manifestations of tuberculosis see the section about tuberculosis in this chapter) Its diagnosis mainly should be based on chest X-ray and findings of tubercule bacillus in sputum or other specimens, or tuberculosis specific pathological changes.

17.4.3.8 Discussion

HIV/AIDS related pulmonary candida albicans is a widespread dimorphism bacteria. The oval shaped budding yeasts and hyphae both can be found in the tissues. Candidiasis is a common disease in AIDS patients. Chest X-ray demonstrates unilateral or bilateral patchy parenchymal changes of the air cavity and nodules with unclear boundaries. Miliary lesions are common. HRCT demonstrates multiple nodular shadows in both lungs, often accompanied with parenchymal changes. Its definitive diagnosis should be based on the findings of candida albicans in the tissues.

17.4.4 HIV/AIDS Related Penicillium Marneffei Infection

Penicillium marneffei (PM) is a newly found penicillium in 1956, which is a special strain with a distribution in South East Asia and Southern China. Rhizomys is its natural host. In 1973, Disalvo et al. [12] reported the first case of natural human PM infection. In 1984, the first case of human PM infection in China was reported in Guangxi Zhuang Autonomous Zone. PM is an opportunistic pathogen and immunocompromised people are susceptible to its infection. Its spreading is along with soil contaminated by Rhizomys feces to invade human body via the respiratory tract, the digestive tract and skin defects. PM infection is believed to be one of the most common opportunistic infections in AIDS patients in Southeast Asia, which has an increasing incidence.

17.4.4.1 Pathogens and Pathogenesis

PM is the only dimorphic fungus in hyphomycetes penicillium, which is a special strain of penicillium. At different culture temperatures, it shows conversion of biphasic forms: fungal phase at 25 °C and yeast phase at 37 °C. The fungal phase is the hyphae of many cells, with certain biological morphology, such as penicillus, conidiophore, chain liked conidiospore and chains between spores. The yeast phase shows unicellular or bicellular form. In the growth process of PM, large quantity bright rosy or dark rosy pigments are produced, which is characteristically PM. The pigment of yeast phase is secondary metabolites of cells with strong hydrophobicity, which can promote the adhesion of conidiums in fungal phase and cells in yeast phase to the alveolar macrophages and other cells surface in the human body. The pigment monoclonal antibody (MAb) can interrupt the pathological process of adhesion. In addition, this pigment can determine the expression of cluster-encoding genes Mbr through diffusion and penetration of drugs to the cell membrane, thus preventing the penetration of hydrophilic antifungal drugs, such as fluconazole. That is to say, it improves the natural antifungal resistance level of PM. The soluble components of the pigment in fungal phase can trigger the generation of anti-conidium antibody (only IgG) in animals to prevent its spreading in the body. The phenomenon proves that, in terms of tissue invasion, fungal phase is less powerful than yeast phase. Conidium in fungal phase is the carrier of pathogen while the cells in yeast phase are the real pathogenic factors.

17.4.4.2 Pathophysiological Basis

When PM spreads to the target organ along with the blood flow, it is engulfed by mononuclear phagocytes. In the cases of replication itself and further spreading, reactive proliferation of phagocytes is caused. Mononuclear phagocyte system has strong defense ability. In the cytoplasm of proliferated mononuclear phagocytes, various amounts of PM can be found. PM mainly invades into the body via the respiratory tract, digestive tract and skin defects. In immunocompetent people, local abscesses form in the invasion site, which is characterized by the thick mucus fluid, with mainly necrosis and liquefaction. Vascular reactions and exudation of neutrophil leukocytes and body fluids is less than abscesses induced by common purulent bacteria. The clinical manifestation is confined suppurative inflammation. When the immunity is compromised, due to the insufficiency of immunologic factors, it is difficult for the immune cells to restrict and digest the engulfed pathogens, which leads to confined suppurative reaction. Therefore, it often presents with diffuse lesions. The pulmonary lesions are principally interstitial exudative inflammation.

17.4.4.3 Clinical Symptoms and Signs

The typical penicillium marneffei disease has acute or subacute onset, along with fever, chills and shivers, cough and expectoration, hemoptysis, shortness of breath, abdominal pain, diarrhea, bloody stool, fatigue, central necrotic papula

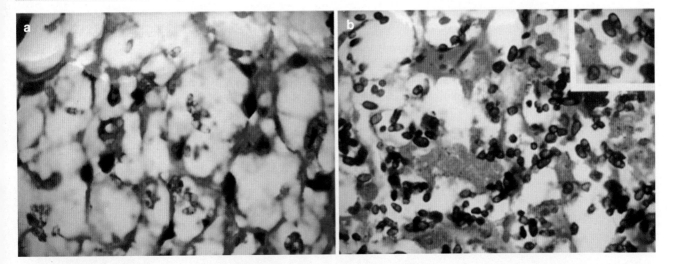

Fig. 17.87 (**a**) HE staining demonstrates lymph nodes, PM in the yeast phase, with sausage liked shape and obvious septa (HE×1000). (**b**) GMS staining demonstrates clearly defined PMs (GMS×1,000)

mainly in the head and face and scattering in the trunk and extremities as well as hepatosplenomegaly.

17.4.4.4 Examinations and Their Selection
Pathogen Examinations
Bone marrow smear and PAS staining can be performed to detect the pathogen. Blood, bone marrow, pleuroperitoneal fluid, phlegm and skin defect tissue are collected for the culture at double temperatures with Sabouraud'Broth medium. At the temperature of 25 °C, the colony is in dark red with villous surface, with surrounding red wine liked pigments to gradually spreading into the medium.

Pathological Examinations
Biopsy of lymph nodes and skin defects with PAS staining and Wright & Gimsa staining can be performed.

Laboratory Tests
WBC count, hemochrome, platelets, AST and CD4 T cell count.

Imaging Demonstrations
CT scanning and routine chest X-ray are the diagnostic imaging examinations of choice, which can facilitate to understand the size, morphology, location, quantity and density of the lesions.

17.4.4.5 Imaging Demonstrations
CT Scanning
It demonstrates multiple small nodular shadows in the lungs, multiple honeycomb liked cavities in both lungs and mediastinal lymphadenectasis. Abdominal scanning demonstrates different degrees of hepatic, splenic and retroperitoneal lymphadenectasis, which can fuse into a huge mass.

Routine Chest X-ray
It demonstrates thickened, deranged and blurry pulmonary markings, small cavities, military nodular shadows, mass liked shadows, spots and patchy shadows, ground glass liked changes, pleuritis and pleural effusion.

Case Study 1

A female patient aged 35 years was confirmatively diagnosed as having AIDS by the CDC. Her husband had a history of drug abuse and she complained of abdominal pain and fever for more than 2 months, with accompanying face rash and diarrhea. Her CD4 T cell count was 5/μl. By examinations, she sustained skin palpula, abdominal tenderness, central concave skin rashes on the face, neck, and upper limbs. There was a palpable mass in the upper left abdomen, hard and tenderness, in a size of 12 × 12 cm. More than 2 months before her admission, she had persistent dull abdominal pain that is commonly in the upper left abdomen, with accompanying fever and face skin rashes that is gradually increasing and spreads to the neck and upper limbs. She also had hepatosplenomegaly, abdominal aortic lymphadenectasis and ascites.

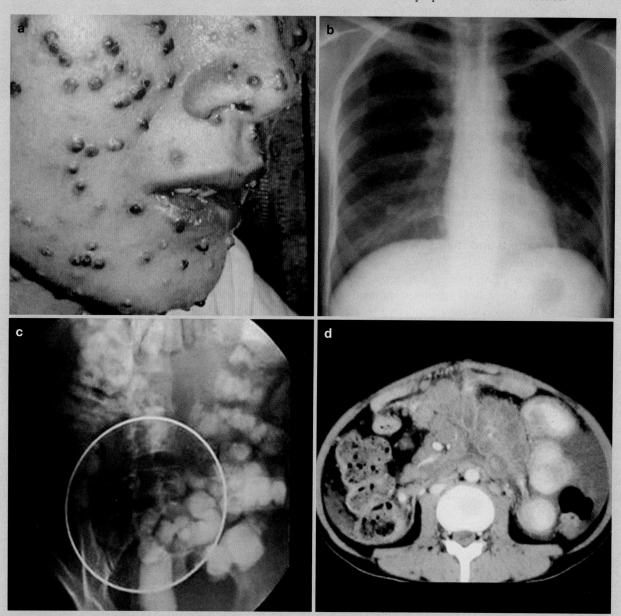

Fig. 17.88 (a–d) HIV/AIDS related penicillium marneffei infection. (a) The gross specimen demonstrates central necrotic pimples on the face. (b) Chest X-ray DR demonstrates cavities in the left upper lung, thickened lung markings in both lower lungs with accompanying multiple spots and flakes shadows. (c) Gastrointestinal barium meal radiology demonstrates left and downwards migration of the intestine due to compression. (d) Enhanced abdominal CT scanning demonstrates retroperitoneal enlarged lymph nodes that fuse into a huge mass, with ring shaped enhancement of the lymph nodes

Case Study 2

A female patient aged 41 years was confirmatively diagnosed as having AIDS by the CDC. She had an unhealthy sexual life, with complaints of fever and cough for more than 1 month, with accompanying concave liked skin rashes in the face and limbs. Her CD4 T cell count was 7/μl.

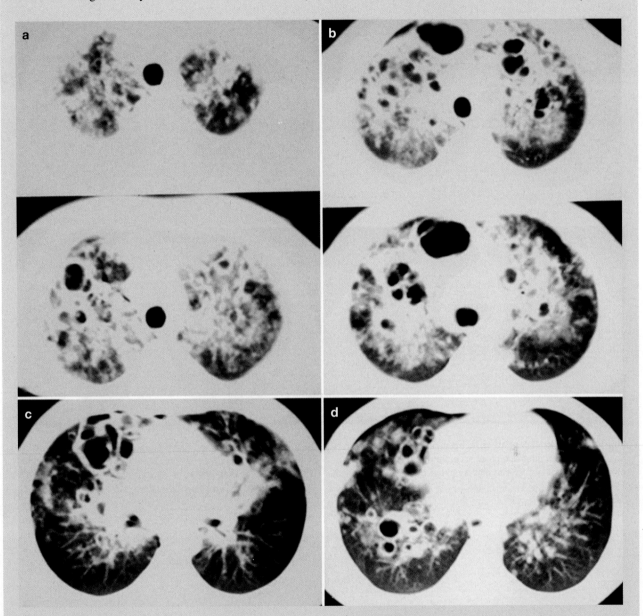

Fig. 17.89 (**a–d**) HIV/AIDS related penicillium marneffei infection. (**a–d**) CT scanning demonstrates multiple small nodular shadows in the lungs that fuse into mass with parenchymal shadows, with the hilum as the center and distributing bilaterally symmetric like butterfly wings. There are also multiple clustering cavities or singular large cavity in both lungs

Case Study 3

A female patient aged 29 years was confirmatively diagnosed as having AIDS by the CDC. She had a history of drug abuse, with complaints of fever and cough for more than 1 month and accompanying concave liked skin rashes in the face and limbs. Her CD4 T cell count was 17/μl.

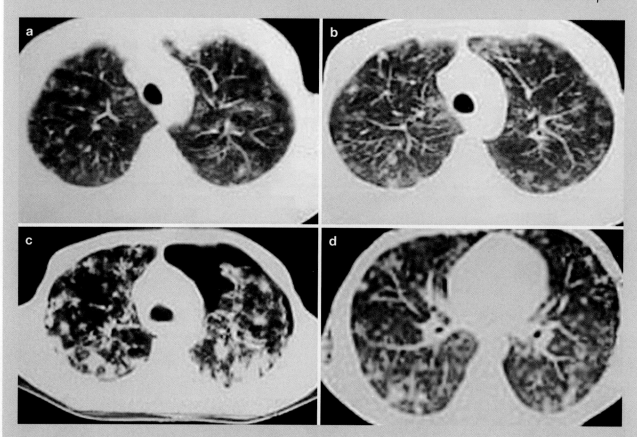

Fig. 17.90 (a–d) HIV/AIDS related penicillium marneffei infection. (a–d) CT scanning demonstrates multiple small nodular shadows in the lungs that fuse into mass in parenchymal shadows, with the hilum as the center and distributing bilaterally symmetric like butterfly wings. There are also multiple clustering cavities or singular large cavity in both lungs

Case Study 4

A female patient aged 51 years was confirmatively diagnosed as having AIDS by the CDC. She had an unhealthy sexual life, with complaints of fever and cough for more than 1 month. Her CD4 T cell count was 7/μl.

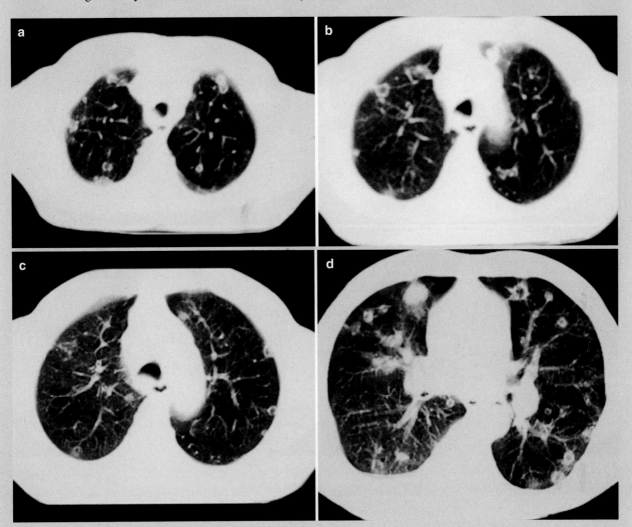

Fig. 17.91 (a–h) HIV/AIDS related penicillium marneffei infection. (a–e) CT scanning demonstrates multiple small nodular shadows and small cavity shadows in the lungs, fusion of some lesions into honeycomb likes cavity shadows or plaque liked dense shadows. (f–h) CT scanning demonstrates large thick-wall cavity shadows in the right lung, surrounding plaque and round liked small cavity shadows and inflammatory infiltrative shadows

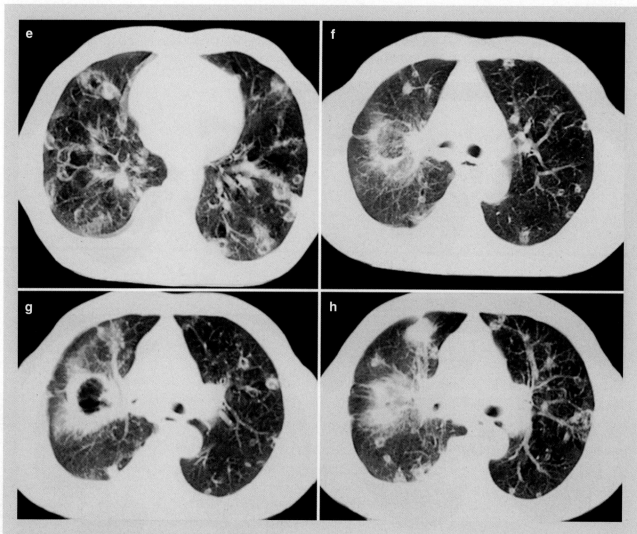

Fig. 17.91 (continued)

Case Study 5

A male patient aged 43 years was confirmatively diagnosed as having AIDS by the CDC. He had a history of drug abuse, with complaints of fever and cough for more than 1 month. His CD4 T cell count was 33/μl.

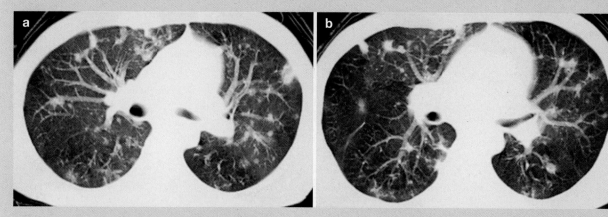

Fig. 17.92 (a–d) HIV/AIDS related penicillium marneffei infection. (a–d) CT scanning demonstrates multiple small nodular shadows and small cavity shadows in the lungs, fusion of the lesions in the right lung into plaque liked shadows with clear boundaries, and multiple round liked small cavity shadows and inflammatory infiltrative shadows in both lungs

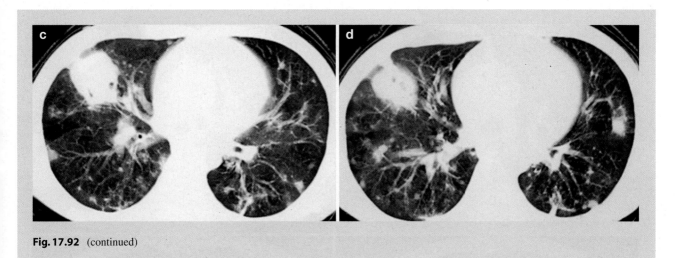

Fig. 17.92 (continued)

Case Study 6

A female patient aged 35 years was confirmatively diagnosed as having AIDS by the CDC. She had a history of extramarital affair, with complaints of fever and cough for more than 1 month. Her CD4 T cell count was 53/μl.

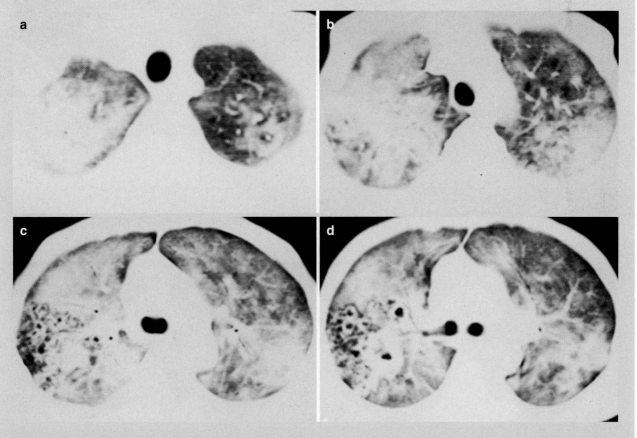

Fig. 17.93 (**a–h**) HIV/AIDS related penicillium marneffei infection. (**a–d**) CT scanning demonstrates diffuse small cavity in honeycomb liked and infiltrative parenchyma shadows, with the hilum as the center to distribute bilaterally symmetric like butterfly wings; multiple honeycomb liked cavity shadows in both lungs. (**e–h**) CT scanning reexamination demonstrates large irregular thick-wall cavities in the right lung, surrounding scattering nodular, honeycomba liked and infiltrative shadows after anti-PM infection treatment for 3 months

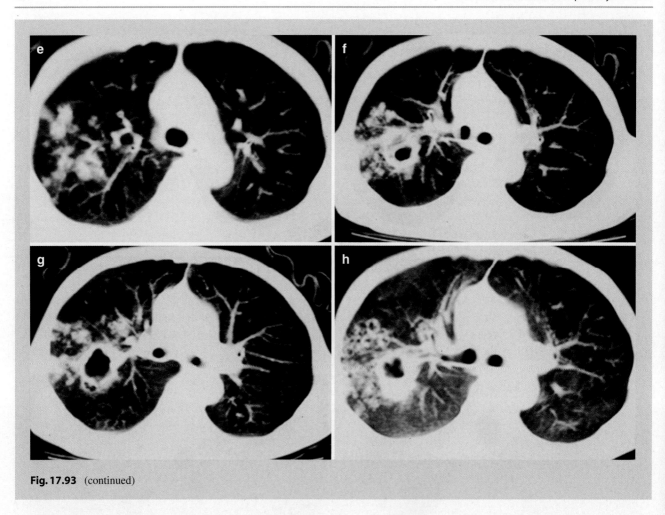

Fig. 17.93 (continued)

Case Study 7
A male patient aged 38 years was confirmatively diagnosed as having AIDS by the CDC. He had a history of extramarital affair, with complaints of fever and cough for more than 1 month. His CD4 T cell count was 93/μl.

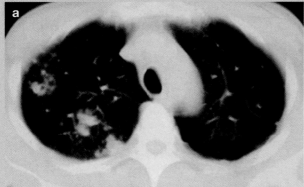
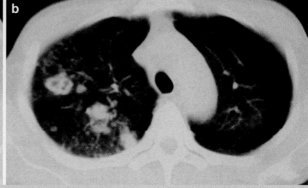

Fig. 17.94 (**a–f**) HIV/AIDS related penicillium marneffei infection. (**a–f**) CT scanning demonstrates multiple nodules and small cavities in honeycomb liked shadows and infiltrative parenchyma shadows in the right lung; flaky transparent areas (bullae of lung) in the right anterior margin of the heart and in the outer zone of the left lung near lateral chest wall

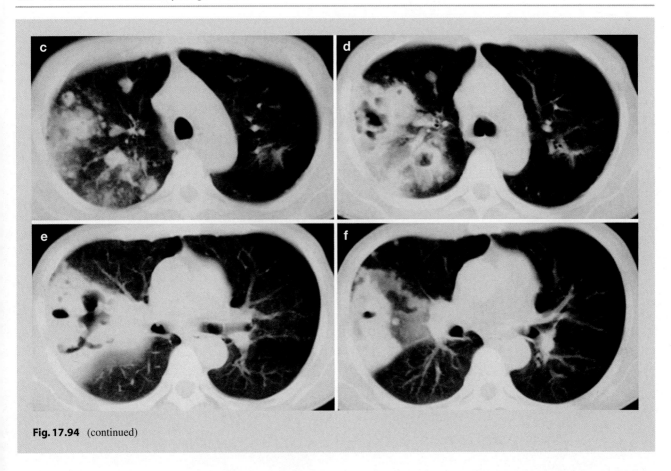

Fig. 17.94 (continued)

Case Study 8

A male patient aged 35 years was confirmatively diagnosed as having AIDS by the CDC. He had been found to be HIV positive for 5 years, with complaints of irregular fever, cough, fatigue and dizziness for 10 days to be hospitalized. By examinations, his CD4 T cell count was 40/μl, HIV positive, Subcultivation of strains demonstrated typical biphasic penicillium. By fungus culture, typical penicillus was found. By bone marrow smear, the round corpuscles mainly located in the macrophages.

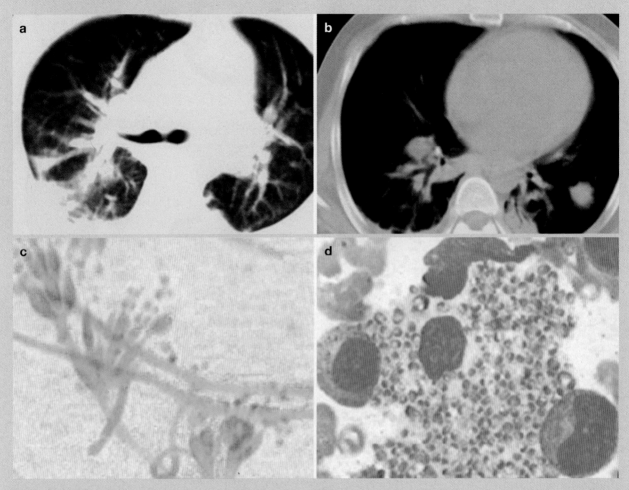

Fig. 17.95 (**a–d**) HIV/AIDS related penicillium marneffei infection. (**a**) CT scanning of the pulmonary window demonstrates irregular large flaky shadows with increased density in the dorsal segment of both lower lobes; enlarged hilum in both lungs, cords liked thickening of the vascular vessels. (**b**) CT scanning of the mediastinal window demonstrates flaky parenchyma shadows in the left lower lung, thickening of both pleura, enlarged hilum shadows in both lungs, thickened right lower bronchial wall. (**c**) Microscopy after culture at 25 °C demonstrates branches and separated hyphae and its string of small spores, with typical penicillus but no sporangium (Medan staining, ×400). (**d**) Bone marrow smear demonstrates round or oval cells like the yeast phase within the macrophages; longer cells like the yeast phase outside the macrophages. The two kinds of cells have slightly curved ends in sausages liked appearance (HE staining, ×400)

Case Study 9

A male patient aged 32 years was confirmatively diagnosed as having AIDS by the CDC. He had a history of extramarital affair, with complaints of fever, cough, chest distress, shortness of breath, fatigue, poor appetite, poor sleep, weight loss and shortness of breath after activities for more than 3 months. His CD4 T cell count was 23/μl. AST 156 μ/L. By B ultrasound, multiple low echo masses adjacent the abdominal aorta, in different sizes. The largest one in size of 13 × 8 mm with clear boundary and even distribution of the inner light spots. All the findings indicated lymphadenectasis adjacent to the abdominal aorta. The signs include a complexion of chronic illness and stool culture with findings of PM.

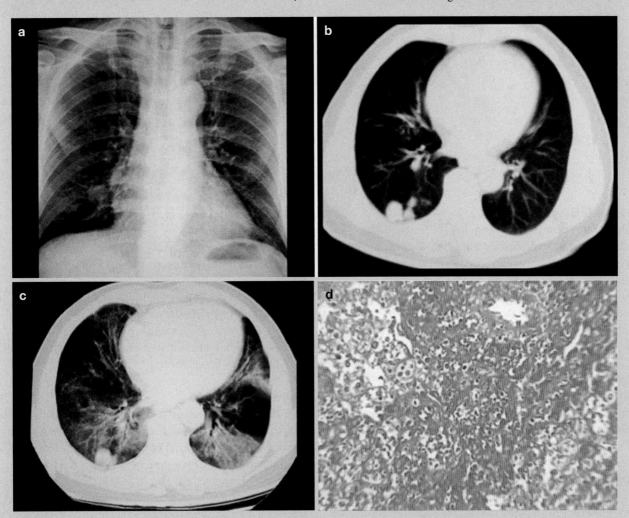

Fig. 17.96 (a–f) HIV/AIDS related penicillium marneffei infection. (a) DR demonstrates flaky blurry dense shadows in the right anterior margin of the heart, with surrounding infiltrative shadows. (b, c) CT scanning of the pulmonary window demonstrates nodular dense shadows in the dorsal segment of the right lower lung, with smooth sharp boundaries; large flaky ground glass liked dense shadows in the dorsal segment of both lungs. (d, e) HE staining demonstrates spores and round liked, long circular or sausage shaped corpuscles in red, in different sizes. (f) HE staining demonstrates spores and round liked, long circular or sausage shaped corpuscles in purplish red, in different sizes

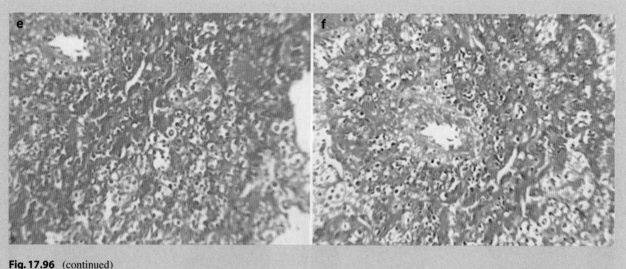

Fig. 17.96 (continued)

17.4.4.6 Diagnostic Basis
Chest X-ray and CT Scanning
Both demonstrate multiple nodules in different sizes and cavity shadows. The cavities cluster into honeycomb liked changes with uneven thickness of the walls, clear boundaries and surrounding inflammatory exudates. Some of the nodules infuse into mass dense shadows. Lesions in both lungs have a symmetrical or asymmetric distribution, with no characteristic leions. Mediastinal lymph nodes are obviously enlarged.

Pathogenic Examinations
Sputum smear for direct microscopy demonstrates candida.

Histopathological Examinations
PMs are found by fibrobronchoscopy lavage smear and biopsy.

Immunological Assays
(1) Candida skin test shows positive. (2) Fluorescent antibody test for PMs is performed in procedures of direct smear, fungal colony culture and histopathological examination of the tissue sections.

Metabolites Test and PCR
Metabolites test of PM and PCR can be performed to determine the gene sequences of PM for the early diagnosis.

17.4.4.7 Differential Diagnosis
HIV/AIDS related penicillium marneffei pneumonia should be differentiated from bronchiectasis and blood borne staphylococcus aureus pulmonary abscess.

Bronchiectasis
Although the cases of bronchiectasis are demonstrated to have clustering round shadows on the cross sections, the wall is thinner and even, accompanying to the spots liked vascular shadows. Some lesions have typical railway liked bronchial dilation signs.

Blood Borne Staphylococcus Aureus Pulmonary Abscess
It is demonstrated to have multiple small cavity lesions in both lungs in line with the evenly distributing blood borne lesions. The lesions are rarely clustering. The wall of the cavities is thick and even with surrounding marginal exudates and blurry boundaries.

17.4.4.8 Discussion
With the steady increasing of HIV infections, reports on the complication of PM disease have also been increasing recently. The disease can be localized but mostly disseminated, with the involvement of lungs, liver, skin, lymph nodes and other tissues and organs. Therefore, it is known as penicilliosis marneffei or disseminated penicillium marneffei infection in literature reports. Due to the insufficient knowledge about the disease, diagnosis is delayed or missed. In Thailand, penicilliosis marneffei has been the indicator disease of AIDS. About 20 % AIDS patients are infected by PM and 70 % have necrotic papula, which is characteristically disseminated penicillium marneffei infection. CT scanning demonstrates HIV/AIDS complicated by disseminated penicillium marneffei infection as flaky parenchyma shadows in the lungs, clustering of cavities and nodular shadows, mediastinal lymphadenectasis and pleural inflammation responses, which can facilitate its clinical diagnosis.

17.4.5 HIV/AIDS Related Mucor Infection

17.4.5.1 Pathogens and Pathogenesis
Mucormycosis is a rare kind of conditional fungal disease, with its pathogen, mucor, distributing widely in the natural world.

It generally fails to cause diseases, but can cause systematic infections in immunocompromised people. Mucor often invades into the human body via the nose to cause paranasal sinuses and orbital infections, which can further invade into the brain to cause meningitis and frontal abscesses. Pulmonary mucormycosis is only second to the nasal-cerebral infection. It can spread via the respiratory tract to cause pulmonary infections. In addition, there are also skin and gastrointestinal mucormycosis as well as disseminated mucormycosis.

17.4.5.2 Pathophysiological Basis
The pathological changes of HIV/AIDS related pulmonary mucormycosis are mainly hemorrhagic necrotic inflammation. The defense mechanism of immunocompetent people is to kill the fungal spores with the phagocytosis of macrophages and oxidation killing mechanism. In immunocompromised or immunodeficient patients, the macrophages are often too weak to restrain the engulfed spores from germinating. Therefore, the disease occurs. Vascular vessels are susceptible to the invasion of mucor, especially the arteries. Mucor can locally multiply to cause the formation of blood clots and embolization, and disseminate to other organs along with the blood flow. The main lesions are hemorrhage and necrosis of local tissues and exudation of neutrophils. The lesions of hemorrhage and necrosis are possibly related to the arteriole lesions caused by hyphae.

17.4.5.3 Clinical Symptoms and Signs
The clinical manifestation of HIV/AIDS related pulmonary mucormycosis is a nonspecific pneumonia. The most common symptoms reported in literatures are persistent high fever, cough, hemoptysis, chest pain and difficulty breathing. It has a rapid progression, with a high mortality rate of 65–96 %. Lung lesions are hemorrhagic infarction or pneumonia, which can cause high fever, cough, expectoration, shortness of breath, chest distress, chest pain, hemoptysis (pulmonary artery involved) and other symptoms. Moist rales can be heard in both lungs and pleural rubs can be heard in the cases of pleura involvement.

17.4.5.4 Examinations and Their Selection
1. Assisted by bronchofibroscopy, lung biopsy can be performed.
2. Histological examinations include bronchial lavage fluid examination, exploratory thoracotomy and puncture of lung tissues for biopsy.
3. Chest X-ray and CT scanning are conventional effective examinations.

17.4.5.5 Imaging Demonstrations
The lesions are frequently found in the dorsal and medial segments of both lungs. Early exudation shows miliary shadows, cavity shadows with no wall or with thin wall and small bronchiectasis shadows. Their further progression may cause fusion infiltration, parenchymal changes, nodules, masses, thick-walled cavities and pleural effusion, with accompanying mediastinal lymphadenectasis.

17.4.5.6 Diagnostic Basis
1. The findings of mucor or their hyphae by sputum and bronchofibroscopic biopsy.
2. The diagnostic imaging demonstrates lesions commonly in the dorsal and medial segments of both lungs. There are diffuse scattering miliary shadows, cavity shadows with no wall or with thin walls and small bronchiectasis shadows. They further progress into fusion infiltration, parenchymal changes, nodules, masses, thick-walled cavities and pleural effusion.
3. Often with accompanying mediastinal lymphadenectasis.

17.4.5.7 Differential Diagnosis
Chest X-ray of pulmonary mucormycosis demonstrates progressive infiltrated parenchymal changes, or masses, nodules, cavities and pleural effusion. It needs to be differentiated from miliary tuberculosis. HIV/AIDS related miliary tuberculosis are commonly demonstrated as chronic blood borne disseminated tuberculosis, with lesions distributing symmetrically in both lungs. Its long term progression causes fusion into masses. Otherwise, it can be cured by anti-TB therapies. The early lesions are no-wall cavities or thin wall cavities and small bronchioectasis shadows, based on which the differential diagnosis can be made.

17.4.5.8 Discussion
Almost all cases of HIV/AIDS related pulmonary mucormycosis are found in immunocompromised patients. Chest X-ray demonstrates parenchyma changes and isolated or multiple nodules or masses. The parenchyma changes are patchy or fuse, with unilateral or bilateral distribution. About 20 % patients have pleural effusion and less than 10 % patients have hilar or mediastinal lymphadenosis. CT scanning demonstrates singular or multiple nodules or masses, commonly with clustering or honeycomb liked cavities.

17.5   HIV/AIDS Related Pulmonary Virus Infection

17.5.1 HIV/AIDS Related Cytomegalovirus Pneumonia

17.5.1.1 Pathogen and Pathogenesis
AIDS patients often sustain pulmonary viral infections, and cytomegalovirus infection is the most common one. Generally, its clinical symptoms are not obvious. Viral pneumonia can be simple, or a part of systemic disseminated infections. Cytomegalovirus pneumonia is caused by cytomegalovirus, which belongs to herpes virus B and is a double-chain DNA virus with exterior capsule and spherical nucleus. Cytomegalovirus has two antigens, complement

fixing antigen and neutralization antigen. Its pathogenesis is the transmission of cytomegalovirus via various routes, with infants commonly via contacts, and adults commonly via sexual contacts. The onset after infection depends on the amount of the invaded viruses and the immunity status of the human body. Due to the important role the cellular immunity plays in anti-cytomegalovirus infection, patients with deficient cellular immunity have more serious conditions after cytomegalovirus infection. In patients with compromised or deficient immunity, the latent CMV infection can be activated to cause diseases. Therefore, patients with AIDS are susceptible to CMV infection.

17.5.1.2 Pathophysiological Basis

Cytomegalovirus pneumonia has extensive pathological changes in the lungs. Pathologically, it shows interstitial pneumonia, with the lesions randomly blood borne distributing in the lungs. The distribution can be diffuse, panlobular or focal. The target cells of pathological changes include alveolar cells and macrophages. Diffused pulmonary interstitial edema and fibrosis as well as alveolar swelling, focal necrosis, bleeding and hyperplasia occur after CMV infections to cause hypoxemia. Gross observation of fresh specimens demonstrates pulmonary surface edema and flaky blooding spots. Fixed specimens demonstrate brown hard lung tissues. Under a microscope, pulmonary interstitial congestion as well as infiltration of lymphocytes and mononuclear cells can be found, with the involved epithelial cells enlarged. In the pulmonary interstitium and alveoli, there are intranuclear inclusions, cytoplasmic inclusions and fluid containing abundant proteins. The classical intranuclear inclusions can be found in the cells, purplish red or purplish blue, round or oval, with surrounding halos in eagle eyes sign. Atypical cytomegalic inclusions in cells are slender, long and round liked with abundant cytoplasm and accentric nucleolus, which are blurry, unclear and atypical (Fig. 17.97a–e). Immunohistochemitry demonstrates HIV P24 antigen positive.

17.5.1.3 Clinical Symptoms and Signs

The systemic symptoms of CMV infection include fever, joint and muscle soreness and pain, abdominal distension and orthostatic hypotension. The respiratory symptoms include paroxysmal dry cough, difficulty breathing, cyanosis and three depressions sign. According to the imaging findings of CMVP, CMV pneumonia can be classified as diffuse,

miliary and mass types, among which the diffuse type is the most common.

17.5.1.4 Examinations and Their Selection

Immunological Assays

Cytomegalovirus can be separated from respiratory secretions culture and urine culture by using human embryonic fibroblasts. By urine sediment smear, giant cell with inclusions can be found. By using immunofluorescence, indirect hemagglutination inhibition and complement fixing test, the antibody titer can be found increased. Indirect immunofluorescence test and immunoenzymic staining test can be applied to detect the anti-CMV-IgG and IgM antibody. In addition, enzyme-linked immuno sorbent assay (ELISA) can also be performed to detect the anti-CMV-IgG and IgM antibody. CMV-IgM antibody positive indicates a recent infection, which has diagnostic value. A single serum CMV-IgG antibody positive indicates a previous infection. And during the acute and recovery phases, double serum CMV-IgG antibody titer being no less than four times increase has diagnostic value, indicating a recent infection.

PCR

PCR can be applied to quantitatively determine the viral load in the whole blood, blood plasma, leukocytes, urine, bronchoalveolar lavage fluid (BALF), cerebrospinal fluid and the tissue specimens, which is believed to be the best way for the diagnosis of invasive CMV infection.

Diagnostic Imaging

Chest X-ray is the most commonly used examination. Chest CT scanning is superior to chest X-ray in terms of resolution and detection rate of the lesions.

17.5.1.5 Imaging Demonstrations

Pulmonary demonstrations by CMVP include diffuse interstitial infiltration and alveolar infiltration to form reticular shadows, nodules and parenchymal changes. The pathological changes of the airway include thickened bronchial wall and bronchiectasis. Necrotic bronchiolitis can cause obstruction of minor airways. CT scanning demonstrates intrapulmonary multiple small nodule shadows and ground glass liked changes. The pathological basis of nodules or masses is hemorrhage and necrosis. The parenchyma changes indicate complications of bacteria infection or fungal infection.

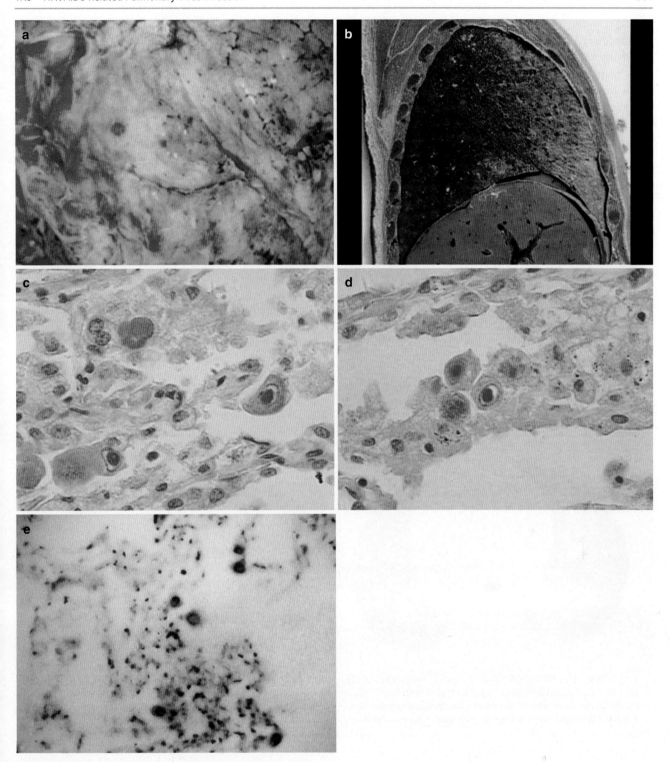

Fig. 17.97 (a) Gross observation of the fresh specimen in autopsy demonstrates pulmonary edema and congestion of cytomegalovirus pneumonia. (b) Gross observation of the formalin fixed specimen in autopsy demonstrates *dark brown* hard pulmonary tissues. (c, d) HE staining demonstrates large quantity cytomegalovirus inclusions in eagle eyes sign. (e) Immunohistochemical demonstrates HIV P24 antigen positive in macrophages of lung tissues (×400)

Case Study 1

A baby boy aged 6 months was confirmatively diagnosed as having AIDS by the CDC. He was infected via vertical transmission from mother to child, with recurrent cough after being born and the most recent cough for 4 days as well as wheezing cough in throat for 1 day before he was hospitalized. He had a past history of premature birth, with primary apnea and bronchial pneumonia and was hospitalized for treatment. Later, he was admitted for three times due to cough, which was diagnosed as interstitial pneumonia. By examinations, WBC 16.3×10^9/L, LYM lymphocyte count 11.7×10^9/L, CMV-Ab weak positive, blood sedimentation 11 mm/h, and tuberculosis antibody negative. After treated by broad-spectrum antibiotic therapy, the therapeutic efficacy is unfavorable.

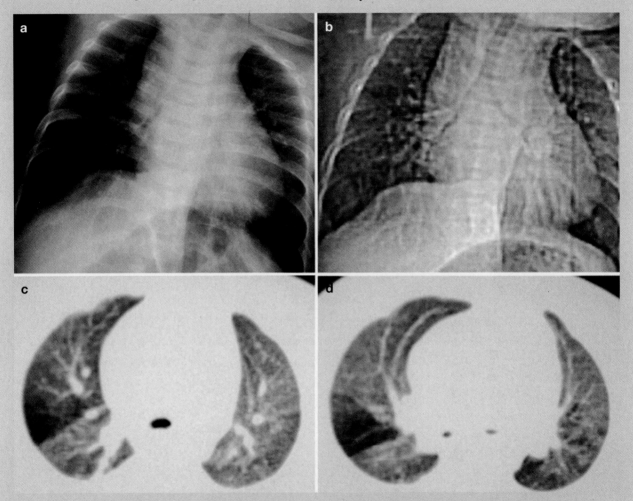

Fig. 17.98 (a–e) HIV/AIDS related cytomegalovirus pneumonia. (a) DR demonstrates thickened lung markings in both lungs, which extend to the outer zone of the lungs. (b) DR demonstrates thickened and deranged lung markings in both lungs with nodular blurry shadows; and cloudy shadows in lung fields. (c, d) CT scanning demonstrates thickened lung markings in both lungs, with diffuse nodular shadows; and cloudy changes in lung fields. (e) HE staining demonstrates cytomegalovirus inclusions

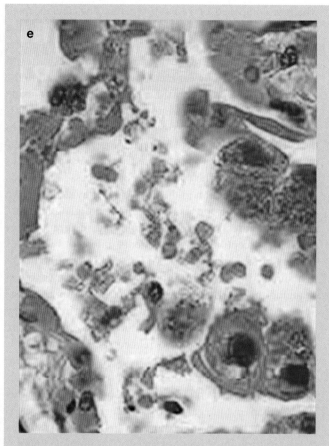

Fig. 17.98   (continued)

Case Study 2

A female patient aged 45 years was confirmatively diagnosed as having AIDS by the CDC. She had a history of paid blood donation in 1995 and was confirmatively diagnosed in Oct. 2003. In Jul. 2005, she sustained symptoms of irregular fever, cough and emaciation for months. Her CD4 T cell count was 56/μl.

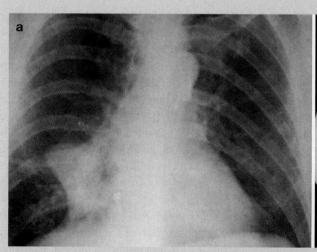
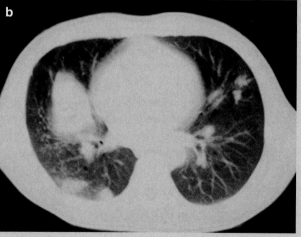

Fig. 17.99 (**a**, **b**) HIV/AIDS related cytomegalovirus pneumonia. (**a**) DR demonstrates enlarged right hilus, thickened and deranged lung markings. (**b**) Plain CT scanning demonstrates mass shadows in the right hilus, spots shadows in the right middle and lower lobes, and patchy shadows in the lingual segment of the left lung

17.5.1.6 Diagnostic Basis

1. CMV antibody positive. When the double serum CMV-IgG antibody titer shows an at least four times increase, reactivation of CMV infection can be considered.
2. PCR and in situ hybridation can be performed to detect CMV-DNA in the lesions tissues.
3. Detection of cytomegalovirus inclusion in the lesion tissues is an important evidence for the diagnosis.
4. Bronchoalveolar lavage fluid, sputum and biopsy tissue can be inoculated into human embryonic fibroblasts for culture; the detection of CMV has more diagnostic value.
5. Imaging examinations demonstrate diffuse interstitial infiltration and alveolar infiltration to form reticular shadows, nodules and parenchymal changes.

17.5.1.7 Differential Diagnosis

1. Mononucleosis caused by pulmonary cytomegalovirus infection is difficult to be differentiated from infectious mononucleosis caused by EBV.
2. Cytomegalovirus pneumonia should be differentiated from pulmonary infections casued by herpes simplex virus, adenovirus and influenza virus.

17.5.1.8 Discussion

Cytomegalovirus (CMV) infection is an important cause of pneumonia in patients with compromised immunity. Imaging findings include nodular shadows with blurry boundaries and bilateral flaky parenchymal changes of the lungs. The nodules tend to be bilaterally symmetric or asymmetric, with centrilobular distribution. Histopathological manifestations are nodular alveolar hemorrhage, necrosis and inflammatory lesions, and diffused alveolar lesions. The nodules tend to have a centrilobular distribution, indicating occurrence of bronchiolitis. In AIDS patients, if the diameter of nodules is under 10 cm, it is most likely to be viral infection. The size of the nodules can facilitate the differential diagnosis of pulmonary infections.

17.5.2 HIV/AIDS Related Herpes Simplex Viral Pneumonia

Herpes simplex viral pneumonia (HSVP) often occurs in the upper respiratory tract, and rarely in the lower respiratory tract. Human herpes simplex virus can be divided into two types, namely herpes simplex virus type I (HSV-I) and herpes simplex virus type II (HSV-II). Herpes simplex viral pneumonia mostly occurs in patients with immunodeficiency.

17.5.2.1 Pathogen and Pathogenesis

Herpes simplex viral pneumonia can be caused by HSV-I and HSV-II, both of which have a nucleocapsid with 20 surfaces. The thickness of the nucleocapsid is about 100 nm,

which is composed of 162 capsomeres. The nucleocapsid contains the core of the virus DNA. The virion gains the phospholipid rich viral envelope when it passes through the nuclear envelope. The nucleocapsid gemmates after it passes through the nuclear membrane and is released to the cell surface. The nucleocapsid can also be released outside the cells or gains its access into the neighbour cells for further reproduction. Herpes simplex virus replicates itself in the cell nucleus to produce histopathologic changes of herpes virus replication, with visible Cowdry A type intranuclear inclusions. The pathogenesis process of herpes simplex virus infection in the body can be divided into five stages: initial skin mucosa infection, acute ganglia infection, latent infections, re-activation, and recurrent infections in susceptible hosts. Patients infected by herpes simplex virus can produce IgM, IgG and IgA antibodies to fight directly against virus protein, which may play a role in changing the severity of the infection. Interferon also participates in the control of herpes simplex infection by inhibiting the virus or regulating the defense mechanism. Genetic factors may be also related to the herpes virus infection. Cellular immunity can confine the infection. Herpes virus cannot reproduce in the alveolar macrophages of human body, which is also the reason why herpes virus is less than cytomegalovirus in lungs. Currently, it is believed that herpes simplex virus is an important pathogen of respiratory infections, especially in immunocompromised patients. Localized herpes simplex viral pneumonia occurs due to the direct spreading of virus in the upper and lower respiratory tract. Diffuse herpes simplex viral pneumonia is caused by the virus spread from the reproductive organs lesions or oral lesions (most possibly blood borne). Viremia caused by HSV-I or HSV-II has been reported, and both are related to diffused infections. But in patients without herpes simplex viral infection in skin mucosa, herpes simplex viral pneumonia can also occur.

17.5.2.2 Pathophysiological Basis

Herpes simplex viral pneumonia is caused by the direct spreading of the virus from the upper and lower respiratory tract. Diffuse herpes simplex viral pneumonia is cause by the spreading of the virus from the reproductive organs lesions or oral lesions (most possibly blood borne). Viremia cause by either HSV-I and HSV-II have been reported, both of which are related to diffuse infections. In such cases, the lung tissues may have inflammatory infiltration, lung parenchyma necrosis, bleeding, cellular swelling and round, diffuse interstitial pneumonia. And in most cases, there are accompanying cellular changes of herpes virus infection such as the intranuclear eosinophilic inclusions, necrotic herpes simplex viral trachitis. Herpes simplex viral bronchitis has demonstrations of mucosa erythema, edema, exudation and ulcer, with coverage of the surface by fibrous purulent membranous secretions.

Fig. 17.100 The structure of herpes simplex virus

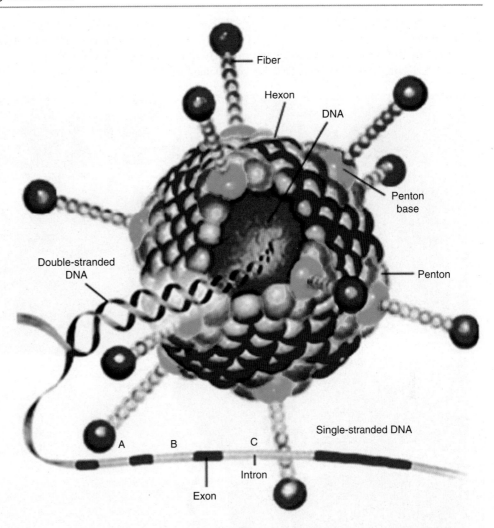

17.5.2.3 Clinical Symptoms and Signs

The common initial clinical symptoms of herpes simplex viral pneumonia are shortness of breath, cough, and fever with a body temperature being higher than 38.5 °C, decreased WBC count, hypoxemia, respiratory dysfunctioning and azotemia. HSV pneumonia may be accompanied by mucocutaneous lesions by HSV, which show earlier than those of pneumonia. There may be concurrent fungus, cytomegalovirus or bacteria infection. Herpes simplex viral tracheobronchitis may show tracheal or bronchial spasm or stenosis.

17.5.2.4 Examinations and Their Selection

Etiological Examinations

HSV can be detected in tracheobronchial secretions, bronchoalveolar lavage fluid and lung tissues. Early sampling should be performed under the guidance of a bronchofibroscope.

Cell Culture

Tissue culture is the most sensitive and specific method for the diagnosis, which can also be used for the classification of the virus.

Virus Detection

Papanicolaou (Pap) or Tzank test is a fast and cheap method for cellular diagnosis.

ELISA

ELISA can be used to detect herpes simplex virus, with a sensitivity of up to 95 % and a high specificity.

Diagnostic Imaging

Chest X-ray demonstrations are less valuable for the differential diagnosis. Pulmonary CT scanning can be applied for the differential diagnosis.

17.5.2.5 Imaging Demonstrations

Herpes simplex viral pneumonia includes three types, namely local, multiple or diffuse interstitial infiltration. In the early stage, typical hilar or diffuse interstitial shadows with increased density can be found, with thickened bronchial wall. As the disease progresses, cloudy or patchy alveolar tamponade and fusion can be found. Chest X-ray may demonstrate negative for herpes simplex viral trachitis and bronchitis.

Case Study

A male patient aged 28 years was confirmatively diagnosed as having AIDS by the CDC. He complained of fever, shortness of breath and cough for 1 week. His CD4 T cell count was 35/μl.

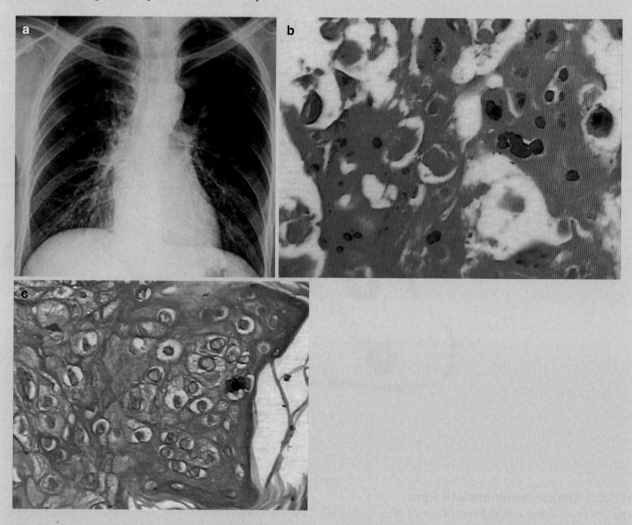

Fig. 17.101 (a–c) HIV/AIDS related Herpes Simplex Viral Pneumonia. (a) DR demonstrates thickened and deranged lung markings in both lungs with accompanying blurry nodular shadows, and cloudy shadows in the lung fields. (b) PAS staining (400×) demonstrates eosinophilic inclusion. (c) Silver methenamine staining demonstrates herpes viral inclusion

17.5.2.6 Diagnostic Basis

1. Clinical and radiological manifestations of HSV pneumonia are non-specific. The diagnosis of herpes simplex viral pneumonia, in addition to the clinical manifestations of pneumonia, should also be based on the histological evidence of pulmonary HSV infection and isolation of virus from the lung tissues.

2. Direct isolation of the virus from the lung tissues can define the diagnosis.

3. Tracheoscopy in combination to the cytologic examination and virus culture has diagnostic value. Bronchofibroscopy demonstrates tracheobronchial mucosa ulcer and(or) coverage by pseudomembrane, which can also be applied to guide the sampling of bronchial lavage fluid or lung tissues for biopsy. Cytological and histological examinations can provide specific evidence for HSV infection: multinucleated giant cells and intranuclear eosinophilic inclusion. In addition, biopsy demonstrates inflammatory infiltration, parenchyma necrosis and bleeding.

4. Immunofluorescence can be applied for the histological examination of herpes simplex virus antigen.

5. The imaging examinations can demonstrate herpes simplex viral pneumonia as localized, multiple or diffuse interstitial infiltration. As the disease progresses, cloudy or patchy alveolar tamponade and fusion can be found.

17.5.2.7 Differential Diagnosis

Herpes simplex viral pneumonia should be differentiated from bacterial pneumonia, CMV pneumonia, and influenza pneumonia.

17.5.2.8 Discussion

HIV/AIDS related herpes simplex viral pneumonia is mostly demonstrated by multiple signs, including small nodules, ground glass liked shadows and patchy parenchymal changes. The nodules are in centrilobular distribution, mostly with accompanying branches liked shadows (tree buds sign). Chest X-ray demonstrates diffuse lung parenchymal changes. Imaging finding are parenchymal change areas with bilaterally blurry boundaries. Generally, the nodules have a diameter of 2–10 mm. CT scanning with high resolution demonstrates nodules with surrouding ground glass liked density lesions.

17.5.3 HIV/AIDS Related Lymphoid Interstitial Pneumonia

Lymphoid/Lymphocytic interstitial pneumonia (LIP) is more common in children with AIDS. The CDC in the United States has defined LIP in children under the age of 13 years as the diagnostic indicator of AIDS. The predictive diagnostic criteria include chest X-ray demonstration reticular nodular changes in pulmonary interstitium of both lungs for no less than 2 months, undetectable pathogens and no responses to the antibiotic therapy.

17.5.3.1 Pathogen and Pathogenesis

Currently, HIV/AIDS related lymphocytic interstitial pneumonia is considered to be related to HIV and Epstein-Barr virus, human T cell leukemia-lymphoma type I virus (HTLV-I) and HIV-I. The infection of the above viruses causes pulmonary lymphatic hyperplasia and other systemic diseases.

17.5.3.2 Pathophysiological Basis

About 22–75 % children with HIV infection sustain LIP, and 3 % in adults. Most cases of non-HIV infected patients with lymphoid interstitial pneumonia are women, at average age of 56 years old, more commonly in the age group of 40–50 years old and above 70 years old. The pathological manifestations are infiltration of small and mature lymphocytes as well as plasma cells in alveolar septum and the alveolus, extensive interstitial fibrosis and non-caseous granuloma. It is characterized by diffuse infiltration of lymphocytes, plasmocytes and histocytes in the pulmonary interstitium. The lymph follicle with germinal center is more common. Hyperplasia occurs in type II alveolar epithelium, and the macrophage increases in the alveolar cavity. There are rare or mild intraalveoli organization and macrophage aggregation. Staining of the immune globulin light chain demonstrates poly-clone B cells.

17.5.3.3 Clinical Symptoms and Signs

The clinical symptoms are in progressive development, with cough and suffocation, rare hemoptysis and Sjogren syndrome commonly in mouth and eyes. By examinations, the signs have slight difference between adults and children. In children, there are lymphadenectasis, hepatosplenomegaly, enlargement of parotid gland, clubbing fingers and wheezing sound. In adults, there are lymphadenectasis, slight fine bubbling rales, as well as hepatosplenomegaly and enlargement of parotid gland in 1/3 patients.

17.5.3.4 Examinations and Their Selection

1. Peripheral hemogram demonstrates increased lymphocytes and eosinophilic granulocytes.
2. Myelogram demonstrates increased lymphocytes, plasmocytes and eosinophils.
3. Blood biochemical examination demonstrates increased immune globulin, predominantly IgM.
4. Blood gas analysis demonstrates hyoxemia.
5. Pathogenic examinations by bronchofibroscopy, bronchial alveolar lavage and biopsy can define the diagnosis.
6. Pulmonary function examinations demonstrate restrictive ventilatory disorder, lower lung compliance and impaired diffusion function. Impaired diffusion function is a more sensitive indicator in monitoring the progress of the disease.
7. Chest X-ray is the most commonly used imaging examination, while chest CT scanning is commonly applied for the differential diagnosis.

17.5.3.5 Imaging Demonstrations

Chest X-ray demonstrates HIV/AIDS related lymphoid interstitial pneumonia as reticular or reticular nodular shadows of lung markings in both lungs. HRCT demonstrates bilateral diffuse ground glass liked density shadows. Perivascular thin-walled pneumatocele is common. Pneumatocele induced by LIP is commonly found in the middle lung field, which probably is due to the valve effects caused by infiltration of cells around bronchioles. Manifestations of pneumatocele, together with ground glass liked density shadows, highly indicate LIP. Centrilobular and subpleural small nodules and thickened intralobular septa can be occasionally found.

Case Study 1
A female patient aged 35 years was confirmatively diagnosed as having AIDS by the CDC. She complained of cough, fever and no sputum. Her CD4 T cell count was 45/ μl.

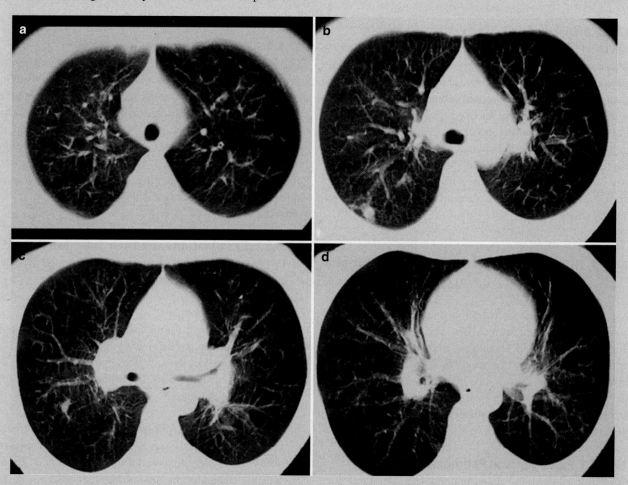

Fig. 17.102 (a–d) HIV/AIDS related lymphoid interstitial pneumonia. (a–d) CT scanning demonstrates thickened and deranged pulmonary markings in both lungs, in reticular appearance; with accompanying multiple small nodular shadows

Case Study 2

A male patient aged 39 years was confirmatively diagnosed as having AIDS by the CDC. He complained of cough and no sputum. His CD4 T cell count was 45/μl.

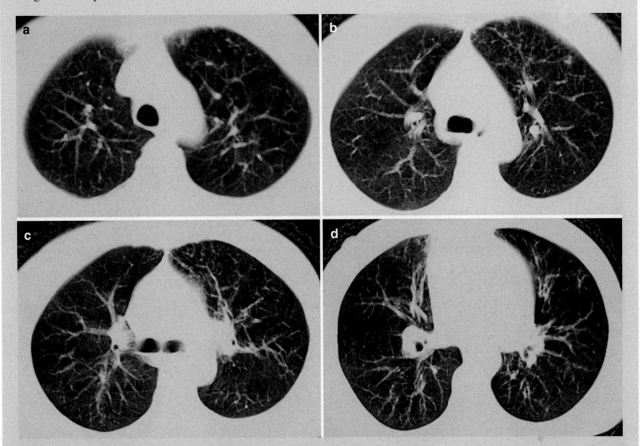

Fig. 17.103 (a–d) HIV/AIDS related lymphoid interstitial pneumonia. (a–d) CT scanning demonstrates thickened and deranged pulmonary markings in both lungs, in reticular appearance; with accompanying multiple small nodular shadows

Case Study 3

A female patient aged 49 years was confirmatively diagnosed as having AIDS by the CDC. She complained of cough and no sputum. Her CD4 T cell count was 7/μl.

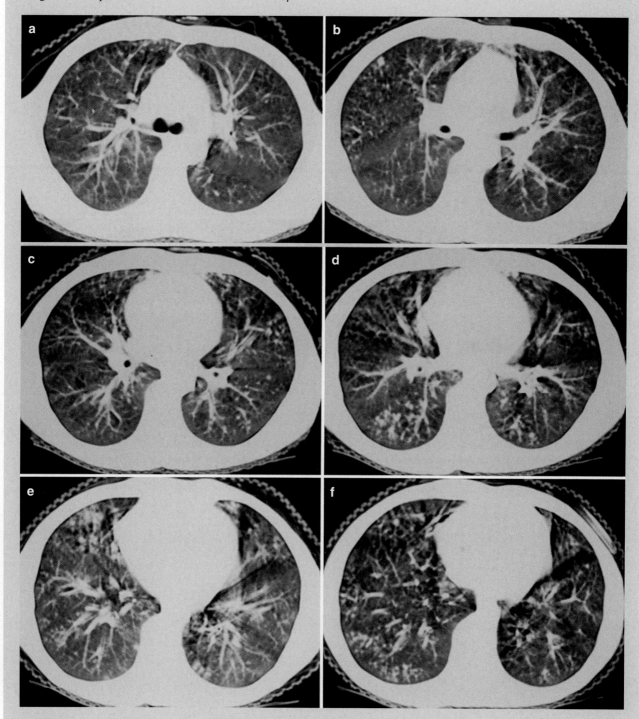

Fig. 17.104 (**a–f**) HIV/AIDS related lymphoid interstitial pneumonia. (**a–f**) CT scanning demonstrates thickened and deranged pulmonary markings in both lungs in reticular appearance, with accompanying multiple small nodular shadows, fusion of some nodules into flaky shadows, and ground glass liked changes in the lung fields

17.5.3.6 Diagnostic Basis

1. Peripheral hemogram demonstrates increased lymphocytes and eosinophilic granulocytes.
2. Myelogram demonstrates increased lymphocytes, plasmocytes and eosinophils.
3. Increased immune globulin, predominantly IgM.
4. Hyoxemia.
5. Pathogenic examination of bronchoalveolar lavage fluids fails to find the pathogen.
6. Pulmonary function examination demonstrates restrictive ventilatory disorder, lower lung compliance and impaired diffusion function.
7. In terms of the diagnostic imaging, chest X-ray demonstrates thickened pulmonary markings or reticular spots shadows, feathery infiltration shadows and nodular shadows in the basal lung and no hilar lymphadenectasis. In the advanced stage, it develops into pulmonary interstitial fibrosis, showing honeycomb liked lung. CT scanning demonstrates small nodular and ground glass liked shadows. Pulmonary function examinations demonstrate reduced lung volume, restrictive ventilatory disorder, lower lung compliance and dysfunctional diffusion. Dysfunctional diffusion is a more sensitive indicator in monitoring the progress of the disease.

17.5.3.7 Differential Diagnosis

HIV/AIDS related lymphoid interstitial pneumonia should be differentiated from allergic pneumonia, carcinomatous lymphangitis and pneumocystis carinii cysts.

17.5.3.8 Discussion

CT scanning with high resolution demonstrates characteristic lesions of HIV/AIDS related lymphoid interstitial pneumonia, including intralobular linear shadows and honeycomb liked changes, with common involvement of the subpleural area and the basal lung. Its characteristic manifestations are clustering gas containing thin-walled cyst in a diameter of 2–10 mm, with clear cyst wall. Shared wall between cysts is its characteristic demonstration. The surrounding ground glass liked density indicates inflammation. Intralobular linear shadows indicate interstitial fibrosis.

17.6   HIV/AIDS Related Pulmonary Parasitic Diseases

17.6.1   HIV/AIDS Related Pulmonary Toxoplasmosis

Pulmonary toxoplasmosis (PT) is caused by the toxoplasma parasitizing in cells. Ludlam et al. firstly proposed the concept of pulmonary toxoplasmosis in 1963 [107], arguing that toxoplasma can cause atypical pneumonia. Later, there are some pathological reports about pulmonary toxoplasmosis or disseminated toxoplasmosis with lung involvement. In recent years, due to the global prevalence of AIDS, the incidence of pulmonary toxoplasmosis is increasing, with most cases being disseminated toxoplasmosis with lung involvement. PT has been one of the important opportunistic infections in patients with immunosuppression, especially AIDS patients.

17.6.1.1 Pathogen and Pathogenesis

HIV/AIDS related pulmonary toxoplasmosis is a zoonotic disease, with cats as its main transmission source, followed by pigs and sheep. People are infected by intake the water or food contaminated by cats' feces or without cooked meat. Immunocompromised AIDS patients are susceptible to this disease, and its occurrence is rare in immunocompetent people. After its invasion into the human body, the sporozoite in the cystozygote and intracystic cystozoite overflows to penetrate the intestinal wall mucosa and spread to the whole body tissues along with blood or lymph flow. The brain, heart, lymph nodes, and lung are the most vulnerable tissues and organs for the infection. Any abnormality in the process of defense mechanism can cause impaired immune functions to eliminate the toxoplasma, which ultimately causes systemic and pulmonary infections. Pulmonary toxoplasma infection may also be caused by the blood borne spreading of reactivated toxoplasma infection in other body parts, with no exclusion of reactivated pulmonary infection or primary pulmonary infection.

17.6.1.2 Pathophysiological Basis

Ludlam et al. generally nominated toxoplasmosis as atypical pneumonia [107]. Catterall et al. divided toxoplasmosis into three types: necrosis, inflammatory infiltration and toxoplasma invasion [109]. It can also be classified as type A: subclinical or occult infection; type B: interstitial and atypical pneumonia; type C: necrotic pneumonia; type D: lobar pneumonia; and type E: granulomas pneumonia (toxoplasmoma). By naked eyes observation, the involved lungs are solid, with congestion and red brown section. The pleura have bleeding spots, with moderate peribronchial lymphadenectasis. Under a light microscope, there is exudation of serous fluids in alveolar cavities, occasional formation of transparent membrane or fibrin purulent exudation, infiltration of small quantity neutrophils, proliferation and shedding of alveolar wall cells, and trophozoite and/or cysts of toxoplasma in epithelial cells and macrophages. The pulmonary interstitium may have infiltration of lymphocytes and plasmocytes as well as visible fibroblasts and macrophages. The granuloma changes are also found in the lung tissues, with central stripes or localized necrosis and surrounding lymphocytes and small quantity multinucleated giant cells. It is difficult to find toxoplasma in granuloma, but it can be found in the normal tissues around or near the granuloma.

17.6.1.3 Clinical Symptoms and Signs

Almost all cases of AIDS complicated by pulmonary toxoplasmosis are caused by disseminated toxoplasmosis with pulmonary involvement. It is commonly diffuse pulmonary inflammation with serious symptoms, including high fever, cough, cyanosis, breathing difficulty, possible occurrence of skin rashes, lymphadenectasis and meningitis. The chronic cases may have long-term low grade fever, cough, and weight loss.

17.6.1.4 Examinations and Their Selection
Pathogen Examinations
Direct light microscopy of the specimen smear and enprint such as blood, cerebrospinal fluid, bone marrow, anterior aqueous humor, phlegm, urine, saliva, and other osmotic solutions, as well as lymph nodes, muscle tissue or other living tissues can be performed for pathogen examinations.

Immunological Assays
Sabin proposed that the staining test have high sensitivity and specificity according to the findings that mixture of fresh toxoplasma with normal serum can be stained deep by alkaline methylene blue staining, while its mixture with immune serum can be stained light or blank by the same staining. Other assays including indirect fluorescent antibody, indirect blood coagulation, and complement fixation test can provide valuable reference for the diagnosis.

Pathological Examinations
Toxoplasm is tested in pathological eaminations that can provide valuable reference for the diagnosis.

Diagnostic Imaging
Chest X-ray is the most commonly used diagnostic imaging examination. And chest CT scanning can be applied for the differential diagnosis.

17.6.1.5 Imaging Demonstrations
Imaging findings of HIV/AIDS related pulmonary toxoplasmosis can be divided into four types: bronchial pneumonia, interstitial pneumonia, pleuritis and complication of cardiovascular disease. The type of bronchial pneumonia is also known as lobular pneumonia, with thickened pulmonary markings that distribute along with the bronchi in the middle and lower lung fields, scattered patchy shadows with uneven density and blurry boundaries, fusion of some shadows into large flaky shadow and widened hilar shadow. The type of interstitial pneumonia is demonstrated as reticular and nodular shadows. The interstitial lesions widen the space between the bronchiole and the alveolar wall, with stripes and flocculent shadows. The type of pleuritis is rare, with signs of pleural effusion. The type of complication of cardiovascular disease is demonstrated as heart failure (acute pulmonary edema), with signs of pericardial effusion.

Case Study

A male patient aged 39 years was confirmatively diagnosed as having AIDS by the CDC. He complained of cough and fever. His CD4 T cell count was 29/μl.

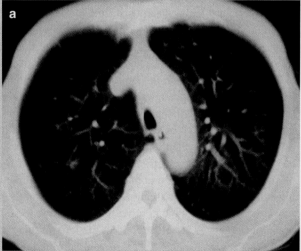
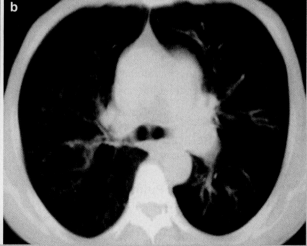
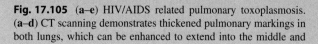

Fig. 17.105 (a–e) HIV/AIDS related pulmonary toxoplasmosis. (a–d) CT scanning demonstrates thickened pulmonary markings in both lungs, which can be enhanced to extend into the middle and outer zones of lungs, in grid liked appearance that is more obvious in the dorsal segment of the lungs. (e) It is demonstrated to have clustering toxoplasma tachyzoites

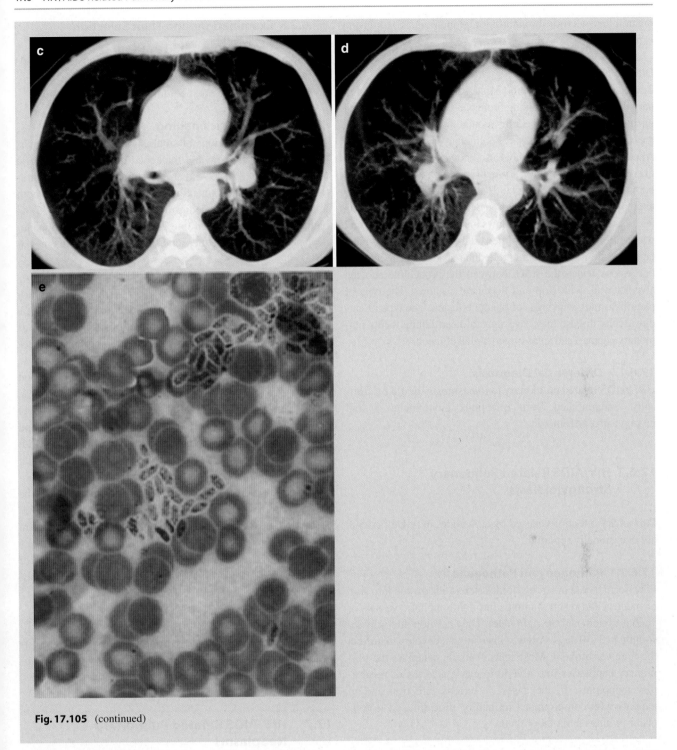

Fig. 17.105 (continued)

17.6.1.6 Diagnostic Basis
Pathogen Examinations

By direct light microscopy, toxoplasma tachyzoites can be found in the specimens such as blood, cerebrospinal fluid, bone marrow, anterior aqueous humor, phlegm, urine, saliva, and other osmotic solutions, as well as lymph nodes, muscle tissues or other living tissues.

Immunological Assays

The fluorescent antibody and complement fixation test are positive.

Pathological Examinations

The biopsy tissue culture and inoculation test are positive. In the lesions and their surrounding tissues of interstitial pneumonia, necrotic bronchitis or granuloma, Toxoplasma can be found.

Diagnostic Imaging

The diagnostic imaging demonstrates any one type of pulmonary toxoplasmosis, including bronchial pneumonia, interstitial pneumonia, pleuritis and cardiovascular disease, can be used as the evidence for the diagnosis of pulmonary toxoplasmosis. The type of bronchial pneumonia is also known as lobular pneumonia, with thickened pulmonary markings with a distribution in both middle and lower lung fields along with the bronchi, scattered patchy shadows with uneven density and blurry boundaries, fusion of some patchy shadows into large flaky shadow and widened hilum. The type of interstitial pneumonia has typical demonstrations of reticular and nodular shadows. The interstitial lesions widen the space between the bronchiole and the alveolar wall, with strip and flocculent shadows. The type of pleuritis is rare, with signs of pleural effusion. The type of cardiovascular disease may have signs of heart failure (acute pulmonary edema), and signs of pericardial effusion.

17.6.1.7 Differential Diagnosis

HIV/AIDS related pulmonary toxoplasmosis should be clinically differentiated from infectious mononucleosis and mycoplasma pneumonia.

17.6.2 HIV/AIDS Related Pulmonary Strongyloidiasis

Pulmonary infections caused by nematodes in AIDS patients are occasionally reported.

17.6.2.1 Pathogen and Pathogenesis

Filariform larvae of strongyloides stercoralis invade into skin or mucosa and reach the lungs through lymphatic vessels or venous system and the right heart. They develop into schistosomula in 3–30 days. A few schistosomula develop mature in the lungs or bronchi. Most schistosomula penetrate the pulmonary capillaries into alveoli to cause a series of respiratory symptoms. In the cases of serious infection and in patients with compromised immunity, disseminated lesions occur in lungs and other organs.

17.6.2.2 Clinical Symptoms and Signs

HIV/AIDS related pulmonary strongyloidiasis can have manifestations of local small bleeding spots, pimples, migratory linear or strips urticaria on skin, as well as manifestations of allergic bronchitis, lobular pneumonia or asthma. AIDS patient may have severe diffuse infection and systemic infection, with symptoms of fever, severe cough, expectoration, hemoptysis, shortness of breath, breathing difficulty, and asthma.

17.6.2.3 Examinations and Their Selection

1. Laboratory tests
2. The pathological examinations include biopsy tissue culture and inoculation test.
3. Chest X-ray is the most commonly used examination.

17.6.2.4 Diagnostic Imaging

There are demonstrations of small spots and flaky shadows, thickened hilar shadow and thickened pulmonary markings. Mitchell reported in 1992 that interstitial or alveolar infiltration in both lungs accounts for 62 %, nodular shadows in both lungs 15 %, hilar or mediastinal lymphadenectasis 26 %, pleural fluids 42 %, septal line 25 %, mediastinal lymphadenectasis and ascites are the important clues for the diagnosis.

17.6.2.5 Diagnostic Basis

1. The clinical manifestations of HIV/AIDS related pulmonary strongyloidiasis are non-specific. Its diagnosis depends on the etiological examinations. The findings of Strongyloides sterocralis in the patient's sputum and feces can define the diagnosis.
2. By laboratory tests, WBC count in peripheral blood increases to 20×10^9/L; eosinophils granulocytes 25–30 %, or even as high as 70–80 %; the serum total lgE level increases by 50 %; 90 % cases with blood serum lgG and lgE of filariform larvae antigen positive. In the cases with femal strongyloides stercoralis parasitizing in the bronchial epithelium, rhabditiform larva, filariform larva, schistosomula, adult strongyloides stercoralis and the eggs can be found in fresh phlegm, which can define the diagnosis.
3. Pathological examinations including biopsy tissue culture and inoculation test are positive.
4. By chest X-ray, the lungs have small spots and flakes of shadows, thickened hilar shadow and thickened pulmonary markings.

17.6.2.6 Differential Diagnosis

HIV/AIDS related pulmonary strongyloidiasis should be differentiated from HIV/AIDS related pulmonary toxoplasmosis, infectious mononucleosis and mycoplasma pneumonia.

17.7 HIV/AIDS Related Pulmonary Neoplasms

17.7.1 HIV/AIDS Related Lymphoma

Pulmonary infiltration of HIV/AIDS related malignant lymphoma commonly has three types: Primary pulmonary lymphoma, which is rare and accounts for 0.5 % of primary pulmonary neoplasms, and 3 % of extranodal lymphomas. Cadranel et al. summarized the characteristics of three typical clonal proliferative diseases in lymphatic system [90],

with primary pulmonary lesions. Pulmonary low malignant B cell lymphoma is the most common primary pulmonary lymphoma which is derived from mucosa related lymphoid tissue. The manifestations include slowly decreased alveolar transparency. Pulmonary high malignant B cell lymphoma is extremely rare, which often occurs with singular lesion and primary disease such as immunodeficiency.

17.7.1.1 Pathogen and Pathogenesis

HIV/AIDS related malignant lymphoma is mostly caused by compromised immunity. HIV/AIDS related Hodgkin's lymphoma is relatively rare. There are also reports about HIV/AIDS related T cell lymphoma with pulmonary involvement.

17.7.1.2 Pathophysiological Basis

HIV/AIDS related malignant lymphomas are mostly highly malignant large cells lymphoma. Cerebral lymphoma is one of the defining diseases of AIDS. It has been reported that the clinical incidence of pulmonary infiltration by malignant lymphoma is 10–20 %, but 29–50 % by autopsy.

17.7.1.3 Clinical Symptoms and Signs

In the early stage, it is commonly asymptomatic. With its progression, symptoms of dry cough, suffocation, and small quantity clear phlegm occur. Mediastinal lymphadenosis includes lymphadenectasis to compress the trachea by, blood vessels and nerves and lead to breathing difficulty, superior vena caval obstruction syndrome, and hoarse voice. The pulmonary parenchyma lesions include reticular structure in the lungs. The clinical symptoms are cough, expectoration, suffocation and breathing difficulty.

17.7.1.4 Examinations and Their Selection

1. Laboratory tests
2. Pathological biopsy, tissue culture and inoculation test.

3. The diagnostic imaging examinations are the most commonly used examinations for the diagnosis.

17.7.1.5 Diagnostic Imaging

The imaging demonstrations of HIV/AIDS related malignant lymphomas include:

1. Mediastinal lymphadenectasis is the most commonly found pulmonary manifestations of malignant lymphoma. The lesions are mainly located in anterior and middle mediastinum, in asymmetric wave liked or lobulated mass. It occurs unilaterally or bilaterally, isolated or fusion.
2. The incidence of pulmonary parenchymal lesions is 20–30 %. Chest X-ray demonstrates mediastinal lymph nodes extending directly into the lungs, which is susceptible to confusion with pneumonia. They are demonstrated as round shadows in the lung fields or distribute in the whole lung fields. Chest X-ray demonstrates the lymphatic spread of lesions as military nodules in different sizes or isolated intrapulmonary nodules or cavities, commonly accompanying with mediastinal hilar lymphadenectasis. In the cases with its occurrence secondary to endobronchial membrane, obstructive pneumonia or atelectasis can be caused. Some patients may have diffuse pulmonary interstitial changes. Pulmonary infiltration by non-Hodgkin's lymphoma can also be divided into four types: (1) Nodular type; (2) Pneumonia-alveolar type; (3) bronchial-vascular-lymphatic type, which can be further divided into the central bronchial-vascular type, and diffuse lymphatic type; (4) diffuse lymphatic type can have lesions of reticular or reticular nodular infiltration and its progression into patchy changes.
3. Miliary-blood borne spreading type is rare.
4. The pleural lesions is mainly pleural effusion, with bloody or serous pleural fluid.

Case Study 1

A male patient aged 43 years was confirmatively diagnosed as having AIDS by the CDC. He complained of chest distress and cough for more than 1 month. His CD4 T cell count was 56/μl.

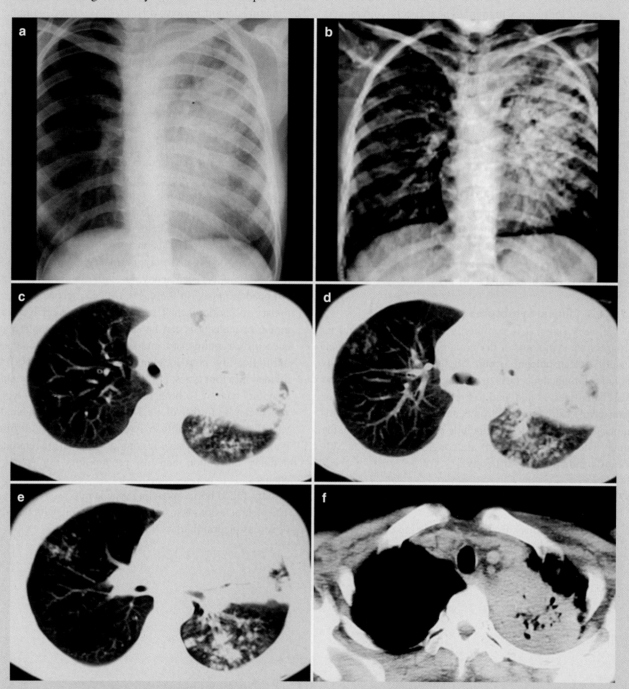

Fig. 17.106 (**a–h**) HIV/AIDS related lymphoma. (**a–b**) DR demonstrates enlarged and thickened left hilum in a huge mass shadow. High KV demonstrates a huge mass shadow in the hilum. (**c–h**) CT scanning of the pulmonary window demonstrates a huge high density mass shadow in the left hilum, surrounding nodular fusion shadows in the lung tissues. CT scanning of the mediastinal window demonstrates a huge high density mass shadow in the left hilum, with air bronchogram sign in the shadow

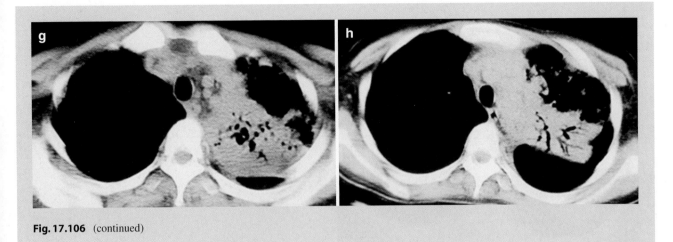

Fig. 17.106   (continued)

Case Study 2

A male patient aged 41 years was confirmatively diagnosed as having AIDS by the CDC. He complained of chest distress and chest pain for more than 2 months. His CD4 T cell count was 36/μl.

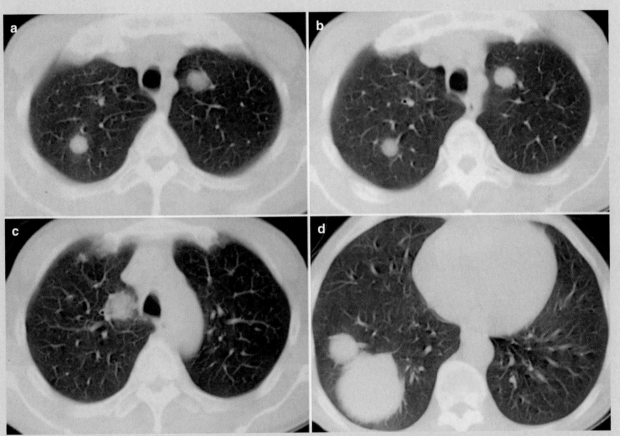

Fig. 17.107   (a–e) HIV/AIDS related lymphoma. (a–e) CT scanning of the pulmonary and mediastinal windows demonstrates multiple round liked nodular shadows with increased density in both lung fields, with clear boundaries; large soft tissue mass shadows in the right lower lung, with slightly lobulated boundaries and spikes. (f–i) CT scanning of the pulmonary and mediastinal windows for reexamination after radiation therapy demonstrates shrinkage of intrapulmonary nodules and masses

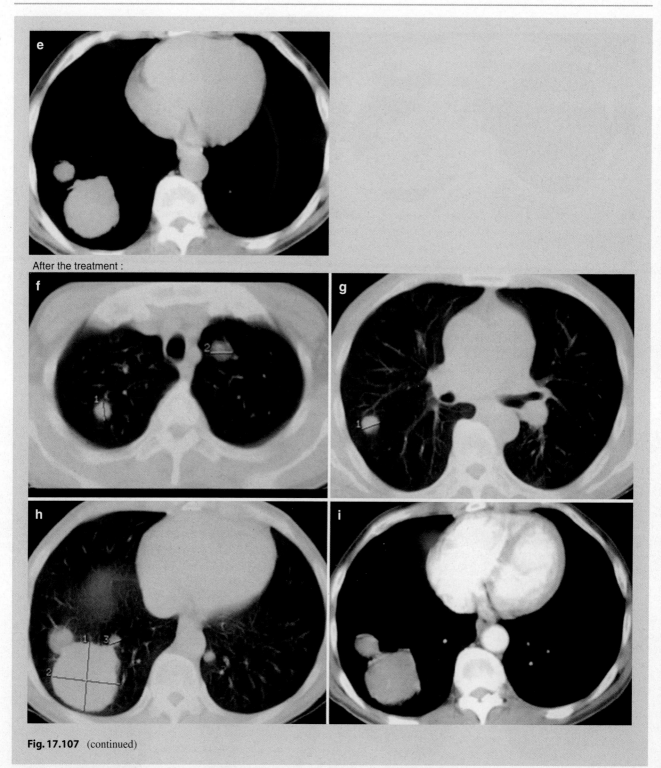

After the treatment :

Fig. 17.107   (continued)

Case Study 3

A male patient aged 35 years was confirmatively diagnosed as having AIDS by the CDC. He complained of chest distress and breathing difficulty for 15 days. His CD4 T cell count was 66/μl.

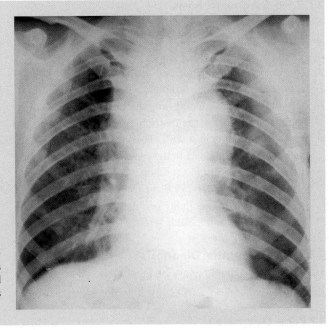

Fig. 17.108 HIV/AIDS related lymphoma. DR demonstrates widened upper middle mediastinum in a dense shadow, enlarged and thickened hilum, thickened and blurry pulmonary markings with diffuse ground glass liked changes

Case Study 4

A male patient aged 26 years was confirmatively diagnosed as having AIDS by the CDC. He had a history of homosexual behaviors and was hospitalized due to a progressively enlarged subaxillary mass for 3 months. HIV antibody was confirmed positive and his CD4 T cell count was 363/μl.

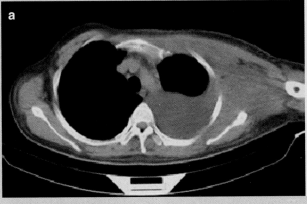
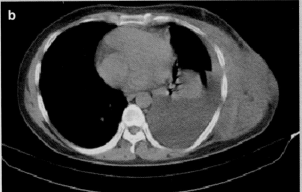

Fig. 17.109 (**a**, **b**) HIV/AIDS related lymphoma. (**a**, **b**) CT scanning demonstrates a huge soft tissue mass shadow in the left lateral chest wall, with a maximal size of about 7.7 × 13.0 cm and occupying 30 sections with 8 mm in thickness of each section and with the upmost to the supraclavicular area and the bottom in the level of thoracic 12th vertebral body in the lower chest wall. There are also large quantity left pleural effusion and parenchymal changes of the left lower lobe with atelectasis. In the left chest cavity, large quantity liquid density shadows can be found, with compressed lung tissues to the hilum. By puncture and biopsy of the subaxillary mass, the diagnosis is defined as diffuse large B cell lymphoma

17.7.1.6 Diagnostic Basis

1. The clinical symptom of difficulty breathing.
2. By pathological examination of lung tissue biopsy, lymphoma cells are found.
3. The imaging demonstrations include interstitial infiltration with mediastinal lymphadenectasis or intrapulmonary mass shadows, being singular or multiple with clear boundaries. The masses distribute in the lungs or in the mediastinum and chest wall. The incidence of lymphadenectasis is about 25 %. In the cases with pleural involvement, tumor occurs in the chest wall. The incidence of pleural effusion is 30–50 %. There are also pulmonary demonstrations of reticular nodular shadows, thickened bronchial walls and lobular septum linear shadows.

17.7.1.7 Differential Diagnosis

HIV/AIDS related pulmonary lymphoma should be differentiated from lung cancer, metastatic tumor and tuberculoma.

17.7.1.8 Discussion

HIV/AIDS related pulmonary lymphoma can be classified into large cells type (Immunoblastic type) and Burkitt liked type. The vast majority of them have the morphology of the B cells, and most are related to Epstein-Barr viral genome. Its occurrence is at a CD4 T cell count being lower than 100/μl. Hodgkin's lymphoma tend to occur in the early stage of AIDS, with a CD4 T cell count being above 200/μl. The most common imaging demonstrations include singular or multiple nodules. The singular lesions have a scattering distribution, with clear boundaries. The smooth nodules should be diagnosed as HIV/AIDS related lymphoma. The larger mass sometimes may have cavities in it. Interstitial infiltration with no masses or nodules is rare. Another rare manifestation of HIV/AIDS related B cell lymphoma is pleural, pericardial or abdominal cavity effusion without scattered masses, which is known as coelom-derived or primary exudative lymphoma.

17.7.2 HIV/AIDS Related Kaposi's Sarcoma

17.7.2.1 Pathogen and Pathogenesis

In the year of 1994, Moore and Chang identified gamma herpes virus in tissues of Kaposi's sarcoma and proved their relationship. Kaposi's sarcoma can be found in any stage of HIV infection, which may occur at even normal level of CD4 T cell count. However, it mostly occurs at a CD4 T cell count being lower than $2,200 \times 10^6/L$. The results of epidemiological studies and the fact of HHV-8 being isolated from Kaposi's sarcoma tissues have demonstrated that Kaposi's sarcoma is closely related to HHV-8 infection. As a result, HHV-8 is known as Kaposi's sarcoma related herpes virus. In patients with HIV/AIDS related Kaposi's sarcoma, its serologic positive rate is 100 %. Kaposi's sarcoma cells can produce IL-6, during which IL-6 plays a role as an autocrine factor to maintain the cell growth, paracrine cytokines, stimulate proliferation of other interstitial cells and induct the vascular growth. Therefore, Kaposi's sarcoma is a kind of tumor with abundant blood vessels. Before the application of HARRT, the incidence of Kaposi's sarcoma in male homosexuals is 21 %. After the clinical application of HARRT treatment, the incidence is decreasing. In addition to HHV-8, some studies indicated that most patients with Kaposi's sarcoma have HIA-DR5 alleles, suggesting a possible relationship between Kaposi's sarcoma and the heredity.

17.7.2.2 Pathophysiological Basis

There is no obvious difference between HIV/AIDS related Kaposi's sarcoma and classic Kaposi's sarcoma in pathological changes. Early pathological manifestations are chronic inflammation or granulomatous inflammation, with formation of new vascular and lymphatic vessels and accompanying edema and bleeding. The findings of large and protruding endothelial cells in granuloma tissue with accompanying erythrocytic exudation and hemosiderin particles have great significance for the early diagnosis. The pathological changes in the advanced stage are significant proliferation of the endothelial cells, and proliferation of fibroblasts around capillaries. In the advanced stage, the lesions are often accompanied by extensive connective tissue hyperplasia, which presents difficulty for its differentiation from common sarcoma. When it is difficult to define the diagnosis by light microscopy, immunohistochemical examinations can be used to define the diagnosis. The pathological changes are characterized by lesions confined to the epithelial lamina propria, gathering of spindle cells with mild heteromorphism around many lacuna vasorum with irregular lumen, erythrocytic exudation and hemosiderin sedimentation. The atypical lacuna vasorum can be compressed by proliferative spindle cells to be absent. Vascular endothelial cells and peripheral spindle cells may have mitotic phase in the advanced stage, with increased heteromorphism cells. The inflammatory cells are mainly plasma cells, with acidophilic corpuscles and PAS staining positive, which can assist the pathological diagnosis.

17.7.2.3 Clinical Symptoms and Signs

Pulmonary Kaposi's sarcoma in AIDS patients rarely has symptoms. It is commonly concurrent with pulmonary opportunistic infections, with symptoms of cough, difficulty breathing and fever. Other symptoms are related with the location of the tumors. The involvement of trachea or bronchi can cause luminal stenosis. The mediastinal tumor can compress and obstruct lymph vessels to cause pulmonary edema or a large quantity pleural fluids, which result in respiratory difficulty, and even respiratory failure.

17.7.2.4 Examinations and Their Selection

(1) Sampling by bronchoscopy or endoscopy to prepare pathological section.
(2) Chest X-ray demonstrates its typical manifestation of pleural effusion.

17.7.2.5 Imaging Demonstrations

DR demonstrates enlarged and deranged hilum in both lungs in bird nest liked appearance. There is light density flaky shadows in the both lower lungs. CT scanning demonstrates multiple rounds liked nodular shadows in the middle and lower lung fields of both lungs with clear boundaries. There are also mediastinal and hilar lymphadenectasis, with common involvement of the pleura and bilateral pleural effusion in a small quantity.

Case Study 1

A male patient aged 33 years was confirmatively diagnosed as having AIDS by the CDC. He had been detected as HIV positive for 5 months, with complaints of recurrent cough and nausea for 10 days and was hospitalized on Jan. 7, 2004. The transmission route was unknown because he denied histories of intraveneous drug abuse, paid blood donation, blood transfusion and unhealthy sexual behaviors. Five months ago, he was diagnosed as AIDS in the stage of AIDS in our hospital, and hospitalized to treat PCP, with a CD4 T cell count of 17/µl. His symptoms were quickly relieved after PCP treatment and he continued the antiviral therapy for almost 5 months after being discharged. By physical examinations, he was in poor spiritual condition, a light blue nodule in size of 0.5×0.5 cm in the left upper chest wall with medium hardness, palpable lymph nodes in size of 1.0×2.0 in the opisthotic area and inguen, no tenderness and being movable. By the digital rectal examination, a palpable prominent nodule with wide base at 4 cm 7 points away from the anus, with flexible texture and smooth surface. By the auxiliary examinations, WBC 3.9×10⁹/L, NEµT 48.3 %, LYM 34.9 %, MON 7.4 %, EOS 9.0 %, RBC 3.27×10¹²/L, HGB 126 g/L, PLT 210×10⁹/L, routine urine test normal, blood sedimentation 16 mm/h. By hepatitis B examinations, HBsAg, Anti-HBe and Anti-HBe positive. His CD4 T cell count was 91/µl. By abdominal B ultrasound, multiple low echo nodules in the abdominal cavity, the largest in size of 1.2×1.0 cm, which are suspected to be enlarged lymph nodes. On Jan. 14, he received inguinal lymph node biopsy, with pathological report of Kaposi's sarcoma. During the treatment and following up, the involvement of lungs, digestive tract, lymph nodes and skin is suspected, with the diagnosis of phase II Kaposi's sarcoma and chemotherapy was recommended. Reexamination by chest X-ray demonstrated normal cardiopulmonary phrenic. Abdominal B ultrasound failed to find enlarged lymph nodes. CT scanning demonstrated shrinkage of lesions in both lungs and mediastinal lymph nodes, with only palpable soybean sized submandibular lymph node. By examinations after chemotherapy, CD4 T cell count 67/µl, viral load 63,000 copies/ml. The patients had multimorphological erythema drug eruptions, which was suspected as drug allergies of chemotherapy, which were absent after symptomatic treatment. The following ups so far show no recurrence of Kaposi's sarcoma, with his CD4 T cell count fluctuating around 400/µl. He can work as usual.

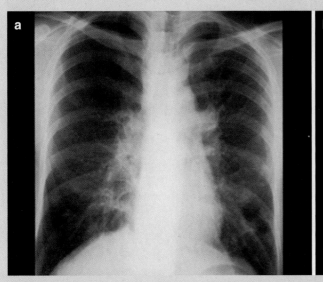
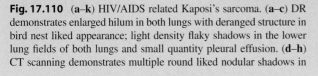
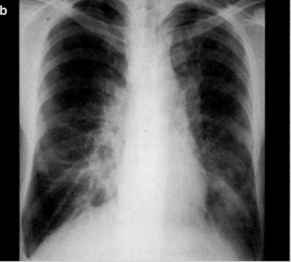

Fig. 17.110 (**a–k**) HIV/AIDS related Kaposi's sarcoma. (**a–c**) DR demonstrates enlarged hilum in both lungs with deranged structure in bird nest liked appearance; light density flaky shadows in the lower lung fields of both lungs and small quantity pleural effusion. (**d–h**) CT scanning demonstrates multiple round liked nodular shadows in the middle and lower lung fields of both lungs with clear boundaries, multiple mediastinal and hilar enlarged lymph nodes. (**i, j**) HE staining demonstrates large quantity spindle cells or fusiform cells as well as thick stained nucleoli also in spindle shape. (**k**) Reexamination after treatment demonstrates no abnormalities in both lungs

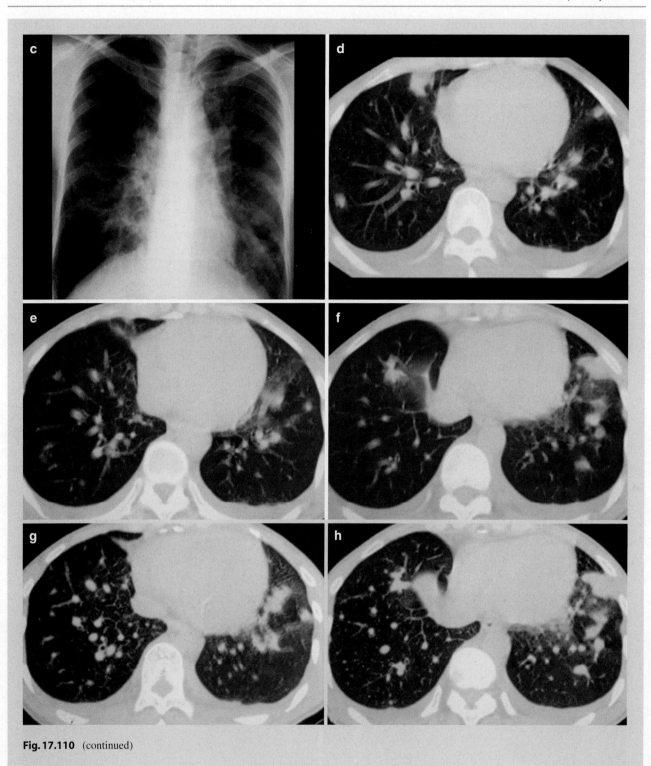

Fig. 17.110 (continued)

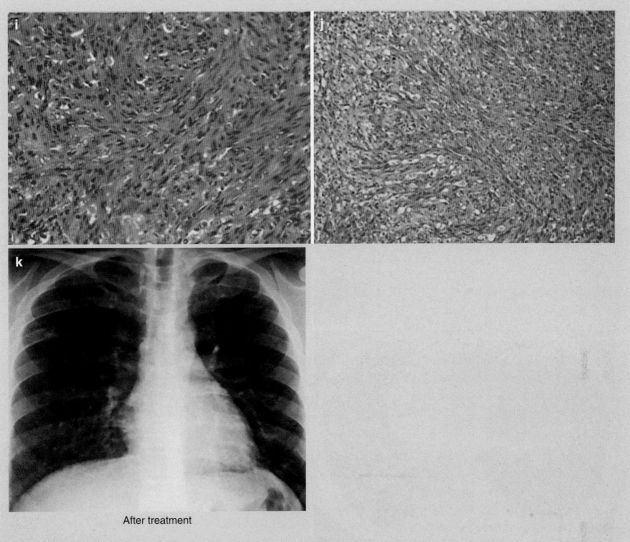

After treatment

Fig. 17.110 (continued)

Case Study 2

A female patient aged 38 years was confirmatively diagnosed as having AIDS by the CDC. She complained of recurrent cough for 10 days and had a history of unhealthy sexual behaviors. Her CD4 T cell count was 35/μl.

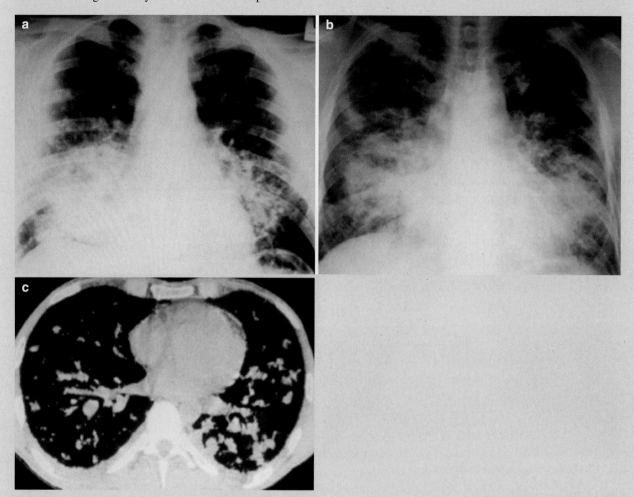

Fig. 17.111 (a–c) HIV/AIDS related Kaposi's sarcoma. (**a, b**) DR demonstrates enlarged hilum in both lungs with deranged structure in bird nest liked appearance, light density flaky shadows in lower lung fields of both lungs. (**c**) CT scanning demonstrates multiple round liked nodular shadows in both middle lower lung fields with clear boundaries, multiple mediastinal and hilar lymphadenectasis, and small quantity pleural effusion in bilateral thoracic cavities

Case Study 3

A male patient aged 39 years was confirmatively diagnosed as having AIDS by the CDC. He complained of recurrent cough for more than 1 month and had a history of unhealthy sexual behaviors. His CD4 T cell count was 55/μl.

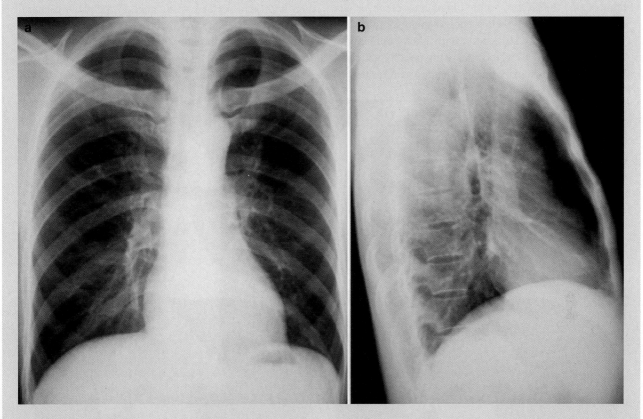

Fig. 17.112 (**a**, **b**) HIV/AIDS related Kaposi's sarcoma. (**a**, **b**) DR demonstrates enlarged hilum in both lungs with deranged structure in bird nest liked appearance

Case Study 4

A male patient aged 36 years was confirmatively diagnosed as having AIDS by the CDC. He had a history of homosexual behaviors, with complaints of fever and cough for 2 months as well as chest distress for more than 20 days. Since, July 2010, fever with a body temperature of about 37.5–37.8 °C occurs, with cough, yellowish bloody sputum, and dark purplish patchy skin rashes.

By examinations, his anti-treponema pallidum antibody positive, multiple dark purplish patchy skin rashes on the face, eyelid, lower jaw, hairline, chest and abdomen with skin surface desquamation, palpable bilateral cervical lymphadenectasis and the largest in size of 10×19 mm. By laboratory tests, WBC 5.98×10^9/L, N 78.74 %, RBC 2.22×10^{12}/L, HGB 71 g/L, PLT 204×10^9/L, CD4 12/μl.

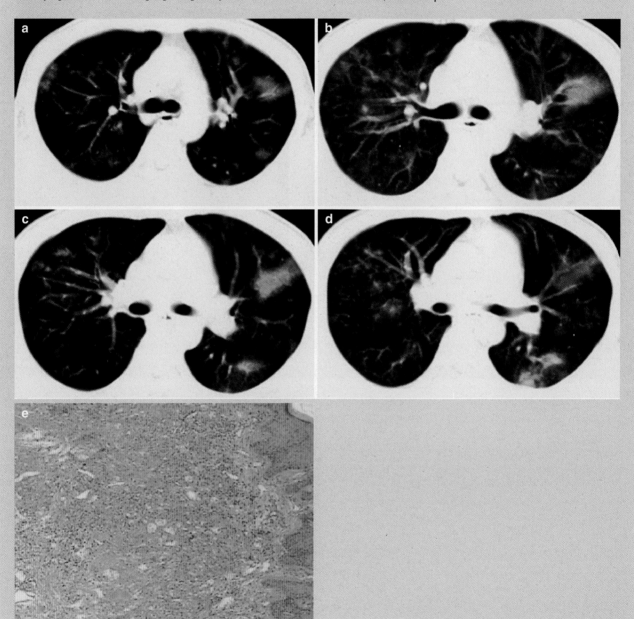

Fig. 17.113 (**a–e**) HIV/AIDS related Kaposi's sarcoma. (**a–d**) Chest CT scanning demonstrates scattered cloudy, mass and flake liked or nodular shadows with increased density. (**e**) Pathological biopsy demonstrates large quantity heteromorphological spindle cells with large thick stained nucleoli, which are in line with the diagnosis of Kaposi's sarcoma. (**f–i**) Cured HIV/AIDS related Kaposi's sarcoma. (**f–i**) Reexamination after treatment demonstrates absent lesions in both lungs, with clear lung fields

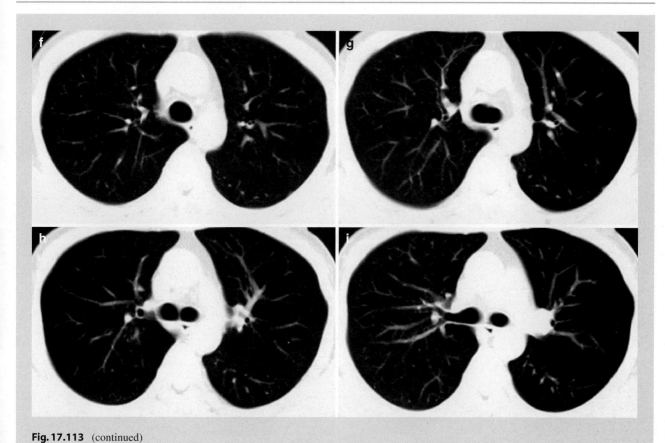

Fig. 17.113   (continued)

Case Study 5

A male patient aged 27 years was confirmatively diagnosed as having AIDS by the CDC. He complained of cough for more than 2 months, chest distress for more than 1 month, and bloody sputum for half a month and was hospitalized. He had a history of homosexual behaviors. By examinations on admission, multiple round purplish blue skin rashes nodules on the limbs. His CD4 T cell count was 9/μl.

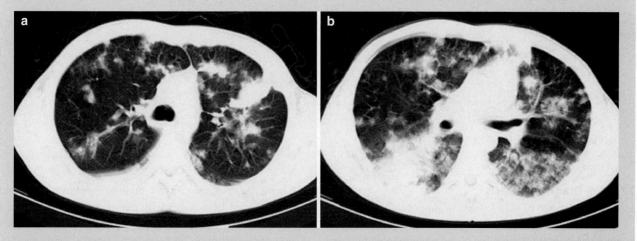

Fig. 17.114   (**a–h**) HIV/AIDS related Kaposi's sarcoma. (**a–d**) CT scanning demonstrates scattered cloudy mass and flakes liked or nodular shadows with increased density in both lungs with uneven density and unclear boundaries, fusion and parenchymal changes of some lesions, more lesions in the lower lobe of both lungs and mostly with parenchymal changes. (**e, f**) Pathological biopsy demonstrates large quantity heteromorphological spindle cells with large and thick stained nucleoli, which are in line with the manifestations of Kaposi's sarcoma. (**g, h**) Immunohistochemical demonstrates positive of C3 and C4

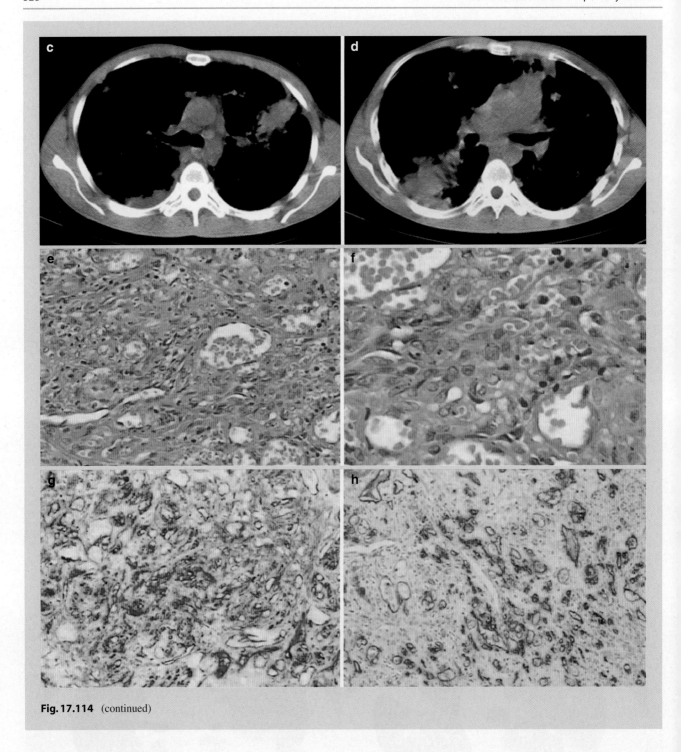

Fig. 17.114   (continued)

17.7.2.6 Diagnostic Basis

1. The appearance of skin lesions of angiosarcoma is gray, grayish black or purplish blue infiltrative nodules or confluent plaques, with possible accompanying bleeding and ulcers. Patients with pulmonary Kaposi's sarcoma are often accompanied with skin involvement, with the common manifestation of difficulty breathing.

2. Chest X-ray demonstrates nodular infiltration around the hilum of both lungs with deranged structure in bird nest liked appearance or infiltration of diffuse reticular nodular infiltration and pleural bloody effusion. CT scanning demonstrates enlarged and blurry hilum of both lungs, multiple intrapulmonary round liked nodular shadows with clear boundaries. The CT scanning

demonstrations can also be flaky flocculent areas with blurry density or parenchymal density areas along with bronchi.

3. Lung puncture for histopathological biopsy demonstrates irregular vascular lumen in the dermis, proliferation of endothelial cell with accompanying heteromorphism. In some cases, there are tumor masses composed of spindle cells and epithelial cells.

17.7.2.7 Differential Diagnosis
Other Sarcoma and Vascular Tumor
HIV/AIDS related Kaposi's sarcoma should be differentiated from other sarcoma and vascular tumor. KS invasion of the digestive mucosa can cause bleeding and upper gastrointestinal symptoms. The pathological lesions can be diagnosed by upper gastrointestinal endoscopy or biopsy. In the cases of no fever and exclusion of infections, the typical imaging demonstrations and bronchoscopy findings can define the diagnosis of pulmonary KS.

Pneumocystis Carinii Pneumonia
HIV/AIDS related Kaposi's sarcoma should be differentiated from Pneumocystis carinii pneumonia. The lesions of PCP are mostly symmetric ground glass liked density shadows extending outwards from the hilum in both lungs. In the middle and advanced stages, nodules, fibrosis and cavities occur, rarely with pleural effusion.

17.7.3 HIV/AIDS Related Lung Cancer

17.7.3.1 Pathogen and Pathogenesis
Lung cancer commonly refers to the cancer in lung parenchyma, usually does not include those mesodermal tumors originating from other pleura, or other malignancies like carcinoid, malignant lymphoma, or metastatic malignancies for other body parts. Therefore, the following lung cancer we are discussing about refers to the malignancies originating from bronchial, or bronchiolar epithelial cells, accounting for 90–95 % of the lung parenchyma malignancies. The cause of lung cancer is still not completely known. Data have indicated that the risk factors of lung cancer include smoking (including second-hand smoke), asbestos, radon, arsenic, ionizing radiation, halogen alkenes, polycyclic aromatic compounds and nickel.

Smoking
Long-term smoking can cause proliferation of the bronchial mucosal epithelial cells and proliferation of squamous epithelium to induce squamous epithelium carcinoma or undifferentiated small cell carcinoma. Non-smokers can also develop lung cancer, but adenocarcinoma is more common among them.

Atmosphere Pollution

Occupational Factors
Long-term exposure to radioactive substances, like uranium and radium, and its derivatives; carcinogenic hydrocarbons, like arsenic, chromium, nickel, copper, tin, ferri, coal tar, bitumen oil, petroleum, asbestos and mustard gas, all can induce lung cancer, which is commonly squamous carcinoma and undifferentiated small cell carcinoma.

Chronic Pulmonary Diseases
Some chronic pulmonary diseases, such as tuberculosis, silicosis and pneumoconiosis, can concurrent with lung cancer. In the cases with these chronic pulmonary diseases, the incidence of cancer is higher than the general population. In addition, bronchopulmonary chronic inflammation and pulmonary fibrous scar lesions may cause metaplasia or hyperplasia of squamous epithelium during their healing processes, based on which some cases can develop into cancer.

Internal Factors of the Human Body
The internal factors of the human body include family heredity, compromised immunity, metabolism and endocrine dysfunction.

17.7.3.2 Pathophysiological Basis
The lung cancers distribute more in the right lung than in the left lung, more in the upper lobe than in the lower lobe. Its locations range from the major bronchus to the bronchioles. The central type of lung cancer has its origination from the major bronchial lobes and locates adjacent to the pulmonary hilum. The peripheral type of lung cancer has its origination from the lower parts of pulmonary segment bronchi and locates in the peripheral areas in the lungs. In the growth process of the lung cancer, it causes the extension and dilation of the bronchial walls, and penetrates the bronchial walls to invade the adjacent lung tissues and form masses. Meanwhile it intrudes into the bronchi to cause luminal stenosis or obstruction. With its further progression and dissemination, it spreads from the lungs and directly extends into the chest walls, mediastinum, heart, major vessels and other adjacent organs and tissues. Lung cancer can also transfer to other parts of the body along with blood and lymph flows or disseminates to other pulmonary lobes via the respiratory tract. The growth rate and transferring paths of lung cancer depend on its histological types, differentiation degree and other biological characteristics.

17.7.3.3 Clinical Signs and Symptoms
Early Symptoms and Signs
Lung cancer has no special symptoms in the early period, only has the common symptoms with common respiratory diseases, including cough, bloody sputum, low grade fever, chest pain and chest distress. Therefore, it is often misdiagnosed.

Symptoms in the Advanced Stage

(1) Face and neck edema; (2) Hoarse voice is the most common symptom; (3) Shortness of breath.

Symptoms of Metastatic Lung Cancer

Lung cancer tends to occur distant metastases in the early stage. In the cases with metastatic lesions to the brain, the patients sustain persistent headache and blurry vision. In the cases with metastatic lesions to the bone, bone destruction may occur to cause fracture.

Signs

(1) Restrictive wheezing sound, mostly occurring in the inspiratory phase and recurring after cough; (2) Hoarse voice, caused by lymph nodes transferring to compress and invade the recurrent laryngeal nerve; (3) Superior vena cava syndrome, caused by the compresses or invasion to the superior vena cava by the mass and venous obstruction, with edema in the head, face, neck, and upper limbs, varicose veins and edema in the upper chest, and accompanying dizziness, chest distress, shortness of breath and other symptoms; (4) Horner's syndrome, with enophthalmos of the affected side, blepharoptosis, shrinkage of the pupils, eye fissure stenosis, increased skin temperature in the upper chest of the affected side and no sweating due to compression or invasion of the apical cancer to the cervical sympathetic ganglia; (5) Should and arm pain, which is radial burning pain in the shoulder and upper limbs of the affected side due to compression or invasion of apical cancer to the brachial plexus nerve; (6) Phrenic nerve paralysis, with symptoms of shortness of breath and chest distress due to invasion to the phrenic nerve; (7) Dysphagia, caused by compressed esophagus by mediastinal lymphadenectasis; and difficulty breathing caused by compressed trachea by mediastinal lymphadenectasis; (8) Pericardial effusion, shortness of breath, arrhythmia and heart dysfunctions due to pericardial invasion; (9) Pleural metastasis, with chest pain and cancerous pleural effusion; (10) Lung cancer metastasis, spreading of lung cancer along with blood flow to the bone, liver, brain, kidney, adrenal gland and subcutaneous tissues. Intrapulmonary metastasis is also common. Metastasis to different locations shows different symptoms and signs. (11) Extrapulmonary signs, commonly including joint pain or joint hypertrophy, clubbing fingers and mental disorders.

17.7.3.4 Examinations and Their Selection

Imaging Examinations

The diagnostic imaging is the most commonly used and an important examination for the diagnosis of lung cancer. It can facilitate to find some specific manifestations in the lesions, which provide clues for the diagnosis of lung cancer. It is also the main basis for the staging of lung cancer, but fails to define the qualitative diagnosis. Chest X-ray is the main examination for the diagnosis of lung cancer. Anteroposterior and lateral chest X-ray are used for preliminary screening. Chest CT is the diagnostic imaging examination of the choice for the diagnosis of lung cancer. For the central type of lung cancer in the early stage, there are direct signs to define the diagnosis. In the early stage, thin layer scanning with a layer thickness of 1.5–4 mm can be performed to observe the bronchial changes. MR imaging can demonstrate intraluminal nodules, luminal thickness and luminal stenosis of the bronchi from the transverse, coronal, and sagittal perspectives. MR imaging demonstrates favorably cancer in the lesions of obstructive pneumonia, and masses covered by the hilum. PET/CT scanning can be used for the screening of lung cancer metastasis and assessing the therapeutic efficacy after treatment. DSA is used for infusion chemotherapy of bronchial artery in the cases of primary lung cancer.

Bronchoscopy

Bronchoscopy is an important examination for the diagnosis of lung cancer. The pathological changes of the endothelium and the lumen of bronchi can be directly observed by using bronchoscopy. For the cases with caner or cancerous infiltration by bronchoscopy, sampling of the tissues under the guidance of bronchoscopy for biopsy can be performed. Otherwise, bronchial secretions can be suctioned under the guidance of bronchoscopy for cytological examinations to define the diagnosis and the histological classification.

Cytological Examinations

In most cases of primary lung cancer, the shed cancer cells can be found in the sputum, which can also facilitate to define its histological classification.

Exploratory Thoracotomy

After several examinations and short-term exploratory therapies, the qualitative diagnosis cannot be defined and the possibility of lung cancer cannot be excluded. Therefore, exploratory thoracotomy can be performed if the patient's physical conditions permit.

17.7.3.5 Imaging Demonstrations

Chest X-ray

Early lesions are confined within the bronchi, causing valve ventilatory disorder and changes of obstructive emphysema. The manifestations include restrictive pulmonary gas increase and sparse lung markings. In the cases with certain degree of bronchostenosis due to unfavorable discharge of the secretions, obstructive pneumonia occurs, showing patchy blurry shadows. In the cases with complete blockage of the bronchi, obstructive atelectasis occurs, showing decreased pulmonary volume, increased density and migration of the mediastinum to the affected side. Obstructive pulmonary bronchiectasis has demonstrations of intrapulmonary cords liked shadows. Lung cancer in the middle and advanced stages are mainly manifested as hilar mass and atelectasis. The mass has a high density with clear boundary. However, the cancer cannot be observed due to its common immersion in the large flaky obstructive pneumonia lesion or large quantity pleural effusion. Atelectasis is commonly manifested as shrinkage of pulmonary segments or shrinkage of unilateral lung, with high density. The shadow of atelectasis widens at the hilum to show prominent mass. In the cases of central type lung cancer in the right upper lobe, a transverse S shape is at the hilum (commonly known as Pancoast cancer). Early diagnosis of central type lung cancer by plain chest X-ray only shows some indirect pulmonary manifestations caused by bronchial obstruction. And these indirect signs are not characteristically lung cancer. In the cases of local obstructive emphysema, these indirect signs can be caused by foreign substances in the bronchi or early inflammation. Obstructive pneumonia is difficult to be differentiated from common pneumonia. Obstructive atelectasis needs to be differentiated from many other conditions.

CT Scanning

(1) Pathological changes in the bronchial lumen including polypoid, nodular or flat papula masses. Benign tumor has smooth boundary and malignant tumor has unsmooth boundary, commonly with wider base and thickened lumen wall. Even the slight bronchial changes caused by the central type of lung cancer can be demonstrated by thin layer CT scanning, including slightly thickened bronchial wall, intraluminal small nodules and lumen stenosis or obstruction. In the middle and advanced stages, the direct signs of the central type lung cancer include thickened bronchial wall, irregular or unsmooth lining of the bronchial lumen. Bronchial obstruction is suddenly truncation or gradual thinning of the lumen to obstruction. (2) Hilar mass locates adjacent or around the bronchi, with smooth or arch shaped boundary. The indirect signs of the central type lung cancer in the middle and advanced stages include secondary changes to bronchial stenosis. Obstructive pneumonia is manifested as patchy blurry shadows or parenchymal changes of the pulmonary segments/lobes, and decreased lung volume.

MR Imaging

MR imaging demonstrates the tumor as long T1 and long T2 signals. In the cases of central type lung cancer with secondary obstructive atelectasis and obstructive pneumonia, enhanced T1 demonstrates the tumor in the lesion of pulmonary atelectasis and obstructive pneumonia. The signal of atelectasis is higher than that of the tumor.

PET/CT Scanning

PET/CT scanning can demonstrates increased and thick stained metabolites of metastatic lesions or residual lesions, which has a diagnostic sensitivity of above 90 %, and a reported specificity of 80–90 %. In addition, it can be applied for the clinical consideration of it hilar, mediastinal lymph node metastasis and extrathoracic distant metastasis, which is an important method to decide clinical stages before lung cancer therapy. But PET has false negative diagnosis in the diagnosis of lung cancer with decreased metabolites, especially the alveolar cell carcinoma. For the diagnosis of pneumonia and pulmonary tuberculosis, it also has false positive results. DSA can demonstrate the blood supply of the tumors.

Case Study

A male patient aged 41 years was confirmatively diagnosed as having AIDS by the CDC. He complained of repeated cough for more than 1 month and reported to have a history of unhealthy sexual behaviors. His CD4 T cell count was 65/ μl.

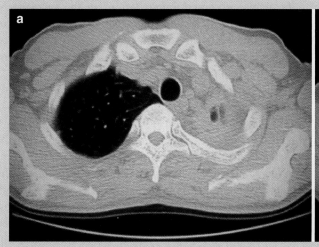
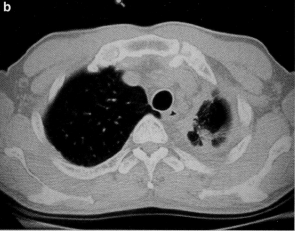

Fig. 17.115 (a–f) HIV/AIDS related lung cancer. (a–f) CT scanning demonstrates diffuse soft tissue density shadows in left upper lung, round liked mass shadows in the middle lung field, thickened pleura in the lateral chest wall with adhesion, and strip liked liquid density shadows

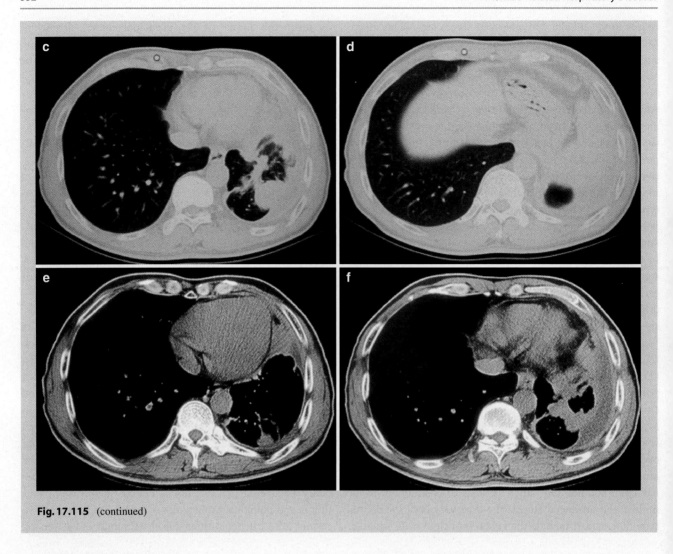

Fig. 17.115   (continued)

17.7.3.6 Diagnostic Basis

1. The case history and related clinical symptoms.
2. By pathological examination, cancer cells can be found in the tissues.
3. The examination for the biomarkers of cancer can detect the serum cancer biomarkers such as cancer embryo antigen (CEA), squamous cell carcinoma (SCC) related antigen and cell keratin 19 fragment (CYFRA21-1) positive.
4. Chest X-ray demonstrations include bronchial obstruction by the cancer to cause obstructive pneumonia or atelectasis, hilar tumor, or widened mediastinal shadow. CT scanning demonstrations include mass shadows intruding into the bronchial lumen, irregular and thickened bronchial wall, and stenosis or obstruction of bronchial lumen. The cases of peripheral type lung cancer have manifestations of nodular or mass shadows around the lung fields, lobulation or incisura with fine and short spikes. The cases of diffuse bronchioloalveolar cell carcinoma have manifestations of infiltrative pathological changes, diffuse scattered nodules and small flake shadows, fusion of

them into large flaky shadows, similar to those of pneumonia. CT scanning with high resolution can define early lung cancer. Enhanced scanning can define hilar and mediastinal lymph nodes metastasis. MR imaging is less favorable in demonstrating lesions in the lung parenchyma than CT scanning. Molecular imaging with fluorodeoxyglucose positron emission tomography computed tomography (^{18}FDG-PET-CT) can demonstrate the increased and thick stained metabolites.

17.7.3.7 Differential Diagnosis
Tuberculosis

(1) Tuberculoma is difficult to be differentiated from the peripheral type of lung cancer. Tuberculoma is more common in young adults, with a long term course of illness. The lesions are commonly found in the apical posterior segment of the upper lobe or dorsal segment of the lower lobe. Chest X-ray demonstrates the lesions with uneven density and satellite lesions. (2) Miliary tuberculosis is difficult to be differentiated from diffuse bronchioloalveolar carcinoma.

Miliary tuberculosis is more common in young adults, with obvious symptoms of systemic toxicity. Anti-tuberculosis drug therapy can relieve the symptoms, with gradually absorbed lesions. (3) Chest X-ray demonstrates hilar lymph node tuberculosis as mass shadows in the hilum of lung, which may be misdiagnosed as the central type lung cancer. Hilar lymph node tuberculosis is more common in teenagers, commonly with symptoms of tuberculosis infection but rarely hemoptysis. Lung cancer can be concurrent with pulmonary tuberculosis.

Pulmonary Inflammations

(1) Bronchial pneumonia; Obstructive pneumonia induced by early lung cancer can be misdiagnosed as bronchial pneumonia. Bronchial pneumonia has an acute onset with more obvious symptoms of infection. Chest X-ray demonstrates patchy or spots shadows, with blurry boundaries and uneven density. The lesions are not confined within one segment or one lobe. (2) Pulmonary abscesses; Central necrosis and liquefaction of the lung cancer results in cancerous cavities. By Chest X-ray, the central type lung cancer can be misdiagnosed as pulmonary abscesses. In the acute period, a pulmonary abscess has obvious symptoms of infection, with large quantity purulent sputum. Chest X-ray demonstrates thin cavity wall, smooth inner wall, liquid level and inflammatory changes in the surrounding lung tissues or pleura.

Other Pulmonary Neoplasms

Pulmonary benign tumors including hamartomas, fibroma and chondroma have slow growth. Chest X-ray demonstrates round liked mass shadow, with homogeneous density without lobation.

Extended Readings

1. World Health Organization (WHO)/Joint United Nations Programme on HIV/AIDS (uNAIDS). Report on the Global AIDS Epidemic, 2008[EB/OL]. (Accessed 15 Apr 2009). Available from URL: http://www.unaids.org/en/KnowledgeCentre/HIVData/GlobalReport/2008/2008_Global_report.asp. 2008.
2. Jones JL, Hanson DL, Dworkin MS, et al. Surveillance for AIDS-defining opportunistic illnesses, 1992–1997. MMWR CDC Surveill Summ. 1999;48:1–22.
3. Song WY, Li HJ. Imaging and pathology of HIV related cytomegalovirus pneumonia. Radiol Pract. 2010;25(1):44–6.
4. Lawrence J, Huang C, George P, et al. Roentgenographic patterns of Pneumocystis Carinii pneumonia in 104 patients with AIDS. Chest. 1987;91(4):323–7.
5. Amorosa JK, Nahass RG, Nosher JL, et al. Radiology distinction of pyogenic pulmonary infection from Pneumocystis Carinii pneumonia in AIDS patients. Radiology. 1990;175(6):721–4.
6. Li H. Atlas of differential diagnosis in HIV/AIDS. Beijing: PMPH; 2009.
7. The National Institutes of Health (NIH) the Centers for Disease Control and Prevention (CDC), and the HIV Medicine Association of the Infectious Diseases Society of America (HIVMA/IDSA). Guidelines for prevention and treatment of opportunistic infections in HIV-infected adults and adolescents [EB/OL]. MMWR, 2009. (Accessed 15 Apr 2009). Available from URL: http://aidsinfo.nih.gov/contentfiles/Adult_OI.pdf.
8. Visnegarwala F, Graviss EA, Lacke CE, et al. Acute respiratory failure associated with cryptococcosis in patients with AIDS: analysis of predictive factors. Clin Infect Dis. 1998;27:1231–7.
9. Meyohas MC, Roux P, Bollens D, et al. Pulmonary cryptococcosis: localized and disseminated infections in 27 patients with AIDS. Clin Infect Dis. 1995;21:628–33.
10. Capponi M, Sureau P. Penicillium de Rhizomys Sinensis. Bull Soc Pathol Exot. 1956;49(4):418–21.
11. Segretain G. Penicillium marneffei agent d'une mycose du system reticuloendothelial. Mycopathol Mycol Appl. 1959;11(4):327–53.
12. Disalvo AF, Fickling AM, Ajello L. Infection caused by Penicillium marneffei description of first natural infection in man. AM J Clin Pathol. 1973;60(2):259–63.
13. Kudeken N, Kawakami K, Saito A. CD4+ T cell-mediated fatal hyperinflammatory reactions in mice infected with Penicillium marneffei. Clin Exp Immunol. 1997;107(3):468–73.
14. Deng Z, Ribas JL, Gibson DW, et al. Infections caused by Penicillium marneffei in China and Southeast Asia: review of eighteen published case and report of our mo re Chinese cases. Rev Infect Dis. 1998;10(3):640–52.
15. Wheat LJ, Connolly-Stringfield PA, Baker RL, et al. Disseminated histoplasmosis in the acquired immune deficiency syndrome: clinical findings, diagnosis and treatment, and review of the literature. Medicine (Baltimore). 1990;69:361–74.
16. Lacombe C, Lewin M, Monnier-cholley L, et al. Imaging of thoracic pathology in patients with AIDS. J Radiol. 2007;88:1145–54.
17. Guilherme FG, Alexandre SM, Cid SF, et al. Clinical and radiographic features of HIV-related pulmonary tuberculosis according to the level of immunosuppression. Rev Soc Bras Med Trop. 2007;40(6):622–6.
18. Dolin PJ, Raviglione MC, Kochi A. Global tuberculosis incidence and mortality during 1990-2000. Bull World Health Organ. 1994;72(2):213–20.
19. Havlir DV, Barnes PF. Tuberculosis in patients with human immunodeficiency virus infection. N Engl J Med. 1999;340:367–73.
20. Batungwanayo J, Taelman H, Dhote R, et al. Pulmonary tuberculosis in Kigali, Rwanda. Impact of human immunodeficiency virus infection on clinical and radiographic presentation. Am Rev Respir Dis. 1992;146:53–6.
21. Jones BE, Young SM, Antoniskis D, Davidson PT, Kramer F, Barnes PF. Relationship of the manifestations of tuberculosis to CD4 cell counts in patients with human immunodeficiency virus infection. Am Rev Respir Dis. 1993;148:1292–7.
22. Awil PO, Bowlin SJ, Daniel TM. Radiology of pulmonary tuberculosis and human immunodeficiency virus infection Gulu, Uganda. Eur Respir J. 1997;10:615–8.
23. Hirschtick RE, Glassroth J, Jordan MC, et al. Bacterial pneumonia in persons infected with the human immunodeficiency virus. Pulmonary Complications of HIV Infection Study Group. N Engl J Med. 1995;333:845–51.
24. Burack JH, Hahn JA, Saint-Maurice D, et al. Microbiology of community-acquired bacterial pneumonia in persons with and at risk for human immunodeficiency virus type 1 infection. Implications for rational empiric antibiotic therapy. Arch Intern Med. 1994;154:2589–96.
25. Hondalus MK, Diamond MS, Rosenthal LA, et al. The intracellular bacterium Rhodococcus equi requires Mac21 to mammalian cells. Infect Immun. 1993;61:2919–29.
26. Walsh RD, Schoch PE, Cunha BA. Rhodococcus. Infect Control Hosp Epidemiol. 1993;14(5):282–7.
27. Takai S, Sasaki Y, Ikeda T, et al. Virulence of Rhodococcus equi isolates from patients with and without AIDS. J Clin Microbiol. 1994;32(2):457–60.

28. Takai S, Sekizaki T, Ozawa T. Association between large plasmid and 15 to 17 kilo dalton antigens in virulent Rhodococcus equi. Infect Immun. 1991;59:4056–60.
29. Tkachuk Saad O, Prescott J. Rhodococcus equi plasmids:Isolation and partial characterization. J Clin Microbiol. 1991;29:2696–700.
30. Marchiori E, Muller NL, de Mendonca RG, Capone D, Souza Jr AS, Escuissato DL, Gasparetto EL, De Cerqueira EM. Rhodococcus equi pneumonia in AIDS: high-resolution CT findings in five patients. Br J Radiol. 2005;78:783–6.
31. Wallace MJ, Hannah J. Cytomegalovirus pneumonitis in patients with AIDS: findings in an autopsy series. Chest. 1987;92:198–203.
32. Moskowitz L, Hensley GT, Chan JC, et al. Immediate causes of death in acquired immunodeficiency syndrome. Arch Pathol Lab Med. 1985;109:735–8.
33. McKenzie R, Travis WD, Dolan SA, et al. The causes of death in patients with humanimmunodeficiency virus infection: aclinical and pathologic study with emphasis on the role of pµlmonary diseases. Medicine. 1991;70:326–43.
34. Geogeann MD, John V, Stuart M, et al. Cytomegalovirus pneumonitis: spectrum of parenchymal CT findings with pathologic correlation in 21 AIDS patients. Radiology. 1994;192:451–9.
35. Scott MA, Graham BS, Verral R, Dixon R, Schaffner W, Tham KT. Rhodococcus equi – an increasingly recognized opportunistic pathogen. Report of 12 cases and review of 65 cases in the literature. Am J Clin Pathol. 1995;103:649–55.
36. Kabani M, Boisrame A, Beckerich JM. A highly representative two hybrid genomic library for the yeast Yarrowia lipolvtica. Gene. 2000;241(2):309–15.
37. Donisi A, Suardi MG, Caasari S, et al. Rhodococcus equi infection in HIV infected patients. AIDS. 1996;10(4):359–62.
38. Harvey RL, Sunstrum JC. Rhodococcus equi infection in patients with and without human immunodeficiency virus infection. Rev Infect Dis. 1991;13(1):139–45.
39. Wicky S, Cartei F, Mayor B, et al. Radiological findings in nine AIDS patients with Rhodococcus equi pneumonia. Eur Radiol. 1996;6:826–30.
40. Sellon DC, Besser TE, Vivrette SL, et al. Comparison of nucleic acid amplification, serology, and microbiologic culture for diagnosis of Rhodococcus equi pneumonia in foals. J Clin Microbiol. 2001;39:1289–93.
41. Kanaly ST, Hines SA, Palmer GH. Cytokine modulation alters pulmonary clearance of Rhodococcus equi and development of granulomatous pneumonia. Infect Immun. 1995;63(8):3037–41.
42. Muller NL, Fraser RS, Lee KS, et al. Diseases of the lung: radiologic and pathologic correlations. Philadelphia: Lippincott Williams & Wilkins; 2003.
43. Reittner P, Ward S, Heyneman L, et al. Pneumonia: high-resolution CT findings in 114 patients. Eur Radiol. 2003;13:515–21.
44. Amorosa JK, Nahass RG, Nosher JL, Gocke DJ. Radiologic distinction of pyogenic pulmonary infection from Pneumocystis carinii pneumonia in AIDS patients. Radiology. 1990;175:721–4.
45. Gruden JF, Huang L, Turner J, et al. High-resolution CT in the evaluation of clinically suspected Pneumocystis carinii pneumonia in AIDS patients with normal, equivocal, or nonspecific radiographic findings. Am J Roentgenol. 1997;169:967–75.
46. Kuhlman JE, Kavuru M, Fishman EK, Siegelman SS. Pneumocystis carinii pneumonia: spectrum of parenchymal CT findings. Radiology. 1990;175:711–4.
47. Sandhu JS, Goodman PC. Pulmonia in patient with AIDS. Radiology. 1989;173:33–5.
48. Schneider MM, Borleffs JC, Stolk RP, Jaspers CA, Hoepelman AI. Discontinuation of prophylaxis for pneumo-cystis carinii pneumonia in HIV-infected patients treated with highly active antiretroviral therapy. Lancet. 1999;353:201–3.

49. White CS, Haramati LB, Elder KH, Karp J, Belani CP. Carcinoma of the lung in HIV-positive patients: findings on chest radiographs and CT scans. Am J Roentgenol. 1995;164:593–7.
50. White DA. Pulmonary complications of HIV-associated malignancies. Clin Chest Med. 1996;17:755–61.
51. Frame PT. Pneumocystis carinii infection and AIDS. In: Crowe S, Hoy J, Mills J, editors. Management of the HIV infected patient. London: Cambridge University Press; 1996. p. 298–308.
52. Naimey GL, Wuerleer RB. Comparison of histologic stains in the diagnosis of Pnemocystis carinii. Acta Cytol. 1995;39(6):1124–9.
53. Barnes PF, Bloch AB, Davidson PT, Snider Jr DE. Tuberculosis in patients with human immunodeficiency virus infection. N Engl J Med. 1991;324:1644–50.
54. Di Perri G, Cazzadori A, Vento S, et al. Comparative histopathological study of pulmonary tuberculosis in human immunodeficiency virus-infected and non-infected patients. Tuber Lung Dis. 1996;77:244–9.
55. Fishman JE, Saraf-Lavi E, Narita M, Hollender ES, Ramsinghani R, Ashkin D. Pulmonary tuberculosis in AIDS patients: transient chest radiographic worsening after initiation of antiretroviral therapy. Am J Roentgenol. 2000;174:43–9.
56. Greenberg SD, Frager D, Suster B, Walker S, Stavropoulos C, Rothpearl A. Active pulmonary tuberculosis in patients with AIDS: spectrum of radiographic findings (including a normal appearance). Radiology. 1994;193:115–9.
57. Haramati LB, Jenny-Avital ER, Alterman DD. Effect of HIV status on chest radiographic and CT findings in patients with tuberculosis. Clin Radiol. 1997;52:31–5.
58. Hocqueloux L, Lesprit P, Herrmann JL, de La BA, Zagdanski AM, Decazes JM, Modaj J. Pulmonary Mycobacterium avium complex disease without dissemination in HIV-infected patients. Chest. 1998;113:542–8.
59. Horsburgh Jr CR. Mycobacterium avium complex infection in the acquired immunodeficiency syndrome. N Engl J Med. 1991;324: 1332–8.
60. Kalayjian RC, Toossi Z, Tomashefski JF, Carey JT, Ross JA, Tomford JW, Blinkhorn Jr RJ. Pulmonary disease due to infection by Mycobacterium avium complex in patients with AIDS. Clin Infect Dis. 1995;20:1186–94.
61. Keiper MD, Beumont M, Elshami A, Langlotz CP, Miller Jr WT. CD4 T lymphocyte count and the radiographic presentation of pulmonary tuberculosis. A study of the relationship between these factors in patients with human immunodeficiency virus infection. Chest. 1995;107:74–80.
62. Sekowitz KA, Raffall J, Riley L, et al. Tuberculosis in the AIDS era. Clin Microbiol Rev. 1995;8(2):180–99.
63. Wolf DA, Wu CD, Medeiros LJ. Mycobacterial pseudotumors of lymph node. Arch Pathol Lab Med. 1995;119(6):811–4.
64. Chen KTK. Mycobacterial spindle cell pseudotumor of lymph node. Am J Surg Pathol. 1992;16(3):276–81.
65. Hoy J. Managenent of the HIV-infected patient. London: Cambridge University Press; 1996. p. 285–97.
66. Sepkowitz KA, Raffall J, Rily L, et al. Tuberculosis in the AIDS era. Clin Microbiol Rev. 1995;8(2):180–99.
67. Uberti-Foppa C, Lillo F, Terreni MR, et al. Cytomegalovirus pneumonia in AIDS patients. Chest. 1998;113(4):919–23.
68. Kida M, Min KW. Atypical cytomegalic cells are diagnostic for cytomegaloviral infection in AIDS. Am J Clin Pathol. 1993;100(3):346–7.
69. Waxman AB, Goldie SJ, Brett-Suith H, Matthay RA. Cytomegalovirus as a primary pulmonary pathogen in AIDS. Chest. 1987;111:128–34.
70. Chuck SL, Sande MA. Infections with Cryptococcus neoformans in the acquired immunodeficiency syndrome. N Engl J Med. 1989;321(12):794–9.

71. Conces Jr DJ. Endemic fungal pneumonia in immunocompromised patients. J Thorac Imaging. 1999;14:1–8.

72. Conces Jr DJ, Stockberger SM, Tarver RD, Wheat LJ. Disseminated histoplasmosis in ADIS: findings on chest radiographs. Am J Roentgenol. 1993;160:15–9.

73. Connolly Jr JE, McAdams HP, Erasmus JJ, Rosado-de-Christenson ML. Opportunistic fungal pneumonia. J Thorac Imaging. 1999;14:51–62.

74. Denning DW, Follansbess SE, Scolaro M, Norris S, Edelstein H, Stevens DA. Pulmonary aspergillosis in the acquired immunodeficiency syndrome. N Engl J Med. 1991;324:654–62.

75. Fish DG, Ampel NM, Galgiani JN, et al. Coccidioidomycosis during human immunodeficiency virus infection. A review of 77 patients. Medicine. 1990;69:384–91.

76. Miller Jr WT, Edelman JM, Miller WT. Cryptococcal pulmonary infection in patients with AIDS: radiographic appearance. Radiology. 1990;175:725–8.

77. Miller Jr WT, Sais GJ, Frank I, Gefter WB, Aronchick JM, Miller WT. Pulmonary aspergillosis in patients with AIDS. Clinical and radiographic correlations. Chest. 1994;105:37–44.

78. Driver JA, Saunders CA, Heinze-Lacy B, et al. Cryptococcal pneumonia in AIDS: is cryptococcal meningitis preceded by clinically recognizable pneumonia. J Acquir Immune Defic Syndr Hum Retrovirol. 1995;9(2):168–71.

79. Chechani V, Kamholz SL. Pulmonary manifestations of disseminated cryptococcosis in patients with AIDS. Chest. 1990;98(5):1060–6.

80. Bani-Sadr F, Hamidou M, Raffi F, Chamoux C, Caillon J, Freland C. Clinical and bacteriological aspects of nocardiasis. Presse Med. 1995;24:1062–6.

81. Furman AC, Jacobs J, Sepkowitz KA. Lung abscess in patients with AIDS. Clin Infect Dis. 1996;22:81–5.

82. Race EM, Adelson-Mitty J, Kitty J, Kriegel GR, Barlam TF, Reimann KA, Letvin NL, Japour AJ. Focal mycobacterial lymphadenitis following initiation of protease-inhibitor therapy in patients with advanced HIV-1 disease. Lancet. 1998;351:251–5.

83. Shapiro JM, Romney BM, Weiden MD, White CS, O'Toole KM. Rhodococcus equi endobronchial mass with lung abscess in a patient with AIDS. Thorax. 1992;47:62–3.

84. Bazot M, Cadranel J, Benayoun S, Tassart M, Bigot JM, Carette MF. Primary pulmonary AIDS-related lymphoma: radiographic and CT findings. Chest. 1999;116:1282–6.

85. Broder S, Karp JE. The expanding challenge of HIV-associated malignancies. CA Cancer J Clin. 1992;42:69–73.

86. Eisner MD, Kaplan LD, Herndier B, Stulbarg MS. The pulmonary manifestations of AIDS-related non-Hodgkin's lymphoma. Chest. 1996;110:729–36.

87. Sider L, Weiss AJ, Smith MD, VonRoenn JH, Glassroth J. Varied appearance of AIDS-related lymphoma in the chest. Radiology. 1989;171:629–32.

88. Mead JH, Mason TE. Lymphoma versus AIDS. Am J Clin Pathol. 1983;80(4):546–7.

89. Haramati LB, Wong J. Intrathoracic Kaposi's sarcoma in women with AIDS. Chest. 2000;117:410–4.

90. Khalil AM, Carette MF, Cadranel JL, Mayaud CM, Bigot JM. Intrathoracic Kaposi's sarcoma. CT findings. Chest. 1995;108:1622–6.

91. Cathomas G, Stalder A, McGandy CE, et al. Distribution of human herpesvirus 8 DNA in tumorous and nontumorous tissue of patients with acquired immunodeficiency syndrome with and without Kaposi's sarcoma. Mod Pathol. 1998;11(5):415–20.

92. Carbone A, Mason TE. Kaposi's sarcoma in lymphnodes concurrent with Hodgkin's disease. Am J Clin Pathol. 1983;80(2):228–30.

93. Safai B, Johnson KG, Myskowski PT, et al. The natural history of Kaposi's sarcoma in the acquired immunodeficiency syndrome. Ann Intern Med. 1985;103(5):744–50.

94. Rabaud C, May T, Lucet JC, Leport C, Ambroies-Thomas P, Canton P. Pulmonary toxoplasmosis in patients in-fected with human immunodeficiency virus: a French National Survey. Clin Infect Dis. 1996;23:1249–54.

95. Li HJ, Gao YQ, Cheng JL, et al. Diagnostic imaging, preautopsy imaging and autopsy findings of 8 AIDS cases. Chin Med J (Engl). 2009;122(18):2142–8.

96. Gao JB, Zhang YG, Li HJ, et al. Analysis on the imaging features of AIDS with pulmonary fungal infection. Chin Med J (Engl). 2010;123(24):3583–6.

97. Li ZC, Li HJ, Dai LL, et al. Liver injury in HIV-1-infected patients receiving non-nucleosides reverse transcriptase inhibitors-based antiretroviral therapy. Chin Med J (Engl). 2010;123(24):3587–90.

98. Li HJ. MRI demonstrations of AIDS complicated by Toxoplasma gondii infection in cervical spinal cord: with 3 cases reports. Chin Med J (Engl). 2010;123(24):3587–90.

99. Li HJ. Diagnostic imaging in AIDS in China: current status and clinical application. Chin Med J. 2011;124(7):963–4.

100. Li HJ, Cheng JL. Imaging and pathological findings of AIDS complicated by pulmonary rhodococcus equi infection. Chin Med J. 2011;124(7):968–72.

101. Wang L, Shi DP, Han X, Zhao QX, Yan B, Li HJ. Magnetic resonance spectroscopy in the diagnosis of cognitive impairment in AIDS patients. Chin Med J. 2011;124(9):1342–5.

102. Li H. CT image demonstrations of HIV-seropositive tuberculosis and their relationship with CD4+ T-lymphocyte count. Chin Med J (Engl). 2010;124(4):124–6.

103. Jones HA, Clark RJ, Schofield JB, et al. Positron emission tomography of 18FDG uptake in localized pulmonary inflammation. Acta Radiol Suppl. 1991;376:148.

104. Capponi MP, Segretain G, Sureau G. Penicilliosisde Rhizomys sinensis. Bull Soc Pathol Exot Filiales. 1956;49:418–21.

105. Zhang Y, Wang M, Li H, et al. Accumulation of nuclear mitochondrial DNA in the frontal cortex cells of patients with HIV-associated neurocognitive disorders. Brain Res. 2012;1458:1–11.

106. Li H, Meng Z, Huang K, et al. Imaging findings of AIDS complicated with pulmonary rhodococcus equi infection and correlated with pathology. Radiol Pract. 2009;24(9):943–7.

107. Ludlam GB, Beattie CP. Pulmonary toxoplasmosis? Lancet. 1963;2(7318):1136–8.

108. Chen S, Ma S. Pathogenesis and prevention of rhodococcus equi infection. J Northwest Minorities Univ (Nat Sci). 2001;22(41):44–8.

109. Catterall JR, Hofflin JM, Remington JS. Pulmonary toxoplasmosis. Am Rev Respir Dis. 1986;133(4):704–5.

Contents

18.1 An Overview of HIV/AIDS Related Cardiac Diseases

Cardiovascular diseases occur in patients with AIDS of its advanced stage. The cardiovascular complications include dilated cardiomyopathy, pericardial effusion, endocarditis, cardiac dysfunction, pulmonary hypertension and arrhythmia. Left ventricular dysfunction is more common in the advanced stage. Since the year of 1981, there has been increasingly clinical and autopsy reports about AIDS complicated by cardiopathy, with the most frequently reported cases of pericarditis or pericardial effusion and occasionally accompanying cardiac tamponade. In adults and children AIDS patients, about 20–40 % is found to have pericarditis. According to the autopsy reports, the incidence of pericardiac lesions is 3–37 %, while its incidence by echocardiography is 30–38 %. HIV/AIDS related cardiopathy is a kind of non-inflammatory heart disease that is related to dysmetabolism. Myocardium is the basic dynamic tissue for the contraction and relaxation of the heart, and it is particularly sensitive to infections, hypoxia, drugs and toxins. Among AIDS patients, dilated and hypertrophic myocardial diseases are more common. By myocardium tissue culture, HIV can be found, although some scholars believed that HIV attacks hemoglobin instead of myocardial tissue. In 5 % cases of myocarditis in AIDS patients by autopsy, only 20 % is pathologically confirmed as having dilated myocardiopathy. By electrocardiography, 30–45 % cases of AIDS complicated by cardiopathy show abnormalities.

Endocardial diseases may occur in AIDS patients. The more commonly endocardial diseases in AIDS patients include non-bacterial endocarditis and infectious endocarditis. Infectious endocarditis can be caused by pathogens of bacteria, fungi, mycobacterium and protozoa, with symptoms of fever, anorexia, upset, chest pain and weight loss.

HIV/AIDS related cardiac diseases include:

H. Li (ed.), *Radiology of HIV/AIDS*,
DOI 10.1007/978-94-007-7823-8_18, © Springer Science+Business Media Dordrecht and People's Medical Publishing House 2014

18.1.1   Pericardial Disease

The pericardium is the most commonly involved part of heart in HIV/AIDS patients. In the early stage of HIV infection, pericardial lesions may occur, but being asymptomatic during his/her life time. HIV/AIDS related pericarditis caused by tuberculous mycobacteria infection is the most common. Staphylococcus and streptococcus are also the common causes of pneumonia and pericarditis. Others pathogens including Nocardia and Listeria can also cause pericarditis. HIV/AIDS related pericarditis has a poor prognosis, with the CD4 T cell count being lower than 100/µl.

18.1.2   Pulmonary Hypertension

AIDS and left ventricular dysfunction, valvular heart disease or cardiac shunt can cause pulmonary hypertension and pulmonary heart disease. Patients with AIDS complicated by pulmonary hypertension mostly sustain serious pulmonary infection, such as Pneumocystis carinii pneumonia and cytomegaloviral pneumonia. Progressive pulmonary pressure in AIDS patients is caused by hyperplasia of pulmonary endothelial cells resulted from stimulation of growth factors to pulmonary endothelial cells. It has been recognized that growth factors can be derived from infected T cells or directly derived from HIV. Therefore, occurrence of dyspnea in AIDS patients shows evidence of right ventricular dysfunction instead of left ventricular dysfunction. In such cases, possible occurrence of pulmonary hypertension should be considered.

18.1.3   Myocarditis

HIV/AIDS related myocarditis plays an important role in progressive left ventricular dysfunction. About 80 % cases of myocarditis is idiopathic and about 20 % is opportunistic. The pathogen usually includes the complex of tubercle bacillus and mycobacterium avium, fungi including cryptococcus, aspergillus, Candida albicans, Histoplasma capsulatum and Coccidiodes, and protozoa including Cytomegalovirus, simplex herpes virus and HIV.

18.1.4   Dilated Cardiomyopathy

HIV/AIDS related dilated cardiomyopathy may be caused by diffuse weakened mobility of myocardium due to myocarditis. The diffuse weakened mobility of myocardium causes compensatory hypertrophy and dilation of the ventricles, and finally progresses into dilated cardiomyopathy.

18.1.5   Cardiac Neoplasm

18.1.5.1 Kaposi's Sarcoma

Kaposi's sarcoma is common in AIDS patients, and usually involves myocardium and epicardium. Generally, cardiac KS is found during autopsy, being asymptomatic during the patient's lifetime. According to data from the autopsy, foci of KS are found in about 28–40 % AIDS patients, involving all parts of heart including heart apex, interventricular septum, pericardium, aortic adventitia and pulmonary artery trunk. The foci of KS can be patchy or nodular.

18.1.5.2 Malignant Lymphomas

Cardiac malignant lymphoma is more common than KS in AIDS patients. For cases with lymphoma with involvement of pericardium, pericardial effusion can be caused. For cases with lymphoma with involvement of myocardium, arrhythmia and conduction block can occur to cause congestive heart failure. Occasionally, lymphoma invades into cardiac chambers to cause blockage of the blood flow. Patients with cardiac lymphoma cannot be pathologically diagnosed during his/her lifetime.

18.1.6   Valvular Heart Disease and Pulmonary Vascular Disease

In AIDS patients, some vascular diseases may occur. HIV/AIDS related cardiopathy is common and dilated cardiomyopathy can also occur as one of the cardiac complications of AIDS. The common cardiovascular diseases that complicate AIDS are myocarditis, cardiomyopathy, pericarditis and pericardial effusion, abnormal heart valves, vascular diseases and neoplasms. In cases of pulmonary infections, the pulmonary vascular intima responds to lesions, mostly caused by HIV under effects of inflammatory mediators and cytokines. The endothelial cells can release vasoactive substances or trigger proliferative response to growth factors to cause the increase of pulmonary vascular resistance. Calabrese et al. reported four cases of AIDS patients, with occurrence of necrotic vasculitis [5]. The lesions were reported to be nodular arteritis and acute inflammation of small and medium-sized blood vessels, resulting in lesions of the skin, muscles and nerve fibers. There were two cases with such lesions occurring in the nervous system, with their clinical and morphological manifestations being in line with those of neurologic granulomatous vasculitis. The pathogenesis of vasculitis is still unknown, and it may be related to the effects of virus (HIV, CNV, HBV and EBV) or immune complexes to cause vascular lesions, opportunistic infections, pulmonary diseases, drugs and nutritional status. Autopsy of AIDS patients found inflammatory and fiber calcified arterial lesions. The inflammatory arterial lesions are vasculitis and peripheral inflammation, while fiber calcified arterial lesions often involve medium sized artery to cause arterial intimal fibrosis, elastic fiber breakage, arterial medial fibrosis and calcification, possibly with accompanying varying degrees of stenosis. In addition, aneurysm can be found in some AIDS patients, with vascular wall fibrosis and calcification as well as endothelial cell proliferation, with accompanying arterial stenosis of different degrees. Changes in the microcirculation have been studied, but the abnormalities and their significance still need clarifying.

18.2 HIV/AIDS Related Pericarditis and Pericardial Effusion

Pericarditis and pericardial effusion are the common complications of AIDS. Pericardial effusion is often ignored in the early stage. For cases of AIDS patients with sinus tachycardia and dyspnea, the possibility of pericardial effusion should be considered. Echocardiography is recommended for the diagnosis and should be performed as early as possible. AIDS complicated by pericardial effusion mostly occurs in those with tuberculous serous cavity effusions, possibly progresses into pericardial tamponade in the advanced stage. Since the first case of AIDS reported in 1981, there were clinical and autopsy reports about the cardiac abnormalities in AIDS patients, among which the most common cardiovascular disease is pericarditis or pericardial effusion, with the symptom of cardiac tamponade. It is estimated that 5–10 % HIV infected patients in America have pericardial effusion, but mostly being asymptomatic and obtaining their definitive diagnosis by echocardiography or autopsy. According to autopsy reports, the incidence of pericardial disease is 3–37 %; and the incidence of pericardial effusion is 30–38 % by echocardiography.

18.2.1 Pathogens and Pathogenesis

In cases of acute pericarditis, infections can be caused by bacteria, parasites, protozoa, viruses and fungi. The pathogens of bacterial infections are commonly streptococcus, staphylococcus and Gram-negative bacilli. The pathogens of virus infections in immunocompromised patients are commonly Echovirus, influenza virus, and Coxsackie B virus. AIDS can be complicated by pericardial effusion due to infections of tuberculous mycobacterium avium, actinomyces, fungi or virus, lymphoma and Kaposi's sarcoma.

The common subtypes of chronic pericarditis are chronic constrictive pericarditis and chronic exudative pericarditis.

Chronic constrictive pericarditis is usually non-specific, but almost all subtypes of acute pericarditis can be its cause. The common cause is tuberculosis or other infection, rheumatoid arthritis, trauma and heart surgery.

Chronic exudative pericarditis is usually non-specific, but can be caused by mycobacterium tuberculosis, fungi or neoplasm. Among inpatients, the most common cause of large quantity pericardial effusion is the metastatic tumors or direct spreading of tumors, such as cancer (especially lung cancer or breast cancer), sarcoma (especially melanoma), leukemia, lymphoma and thoracic tumors.

18.2.2 Pathophysiological Basis

Acute pericarditis can be serous, fibrinous, hemorrhagic or suppurative. It may involve surface of the sub-picardial myocardium. The quantity and quality of the cellular responses are determined by pathogens.

Chronic pericarditis can be serous, chylous or blood exudative. Alternatively, chronic pericarditis can be fibrinous, adhesive or calcified. And it can be constrictive and asymptomatic. In cases of chronic exudative pericarditis, the pericardial effusion fluid is about 50–1,000 ml (normally less than 25 ml). In the cases of less but rapid pericardial effusion, more but slow pericardial effusion, decreased accommodation of the pericardium due to fibrosis, calcification and neoplasm, the ventricular filling during its diastole can be restricted. Under such conditions, the terminal pressure of the left ventricular diastole is determined by the quantity of pericardial effusion and the thickness of the thickened pericardium. The diastolic pressures of ventricles, atria and venous bed are close, usually being 13–32 mmHg. Occurrence of venous congestion of systemic circulation causes too much body fluid effusion from the capillaries, resulting in postural edema and later ascites. The sign of surrounding tissue congestion is more obvious than that of pulmonary congestion, but pulmonary edema with obvious clinical symptoms is not common. However, pericardial effusion gradually progresses and the quantity of effusion being up to more than 1,000 ml may fail to cause pericardial tamponade due to its elasticity for adaptation.

Pathologically, pericarditis can be divided into two stages of the fibrinous stage and the serofibrinous stage. In the early stage of pericarditis, parietal and visceral pericardium has congestion, swelling and effusions of fibrin, leukocyte and some endothelial cells. The thick exudates can be restricted to a certain part of pericardium or diffuse across the entire surface of the heart. The surface of the pericardium can be coarse. In the cases of increased exudates, the effusion fluid can be serofibrinous effusions, with its quantity varying from 100 to 2,000–3,000 ml. The sub-epicardial myocardium often has inflammatory changes. After being cured, the exudates can be reabsorbed within 2–3 weeks or shorter time period. But in some cases, the exudates may remain for several days or even years, such as in the cases of tuberculous pericarditis. When pericardium recedes, varying degrees of adhesion may remain. Sometimes, both layers of pericardium can be obviously thickened and adhesive to completely fill the pericardial cavity. Therefore, thick and hard scars form to compress the heart and the major vascular roots. The cardiac diastole is therefore affected to develop into chronic constrictive pericarditis.

18.2.3   Clinical Symptoms and Signs

Acute pericarditis is manifested with symptoms of chest pain, difficulty breathing, fever, pericardial friction sound, pericardial tamponade, chest or retrosternal dull or sharp pain that radiates to the neck, trapezius (especially the left side) or the shoulder. The severity of the pain varies, commonly aggravating at conditions of chest motion, coughing and breathing and alleviating at the postures of standing up from sitting and leaning forward. Fever, chills and fatigue are very common. And the most important sign is three-phase or two-phase (systolic and diastolic) pericardial friction sound. For cases of large quantity pericardial effusion, the heart sound is low, with enlarged range of dullness sound. In such cases, the lungs can be compressed to cause dyspnea. About 8–30 % patients with pericarditis have symptoms of heart tamponade, with accompanying increased central venous pressure. Cardiac

tamponade is fatal. Chronic pericarditis has symptoms of fever but with no chest pain.

18.2.4   Examinations and Their Selection

18.2.4.1 Echocardiography
Echocardiography is the examination of choice for HIV/AIDS related pericarditis and pericardial effusion. The demonstrations include liquid dark area within pericardial cavity. It is a diagnostic method with accuracy, safety and simple manipulations.

18.2.4.2 Electrocardiography
For the cases with pericardial effusion, QRS waves group is in low voltage.

18.2.4.3 Pericardiocentesis
Pericardiocentesis facilitates to clarify the quality of pericardial effusion. Its combination with smear and culture can detect the pathogens of the infection. For cases of neoplastic pericardial effusion, tumor cells can be detected.

18.2.4.4 Diagnostic Imaging
CT scanning and MR imaging are the effective assistant examinations, with accurate localization.

18.2.5   Imaging Demonstrations

For the cases of pericardial effusion, the imaging demonstrations include enlarged heart shadow in shape of a flask, the increased ratio of heart to chest, and the absence of outer line of the heart. Generally, when pericardial effusion reaches up to 300–500 ml or above, the heart shadow commonly expands to both sides, with different morphology of the heart shadow due to different posture. Superior vena cava obviously expands and the cardiophrenic angle becomes blunt. When pericardial effusion exceeds 1,000 ml, the heart shadow obviously expands in a shape of triangle or flask. In addition, normal limits of heart arches are absent, with weakened or no heart beat by X-ray.

Case Study 1

A male patient with AIDS aged 15 years. He was confirmatively diagnosed by CDC. He complained of fever for 1 month, with history of blood donation and symptoms of fever, cough and chest distress. His CD4 T cell count was 69/ μl.

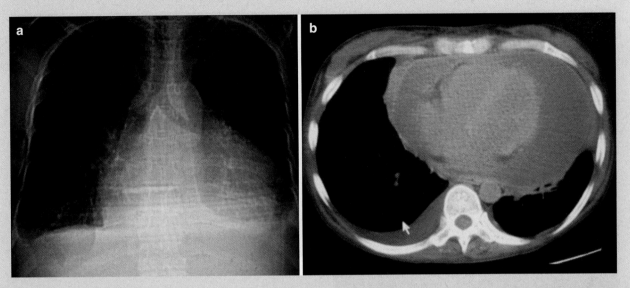

Fig. 18.1 (a, b) HIV/AIDS related pericardial effusion. (a) DR demonstrates enlarged heart shadow in shape of a flask, increased ratio of the heart to the chest, closed bilateral costophrenic angles with adhesion. (b) CT scanning demonstrates stripe liked fluid density shadow in the pericardial cavity and fluid density shadow in posterior chest wall of the right chest cavity

Case Study 2

A female patient aged 33 years was confirmatively diagnosed as having AIDS by CDC. She had a history of blood transfusion in 1996, with chief complaints of fever, cough and chest distress in 2007. Her CD4 T cell count was 46/μl.

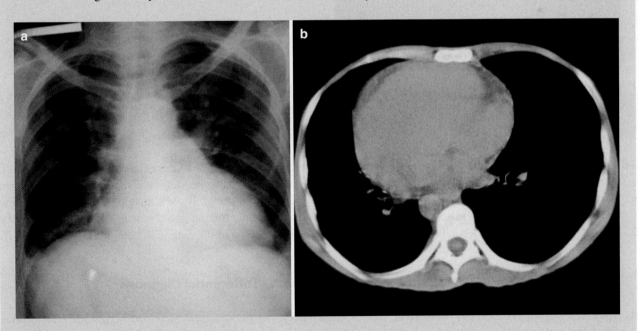

Fig. 18.2 (a, b) HIV/AIDS related tuberculous pericarditis. (a) DR demonstrates enlarged heart shadow in shape of a flask and increased ratio of the heart to the chest. (b) CT scanning demonstrates stripe liked fluid density shadow in the pericardial cavity

Case Study 3

A female patient aged 38 years was confirmatively diagnosed as having AIDS by CDC. She had a history of blood transfusion in 1995, and complained of fever, cough, expectoration and chest distress in 2007. Her CD4 T cell count was 46/μl.

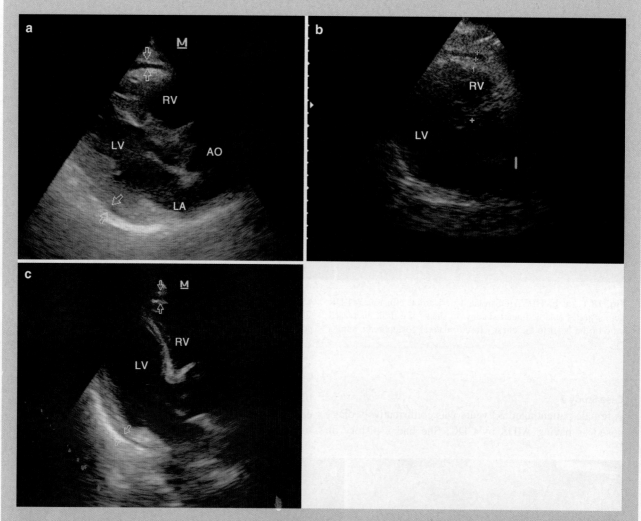

Fig. 18.3 (**a–c**) HIV/AIDS related pericardial effusion. (**a–c**) Color Doppler ultrasound demonstrates long axis cross section of the left ventricle: fluid dark area of 7 mm in width in the pericardial cavity and the posterior wall of the left ventricle, fluid dark area of 5 mm in width in the anterior wall of the right ventricle, with favorable echoes. *AO* aorta opening , *LA* left atria, *LV* left ventricle, *RV* right ventricle

18.2.6   Criteria for the Diagnosis

1. In combination of the clinical manifestations to pericardial effusion examination and history of tuberculosis.
2. The detection rate of tubercle bacillus in pericardial effusion and positive rate by pericardial effusion culture is low. By OT test, only 60 % patients can be found moderately or strongly positive.
3. By PCR, the positive rate can be increased.
4. Echocardiographic findings are non-specific, but it can define the quantity of pericardial effusion and adhesive or thickened pericardium. Thus it provides valuable data for the pathogenic diagnosis. Meanwhile it can be used to evaluate the therapeutic efficacy.
5. Electrocardiography shows low voltage of QRS wave groups and inverse T wave.
6. Chest X-ray demonstrates enlarged heart shadow. By CT scanning, the findings include liquid density shadow in pericardial cavity. By MR imaging, the findings include pericardial effusion liquid in stripes of long T1 and long T2 signals and the diagnosis is reliable.

18.2.7   Differential Diagnosis

AIDS patients can have increased pericardial effusion due to bacterial infection, virus infection, autoimmunity and dysmetabolism. The effusion can be transudative, exudative, bloody and purulent. In the cases of a rapid increase of pericardial effusion fluid, the diastolic filling of the heart is limited to show the sign of pericardial tamponade. Two-dimensional echocardiography provides valuable information for the quantitative and qualitative diagnosis of pericardial effusion. Currently, pericardial effusion can be quantitatively divided into 5°: (1) minimal pericardial effusion (less than 50 ml), with demonstrations of echo-free dark area in width of 2–3 mm in the pericardial cavity of the atrioventricular groove; (2) small quantity of pericardial effusion (50–100 ml), with demonstrations of echo-free dark area in width of 3–5 mm limited in the atrioventricular groove and in the pericardial cavity of the left posterior ventricular wall; (3) Moderate quantity of pericardial effusion (100–300 ml), with demonstrations of echo-free dark area in width of 5–10 mm in pericardial cavity at the posterior wall of the left ventricle, the heart apex and the anterior wall of the right ventricle; (4) Much pericardial effusion (300–1,000 ml), with demonstrations of the dark area in width of 10–20 mm surrounding the whole heart, with accompanying heart shrinkage and the heart swinging sign; (5) Maximal quantity of pericardial effusion (1,000–4,000 ml), with demonstrations of echo-free dark area in width of 20–60 mm in the pericardial cavity at the posterior wall of the left ventricle; and echo-free dark area in width of 20–40 mm in the pericardial cavity at the anterior wall of the right ventricle, with obvious heart swinging sign and heart striking sign. Clinically, it should be differentiated from following diseases: (1) It should be differentiated from neoplastic pericarditis. Primary pericardial tumor is commonly interstitial tumor, which rarely occurs. Metastatic tumor is more common, with originations from bronchial and breast malignant tumors. In addition, lymphoma and leukemia can also involve the pericardium to cause friction sound and effusions. The effusion is mostly bloody, with no obvious chest pain. (2) With the development and widespread application of interventional cardiology, it also should be differentiated from catheterization induced bloody pericardial effusion. (3) Trauma can also cause bloody pericardial effusion.

18.3 HIV/AIDS Related Myocarditis and Cardiomyopathy

18.3.1 HIV/AIDS Related Myocarditis

AIDS-related myocarditis is localized or diffuse inflammation of the myocardium caused by various pathogenic factors. Based on these pathogenic factors, myocarditis can be divided into viral type, bacterial type, parasitic type and fungal type. There have also been reports about metabolic and toxic myocardiopathies in AIDS patients. About more than 20 kinds of virus can cause viral myocarditis, mostly occurring in the advanced stage of AIDS.

18.3.1.1 Pathogens and Pathogenesis
There are many pathogenic factors contributing to the occurrence of myocarditis, such as viruses, bacteria, fungi, parasites, immune responses and physical and chemical factors. The classification of myocarditis varies greatly. Based on the pathogenic factors, it can be divided into the following types:

Viral Myocarditis
It is primary myocardial inflammation caused by virus, commonly involving pericardium to cause perimyocarditis. Virus HIV-1 infection can lead to myocarditis. Sensitized cytotoxic T cells can destroy the virus infected myocardial cells.

Bacterial Myocarditis
After HIV/AIDS related bacterial infections, the bacteria or toxin produced by bacteria can infect the myocardium. Alternatively, allergic response induced by bacteria produced substances can also cause myocarditis, such as myocardial abscess caused by pyogenic bacteria. Streptococcal infection of the upper respiratory tract is a non-specific (interstitial) myocarditis caused by streptococcal toxin.

Parasitic Myocarditis
The most commonly parasitic myocarditis is toxoplasma myocarditis, which is caused by infection of rat toxoplasma gondii.

18.3.1.2 Pathophysiological Basis
HIV/AIDS related viral myocarditis mostly involves atrial posterior wall, interventricular septum and heart apex, and sometimes involves the conduction system. Under a microscope, the common pathological change is necrotic myocarditis. Diffuse infiltration of lymphocytes and necrosis of myocardial histocytes can be found in the myocardial interstitium of viral myocarditis. In the advanced stage, obvious myocardial interstitial fibrosis can be found, with accompanying compensatory myocardial hypertrophy and dilation of heart chambers (congestive cardiomyopathy). For the cases of HIV/AIDS related bacterial myocarditis, multiple yellow small abscesses can be found on the surface or cross section of the heart by observation with naked eyes, with surrounding congestion stripes. Microscopically, necrosis and liquefaction of myocardial cells can be found in the abscesses, as well as large quantity of pyocytes and different quantities of bacterial colonies in the abscess cavity. The myocardial tissues surrounding the abscesses are found to have degenerative and necrotic changes of different degrees, with infiltration of neutrophils and mononuclear cells in the interstitium. The foci are commonly found in the right ventricular wall. After healed, fine network liked small scars occur. In some cases, diffuse myocardial necrosis occurs, possibly leading to cardiac sudden death. In cases of HIV/AIDS related parasitic myocarditis, toxoplasma gondii gains access to the human body to infect the mononuclear macrophage system and various tissues along with blood flow, and replicates themselves in the cells to form toxoplasma gondii group, which is also known as pseudocysts. The rupture of the pseudocyst causes the access of toxoplasma gondii to the surrounding tissues. There is infiltration of lymphocytes and mononuclear cells around the myocardial cells.

18.3.1.3 Clinical Symptoms and Signs
The clinical manifestations include fatigue, shortness of breath, palpitation and precordial upset. There are also

weakened first heart sound, and strengthened third and/or fourth heart sound to cause atrial or ventricular gallop rhythm and heart murmur.

18.3.1.4 Examinations and Their Selection
Electrocardiography

By electrocardiography, the positive rate is high. Therefore, it is the examination of choice and also important basis for the diagnosis. The demonstrations by ECG include inferior migration of the ST segment wave, low and constant or inverse T wave.

Echocardiography

It facilitates to understand the morphologic and functional changes of the heart.

Laboratory Blood Tests

In the cases of viral myocarditis, leukocyte count may be within the normal limits. GOT, GPT, LDH and CPK are with the normal limits or increased. In the cases of chronic myocarditis, these indices are commonly within the normal limits.

Diagnostic Imaging

CT scanning and MR imaging can directly demonstrate the morphological changes of the myocardium and cardiac chambers.

18.3.1.5 Imaging Demonstrations

The imaging demonstrations include myocardial hypertrophy and enlarged heart shadow. By ultrasound of the heart, liquid dark area can be found in the ventricular wall, with decreased heart functions in contracting and relaxing.

Case Study 1

A male patient aged 14 years was confirmatively diagnosed as having AIDS by CDC. He was found to be HIV positive 5 years ago and paid his clinic visit due to the initial symptom of diarrhea. His CD4 T cell count was 7/μl. By routine blood test, the findings include WBC 3.09×10^9/L, RBC 2.09×10^{12}/L. By liver function examination, the findings include ALT 21 U/L and ALT 56 U/L.

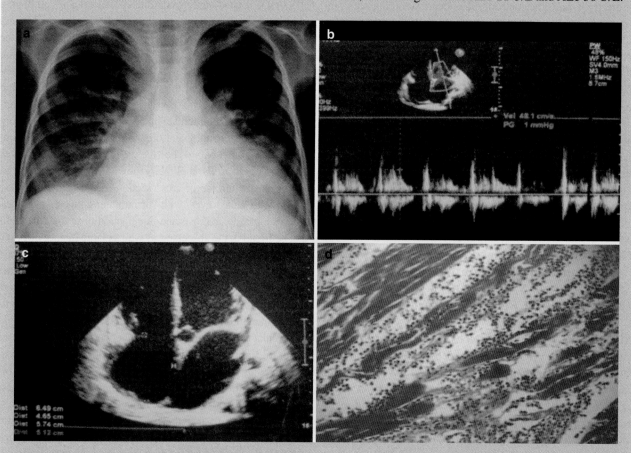

Fig. 18.4 (a–d) HIV/AIDS related myocarditis. (a) DR demonstrates enlarged heart in shape of a flask, and increased ratio of the heart to the chest. (b, c) Ultrasound demonstrates enlarged heart, the left antrum in size of 65×46 mm, the right antrum in size of 57×55 mm. CDFI demonstrations of reflux signals in all valvular ports, large quantity of reflux signals at the tricuspid port, fluid dark areas at the left ventricular wall and the posterior wall in thickness of 6 and 9 mm respectively, decreased heart functions in contracting and relaxing, fluid dark area in thickness of 5 mm at the anterior wall of right ventricle. (d) It is demonstrated to have myocardial interstitial edema, numerous infiltrations of neutrophile granulocytes, pyogenic bacteria induced degeneration and necrosis of partial myocardium

Case Study 2

A patient was confirmatively diagnosed as having AIDS by CDC. He sustained myocardial aspergillus infection.

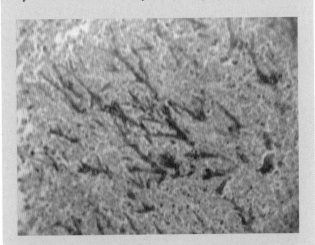

Fig. 18.5 Myocardial aspergillus infection. It is demonstrated to have focal necrosis of the myocardial cells, many hyphae of aspergillus in the focus, and branch and radiation liked distribution of the hyphae

Case Study 3

A patient was confirmatively diagnosed as having AIDS by CDC. He was found to have toxoplasma gondii cysts in the epicardium.

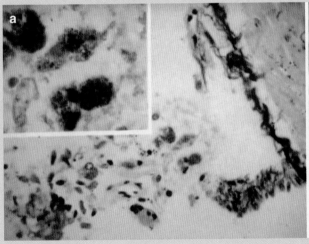
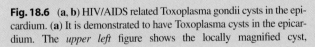
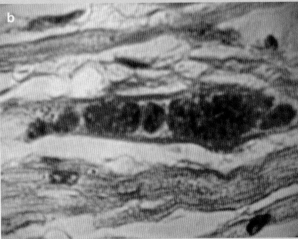

Fig. 18.6 (**a, b**) HIV/AIDS related Toxoplasma gondii cysts in the epicardium. (**a**) It is demonstrated to have Toxoplasma cysts in the epicardium. The *upper left* figure shows the locally magnified cyst, HE ×400. (**b**) It is demonstrated to have multiple Toxoplasma cysts within myocardial cells. The cysts are in round or oval shapes, with particle substances in them, which as tachyzoites of Toxoplasma gondii

18.3.2   HIV/AIDS Related Cardiomyopathy

Cardiomyopathies are myocardial diseases with no known reasons. Generally, it is believed that cardiomyopathies are related to viral infections, autoimmune responses, heredity, drug poisoning and dysmetabolism. Cardiomyopathies exclude those specific myocardial diseases with known reasons and secondary to general diseases. The causes of cardiomyopathies are still unknown.

By ultrasound, HIV/AIDS related cardiomyopathies are demonstrated as dilated cardiomyopathy, specifically including dilated ventricles, strengthened and thinner myocardial echo, and abnormal heart functions. Ronald et al. reported 25 cases of HIV/AIDS related cardiomyopathies including eight cases of dilated cardiomyopathy [4]. The imaging demonstrations are characterized by enlarged ventricles and predominantly enlarge left ventricle, crescent shaped interventricular septum protruding toward the right ventricle, with accompanying diffuse decreased motion of the ventricular wall. The incidence rate of the pathological changes in the right ventricle is found to be 20–40 %. It has been also reported that the severity of the right ventricular dilation is related to active pneumocystis carinii pneumonia, a defining pulmonary disease of HIV/AIDS. Therefore, it has been speculated that the dilation of the right ventricle may be related to pulmonary oxygen saturation, which is resulted from pulmonary hypertension. Generally, cardiomyopathy is believed to be caused by HIV-1 direct infection of the myocardium to result in myocarditis. The possibility of ECHO virus or Coxsackie virus infection cannot be excluded, which has been proved in some autopsy and biopsy reports.

Case Study 1

A male patient aged 56 years was confirmatively diagnosed as having AIDS by CDC. He has a history of blood donation in 1991, and complained of fever, shortness of breath after physical activities in 2008. His CD4 T cell count was 41/μl.

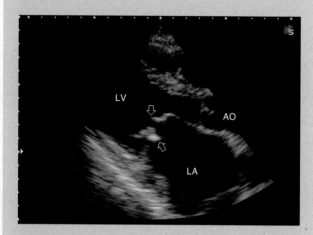

Fig. 18.7 HIV/AIDS related dilated cardiomyopathy. Color Doppler ultrasound demonstrates enlarged heart, especially the left ventricle; diffuse decrease of the motion range of left ventricular wall; obviously decreased thickening rate in contraction period of the ventricular wall; normal morphology of the mitral valve with decreased opening width, inferior migration of the closing point and dysraphism, obviously enlarged EPSS; no obvious morphological and structural abnormalities of other heart valves; decreased heart functions. Doppler ultrasound demonstrates reflux blood flow bundles originating from mitral and tricuspid ports in the right and left atria during their systolic period. *AO* aorta opening, *LA* left atria, *LV* left ventricle

Case Study 2

A female patient aged 36 years was confirmatively diagnosed as having AIDS by CDC. She had a history of blood transfusion in 1995, and complained of fever, cough, expectoration and shortness of breath in 2009. Her CD4 T cell count was 66/μl.

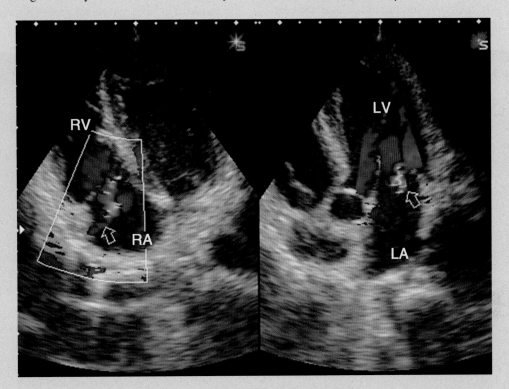

Fig. 18.8 Color Doppler ultrasound demonstrates cross sectional four chambers of the heart: slight reflux signals in mitral valve and tricuspid valve, and normal sizes of the heart chambers. Diagnosis: HIV/AIDS complicated by mitral and tricuspid regurgitation. *LA* left atria, *LV* left ventricle, *RA* right atria, *RV* right ventricle

Case Study 3

A male patient aged 43 years was confirmatively diagnosed as having AIDS by CDC. He had a history of blood donation in 1993, and complained of fever and progressive emaciation in 2006. His CD4 T cell count was 32/μl.

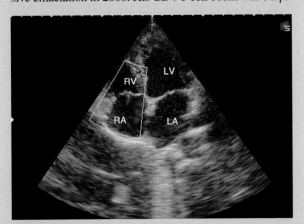

Fig. 18.9 HIV/AIDS related tricuspid regurgitation. Color Doppler ultrasound demonstrates cross sectional four chambers of the heart: slight reflux signals in tricuspid valve, normal sizes of the chambers of the heart. *LA* left atria, *LV* left ventricle, *RA* right atria, *RV* right ventricle

Case Study 4

A male patient aged 26 years was confirmatively diagnosed as having AIDS by CDC. He had a history of unhealthy sexual life, and complained of fever and oral ulcers in 2008. His CD4 T cell count was 61/µl.

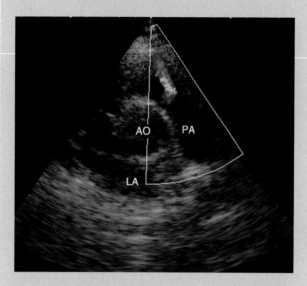

Fig. 18.10 HIV/AIDS related dilated cardiomyopathy and moderate pulmonary valve regurgitation. Color Doppler ultrasound demonstrates cross sectional blood vessels in short axis view: moderate reflux signal in pulmonary arterial valve and normal sizes of the heart chambers. *AO* aorta, *LA* left atria, *PA* pulmonary artery

Case Study 5

A female patient aged 50 years was confirmatively diagnosed as having AIDS by CDC. She had a history of blood donation in 1992, and complained of fever, shortness of breath and cyanosis in 2004. Her CD4 T cell count was 33/ µl.

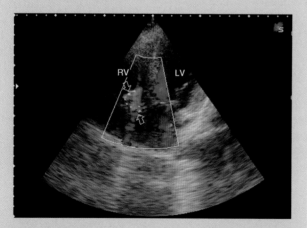

Fig. 18.11 AIDS complicated by pulmonary hypertension (moderate), moderate -severe tricuspid regurgitation. Color Doppler ultrasound demonstrates cross sectional view of the heart chambers: moderate -severe reflux signals in tricuspid valve, and the estimated pulmonary arterial pressure being 55 mmHg, enlarged right ventricle and increased root diameter of the pulmonary artery. *LV* left ventricle, *RV* right ventricle

Case Study 6

A male patient aged 57 years was confirmatively diagnosed as having AIDS by CDC. He had a history of blood transfusion in 1993, and complained of fever, emaciation and fatigue in 2007. His CD4 T cell count was 39/µl.

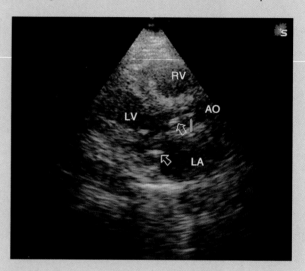

Fig. 18.12 AIDS complicated by rheumatic heart disease (mitral and aortic valve stenosis). Color ultrasound demonstrates cross sectional left heart along the long axis: thickened mitral valve, strengthened echo, obvious calcification of the cusp, adhesion of their junction, limited opening. Doppler ultrasound demonstrations of increased speed of blood flow in diastolic period of mitral valve, slightly thickened and calcified aortic valvular margins, limited opening but quite good opening and closure; enlarged left atrium. *AO* aorta, *LA* left atria, *LV* left ventricle, *RV* right ventricle

18.3.3 Discussion

Valvular heart disease is the functional or structural abnormalities of singular or multiple valves (including valve cusp, valve ring, tendon or papillary muscles) due to inflammation, mucoid degeneration, congenital malformation, ischemic necrosis and trauma. The pathological process results in valvular stenosis or incomplete closure. Severe dilation of the ventricles and the roots of the aorta and pulmonary artery can also cause relative incomplete closure of the corresponding atrioventricular valve and semilunar valve. Mitral valve is the most commonly involved, followed by the aortic valve. The pathological changes of valves have the following manifestations: (1) Restricted opening of the valve, with narrowed valvular orifice and obstructed blood flow; (2) Incomplete valvular closure, with regurgitation of the blood flow; (3) Concurrent of the above two conditions. In AIDS patients, valvular heart diseases commonly include tricuspid incompetence, mitral incompetence and pulmonary valvular incompetence.

18.4 HIV/AIDS Related Endocardial Diseases

Endocarditis in HIV positive patients can be divided into two types, namely marantic endocarditis (also known as non-bacterial thrombotic endocarditis) and infectious endocarditis (including bacterial endocarditis and fungal endocarditis). Infectious endocarditis is more common in AIDS patients who are intravenous drug abusers. The excrescence of these two types of endocarditis is similar to each other, and the incidence of such disease varies from 6.3 to 34 % according to international reports. A research report from China by Zhu and Yuan, et al. indicated an incidence of 0.76 %, which is lower than that internationally reported. It has been speculated that the difference of the reported incidence may be related to the different routes of transmission. It was reported that 21 cases with left ventricular diastolic dysfunction (the incidence is 16.03 %) and 18 cases with left ventricular systolic dysfunction (the incidence is 13.74 %), indicating that diastolic dysfunction may occur earlier than systolic dysfunction. Among the 18 cases with left ventricular systolic dysfunction, the CD4 T cell count in 12 cases (66.67 %) is lower than 400×10^6/L, and in 8 cases (44.44 %) is lower than 200×10^6/L. The results indicate that left ventricular systolic dysfunction occurs more commonly in AIDS patients with lower CD4 T cell count, especially those in the advanced stage of AIDS, which is in consistency with the results in international reports. endocardial diseases commonly occur secondary to cardiopathies. However, endocardial diseases can be primary and singular in AIDS patients. The common endocardial diseases in AIDS patients include non-bacterial thrombotic endocarditis and infectious endocarditis. Non-bacterial thrombotic endocarditis occurs based on cachexia, blood coagulation disorder and endocardiosis, with involvement of any valve. The damage to endothelial cells may induce thrombosis. In the cases with accompanying thrombus shedding, symptoms of embolism occur. By echocardiography, heart valvular excrescence can be found. Infectious endocarditis is caused by infections by bacteria, candida and aspergillus. Aspergillus endocarditis can cause myocarditis and pericarditis. And aspergillus on the endocardium can shed to cause cerebral thrombosis. Echocardiography, especially transesophageal echocardiography, is sensitive to valvular excrescence and complicated valvular lesions and facilitates the differential diagnosis of the two types endocarditis.

Case Study

A male patient aged 36 years was confirmatively diagnosed as having AIDS by CDC. He had a history of blood donation in 1994, and complained of fever, chest distress after physical activities and shortness of breath. His CD4 T cell count was 41/µl.

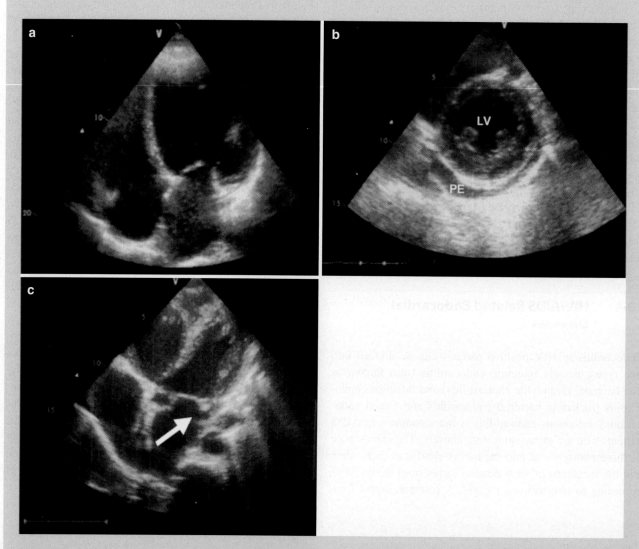

Fig. 18.13 (**a–c**) HIV/AIDS related pericardiopathy, myocardiopathy and endocardiopathy. (**a**) Ultrasonogram of dilated myocardiopathy in the patient with AIDS. (**b**) Ultrasonogram of pericardial effusion in the patient with AIDS. (**c**) Ultrasonogram of endocarditis in the patient with AIDS (excrescence pointed with a *white arrow*). *LV* left ventricle, *PE* pericardial effusion

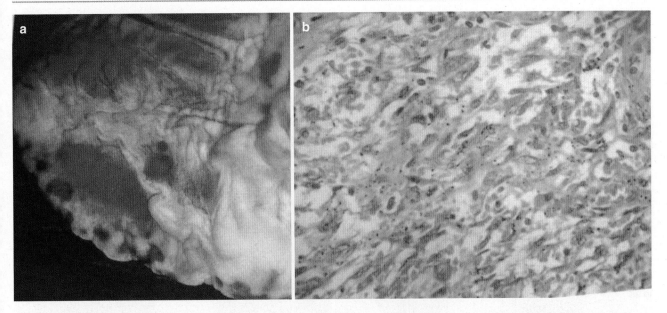

Fig. 18.14 (**a, b**) HIV/AIDS related cardiac Kaposi's sarcoma. (**a**) Multiple flakes of purple prominences on the surface of the heart. (**b**) There is large flakes of spindle cells in braided liked arrangement in different sizes, intercellular leakage of many erythrocytes

18.5   HIV/AIDS Related Cardiac Tumors

HIV/AIDS related cardiac neoplasm refers to occurrence of tumors caused by compromised immunity due to HIV infection, among which Kaposi's sarcoma is more common, especially common in homosexual AIDS patients. Kaposi's sarcoma is mostly restricted in visceral layer of the pericardium, with possible invasion to the myocardium, parietal layer of the pericardium and the coronary artery. There have been also reports about HIV/AIDS related myocardial and pericardial lymphomas. Both of Hodgkin lymphoma and non-Hodgkin lymphoma can involve endocardium and myocardium, with more commonly involved epicardium. The clinical symptoms are similar to those of pericardial effusion. For cases with lymphoma and involved pericardium, pericardial effusion may occur. For cases with lymphoma and involved myocardium, arrhythmia, conduction block and congestive heart failure may occur. For cases with lymphoma and its invasion into the cardiac chambers, blockage of blood flow may occur. Generally, patients with HIV infection are rarely found to have severe cardiac diseases. HIV/AIDS related cardiac neoplasms may be asymptomatic, or with similar symptoms to other cardiopathies including life threatening cardiac dysfunction. The symptoms include sudden heart failure, arrhythmia and sudden decrease of blood pressure caused by blood flowing into pericardium (the sack that wraps up the heart). Because cardiac neoplasm rarely occurs with its symptoms similar to those of other types of cardiopathies, its diagnosis is difficult. And patients with such disease usually fail to obtain the pathological diagnosis during their lifetime.

18.6   HIV/AIDS Related Vascular Diseases

18.6.1   Venous Thrombosis and Pulmonary Embolism

AIDS may be complicated by venous thrombosis and pulmonary embolism. Pulmonary embolism can be caused by shedding of deep vein thrombus.

Case

A male patient aged 27 years was confirmatively diagnosed as having AIDS by CDC. He complained of shortness of breath and chest distress. His CD4 T cell count was 35/μl.

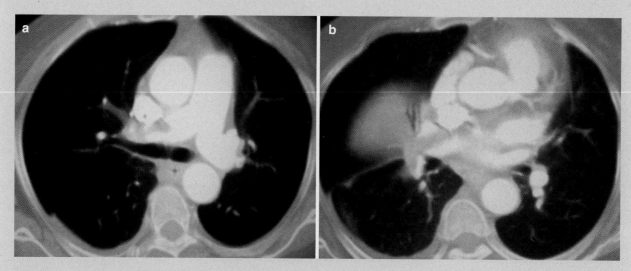

Fig. 18.15 (**a**, **b**) HIV/AIDS related pulmonary embolism. (**a**, **b**) Enhanced scanning demonstrates filling defects in the right pulmonary trunk and left upper pulmonary artery

18.6.2 Pulmonary Hypertension

HIV infection complicated by pulmonary hypertension (HIV-PAH) is one of the non-infective complications of HIV infection, with an incidence of about 0.5 %. Its pathogenesis is still unknown. The common pathogenic causes include pneumocystis carinii pneumonia, recurrent thromboembolism of minor pulmonary arterial branches caused by pulmonary infection due to inflammatory mediators or cytokines, and intrapulmonary venous occlusion. The resulted pulmonary fibrosis and minor artery occlusion result in the increase of pulmonary vascular resistance and the increased pulmonary arterial pressure. It may also be related to HIV envelope protein and hereditary susceptibility. The pathological changes of lung tissue in cases of HIV-PAH are similar to those of idiopathic pulmonary hypertension (IPAH). The clinical manifestations are nonspecific, and the most common symptom is progressive dyspnea. The treatment commonly is against pulmonary hypertension and anti-retroviral therapy. HIV-PAH is the single risk factor that may cause the death of HIV-infected patients. When HIV-infected patients complain of cardiopulmonary symptoms of inexplicable reasons, HIV-PAH should be considered. Pulmonary arterial lesions caused by the immune effects of HIV infection, thrombus and pulmonary microvascular embolism caused by contaminated intravenous infusion drugs all may lead to pulmonary hypertension. In China, Zhu et al. reported the incidence of pulmonary hypertension in AIDS patients is 2.29 %, with all three cases with slight pulmonary hypertension and their systolic pressure being no higher than 50 mmHg. In addition, the chest X-ray indicated thickened and deranged pulmonary markings, which came into the conclusion that patients with AIDS complicated by pulmonary infections are more susceptible to pulmonary hypertension. By echocardiography, the diagnosis can be non-invasively made based on the pressure discrepancy of tricuspid regurgitation. Other cardiac complications, such as ischemic cardiomyopathy, may be due to atherosclerosis caused by viral infection of monocytes and macrophages. It may also be due to adhesive changes of leukocytes or arteritis. Two cases ischemic changes by ECG have been reported, with an incidence of 1.53 %. Abnormalities in the conduction system may be caused by lymphocytic myocarditis, opportunistic infections, myocardium toxicity of drugs and local existence of HIV in cardiac conduction tissues, with the reported incidence of 4.58 %. Generally, echocardiography demonstrates hypertrophy or dilation of the right ventricle but normal findings of the left ventricle, which can be diagnosed as having pulmonary hypertension. Indicators of dyspnea and hypertrophy of the right ventricle in AIDS patients can be diagnosed as having pulmonary hypertension.

18.6.3   Vasculitis

The pathogenesis of HIV/AIDS related vasculitis and perivasculitis is still unknown, which may be related to vascular wall lesions directly caused by HIV itself or to vascular lesions due to the formation of immune complex. The lesions are manifested as nodular arteritis and acute inflammation of small or medium sized blood vessels, leading to lesions of skin, muscle and nerve fibers. Perivasculitis usually involves small and medium sized arteries, with manifestations of arterial intimal fibrosis, elastic fiber breakage, arterial medial fibrosis, accompanying varied degrees of vascular stenosis, and possible occurrence of necrotic vasculitis.

Case Study
A male patient aged 31 years was confirmatively diagnosed as having AIDS by CDC. He complained of progressive dyspnea, shortness of breath and chest distress. His CD4 T cell count was 75/μl.

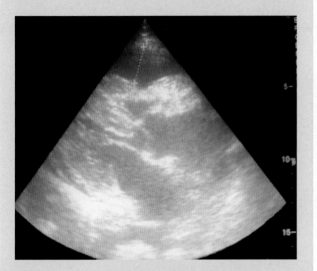

Fig. 18.16 HIV/AIDS related pulmonary hypertension. It is demonstrated to have widened pulmonary artery segment

Case Study 1
A male patient aged 27 years was confirmatively diagnosed as having AIDS by CDC. He complained of lower extremities numbness and pain. And his CD4 T cell count was 15/μl.

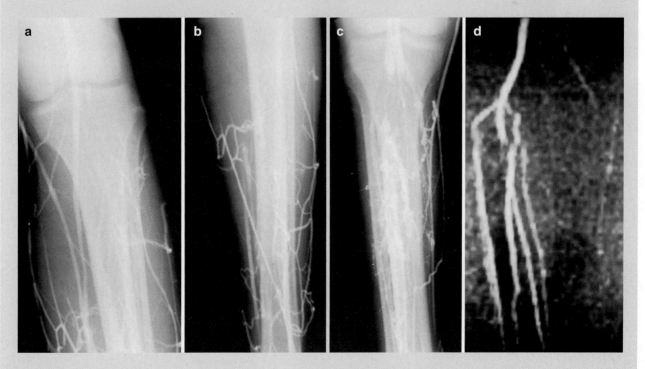

Fig. 18.17 (**a–d**) HIV/AIDS related vasculitis. (**a–d**) It is demonstrated to have circuity and stenosis of popliteal vein

Case Study 2

A female patient aged 31 years was confirmatively diagnosed as having AIDS by CDC. Her CD4 T cell count was 5/ μl.

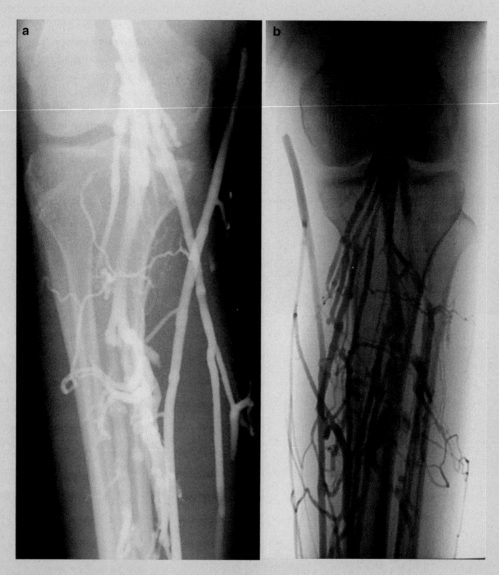

Fig. 18.18 (**a, b**) HIV/AIDS related stenosis and phlebangioma of the popliteal artery. (**a, b**) It is demonstrated to have stenosis, circuity and aneurysmoid dilatation of the popliteal artery

Case Study 3

A male patient aged 30 years was confirmatively diagnosed as having AIDS by CDC. He complained of lower extremities numbness, and his CD4 T cell count was 21/μl.

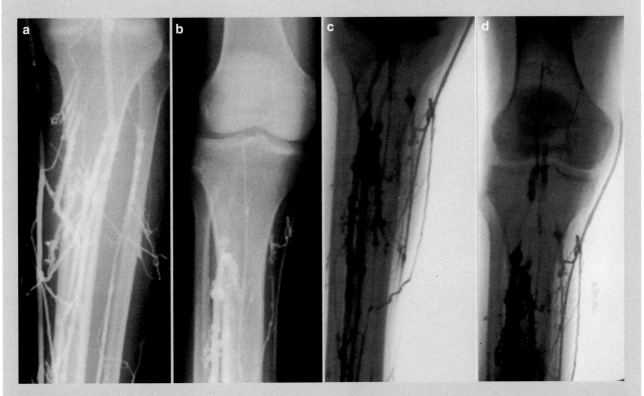

Fig. 18.19 (a–d) HIV/AIDS related stenosis and phlebangioma of the popliteal vein. (a–d) It is demonstrated to have distal stenosis of the genicular artery, varying degrees of stenosis of the peroneal artery, the anterior and posterior tibial arteries, venous bead string liked stenosis and breakage of the foot dorsal vein

Case Study 4

A boy aged 5 years was confirmatively diagnosed as having AIDS by CDC. He complained of lower extremities numbness and pain, and his CD4 T cell count was 13/μl.

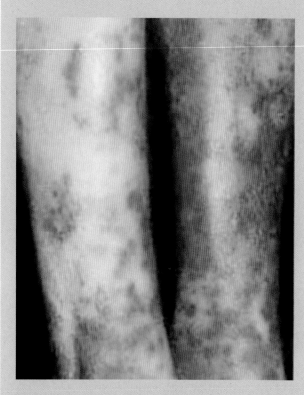

Fig. 18.20 HIV/AIDS related leukocytoclastic vasculitis. It is demonstrated to have multiple patchy congestion plaques in bilateral lower extremities, with some fusing in color of purplish brown

Extended Reading

1. Barbaro G. Cardiovascular manifestations of HIV infection [J]. Circulation. 2002;106(11):1420–5.
2. Barbaro G, Barbarini G, Pellicelli AM. HIV associated coronary arteritis in a patient with fatal myocardial infarction [J]. N Engl J Med. 2001;344(23):1799–800.
3. Barbaro G, Fisher SD, Lipshultz SE. Pathogenesis of HIV associated cardiovascular complications [J]. Lancet Infect Dis. 2001;1(2):115–24.
4. Braithwaite RS, Concato J, Chang CC, et al. A framework for tailoring clinical guidelines to comorbidity at the point of care [J]. Arch Intern Med. 2007;167(21):2361–5.
5. Calabrese LH. Infection with the human immunodeficiency virus type 1 and vascular inflammatory disease [J]. Clin Exp Rheumatol. 2004;22(6 Suppl 36):S87–93.
6. Chaves AA, Mihm MJ, Schanbacher BI. Cardiomyopathy in a murine model of AIDS: evidence of reactive nitrogen species and corroboration in HIV/AIDS cardiac tissues [J]. Cardiovasc Res. 2003;60(1):108–18.
7. Cotter BR. Epidemiology of HIV cardiac disease [J]. Prog Cardiovasc Dis. 2003;45(4):319–26.
8. Herskowitz A, Vlahov D, Willoughby S, et al. Prevalence and incidence of left ventricular dysfunction in patients with human immunodeficiency virus infection [J]. Am J Cardiol. 1993;71(11):955–8.
9. Herskowitz A, Willoughby SB, Baughman KL. Cardiomyopathy associated with anti-retroviral therapy in patients with human immunodeficiency virus infections: a report of six cares. Ann Intern Med. 1992;116:311.
10. Maserli R, Parsi A. Rapidly reversible cardiomyopathy in an AIDS patients. AIDS. 1991;5:1145.
11. Miller RF, Howling SJ, Reid AJ, et al. Pleural effusions in patient s with AIDS [J]. Sex Transm Infect. 2000;76(2):122–5.
12. Nzuobontane D, Blackett KN, Kuaban C. Cardiac involvement in HIV infected people in Yaounde Cameroon [J]. Postgrad Med J. 2002;78(925):678–81.
13. Pellicelli A, Barbaro G, Palmieri F, et al. Primary pulmonary hypertension in HIV disease: a systematic review [J]. Angiology. 2001;52(1):31–41.
14. SilvaCardoso J, Moura B, Martins L, et al. Pericardial involvement in human immunodeficiency virus infection [J]. Chest. 1999;115(2):418–22.
15. Wang XF. Echocardiography [M]. 3rd ed. Beijing: People's Medical Publishing House, PMPH; 1999. p. 283–553.

Contents

H. Li (ed.), *Radiology of HIV/AIDS*,
DOI 10.1007/978-94-007-7823-8_19, © Springer Science+Business Media Dordrecht and People's Medical Publishing House 2014

19.1   An Overview of HIV/AIDS Related Gastrointestinal Diseases

The gastrointestinal tract is one of the most involved organs by HIV/AIDS, with lesions in the mesentery, peritoneum and retroperitoneum. HIV/AIDS related gastrointestinal diseases can be divided into two types, including inflammations and neoplasms, such as CMV infection and KS. These diseases can involve all kinds of tissues in the digestive system. For instances, Candida mainly invades oral cavity and esophagus, while protozoa infection often involves colon to cause chronic diarrhea. KS commonly occurs in esophagus, followed by the small intestine and colon in frequency of occurrence. Lymphomas mostly occur in small intestine and colon.

The common inflammatory diseases include:

1. Candida infections

   Candida albicans is the most common pathogen for esophageal infections in HIV/AIDS patients, with typical symptoms of swallowing pain and difficulty swallowing, progressive chest pain that may be severe. In the early stage, the lesions include small patchy filling defects in esophageal mucosa that distribute along the long axis of the esophagus, mucosal edema, and further brush liked change of the esophagus wall. Deep ulceration and mucus shedding are causes of irregular esophageal wall in its progressive stage.

2. Spastic esophagitis

   Clinically, based on esophageal spasm, spastic esophagitis can be diagnosed. It is favorably demonstrated by esophageal contrast radiography. The common demonstrations include multiple scattering superficial ulcers that distribute between normal mucosa.

3. Cytomegalovirus infections

   Cytomegalovirus esophagitis is a common complication in AIDS patients, with involvements of almost all segments of gastrointestinal tract. Infections of colon and small intestine are more common than infections of esophagus and stomach. Ulcer occurs due to local tissue ischemia induced by CMV. CMV esophagitis has common manifestations of discontinuous ulcers between normal esophageal mucosa. The definitive diagnosis depends on biopsy. CMV gastritis commonly involves gastric sinuses. By barium meal radiography, the gastric sinus wall is demonstrated to have nodular thickening, ring shaped stenosis of the gastric sinus cavity, and accompanying weakening dilation. CMV colonitis firstly is demonstrated as superficial ulcers. But with the occurrence of edema, mucosal folds are thickened, with enlarged and deepened ulcers.

4. Tuberculous esophagitis

   Tuberculous esophagitis is often derived by expanding of necrotic lymphoid tuberculosis within the mediastinum adjacent to the middle esophageal segment. Esophageal X-ray and CT scanning demonstrate local external lump impression, deep ulcer, sinus tract and fistula formation. Intestinal tuberculosis commonly involves ileocecus. By barium double contrast and radiography, there are ring shaped stenosis and ring shaped thickening of the ileocecus wall. In some cases, there is also formation of sinus tract, such as occurrence of urethrorectal fistula.

5. Kaposi's Sarcoma (KS)

   KS is a kind of tumor derived from lymphatic reticuloendothelial cells. KS often occurs in homosexual/bisexual AIDS patients, with an incidence of up to 50 %. A KS related herpes virus (KS-HV) has been isolated from KS in patients of different ethnic groups, indicating its existence in KS. It involves different organs including, in frequency order, skin, lymph nodes, gastrointestinal tract, lungs, liver and spleen. The gastrointestinal tract is one of the most commonly involved organs, with typical manifestations of smooth submucosal nodules and accompanying/absent navel liked depression.

6. HIV/AIDS related lymphomas

   In patients with AIDS, about 10 % sustains NHL, which often occurs in superficial lymph nodes and mediastinal lymph nodes, especially in the esophagus, skeleton and abdominal organs, with no peripheral lymphadenectasis. Cases of gastric, intestinal or rectal lymphoma are demonstrated to have irregular thickening of the mucosal folds by barium meal radiography.

General introduction to HIV/AIDS related intestinal diseases:

1. Small intestinal diseases

   HIV/AIDS related small intestinal disease is commonly enteritis caused by opportunistic infection. The pathogen is cryptozoite and mycobacterium avium. And small intestinal infections caused by tubercle bacillus, salmonella and campylobacter jejuni are also common. The common symptoms include diarrhea or chronic diarrhea for four to five times a day, abdominal distension, nausea and spastic pain. Cryptozoite can only cause slight diarrhea among people with normal immunity that is self restraint lasting for 2–3 days. But in AIDS patients, it can cause severe diarrhea, such as cholera liked diarrhea. Mycobacterium avium can gain its access to the digestive tract via oral cavity to invade the small intestines, leading to fever and diarrhea.

2. Colon and rectal diseases

   The pathogens that cause colon and rectal infections in AIDS patients are commonly histolytic amebic protozoa, Giardia lamblia and herpes simplex (HSV). The other pathogens include cryptosporidium and cytomegalovirus, whose infections can cause colonitis that is common in AIDS patients. Cryptosporidium/cytomegalovirus infection induced colonitis is especially common in AIDS patients who are receiving antibiotic therapy. The clinical manifestations of colon and rectal diseases in AIDS patients are inflammation and perianal pain. Intestinoendoscopy demonstrates mucosal ulcers. The colon infection caused by cytomegalovirus (CMV) can lead to ulcer and perforation. Other related intestinal lymphomas and KS are more common in male homosexual patients with AIDS.

19.2 HIV/AIDS Related Viral Esophagitis

19.2.1 HIV/AIDS Related CMV Esophagitis

Cytomegalovirus infection, a common complication of HIV/AIDS, can lead to death. About 2–13 % AIDS patients have involvement of the gastrointestinal tract by CMV infection, leading to esophagitis, gastritis and colonitis. According to autopsy of CMV infected AIDS patients, about 90 % has explicit CMV infection and the cause of death is CMV infection in 40 % such patients. Studies have demonstrated that about 24 % AIDS patients have severe CMV infection within 2 years after the onset, which leads to occurrence of earlier death in AIDS patients. CMV infection in HIV/AIDS patients can involve all organs of the body, even the skin. But the commonly involved are the lungs, the central nervous system and the gastrointestinal tract. CMV pneumonia often causes death in patients with HIV/AIDS.

19.2.1.1 Pathogens and Pathogenesis

CMV belongs to the herpes virus family, and it can invade human body via various routes, including placenta, contacts, injection, blood transfusion, breathing, digestion, sexual intercourse and organ transplantations. AIDS patients are susceptible to CMV infection, with an incidence of up to 95 % in homosexual patients with AIDS. Generally, CMV remains a long-term incubation in the human body. CMV infection commonly occurs in immunocompromised population, with more than 90 % patients having CMV antibody positive and more than 50 % patients having virusemia. The compromised immunity occurs in AIDS patients due to HIV infection, while CMV can also have inhibitory effect on cellular immunity which worsens the immunity of AIDS patients.

19.2.1.2 Pathophysiological Basis

CMV infection often involves the adrenal gland, lungs and digestive tract, and it can also invade the spleen, lymph nodes, heart, thyroid gland, brain, pancreas, retina, liver, gall bladder, meninges, saliva gland, peripheral nerves, bladder, respiratory tract, larynx and other body organs. Klatt et al. retrospectively reviewed clinical data of 565 cases of AIDS [11]. It has been reported that CMV infection involved alimentary tract segments occurs in 165 cases (57.7 %), including 41 cases with esophageal involvement, 34 cases with gastric involvement, 40 cases with small intestine involvement and 43 cases with colorectal involvement. During the progression of HIV/AIDS, most patients sustain complications of active infections, with about 1/4 having life threatening serious infection. The characteristic pathology of CMV infection includes formation of cytomegaly and intranuclear virus inclusion bodies in owl's eye sign. CMV antibody can be immunohistochemically marked for its demonstration. Atypical

Table 19.1 Alimentary diseases caused by CMV infection

Common diseases	Clinical manifestations
Esophagitis	Difficulty swallow, retrosternal pain
Gastritis	Epigastric pain, gastric ulcer
Colorectal inflammation	Abdominal pain, diarrhea, poor appetite, weight loss and fever

giant cells also have diagnostic value, which constitutes the criteria for the early diagnosis. In addition, there are also necrosis and shedding of local alimentary mucosal epithelial cells, degeneration and necrosis of tissues as well as mononuclear cells infiltration with accompanying necrotic focus.

19.2.1.3 Clinical Symptoms and Signs

The common clinical symptoms are fever and fatigue. Within 1–2 weeks after occurrence of fever, the absolute value of lymphocyte count in the blood increases, with heteromorphic changes and skin maculopapule. Esophagitis, gastroenteritis, splenomegaly and lymphadenitis (Table 19.1) can also occur.

19.2.1.4 Examinations and Their Selection

1. The definitive diagnosis of the disease depends on cytological and pathological examinations as well as virus culture. Brush cytology can be applied to collect samples for detection of inclusion bodies in the squamous epithelial cells. Using such procedure, the results can be obtained within 24 h. The positive rate is high in biopsy of specimens obtained by fibergastroscopy from the ulcers margin. In the advanced stage of the disease, it is difficult to harvest specimens. By virus culture, the results can be obtained within 24–72 h.

2. By immunohistochemistry and in situ hybridization, the diagnosis can be made. By immunohistochemistry, the cytoplasm, nucleus and cytomegalic inclusion in the epithelial cells from lesions can be stained to show strong positive. In situ hybridization demonstrates the nucleus positively stained.

3. The findings of serum anti-CMV antibody positive and IgM antibody positive can confirm the reactivation of current infection or latent infection. But the finding of serum IgG positive indicates a past infection.

4. Using human fibroblasts to culture the patient's specimens from surgical operation, blood, secretions and excretions, CMV can be isolated within about 4 weeks.

5. Using the patient's specimens from surgical operation, blood, secretions and excretions, CMV antigen can be detected. Its sensitivity to immunofluorescence can be up to 100 %.

6. The finding of isolated ulcer in normal mucosa is characteristic by barium swallow examination. In the early stage, the ulcer is in shape of shallow round or oval. But in the advanced stage, the ulcer fuses to form plaque.

7. In the early stage, gastroscopy demonstrates superficial and isolated small ulcers in the mucosa.

19.2.1.5 Imaging Demonstrations
Gastrointestinal Radiography

The direct signs include local or extensive CMV infection, with involvement of any segment of gastrointestinal tract to cause various lesions. The lesions include small and superficial erosion as well as deep ulcer and perforation. The indirect signs include esophageal irritation.

Direct Signs by Esophagoscopy

There are obvious congestion and edema in the mucosa of esophageal wall as well as crisp mucosa that tends to bleed when touched. There are also erosion or different sizes of ulcers, and even perforation.

Case Study

A male patient aged 34 years was confirmatively diagnosed as having AIDS by the CDC. He complained of retrosternal intermittent unsmooth swallowing for half a year, burning and progressive odynophagia for 6 weeks. His CD4 T cell count was 9/μl

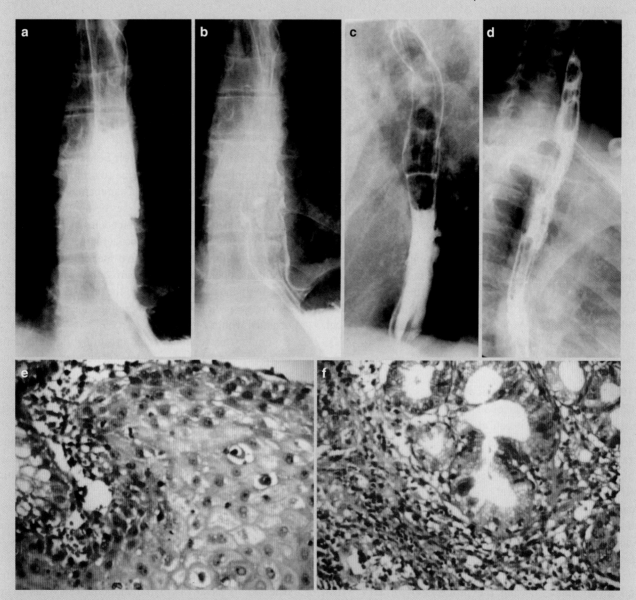

Fig. 19.1 (a–f) HIV/AIDS related CMV esophagitis. By esophageal barium meal radiology: (a, b) It is demonstrated to have normotopic barium meal filling sign and mucosa sign, indicating a niche liked filling defect and barium plaque in the lower part of the esophagus. (c) It is demonstrated to have right anterior oblique view of barium meal filling sign and mucosal niche liked barium plaque protrusion, with small burr shaped barium shadow. (d) It is demonstrated to have left anterior oblique view of coarse and unsmooth mucosa in middle and lower segments of the esophagus. (e) HE staining demonstrates cytomegalovirus inclusion bodies in the esophageal squamous epithelium (HE ×200). (f) HE staining demonstrates to have cytomegalovirus inclusion bodies in the mucosa of the lower segment of the esophagus (HE ×200)

19.2.1.6   Criteria for the Diagnosis
Clinical Symptoms
CMV esophagitis has common symptoms of retrosternal foreign sense, retrosternal pain, odynophagia and dysphagia as well as esophageal bleeding. Slight infection commonly is asymptomatic.

Endoscopy
At the dismal esophagus, there are small blisters, hole liked ulcers of various sizes, obvious congestion and edema in the fundus, crisp mucosa that tends to bleed when touched.

Biopsy
Biopsy of ulcers demonstrates acute/chronic inflammation, with findings of cytomegalovirus inclusion bodies. Biopsy in the early stage for virus culture has positive findings.

Esophageal Barium Meal Radiology
It demonstrates multiple scattered superficial ulcers, in manifestations of multiple patch liked filling defect and spike liked small ulcers.

Cytomegalorirus
There is increased titer of cytomegalovirus antibody in AIDS patients.

19.2.1.7 Differential Diagnosis
HIV/AIDS related CMV esophagitis should be differentiated from HSV esophagitis, candidal esophagitis and esophageal burn lesions.

19.2.2 HIV/AIDS Related HSV Esophagitis

19.2.2.1 Pathogens and Pathogenesis
The pathogen of viral esophagitis is herpes viruses. Therefore, viral esophagitis is also known as herpetic esophagitis. Currently, it is believed that the pathogens are commonly herpes simplex virus I and II, herpes zoster virus (HZV), CMV and EBV, in which HSV is more common. HSV can reach the esophagus along the vagus nerve to cause mucosal herpes lesions, which is common in immunocompromised and AIDS patients. The pathogenesis of herpes virus induced esophagitis is still in disagreement. Some scholars believe that the virus causes subintimal inflammation of the capillaries, arterioles and venules, with occurrence of thrombus to cause local necrosis and the resulted mucosal ulcers.

19.2.2.2 Pathophysiological Basis
HSV can reach esophagus along the vagus nerve to cause mucosal herpes lesions. The earliest pathological changes include focal ulcers. Generally, the disease can be divided into three stages. In the first stage, multiple small blisters occur at the distal esophagus. In the second stage, the small blisters fuse into swelling in size of 0.5–2 cm.

Table 19.2 Digestive diseases caused by HSV infection

Common diseases	Manifestations
Pharyngitis and esophagitis	Dysphagia, substernal pain
Colon and rectal inflammation	Anus and rectum pain, abdominal pain, diarrhea, poor appetite, weight loss , tenesmus, constipation, sacral abnormal feeling

19.2.2.3 Clinical Symptoms and Signs
The common symptoms include retrosternal foreign sense and pain, odynophagia and dysphagia as well as occasional esophageal bleeding. Slight infections are usually asymptomatic. During the epidemic of the virus, cases with general soreness and pain, sore throat and accompanying esophageal symptoms should be diagnosed as having virus esophagitis (Table 19.2).

19.2.2.4 Examinations and Their Selection
1. The definitive diagnosis of the disease depends on cytological and pathological examinations as well as virus culture.
2. By immunohistochemistry and in situ hybridization, the diagnosis can be made.
3. In situ hybridization should be performed with DNA probe of the herpes simplex virus. By immunohistochemistry, the cytoplasm, nucleus and cytomegaly inclusion of lesions epithelial cells are all stained strongly positive. By in situ hybridization, the nucleus is positive.
4. By esophageal barium swallowing examination, isolated superficial ulcers are characteristic findings.
5. By gastroscopy, small isolated superficial ulcers can be found in mucosa in the early stage of the disease, in sizes ranging from several millimeters to several centimeters.
6. Biopsy.

19.2.2.5 Imaging Demonstrations
Gastrointestinal Radiography
The direct signs include characteristic isolated ulcers by double contrast esophageal radiography, in shallow round or oval shape in the early stage and fusion of ulcers into plaques in the advanced stage. The indirect signs include esophageal irritation.

Esophagoscopy
Esophagoscopy demonstrates hole liked ulcers of different sizes in the distal segment of the esophagus, and normal mucosa between ulcers. There are obvious congestion and edema in the mucosa in the early stage of the disease, and fusion of ulcers in the advanced stage. The mucosa is crisp, with diffuse damages and bleeding.

19.2.2.6 Criteria for the Diagnosis
1. Clinical symptoms include general soreness and pain, sore throat and upper gastrointestinal tract symptoms with accompanying esophageal symptoms.

2. By endoscopy, there are small blisters in the distal esophagus, hole liked ulcers of different sizes and normal mucosa between ulcers.
3. Scattering and multiple superficial ulcers by esophageal barium radiology of double contrast.
4. Biopsy and culture can confirm the diagnosis.

19.2.2.7 Differential Diagnosis
Cytomegalovirus Esophagitis
CMV infection is commonly complicated by infections of HSV, fungus and bacteria.

HZV Infection
VZV can cause necrotic esophagitis, and it can also lead to disseminated visceral infections.

HIV/AIDS Related Virus Esophagitis
The infected localizations have multiple ulcers, with symptoms of fever, diarrhea and odynophagia.

Papilloma Virus Infection
It can cause wart and flat condyloma of the squamous epithelium.

19.2.3 HIV/AIDS Related Esophagitis

Some chronic inflammation of the gastrointestinal tract and diarrhea show no evidence of pathogenic infection. It has been speculated that HIV may directly affect the intestinal environmental balance, which are known as idiopathic HIV/AIDS related intestinal diseases.

19.3 HIV/AIDS Related Candida Esophagitis

19.3.1 Pathogens and Pathogenesis

Candida albicans is a kind of conditional pathogenic fungi. The weakened immunity or the dysfunctional bacterial colonies cause candida albicans to be pathogenic fungi to cause candida infection. The incidence of candida infection is 80–90 %. The lesions commonly are found in the oral cavity, throat, esophagus and lungs. In AIDS patients, about 20 % has candida esophagitis. It is ulcerative pseudomembranous esophagitis caused by invasion of candida albicans to the esophageal mucosa. Such patients' CD4 T cell count are commonly lower than 350/μl.

19.3.2 Pathophysiological Basis

Candida is a kind of conditional pathogen and Candida albicans is the main pathogenic type. Candida invades into the blood to cause candidemia, and then disseminated to visceral tissues and organs to cause multiple abscesses and chronic inflammation. The esophageal mucosa is found to have congestion, swelling, necrosis and even ulceration.

19.3.3 Clinical Symptoms and Signs

Clinical symptoms are pharyngalgia, odynophagia and dysphagia. Most patients have accompanying epigastric distention, hiccups, poor appetite and other gastrointestinal symptoms.

19.3.4 Examinations and Their Selection

1. By digestive endoscopy, there are irregular ulcers and white pseudomembrane in the esophageal mucosa.
2. Among various imaging examinations, barium meal radiography is of choice.
3. Digestive endoscopy.
4. Biopsy for pathological examination.

19.3.5 Imaging Demonstrations

19.3.5.1 Digestive Radiography
Esophageal X-ray of double contrast demonstrates (1) A wide range of involvement with different degrees of severity, increasingly serious involvements from the top to the bottom of the esophagus; (2) Abnormal dynamic changes including reduced tension and weakened peristalsis of all involved esophagus segments that are more obvious in lower esophagus, and delayed emptying; (3) Contour profile abnormalities including slight stenosis of the involved esophageal lumen as well as rough and irregular esophageal wall with brush liked sign; (4) Mucosal abnormalities including unevenly thickened mucosa, and scattering irregular filling defects of varying sizes on the surface of the thickened mucosa in cobblestone liked sign.

19.3.5.2 Digestive Endoscopy
It demonstrates congestion and edema of the involved esophagus, unevenly scattering irregular yellowish white pseudomembranous plaques of different sizes covering the mucosal surface that are more obvious in the lower segment.

Case Study 1

A male patient aged 36 years was confirmatively diagnosed as having AIDS by the CDC. He had symptoms of fever, fatigue, emaciation, throat irritation, dysphagia or odynophagia and feeling of retrosternal burning. His CD4 T cell count was 145/μl

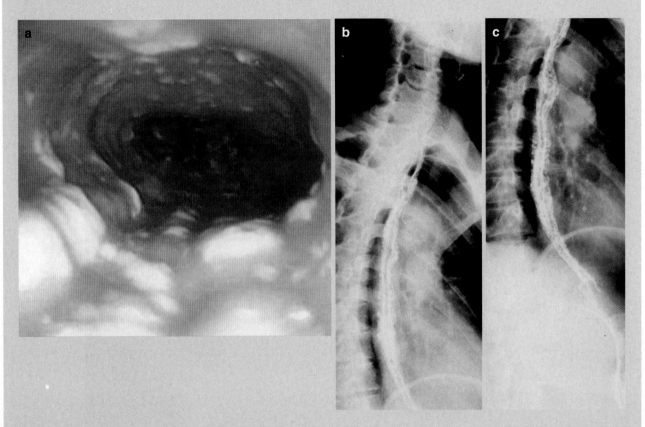

Fig. 19.2 (**a–c**) HIV/AIDS related candida esophagitis. (**a**) Digestive endoscopy demonstrates mucosal congestion and edema in all segments of the esophagus, scattering yellowish white pseudomembranous plaques of different sizes adhering to the mucosa that is unable to be detached. (**b–c**) Esophagus barium meal radiology demonstrates thickened esophageal barium meal mucosa, narrowed lumen and blurry borderlines in lace liked sign or sawtooth liked sign

Case Study 2

A male patient aged 38 years was confirmatively diagnosed as having AIDS by the CDC. He had symp-toms of fever, fatigue, emaciation, throat foreign sense, dysphagia or odynophagia, and retrosternal burning sense. His CD4 T cell count was 85/μl

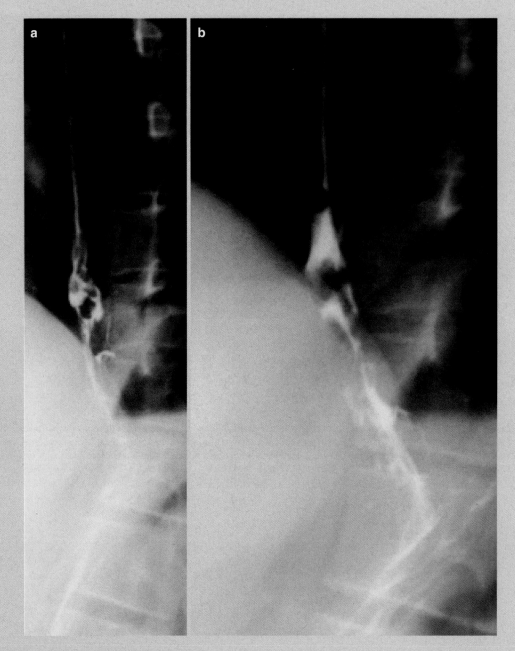

Fig. 19.3 (**a**, **b**) HIV/AIDS related candida esophagitis. (**a**, **b**) Esophagus barium meal radiology demonstrate thickened mucosa of the middle and lower segments of the esophagus, plaque liked filling defects, narrowed lumen, blurry and irregular borderline

Case Study 3

A male patient aged 17 years was confirmatively diagnosed as having AIDS by the CDC. He had symp-

toms of fever, sense of foreign substance in the throat, dysphagia and retrosternal sense of burning. His CD4 T cell count was 40/ μl

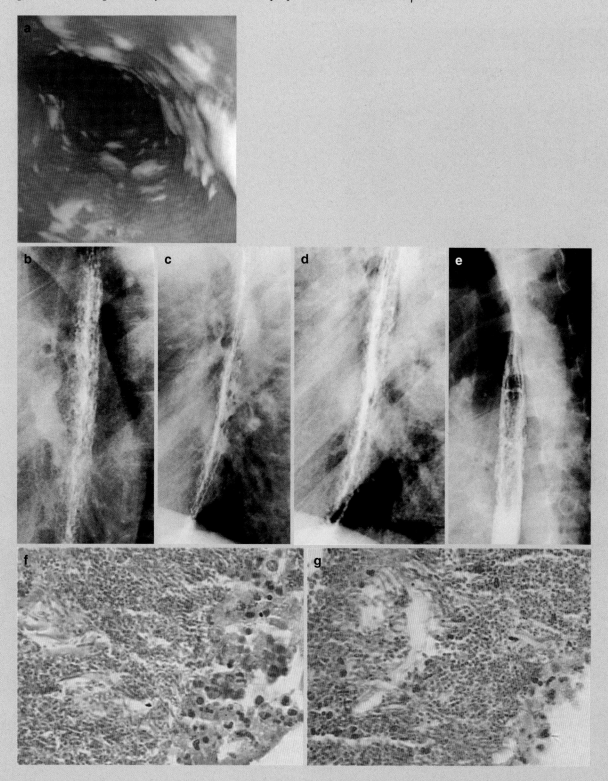

Fig. 19.4 (a–g) HIV/AIDS related candida esophagitis. (a) Gastroscopy demonstrates mucosal congestion and edema of all segments of the esophagus, and scattered yellowish white pseudomembranous plaques of varying sizes adhering to the mucosa. (b–e) Esophagus barium meal radiology demonstrate thickened esopha-geal mucosa, narrowed lumen, blurry and irregular borderline, with lace liked sign or snake skin liked sign. (f–g) Biopsy and pathological tissue analysis demonstrate growth of large quantity cadida that is consistent with cadida infection

Case Study 4

A female patient aged 45 years was confirmatively diagnosed as having AIDS by CDC. She had symptoms of fever, emaciation and dysphagia. Her CD4 T cell count was 80/μl.

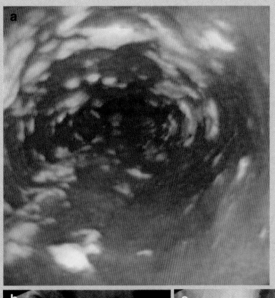

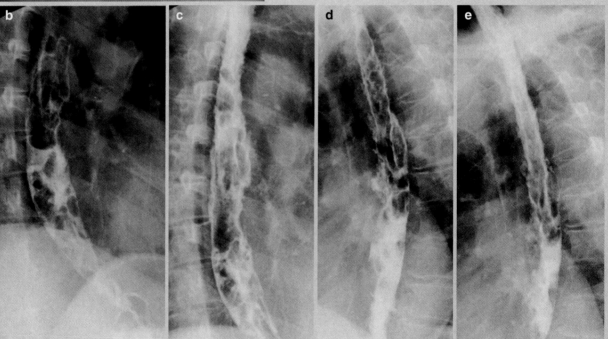

Fig. 19.5 (a–e) HIV/AIDS related candida esophagitis. (a) Gastroscopy demonstrates mucosal congestion and edema in all segments of the esophagus, and scattered yellowish white pseudo-membranous plaques of varying sizes adhering to the musosa. (b–e) Esophagus barium meal radiology demonstrate thickened esophageal mucosa, multiple flaky filling defects in the lumen, blurry and irregular borderline

Case Study 5

A female patient aged 30 years was confirmatively diagnosed as having AIDS by CDC. She had symptoms of fever, Sense of foreign substance in the throat, dysphagia and retrosternal sense of burning. Her CD4 T cell count was 115/ μl.

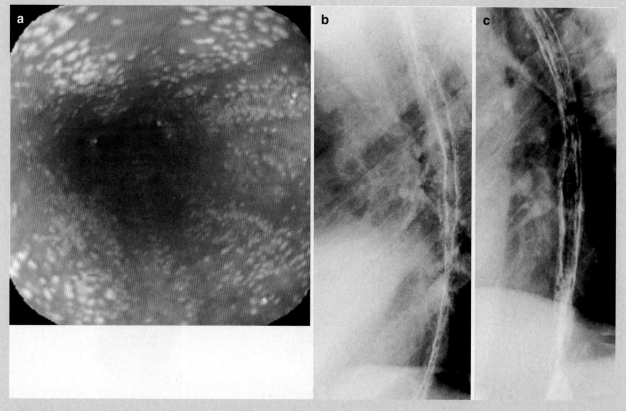

Fig. 19.6 (a–c) HIV/AIDS related candida esophagitis. (a) Gastroscopy demonstrates mucosal congestion and edema of all segments of the esophagus, and scattered yellowish white pseudomembranous plaques of varying sizes adhering to the mucosa. (b, c) Esophagus barium meal radiology demonstrate thickened esophageal mucosa, multiple spots filling defects, narrowed lumen, blurry and irregular borderline in lace liked sign or snake skin liked sign

Case Study 6

A female patient aged 39 years was confirmatively diagnosed as having AIDS by CDC. She had symptoms of fever, emaciation, sense of foreign substance in the throat, odynophagia, and retrosternal sense of burning. Her CD4 T cell count was 115/μl.

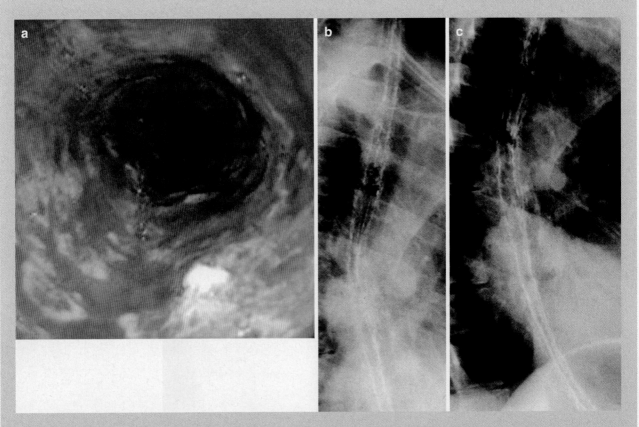

Fig. 19.7 (a–c) HIV/AIDS related candida esophagitis. (a) Gastroscopy demonstrates mucosal congestion and edema of all segments of the esophagus, and scattered yellowish white pseudo-membranous plaques of varying sizes adhering to the mucosa. (b, c) Esophagus barium meal radiology demonstrate thickened esophageal barium meal mucosa, multiple spots filling defects, narrowed lumen, blurry and irregular borderline in lace liked sign or snake skin liked sign

Case Study 7

A female patient aged 50 years was confirmatively diagnosed as having AIDS by CDC. She had symptoms of high fever, fatigue, sense of foreign substance in the throat, dysphagia and odynophagia. Her CD4 T cell count was 15/μl.

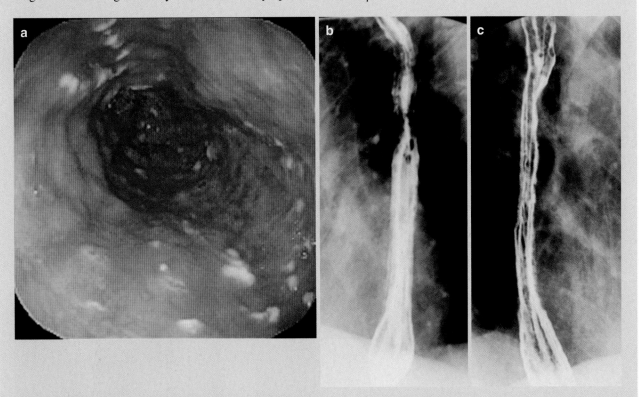

Fig. 19.8 (a–c) HIV/AIDS related candida esophagitis. (a) Gastroscopy demonstrates mucosal congestion and edema of all segments of the esophagus, and scattered yellowish white pseudomembranous plaques of varying sizes adhering to the mucosa. (b, c) Esophagus barium meal radiology demonstrate thickened esophageal barium meal mucosa, multiple spots filling defects, narrowed lumen, blurry and irregular borderline, with lace liked sign or snake skin liked sign

Case Study 8

A male aged 38 years was confirmatively diagnosed as having AIDS by CDC. He had symptoms of fever, sense of foreign substance in the throat, dysphagia and retrosternal sense of burning. His CD4 T cell count was 55/μl.

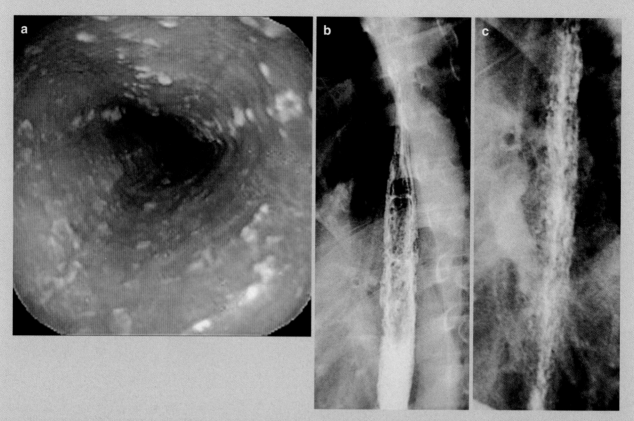

Fig. 19.9 (a–c) AIDS-related Candida esophagitis. (a) Gastroscopy demonstrates mucosal congestion and edema of all segments of the esophagus, and scattered yellowish white pseudomembranous plaques of varying sizes adhering to the mucosa. (b, c) Esophagus barium meal radiology demonstrate thickened esophageal mucosa, multiple spots filling defects, narrowed lumen, blurry and irregular borderline, with lace liked sign or snake skin liked sign

Case Study 9

A female patient aged 42 years was confirmatively diagnosed as having AIDS by CDC. She had symptoms of high fever, sense of foreign substance in the throat and dysphagia. Her CD4 T cell count was 85/μl.

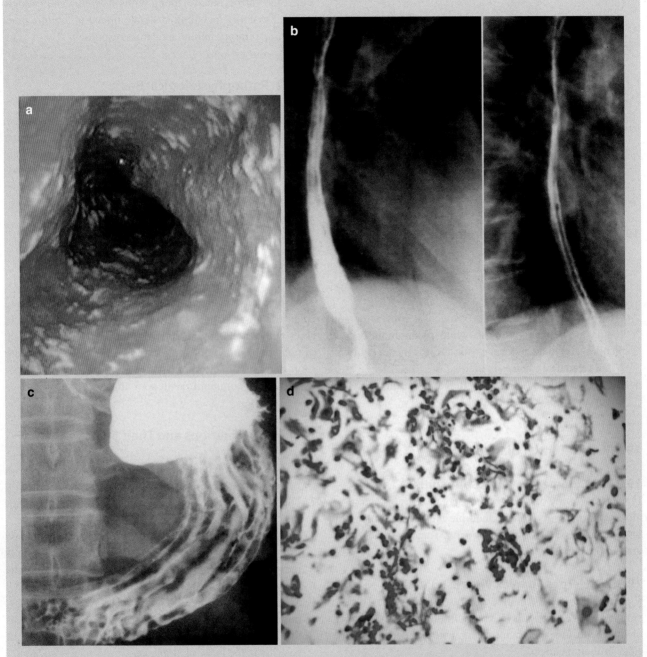

Fig. 19.10 (a–c) HIV/AIDS related candida esophagitis. (a) Gastroscopy demonstrates mucosal congestion and edema of all segments of the esophagus, and scattered yellowish white pseudomembranous plaques of varying sizes adhering to the mucosa. (b) Esophagus barium meal radiology demonstrates thickened esophageal mucosa, multiple spots filling defects, narrowed lumen, blurry borderline with lace liked sign or snake skin liked sign. (c) Esophagus barium meal radiology demonstrates coarse gastric mucosa, and multiple round filling defects gastric body and antrum. (d) HE staining demonstrates candida albicans in gastric mucosa (HE ×400). (e) PAS staining of the candida albicans in gastric mucosa demonstrates red spores and pseudohyphae of Candida albicans (×1,000)

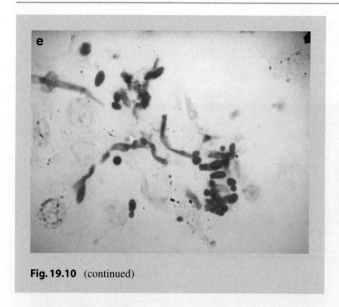

Fig. 19.10 (continued)

19.3.6 Criteria for the Diagnosis

1. The sensitivity of digestive radiography to pseudomembranous plaques is up to 90 %, with cobblestone liked filling defects.
2. Gastroscopic demonstrations of mucosal congestion and edema as well as yellowish white pseudomembranous plaques are main evidences for the diagnosis of HIV/AIDS related candida esophagitis.
3. Biopsy finding of yeast liked fungal pseudohypha is an important evidence for the diagnosis.

19.3.7 Differential Diagnosis

19.3.7.1 Cytomegalovirus Esophagitis
Esophageal X-ray of double contrast demonstrates cytomegalovirus esophagitis to have multiple flat mucosal ulcers in large diameters. Low density edema rings can be found around the ulcers.

19.3.7.2 Herpes Simplex Virus Esophagitis
Esophageal X-ray of double contrast demonstrates herpes simplex virus esophagitis to have multiple spots, ring shaped or linear mucous superficial ulcers, and low density edema rings around the ulcers.

19.4   HIV/AIDS Related Gastritis

19.4.1 Pathogens and Pathogenesis

Some chronic inflammation and diarrhea have no evidence of pathogen infections, which has been speculated to be related to direct effects of HIV on intestinal environmental balance. Such diseases are known as idiopathic HIV/AIDS related intestinal diseases. The causes of HIV/AIDS related gastritis can be divided into exogenous and endogenous.

Generally, the pathogens that gain their access to the stomach to cause gastritis are exogenous, commonly including chemical factors, physical factors, bacteria (especially the Helicobacter pylori), virus and toxins. The pathogens that infect the gastric mucosa along with blood flow are endogenous, commonly including systemic infection, uremia, liver failure, respiratory failure and stress responses.

19.4.2 Pathophysiological Basis

Most foci of acute gastritis occur from the gastric fundus in appearance of petechia or ecchymosis that fuse into irregular small ulcers in sizes of 2–20 mm. The histologic lesions are restricted to the mucosa. The focus continuously progresses to involve the submucosa, even penetrate the serosa, leading to multiple hemorrhage of the gastric fundus and involvement of the gastric antrum.

19.4.3 Clinical Symptoms and Signs

The common clinical manifestations of acute gastritis are epigastric upset, pain, nausea, vomiting and poor appetite. In cases with accompanying enteritis, diarrhea occurs. Physical examinations may find epigastric slight tenderness, with short duration of several days. Chronic gastritis has no specific findings, commonly with poor appetite.

19.4.4 Examinations and Their Selection

1. Gastroscopy in combination with direct vision biopsy is the main method for the diagnosis of chronic gastritis.
2. Digestive tract radiography demonstrates no specific findings in most cases of chronic gastritis.
3. Gastric juice analysis demonstrates chronic atrophic gastritis with dysfunctioning gastric acid secretion, which is more serious in cases with chronic atrophic gastritis in the body of stomach.
4. Serum parietal cell antibody test and serum gastrin determination demonstrate serum parietal cell antibody positive and increased level of serum gastrin in most cases of gastritis in the body of stomach.

19.4.5 Imaging Demonstrations

19.4.5.1 Digestive Radiography
The direct signs include thickened gastric mucous, poor adhesion of barium. The indirect signs include accelerated gastric peristalsis or irritation signs.

19.4.5.2 Gastroscopic Demonstrations
Mucosal congestion and edema of the stomach, possibly with superficial ulcers.

Case Study 1
A male aged 28 years was confirmatively diagnosed as having AIDS by CDC. He has symptoms of epigastric upset, pain, nausea, vomiting and poor appetite. His CD4 T cell count was 34/μl.

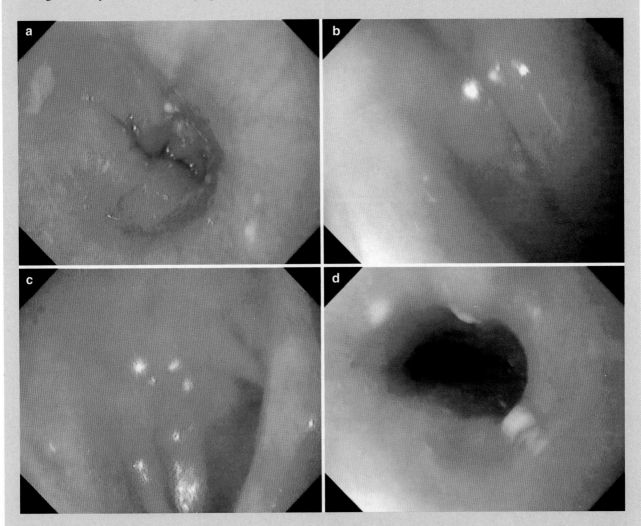

Fig. 19.11 (**a–j**) HIV/AIDS related gastritis and duodenitis. (**a**) Gastroscopy demonstrates smooth esophageal mucosa, favorable peristalsis and mucosal edema. (**b**) Gastroscopy demonstrates measles liked changes of mucosa in the body of stomach, antral mucosa commonly in red and white with dominant color of red, multiple swelling lesions with central depression, smooth surface, favorable peristalsis, round pyloric ostium with favorable opening. (**c–e**) Gastroscopy demonstrates multiple flaky congestion of varying sizes in the duodenal lumen, and no erosion. (**f**) Gastroscopy demonstrates clearly defined dentate line in size of 0.1 cm×0.2 cm, no varicosis at the esophageal gastric fundus, large quantity of turbid mucous fluid in the mucus pool. (**g**) PAS staining demonstrates HIV inflammation with infiltration of inflammatory cells and gland atrophy (PAS ×10). (**h–i**) PAS staining demonstrates dilated glandular cavity, mucosal hemorrhage, and infiltration of inflammatory cells in the muscularis mucosa, which is serious inflammation (PAS ×20). (**j**) Immunohistochemistry demonstrates lymphocyte HIV-1GP120 antigen positive in the gastric mucosa in yellowish brown (×200)

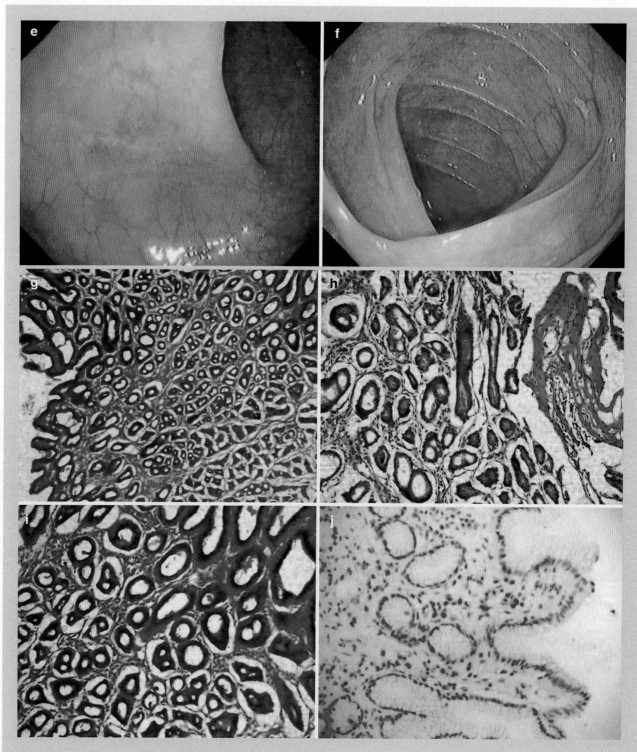

Fig. 19.11 (continued)

Case Study 2
A male patient aged 47 years was confirmatively diagnosed as having AIDS by CDC. He complained of epigastric upset, epigastric distention and poor appetite. His CD4 T cell count was 84/μl.

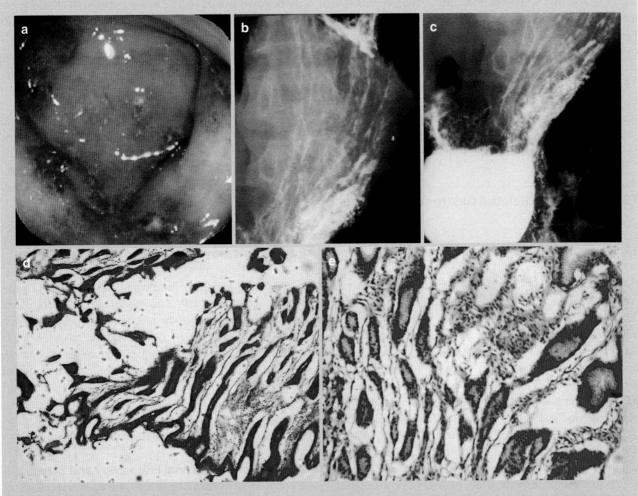

Fig. 19.12 (a–e) HIV/AIDS related gastritis. (a) Gastroscopy demonstrates multiple flaky milky white ulcers in the gastric mucosa, with flaky hemorrhagic plaques; (b, c) Esophagus barium meal radiology demonstrates thickened and coarse gastric mucosa; (d) PAS staining demonstrates dilated glandular cavities, mucosal hemorrhage, infiltration of inflammatory cells in the muscularis mucosa, which is severe inflammation (PAS ×10); (e) HE staining demonstrates dilated glandular cavities, mucosal hemorrhage, and infiltration of the inflammatory cells in the muscularis mucosa, which is severe inflammation (HE ×40)

19.4.6 Criteria for the Diagnosis

1. The symptoms of chronic gastritis are nonspecific, with few signs.
2. X-ray facilitates to diagnose the space occupying diseases of the stomach. The definitive diagnosis depends on gastroscopy and gastric mucosa biopsy.
3. The diagnosis of chronic gastritis depends on histological changes and anatomic localization, with reference to immunological indices. The conference on chronic gastritis held in Chongqing, China in 1982 proposed a simple classification of gastritis: (1) superficial gastritis, with involvements of the surface and epithelium of the gastric mucosa, including symptoms of erosion and bleeding. Diffuse or confined should be defined. For cases of confined chronic gastritis, the localization of the lesions should be indicated. (2) Atrophic gastritis, with involvements of the glands in the deep mucosa to cause atrophy. (3) Hypertrophic gastritis. Its occurrence is still in controversy because there lacks supports by evidence of epithelial cells hypertrophy.

19.4.7 Differential Diagnosis

19.4.7.1 Peptic Ulcer

Both have chronic epigastric pain. Peptic ulcer has symptoms of epigastric regular periodic pain, while chronic gastritis has no regular pain, with common symptom of dyspepsia. Their differential diagnosis depends on barium meal radiology and gastroscopy.

19.4.7.2 Chronic Biliary Diseases

Chronic cholecystitis and cholelithiasis have symptoms of chronic right epigastric and abdominal distension, belching and some other symptoms of dyspepsia, which can be misdiagnosed as chronic gastritis .

19.5 HIV/AIDS Related Gastroduodenal Ulcer

19.5.1 Pathogens and Pathogenesis

HIV infection causes gastric mucosal inflammation and epithelial cell apoptosis. Studies have demonstrated that apoptosis may play an important role in the pathogenesis of HIV/AIDS related digestive diseases and gastric mucosal apoptosis index may not be related to local inflammation and Hp infection but to HIV itself and environmental changes of mucosal immune. Generally, it is believed that HIV/AIDS related gastroduodenal ulcer is caused by compound factors leading to vascular and muscular spasm of the gastroduodenal wall. The resulted cellular malnutrition of gastrointestinal wall and decreased defense of gastrointestinal mucosa cause the gastrointestinal mucosa being susceptible digestion by gastric juice to lead to ulcers.

19.5.2 Pathophysiological Basis

The lesions of HIV/AIDS related gastroduodenal ulcer are commonly found in similar localizations to typical duodenal ulcer in patients with normal immunity. The pathogenic process can be divided into three stages, including erosion, acute ulcer and chronic ulcer.

19.5.2.1 Erosion

Erosion is the shallow depression of the mucosa, and usually does not penetrate the muscularis mucosa. By naked eyes, erosion is the red spots with shallow depression, in diameters of less than 0.5 cm. By microscopy, the shallow erosion only involves the gland neck and sometimes muscularis mucosa. On the erosion fundus, there are few necrotic tissues and large quantity infiltration of neutrophils.

19.5.2.2 Acute Ulcer

Acute ulcers refer to those ulcers that penetrate the muscularis mucosa and involve the inferior layer of the mucosa. It can be derived from erosion, in diameters of less than 1 cm with clearly defined borderline. By microscopy, mucosa and muscularis mucosa are all destroyed and absent. The fundus of the ulcers is attached with small quantity necrotic tissues and small quantity fibrins and infiltration of many neutrophilic granulocytes.

19.5.2.3 Chronic Ulcer

About 15 % cases of duodenal ulcer are multiple, with accompanying gastric ulcer. By naked eyes, the ulcer fundus is attached by few exudates and necrotic tissues. Under a microscope, the ulcer is composed of 4 layers, namely inflammatory exudates, coagulative necrotic tissue, granuloma tissue and scar tissue.

19.5.3 Clinical Symptoms and Signs

HIV/AIDS related ulcers have common symptoms of pain, which is induced by HIV and other related factors. Pains from lesser gastric curvature ulcers mostly occur after the meals. Pains from duodenal ulcer and helicobacter pylori gastric ulcer usually occur in hunger and relieves after meals, which are similar to patients with gastric ulcers and normal immunity.

19.5.4 Examinations and Their Selection

19.5.4.1 Gastrointestinal Endoscopy and Biopsy

They can directly demonstrate the size and morphology of the lesions, and facilitate their qualitative diagnosis.

19.5.4.2 Diagnostic Imaging

Digestive radiography is a common examination for the diagnosis of ulcers. It can directly demonstrate the ulcer niche of the stomach and duodenum as well as its secondary organic and functional changes. It can also demonstrate different manifestations in different stages of ulcers, including its active stage and its healing stage. Virtual endoscopy by CT scanning or MR imaging has a limited application.

19.5.5 Imaging Demonstrations

19.5.5.1 Digestive Radiography

Gastric ulcer and duodenal bulbar ulcer are characterized by (1) Niche shadow, which is a direct X-ray demonstration for the diagnosis of duodenal ulcer. Duodenal bulbar ulcer mostly occurs in the anterior and posterior wall adjacent to the duodenal bulbar fundus, with surrounding transparent edema stripes that is gradually blurry towards the periphery, sometimes with short and fine mucosal markings whipping together. In cases of concurrent anterior and posterior wall ulcers in duodenal bulb, slight rotation can demonstrate two isolated barium plaques, known as kissing ulcers. (2) Deformity due to functional or organic changed caused by ulcer. The duodenal bulb commonly loses its normal morphology of triangular shape, and a variety of malformations occur, which is the common and important sign of bulbar ulcers. When the overall bulb spasm occurs, it demonstrates an irritative phenomenon. (3) Mucosal changes including the mucosal patterns in radial shape, whipping together towards the niche shadow. (4) Other changes including pyloric spasm, and duodenal ulcer lesions. Duodenal ulcer may progress into deep or surrounding tissues to penetrate the duodenal wall, leading to peripheral duodenal adhesion, narrowed and even obstructed passage, and other complications.

19.5.5.2 Gastroscopy

The lesions and their severity of gastric and duodenal ulcers can be determined by gastroscopy. From the most serious to slight, the disease can be divided into three stages and each stage can be subdivided into two periods. They are represented by A1, A2; H1, H2; and S1, S2.

1. Acute stage can be subdivided into A1 and A2 periods. In A1 period, there are necrosis of the ulcer surface with coverage of thick white/yellow mosses, and obvious peripheral congestion and edema. In A2 period, there are necrosis of the ulcer surface with thinner coverage of the moss, and obvious peripheral congestion and edema.

2. Healing stage can be subdivided into H1 and H2 periods. In H1 period, there is no necrosis on the ulcer surface with thinner or absent coverage of the white moss, erosion, alleviated or absent peripheral congestion and edema, and regeneration of the epithelium. In H2 period, there are absent erosion, slight peripheral congestion or absent peripheral congestion and edema, obvious regeneration of epithelium and mild mucosal concentration.

3. Scar stage can be subdivided into S1 and S2 periods. S1 period is also known as the red scar period, with red scar, no peripheral congestion and edema, regenerated epithelium and concentrated mucosa. In S2 period is also known as the white scar period, with white scar at the locations of ulcers and obvious concentrated mucosa.

Its staging can facilitate the description in the clinical diagnosis. However, the borderlines between stages and periods are difficult to be defined.

Case Study 1

A male patient aged 26 years was confirmatively diagnosed as having AIDS by the CDC. He had symptoms of epigastric pain for several months. His CD4 T cell count was 85/μl.

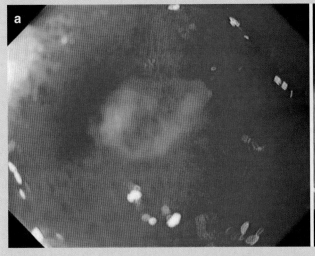
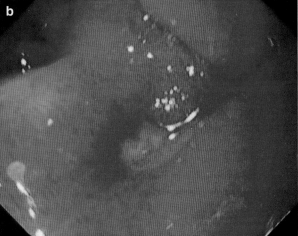
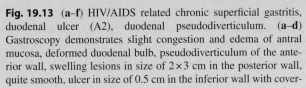

Fig. 19.13 (**a–f**) HIV/AIDS related chronic superficial gastritis, duodenal ulcer (A2), duodenal pseudodiverticulum. (**a–d**) Gastroscopy demonstrates slight congestion and edema of antral mucosa, deformed duodenal bulb, pseudodiverticulum of the anterior wall, swelling lesions in size of 2×3 cm in the posterior wall, quite smooth, ulcer in size of 0.5 cm in the inferior wall with coverage of white moss, and peripheral mucosal congestion and edema by gastroscopy. (**e, f**) The histopathological analysis demonstrates atrophic and loosened gastric interstitium, dilated gland lumen, infiltration of large quantity inflammatory cells, and severe inflammation

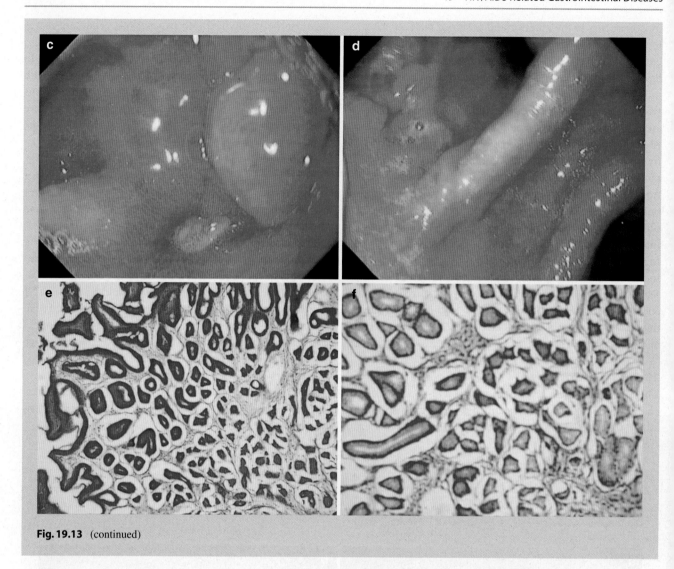

Fig. 19.13   (continued)

19.5.6 Criteria for the Diagnosis

1. Clinical symptoms include acid reflux, chronic epigastric pain and other symptoms.
2. By gastroscopy, there is mucosal erosion or ulceration of the stomach and duodenum.
3. Digestive radiology demonstrates niche shadow of the duodenal bulb, gathered mucosa and irritation sign.
4. Biopsy for pathology demonstrates infiltration of large quantity inflammatory cells.

19.5.7 Differential Diagnosis

1. Various lesions of gastritis, functional gastrointestinal diseases.
2. Benign ulcers and malignant ulcers.
3. Gastric cancer, hepatobiliary tumor and pancreatic head carcinoma.
4. Colonic irritation syndrome.

19.6   HIV/AIDS Related Ileocecal Tuberculosis

19.6.1 Pathogens and Pathogenesis

HIV/AIDS-related ileocecal tuberculosis generally is caused by the mycobacterium tuberculosis along with blood flow, and it can also be caused by drinking contaminated milk or dairy products. People with bovine tuberculosis can also spread the disease. Its spreading routes include (1) gastrointestinal infections are the main spreading routes of ileocecal tuberculosis. After the oral intake of mycobacterium tuberculosis, they cannot be killed by gastric acid due to its adipose enveloping membrane. When the bacteria reaches the ileocecus, the food containing mycobacterium tuberculosis has been chyme, which has a greater chance to directly contact with the intestinal mucosa. Simultaneously, due to the physiological retention and reverse peristalsis of the ileocecus, the chance of infection increases. In addition to the abundant lymphoid tissues in the ileocecus, its susceptibility to tuberculosis increases its chance of infection. Therefore, intestinal tuberculosis mostly occurs in the ileocecus. (2) Spreading along with blood flow is also an infection route of intestinal tuberculosis. HIV/AIDS related miliary tuberculosis invades the intestinal tract via spreading along with blood flow. (3) Intestinal tuberculosis can also be caused by the direct spread of intra-abdominal tuberculosis, such as fallopian tuberculosis, tuberculous peritonitis and mesenteric lymph nodes. And such infections are spread along with lymph flow.

19.6.2 Pathophysiological Basis

Ileocecus is a predispose site of HIV/AIDS related intestinal tuberculosis. It commonly occurs in young and middle aged populations, with female patients slightly more than male patients. After invasion of TB bacteria, its pathological changes vary with the immunity and allergic responses to mycobacterium tuberculosis. In the cases of large quantity bacteria invasion with high toxicity, and strong allergic reactions of human body, the lesions are commonly exudative, possibly with caseous necrosis and ulceration. In the cases of mild infection but strong immunity (mainly cellular immunity) of the human body, the lesions are often hyperplastic, with tuberculous nodules and further fibrosis, known as hyperplastic intestinal tuberculosis. Mixed intestinal tuberculosis sometimes occurs.

19.6.2.1 Ulcerative Intestinal Tuberculosis
After invasion of mycobacterium tuberculosis to the intestinal wall, firstly the concentrated lymphoid tissue in the intestinal wall causes congestion, edema and exudative lesions, which further develop into caseous necrosis. After that, ulceration occurs to spread peripherally. The borders of the ulcers may be irregular with different depth, sometimes to the muscular layer or serosa layer of the intestinal wall, and even involve the peritoneum or adjacent mesenteric lymph nodes. Ulcers of intestinal tuberculosis can spread with lymph flow of the intestinal wall, mostly in ring shape. Ulcerative intestinal tuberculosis is often demonstrated as having adhesion with abenteric tissues, and therefore low incidence of intestinal perforation. In the repairing process, due to large quantity fibrous tissue hyperplasia and scar formation, ring shaped stenosis of intestinal lumen can occur.

19.6.2.2 Hyperplastic Intestinal Tuberculosis
In the early stage, there are local edema and lymphangiectasia. In the chronic period, there are hyperplasia of large quantity tuberculous granulation tissue and fibrous tissue, commonly in the inferior layer of mucosa with nodules of varying sizes. In the serious cases, there are tumor liked masses protruding into the intestinal lumen to cause intestinal stenosis, and even intestinal obstruction.

19.6.3 Clinical Symptoms and Signs

Most patients have a history of pulmonary tuberculosis, with symptoms of the lower right abdominal pain. By palpation, there are restricted tenderness point and abdominal mass of medium hardness, possibly with slight tenderness and limited mobility. Ulcerative intestinal tuberculosis is often accompanied by tuberculosis toxemia, with symptoms of low fever after noon, irregular fever, remittent/continued fever, accompanied by night sweating as well as fatigue, emaciation, anemia and malnutritional edema and other symptoms and signs.

19.6.4 Examinations and Their Selection

19.6.4.1 Tuberculin Test
The finding is an important indicator for the definitive diagnosis.

19.6.4.2 Hemogram Erythrocyte Sedimentation Rate
The cases of ulcers commonly have normal or lower WBC count, higher lymphocyte count, with signs of slight and moderate anemia. In patients in active phase of TB, the erythrocyte sedimentation is often accelerated.

19.6.4.3 Stool Examination
In cases of hyperplastic intestinal tuberculosis, the stool has no significant changes. In cases of ulcerative intestinal tuberculosis, microscopic examination of the stool demonstrates small quantity of pyocytes and erythrocytes.

19.6.4.4 Colon Endoscopy
It can be applied for the direct observation of ileocecal lesions. And it can also be used for the collection of specimens for biopsy and bacteria culture.

19.6.4.5 Diagnostic Imaging
Barium meal radiography or barium enema examination is of great significance for the diagnosis of intestinal tuberculosis. Patients with complication of intestinal obstruction should avoid barium enema, otherwise, barium enema can aggravate the obstruction.

19.6.5 Imaging Demonstrations

19.6.5.1 Digestive Radiology
(1) Leaping sign or irritation sign, accelerated intestinal movements, poor local adhesion of barium; (2) Thickened and deranged intestinal mucosal folds, with sawtooth liked borders and small niche shadow; (3) multiple polypoid hyperplasia; (4) thickened intestinal wall, irregular stenosis of intestinal lumen or perforation and adhesion.

19.6.5.2 CT Scanning

It demonstrates edema and thickening of the intestinal wall, irregular stenosis of intestinal lumen or perforation and adhesion.

19.6.5.3 Gastroscopy

It can be applied for the direct observation of the lesions in the entire colon, the cecum and ileocecus. It can also be used for the collection of specimens for biopsy and bacteria culture to find the mycobacterium tuberculosis.

Case Study 1

A female patient aged 53 years was confirmatively diagnosed as having AIDS by CDC. She had a history of paid blood donation and had been HIV positive for 5 years. She complained of fatigue and night sweat for 2 months, intermittent fever for 1 month, with right lower abdominal pain. Her CD4 T cell count was 85/μl.

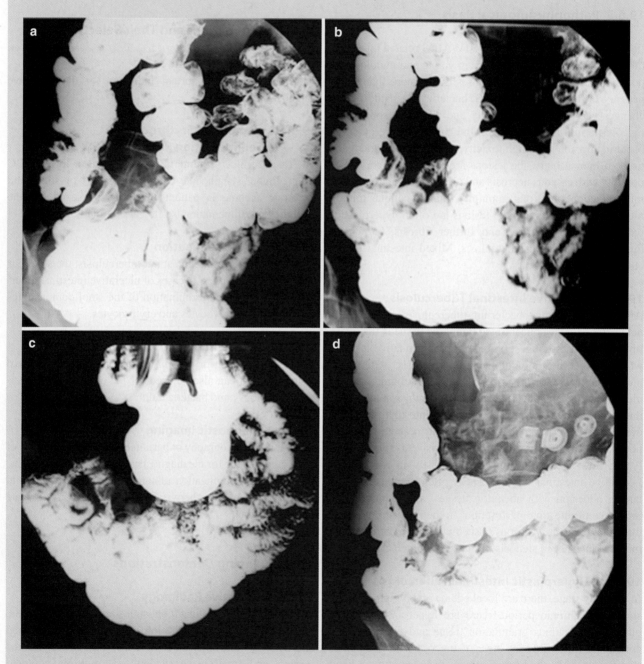

Fig. 19.14 (a–d) HIV/AIDS related ileocecal tuberculosis. (a–d) Barium meal radiography demonstrates right ileocecal stenosis, poor filling, irregular intestinal wall and fine ulcers

Case Study 2

A male patient aged 39 years was confirmatively diagnosed as having AIDS by CDC. He had a history of paid blood donation and had been HIV positive for 4 years. He complained of fatigue and night sweat for 2 months, intermittent fever for 1 month, with body temperature sometimes up to 40 °C, and right lower abdominal pain. His CD4 T cell count was 113/μl.

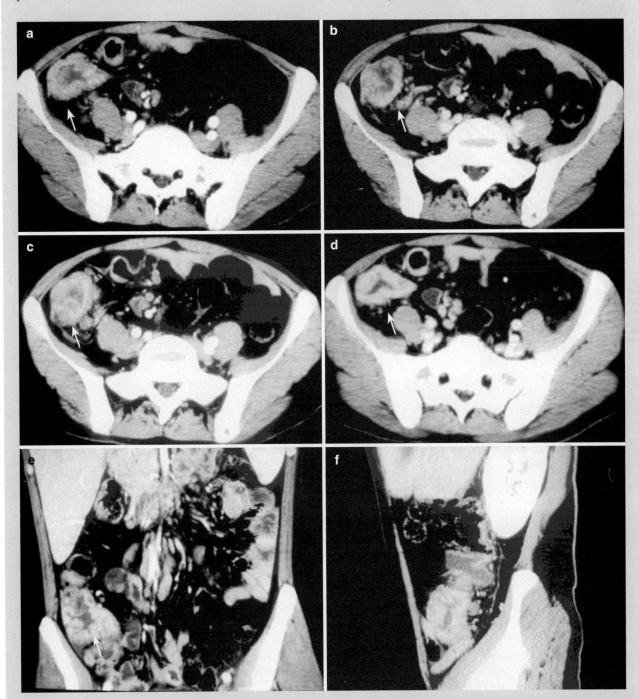

Fig. 19.15 (**a–m**) HIV/AIDS related ileocecal tuberculosis. (**a, b**) CT scanning demonstrates irregularly thickened right intestinal wall and intestinal stenosis (*arrow*). (**c, d**) Enhanced CT scanning demonstrates abnormal enhancement of the intestinal wall (*arrow*). Enhanced delayed (**e, f**) CT scanning and 3-dimensional reconstruction demonstrate irregularly thickened right intestinal wall (*arrow*), stenosis of the intestinal lumen, with abnormal enhancement of the intestinal wall and no surrounding adhesion. (**g**) Abdominal plain scanning demonstrates multiple fluid levels of different sizes. (**h**) Chest X-ray demonstrates large quantity free gas below the right diaphragm, and small quantity free gas in the left subdiaphragmatic lobe. (**i, j**) It is demonstrated to have intestinal disruption, with interconnected mesentery after surgical removal. (**k, l**) It is demonstrated to have local tissue necrosis of the intestinal wall, fibrous connective tissue hyperplasia, and the formation of tuberculous granuloma. (**m**) It is demonstrated to have multiple multinucleated maglocytes and epithelialoid cells gathering into floral hoop sign

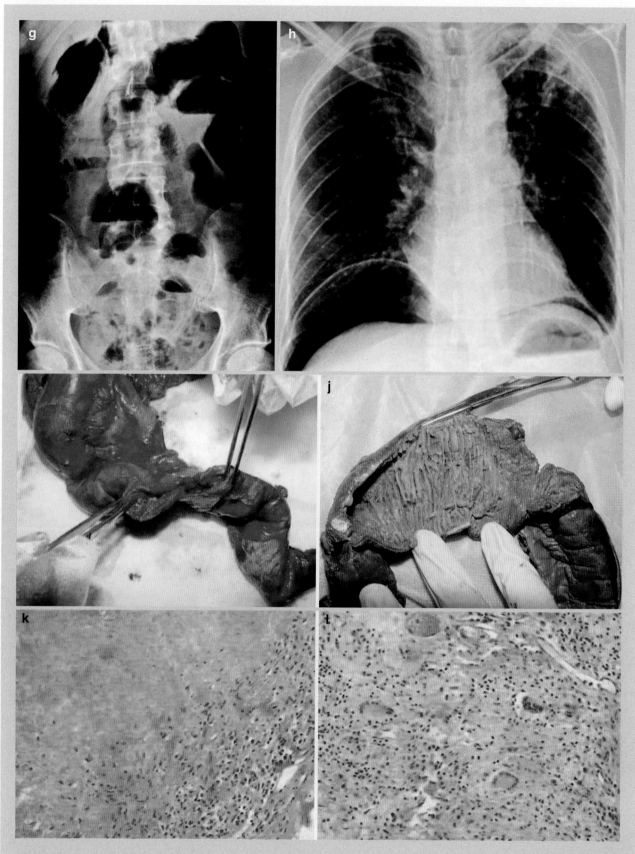

Fig. 19.15 (continued)

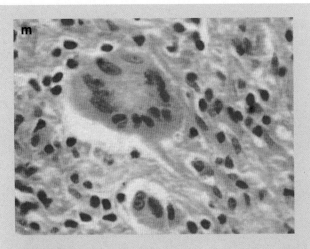

Fig. 19.15 (continued)

Case Study 3

A female patient aged 38 years was confirmatively diagnosed as having AIDS by CDC. She received periappendicural abscess incision for its drainage on Aug. 15, 2007 (with no findings of the appendix tissue during the operation, but only receiving incision and drainage) and was cured and discharged on Sep. 5, 2007. During Oct. 12–24, 2007, she was hospitalized due to right lower abdominal mass and fever and received anti-inflammatory therapy. After she was discharged, the right lower abdominal mass still progressively enlarged, with accompanying fever, fatigue and anorexia and she received intermittent anti-inflammatory and symptomatic treatment. On Nov. 27, 2008, she was hospitalized again due to progressively enlarging right lower abdominal mass and its rupture. Presently, the right lower abdominal mass was 18 × 19 cm in size, being hard and fixed with no obvious tenderness. She also had lumbosacral soreness and pain, radiating to the right lower extremity. She was found to have moderate edema of the right lower extremity and limited knees bending. Palpation of the right groin can find funicular liked swollen lymph nodes groups.

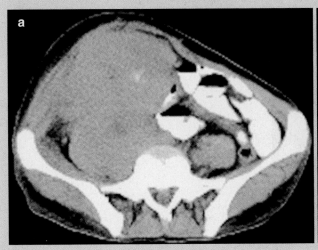

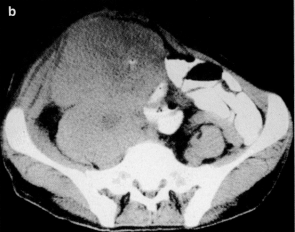

Fig. 19.16 (a–g) TB abscesses of the intestinal lumen with accompanying intra-abdominal infective abscesses, intestinal lymphoma complicated by intra-abdominal infection and intra-abdominal multi-pathogens infections. (**a–e**) CT scanning demonstrates a space occupying lesion in the right lower quadrant of the abdomen, obviously thickened intestinal wall, stenosis of the intestinal lumen, migration of bladder and uterine due to compression. (**f, g**) CT scanning demonstrates a huge mass under the right psoas muscle, and when the psoas muscle lifed, the mass can be found in the right iliac fossa

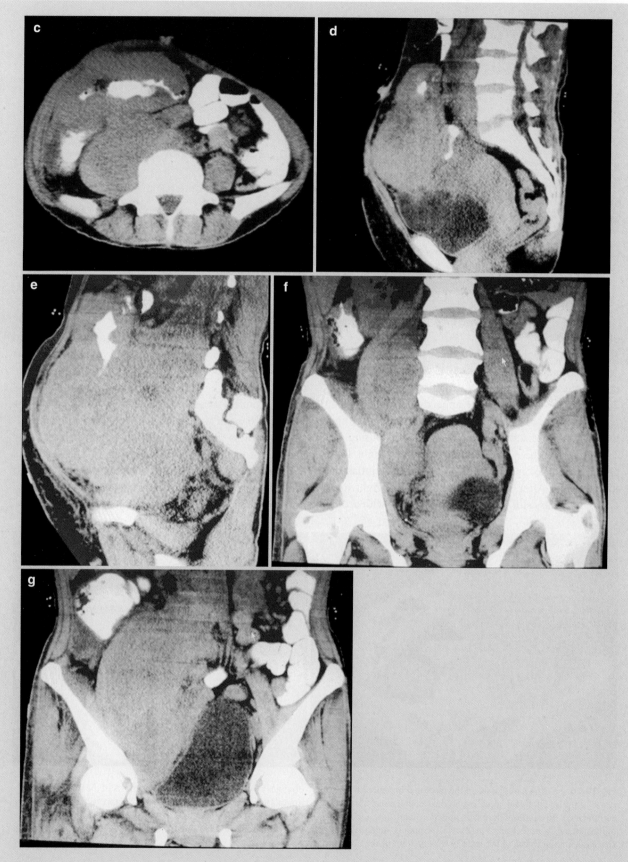

Fig. 19.16 (continued)

19.6.6 Criteria for the Diagnosis

1. AIDS patients with abenteric tuberculosis, especially patients with open pulmonary tuberculosis have gastrointestinal symptoms.
2. The clinical manifestations include diarrhea, abdominal pain, right lower quadrant tenderness, possible abdominal mass, intestinal obstruction with unknown cause, and accompanying fever, night sweating and other symptoms of tuberculous toxemia.
3. Barium meal radiology demonstrates ileocecal irritation, stenosis of intestinal lumen, filling defects, shortened and deformed intestinal tract.
4. Tuberculin test positive.

19.6.7 Differential Diagnosis

19.6.7.1 Differential Diagnosis from Crohn's Disease

The X-ray demonstrations of Crohn's disease are similar to those of intestinal tuberculosis, and both mostly occur in the ileocecus. However, Crohn's disease has a segmental occurrence, with clearly defined interface, while tuberculosis infiltration is migrational, with no clearly defined interface. The mucosal lesions of Crohn's disease are longitudinal crack liked ulcers and pebble liked changes, with occurrence of intestinal fistula. Some large granulomas in cases of tuberculosis can cause filling defects. Therefore, the differential diagnosis can be made.

19.6.7.2 Differential Diagnosis from Ileocecal Tumor

In the cases of ileocecal tumor, the intestinal wall is irregular, with intact borders and ulceration. The lesions are restricted with clearly defined borders. In the cases of ulcerative cancers, the apple core sign can be found, while multiple ulcers can be found in the cases of intestinal tuberculosis in a large rang, which helps the differential diagnosis. The cases of intestinal lymphoma have similar demonstrations in the mucous membrane, the range is longer, with thickening of the involved intestinal wall in the sense of hard rubber and stenosis.

19.6.7.3 Differential Diagnosis from Ulcerative Colitis

Ulcerative colitis occurs more common in the left colon, mostly progressing from the rectum upwards. In some serious cases, it can invade the whole colon, even involve the terminal ileum. The demonstrations include rectal spasmodic contraction, shallow or absent colon bags, rough borders and shallow sawtooth liked ulcers, larger ulcers in button liked sign. In chronic cases of advanced stage, intestinal wall fibrosis occurs, with demonstrations of continuous concentric stenosis of the intestinal lumen, and stiff borders. All the demonstrations facilitate the differential diagnosis.

19.7 HIV/AIDS Related Vesicorectal Fistula

19.7.1 Pathogens and Pathogenesis

HIV/AIDS related abdominal infections are an important factor for the occurrence and development of intestinal fistula, also being one of the common clinical manifestations. Abdominal infections, especially the intra-abdominal abscess, can cause intestinal fistula. In the early stage of intestinal fistula, the leakage of intestinal fluid can cause varying degrees of abdominal infections and abdominal abscesses. Further progression of the conditions may cause diffuse peritonitis, sepsis and other clinical manifestations. AIDS complicated by intestinal fistula mostly has manifestations of malnutrition, hypoproteinemia, edema, emaciation and other clinical manifestations. According to the location of the intestinal fistula and the different flow volumes, there is varying degrees of homeostatic imbalance, with manifestations of hypokalemia, hyponatremia and metabolic acidosis.

19.7.2 Pathophysiological Basis

HIV/AIDS related vesicorectal fistula refers to occurrence of abnormal passages of bladder and rectum, with intestinal contents gaining access to the bladder and discharged via the urethra, and the resulted infections, loss of body fluid, homeostasis imbalance, organ dysfunction and malnutrition.

19.7.3 Clinical Symptoms and Signs

Feces can cause infections of bladder and urinary tract, with symptoms of frequent urination, urgent urination and dysuria. The feces and gas can be discharged from the urethra, and the urination with bowel movements. By digital rectal examination, the fistula hole can be touched in the anterior rectal wall.

19.7.4 Examinations and Their Selection

19.7.4.1 Cystoscopy

Visible bladder fistula hole, and feces and gas in the bladder.

19.7.4.2 Colonoscopy

Visible fistula hole in the anterior rectal wall, outflows of urine from the fistula, qualitative diagnosis by biopsy.

19.7.4.3 Cystography

Flowing of the contrast agent into the rectum.

19.7.5 Imaging Demonstrations

By cystography, the contrast agent flows like a river into the rectum. By cystoscopy, there are bladder fistula hole, feces and gas in the bladder. By colonoscopy, fistula hole can be found in the anterior rectal wall and outflows of urine from the fistula.

Case Study

A male patient aged 37 years was confirmatively diagnosed as having AIDS by CDC. He had a history of blood donation in 1995, and was definitively diagnosed in Jun., 2005. He had initial symptoms in Aug. 2008, with left testicular swelling and right scrotal blister and deep ulceration for more than 2 months that could not be cured. Ulcer secretions smear was Gram stained to show demonstrations of large quantity Gram-negative short bacillus and small quantity Gram-positive bacillus. There are also small quantity Gram-negative diplococci and more Gram-positive cocci. By acid-fast staining, there are small quantity acid-fast bacilli. In the past few days, urine is discharged from bowel movements. His CD4 T cell count was 35/μl.

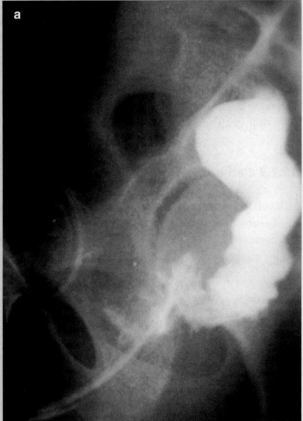
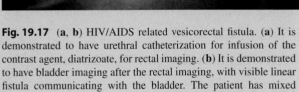
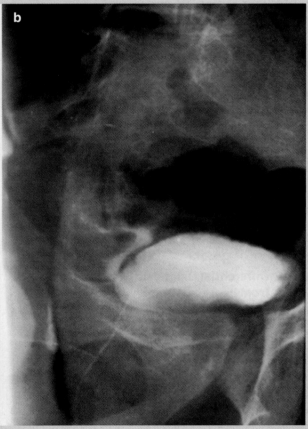

Fig. 19.17 (**a**, **b**) HIV/AIDS related vesicorectal fistula. (**a**) It is demonstrated to have urethral catheterization for infusion of the contrast agent, diatrizoate, for rectal imaging. (**b**) It is demonstrated to have bladder imaging after the rectal imaging, with visible linear fistula communicating with the bladder. The patient has mixed bacterial infections of the urinary system secondary to the scrotal ulcers and herpes, whose progression to involve the rectal wall and cause fistula. In combination with the case history, the diagnosis can be defined

19.7.6 Criteria for the Diagnosis

19.7.6.1 Irritative Symptoms of the Bladder
The bladder and urinary tract infections caused by feces, with frequent urination, urgent urination and dysuria.

19.7.6.2 Clinical Symptoms and Signs
The clinical symptoms and signs include fever, abdominal pain, constipation and hematuria, palpable abdominal mass, discharge of feces and gas during urination.

19.7.6.3 Cystography
After infusion of the contrast agent, lateral radiograph demonstrates access of the contrast agent into the intestinal tract. By barium meal radiology or barium enema, the access of the barium into the bladder helps to find the primary lesion and the location of the fistula hole.

19.7.6.4 Cystoscopy
Cystoscopy demonstrates mucosal edema and congestion of the bladder in inflammatory changes, with fistula hole. In the cases of small fistula hole, the oral intake of carbon powder demonstrates black precipitating substance in the bladder.

19.7.6.5 Colonoscopy
Colonoscopy demonstrates the size and location of the fistula hole. Qualitative diagnosis can be made by biopsy.

19.7.7 Differential Diagnosis

Rectourethral fistula
   Rectourethral fistula is the abnormal passage between urethra and rectum. The fistula hole can be found between the prostatic urethra and the rectum. During urination, urine flows into the rectum, Urine is discharged by bowel movement. And feces and gas are discharged by urination. By urethrography, the contrast agent gains its access in the rectum. By urethroscopy, the fistula hole is found to be in the posterior urethra instead of the bladder. By rectoscopy, there is fistula hole in the rectum, and the catheterization via the fistula hole to communicate with the urethra. The disease can be misdiagnosed as vesicorectal fistula.

19.8 HIV/AIDS Related Gastrointestinal Viral Infections

19.8.1 HIV/AIDS Related Gastrointestinal Cytomegalovirus Infection

19.8.1.1 Pathogens and Pathogenesis
Cytomegalovirus belongs to beta subfamily of the human herpes virus family, with obvious specificity to species of the host. It is the largest virus with the most complex structure in human herpes virus family. CMV is in spherical shape, with

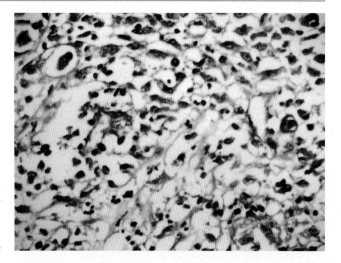

Fig. 19.18 HIV/AIDS related cytomegalovirus enteritis. HE staining demonstrates cytomegalovirus inclusion bodies in submucosal intestine (HE ×200)

a diameter of about 300 nm. CMV has only one serotype, and commonly AD169 is used as the representative strain for serological test. After cytomegalovirus infection, the virus is restricted within the salivary gland. It can be found in all organs and tissues of the human body and directly leads to the damage of the infected host cells. Alternatively, it has pathogenic effects through the immune pathogenesis, mainly targeting to epithelial cells. The infected targeting cells are assimilated to cytomaglovirus, with inclusion bodies in the cytoplasm and nucleus in appearance of an owl's eyes. The disease is also known as cytomegalic inclusion disease (CID). Secondarily, the infected cells degenerate, with enlarged volumes and disintegration, resulting in local necrosis and inflammation. Therefore, gastrointestinal tract infections occur to cause mucosal lesions, and even ulceration.

19.8.1.2 Pathophysiological Basis
Cytomegalovirus can invade any part of the gastrointestinal tract, but the colon is the most commonly invaded. And occasionally, cytomegalovirus can affect the entire gastrointestinal tract. Cytomegalovirus gastritis has demonstrations of swollen mucosal folds and superficial ulceration or erosion. CMV colitis has 2 types, the scattered lesions type and the segmental lesions type. The scattered lesions invade the entire gastrointestinal tract, with absent colon bags, slight stenosis of the intestinal lumen, and granuloma erosion and superficial ulceration in the intestinal mucosa. Segmental lesions mainly involve the cecum and terminal ileum, with cecal spasm, irregularly thickened mucosal folds and superficial thrush liked ulcers. The ulceration in the intestinal mucosa is a result of intestinal mucosal ischemic necrosis caused by CMV induced vasculitis.

19.8.1.3 Clinical Symptoms and Signs
HIV/AIDS related gastrointestinal CMV infection is an acquired infection, with an incidence of 5–10 %. It has

manifestations of diarrhea, abdominal pain, weight loss, loss of appetite and fever. The CD4 T cell count is less than 100/ μl, CMV infection is the major cause of onset and death in immunocompromised patients. In advanced stage of AIDS, CMV infection often causes retinitis and colon/esophagus ulcers, mostly occurrence of sigmoid colon ulcer and rectum ulcer. In some serious cases, mucosal ulceration, bleeding, perforation and peritonitis occur. CMV infection is mostly subclinical, and patients with explicit infection have diverse clinical manifestations. Death may occur in some serious cases.

19.8.1.4 Examinations and Their Selection
1. Typical intranuclear inclusions can be found by shedding cells test and histopathological examination.
2. Virus isolation and antigen detection.
3. Application of enzyme marked human cytomegalovirus.
4. Molecular hybridization test can identify DNA components of CMV.
5. Serological tests
6. Gastrointestinal imaging
7. Gastroscopy and enteroscopy.

19.8.1.5 Imaging Demonstrations
Digestive Radiology
Digestive radiology can demonstrate ulceration in the gastrointestinal tract, cobble stone appearance and peristalsis disorder.

Digestive Endoscopy
The demonstrations include obvious red plaque edema on the surface of the mucosa, mostly with spots bleeding and possible occurrence of esophageal ulcerations.

19.8.1.6 Criteria for the Diagnosis
Cytology of Shedding Cells
The characteristic giant cell can be detected in urinary sediment of CMV patients. Such cells can be found by H&E staining of the gastrointestinal specimens biopsy.

Application of Enzyme Labeled Human Cytomegalovirus (HCMV)
The monoclonal antibody of early antigen can be used for direct immunoenzyme staining for specimen inoculated tissue and cell cultures. After 12–24 h, a positive result can be obtained, which is rapid and specific.

Molecular Hybridization Test
32P marked HCMV-DNA/HCMV-RNA probe or biotin labeled HCMV-DNA probe is used for molecular hybridization test, which has favorable sensitivity and specificity. homologous sequences of 3.2–10 pg can be detected.

Serological Tests
For cases with anti-CMV IgM antibody positive or total antibody (anti-CMV) conversion from negative to positive, the diagnosis of primary CMV infection can be made. For cases with anti-CMV IgM antibody positive or total antibody have an at least four times increase, it can be defined as the current illnesses. In combination of clinical manifestations, the diagnosis can be made.

Gastrointestinal Radiology
Demonstrations include mucosal irritation of gastrointestinal tract, bleeding or ulcerations. By biopsy and pathological analysis, an owl's eyes sign can be found.

19.8.1.7 Differential Diagnosis
1. Toxoplasmosis
2. Rubella virus infection
3. Herpes simplex virus infection
4. Other possible pathogens infection (such as Treponema pallidum)

19.8.2 HIV/AIDS Related Gastrointestinal Herpes Simplex Virus Infection

19.8.2.1 Pathogens and Pathogenesis
In AIDS population, incidence of HSV infection and its recurrence are obviously increasing, with a seropositive rate of up to more than 80–90 %. HSV is a virus with double-stranded DNA, with enveloped lipoprotein in a diameter of 150–200 nm. HSV has HSV-1 and HSV-2 serotypes. HSV invades the human body via the oral cavity, respiratory tract, genital mucosa or ruptured skin. The AIDS patients are more vulnerable to HSV infection due to their compromised immunity, and they commonly have serious symptoms and organ damages.

19.8.2.2 Pathophysiological Basis
Herpes simplex virus infection firstly is skin mucosa infection and acute ganglion infection. The susceptible hosts have latent and recurrent infection. The inoculation of pathogenic virus to the skin mucosa triggers the initial infection. The skin can defense against the infection of herpes simplex virus, with mucosa and conjunctiva being more vulnerable to HSV invasion. Patients infected by herpes simplex virus have the blast cell assimilation reactions, antibody dependent/independent cytotoxicity and natural killer cells activities. Cellular immunity can confine infection, but fails to inhibit the latent infection and its reactivation. In particular, the functions and amount of T lymphocytes in AIDS patients have varying degrees of inhibition or decrease. Therefore, AIDS patients are susceptible to HSV infection. Occurrence of HSV-1 and HSV-2 viremia is related to diffuse infection.

Table 19.3 Symptoms of HSV infection in AIDS patients

HSV infection	Local symptoms
Herpetic stomatitis	Oral ulcers, herpes
Pharyngitis, esophagitis	Difficulty swallowing, swallowing pain, retrosternal pain
Rectitis	Anorectal pain, liquid outflow, tenesmus, constipation, abnormal sense of sacrum

And its pathological basis is diffuse inflammation of the gastrointestinal tract, with manifestations of mucosal red plaques, edema, exudates and ulceration that has coverage of fiber purulent membranous secretions. The histocytes have characteristic intranuclear eosinophilic inclusions, with manifestations of necrotic and herpes simplex viral esophagitis.

19.8.2.3 Clinical Symptoms and Signs

AIDS patients commonly have severe symptoms of HSV infection (Table 19.3), with possible occurrence of disseminated infection. Generally, HSV infection is widespread, but mostly being asymptomatic. The clinical manifestations are related to the localization of infection, age, immunity, antigen type and other factors. In initial infection, the body has no antibodies, with symptoms of fever, upset, local lymphadenectasis, muscular pain and other symptoms.

19.8.2.4 Examinations and Their Selection
HSV Antibody Determination

Using neutralization reaction and complement fixation test, serum HSV antibody titer can be detected. For the cases with the antibody titer being with more than four times increase, recurrence of HSV infection is indicated.

Virus Isolation

The excretions are collected for tissue culture and virus isolation, based on which the diagnosis can be made.

In Situ Hybridization

By using DNA probe of HSV, DNA in situ hybridization is performed to detect the DNA of HSV, with strong sensitivity.

Polymerase Chain Reaction (PCR)

The exudates from the involved cells or herpes contain DNA components of HSV. PCR can be performed with in vitro amplification, which has a strong sensitivity.

Pathological Examination

Biopsy of pathological tissues can be performed to observe the morphology and characteristics of lesions. The findings of intranuclear inclusions in the multi-nucleus have important diagnostic value.

19.8.2.5 Imaging Demonstrations
Gastrointestinal Radiology

X-ray demonstrates gathering or scattering spots superficial ulcers in the middle segment of the esophagus, with surrounding stripes of edema (halo sign).

Gastrointestinal Endoscopy

Gastrointestinal endoscopy demonstrates obvious erythema and edema in the mucosal surface, half with esophageal ulcers. Especially its concurrence with CMV infection makes the oral ulcers difficult to heal.

19.8.2.6 Criteria for the Diagnosis
1. The antibody titer is more than four times by HSV antibody detection.
2. HSV virus can be isolated by virus isolation.
3. In situ hybridization demonstrates DNA of the HSV.
4. Polymerase chain reaction (PCR) demonstrates DNA components of the HSV.
5. Pathology demonstrates intranuclear inclusions in the multi-nucleus.
6. X-ray demonstrates gathering or scattering spots superficial ulcers in the middle segment of the esophagus, with surrounding stripes of edema (halo sign).
7. Digestive endoscopy demonstrates obvious erythema and edema on the mucosal surface, half with esophageal ulcers.

19.8.2.7 Differential Diagnosis
1. CMV infection should be differentiated from HSV infection.
2. Concurrence of HSV infection and CMV infection should be differentiated from HSV infection.

19.8.3 HIV/AIDS Related Gastrointestinal Adenovirus Infection

19.8.3.1 Pathogens and Pathogenesis

Adenovirus contains double-stranded linear DNA, with an average diameter of 70 nm. Its core components have a capsid, with no adipose envelope. Currently its 41 serotypes are known, in addition to some adenovirus that cannot be typed. Generally, adenovirus can grow in ordinary cell culture, but adenovirus in the feces only grow in selectively some cells. Therefore, it is known as the intestinal adenovirus.

19.8.3.2 Pathophysiological Basis

In AIDS patients with chronic diarrhea, intestinal adenovirus mainly infects the jejunum and ileum. Villi of the intestinal mucosal epithelial cells are smaller and shorter, with cellular degeneration and lysis as well as mononuclear cells infiltration in intestinal lamina propria. Therefore, intestinal absorption dysfunction occurs to cause osmotic diarrhea. The CD4 T cell count is commonly lower than 50/µl.

19.8.3.3 Clinical Symptoms and Signs

The incubation period of adenovirus gastroenteritis is about 10 days, with clinical manifestations of diarrhea, in small/large quantity and being watery or loose. In some cases, mucous fluid may be discharged. The duration of the illness is usually 4–8 days, often accompanied by vomiting. In some serious cases, dehydration occurs, and even death. Some patients have respiratory symptoms, and a few patients may have fever, with self-limited duration. The detoxification period is about 1 week. About 68–85 % AIDS patients have intestinal pathogens infection, including adenovirus (Adv) infection.

19.8.3.4 Examinations and Their Selection

Virus Particles Detection

The conventional electron microscopy can define the existence of adenovirus. And immune electron microscopy can define its subtype.

Tests and Assays

Hemagglutination inhibition test or ELISA findings of adenovirus antigen positive can define the diagnosis.

Molecular Biology Test

Polyacrylamide gel electrophoresis can detect adenovirus antigen in feces. Its positive rate is higher than that detected by electron microscopy.

Diagnostic Imaging

It demonstrates the functions and lesions range in the intestinal tract.

Digestive Endoscopy

Digestive endoscopy can be applied to observe the intestinal mucosal lesions and to collect tissues from lesions for biopsy.

19.8.3.5 Imaging Demonstrations

1. No characteristic findings by gastrointestinal radiology
2. No characteristic findings by gastrointestinal endoscopy

19.8.3.6 Criteria for the Diagnosis

1. Findings of adenovirus particles by conventional electron microscopy, with its subtype defined by immune electron microscopy.
2. Adenovirus antigen positive by hemagglutination inhibition test or ELISA.
3. Fecal adenovirus positive by molecular biology test
4. Findings of DNA components of adenovirus by in situ hybridization
5. Intestinal dysfunction signs by gastrointestinal radiography
6. Mucosal congestion, edema, or spots erosion by digestive endoscopy

19.8.3.7 Differential Diagnosis

It should be differentiated from infections of CMV, HSV and other pathogens.

19.9 HIV/AIDS Related Gastrointestinal Bacterial Infections

19.9.1 HIV/AIDS Related Gastrointestinal Mycobacterial Infection

19.9.1.1 Pathogens and Pathogenesis

Infections of mycobacterium, Salmonella, Shigella, Campylobacter jejuni often occur in gastrointestinal tract of AIDS patients. In addition, bacteremia and drug resistance occur more frequently than those in common people.

19.9.1.2 Pathophysiological Basis

Intestinal mycobacterium tuberculosis infection in AIDS patients is commonly secondary to pulmonary tuberculosis. Pathologically, intestinal tuberculosis can be divided into ulcerative and proliferative. Ulcerative intestinal tuberculosis is more common in AIDS patients due to their compromised or loss of immune mediation. Its pathological basis is the collection of lymph nodes in the intestinal wall and invaded lymphoid follicles to cause caseous lesions, followed by ulcerations. And the lesions can spread along the intestinal wall or progress into deep tissues to invade the serosa, resulting in adhesions or fistula formation. Proliferative intestinal tuberculosis is less common in AIDS patients. It firstly invades the cecum, and then spreads to the ascending colon and terminal ileum, characterized by large quantity granulation tissue, thickened intestinal wall, narrowed intestinal lumen and local formation of lumps. In the cases with involvements of peritoneum and mesentery, peritonitis, intestinal adhesions and ascites can occur.

19.9.1.3 Clinical Symptoms and Signs

Mycobacterium can cause colorectal inflammation, leading to invasive and hemorrhagic ulcers. Infection of mycobacterium avium complex (MAC) commonly occurs in the small intestines and the rectum. The clinical manifestations include lower abdominal pain and upset, nausea, watery or bloody diarrhea, accompanied by fever, chills and muscular soreness and pain. Occasionally, there are bleeding, perforation and obstruction.

19.9.1.4 Examinations and Their Selection

1. Digestive radiology can demonstrate spasm and contraction of the diseased intestine as well as deranged mucosa folds.
2. Digestive endoscopy is applied for direct observation and biopsy.

3. The pathological analysis can demonstrate tuberculous granuloma.
4. Acid-fast staining of tissues can be applied to detect mycobacterium tuberculosis.
5. Gastrointestinal radiology can demonstrate the localization, range and functions of the diseased intestine as well as its relationship with the surrounding tissues.
6. Digestive endoscopy can demonstrate the lesions on intestinal mucosa and can be applied to collect specimens for biopsy.

19.9.1.5 Imaging Demonstrations
Gastrointestinal Radiography
It demonstrates intestinal spasm and contraction, and deranged mucosal folds. When the barium reaches the lesions, a small quantity barium is filling in a linear shape. The mass shaped barium goes smoothly through the intestine, which is known as the irritative sign and is a typical manifestation in cases of ulcerative intestinal tuberculosis. By barium enema, there are deranged or destroyed mucosal folds, with small spots or spikes liked niche shadows and fast intestinal movements.

Digestive Endoscopy
The gastrointestinal mucosa has characteristic patches of yellowish white pseudomembrane, which is caused by large quantity of mycobacteria in the mucosal macrophages.

19.9.1.6 Criteria for the Diagnosis
1. By Colonoscopy biopsy and acid-fast staining to find mycobacterium tuberculosis.
2. Stool culture to find Mycobacterium positive.
3. X-ray demonstrates intestinal spasm and contraction, deranged mucosal folds and small ulcers.
4. Findings of yellowish white pseudomembrane by gastroscopy and colonoscopy.

19.9.1.7 Differential Diagnosis
1. Gastrointestinal CMV infection.
2. Gastrointestinal HSV infection.
3. Other neoplastic lesions.

19.9.2 HIV/AIDS Related Gastrointestinal Salmonella Infection

19.9.2.1 Pathogens and Pathogenesis
Salmonella has more than 1,800 kinds of serotypes, among which about 20 kinds are pathogenic, including Eberthella typhi and Salmonella enteritidis. Salmonella inflammation is a result of dietary intake of foods contaminated by intestinal Salmonella infection (such as cattle and poultry).

Generally, the invaded Salmonella can be killed by human cellular immunity. Among AIDS patients, due to decreased or loss of immunity, the incidence of Salmonella bacteremia is high.

19.9.2.2 Pathophysiological Basis
Typical typhoid in AIDS patients is that after the access of bacteria to the small intestines, they penetrate the intestinal mucosal epithelium to invade the lymphoid tissues in the intestinal wall. The bacteria also spread along with lymph flow to the mesenteric lymph nodes and other lymphoid tissues to reproduce there. Their flow into blood along thoracic duct causes the first bacteremia. The duration is the first week of the whole illness course, known as the prodromal period. Then the bacteria along with the blood flow reach the bone marrow, liver, spleen, kidney, gall bladder and skin, reproducing there. The bacteria that have been engulfed by phagocytes in the organs re-enter the bloodstream to cause the second bacteremia. This period has obvious clinical symptoms, being equal to the 2nd–3rd weeks of the illness course. The bacteria can invade the intestinal lymphoid tissue again to cause allergic responses and the resulted local necrosis and ulcerations. In the serious cases, intestinal bleeding and perforation occur. Bacteria in the kidney can be discharges along with urination. In the 4th week, the patients are in the recovery period, with gradual healing.

19.9.2.3 Clinical Symptoms and Signs
Immunocompromised people are the most susceptible groups to Salmonella infection. It has been reported that the incidence of Salmonella infection in AIDS patients is 100 times as high as that in common people. It has been also reported that the incidence of Salmonella infection in male homosexual AIDS patients is 20 times as high as that in common people. Salmonella infection mostly occurs in the early stage of AIDS, and causes infections of stomach and intestines. Its symptoms include diarrhea, headache, nausea, stomach cramps and fever, with a duration of 1–2 days or even longer. Death may occur due to salmonella bacteremia or sepsis.

19.9.2.4 Examinations and Their Selection
1. Staphylococcal protein A coagglutination test, enzyme-linked immunosorbent assay and radioimmunoassay (RIA) can detect the serum or urine soluble antigens of bacilli typhi and bacilli paratyphoid in the patients.
2. Widal's test can facilitate the diagnosis of Salmonella infection.
3. Gastrointestinal radiology can be applied to observe the intestinal dysfunctioning disorders and ulcerations.
4. Digestive endoscopy can demonstrate the mucosal congestion, edema, or spots erosions.

19.9.2.5 Imaging Demonstrations
Gastrointestinal Radiology

By gastrointestinal radiology, the demonstrations include intestinal dysfunctioning disorders and ulceration.

Digestive Endoscopy

By digestive endoscopy, the demonstrations include intestinal mucosal edema, erosion and ulcerations.

19.9.2.6 Criteria for the Diagnosis
Rapid Diagnostic Test

In recent years, the application of staphylococcal protein A coagglutination test, enzyme-linked immunosorbent assay and radioimmunoassay (RIA) are commonly applied for the detection of the soluble antigens of bacilli typhi and bacilli paratyphoid in patients' serum or urine to assist the early clinical diagnosis of such infections.

Widal's Test

It facilitates the diagnosis of Salmonella infection

Gastrointestinal Radiology

It demonstrates the intestinal function disorders and ulcerations.

Digestive Endoscopy

It demonstrates intestinal inflammations and can be used to collect specimens for the biopsy for the confirmative diagnosis.

19.9.2.7 Differential Diagnosis
1. Mycobacterium.
2. Shigella.
3. Other pathogens.

19.9.3 HIV/AIDS Related Gastrointestinal Shigella Infection

19.9.3.1 Pathogens and Pathogenesis

Shigella belongs to the genus of Shigella, the family of enterobacteria, which is also known as dysentery bacillus. The bacterium is a small and short Gram-negative bacillus with no power and no gas. It is empowered with pathogenicity under three conditions: (1) with smooth lipopolysaccharide O antigen; (2) with the gene encoding that enables them to invade the epithelial cells and replicate there; (3) producing toxins after its invasion. The prognosis of Shigella invasion into the human body depends on the result of the interactions between the immunity of the human body and the virulence of the bacterium.

19.9.3.2 Pathophysiological Basis

Intestinal lesions by dysentery mostly occur in the sigmoid colon and rectum. But in some serious cases, the entire colon, ileocecus, and even the terminal ileum can be involved. The basic pathological changes include diffuse fibrin exudative inflammation in the intestinal mucosa, and multiple superficial ulcers. Microscopic examination demonstrates diffuse congestion and edema of intestinal mucosa and mucous bloody exudation of intestine mucus in the slightly ill cases; large flaky shedding of the intestinal mucosa, and grayish white fibrous pseudomembrane composed of necrotic shedding epithelial cells, fibrin, neutrophils, and Shigella bacteria in the severely ill cases. The following demonstrations include mesenteric lymphadenectasis, toxic and degenerative changes of the liver, kidney and other parenchymal organs. In the cases of chronic dysentery, there are intestinal mucosal edema and thickening, formation of depressed scar, intestinal mucosal cysts and intestinal polyps.

19.9.3.3 Clinical Symptoms and Signs

There are 32 serotypes of Shigella, transmitted via routs of contacts between humans and from fecal to oral. It is one of the causes for occurrence of diarrhea in male homosexuals and in AIDS patients. Its clinical symptoms include fever, tenesmus, abdominal pain, bloody stools, and other dysentery symptoms. Bacteremia can also occurs.

19.9.3.4 Examinations and Their Selection
1. Stool examination provides important information for the clinical diagnosis and treatment.
2. Digestive endoscopy is a commonly used examination, with a high positive rate in the following biopsy.
3. Gastrointestinal radiology is a commonly used examination for the diagnosis.

19.9.3.5 Imaging Demonstrations
Gastrointestinal Radiography

It demonstrates intestinal functional disorders, ulcers and polypoid filling defects.

Digestive Endoscopy

It demonstrates grayish white fibrous pseudomembrane and ulceration.

19.9.3.6 Criteria for the Diagnosis
1. Stool examination findings of the Shigella.
2. Dysentery bacilli positive by biopsy after digestive endoscopy.
3. Stomach spasms and intestinal functional disorders by gastrointestinal radiology.

19.9.3.7 Differential Diagnosis
1. Salmonella infection
2. Mycobacterium infection

3. Viral gastroenteritis
4. Campylobacter jejuni infection

19.9.4 HIV/AIDS Related Campylobacter Jejuni Infection

19.9.4.1 Pathogens and Pathogenesis

The vast majority of pathogens to human body are Campylobacter jejuni and the fetus subspecies of Campylobacter fetus, followed by Campylobacter coli. Campylobacter coli is micro-aerophilic gram-negative bacilli, with a length of 1.5–5 um and a width of 0.2–0.5 um. It is in a shape of curve, S or spiral, with 3–5 Campylobacter coli in a string or singular arrangement. The bacteria has two pointed ends with polar flagellum, which can move fast in a straight or spiral line. It has no capsule, transmitting via the route from feces to mouth. The mechanism of Campylobacter jejuni induced human enteritis has not completely known. It has bee speculated that it may be related to its pathogenicity, endotoxins and exotoxins.

19.9.4.2 Pathophysiological Basis

By intestinal mucosal pathology, it is non-specific colitis, with infiltrations of neutrophil leukocytes, monocytes, and eosinophilic granulocytes in the lamina propria; degenerated and atrophic intestinal gland, loss of mucous fluid; crypt abscesses; mucous epithelial cell ulceration, ulcerative colitis and Crohn's disease.

19.9.4.3 Clinical Symptoms and Signs

Early clinical symptoms include headache, fever, muscular soreness and pain, and other prodromal symptoms, followed by diarrhea, nausea and vomiting. Patients with an acute onset have fever, abdominal pain, diarrhea and general upset. Generally, the patient firstly excretes watery loose stools, followed by mucous or bloody mucous stools, or even bloody stool. The lesions may involve the rectum and sigmoid colon, possibly with accompanying tenesmus. In the slightly ill cases, patients have intermittent diarrhea, and sometimes bloody stools. In the severely ill cases, patients have persistent high fever with severe bloody stools. In some severe cases, there are toxic giant colitis, or pseudomembranous colitis and lower gastrointestinal bleeding.

19.9.4.4 Examinations and Their Selection
Routine Stool Test

It appears to be mucous or watery. By microscopy, there are more leukocytes or more erythrocytes.

Bacteria Culture

It is a commonly used examination, with a positive rate of 5–30 %.

Diagnostic Imaging

Angiography shows intestinal digestive disorders, ulcers and polypoid filling defect.

Gastrointestinal Endoscopy

There are white fiber psedomembrane and ulcers.

19.9.4.5 Imaging Demonstrations

1. Gastrointestinal radiology has non-specific demonstrations.
2. Digestive endoscopy has non-specific demonstrations.

19.9.4.6 Criteria for the Diagnosis

1. Routine stool test findings of Campylobacter jejuni in 20 % AIDS patients.
2. Bloody diarrhea and more leukocytes indicate Campylobacter jejuni enteritis.
3. Bacteria culture findings of Campylobacter jejuni positive. The positive rate is about 5–30 %.
4. Campylobacter jejuni is sensitive to erythromycin, aminoglycoside and some other antibiotics.
5. Imaging demonstrations are non-specific.
6. Gastrointestinal endoscopy demonstrations are non-specific.

19.9.4.7 Differential Diagnosis

1. Salmonella infection
2. Mycobacterium infection
3. Viral gastroenteritis

19.9.5 HIV/AIDS Related Gastrointestinal Histoplasmosis

19.9.5.1 Pathogens and Athogenesis

Histoplasmosis (HP) in AIDS patients is disseminating. The patients have skin and oral lesions. Histoplasma capsulatum invasion can involve the gastrointestinal tract and other tissues and organs, which commonly invades the mononuclear phagocytes. Under a microscope, Histoplasma capsulatum specimens are yeast type in mononuclear cells or neutrophils in a round or oval shape with a diameter of 1–5 um. It reproduces by budding, surrounded by nonstaining capsule liked substance. Histoplasma capsulatum is a pathogenic dimorphic fungus. People with normal immunity have no such fungi in their bodies and their histoplasmosis is self-healing. But in people with immunodeficiency, histoplasma capsulatum is pathogenic.

19.9.5.2 Pathophysiological Basis

Histoplasmosis (HP) is closely related to the immunity. Its basic pathological change is hyperplasia of the macrophages. After invasion of Histoplasma capsulatum into human body, it grows and replicates in the mononuclear

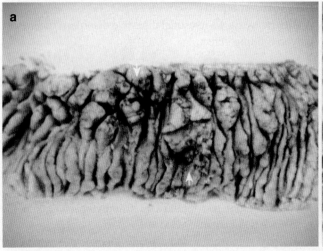
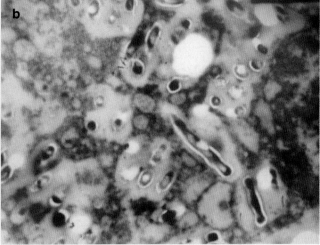

Fig. 19.19 (**a**, **b**) HIV/AIDS related intestinal histoplasmosis. (**a**) Gross observation of the specimen obtained by surgical removal demonstrates foci of intestinal histoplasmosis. (**b**) Electron microscopic examination of intestinal mucosa demonstrates capsular spores of histoplasma capsulatum (The figures provided by Lang ZW)

macrophages to cause hyperplasia of the giant cell and further result in granuloma. Caseous necrosis can occur in local lesions, being dissolved and absorbed. Or caseous necrosis is followed by fibrosis and calcification that is self healing. But in AIDS patients, the mononuclear macrophage system fails to control the infection due to their lack of immune mediation. Therefore, histoplasma capsulatum disseminates extensively in tissues containing abundant macrophages, which presents difficulties for the granulation tissues to grow with following fibrosis and even calcification.

19.9.5.3 Clinical Symptoms and Signs

The common clinical manifestations are long-term fever, upset, cough, weight loss, swollen lymph nodes, enlarged liver and skin defects. AIDS patients have consuming and febrile diseases, weight loss, hepatosplenomegaly and skin mucus lesions.

19.9.5.4 Imaging Demonstrations
Gastrointestinal Radiology
There are intestinal functional disorders, thickened mucosal folds and multiple round liked filling defects.

Gastrointestinal Endoscopy
There are intestinal mucosal inflammations and multiple polypoid lesions.

19.9.5.5 Criteria for the Diagnosis
Pathologic Examination
By direct microscopic examination, there are round or oval yeast liked budding bacteria within and out of the mononuclear or multinucleated macrophages. For the cases with surrounding halo, the diagnosis can be made.

Immunological Assays
The applicable immunological assays include complement fixation test (CF), radioimmunoassay (RIA), enzyme-linked immunosorbent assay determination (ELISA) and Western blot (WB), molecular cloning and recombinant antigen. Because of weakened or loss of immune responses in AIDS patients, the immunological examinations have a high false negative rate.

Histological Examination
By oil microscopy, histoplasma capsulatum can be found.

Fungi Culture
By fungi culture, histoplasma capsulatum can be found.

Gastrointestinal Radiology
By gastrointestinal radiology, the demonstrations are multiple round filling defects.

Gastrointestinal Endoscopy
By gastrointestinal endoscopy, the demonstrations are multiple intestinal polypoid lesions.

19.9.5.6 Differential Diagnosis
1. Salmonella infection.
2. Mycobacterial infection.
3. Viral gastroenteritis.
4. Campylobacter jejuni infection.
5. Crohn's disease.

19.10 HIV/AIDS Related Gastrointestinal Parasitosis

19.10.1 HIV/AIDS Related Gastrointestinal Cryptosporidiosis

19.10.1.1 Pathogens and Pathogenesis

Gastrointestinal cryptosporidiosis is the common cause diarrhea in AIDS patients, which is mainly cryptosporidium infection. Cryptosporidium species (CS) infects both human and animals. The cryptosporidium oocyst is in a diameter of 2–6 um, in a shape of round or oval containing four bare banana shaped sporozoites and one residuum. After the invation of cryptosporidium into the human body, its capsule is dissolved by digestive fluid to expose the sporozoite, which is attached to the intestinal mucosa and grows there into trophozoites in the epithelial cells. The trophozoite then develops into schizonts, whose rupture causes its invasion into other epithelial cells. Alternatively, the schizont develops into gametophyte to form the oocyst. The oocysts with thick walls can be discharged with the stool, while the occysts with thin walls can release sporozoites to invade the intestinal epithelial cells and they can also be discharged with the stool. The oocysts of cryptosporidium parasitize in the microvilli of the epithelial cells of the small intestines, and its pathogenicity is closely related to immunity. Generally, its infection of common populations is self-limited, but its infection of AIDS patients can be serious. Cryptosporidium can infect the gastrointestinal tract of AIDS patients and reproduce there to cause serious formidable fatal diarrhea. The pathogenic mechanism of cryptosporidium is still unknown, and it is speculated that it might be a result of multiple pathogenic factors.

19.10.1.2 Pathophysiological Basis

Cryptosporidium parasitize in the surface of intestinal mucosa to cause the dysfunction of intestinal villi. It leads to large quantity reproduction of the intestinal bacteria and production of toxins, resulting in decreased or loss of disaccharidase and other mucosal enzymes in the intestines, and the dysfunction of adipose digestion and absorption are all causes of severe diarrhea. The lesions are commonly found in the small intestines and colon. When pathological biopsy or autopsy is performed, cryptosporidia can be found in the entire gastrointestinal tract. By microscopy, there are atrophy or absence of the small intestinal villi in the lesions, enlarged epithelial cells in crypts and deepened crypts. The epithelial cells of the intestinal mucosa are flat. There is infiltration of lymphocytes, neutrophils, plasma cells and microphages in the villus epithelial cells and lamina propria. The pathological changes of colon mucosa are similar to those of small intestines.

19.10.1.3 Clinical Symptoms and Signs

The clinical symptoms is commonly chronic diarrhea, with an latent period of about 4–14 days. Its onset is chronic, commonly with accompanying abdominal pain, long term diarrhea that cannot heal and watery stools. The patients are susceptible to dehydration, acidosis, hypokalemia, and vitamins deficiency.

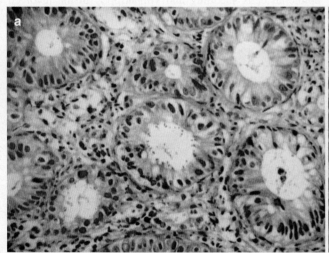
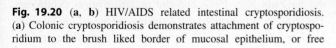
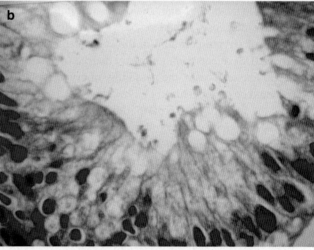

Fig. 19.20 (**a**, **b**) HIV/AIDS related intestinal cryptosporidiosis. (**a**) Colonic cryptosporidiosis demonstrates attachment of cryptosporidium to the brush liked border of mucosal epithelium, or free cryptosporidium in the glandular cavity (HE ×200). (**b**) Oil microscopy demonstrates morphology of Cryptosporidium (HE ×1,000) (Provided by Lang ZW)

19.10.1.4 Examinations and Their Selection
Stool Examination
Microscopy demonstrates stool contents of leukocytes and pyocytes.

Pathogen Examination
The patients' stool or vomitus are collected to detect oocysts of Cryptosporidium, which is a commonly used examination.

Immunological Assays
Both immunofluorescence assay (IFA) and monoclonal antibody test have favorable specificity and sensitivity, being up to 100 %.

Diagnostic Imaging
Gastrointestinal radiology is a commonly used examination.

Gastrointestinal Endoscopy
It is a more commonly used examination and can be applied to collect specimens for biopsy.

19.10.1.5 Imaging Demonstrations
Gastrointestinal Radiology
The demonstrations are non-specific, with intestinal functional disorders, irritative sign, and thickened mucosal folds.

Gastrointestinal Endoscopy
The demonstrations are non-specific, with inflammations of intestinal mucosa.

19.10.1.6 Criteria for the Diagnosis
1. The diagnosis of cryptosporidiosis is mainly based on the epidemiologic history and clinical manifestations. The definitive diagnosis should be based on findings of the oocysts of Cryptosporidium in the stool or other specimens. AIDS patients commonly have diarrhea of unknown causes. For such cases, the possibility of cryptosporidiosis should be considered.
2. After the invasion of Cryptosporidium to human body, specific antibodies can be produced. The specific antibody can be detected by immunological assays and serological tests to define the diagnosis.
3. Due to the suppressed immunity, AIDS patients have declined ability to produce antibodies. Therefore, the antibody titer should be objectively assessed. PCR has both high rates of sensitivity and specificity, and Cryptosporidium can be found by gene amplification.

19.10.1.7 Differential Diagnosis
When intestinal symptoms occur in the cases of cryptosporidiosis, it should be differentiated from other common enteric pathogens infections, including bacillus typhi, pathogenic Salmonella, Campylobacter, Clostridium difficile, Giardia lamblia, Entamoeba histolytica. In addition, some less common pathogens should be considered, especially CMV, Mycobacterium avium, cryptosporidium parvum, and round cryptosporidium.

19.10.2 HIV/AIDS Related Gastrointestinal Isosporiasis

19.10.2.1 Pathogens and Pathogenesis
Isosporiasis is a kind of Isospora belli infection that can cause diarrhea. The oocysts of Isospora belli are pathogenic after their sporulation. In tropical and subtropical regions, human isosporiasis is very common, and it infects people via fecal-oral route due to contaminated foods or drinks. Dogs and other mammals are believed to be the reservoir hosts of the Isospora belli. Its pathogenic mechanism has not been clarified. The parasites invade the intestinal epithelium and divide repeatedly, which can lead to mucosal damage, erosion and absorptional dysfunction. The metabolites of parasites may also have toxic effects.

19.10.2.2 Pathophysiological Basis
The studies of AIDS patients in the United States have demonstrated that its incidence is 15 %. After sporozoites gain their access to the intestinal cells, they begin to divide and their amount increases by several times. In the process of Isospora proliferation, the intestinal mucosa is damaged. In the chronic cases, there are shortened intestinal mucosal villi, deepened crypts, with infiltration of eosinophils and neutrophils in the lamina propria. There are also mucosal epithelial cells shedding and villi atrophy in the involved small intestines (jejunum and ileum). The cortex is extensively damaged, with severely affected functions of digestion and absorption.

19.10.2.3 Clinical Symptoms and Signs
Due to impaired T cells participated immune functions, the immunity is incapable of eliminating the protozoa. The infection of coccidia can cause severe diarrhea, gastroenteritis, nausea, anorexia, or even diffuse abdominal cramps, and it can also lead to long-tem chronic diarrhea and weight loss. HIV/AIDS related isosporiasis and cyclospora cayetanensis can cause similar refractory diarrhea to that in cases of cryptosporidiosis. Studies have shown that diarrhea induced cryptosporidiosis ranks the first in the incidence of HIV/AIDS related parasitic diarrhea. Occasionally, the patients may have chronic malabsorption syndrome. The disease is generally self-limiting; with self heal lesions in short period of time. Death may occur in the serious cases.

19.10.2.4 Examinations and Their Selection
Pathogen Examination
The disease can be definitively diagnosed by findings of Isospora oocysts in the stool specimen.

Diagnostic Imaging
Gastrointestinal radiography is a commonly used examination.

19.10.2.5 Imaging Demonstrations
1. Non-specific demonstrations by gastrointestinal radiography.
2. Non-specific demonstrations by gastroscopy.

19.10.2.6 Criteria for the Diagnosis
1. Microscopic findings of characteristic oocysts can define the diagnosis. The stool examination should be performed for several times and the oocysts can be found by improved acid-fast staining. For patients with Isospora belli infection, their stools usually contain eosinophils derived enzyme, Charcot-Leyden crystals. The peripheral blood is demonstrated to have increased eosinophils.
2. Sometimes when the protozoa is in the cells, the definitive diagnosis depends on intestinal biopsy. Intestinal mucosal biopsy demonstrates shortened microvilli, and the infiltration of lymphocytes, plasma cells and eosinophils in the lamina propria.
3. Non-specific demonstrations by gastrointestinal radiology.
4. Non-specific demonstrations by gastroscopy.

19.10.2.7 Differential Diagnosis
1. Histolytic amebiasis.
2. Cryptosporidiosis.
3. Giardiasis.

19.10.3 HIV/AIDS Related Gastrointestinal Entamoebiasis Histolytica

19.10.3.1 Pathogens and Pathogenesis
Entamoeba histolytica Schaudim (1903) belongs to the family of Entamoeba and species of Entamoeba. In 1928, Brumpt proposed that there are two types of Entamoeba histolytica schaudim, with one being able to cause amebiasis and the other is non-pathogenic in spite of their similar morpholgy and life history, which is known as Entamoeba dispar. Amoebiasis is caused by Entamoeba histolytica Schaudim, while Entamoeba dispar has no pathogenicity. Enteric E. histolytica disease is a kind of transmitted gastrointestinal disease dominated with dysentery symptoms, which is caused by the pathogenic invasion of Entamoeba histolytica protozoon to the colon wall. It has a high incidence in AIDS patients (especially homosexual AIDS patients). It might be caused by direct swallowing of amoebic cysts during sexual mouth-anal intercourse. The cystic wall has anti-gastric acid effect, which renders its passing through the stomach intactly to the colonic ileocecum. Under the effects of intestinal digestion, the oocysts is exposed to the intestinal environment and grows there into small trophozoites, in a diameter of 3–12 um. The small trophozoite is in binary division to reproduce, supplied by swallowing intestinal contents and bacteria as their nutrients. But it cannot swallow erythrocytes. The large trophozoite is in a diameter of about 20–30 um and can actively swallow erythrocytes and tissue fragments, which are also known as the pathogenic or tissue trophozoites. Due to the decreased immunity of AIDS patients, small trophozoites can invade the tissues to cause disease. They invade the intestinal wall by their adhesion to colon epithelium and the mechanical movements of their pseudopodium as well as the solubility of their enzymes. Their subsequent growth into large trophozoites and proliferation in a large quantity cause solution, necrosis and ulceration of local intestinal mucosa.

19.10.3.2 Pathophysiological Basis
The incidence is higher in homosexual AIDS patients, and it has been reported that HIV/AIDS complicated by amoebiasis has an incidence of 1–40 % in AIDS patients of the United States. The lesions are commonly found in the cecum and ascending colon, followed by sigmoid colon and rectum. In the serious cases, the whole colon and lower part of small intestines can be involved. In the early stage, multiple prominent grayish yellow spots necrosis or superficial ulceration in size of a cap pinhead can be found on the surface of the intestinal mucosa. With the progression of the disease, the necrotic foci enlarge in a shape of round button, with surrounding bleeding stripes. Due to the continual reproduction of trophozoites in the intestinal mucosa, they penetrate the muscularis mucosa to the submucosa to cause tissue necrosis, liquefaction and shedding. Subsequently, a flask-shaped ulcer occurs with a small opening and a large bottom, with superficial borderline that has diagnostic significance. The mucosa between the ulcers is normal or only is demonstrated as having slight catarrhal inflammation. In the serious cases, adjacent ulcers can communicate each other in the submucosa to form a huge ulcer with superficial borderline, whose diameter can be up to 8–12 cm. Under a microscope, the liquefaction necrosis caused by amoebiasis is stained light red, with no demonstration of the structure. And the inflammatory responses of the adjacent tissues are slight, only with congestion, hemorrhage, and small quantity infiltration of lymphocytes and plasma cells. In the chronic stage, the demonstrations are complex due to the altering occurrence of old and new ulcerations, with concurrent necrosis, ulceration, granulation tissue hyperplasia and scar formation. The intestinal wall may be thickened and hard due to fibrous tissue proliferation, even with intestinal stenosis. Sometimes a limited mass can be formed due to the excessive hyperplasia of

granulation tissue, which is known as amoeboma. Amoeboma is more common in the cecum.

19.10.3.3 Clinical Symptoms and Signs

The intestinal symptoms dominate the acute phase, with abdominal pain, diarrhea, increased bowel movements in purple red or dark red paste due to its contents of mucus, much blood and necrotic dissolved intestinal tissues, with stench smells. Amoebic trophozoites can be found by stool examination.

The chronic stages is demonstrated by alternative occurrence of diarrhea and constipation. Therefore, the clinical symptoms recur, being unhealed for more than 2 years.

19.10.3.4 Examinations and Their Selection

Stool Examination

Microscopic findings of E. histolytica is an important basis for the definitive diagnosis.

Immunological Assay

A variety of modified enzyme-linked immunosorbent assay (ELISA) are more commonly used.

Culture

Artificial culture shows E. histolytica.

Gastrointestinal Endoscopy

It demonstrates intestinal ulcers, which helps to define the location of the biopsy.

Diagnostic Imaging

Gastrointestinal radiology can provide valuable information for the diagnosis due to its demonstrations of intestinal ulcers, stenosis and amebic abscesses.

19.10.3.5 Imaging Demonstrations

Gastrointestinal Radiology

The demonstrations are non-specific, with mucosal ulceration and intestinal stenosis.

Gastrointestinal Endoscopy

The demonstrations include mucosal edema, necrosis, ulceration, granulation tissue hyperplasia and scar formation. There are scattered small yellowish particles on the intestinal mucosa. Biopsy with the tissues obtained from the lesions can find eggs of parasites.

19.10.3.6 Criteria for the Diagnosis

1. Stool examination findings of amoebic cysts or trophozoites can define the diagnosis.
2. The detection rate is the highest by biopsy of intestinal mucosal ulcer lesions or smear of intestinal mucosal ulcer scratches facilitated by flexible sigmoidoscopy or fibercolonoscopy, being approximately 85 % in patients with

dysentery. The specimens for biopsy should be collected from the borderline of the ulcers. Specimens from abscesses puncture should also be collected from the intestinal wall. The properties of the collected fluid should be closely observed.
3. Currently, various modified enzyme-linked immunosorbent assay (ELISA) have gained a common application in the clinical practice. Serological test demonstrates a high titer.
4. Barium meal radiography demonstrates deranged and rough intestinal mucous membrane, with ulcerations or intestinal stenosis.
5. Gastrointestinal endoscopy demonstrates localized or diffuse hemorrhage or edema, ulcers, or even polyps of the colonic mucosa.

19.10.3.7 Differential Diagnosis

E. histolytica colitis should be differentiated from acute/chronic enteritis/dysentery, nonspecific ulcerative colitis and colon cancer. And it should also be differentiated from enteritis caused by other parasites.

19.10.4 HIV/AIDS Related Gastrointestinal Giardiasis

19.10.4.1 Pathogens and Pathogenesis

Giardia lamblia stiles is shortened as Giardia lamblia, living in the gastrointestinal tract in two forms, namely trophozoites and cysts. Giardiasis commonly occurs in male homosexual AIDS patients, with a common transmission route of swallowing mature cysts. The swollen cysts are ingested by gastric acid to excyst in the duodenum and grow into trophozoites there. Trophozoites commonly parasitize in the human duodenum and the upper jejunum. The pathogenic mechanism of Giardia lambia has not been completely clarified. Generally, it is believed that the pathogenesis is related to the pathogenicity of the parasite strain, symbiotic environment, the host immunity, irritation and damage of intestinal mucosa caused by trophozoites and synergy of intestinal bacteria, which can cause intestinal functions disorders. Especially immunocompromised AIDS patients are more susceptible to serious infections.

19.10.4.2 Pathophysiological Basis

The swallowed cysts of Giardia lamblia change into oocysts, which grow into active trophozoites in the upper small intestines and parasitize in the jejunum. AIDS patients are more vulnerable to infection of Giardia lamblia due to their compromised immunity. Infection of Giardia lamblia is more common in male homosexual AIDS patients.

19.10.4.3 Clinical Symptoms and Signs

After infection of Giardia lamblia, the average incubation period is 7–14 days, and the longest is 45 days. The symptoms of the acute stage include upper abdominal upset, diarrhea, malabsorption, weight loss, and accompanying spastic abdominal pain, abdominal distention, nausea and other symptoms. Symptoms of the chronic stage include intermittent loose stools, poor appetite, malnutrition, abdominal distention or spastic abdominal pain.

19.10.4.4   Examinations and Their Selection
Pathogenic Examination
The examination to find trophozoites or cysts in the stool is commonly used in clinical diagnosis. The detection rate can be increased in duodenal fluid or bile examination.

Immunological Assay
ELISA is simple to perform, with a detection rate of up to 92–98.7 %, which is feasible for epidemiological survey.

Gastrointestinal Endoscopy
For biopsy of intestinal mucosa.

Gastrointestinal Radiography
With findings of intestinal spasms with functional disorders.

19.10.4.5   Imaging Demonstrations
Gastrointestinal Radiography
With demonstrations of intestinal spasms and functional disorders.

Gastrointestinal Endoscopy
With demonstrations of non-specific inflammation.

19.10.4.6   Criteria for the Diagnosis
The findings of cysts or trophozoites in specimens of stool, duodenal fluid or bile can define the diagnosis.

19.10.4.7   Differential Diagnosis
Due to commonly mixed infection of Giardia lamblia together with cytomegalovirus, Pneumocystis carinii and Mycobacterium, the differential diagnosis should be made. Due to the currently applied effective drugs therapy, long-term infection of Giardia lamblia is rarely found.

19.10.5   HIV/AIDS Related Gastrointestinal Microsporidiosis

19.10.5.1   Pathogens and Pathogenesis
Microsporidium is one of the common pathogenic protozoa in patients with HIV infection, whose diameter is only 1–2 um. It is an intracellular protozoan parasite. Gastrointestinal microsporidium infections are commonly caused by invasion of mature spores to the cells in the intestinal wall after being swollen. The common target of microsporidium infection is the intestinal epithelial cells, which

commonly is a restricted infection. Microsporidium is the most common enteric pathogens in AIDS patients.

19.10.5.2   Pathophysiological Basis
The occurrence of Microsporidium infection is related to decreased CD4 T cell count. Jejunum is the most susceptible to Microsporidium infection, followed by the distal duodenum. The typical specific lesions are focal granuloma, vasculitis and perivascular inflammation.

19.10.5.3   Clinical Symptoms and Signs
The common symptoms of intestinal microsporidiosis are emaciation and chronic watery diarrhea with increased frequency of daily bowel movements, accompanied by nausea, poor appetite or abdominal pain.

19.10.5.4   Examinations and Their Selection
1. Gastrointestinal radiology
2. Gastrointestinal endoscopy
3. Biopsy and electron microscopy for pathogens are the most reliable examinations for the diagnosis.

19.10.5.5   Imaging Demonstrations
Gastrointestinal Radiology
With demonstrations of intestinal cramps and functional disorders.

Gastrointestinal Endoscopy
With demonstrations of non-specific inflammation.

19.10.5.6   Criteria for the Diagnosis
1. Electron microscopic finding of Microsporidium ultrastructure in the epithelial cells of the small intestines is the basis of definitive diagnosis.
2. Histopathological findings of slight infiltration of inflammatory cell in the small intestine, and infected intestinal cells in flakes distribution.
3. PCR has a sensitivity to microsporidium of up to 93 %.
4. Gastrointestinal radiography demonstrates intestinal cramps and functional disorders.

19.10.5.7   Differential Diagnosis
Due to the common occurrence of mixed infections by microsporidium together with cytomegalovirus, Pneumocystis carinii and Mycobacterium, the differential diagnosis should be made.

19.10.6   HIV/AIDS Related Gastrointestinal Toxoplasmosis

19.10.6.1   Pathogens and Pathogenesis
Toxoplasmosis is a zoonotic disease, commonly a latent infection in humans. Human toxoplasmosis is more

common in immunocompromised pregnancies and infants with congenital infections. After the pregnant women are infected, the pathogen can pass through the placenta to infect the fetus and directly affect the fetal development to cause serious deformation. The damage to the fetus is ten times as serious as that to the uninfected pregnant women, which renders it to be one of the most serious congenital infections. Both WHO and the CDC of the United States have listed it as the definitive disease of AIDS (immunodeficiency). Mammals and some poultries can be the reservoir hosts of T. gondii, and the most common reservoir host is the incompletely cooked pork, beef and mutton. Congenital toxoplasmosis infection is spread through the placenta. The initial infection of the pregnant woman, explicit or implicit, can spread to the fetus. The acquired toxoplasmosis is spread through the mouth, due to intake of contaminated food and water by oocysts, undercooked meat and eggs containing cysts and pseudocysts and unsterilized milk.

19.10.6.2 Pathophysiological Basis

After the infection of Toxoplasma gondii to human body, it gains access to the organic or tissue cells to reproduce. The escaped protozoa (tachyzoite) repeatedly invade its neighboring cells to cause focal necrosis of local tissue and inflammatory response of the surrounding tissue, which are the basic changes in the acute stage. In patients with normal immunity, the infection turns latent. In patients with AIDS, due to their compromised immunity, the protozoa reproduce in a large quantity to cause allergic responses and formation of granulation tissues. The systemically disseminated lesions can also occur.

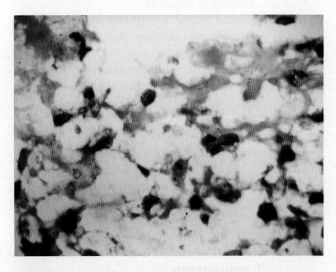

Fig. 19.21 HIV/AIDS related intestinal lymph nodes infection by Toxoplasma gondii. HE staining demonstrates Toxoplasma gondii cysts in the intestinal lymph nodes (HE ×400) (Provided by LANG ZW)

19.10.6.3 Clinical Symptoms and Signs

Generally, toxoplasmosis can be divided into two types, congenital and acquired. The most clinical symptoms are caused by reactivation of recent acute infection or latent infection. Pregnant women with toxoplasmosis during early pregnancy can cause congenital infection in 10–25 % fetuses to cause spontaneous abortion, stillbirth, premature delivery and severe neonatal infection. Most infected babies may be asymptomatic. Acquired toxoplasmosis can be divided into localized and systemic. The localized infection is commonly lymphadenitis, accounting for about 90 %, with common involvement of neck or axillary. In the cases with involvement of retroperitoneal or mesenteric lymph nodes, the symptoms include abdominal pain, high fever, macula and papula as well as gastroenteritis.

19.10.6.4 Examinations and Their Selection

1. Gastrointestinal radiology.
2. Gastrointestinal endoscopy.
3. Biopsy and electron microscopy to detect pathogens is the most reliable examinations for the diagnosis.
4. Toxoplasma antibody detection.

19.10.6.5 Imaging Demonstrations
Gastrointestinal Radiology

With demonstrations of intestinal spasm and functional disorders.

Gastrointestinal Endoscopy

With non-specific demonstrations of mucosal bleeding, erosions or superficial ulcers.

19.10.6.6 Criteria for the Diagnosis

1. Findings Toxoplasma gondii by tissue culture.
2. The diagnosis can be made based on findings of PCR. PCR has been demonstrated to be faster, with higher specificity and sensitivity, compared to probe hybridization, animal vaccination and immunological assays.
3. The applied antigens include tachyzoite soluble antigen (cytoplasmic antigen) and membrane antigen in antibody detection.
4. Demonstrations of intestinal function disorders by gastrointestinal radiology.
5. Demonstrations of mucosal bleeding, erosion or superficial ulcers, chronic inflammatory cell infiltration, or even necrotic lesions by gastrointestinal endoscopy and biopsy.

19.10.6.7 Differential Diagnosis

Due to the occurrence of mixed infection of toxoplasma together with cytomegalovirus, Mycobacterium and other protozoa, the differential diagnosis should be performed.

19.10.7 HIV/AIDS Related Strongyloidiasis

19.10.7.1 Pathogens and Pathogenesis

Strongyloides stercoralis belongs to facultative parasites, with a complex life cycle. Generally, it parasitizes in the upper small intestines of humans, commonly with chronic asymptomatic infection. Severe self-infection can often lead to serious failure and death. Infection of Strongyloides stercoralis rarely occurs in AIDS patients.

19.10.7.2 Pathophysiological Basis

After the invasion of Strongyloides stercoralis into the human body, it gains its access to the organ or tissue cells to reproduce, resulting in focal necrosis of local tissue and inflammatory responses in the surrounding tissues. The infection can be divided into mild, moderate, and severe cases according to its severity. The mild cases are characterized by changes of catarrhal enteritis, intestinal mucosal congestion, small bleeding spots and ulcers. Light microscopically, there are infiltrations of eosinophilic granulocytes and mononuclear cells, and stercoralis in the intestinal glands concave. The moderate cases are characterized by edema enteritis, thickening and edema of the intestinal wall and reduced mucosal folds. Light microscopically, there are enlarged intestinal villi, mucosal atrophy and submucosal edema. In addition, the parasite can be found in each layer of the intestinal wall. The severe cases have bleeding, erosions, ulcers, swollen lymphoid follicles, and even intestinal perforation. Due to edema and fibrosis, the intestinal wall is thickened and hardened, partially with tetanus. There are also mucosal atrophy and multiple ulcers, whose diameters range from 2 to 50 mm. Light microscopically, there are fibrosis, submucosal edema, muscular layer atrophy, and the parasites throughout the thickened intestinal wall.

19.10.7.3 Clinical Symptoms and Signs

The intestinal symptoms are commonly right upper quadrant abdominal pain, long-term chronic diarrhea, frequent diarrhea with watery stools or mucus bloody stools, tenesmus, occasional constipation. In some serious cases, there are nausea, vomiting, and paralytic intestinal obstruction. Even intestinal perforation, systemic failure and death may occur.

19.10.7.4 Examinations and Their Selection
Pathogen Examination

Findings larva in the stool or culture findings of filariform larva can define the diagnosis.

Immunological Assay

ELISA can be applied to detect specific serum antibodies, which can assist the diagnosis for the mild to moderate cases.

Gastrointestinal Radiography

It can demonstrates intestinal function disorders.

Gastrointestinal Endoscopy

Gastrointestinal endoscopy can be applied for gastric and duodenal fluid drainage to detect the pathogens. It has greater diagnostic value than stool examination.

19.10.7.5 Imaging Demonstrations
Gastrointestinal Radiology

With demonstrations of intestinal function disorders.

Gastrointestinal Endoscopy

With demonstrations of mucosal bleeding, erosions or superficial ulcers.

19.10.7.6 Criteria for the Diagnosis

The diagnosis is based on rod-shaped larva found in the stool. By Gastrointestinal radiology, there are signs of intestinal function disorders. By gastrointestinal endoscopy, there are mucosal bleeding, erosions or superficial ulcers.

19.10.7.7 Differential Diagnosis

The differentiation of various intestinal protozoa.

19.11 HIV/AIDS Related Intestinal Tumors

19.11.1 HIV/AIDS Related Intestinal Lymphoma

19.11.1.1 Pathogens and Pathogenesis

Receiving immunosuppressive therapy to cure inflammatory intestinal diseases has an five times increase of risk for occurrence of intestinal lymphoma. The risk for patients with immunodeficiency to sustain lymphoma is 100 times as high as that for people with normal immunity. There are other risk factors of lymphoma, including intravenous drug abuse, homosexuality, Epstein-Barr virus infection, genetic changes, decline in CD4 T cell count, and opportunistic infections. It has been reported that the incidence of NHL in patients with CD4 T cell count being lower than 50/µl is 12 times as high as those with their CD4 T cell count above 350/µl. These neoplasms are generally rare in children. But due to HIV infection, lymphoma is the most common neoplasm in the gastrointestinal tract of Children, with higher incidence of B cell lymphoma but lower incidence of T cell lymphoma. Lymphomas can be divided into in lymphonodus, extranodal and extranodal with accompanying in it. Hodgkin lymphoma (HL) commonly involves the lymph nodes, with an incidence of extranodal lesions being lower than 1 %. Primary extranodal lesion is rare. Non-Hodgkin's lymphoma (NHL) can involve lymph nodes, extranodal lymphoid tissues, extranodal non-lymphoid tissue or concurrent involvement of all the above, with simple lymph node lesions accounting for 1/3. Therefore, most extranodal lymphoma is NHL, with an incidence of 5–30 % in all cases of lymphomas. In that, 25 % is gastrointestinal lymphomas and another 25 % is respiratory lymphomas. Mucosa related lymphomas are commonly B cell lymphoma with low malignancy derived from the gastrointestinal tract and other mucosal tissues. Gastrointestinal mucosa related lymphomas has 50 % gastric lymphomas, 20–54 % small intestinal lymphomas and 4–6 % colonic lymphomas. Gastrointestinal mucosa related lymphomas is originated from the gastrointestinal lamina propria and submucosal lymphoid tissue, mostly being NHL and rarely being HL. Lymphoma generally is derived from B cells. Intestinal lymphomas can be derived from T cells. Gastrointestinal mucosa related lymphoma is derived from B cells lymphoma in the mucosa related extranodal marginal areas.

19.11.1.2 Pathophysiological Basis

NHL is generally grayish white parenchymal mass. Histologically, NHL is divided into T cells, B cells and histocytes based on its origination cells. Most AIDS patients sustain B cells lymphoma. About 2/3 is large cells lymphoma, including the highly malignant immunoblastic cells lymphoma and moderately malignant diffuse large cells lymphoma. About 1/4 is small non-cleaved lymphoma (belonging to Burkitt). Cases of T cells lymphoma are rarely reported. Finding of RS Mirror cells is the most valuable for the diagnosis, which can express CD15 or CD30.

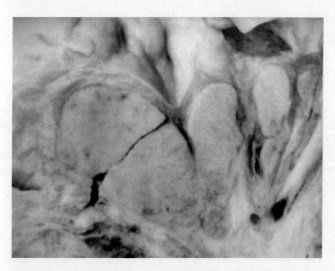

Fig. 19.22 Malignant lymphoma of the mesenteric lymph nodes, and the cross section of the enlarged lymph nodes in grayish white (Provided by LANG ZW)

19.11.1.3 Clinical Symptoms and Signs

HIV/AIDS related lymphoma commonly involves the lymph nodes to cause lymphadenectasis. It is common in extranodal tissues including bone marrow, tonsils, liver and spleen, with corresponding clinical symptoms.

19.11.1.4 Examinations and Their Selection

1. By gastrointestinal radiology, the localization and range of the lesions can be defined as well as their relationship with surrounding tissues.
2. By CT scanning, the localization and range of the lesions can be observed from the cross sections. Their blood supply and the relationship with surrounding tissues can be also observed.
3. By gastrointestinal endoscopy, the range of lesions can be directly observed. It can also be used to collect specimens for biopsy.
4. By pathological analysis, the type of involved tissues can be determined, which is used to define the qualitative diagnosis.

19.11.1.5 Imaging Demonstrations

Gastrointestinal Radiology

(1) Thick mucosal lymphoma lesion spreads under the mucosa vertically. By gastrointestinal barium meal radiology, there are irregular thickening of the mucosa to above 10 mm. (2) Nodules or masses, with the nodule being smaller than 2 cm and the mass being larger than 2 cm. The lesions can be singular or multiple. Barium meal radiology demonstrates the lesions to be filling defects with smooth and intact borders. In the cases with ulcers on the surface, a target sign or a bull's-eye sign is demonstrated. (3) In the cases of the whole stomach infiltration, barium meal radiology demonstrates leather liked stomach, with a certain degree of dilation and flexibility.

CT Scanning

With demonstrations of thickened gastric wall with smooth and intact contour, niche shadow and ring dike sign, which is obviously exterior invasion.

Gastrointestinal Endoscopy

With demonstrations of lymphoma or stomach carcinoma lesions of varicose veins and ulcers in the gastric wall.

Pathological Analysis

With demonstrations of lymphoma cells, B cells type.

Case Study 1

A male patient aged 28 years was confirmatively diagnosed as having AIDS by the CDC. He had symptoms of abdominal distention, abdominal pain, vomiting, no gas discharge for 24 h. By physical examination, he was found to be in failure liked conditions and have prominent abdomen, with tenderness and obvious rebound tenderness and weakened bowel sounds. The clinical diagnosis was intestinal obstruction. His CD4 T cell count was 1/μl.

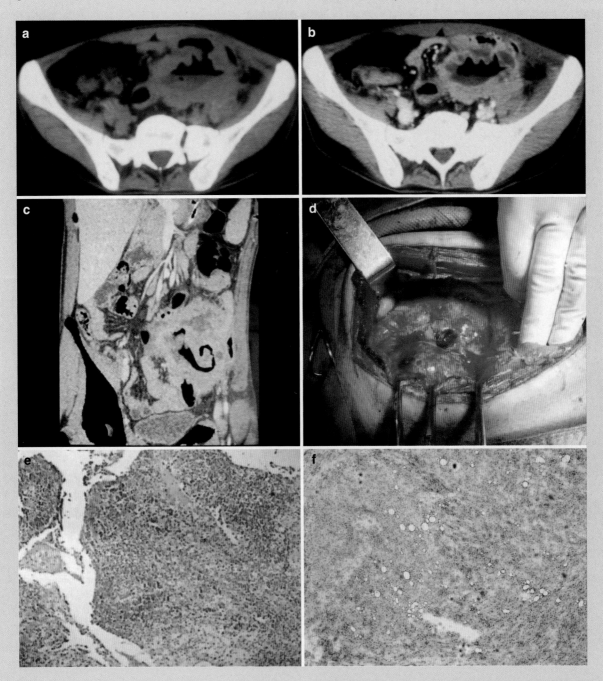

Fig. 19.23 (**a–f**) HIV/AIDS related intestinal B cell lymphoma. (**a**) CT scanning demonstrates thickened left intestinal wall, with mass liked border as well as smooth and intact interior intestinal wall. (**b**) Enhanced CT scanning demonstrates enhancement of the thickened intestinal wall. (**c**) Coronal reconstruction demonstrates thickened left intestinal wall. (**d**) Abdominal incision demonstrates the milky white mesenteric lymph nodes in the left colon, right intestinal adhesions and fixation that cannot be totally removed but collection of two intestinal wall specimens in size of about 1×1 cm. (**e**) Histopathology analysis demonstrates obvious decrease and atrophy of lymphoid follicles. According to data analysis, intestinal lymphoma generally does not invade the mesenteric lymph nodes. Microscopically, there are obviously decreased lymph node follicles in amount and volume, relative hyperplasia of mature small lymphocytes, obvious hyperplasia of small follicular blood vessels and histocytes, with changes being in line with follicular resolution stage of HIV/AIDS related lymphadenopathy. (**f**) Histopathology analysis demonstrates changes in line with intestinal B cell lymphoma

Case Study 2

A boy aged 8 years was confirmatively diagnosed as having AIDS by the CDC. He was infected by vertical transmission from mother to infant and complained of abdominal distension and enlarged liver. His CD4 T cell count was 34/μl. CT scanning was performed 1 month before his death.

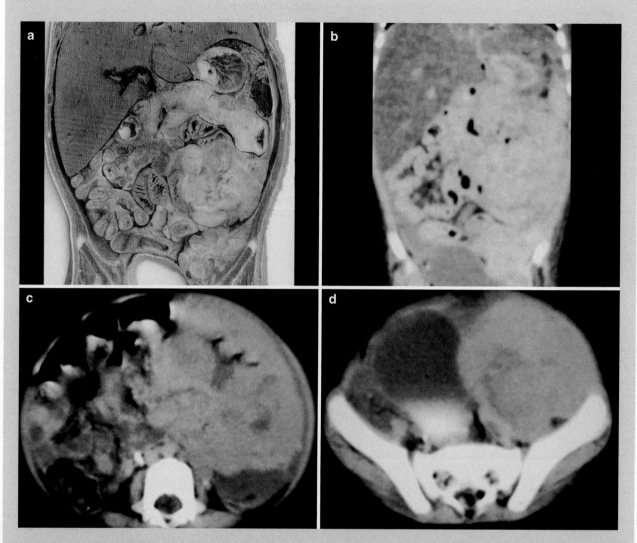

Fig. 19.24 (**a–i**) HIV/AIDS related intestinal B cell lymphoma. (**a**) Gross specimen demonstrates enlarged liver, disproportional ratio of the left to the right liver, diffuse swelling of the liver with unclearly defined borderline; unclearly defined left intestines, obviously thickened intestinal wall and unclearly defined interface between intestinal wall and gastric wall, obviously thickened gastric wall, left colon wall and the ileum wall. (**b–d**) CT scanning demonstrates enlarged liver, diffuse increase of density in the left abdominal cavity and absent of the intestinal interface. (**e, f**) Intestinal barium radiology demonstrates embracing ball sign in the distal ileum, with impression; intestinal wall defects, absent normal mucosa, sea horse liked intestines, thickened mucosal folds, bracing sign of the intestines. (**g–i**) Autopsy demonstrates lymphoma invasion into each layer of intestinal wall, extensive infiltration and tumor cells invasion into parenteral adipose tissue

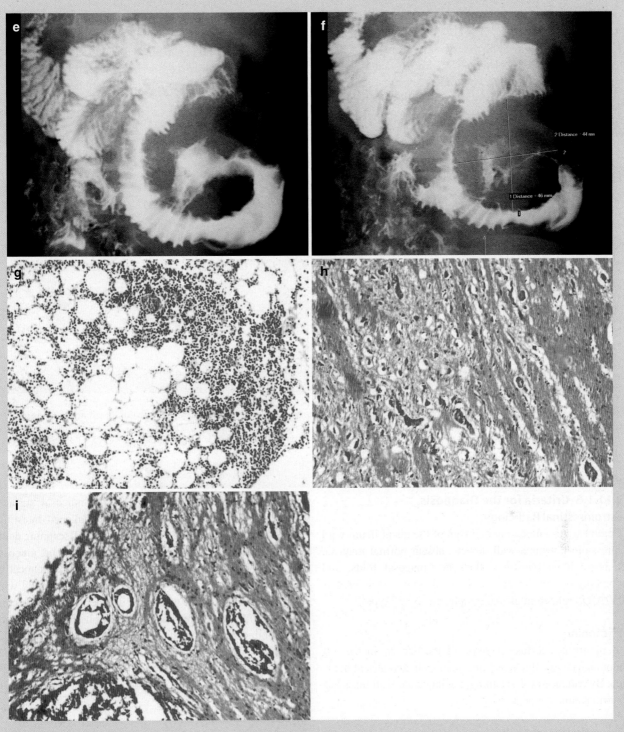

Fig. 19.24 (continued)

Case Study 3 HIV/AIDS Related Body Cavity Based Lymphoma (BCBL)

A female patient aged 53 years was confirmatively diagnosed as having AIDS by the CDC. She sustained abdominal mass and ascites. By ascites examination: light yellow, clear, no clots, Rivalta test (++), WBC 0.65×10^9/L, sg 0.38, L cells 0.57 and mesothelial cells 0.05. Her CD4 T cell count was 25/μl.

A highly malignant body cavity based lymphoma (BCBL) or effusion based lymphoma (primary effusion lymphoma) is found in patients with advanced AIDS. The disease is characteristic both clinically and biologically, and has its own morphologic, immunophenotypic and genetic properties.

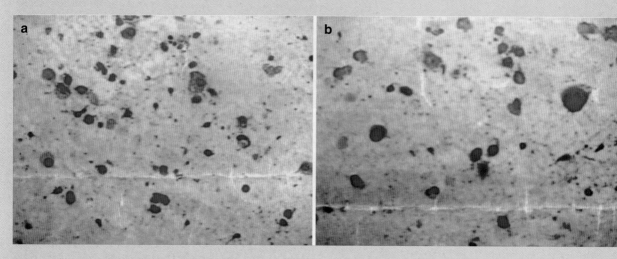

Fig. 19.25 (**a, b**) HIV/AIDS related body cavity based lymphoma. (**a, b**) Shedding cytological examination of ascites demonstrates multiple degenerated nuclear heterogeneous cells

19.11.1.6　Criteria for the Diagnosis
Gastrointestinal Radiology

It demonstrates embracing ball sign of the distal ileum with impression, intestinal wall defects, absent normal mucosa, sea horse liked intestines, thickened mucosal folds, and embracing sign of the intestines. The diagnosis is defined as HIV/AIDS related intestinal lymphoma (B cell type).

CT Scanning

It demonstrates diffuse increase of the density in the left abdominal cavity, thickened intestinal wall, and absent interface. By enhanced CT scanning, the intestinal wall mass has abnormal enhancement.

Histopathological Analysis

It demonstrates lymphoma invasion into each layer of the intestinal wall, with extensive infiltration. Tumor cells invade the parenteral adipose tissue.

19.11.1.7　Differential Diagnosis
Intestinal Adenocarcinoma

Lymphoma with ring shaped thickening of the intestinal wall should be differentiated from intestinal adenocarcinoma. The demonstrations of intestinal adenocarcinoma by CT scanning include irregular thickening of the intestinal wall in circular or eccentric, necrosis and ulceration of the intestinal

wall, sharp and unsmooth edge of the mucosal surface, clearly defined boundary between the thickened intestinal wall and normal intestinal wall. Enhanced CT scanning demonstrates obvious enhancement of and thickened mucosa, which often leads to lumen stenosis. Intestinal adenocarcinoma is prone to direct invade extra-serosa, but rarely with lymphadenectasis in the mesentery and peritonium. The confined HIV/AIDS related intestinal lymphoma has a larger range of thickened intestinal wall. In the cases with multiple, segmental and extensive intestinal wall lesions or intestinal wall lesions acrossing the ileocecal valve and intussusception, lymphoma should be considered.

Interstitial Tumor

Lymphoma with intraluminal mass should be differentiated from interstitial tumor. The interstitial tumor of the small intestines is more common than interstitial tumor of the colon, mostly being malignant. When it is found, the mass is large, with manifestations of eccentric round liked mass in the intestinal wall that can grow inward, outward or concurrent inward and outward the intestinal lumen. By enhanced imaging, it is demonstrated to have obvious enhancement. In some foci, there are obviously thickened and deranged supplying blood vessels, with inner irregular necrotic areas and with no accompanying mesenteric or retroperitoneal lymphadenectasis. Intestinal mass type of HIV/AIDS related intestinal lymphoma has common manifestations of intralumen mass with even density. By enhanced imaging, the mass is demonstrated to have even enhancement. There is a thick blood vessel wrapping inside, being different from obviously thickened and deranged supplying blood vessels in the cases of interstitial tumor. The intralumen mass type of HIV/AIDS related intestinal lymphoma commonly has accompanying mesenteric and retroperitoneal lymphadenectasis with moderate even enhancement by enhanced imaging. In the cases with necrosis, ring shaped enhancement can be demonstrated, with no enhancement of central low density area. Therefore, it is believed that the two diseases have obvious differences for the differential diagnosis.

19.11.1.8   Discussion

Lymphoma is a malignant tumor of lymphoid tissue. Its etiology is related to autoimmune diseases and genetic defects. Some scholars believe that the occurrence of lymphoma can be partially (90 %) attributed to the environment and partially (10%) to the mechanisms and genetic factors. Immunodeficient patients due to HIV infection are the high risk population. LI et al. reported a group of cases with HIV/AIDS related intestinal lymphoma [15], two cases having extensive involvement of the ileum that across the ileocecus to involve the left colon, the mesentery adhesion into pie shape and another one case having lesions in the jejunum. Their CT scanning demonstrations are characterized by irregular ring shaped thickening of the intestinal wall, intestinal lumen stenosis, smooth inner wall, gradual migration of the thickened intestinal wall and the normal intestinal wall. By enhanced scanning, the thickened intestinal wall and the swollen lymph nodes are demonstrated to have moderate even enhancement. The swollen lymph nodes can be demonstrated to have ring shaped enhancement, with no enhancement of a mass supplied by obviously thickened and deranged blood vessels. Cords liked or nodule liked thickening of the mesentery and the omentum majus as well as abdominal effusions are also CT demonstrations of HIV/AIDS related intestinal lymphoma, which are important reference for clinical decision making. Under a microscope, there are diffuse invasion of lymphocytes into each layer of the intestinal wall, obviously decreased amount and volume of lymph node follicles, relatively hyperplasia of small mature lymphocytes in the cap zone, apparent hyperplasia of follicular small blood vessels and histocytes. These are changes of follicular resolution stage in cases of immunodeficiency related lymphadenosis.

19.11.2   HIV/AIDS Related Intestinal Kaposi's Sarcoma (KS)

19.11.2.1   Pathogens and Pathogenesis

Kaposi's sarcoma (KS) is a kind of vascular tumor that originates from the endothelial cells and pericytes. Studies have demonstrated that KS is commonly in the skin and lungs, and no cases of rectal KS has been reported in China. Its etiology remains unknown and is generally believed to be related to the following factors: genetic predisposition, environmental factors, endocrine disorders, viral infection, cellular immune deficiency. KS cells may be originated from blood vessels derived from mesenchymal precursor cells or from abnormally developed endothelial cells. These cells may undergo convertion due to their exposure to an infectious agent. In vitro culture, reverse stimulation of Tat gene and its products, Tat protein, by HIV-1 stimulates the growth of KS cells, which may change the cell receptors and lead to expressions of oncostatin-M and IL-6 receptor. KS cells can produce IL-6. In the process, IL-6 maintains the cell growth as an autocrine factor, and can paracrine cytokines to stimulate other mesenchymal cells for proliferation and to induce the growth of blood vessel.

19.11.2.2   Pathophysiological Basis

Skin lesions of KS originate from the middle layer of the dermis and extend to the epidermis. Histopathologically, the spindle cells and the vascular structures have different degrees of fusion. By special factor VII staining, the cells originate from the endothelial cells, tumor cells and smooth muscular cells. The fibroblasts are similar to myoblasts. Painless KS has manifestations of nodule or plaque liked skin lesions. KS with lymphadenopathy is metastatic and infiltrative, with involvement of lymph nodes and organs. Occasionally, KS with lymphadenopathy can invade the gastrointestinal tract. AIDS complicated by KS has less skin lesions or extensive lesions in the skin, mucosa, lymph nodes and organs.

19.11.2.3   Clinical Symptoms and Signs

It is more common in male homosexual AIDS patients. In early stage, the skin lesions are red or purple red macula or papula, surrounded by a pale halo. The lesions further progress to large nodules or plaques. The skin lesions are multiple, commonly in the body trunk, head and face, oral cavity, gastrointestinal tract and conjunctiva.

19.11.2.4   Examinations and Their Selection
Gastrointestinal Radiology
With demonstrations of the size, location and amount of the lesions.

Gastrointestinal Endoscopy
With demonstrations of the amount and location of the space occupying lesions. The collected specimens can be performed biopsy.

Biopsy and Pathology
There are multiple regular cracks in the tumor, with lining of fine, long and slightly atypical cells. In the cracks, there are erythrocytes and phagocytes engulfing hemosiderin. There are also varying amounts of spindle cells. Some cells have large nuclei, being irregular in shape and heterologous.

Screening
In the high risk populations, HIV related KS should be screened.

19.11.2.5 Imaging Demonstrations
Gastrointestinal Radiology

Barium meal radiography can demonstrate the space occupying lesions in the lumen, which are in round liked or oval filling defects.

Gastrointestinal Endoscopy

With demonstrations of proliferative neoplasms, normal surface mucosa, wide fundus; erosion and defects of the mucosal tissues, tumor tissue is unclearly defined from its surrounding tissues.

Case Study 1

A male patient aged 30 years was confirmatively diagnosed as having AIDS by CDC. His was a homosexual and was hospitalized due to complaints of cough, sputum and fever for 2 months, difficulty breathing and swallowing pain for 20 days. His CD4 T cell count was 105/μl.

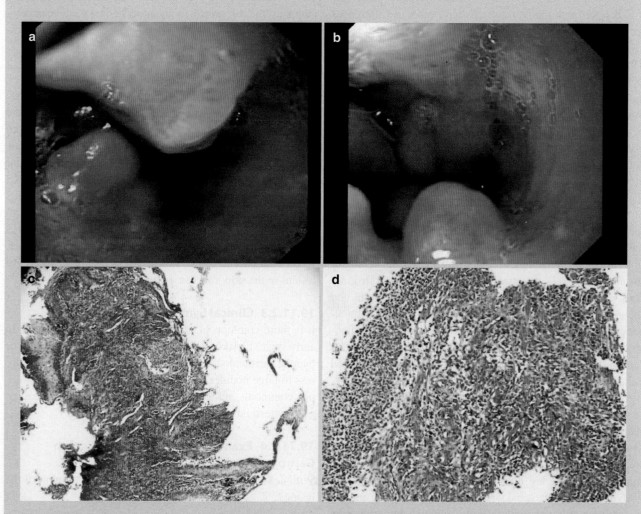

Fig. 19.26 (a–g) HIV/AIDS related intestinal Kaposi's sarcoma. (**a, b**) Gastrointestinal endoscopy demonstrates a proliferative neoplasm, normal mucosal surface and wide fundus. (**c**) Biopsy tissue analysis demonstrates the mocosa tissue of the covered stratified squamous epithelium, and erosion and defect of the epithelial tissue, tumor tissue being unclearly defined with the surrounding tissues. (**d**) It is demonstrated to have inferior interstitial edema of the mucosa, hyperplasia of a large quantity fibrous tissue and infiltration of large quantity inflammatory cells. (**e**) It is demonstrated that tumor tissues being dominated by hyperplasia of a large quantity spindle cells, with visible immature round cells. (**f**) It is demonstrated to have mixed growth of spindle cells and angioma liked lesions in local area of the tumor. (**g**) It is demonstrated to have occasional crack liked structure containing erythrocytes within the spindle cells. The demonstrations are in line with the manifestations of KS

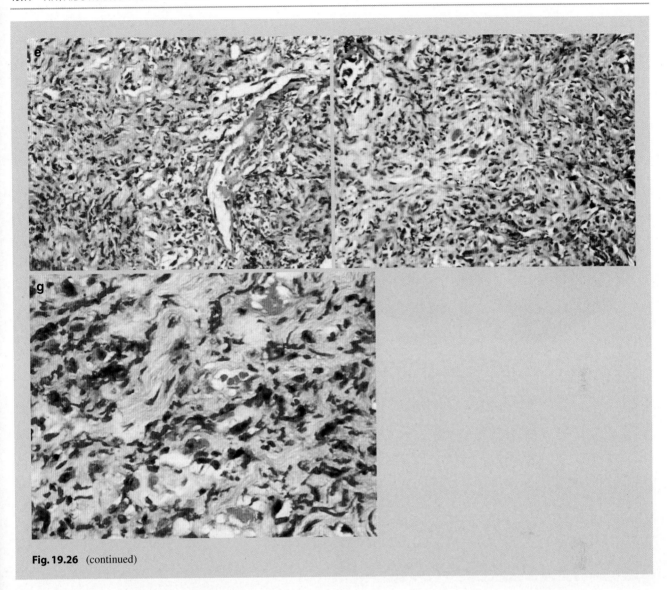

Fig. 19.26   (continued)

Case Study 2

A male patient aged 29 years was confirmatively diagnosed as having AIDS by the CDC. He had a history of homosexuality for 7 years. In recent 1 month, he had recurrent difficulty in bowel movements, with pus and blood in the stool. He also had abdominal distention and paroxysmal abdominal pain. His CD4 T cell count was 48/μl.

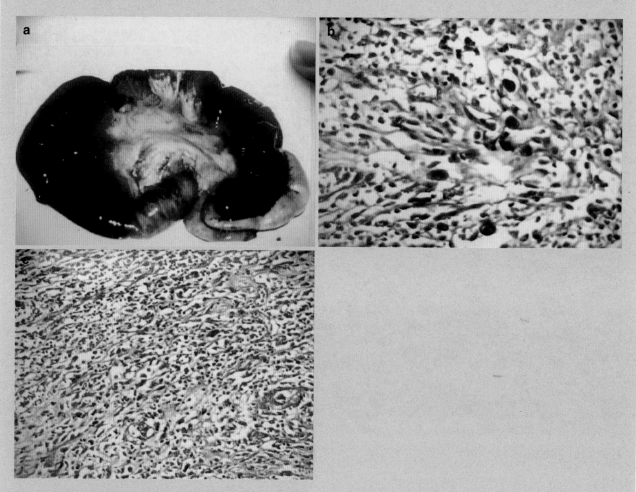

Fig. 19.27 (**a–c**) HIV/AIDS related intestinal Kaposi's sarcoma. (**a**) The gross observation after its surgical removal demonstrates purplish red or purplish black Kaposi's sarcoma in the small intestinal wall. (**b**) HE staining demonstrates the small intestinal KS, with crack liked blood vessels in large quantity of heterologous spindle cells, complicated by CMV infection, intranuclear inclusions in the giant cell (HE ×400). (**c**) HE staining demonstrates the small intestinal Kaposi's sarcoma, with crack liked blood vessels in large quantity of heterologous spindle cells, complicated by CMV infection, an intranuclear inclusion in giant cell at the left bottom (HE ×200) (Figures provided by Lang ZW)

Case Study 3

A male patient aged 27 years was confirmatively diagnosed as having AIDS by CDC. He had a history of homosexuality for 7 years and had been hospitalized and diagnosed as having AIDS and PCP. He denied a past history of hepatitis, tuberculosis and other infectious diseases. And his family history had no speciality. In recent 1 month, the patient had a recurrent bowel movements difficulty, with a sense of incomplete bowel movement, and occasionally with pus and blood. He occasionally had abdominal distention, no paroxysmal abdominal pain, no tenesmus, no alternating diarrhea and constipation. Physical examinations found: body temperature 36.2 °C, pulse 90 beats/min, respiration 20/min, blood pressure 120/80 mmHg (1 mmHg=0.133 kPa), perianal small papillary neoplasms in the marginal anal skin. Digital examination found anal canal narrowed, palpable mass in the bottom of the rectum, and no other abnormalities. Laboratory tests found anti-HIV antibody positive. His CD4 T cell count was 58/μl.

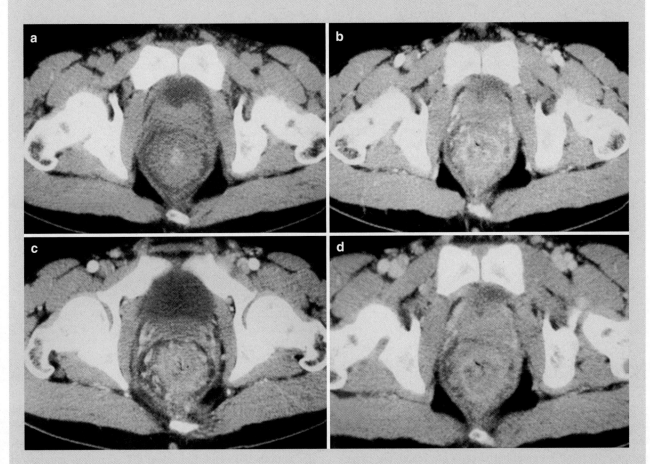

Fig. 19.28 (a–d) Plain CT scanning and enhanced scanning demonstrate obviously thickened rectal wall, with the thickest wall in thickness of about 2.0 cm, even density, CT value of approximately 33–42 HU, significantly thinner and narrowed intestinal lumen, regular and intact intestinal exterior wall, adipose space in surrounding tissues of the left, right and posterior rectal wall; enhanced scanning demonstrates the arterial phase with uneven obvious enhancement of the thickened rectal wall, large quantity small spots and thin strip of enhanced vascular shadow that is slight lower than the major arteries in the same plane, with CT value of about 110–125 HU and clearly defined borderline. In its surrounding tissues, there are mixed irregular soft tissue density shadows, with CT value of about 50–60 HU, whose degree of enhancement is similar to that of pelvic wall soft tissues (55–63 HU); enhanced scanning demonstrates the venous phase to have enhanced vascular shadow, with blurry borderline; anterior migration of the seminal vesicle due to compression, the rectal anterior wall being unclearly defined from the prostate posterior margin. (e–g) HIV/AIDS related rectal Kaposi's sarcoma. (e–g) It is demonstrated that dense staining of nucleolus of a large quantity spindle cells. (h) Immunohistochemistry demonstrates CD117(−), CD34(++), CD31(−) and SMA(−). The demonstrations are in line with manifestations of Kaposi's sarcoma (Provided by Yunnan Hospice of AIDS)

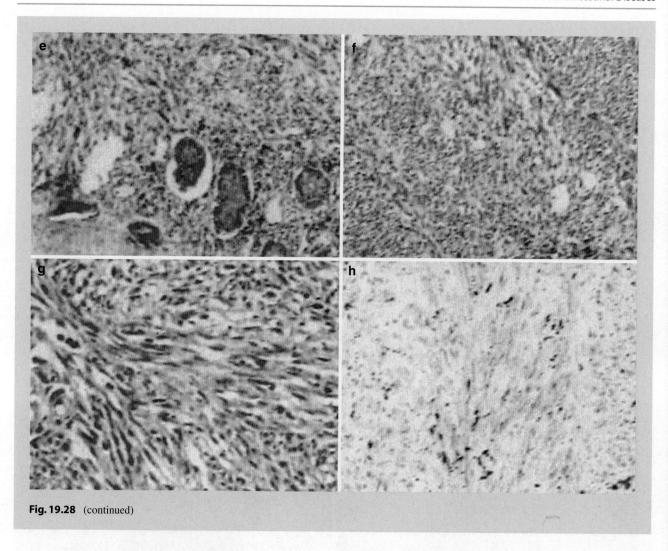

Fig. 19.28 (continued)

19.11.2.6 Criteria for the Diagnosis

KS is a disease composed of hyperplastic blood vessels and spindle cells. Simonart et al. observed the phenotypic properties of KS cells cultured from different lesions [21]. Based on the observation, they believed that the spindle cells are KS tumor cells, and the endothelial cells are reactively hyperplastic. In early stage, KS is composed of hyperplastic vascular structures. With the progression of the lesion, the spindle cell gradually increases, but with no obvious heterotype and with rare mitotic phase. KS can be divided into 3 types, with the classification corresponding to the staging. That is angioma type (early stage), spindle cell type (advanced stage) and mixed type (intermediate or transitional stage). The pathological findings of this case include: CD117(−), CD34(++), CD31(−) and SMA(−). CD117 is currently believed to be one of the major markers for the diagnosis of GIST. CD31 is commonly used as an indicator for the diagnosis of angiosarcoma. SMA contributes to the assistant differentiation of myogenic sarcoma. CD34 expression is positive in the capillary liked region and the crack liked structure; is strongly positive in more maturely differential

blood vessels. Both the spindle cells and vascular endothelial cells in the lesion tissues can express CD34, with different degrees of positive expression. In healthy people, CD34 expression should be negative in lymphatic vessels, but the results show CD34(++), suggesting its origination from vascular endothelial cells. Enhanced CT scanning demonstrations in combination with the pathological classification of KS, the mixed type is indicated. The comparison of CT demonstrations and pathological findings indicate that (1) plain scanning demonstrates the thickened rectal wall and unclearly defined internal structure in the lesions distinguished; (2) enhanced scanning in the arterial phase demonstrates a large quantity enhancement of vascular shadow, which is pathologically hyperplastic capillaries; (3) soft tissue density shadow around the vascular enhancement is pathologically spindle cell. Kaposi's sarcoma rarely occurs in the rectum. The degree of tumor vascular differentiation and percentage of the spindle cells, from the most to the least, is angioma type, mixed type, spindle cell type. Plain CT scanning cannot distinguish the tissue structure of the lesions, but enhanced scanning demonstrations of the foci are characteristic.

19.11.2.7 Differential Diagnosis

Lymphatic Sarcoma

Lymphatic sarcoma commonly occurs in females after their breast cancer surgery, with skin lesions of blue or red nodules. Pathological examination demonstrates lumen with hyperplasic endothelium and surrounding focal infiltration of inflammatory cells, and the erythrocytic overflow from the dermis.

Angiosarcoma

Skin lesions are gray, grayish black or purplish blue infiltrative nodules or fusive plaques, possibly with accompanying bleeding and ulcers. Histopathological examination demonstrates irregular vascular lumen, hyperplasic endothelial cells, accompanied by heterotypic cells. In some cases, there are tumor mass composed of spindle cells and epithelial cells.

19.11.3 HIV/AIDS Related Other Gastrointestinal Tumors

19.11.3.1 HIV/AIDS Related Antrum of Stomach Moderately-Poorly Differentiated Adenocarcinoma (Ulcerative Type)

Case Study

A male patient aged 53 years was confirmatively diagnosed as having AIDS by the CDC. He complained of abdominal distention with unknown causes 1 month ago, especially severe after meals, with accompanying acid reflux and no heartburn. He had a history of blood transfusion twice in 1995 and in Jun. 2010. About 15 years ago, he was diagnosed as having gastric ulcer and was treated with blood transfusion. Six months ago, due to upper gastrointestinal bleeding, he was detected to be HIV positive. The findings by examinations include: (1) endoscopic demonstrations of esophagitis, gastric retention and gastric ulcer (A2); (2) pathological examination demonstrates (antrum) moderately-poorly differentiated adenocarcinoma; (3) laboratory tests demonstrate CEA 6.520 ng/ml, RH blood type positive.

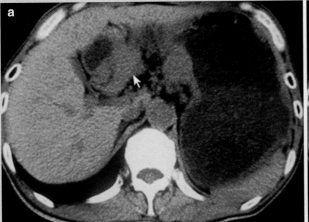 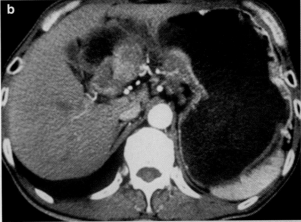

Fig. 19.29 (a–n) HIV/AIDS related moderately-poorly differentiated adenocarcinoma (ulcerative type). (**a**) Plain CT scanning demonstrates round liked soft tissue dense shadow at the lateral gastric lesser curvature, with clearly defined boundary. (**b**) Enhanced CT scanning demonstrates slight enhancement of the round liked soft tissue dense shadow at the lateral gastric lesser curvature. (**c**) Enhanced CT scanning demonstrates thickened wall of the gastric lesser curvature with obvious enhancement. (**d**, **e**) Enhanced delayed CT scanning demonstrates multiple round liked nodular enhancement of the gastric lesser curvature, thickening and obvious enhancement of the local gastric wall. (**f**–**i**) Enhanced delayed CT scanning and coronal reconstruction demonstrate multiple nodular abnormal enhancement of the gastric lesser curvature with unclearly defined boundary, thickening and enhancement of the local gastric wall. (**j**, **k**) Microscopy and routine H&E staining demonstrate heterotypic and hyperplastic tumor tissue in gastric mucosa, with large and deeply stained nuclei, basophilic cytoplasm, cord liked arrangement and luminal liked appearance. (**l**–**n**) Immunohistochemistry demonstrates CK8/18(+), CK20(−), AE1/AE3(+) and Ki67(+, 80 %), CgA(−), Syn(−), S-100(+). The demonstrations are in line with the manifestations of antral moderately-poorly differentiated adenocarcinoma

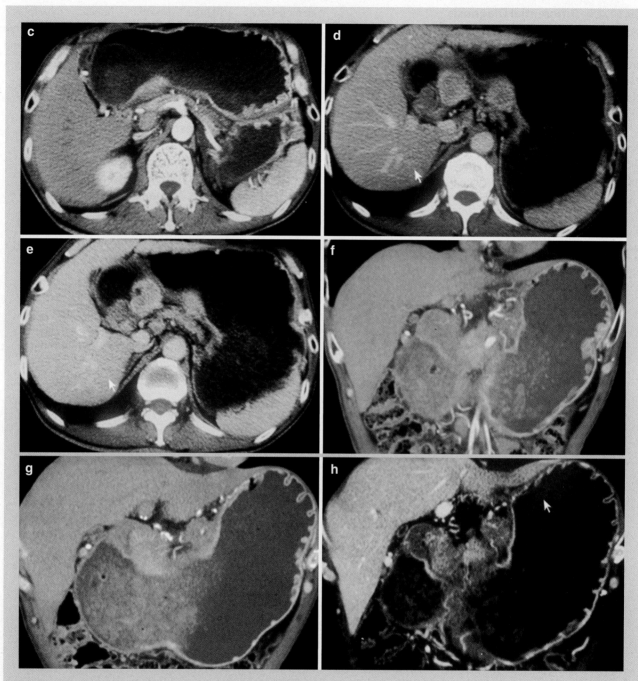

Fig. 19.29 (continued)

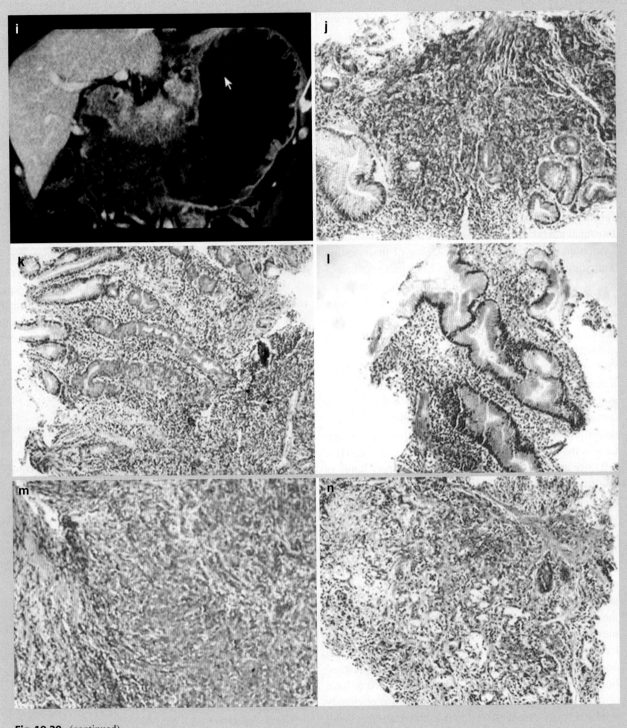

Fig. 19.29 (continued)

Criteria for the Diagnosis

1. Barium meal radiology demonstrates filling defects of the gastric lumen and stiff antral wall.
2. CT scanning demonstrates round liked soft tissue dense shadow at the lateral gastric lesser curvature and thickened gastric wall. Enhanced CT scanning demonstrates slight enhancement of the round liked soft tissue dense shadow at the lateral gastric lesser curvature.
3. Pathological analysis and H&E staining demonstrate heterotypic and hyperplastic tumor tissue in the gastric mucosa. Immunohistochemistry demonstrates CK8/18(+), CK20(−), AE1/AE3(+) and Ki67(+, 80 %).

Differential Diagnosis

1. Intestinal adenocarcinoma
   Lymphoma with ring shaped thickening of the intestinal wall should be differentiated from intestinal adenocarcinoma. The demonstrations of intestinal adenocarcinoma by CT scanning include irregular thickening of the intestinal wall in circular or eccentric, necrosis and ulceration of the intestinal wall, sharp and unsmooth edge of the mucosal surface, clearly defined boundary between the thickened intestinal wall and normal intestinal wall. Enhanced CT scanning demonstrates obvious enhancement of and thickened mucosa, which often leads to lumen stenosis. Intestinal adenocarcinoma is prone to direct invade extra-serosa, but rarely with lymphadenectasis in the mesentery and peritonium. The confined HIV/AIDS related intestinal lymphoma has a larger range of thickened intestinal wall. In the cases with multiple, segmental and extensive intestinal wall lesions or intestinal wall lesions acrossing the ileocecal valve and intussusception, lymphoma should be considered.
2. Interstitial tumor
   Lymphoma with intraluminal mass should be differentiated from interstitial tumor. The interstitial tumor of the small intestines is more common than interstitial tumor of the colon, mostly being malignant. When it is found, the mass is large, with manifestations of eccentric round liked mass in the intestinal wall that can grow inward, outward or concurrent inward and outward the intestinal lumen. By enhanced imaging, it is demonstrated to have obvious enhancement. In some foci, there are obviously thickened and deranged supplying blood vessels, with inner irregular necrotic areas and with no accompanying mesenteric or retroperitoneal lymphadenectasis. Intestinal mass type of HIV/AIDS related intestinal lymphoma has common manifestations of intralumen mass with even density. By enhanced imaging, the mass is demonstrated to have even enhancement. There is a thick blood vessel wrapping inside, being different from obviously thickened and deranged supplying blood vessels in the cases of interstitial tumor. The intralumen mass type of HIV/AIDS related intestinal lymphoma commonly has accompanying mesenteric and retroperitoneal lymphadenectasis with moderate even enhancement by enhanced imaging. In the cases with necrosis, ring shaped enhancement can be demonstrated, with no enhancement of central low density area. Therefore, it is believed that the two diseases have obvious differences for the differential diagnosis.

19.11.3.2 HIV/AIDS Related Anal/Rectal Carcinoma

HIV/AIDS related anal infiltrating cancer is insufficiently studied, which has an increasing incidence in AIDS patients. Studies in San Francisco during 1985–1987 indicated that the incidence of anal/rectal carcinoma in single male young adults is six times as high as that during the period of 1973–1978. The tissue type of anal/rectal cancer is squamous cell carcinoma, mostly with poor differentiation. In some cases, there are transitional cell carcinoma, mucoepidermoid carcinoma and adenocarcinoma, which is related to the differentiation of cloaca components.

Extended Reading

1. Aithal GP, Mansfield JC. Review article: the risk of lymphoma associated with inflammatory bowel disease and immunosuppressive treatment. Aliment Pharmacol Ther. 2001;15:1101–8.
2. AliMohamed F, Lule GN, Nayo J. Prevalence of Helicobacter pylori and endoscopic findings in HIV seropositive patients with upper gastrointestinal tract symptoms at Kenyatta National Hospital, Nairobi. East Afr Med J. 2002;79(5):226–31.
3. Clarke CA, Glaser SL. Changing incidence of non-Hodgkin lymphomas in the United States. Cancer. 2002;94:2015–23.
4. Dieterich DT, Rahmin M. Cytomegalovirus colitis in AIDS: presentation in 44 patients and a review of the literature. J Acquir Immune Defic Syndr Hum Retrovirol. 1991;4:s29–35.
5. Diotallevi P, Montella F, Di-Sora F. Double-contrast esophagography in the diagnosis of esophagitis due to candida: a study on HIV-seropositive patients. Radiol Med. 1992;84:59–63.
6. Dodd GD. Lymphoma of the hollow abdominal viscera. Radiol Clin North Am. 1990;28:771–83.
7. Ha CS, Cho MJ, Allen PK, et al. Primary Non-Hodgkin lymphomas of the small bowel. Radiology. 1999;211:183.
8. Hollandgn GN, Sison RF, Jatulis DE, et al. Survival of patients with the acquired immune deficiency syndrome after development of cytomegalovirus retinopathy. UCLA CMV Retinopathy Study Group. Ophthalmology. 1990;97:204–11.
9. Jaffe ES, Harris NL, Diebold J. Word Heath Organization classification of neoplastic diseases of the hematopoietic and lymphoid tissues. Am J Clin Pathol. 1999;111:8.
10. Jaffy ES, Harris NL, Stein H, et al., World Health Organization Classification of Tumours. Pathology and genetics of tumours of haematopoietic and lymphoid tissues. Lyon: IARC Press; 2001. p. 111–235.
11. Klatt EC, Nichols L, Noguchi T, et al. Evolving trends revealed by autopsies of patients with the acquired immunodeficiency syndrome. Arch Pathol Lab Med. 1994;118(8):884–7.

12. Koh PK, Horsman JM, Radstone CR, Hancock H, Goepel JR, Hancock BW. Localised extranodal non-Hodgkin's lymphoma of the gastrointestinal tract: Sheffield Lymphoma Group experience (1989–1998). Int J Oncol. 2001;18:743–8.

13. Levine MS, Rubesin SE, Ott DJ. Update on esophageal radiology. AJR Am J Roentgenol. 1990;155:933–41.

14. Levine MS, Woldenberg R, Herlinger H. Opportunistic esophagitis in AIDS: radiographic diagnosis. Radiology. 1987;165:815–20.

15. Li H, Cheng JL. AIDS complicated by intestinal canal lymphoma: X-ray radiology, CT scanning and pathological findings. Chin Med J (Engl). 2011;124(9):1427–30.

16. Li YJ, Lu XH. Digestive endoscopy. Beijing: Science publishing house; 1995. p. 149–51.

17. Mendelson RM, Fermoyle S. Primary gastrointestinal lymphomas: a radiological-pathological review. Part1: stomach, oesophagus and colon. Australas Radiol. 2005;49:353.

18. Ney KA, Cartwright RA. Increasing incidence and descriptive epidemiology of extranodal non-Hodgkin lymphoma in parts of England and Wales. Hematol J. 2002;3:95–104.

19. Scutellair PN, Borgati L, Spanedda R. Non-Hodgkin's lymphomas of extranodal localization. Strategies for imaging diagnosis. Radiol Med (Torino). 2000;100:262.

20. Shang KZ, Chen JR. Principle and diagnosis of gastrointestinal radiography. Shanghai: Shanghai Scientific and Technological Literature Publishing House; 1995. p. 147–8.

21. Simonart T, Debussher C, Liesnard C, et al. Cultured Kaposi's sarcoma tumor cells exhibit a chemokine receptor repertoire that does not allow infection by HIV-1. BMC Dermatol. 2001;1:2.

22. Smedby KE, Akerman M, Hilderbrand H, Glimelius B, Ekbom A, Askling J. Malignant lymphomas in celiac disease: evidence of increased risks for lymphoma types other than enteropathy-type T cell lymphoma. Gut. 2005;54:54–9.

23. Vazquez JA. Therapeutic options for the management of oropharyngeal and esophageal candidiasis in HIV/AIDS patients. HIV Clin Trials. 2000;1:47–59.

24. Wang CY, Snow JL, Daniel Su WP. Lymphoma associated with human immunodeficiency virus infection. Mayo Clin Proc. 1995;70:665–72.

25. Weber AL, Rahemtullah A, Ferry JA. Hodgkin and Non-Hodgkin lymphomas of the head and neck: clinical, pathologic, and imaging evaluation. Neuroimaging Clin N Am. 2003;13:371.

26. Zalar AE, Olmos MA, Piskorz EL, Magnanini FL. Esophageal motility disorders in HIV patients. Dig Dis Sci. 2003;48:962–7.

Contents

20.1 General Introduction to HIV/AIDS Related Hepatobiliary, Pancreatic and Splenic Diseases

The liver, gallbladder, pancreas and spleen are the commonly involved organs in AIDS patients and it has been reported that 60–84 % AIDS patients have hepatomegaly and hepatic dysfunction, with accompanying jaundice and 60 % AIDS patients have increased aminotransferase and serum alkaline phosphatase.

20.1.1 Hepatic Diseases

The opportunistic infections of the liver are due to cellular immunodeficiency, and some opportunistic infections can suppress the immune functions.

(1) CMV infection. It is common and often disseminated. In the hepatic parenchyma, there are diffuse microabscesses but no diffuse fused necrotic foci. (2) Mycobacteria infection. The incidence of mycobacteria infection is about 46–57 % in AIDS patients, mostly of M. avum complex (MAC) infection. Abdominal CT scanning or US examination demonstrates focal lesions in the liver parenchyma, with characteristic changes of granulomatosis formation with histocyte proliferation and sometimes abscesses formation. (3) Parasitic infection. Toxoplasma infection can result in degeneration and necrosis of hepatic cells,

H. Li (ed.), *Radiology of HIV/AIDS*,
DOI 10.1007/978-94-007-7823-8_20, © Springer Science+Business Media Dordrecht and People's Medical Publishing House 2014

lymphocytes infiltration and formation of granuloma. Leishmania infection can also spread to the liver. AIDS complicated by Leishmania infection has a high morbidity. (4) Fungal infection. It usually leads to hepatomegaly and hepatic granuloma. Candida infection with accompanying microabscess in the liver is occasionally reported. (5) Carinii infection. Pneumocystis carinii pneumonia is an important diagnostic indicator of AIDS. Moreover, Carinii can involve extra-pulmonary tissues such as esophagus, gastrointestine, liver and spleen, and kidney, about 35 % with hepatic lesions. The diagnostic imaging demonstrates diffuse nodules in the liver, spleen and kidney, often accompanied by dystrophic calcification. (6) Bacterial infection. It is relatively rare. (7) Hepatic tumor. The most common hepatic tumor is KS, followed by non-Hodgkin's lymphoma (NHL). About 30 % male homosexual AIDS patients have initial clinical manifestations of KS. CT scanning or liver scintigraphy demonstrates KS as multiple intrahepatic nodules which are non-specific changes. Moon et al. reported 19 % KS is demonstrated as hepatomegaly and only 3 % with focal lesions by abdominal CT scanning [12]. The incidence of HIV/AIDS related NHL is 6–8 %, with clinical manifestation of hepatomegaly. Abdominal imaging demonstrates intrahepatic focal lesions. (8) HIV/AIDS related hepatic hemangioma. AIDS complicated by hemangioma is not necessarily related to HIV infection but may be accompanying lesions. Trojan et al. reported its incidence of about 3 % [17].

20.1.2 Gallbladder and Biliary Diseases

Gallbladder and biliary diseases can also occur in AIDS patients, usually manifested as acalculous cholecystitis and AIDS cholangiopathy. CT scanning and MR imaging demonstrate thickened and coarse gallbladder wall. Recent studies have demonstrated that parasitization of Cryptosporidium on biliary epithelium can cause cholangitis and cholecystitis, with an incidence of 10 % in AIDS patients. Its principal clinical symptoms include nausea, vomiting, and abdominal confined pain of the right upper quadrant. X-ray demonstrates sclerotic cholangitis signs such as thickened gallbladder wall, proximal cholangiectasis, distal biliary stenosis and irregular biliary lumen.

20.1.3 Splenic Diseases

AIDS can involve spleen throughout its progression. In the acute period of HIV infection, some patients have splenomegaly. In the AIDS associated syndrome period, spleen changes along with lymph nodes from primary proliferation to lymphopenia. In the typical AIDS period, malignant lymphoma can also involve the spleen.

20.1.4 Pancreatic Diseases

AIDS patients have 35–800 times risk for developing acute pancreatitis than the general population. In other words, about 5–14 % HIV-infected patients experience acute pancreatitis and pancreas swelling, which can be caused by drugs, immunodeficiency, opportunistic infections and alcohol abuse. Infiltration of pancreatic lymphoma and KS can lead to pancreatic duct obstruction, which would trigger pancreatitis. By autopsy, pancreatic lymphoma and KS have an incidence of about 8 % in AIDS patients but usually without clinical symptoms. After the occurrence of AIDS complicated by pancreatitis, the further complications of pancreatic pseudocyst, acute respiratory distress syndrome and multiple organs failure may also occur.

20.1.4.1 Imaging Demonstrations Review

CT scanning, MR imaging or US examination should be the diagnostic imaging of choice for the diagnosis of hepatic lesions or cholangiectasis. However, the diagnostic imaging demonstrates no abnormalities in AIDS patients with biliary disease, with failed detection of choledocholith. Endoscopic retrograde cholangiography can facilitate diagnose of highly suspected biliary disease. Patients with hepatic focal lesions, biopsy guided by CT scanning or US examination can provide valuable diagnostic information. Focal lesions are not necessarily malignancies. In AIDS patients, opportunistic infections are sometimes suspected as metastatic tumors while histological examinations demonstrate as curable diseases such as tuberculosis or Carinii infection.

20.2 HIV/AIDS Related Liver Tumor

20.2.1 HIV/AIDS Related Lymphoma

Non-Hodgkin lymphoma (NHL), HIV/AIDS related lymphoma, is following KS to be the second commonly malignancy in AIDS patients. HIV infected people are at a significantly higher risk of developing lymphoma, especially senior B-cell lymphomas occurring at a CD4 T cell count of less than 100/mm^3. The proportion of extranodal lymphoma is higher than HIV negative patients.

Meanwhile, the incidence of HIV/AIDS related hepatic NHL is 6–8 %.

20.2.1.1 Pathogens and Pathogenesis

The classical model of ARL occurrence is as the following. B lymphocytes, under the violent stimulations by HIV, Epstein Barr Virus (EBV) and other infectious agents, induce continuous release of growth factors and cytokines to increase the risk of genetic mutations in the proliferative cells groups which accelerates B cell malignancy. The commonly found mutated genes include proto-oncogene c-myc (found in Burkitt lymphoma), bcl-6 (found in diffuse large B-cell lymphoma) and some anti-oncogenes. Studies have demonstrated a constant relationship between the occurrence of EBV infection and some diffuse large B-cell lymphoma (DLBCL).

20.2.1.2 Pathophysiological Basis

ARL can be categorized into three types by naked eyes observation. (1) Singular nodule/mass. An isolated large nodule/mass in the liver, commonly with a diameter of above 3 mm. (2) Multiple nodules. Multiple small nodular foci in the liver, commonly in a diameter of less than 3 mm. (3) Diffuse infiltration or hepatomegaly. With unclearly defined foci and with no distinct nodules or masses.

Histologically, DLBCL and Burkitt lymphoma are the most common ARL, accounting for about 90 %. According to cellular origins, DLBCL can be divided into two subtypes: centroblast type (originated from B cell of germinal center) and immunoblast type (originated from B cell after germinal center)

20.2.1.3 Clinical Symptoms and Signs

The clinical manifestations include abdominal pain, abdominal distension, emaciation, fatigue, superficial lymphadenectasis as well as hepatomegaly and splenomegaly.

20.2.1.4 Examinations and Their Selection
US Examination, CT Scanning and MR Imaging

They have high detection rate of nodular and mass lymphoma but low detection rate of diffuse and infiltrative lesions.

PET

It can be applied to detect lymphoma or to screen residual foci of lymphoma.

Liver Biopsy

It is the primary basis for the definitive diagnosis.

20.2.1.5 Imaging Demonstrations
Ultrasound Examination

Singular nodule type or mass type is demonstrated as low echo, few even no echo. Sometimes, US demonstrates a target sign, namely central high echo of the focus and marginal low echo, with low echo infiltration shadow of the unclear tumor border. Multiple nodule type usually involves several organs, demonstrated as multi-focal low echo nodules. Diffuse infiltration type shows liquid or gel liked lesions between abdominal organs and mesentery. Although the lymphoma infiltration is parenchymal, there is almost no echo by US.

CT Scanning

For the singular nodule/mass type, plain CT scanning demonstrates singular or multiple masses or nodules with low density in the liver, mostly with clear boundary. The singular lesion may be lobular but the multiple lesions are round or oval. The large nodule commonly has central necrosis in much lower density, occasionally with calcification. Enhanced scanning demonstrates no enhancement or only light enhancement in the artery phase, whereas clearly defined focus in the vein phase, with no enhancement or merely slight even enhancement of the tumor. The focus has a lower density than liver parenchyma.

For the diffuse infiltration type, plain CT scanning demonstrates general decrease of liver density, with extended liver contour in disproportion. Enhanced scanning demonstrates no masses or nodules. Apicella et al. [1] believed that no matter which type the lesions are, the peripheral blood vessels have demonstrations of stenosis due to compression, migration due to push and pull, deformation, but mostly no invasive obstruction, interruption and destruction. Enhanced scanning demonstrates continuous blood vessels shadow in the peritumor tissues or in the tumor, which is the characteristic demonstration of the disease.

MR Imaging

For the nodule/mass type, T1WI demonstrates low signal foci in the liver parenchyma, with clear boundary, in round or lobular shape. T2WI demonstrates slightly higher to high signal, with clear boundary, with central much higher or no signal. For the diffuse infiltration type, T1WI demonstrates decreased liver signal in the liver while T2WI increased liver signal, including demonstrations of enlarged liver and disproportional liver, but with no findings of nodule/mass foci. Enhanced imaging demonstrates the same as CT scanning, with no obvious enhancement or slight marginal enhancements of the foci in arterial/venous phases. There are continuous blood vessels surrounding or in the tumors.

Case Study 1

A female patient aged 37 years was confirmatively diagnosed as having AIDS by CDC. She complained of fever for more than 1 month and fatigue for 1 week. She had a history of intravenous drug abuse, with physical examinations findings of LDH 1,787 U/L, AFP <50 U/L and enlarged liver. Her CD4 T cell count was 85/μl.

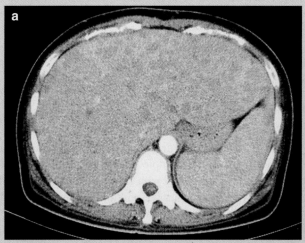
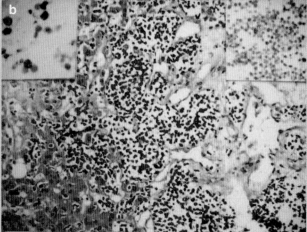

Fig. 20.1 (**a**, **b**) HIV/AIDS related hepatic lymphoma. (**a**) CT scanning demonstrates enlarged liver with regular border. Plain scanning demonstrates uneven density in the liver parenchyma. Enhanced scanning demonstrates diffuse nodular low density shadows of various sizes at the arterial phase in the liver parenchyma, with clear borders. In addition, there are fusion of some foci with marginal uneven ring shaped enhancement, low density foci at the portal and delayed phases. (**b**) HE staining demonstrates hepatic T cell lymphoma, with diffuse distribution of the tumor cells in the hepatic sinus. Immunohistochemistry findings of tumor cell CD3 positive demonstrated in the left upper corner and tumor cell CD45RO positive demonstrated in the right upper corner, HE ×100 (Figs provided by LANG, ZHW)

Case Study 2

A male patient aged 27 years was confirmatively diagnosed as having AIDS by CDC. He found a cervical mass that was progressively enlarging for 5 months, with no symptoms of fever and pain. He had a past history of intravenous drug abuse. On admission, he was found HIV antibody (+), CD4 T cell count 420/μl. By physical examination, multiple lymphadenectasis in the left side of neck, hard, poor mobility, with multiple foci fusion into a mass in size of 4×5 cm.

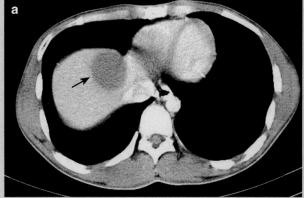
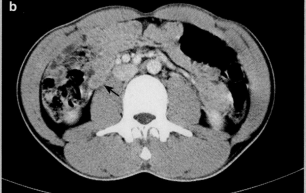

Fig. 20.2 (**a–f**) HIV/AIDS related hepatic lymphoma. (**a**) CT scanning demonstrates round liked low density shadow in the right hepatic lobe, in size of 4.0×3.5×2.4 cm, with homogeneous density and a CT value of about 47 HU (*arrow*). Enhanced scanning demonstrates slight enhancement of the foci at the arterial and portal vein phases, with clear boundary and a CT value of about 55 HU. (**b**) CT scanning demonstrates retroperitoneal multiple lymphadenectasis (*arrow*). (**c**, **d**) Cervical lymph nodes puncture for biopsy demonstrates pathologically and immunohistochemical confirmed diffuse giant B cell lymphoma. (**e**, **f**) Immunohistochemistry demonstrates CD20 (+) and CD79a (+)

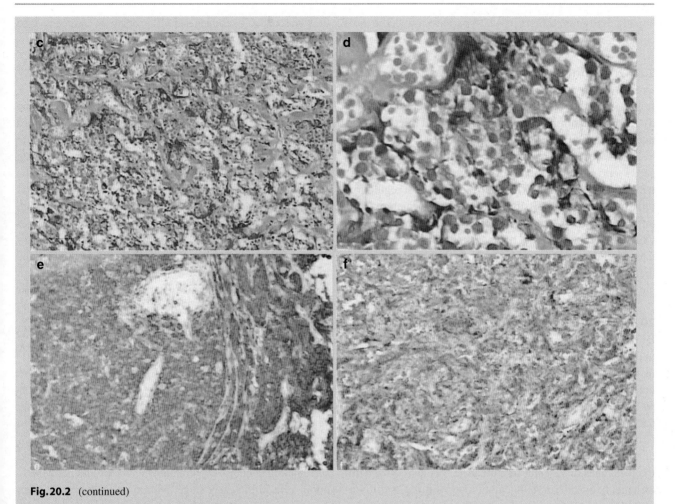

Fig. 20.2 (continued)

20.2.1.6 Evidence for the Diagnosis

Imaging demonstrations of hepatic lymphoma are non-specific, whose accurate diagnosis should be made in combination with clinical data. The diffuse infiltration type can be misdiagnosed by CT scanning or MR imaging, which should be paid enough attention. Nodular hepatic lymphoma is demonstrated as multiple low density foci in the liver, with a tendency to fuse and no/slight enhancement by enhanced imaging.

20.2.1.7 Differential Diagnosis
Diffuse Hepatic Cancer

Diffuse infiltration hepatic lymphoma should be differentiated from diffuse hepatic cancer. The former merely results in thinner vein due to compression but with no involvements of the vascular wall and cavity, while the latter is prone to cause portal vein embolus and coarse venous wall in the liver. In addition, diffuse hepatic cancer has the foci of relatively even density while diffuse infiltration hepatic lymphoma has the foci of uneven density.

Hepatic Metastatic Tumor and Nodular Hepatocellular Carcinoma

The imaging demonstrations of nodular hepatic lymphoma are quite similar to those of hepatic metastases and nodular hepatocellular carcinoma. For primary hepatic lymphoma, extrahepatic organs and tissues generally present no changes. Delayed scanning of hepatic lymphoma in the arterial and port vein phases shows no obvious enhancement, with relatively even density and rare necrosis in the foci, which is different from the enhancement features of hepatic cancer and metastases. Occasionally, biopsy should be performed to differentiate hepatic lymphoma from hepatic metastases and nodular hepatocellular carcinoma.

20.2.2   HIV/AIDS Related Kaposi Sarcoma (KS)

Kaposi sarcoma is an indicative disease of AIDS, being commonly multiple and terminally involving the liver with an incidence of 14–18 %. KS is the most common hepatic malignant tumors in AIDS patients and is the most common reason of death in AIDS patients.

20.2.2.1 Pathogens and Pathogenesis

Until now, the pathogen of KS has not been fully unveiled. It is presumed to be associated with viral infections, heredity factors and hormones, among which viral infection, particularly KS associated virus (KSHV) infection is assumed to be a necessary factor for the occurrence of KS. KSHV genes encodes are similar to many cytokine analogues which make cellular growth independent of host regulation, thus increasing the possibility of tumors formation. HIV infection is an essential cofactor for the occurrence of KS, which impairs the defense mechanism of the hosts to facilitate KSHV replication. Moreover, some experts believe that EBV, CMV and HIV are all helper viruses that contribute to the occurrence of KSHV infection.

20.2.2.2 Pathophysiological Basis

By naked eyes observation, there are dark red tumor nodules in diameter of 5–10 mm on the liver envelope, radial growth of KS in the portal area and its infiltration along the biliary branches on the cross sections. Multiple dark red spots can be found in the liver parenchyma. Histologically, the typical pathological changes include infiltration of the tumor into portal area, enlarged portal area, focal concentration of large quantity hyperplasia of the vascular vessels in angioma liked changes or vascular fracture. The foci also show hemorrhage, hemosiderin sedimentation and infiltration of lymphocytes and plasmacytes. Meanwhile acidophilic inclusion bodies can be found in the tumor cytoplasm.

20.2.2.3 Clinical Symptoms and Signs

Its clinical manifestations are non-specific, generally with liver involvement as a part of skin and organs diffuse lesions. The clinical manifestations are fever, emaciation, anemia and increased serum alkaline phosphatase.

20.2.2.4 Examinations and Their Selection

1. Laboratory tests demonstrate slightly increased serum alkaline phosphatase.

2. Ultrasound, CT scanning and MR imaging are commonly used diagnostic imaging, with non-specific demonstrations of KS.

20.2.2.5 Imaging Demonstrations
Ultrasound

Disseminated KS can involve almost all parts of human body. However, abdominal ultrasound rarely detects lesions in the liver, spleen and pancreas, because its involvement in the advanced stage of KS and KS grows in infiltration along portal vessels rather than mass growth. By ultrasound, the only finding is low echo changes at the marginal hepatic artery, portal vein and bile duct, namely the portal triad, while abnormal high echo of intrahepatic multiple nodules (5–12 mm) is rarely found. In the cases of skin or gastrointestinal KS, the following ultrasound signs can indicate the intrahepatic KS. (1) hepatic pedicle infiltration; (2) high echo foci in the liver parenchyma; (3) intrahepatic bile duct dilation but no extrahepatic bile duct dilation. The high echo area in the liver may be consistent with the spreading of KS.

CT Scanning

The demonstrations are multiple low density small nodules foci, with a distribution tendency of adjacent to hepatic portal, liver envelope and surrounding the perihepatic portal vein. There is also irregular enlargement of the portal vein branches shadows in the liver parenchyma. Enhanced scanning demonstrates multiple low density small nodules foci surrounding the hepatic portal, liver envelope and perihepatic portal vein in the early stage, with more amount than plain scanning. Delayed scanning for 4–7 min demonstrates enhancement of most nodular shadows, with equal or slightly higher density. Sometimes, the small nodules shadows are in ring shaped enhancement. In some cases, there are accompanying splenomegaly, lymphadenectasis of retroperitoneum, mesentery and peripancreas and high density of the involved lymph nodes.

MR Imaging

The demonstrations include high signal by PDWI, and high signal tumor focus with perivascular infiltration in a shape of grape cluster.

Case Study 1

A male patient aged 33 years was confirmatively diagnosed as having AIDS by CDC. He was found HIV antibody (+) 5 months ago, with present symptoms of cough, expectoration, nausea and diarrhea for 10 days. By physical examination, he was found to have emaciation, palpable enlarged hard lymph nodes without tenderness behind ears and at the bilateral groins, in size of about 10 × 20 mm. His CD4 T cell count was 87/μl.

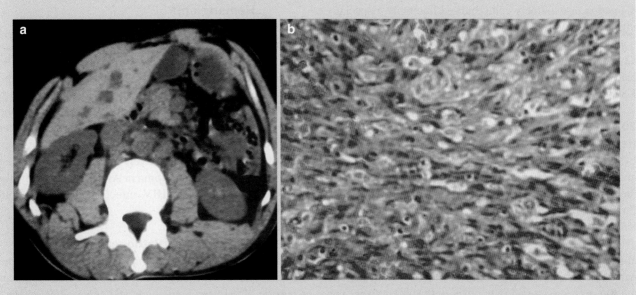

Fig. 20.3 (**a, b**) HIV/AIDS related KS carcinoma. (**a**) CT scanning demonstrates multiple low density nodular foci in the liver, multiple low density foci of various sizes in the abdominal cavity, with clear boundaries. (**b**) Biopsy demonstrates groin lymph nodes with abundant blood vessels like fissures and obvious proliferation of spindle cells

Case Study 2

A male patient aged 43 years was confirmatively diagnosed as having AIDS by CDC. His CD4 T cell count was 77/μl.

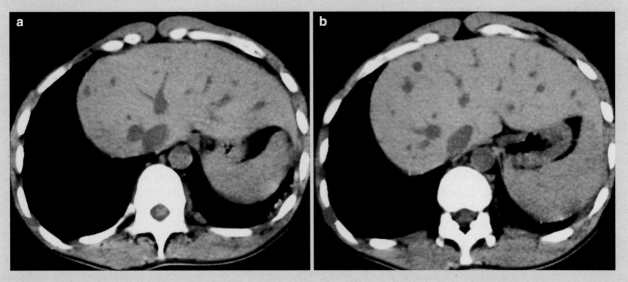

Fig. 20.4 (**a, b**) HIV/AIDS related Kaposi carcinoma. CT scanning demonstrates enlarged liver and spleen, multiple round low density foci of various sizes in the liver, with clear boundaries

20.2.2.6 Diagnostic Basis

Hepatic KS has no characteristic demonstrations by diagnostic imaging. The findings of hepatomegaly and multiple low density nodules in the liver with a distribution tendency around the portal area, liver envelope and peripheral portal veins, the clinical data indicates patients of HIV, organ transplantation or extremely compromised immunity. Especially in the cases with accompanying typical skin lesions (skin nodules and infiltrative spots in a bilaterally symmetric development in purplish brown or reddish blue with accompanying edema) and multiple organs lesions, the diagnosis of KS should be considered.

20.2.2.7 Differential Diagnosis

Hepatic Metastases

Both hepatic KS and hepatic metastases exhibit multiple nodular lesions. However, the lesions of KS are close to the portal area, liver envelope and perihepatic portal veins. Enhanced and delayed scanning demonstrate the lesions of KS as higher or equal enhancement comparing to the liver parenchyma, with rarely peripheral enhancement. The clinical data indicates compromised immunity and accompanying characteristic skin lesions. The lesions of hepatic metastases are scattered in the liver with similar sizes. The enhanced scanning demonstrates the foci mostly in marginal enhancement which is generally lower than normal liver parenchyma. In addition, the cases of hepatic metastases should have a past history of primary tumors.

Hepatic Lymphoma

Nodular hepatic lymphoma is demonstrated to have multiple low density foci in the liver with a fusion tendency. Enhanced scanning demonstrates no enhancement or slight enhancement. It is relatively difficult to be differentiated from KS. In combination with clinical manifestations and case history, the differential diagnosis can be made. The final definitive diagnosis depends on the biopsy.

Hepatic Schistosomiasis

Hepatic schistosomiasis shows subcapsular fibrosis and peripheral fibrosis of the portal vein. By the diagnostic imaging, it is similar to the distribution of KS nodules adjacent to the liver envelope and portal vein. However, hepatic schistosomiasis has characteristic envelope and septal calcification, resulting in map liked changes of the liver parenchyma. Meanwhile, the liver envelope and the septum are enhanced but no enhancement of the fibrosis foci by enhanced and delayed scanning, which are different from the findings of hepatic KS. In addition, the cases of KS commonly have impaired immunity, with accompanying characteristic skin lesions, while hepatic schistosomiasis usually has manifestations of hepatocirrhosis.

20.2.3 HIV/AIDS Related Hepatic Hemangioma

Hepatic hemangioma is the most common hepatic benign tumors, with an incidence of 0.4–7.3 % by autopsy. The diseases can be found in all age groups, but mostly in the middle aged females, with an incidence six times as high as that of males. About 90 % tumors are singular and the other 10 %, multiple. It occurs mostly below the liver envelope near the diaphragmatic surface, with involvement of both right and left liver lobes, but more in the right lobe. Hepatic hemangioma in AIDS patients may not necessarily be related to HIV infection but may be an accompanying lesion.

20.2.3.1 Pathogens and Pathogenesis

The cause of hepatic hemangioma remains unclear. Some scholars believe that it is caused by abnormal development of hepatic blood vessel structures and some other scholars believe that it is related to estrogen level.

20.2.3.2 Pathophysiological Basis

Histologically, hepatic hemangioma can be divided into cavernous hemangioma, sclerotic hemangioma, hemangioendothelioma and capillary hemangioma. Cavernous hemangioma is the most commonly seen in clinical practice.

Cavernous Hemangioma

By naked eyes observation, cavernous hemangioma is in blue or purplish red nodules with clear boundaries, mostly without capsules. Its cross section is honeycomb liked, with fibrosis, calcification and thrombus. Microscopy demonstrates tumors with components of vascular lumens and connective tissues of various sizes. The inner surfaces of the vascular lumens are covered by a single layer of flat endothelial cells.

Sclerotic Hemangioma

The tumor body is completely or mostly occupied by fibrous scar tissues or organized thrombus, usually with accompanying calcification. Lesions usually are small, with a diameter of less than 4 cm.

Hemangioendothelioma

The proliferation of vascular endothelial cells is active, which can readily cause malignant degeneration.

Capillary Hemangioma

It presents vascular stenosis and increased fibrous septal tissues.

20.2.3.3 Clinical Symptoms and Signs

Patients with hepatic hemangiomas in diameter less than 4 cm are usually asymptomatic, usually discovered occasionally in physical examination. About 40 % patients with hepatic hemangiomas in diameter more than 4 cm have abdominal irritation, hepatomegaly, poor appetite and indigestion. Huge hemangiomas can lead to significant enlargement of the liver and their rarely seen syndrome includes consumptive coagulation defect, thrombocytopenia and hypo-fibremia.

20.2.3.4 Examinations and Their Selection

CT Examination

It is an effective diagnostic imaging for the diagnosis and differential diagnosis of hepatic hemangioma.

MRI Examination

It can be applied for the diagnosis and differential diagnosis of hepatic hemangioma, with higher sensitivity and specificity than CT scanning. It can define the diagnosis without enhanced imaging.

Ultrasound

It is commonly used for screening and following up. For some cases of cavernous hemangioma, it can be performed for the qualitative diagnosis.

20.2.3.5 Imaging Demonstrations

Ultrasound

The tumors are round or round liked masses, with clear boundaries. On its margin, there are fracture sign, vascular accessing or penetrating sign. Tumors are commonly demonstrated as strong echo and rarely weak echo or uneven mixed echoes. For the cases of huge tumors, the pressing to the tumor by the probe during scanning may show deformation of the tumor.

CT Scanning

Plain scanning demonstrates mostly round or round liked low density foci with some few foci in lobular appearance with even inner density. In the comparatively larger tumors, there are commonly complications of high density calcification or low density degeneration and necrosis. In the cases with complicated hepatic adipose infiltration, the foci show slight high or high density. Tumors are clearly defined from their surrounding normal hepatic tissues, without peritumor edema. Dynamic enhanced scanning demonstrates the following four types of enhancement of the hemangioma. (1) Even enhancement of the tumor at the arterial phase, with an enhancement degree close to the aortic artery density, and a higher enhancement of the tumor than the liver parenchyma density at both the portal and delayed phases. This type of enhancement is usually found in the cases of hemangioma with a diameter less than 1.5 cm. (2) C or flower ring shaped, or nodular enhancement at the peripheral area of the tumor at the arterial phase, or a marginal spot liked enhancement (with varying shapes due to different perspectives sections) that is similar to the aortic artery density. Subsequently, along with the contrast agent spreading gradually toward the center, the tumor is completely filled at the delayed phase to demonstrate high or equal density, with findings of central necrosis and no enhancement of the scar tissues. Such findings are found in the cases of hemangioma with a diameter of above 3 cm. These are typical enhancement demonstrations of hemangioma and are the most common demonstrations. (3) No enhancement at the arterial phase and peritumor nodular enhancement at portal or delayed phase. The tumor is slowly filled by the contrast agent, with long term duration up to 10 min. (4) No enhancement of the tumor by dynamic scanning at the arterial phase. This type of demonstration is extremely rare and commonly found in the cases of sclerotic hemangioma.

MR Imaging

Low or equal signal of the tumor is demonstrated by T1WI; bright high signal by T2WI, which is highly similar to the demonstrations of hepatic cysts. However, hemangioma presents a higher T2 signal, in characteristic bulb sign. With the prolonging of TE, the signal of the tumor gradually increases in intensity, in contrast with the low signal of the liver parenchyma. Under the condition of TE 120–180 ms, hemangioma demonstrates similar signal to the cerebrospinal fluid. Hemangiomas with a diameter less than 3 cm have a homogenous signal while hemangiomas with a diameter above 3 cm show a heterogeneous signal in the tumor body. The central necrosis shows a higher signal than the peritumor tissues by T2WI. Fibrous scars always present low signal by both T1WI and T2WI.

The specificity of MR imaging to hemangiomas is up to 92–95 %. MR imaging can define the diagnosis without enhanced imaging. However, for some cases of atypical hemangioma or suspected with complications of other malignancies, dynamic enhanced imaging with Gd-DTPA can provide further information for differential diagnosis, with consistent enhancements with enhanced CT scanning. Degenerations, necrosis and thrombus in the tumors present no enhancement in low signal.

By enhanced imaging with SPIO, due to the contents of Kupffer cells in the hemangiomas, the foci are demonstrated low signal by T2WI, being still high comparing to that of the normal hepatic parenchyma.

Case Study 1

A female patient aged 43 years was confirmatively diagnosed as having AIDS by CDC. Her CD4 T cell count was 80/µl.

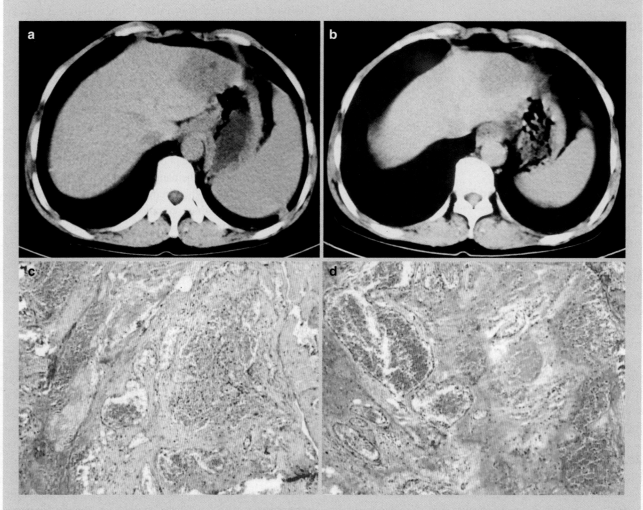

Fig. 20.5 (a–d) HIV/AIDS related hepatic hemangioma. (a, b) CT scanning demonstrates round low density foci in the lateral segment of the hepatic lobe, with clear boundaries. Enhanced scanning demonstrates even enhancement of the foci at the venous phase, with clear boundary and lower density than surrounding hepatic parenchyma. (c, d) HE staining demonstrates cystic enlarged space with accumulation of large quantity erythrocytes in it

Case Study 2

A male patient aged 29 years was confirmatively diagnosed as having AIDS by CDC. His CD4 T cell count was 117/µl.

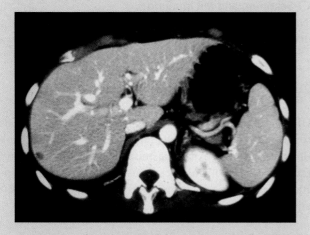

Fig. 20.6 HIV/AIDS related hepatic hemangioma. Enhanced CT scanning demonstrates round low density foci at the arterial phase under the envelope in the posterior segment of the right hepatic lobe, in size of 8×6 mm with clear boundaries, and marginal nodular enhancement of the foci

20.2.3.6   Criteria for the Diagnosis

CT scanning, MR imaging and ultrasound are all of great value for the diagnosis, with typical demonstrations of the hepatic tumors presenting less difficulties for the diagnosis. CT scanning can define the diagnosis of up to 90 % cases of cavernous hemangioma. For the cases with concurrent bulb sign by MR imaging; marginal fracture sign, vascular accessing or penetrating sign, the accuracy rate of diagnosis can be increased.

20.2.3.7   Differential Diagnosis

For hemangiomas with non-specific imaging demonstrations, it should be differentiated from other hepatic neoplastic lesions.

Primary Hepatocellular Carcinoma

Patients with primary hepatocellular carcinoma commonly have a history of hepatitis and hepatocirrhosis, AFP positive and peritumor edema, with involvement of adjacent portal veins and bile ducts. Its adjacent hepatic envelope shrinkage is more common. By MR imaging, weighted T2WI of hemangiomas presents bulb sign while hepatocellular carcinoma presents slightly high or equal signal. By enhanced imaging, hemangioma manifests enhancement of "early in and late out" or "late in and late out" while hepatocellular carcinoma presents "early in and early out" sign. In addition, hepatic

carcinoma has pseudocapsule but hepatic hemangioma has no capsule. Especially by enhanced imaging at the delayed phase, the pseudocapsule of the hepatocellular carcinoma can be well defined.

Hepatic Metastases

Metastatic foci with abundant blood supply like nasopharyngeal carcinoma, leiomyosarcoma, carcinoid and neuroendocrine tumors have similar signal to hemangioma by T2WI. And the metastatic foci are demonstrated as low density by CT scanning. All these demonstrations present difficulty for their differential diagnosis. Enhanced scanning of these foci demonstrates even or uneven enhancement at the arterial phase, equal or slight low density of the decreased enhancement at the portal vein phase, which is obviously different from demonstrations of hemangioma, including nodular enhancement, slow filling and persistent enhancement. In addition, small liquefaction and necrosis foci in the tumor nodules are also facilitative for their differential diagnosis. Hepatic metastases are usually multiple. The case history and relevant laboratory tests findings can also be referred for the differential diagnosis.

Focal Nodular Hyperplasia (FNH)

Plain CT scanning demonstrates poorly defined slightly low density shadows. Dynamic enhanced scanning demonstrates obvious enhancement at the arterial phase, with slightly high or equal density signal. Delayed scanning demonstrates equal or slightly low signal. These demonstrations should be differentiated from hemangioma. The key points for the differential diagnosis are the enhancements by enhanced scanning: (1) Hepatic hemangioma usually presents nodular or cotton wool liked enhancement starting from the focus border toward the center, while FNH presents enhancement of the foci starting from the center towards the peripheral area like a spring or at the arterial phase presents a gradual decreasing enhancement to the peripheral area. (2) Central scar of hepatic hemangioma presents no delayed enhancement while some cases of FNH can have delayed enhancement of the central scar (FNH with thrombus in the blood vessels of central scar presents no delayed enhancement). (3) FNH usually shows distorted and thickened arteries at the focus center or its peripheral area while hepatic hemangioma rarely presents such a sign.

20.3   HIV/AIDS Related Viral Hepatitis

HIV/AIDS can also be complicated by various virus hepatitis. Even HIV and hepatitis virus can infect the same cell. Coinfection or interaction between cytokine and viral protein can make the conditions complex and progress rapidly.

20.3.1   HIV/AIDS Related Viral Hepatitis A

20.3.1.1 Pathogens and Pathogenesis

Studies on the pathogenesis of hepatitis A are rarely reported, hence, it has not been full clarified. After infection of hepatitis A virus (HAV) via the oral cavity, the patients show a short term temporary viremia before its onset. After that, the virus is located in the liver. It was believed that HIV has direct destructive effects on the hepatic cells. However, recent studies have demonstrated that its pathogenesis is mainly predisposed to be immune responses of the host. In the early stage after its onset, HAV proliferates in large quantity in the hepatic cells, together with the toxic effects of CD8 on T cells, the hepatic cells are damaged. In the later stage after its onset, the lesions are predominantly pathological changes of the defense mechanism.

20.3.1.2 Pathophysiological Basis

Hepatitis A mainly presents acute hepatitis lesions and can also cause cholestatic hepatitis and severe hepatitis. Its principal pathological changes are as the following. (1) Degeneration and necrosis of the hepatic cells. The most common is early swelling of the hepatic cells in balloon sign, with accompanying hepatocyte acidophilic degenerations and formation of acidophilic bodies, which leads to loss of hepatic sinuses. Subsequently, the hepatocytes in the hepatic lobules are disorderly arranged, with lytic necrosis of the hepatocytes around central veins of hepatic lobules. (2) Inflammatory cells infiltration is found in the portal area, mostly large monocytes and lymphocytes. (3) Kupffer cell hyperplasia in the sinusoid wall. The above pathological changes are reversible, which may recover to normal in 1–2 months after receding of jaundice. The lesions of jaundice hepatitis A and non-jaundice hepatitis A are similar lesions, but the cases of non-jaundice hepatitis A having relatively mild symptoms.

20.3.1.3 Clinical Symptoms and Signs

After infection of hepatitis A virus, generally there is about 1 month asymptomatic incubation period. Subsequently, symptoms of unknown causes occur, including fever, fatigue, poor appetite, nausea, vomiting and yellow skin. In some cases, there are also abdominal distension or diarrhea. The urine is in brown and the stool light-colored. Liver examination shows hepatomegaly and tenderness or percussion pain.

20.3.1.4 Examinations and Their Selection
Blood Test
Leukocyte count decreases slightly or remains normal, while lymphocyte count increases comparatively.

Urine Test
Urobilinogen and bilirubin are positive.

Serum HAV Antibody
With positive finding.

Liver Function Test
It is the basis for the diagnosis, with increased serum GPT which can be normal in the third to fourth week, and increased serum AKP and γ-GT.

CT Scanning and MR Imaging
They are commonly used imaging examinations for the diagnosis.

20.3.2   HIV/AIDS Related Viral Hepatitis B

HIV and hepatitis B virus (HBV) have similar transmission routes, including intravenous drug abuse, hemophilia, multiple transfusions, sexual transmission and perinatal vertical transmission, all of which can cause overlapping infections. Biological behavioral changes thus occur, to complicate the clinical manifestations.

20.3.2.1 Pathogens and Pathogenesis

Although HBV is a hepatotrophic virus and HIV is a non-hepatotrophic virus, studies have demonstrated that HBV can also infect T lymphocytes. Thereby these viruses can intracellularly meet in the infected patients. Consequently, mutual promotion of genetic transcription and replication between these two species of viruses can accelerate their progressions and aggravate the conditions. The HBV infection by HIV positive patients presents a poorer prognosis. Patients with HBV infection are more susceptible to HIV infection.

20.3.2.2 Pathophysiological Basis

In HBV infected patients, the histological changes include characteristic ground glass liked hepatocytes and cytoplasm containing HBsAg. The disease commonly has chronic hepatitis manifestations, with non-specific reactive hepatitis in the slight cases but fragmental necrosis and bridging necrosis in the severe cases. There are also portal fibrosis and its peripheral septal fibrosis, infiltration of lymphocytes, plasmocytes and histocytes in the portal area, as well as balloon like changes of the hepatocytes and acidophilic necrosis of the hepatocytes. In the advanced stage, the typical changes are formation of pseudolobule and even fibrosis.

20.3.2.3 Clinical Symptoms and Signs

The clinical manifestations are predominantly chronic hepatitis, with the symptoms of fatigue, poor appetite, jaundice and hepatalgia. By physical examinations, there is enlarged hardened liver. With its progression, hepatocirrhosis related symptoms and signs occur.

20.3.2.4 Examinations and Their Selections
Liver Function Test
The result is the important basis for the definitive diagnosis.

CT Scanning and MR Imaging
Both are commonly used imaging examinations.

Ultrasound
It is a commonly used diagnostic examination and can be applied for screening and follow-up examination but it fails to define the qualitative diagnosis.

Pathological Examination of Liver Tissues
The pathological findings are the golden criteria for its definitive diagnosis. In addition, it also provides information as the golden criteria for accessing the inflammation activity, fibrosis degree and therapeutic efficacy.

20.3.2.5 Imaging Demonstrations
CT scanning and MR imaging are ordered for patients with hepatitis to detect hepatocellular liver cancer. Imaging demonstrations of hepatitis are non-specific. CT scanning demonstrates acute hepatitis as hepatomegaly, diffuse adipose degenerations, thickened biliary wall and low density area around the portal veins due to edema. MR imaging demonstrates hepatitis as high signal by T2WI and prolonged relaxation of hepatic T1 and T2 due to peripheral edema of the portal veins. In the cases of chronic hepatitis, enhanced MR imaging with injection can distinguish fibrosis from concurrent or recent occurrence of hepatocellular lesions. About 70 % patients present early flaky enhancement, which is histologically confirmed as liver inflammation. About 95 % patients show late linear enhancement, which is histologically confirmed as fibrosis.

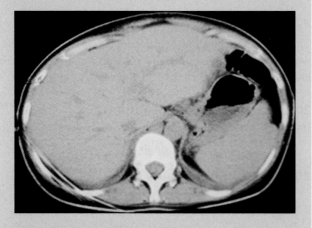

Case Study
A male patient aged 43 years was confirmatively diagnosed as having AIDS by CDC. His CD4 T cell count was 76/μl.

Fig. 20.7 HIV/AIDS related hepatitis B. CT scanning demonstrates enlarged liver with smooth border and homogeneous density in the hepatic parenchyma

20.3.3   HIV/AIDS Related Viral Hepatitis C

Since HIV and hepatitis C virus (HCV) have the same transmission routes, including blood transmission, sexual contracts and perinatal vertical transmission, overlapping infection of HIV and HCV is relatively common.

20.3.3.1 Pathogens and Pathogenesis
HIV is a member of Retroviridae family and Lentivirus genus and HCV belongs to the Flaviviridae family and Hepacivirus genus. Both are RNA viruses. Concurrent infections of both viruses to hepatocytes, they can interact at the molecular level. HIV infection can change the natural history of HCV infection by decreasing the spontaneous virus clearance rate of HCV infection. Overlapping infection of HIV/HCV may progress into hepatocirrhosis, liver failure and primary liver cancer with accelerated rate. In addition, HIV infection induced immunorepression is favorable to HCV replication to disrupt the immune mediated HCV clearance. The effects of HCV infection on HIV infection remain controversial. Some studies have demonstrated that overlapping infections of HIC/HCV progress more rapidly to AIDS or death. However, most scholars believe that HCV infection is of litter impact on the progression of HIV infection.

20.3.3.2 Pathophysiological Basis
Overlapping hepatic infections of HIV/HCV is pathologically characterized predominantly by interstitial inflammation. The hepatic lesions are changed into lymphocytes infiltration, with accumulated lymphocytes into mass and formation of lymph follicles. In some cases, there are swelling and proliferation of endothelial cells and Kupffer cells. In the cases with serious intralobular inflammation, fragmental necrosis can be found, with diffuse hepatocellular adipose degeneration.

20.3.3.3 Clinical Symptoms and Signs
It is clinically mainly manifested as chronic hepatitis. Compared to the overlapping infections of HIV/HBV, viral hepatitis C more commonly progresses into post-hepatitis hepatocirrhosis.

20.3.3.4 Examinations and Their Selections
Liver Function Test
The findings are the principal basis for definitive diagnosis.

CT Scanning and MR Imaging
They are commonly used in the clinical practice for the diagnosis.

Ultrasound
It is a commonly used diagnostic examination for screening and following up examinations. But it fails to provide

evidence for the qualitative diagnosis. It has high diagnostic value for hepatocirrhosis.

Pathological Examination of Hepatic Tissues

The findings are the gold criteria for defining the diagnosis as well as assessing the inflammation activity, fibrosis degree and therapeutic efficacy.

20.3.3.5 Imaging Demonstrations

The imaging demonstrations are non-specific. In patients with chronic active hepatitis, most have lymphadenectasis of hepatic portal, hepatogastric ligament and retroperitoneum. The size, quantity and signal of perihepatic lymph nodes are related to the activity of the disease. In patients with viral hepatitis C that progresses into hepatocirrhosis, there are nodules at the surface of the liver, with ascites and portal hypertension.

20.3.4   HIV/AIDS Related Viral Hepatitis D

Viral hepatitis D is an infection caused by HDV and HBV infection. It is transmitted via transfusion of blood and blood products, which is similar to those of HBV. The overlapping infections of HDV and HBV can exacerbate hepatic lesions, which promote its progression into chronic active hepatitis, hepatocirrhosis and severe hepatitis.

20.3.4.1 Pathogens and Pathogenesis

Its pathogenesis has not been fully elaborated. Currently, it is believed that HDV exerts a direct damage effect on hepatocytes, which can also be mediated by the host immune responses.

20.3.4.2 Pathophysiological Basis

The pathological changes of HDV infection are characterized by acidophilic changes of hepatocytes and vesicular adipose degeneration, with accompanying inflammatory cells infiltration and portal inflammation responses. The overlapping of chronic HBV infection and HDV infection can exacerbate the lesions of the hepatic tissues.

20.3.4.3 Clinical Symptoms and Signs

The clinical manifestations of HDV infection are determined by original HBV infection conditions. It has an incubation period of 4–20 weeks, which can be divided into following two types. (1) Concurrent infections of HDV and HBV. It is found in patients without a past history of HDV infection, but concurrence of HDV and HBV infections, with manifestations of acute HDV. Its clinical symptoms are similar to those of acute HBV, presenting twice increases of bilirubin and ALT the disease course. After findings of serum HBsAg,

intrahepatic HDAg shows positive. Patients in the acute phase have their serum HDAg being positive for several days before conversion into negative, followed by anti-HD IgM positive which has a short duration and low titer. However, anti-HD IgG remains negative. (2) The overlapping infection of HDV and HBV. Its clinical manifestations are diverse, in some cases being similar to those of acute hepatitis and in some other cases being similar to those of chronic hepatitis or severe hepatitis. It is commonly found in patients with chronic HBV infection, whose symptoms are principally determined by the past history of chronic HBsAg carriers or chronic HBV disease before HDV infection. In the case with a past history of HBsAg carrier, patients with HDV infection present symptoms similar to acute HBsAg positive hepatitis, with negative anti-HBV IgM and more severe conditions that those with simple HBV. In the cases with a past history of chronic HBV diseases, HDV continuously replicates itself due to the persistent HBV infection to exacerbate the hepatic lesions. Sometimes, an acute attack of hepatitis or its accelerated progression to chronic active hepatitis and hepatocirrhosis is resulted in. Therefore, in the cases of chronic HBV with original stable conditions, a sudden exacerbation and even liver failure like severe hepatitis, the possibility of overlapping infection of HDV and HBV should be considered.

20.3.4.4 Examinations and Their Selection

Liver Function Test

The findings are the principal basis for the definitive diagnosis.

CT Scanning and MR Imaging

They are commonly used diagnostic imaging.

Ultrasound

It is a widely applied examination for screening and following up examinations. But it fails to provide information for the qualitative diagnosis.

Pathological Examination of Hepatic Tissues

The findings are the golden criteria to define the diagnosis as well as to assess the inflammation activity, fibrosis degree and therapeutic efficacy.

20.3.4.5 Imaging Demonstrations

Imaging examination shows non-specific features.

20.3.5   HIV/AIDS Related Cirrhosis

20.3.5.1 Pathogens and Pathogenesis

HBV and HCV infections via haematogenous spreading or sexual contact in AIDS patients can result in hepatocellular lesions, which finally progress into hepato-cirrhosis. Hepatocirrhosis can be of many causes like HBV hepatocirrhosis, HCV hepatocirrhosis, HEV hepatocirrhosis, HDV hepatocirrhosis, drug induced hepatocirrhosis, auto-immune hepatocirrhosis, alcoholic hepatocirrhosis and hepatic veno-occlusive cirrhosis. In China, post-hepatitis cirrhosis is the most common, which is followed by alcoholic hepatocirrhosis.

20.3.5.2 Pathophysiological Basis

According to the morphology of the lesions, HIV/AIDS related hepatocirrhosis can be divided into four types. (1) small nodular hepatocirrhosis; (2) large nodular hepatocirrhosis; (3) Mixed hepatocirrhosis; and (4) incomplete septal hepatocirrhosis.

20.3.5.3 Clinical Symptoms and Signs

In its early stage, it can be asymptomatic. But later, it has different degrees of abdominal distention, indigestion, emaciation, fatigue and jaundice. In the cases with the complication of portal hypertension, there are symptoms of abdominal wall vein engorgement, hepatomegaly, spleno-megaly and ascites. Laboratory tests demonstrate increased serum transaminase, inverted ratio of albumin/globulin.

20.3.5.4 Examinations and Their Selection
Liver Function Test
The findings are the principal basis for the definitive diagnosis.

CT Scanning and MR Imaging
They are the commonly used diagnostic imaging examinations.

Ultrasound
It is a widely applied examination for screening and following up examinations. But it fails to provide information for the qualitative diagnosis.

Pathological Examination of Hepatic Tissues
The findings are the golden criteria to define the diagnosis.

20.3.5.5 Imaging Demonstrations
Ultrasound
Ultrasound can demonstrate the size, shape, abnormal echo of the liver as well as abnormal changes of the liver including splenomegaly and portal hypertension. In the cases with serious hepatic atrophy, the liver is demonstrated to have thinner, rigid and circuitous portal veins, which are blurry or even no demonstration of the terminal portal veins. These demonstrations suggest hepatic fibrosis and decreased hepatic blood flow.

CT Scanning
In the early stage, the liver may show enlargement. But CT scanning demonstrations are non-specific. In the middle and advanced stages, hepatocirrhosis progresses with enlargement and atrophy of the liver lobes, with manifestations of general hepatic atrophy but more commonly enlargement of the cau-date lobe and left lateral lobe as well as atrophy of the right lobe and left lobe. In some cases, there is also enlargement of the right lobe and atrophy of the left lobe or atrophy of the caudate lobe. The result is disproportional hepatic lobes. The liver border is demonstrated to be uneven. There are also widened hepatic portal and hepatic fissure, decreased or increased hepatic density and signs of portal hypertension including sple-nomegaly, ascites and esophageal and gastric basal varices.

MR Imaging
MR imaging demonstrates similar signs to CT scanning in terms of liver size, shape, splenomegaly and portal hypertension. By T1WI, the thinner vascular vessels and inflammatory fibrous tissues are manifested as a fine and chaotic network with a high signal in the liver parenchyma. By T1WI, the regenerative nodule generally is demonstrated as equal signal and by T2WI, homogeneous low signal with no capsules. Enhanced imaging demonstrates obvious enhancement. SPIO imaging demonstrates enhanced contrast. Due to the contents of Kupffer cells in the regenerative nodules, SPIO contrast agent is devoured to show a decreased signal by T2WI.

Case Study 1
A male patient aged 35 years was confirmatively diagnosed as having AIDS by CDC. His CD4 T cell count was 65/μl.

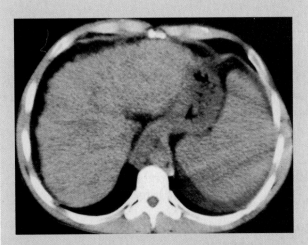

Fig. 20.8 HIV/AIDS related hepatocirrhosis, hepatomegaly and hepatolithiasis. CT scanning demonstrates the liver with irregular wave liked borderline, slightly decreased volume as well as thickened and enlarged spleen

Case Study 2

A male patient aged 45 years was confirmatively diagnosed as having AIDS by CDC. His CD4 T cell count was 116/μl.

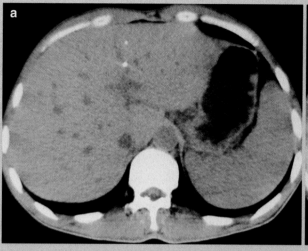 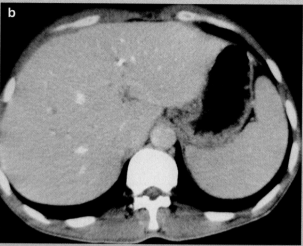

Fig. 20.9 (**a, b**) HIV/AIDS related hepatocirrhosis, splenomegaly and hepatolithiasis. (**a**) Plain CT scanning demonstrates enlarged liver, multiple bile duct dilations in the liver, calculus shadows in the dilated bile ducts and splenomegaly. (**b**) Enhanced CT scanning demonstrates homogeneous enhancement of the liver and the spleen

20.3.5.6 Diagnostic Basis

Hepatocirrhosis has early manifestation of simply hepatomegaly. Its imaging demonstrations are non-specific. In the middle and advanced stages, hepatocirrhosis has typical abnormalities in size, shape, echo, density, signal and contour of the liver. There are also signs of splenomegaly and portal hypertension. Ultrasound, CT scanning and MR imaging can define the diagnosis.

20.3.5.7 Differential Diagnosis

The regenerative nodules should be differentiated from liver cancer. Dynamic enhanced CT scanning demonstrates the regenerative nodules with no obvious enhancement. MR imaging demonstrates low T2WI signal, which can serve for its differential diagnosis.

20.4   HIV/AIDS Related Hepatic Opportunistic Infections

20.4.1 HIV/AIDS Related Hepatic CMV Infection

CMV is the most common opportunistic causative virus in AIDS patients. Clinically 5–25 % AIDS patients have hepatic CMV infection. Its incidence can be up to 33–44 % by autopsy.

20.4.1.1 Pathogens and Pathogenesis

Hepatic CMV infection is usually a part of general CMV infection, which is caused by reactivated latent infection. Simple CMV hepatitis rarely occurs.

20.4.1.2 Pathophysiological Basis

By naked eyes observation, there is hepatomegaly. In rare cases, multiple or single grayish white adipose infiltration foci can be found. Under a microscope, CMV inclusion bodies can be found in the hepatocytes, Kupffer cells and endothelial cells, with small focal necrosis, microabscesses, and occasionally massive hepatocellular necrosis.

20.4.1.3 Clinical Symptoms and Signs

AIDS patients mostly have clinical symptoms of general CMV infection, with accompanying hepatomegaly and increased ALT.

20.4.1.4 Examinations and Their Selection
Ultrasound and CT Scanning

They are commonly used diagnostic imaging examinations.

Liver Biopsy

The findings are the principal basis to define the diagnosis.

20.4.1.5 Imaging Demonstrations
Ultrasound

Demonstrations of multiple focal fine high/low echo.

CT Scanning

Plain CT scanning demonstrates hepatomegaly, diffuse small low density foci in the liver parenchyma. Enhanced scanning demonstrates no obvious enhancement of the foci. In some rare cases, there are several low density foci in the liver parenchyma with different sizes. Dynamic enhanced scanning demonstrates no enhancement.

20.4.1.6 Diagnostic Basis

The clinical manifestations include slight liver lesions. Liver biopsy demonstrates non-specific inflammatory lesions. Detection of intranuclear inclusion bodies in the lesion tissues can define the diagnosis.

20.4.1.7 Differential Diagnosis

HIV/AIDS related hepatic CMV infection should be differentiated from hepatic metastases. Enhanced CT scanning demonstrates hepatic metastases with enhancement of the focus border, with bull's eyes sign. The patients with hepatic metastases usually have a past history of primary cancer or its surgical removal. Whereas, patients with HIV/AIDS related hepatic CMV infection should have CMV infection and HIV antibody positive, with evidence of general CMV infection. Its definitive diagnosis can be made by biopsy findings of CMV inclusion body.

20.4.2   HIV/AIDS Related Hepatic Tuberculosis

Hepatic tuberculosis is extremely rare extrapulmonary tuberculosis. However, with the widespread application of organ transplantation and the increasing AIDS prevalence, the incidence of hepatic tuberculosis is gradually increasing.

20.4.2.1 Pathogens and Pathogenesis

Hepatic tuberculosis is not a primary lesion but secondary to blood-borne dissemination (hepatic arteries or portal veins) of mycobacteria bacilli into the liver from other organs, or direct TB infection of the liver via lymphoid duct, bile duct or adjacent foci. Due to the abundant mononuclear phagocytes system and powerful regenerative repair ability, together with suppression of MTb growth by the bile, the liver is not predisposed to occurrence of the hepatic disease in immunocompetent people despite of MTb invasion into the liver. But due to the compromised immunity in AIDS patients, they are susceptible to hepatic tuberculosis.

20.4.2.2 Pathophysiological Basis

Hepatic tuberculosis can be pathologically divided into following five types.

Miliary Tuberculosis

It is commonly caused by spreading of abdominal tuberculosis foci to the portal veins, with manifestations of diffuse solitary nodules in the liver which cannot be distinguished by naked eyes, fusion of multiple nodules to form a gray or grayish yellow nodule that is visible to naked eyes. Histologically, hepatocellular damages are demonstrated, with regional focal necrosis, migration of Kupffer cells and pylephlebitis; focal proliferation of Kupffer cells, formation of epithelioid nodules and small focal caseous necrosis. This type is clinically common and can be further categorized into subtypes of acute and chronic.

Singular Hepatic Tuberculoma

Hepatic tuberculoma is a tuberculous nodule with a diameter of more than 2 cm, which is also known as tuberculous granuloma. AIDS patients usually show typical granuloma, manifested as nodules or huge masses of various sizes and follicular foci composed of epithelioid cells and giant cell, with accompanying lymphocytes infiltration, Kupffer cells proliferation, hepatocellular fatty degeneration and amyloidosis. Large tuberculous granulomas or caseous materials can form tuberculoma.

Tuberculous Liver Abscess

It occurs due to liquefaction necrosis of caseous materials, which can be singular or multiple, in unilocular or multilocular. The abscesses can reach a size of 20 cm in the diameter, but mostly are small.

Hepatic Envelope Tuberculosis

The cases of hepatic envelope tuberculosis have an extensively thickened hepatic envelope or have nodular lesions, which is mostly a part of peritoneal tuberculosis.

Tuberculous Cholangitis

It is caused by penetrating of caseous tuberculoma or tuberculous abscess into the bile duct, which can be restricted in a part of the biliary system or spread to involve the whole biliary system.

The above types of hepatic tuberculosis can concur in just one patient.

20.4.2.3 Clinical Symptoms and Signs

Hepatic tuberculosis generally has non-specific clinical symptoms, commonly with a chronic onset. In the serious cases, there are symptoms of low grade fever, fatigue, night sweating, emaciation, hepatic area pain and hepatosplenomegaly.

20.4.2.4 Examinations and Their Selection
Routine Blood Test

Most patients have anemia of different degrees and lower or normal WBC count. In some rare cases, there is thrombocytopenia, with the lowest being 5×10^9/L. Moderately or significantly accelerated blood sedimentation is also common.

Liver Function Test

More than half patients have decreased albumin and increased globulin. About 1/3 patients have increased SGPT, TTT, ZnTT and AKP and less patients have increased bilirubin.

Tuberculin Test

Mostly negative.

Pathological Biopsy of the Liver

Hepatic puncture or laparoscopy can be performed to obtain liver tissues for pathological biopsy. Specific lesions of miliary hepatic tuberculosis can be found. The positive detection rate in patients with non-miliary hepatic tuberculosis is low. Sometimes, the findings are only non-specific inflammations to present difficulty for the diagnosis.

Ultrasound

For the cases with miliary hepatic tuberculosis, diffuse strong echo and hepatomegaly can be detected. For the cases with tuberculoma and tuberculous abscess, the ultrasound indicates space occupying lesions, which fails to provide information for its qualitative diagnosis.

Liver Scanning and Hepatic Angiography

They can demonstrate hepatomegaly and space occupying lesions, but the qualitative diagnosis cannot be defined.

CT Scanning and MR Imaging

Both are commonly used diagnostic imaging examinations.

20.4.2.5 Imaging Demonstrations
Miliary Tuberculosis

Ultrasound demonstrates early hepatomegaly, diffuse strong echo in the liver parenchyma with an uneven distribution, blurry hepatic veins, lymphadenectasis of the hepatic portal and ascites. In the advanced stage, caseous necrosis and calcium salt deposition are demonstrated, with multiple strong crescent shaped echo in the liver parenchyma and its posterior acoustic shadow, which is extremely similar to hepatolithiasis but with no intrahepatic cholangiectasis. Plain CT scanning fails to demonstrate the small non-calcified miliary foci (in a diameter of <0.5 cm), with only abnormality of hepatomegaly; the large miliary foci (in a diameter of >0.5 cm) in low density complicated by sand liked calcification. Enhanced CT scanning demonstrates no enhancement of the foci. MR imaging demonstrates low T1WI signal in multiple scattering distribution and different sizes; high T2WI signal of the foci, with clearly defined boundaries; uneven T1 and T2 signals of the larger foci. Enhanced MR imaging demonstrations are similar to those by CT scanning, with no enhancement of the foci.

Singular Hepatic Tuberculoma

Ultrasound demonstrates low echo nodules in the liver parenchyma with relatively smooth and intact boundaries. The echo in the foci is uneven, with complicated calcification at the center or margin of the foci and with blurry boundaries. The peripheral bile ducts and vascular vessels are compressed. Plain CT scanning demonstrates solitary low density foci with a diameter of 2–4 cm and intact smooth boundaries in the liver parenchyma. The interior density is uneven, with spots, clustering or powder liked calcification. Enhanced scanning demonstrates no enhancement at the arterial phase, no enhancement or slight ring shaped enhancement of the focus boundaries at the venous and delayed phase. MR imaging demonstrates nodular low T1WI signal with smooth and clear boundaries or shallow lobular signal with spots or sand liked no signal area. There are slightly high T2WI signal of the foci, with uneven interior signal. Enhanced MR imaging demonstrates the same as the CT scanning. CT scanning of hepatic tuberculoma demonstrates intrahepatic solitary space occupying lesion, with even density by plain scanning, with accompanying central necrosis and a very thin smooth envelope. Enhanced scanning demonstrates slight enhancement of the envelope.

Tuberculous Liver Abscess

Ultrasound demonstrates round or round liked no echo nodules in the liver, with smooth and clear boundaries and interior spots strong echo. The echo in posterior nodules is strong. Plain CT scanning demonstrates cystic low density foci and sometimes liquid-liquid level or cystic wall with complicated high density calcification. Peripheral accompanying satellite foci can be found. Enhanced scanning demonstrates no enhancement of the foci, or slight ring shaped enhancement of the foci borders. Some cystic wall has demonstrations of multi-layered or honeycomb liked septal enhancement. MR imaging demonstrates round or round liked low T1WI signal and obviously high T2WI signal. In the cases with focus septa or cystic wall calcification, the interior signal is generally uneven. Enhanced imaging demonstrates slight to moderate enhancement of the abscess walls and the septa.

Hepatic Envelope Tuberculosis

Simple hepatic envelope tuberculosis is extremely rare. As for tuberculosis of the liver parenchyma frequently occurs in the liver margin, hepatic envelope tuberculosis generally concurs with tuberculosis of the liver parenchyma. Ultrasound demonstrates thickened liver envelope with strong echo, subcapsular liquid echo and irregular low echo in the local liver parenchyma. Plain CT scanning demonstrates thickened liver envelope strip or arch liked calcification in the cases with increased density. The continuous liver margin has round liked irregular low density area, which is actually subcapsular effusion. Enhanced scanning demonstrates different slight enhancement of the liver envelope and the peripheral area around the foci in the liver parenchyma. MR imaging demonstrates irregular thickening of the liver envelope in equal T1WI signal and no signal for the cases with envelope calcification. The subcapsular effusion is in low signal and local liver parenchyma lesions are in low signal. Meanwhile, the thickened or calcified liver envelope is in low or no T2WI signal, subcapsular effusion in obviously high signal, the foci in low signal and the marginal inflammatory responses in high signal. Enhanced imaging demonstrates slight enhancement of the peripheral area around intrahepatic foci and no enhancement of the subcapsular effusion and the foci in the liver parenchyma.

Tuberculous Cholangitis

It is extremely rare, with main manifestations of irregular intrahepatic cholangiectasis, spots calcification at the hepatic portal or spots calcification along the biliary wall, which are characteristic demonstrations of the diseases.

Case Study 1
A female patient aged 36 years was confirmatively diagnosed as having AIDS by CDC. Her CD4 T cell count was 56/μl.

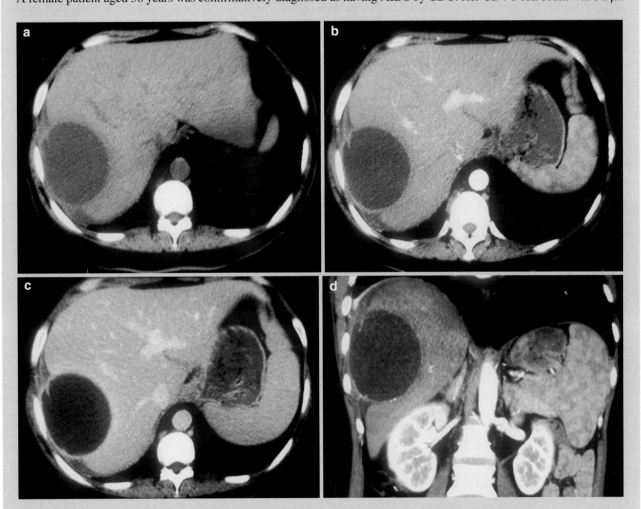

Fig. 20.10 (**a–h**) HIV/AIDS related subenvelope tuberculous abscess of the liver. (**a–d**) Before administering the therapies, plain CT scanning demonstrates round liked low density cystic foci in the posterior segment of the right hepatic lobe, with clear boundaries, and halo sign around the foci. Enhanced scanning demonstrates no enhancement of the foci at the arterial phase, slight marginal enhancement of the foci at the venous phase, obvious enhancement of the surrounding liver parenchyma. By coronal scanning, there are multiple calcification spots at the margin of the foci. (**e, f**) After administering the therapy, the reexamination demonstrates high density shadow in the focus, possibly hemorrhage. (**g**) HE staining demonstrates tuberculosis bacilli. (**h**) PAS staining demonstrates tuberculosis bacilli

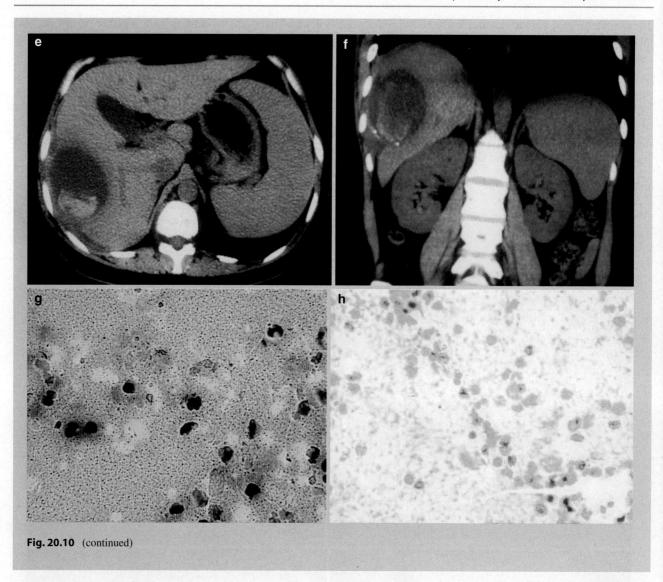

Fig. 20.10 (continued)

Case Study 2

A male patient aged 47 years was confirmatively diagnosed as having AIDS by CDC. His CD4 T cell count was 76/μl.

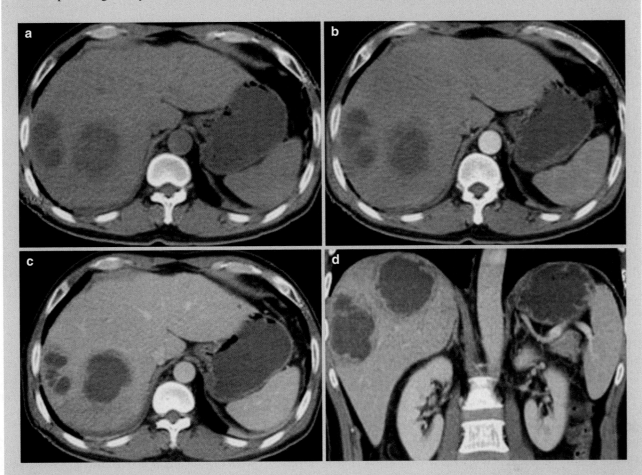

Fig. 20.11 (**a–d**) HIV/AIDS related hepatic tuberculous abscess. (**a**) CT scanning demonstrates two irregular low density foci in the right hepatic lobe, with blurry boundaries, and surrounding low density stripe of edema. In the lateral foci, there are septa. (**b**) Enhanced scanning demonstrates no enhancement of the foci and edema stripe at the arterial phase. (**c**) It is demonstrated to have slight ring shaped enhancement of the foci borders, enhancement of the septa and no enhancement of the edema stripes at the delayed phase. (**d**) Coronal scanning

Case Study 3

A male patient aged 31 years was confirmatively diagnosed as having AIDS by CDC. His CD4 T cell count was 86/μl.

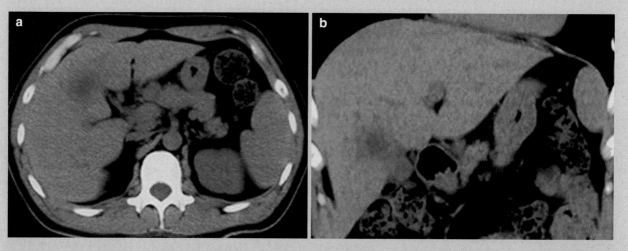

Fig. 20.12 (**a, b**) HIV/AIDS related hepatic tuberculous abscess. (**a**) CT scanning demonstrates round liked low density foci in the V segment of the liver in size of 27×24×31 mm, with quite clear boundary and a CT value of about 36 HU. (**b**) Coronal scanning

20.4.2.6 Diagnostic Basis

Hepatic tuberculosis is relatively rare. Its clinical manifestations are non-specific and imaging demonstrations are diverse and non-specific.

20.4.2.7 Differential Diagnosis

Primary Hepatocellular Carcinoma

Hepatic solitary tuberculosis is extremely rare, which should be differentiated from primary hepatocellular carcinoma. Hepatic solitary tuberculosis shows no obvious enhancement at the arterial phase while primary hepatocellular carcinoma presents evident enhancement due to the supplying by the hepatic arteries in a typical "quick in and quick out" sign. Moreover, hepatic solitary tuberculosis shows smooth and very thin capsule and primary hepatocellular carcinoma presents pseudocapsule which is caused by hepatic tissue hyperplasia and liver fibrosis triggered by tumor compression. The pseudocapsule is with uneven thickness and blurry boundaries. Patients with primary hepatocellular carcinoma generally have a past history of chronic hepatitis, with an AFP positive rate of 70–90 %.

Atypical Mycobacterium Avium Intracellular (MAI) Infection

The imaging demonstrations of these two diseases are similar. However, MAI infected patients present more serious hepatosplenomegaly than those with mycobacterium tuberculosis bacillus (MTb) infection. Homogeneous lymphadenectasis is more commonly found in MAI infection, while lymph nodes liquefaction and necrosis are principally found in MTb infection. Moreover, typical MTb infection occurs earlier than MAI infection, but clinically these two diseases usually are concurrent. Ultrasound guided puncture for biopsy can be performed to facilitate the diagnosis.

Hepatic Metastatic Tumors

Central powder liked calcification at the center of nodular hepatic tuberculosis can contribute to their differentiation. However, a past history of primary tumors is more important for the differential diagnosis.

Intrahepatic Multiple Hemangiomas

Dynamic enhanced scanning of nodular hepatic tuberculosis presents obvious ring shaped enhancement at the venous phase, while dynamic enhanced scanning of hemangiomas shows a typical "quick in and slow out" sign.

Bacterial Liver Abscess

Tuberculous hepatic abscess has a similar CT value to bacterial hepatic abscess, which presents difficulty for their differential diagnosis. Bacterial hepatic abscess presents smooth borders and more obvious peripheral enhancement, while tuberculous hepatic abscess is commonly formed by fused nodules with irregular borders and clustering nodular shadows. Patients with bacterial hepatic abscess manifest violent general bacteremic responses but patients with tuberculous hepatic abscess commonly present obvious clinical symptoms due to their compromised immunity.

20.4.3 HIV/AIDS Related Hepatic Non-tuberculosis Mycobacteria Infection

In AIDS patients, mycobacterium avium complex (MAC) infection is the most common opportunistic infection of the liver, with an incidence of 20–55 % by autopsy. It is commonly found in the advanced stage of HIV infection, which is a main cause of death in AIDS patients.

20.4.3.1 Pathophysiology

The liver parenchyma presents miliary nodules. Microscopy indicates epithelioid granuloma, with no caseous necrosis. MAC lives in the cytoplasma of macrophages. The largest macrophage is up to 50 um. Large quantity MACs can be demonstrated by H&E staining and other particular stainings including Ziehl-Neelsen, PAS, Giemsa, Methenamine and Silver.

20.4.3.2 Clinical Symptoms and Signs

MAC infection usually occurs in the advanced stage of HIV infection, with accompanying symptoms of fever or weight loss. Physical examination demonstrates hepatomegaly and slight increases of bilirubin and transaminase.

20.4.3.3 Examinations and Their Selection

CT Scanning and Ultrasound

It presents focal lesions in the liver parenchyma, with typical pathological changes of proliferation of histocytes to for granulomatous lesions.

Liver Puncture for Biopsy

It demonstrates atypical granulomas formed by foam liked histocytes and relatively slight inflammatory response.

Cell Culture

Cell culture facilitates the detection of pathogens and differentiation of its types.

20.4.3.4 Imaging Demonstrations

Ultrasound

With findings of multiple Low echo foci in the liver.

CT Scanning

The liver and spleen are found in normal size or in slight enlargements. But in some rare patients, moderately or seriously enlarged liver and spleen (the hepatic head and caudate lobe in a diameter of ≥21 cm, the splenic head and caudate lobe with a diameter of ≥16 cm) may be found. There are fine low density areas in the liver, spleen, kidney and pancreas, and abdominal lymphadenectasis with homogeneous soft tissue density.

Case Study

A female patient aged 37 years was confirmatively diagnosed as having AIDS by CDC. Her CD4 T cell count was 46/μl.

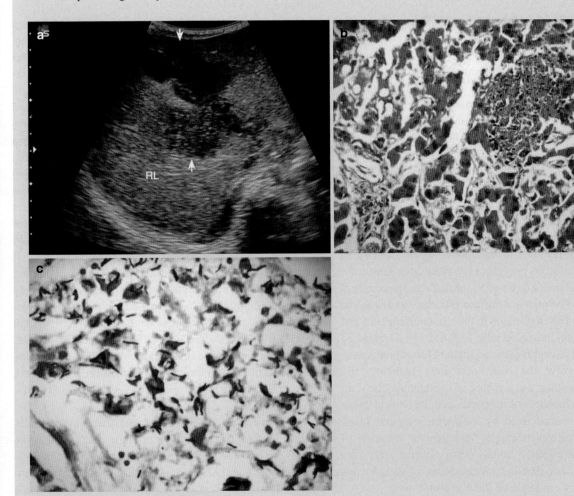

Fig. 20.13 (a–c) HIV/AIDS related hepatic MAC abscess. (a) Liver ultrasound demonstrates low echo in the liver parenchyma (*arrows*). (b) HE staining demonstrates hepatic MAC infection in non-typical tuberculosis nodular changes, HE ×200. (c) HE staining demonstrates hepatic MAC infection, foam liked cytoplasms of histocytes and epithelioid cells in the non-typical tuberculosis nodules, HE ×200. *RL* right liver

20.4.3.5 Diagnostic Basis

MAC induced hepatic lesions have non-specific clinical manifestations. Significant increase of serum alkaline phosphatase is an sensitive indication of disseminated MAC disease.

20.4.3.6 Differential Diagnosis

This disease should be differentiated from hepatic tuberculosis. The imaging manifestations of the two diseases are extremely similar, both presenting multiple low density (echo) lesions in the liver. Mycobacterium bacilli infection occurs earlier than MAC infection due to its stronger virulence, therefore, lesions occurrence time sometimes can serve for their differentiation. Meanwhile, hepatomegaly and splenomegaly degrees as well as necrosis of the swollen lymph nodes are important signs for their differentiation. MAC infection presents significant liver and spleen swelling (the hepatic head and caudate lobe with a diameter $\geq$21 cm, the splenic head and caudate lobe with a diameter $\geq$16 cm), while mycobacterium bacilli infection generally shows lymph node liquefaction and necrosis. Imaging guided puncture for biopsy can facilitate the diagnosis.

20.4.4 HIV/AIDS Related Hepatic Parasitic Infection

Leishmaniasis is caused by leishmania infection, which, according to its clinical symptoms, can be divided into visceral leishmaniasis (VL), an opportunistic infection usually found in HIV infected patients when their CD4 T cell count is less than 200/mm^3 and cutaneous leishmaniasis. Both pathogens of leishmania and HIV can infect the mononuclear macrophages. In vitro experiments have demonstrated that HIV infection can promote leishmania growth in macrophages. Th2 cytokines produced by HIV infection, such as IL-4, IL-6 and IL-10 can damage Th1 cellular functions and killing capability of the macrophages. Since Th1 mediated immune response is indispensable to the controlling of Leishmania infection, HIV infection provides a favorable environment for Leishmania infection. Likewise, VL also affects the course of HIV infection. The principal surface proteins of Leishmania can up-regulate HIV replication in the mononuclear cells and CD4 T cells. Cytokines (especially TNF-a and IL-6) produced by activated polyclonal B cells can trigger HIV expression.

VL can involve the liver, presenting pathologically Kupffer cells swelling and presence of Leishmania donovani body in the macrophages of the portal area. Its clinical manifestations are characterized by long-term irregular fever, emaciation, hepatosplenomegaly and general decrease of blood cells. The infection usually occurs several years after the first contact and detailed understanding of the patient's travelling history can facilitate the diagnosis.

Occasionally, toxoplasma infection is found in the liver, which results in hepatocellular degeneration and necrosis, lymphocyte infiltration or formation of granuloma. Meanwhile, toxoplasma cysts or tachyzoite can be detected in the liver tissues, which should be confirmed by immunohistochemistry if necessary. Moreover, toxoplasmas can also sometimes be found in the lesions of hepatocirrhosis and hepatic necrosis.

20.4.5 HIV/AIDS Related Hepatic Fungal Infection

Fungal infections can readily be found in AIDS patients but disseminated fungal infections involving the liver and spleen are relatively rare and principally occur in the advanced stage of AIDS. Histoplasma, Cryptococcus, Candida and Coccidioides can cause liver infection. As fungal infections are generally controlled by cellular immunity, the first opportunistic infection of HIV infected patients with T cell dysfunction are mostly caused by one of the above mentioned fungi. Its clinical symptoms include general infection, accompanying hepatomegaly and liver dysfunction of various degrees.

AIDS complicated by disseminated histoplasmosis is a result of endogenic reaction rather than primary infection, which, however, lacks radiological evidence of previous infections. CT scanning demonstrates abnormal manifestations of the liver and spleen, which nevertheless are non-specific. About 2/3 patients present hepatomegaly and splenomegaly, with an incidence of moderate or serious hepatosplenomegaly being less than 20 %. Serious splenomegaly commonly presents obviously enlarged or huge spleen (16–25 cm in diameter of the head and caudate spleen lobes) in nodular appearance. A rarely seen but significant CT sign is diffuse splenic density decrease. Although its incidence is only 20 %, it is generally believed to be a specific demonstration of histoplasmosis. In addition, there is commonly abdominal lymphadenectasis.

Although Mucocutaneous candidiasis is quite common among AIDS patients, disseminated candidiasis is extremely rare, especially in the early stage of AIDS, because it is usually related with neutropenia or neutrophil dysfunction but not related to T cell dysfunction. CT scanning of patients with disseminated candidiasis presents multiple fine low density nodules (diameter <5 mm) in the liver parenchyma. Ultrasound demonstrates typical low echo foci and bulls' eyes sign.

AIDS patients usually develop disseminated coccidioidomycosis because of reactivation of static infection that the patients are infected with during stay or traveling in the epidemic area. CT scanning demonstrates slight hepatosplenomegaly, small low density area in the spleen and splenic lymphadenectasis. The enlarged lymph nodes are in homogeneous soft tissue density or with central low density area.

Most cases of AIDS complicated by Cryptococcus infection can commonly involve the brain or lungs, rarely the abdomen. Pathologically, granulomas do not occur but the formation of small abscesses encompassed by massive macrophages. Its clinical manifestations include non-specific hepatosplenomegaly, lymphadenectasis, an increase of serum alkaline phosphatase activity, and a slight increase of transaminase. Liver puncture for biopsy can facilitate the diagnosis.

20.4.6 HIV/AIDS Related Hepatic Pneumocystis Carinii Infection

The incidence of extra-pulmonary Pneumocystis carinii infection is 0.5–3.0 %, with common involvements of the liver (35 %), spleen and kidney. Liver lesion is a sign of general dissemination of Carinii.

20.4.6.1 Pathophysiological Basis
By naked eyes observation, there are multiple unclean white foci of bean size in the liver. Microscopically, there are necrotic foci with clear boundaries filled by particles, or foam liked nodules with abundant pathogens but no accompanying inflammatory cells, or presence of granuloma lesions with multinuclear giant cell and accompanying calcium salt deposition. Hepatic necrotic foci with accompanying typical calcium salt deposition are suggestive of sporozoan infection. GMS staining shows round and central hollow Pneumocystis.

20.4.6.2 Clinical Symptoms and Signs
Clinical manifestations are non-specific, including cough, dyspnea, pulmonary shadows and hepatosplenomegaly.

20.4.6.3 Examinations and Their Selection
1. Ultrasound and CT scanning are commonly used examinations for the diagnosis.
2. Laboratory tests can detect Pneumocystis carinii in the ascites or liver tissues, which is the essential evidence for the definitive diagnosis.

20.4.6.4 Imaging Demonstrations
Ultrasound
The early foci are low-echo liquid dark area and late foci of high-echo calcification. The foci usually are small (2–5 mm), in numerous abnormal spots echoes in the abdominal parenchymal organs. They can be found weeks or months before abnormalities demonstrated by CT scanning. The lesions can also involve lymph nodes, pancreas, omentum and peritoneum.

CT Scanning
CT scanning demonstrates calcification of the foci in the abdominal organs and lymph nodes, commonly involving the spleen, liver and kidney. It can also occur in the lymph nodes, adrenal gland, retroperitoneum and intestinal wall. The calcification is usually multiple, in appearance of fine, patchy, coarse, and irregular or ring shape. The involvement of the liver, spleen and lymph nodes is focal, multifocal, fused or diffuse, with normal or decreased volumes. Occasionally, plain scanning demonstrates clearly defined hepatic and splenic calcification by less obvious by enhanced scanning. The visceral multifocal lesions of low density are mostly found in the spleen. The sizes of foci range from several millimeters to 8 cm or even larger, which may be the only CT sign of sporozoan infection, or with accompanying spleen and other visceral calcification. The following up by CT scanning demonstrates shrinkage or absorbed focal lesions, with occurrence or progression of calcification.

20.4.6.5 Diagnostic Basis
The diagnostic imaging demonstrates low density and calcification in the abdominal organs. A case history of PCP infection can indicate the diagnosis. But the key point for the diagnosis is to find Carinii sporozoan in the body fluid or tissues.

20.4.6.6 Differential Diagnosis
This disease should be differentiated from lesions caused by disseminated Candida, Aspergillus and Mycobacterium bacilli infections, which can simultaneously involve the liver, spleen, lymph nodes, pancreas, omentum and peritoneum. Calcification has long been believed to be the typical presentation of Carinii sporozoan infection, but recently is also found in MAC and CMV infections. Ultrasound or CT scanning guided puncture for biopsy can facilitate the diagnosis.

20.4.7 HIV/AIDS Related Hepatic Bacterial Infection

In AIDS patients, hepatic opportunistic suppurative infections are quite rare, among which Salmonella infection is the more common and is prone to recur, with accompanying bacteremia. The clinical manifestations include fever, abdominal pain and diarrhea. The cases with accompanying liver dysfunction are usually Salmonella invasion of the liver. Its diagnosis mainly depends on blood and stool culture.

20.4.7.1 Imaging Demonstrations
Ultrasound
Bacterial hepatic abscess is firstly demonstrated to have small low echo nodules, which gradually enlarge with central liquefaction. Patients with compromised immunity may

have an incomplete or even interrupted development course of hepatic abscess. There are actually no central liquefaction in the abscess but a malformation of the abscess wall to produce confusing ultrasound demonstrations. The abscess center can show no low echo, which can even be similar to parenchymal mass.

CT Scanning
Characteristic CT scanning demonstrations include round or irregular low-density lumps and their peripheral capsules may present enhancement by enhanced scanning.

MR Imaging
The demonstrations include singular or multiple rounds, oval or lobular mass with clear boundary. Compared to the liver tissues, MR imaging demonstrates lower T1WI signal and obviously high T2WI signal. About 1/3 foci are surrounded by slightly higher T2WI signal, representing peripheral edema of the foci. Most foci are demonstrated to have peripheral enhancement. Meanwhile, a minority of abscesses contain septa, with enhancement by enhanced imaging.

20.4.7.2 Examinations and Their Selection
Laboratory Tests
With increased WBC count and neutrophil count and liver dysfunction such as increased ALT and ALP. Liver abscess puncture for fluid culture and biopsy can detect the pathogenic bacteria.

Ultrasound and CT Scanning
Both are of certain value in defining the liver abscess and its location, which also provide a clear and visualized image for abscess puncture and surgical drainage.

20.4.7.3 Diagnostic Basis
As large doses of antibiotics are administered to AIDS patients for other reasons, blood culture and liver biopsy can hardly detect the growth of bacteria. Thereby, for the cases with demonstrations of large low density/echo foci in the liver of AIDS patients, the diagnosis of liver abscess should be considered.

20.4.7.4 Differential Diagnosis
Atypical liver abscess should be differentiated from hepatic metastases. Metastases focus is commonly multiple and the patients usually have a past history of primary tumors. Although peritumor edema may also be found, its range is much smaller than that of liver abscess. Abscess usually contains septa but metastases rarely do. Enhanced

scanning demonstrates transient enhancement of the peripheral area of liver abscess but rarely found in metastases. The findings of gas content in the focus support the diagnosis of liver abscess.

20.5 HIV/AIDS Related Biliary Inflammation

Biliary inflammation occurs in AIDS patients commonly 1–8 months after the onset of AIDS.

20.5.1 Pathogens and Pathogenesis

Pathogens of Biliary inflammation are commonly CMV, Cryptococcus and microspore cocci and rarely Candida albicans. Its secondary bacterial infections also commonly occur. Concurrent infections of two pathogens can also occur. In addition to infections, biliary lesions (such as sclerotic cholangitis) are also related to immunorepression induced by HIV infection.

20.5.2 Pathophysiological Basis

Lesions most frequently involve the general bile duct, manifested as lumen stenosis due to diffuse thickening of the bile duct wall. The bile duct wall can be eight times as thick as the normal one, with the lumen in a diameter of just 3–5 mm. And in some cases, the whole biliary system can be involved to cause cystic changes. The bile is straw yellow or like thick silt. The lymph nodes adjacent to the general bile duct usually enlarge with dense adhesions. Histological examination shows inflammation and fibrosis in the submucosa and subserosa, with edema between them and intact biliary mucosa. HIV/AIDS related sclerotic cholangitis (ASC) refers to biliary sclerosis and stenosis accompanied by papillary stenosis to cause proximal cholangiectasis in AIDS patients.

20.5.3 Clinical Symptoms and Signs

This disease is mostly found in the middle aged adults, presenting with severe pain at the right hypochondriac region or the epigastric area, accompanied by fever, or with diarrhea. It is usually caused by CMV or Cryptococcus infection, especially when CD4 T cell count is less than 50/mm^3. There are also cases reports of biliary infection of Microsporum coccus. Laboratory tests demonstrate increases of serum alkaline phosphatase and γ-GT, normal or a slight increase of aminotransferase and normal bilirubin. Anicteric cholestasis syndrome is relatively common in AIDS patients, which is induced by many factors and has similar manifestations to those of acalculous cholecystitis such as pain, fever, an increase of serum alkaline phosphatase, normal bilirubin. About 77 % patients show abnormalities by ERCP.

Sclerotic cholangitis is principally manifested with nausea, vomiting and abdominal pain in the right upper quadrant, accompanied by an increase of the alkaline phosphatase, or painless obstructive jaundice which is persistent or intermittent and results in skin scratches in addition to yellowish skin and sclera as well as dark colored urine and light colored stool. Physical examination suggests a palpable soft liver, light tenderness of the epigastric area or the upper right quadrant, no enlargement of the gallbladder and a common sized spleen. Palpable enlargement of the liver indicates hepatocirrhosis. Acalculous cholecystitis usually occurs after Campylobacter jejuni and Salmonella enteritis or in Cryptococcus and CMV infected patients. The occurrence of biliary lesions has manifestations of pain in the right ribs area, fever and an increase of the serum alkaline phosphatase.

20.5.4   Examinations and Their Selection

20.5.4.1   Ultrasound

It is convenient and simple to manipulate, which is the diagnostic imaging of choice for the diagnosis of HIV/AIDS related biliary lesions.

20.5.4.2   CT Scanning

In addition to the demonstration of the bile duct, it can also demonstrate abnormalities of organs and structures apart from the bile duct.

20.5.4.3   MR Imaging

It can favorably provide information about anatomic details and contrast resolutions. Moreover, MPCP has partly replaced ERCP to be an important examination for the diagnosis of biliary diseases.

20.5.4.4   Endoscopic Retrograde Cholangiopancreatography (ERCP)

Endoscopic retrograde cholangiopancreatography (ERCP) can be performed to directly assess the bile duct, which can be applied for pathological diagnosis. Although being invasive, it can provide better anatomic details of the bile duct and mucosa details.

20.5.5   Imaging Demonstrations

20.5.5.1   Ultrasound

Common signs of HIV/AIDS related biliary infections include thickened mucosa of the gallbladder and bile duct, intrahepatic and extrahepatic bile duct dilation, cholestasis and low echo nodules at the ends of the general bile duct as a result of sphincter edema. Dilation of the general bile duct has a high incidence, usually with no obvious irregular enlargement of intrahepatic bile ducts but of various degrees in the liver, which is suggestive of the irrelevance among intrahepatic bile duct dilation. The gallbladder usually shows dilation accompanied by thickened wall. Acalculous cholecystitis presents thickened gallbladder wall and gallbladder dilation.

20.5.5.2   CT Scanning

CT demonstrations are similar to ultrasound, showing irregular intrahepatic biliary dilation, thickened biliary mucosa, thickened gallbladder wall as well as abnormal enhancement shadows of the foci.

20.5.5.3   ERCP

HIV/AIDS related biliary lesions are similar to sclerotic cholangitis in intrahepatic biliary changes, with manifestations of local stenosis and segmental dilation in beads string liked appearance, decreased biliary branch terminals in withered twigs sign. However, the extrahepatic biliary changes are different from sclerotic cholangitis, with less common manifestations of diverticular and cystic dilations and terminal stricture but more common manifestations of moderate dilation of the bile duct with nodular irregular borders. These manifestations show the focal conditions of the inflammation. About 50 % patients have ampulla stenosis with accompanying pancreatic duct dilation, 25 % have ampulla stenosis without intrahepatic biliary dilation and even less cases have proximal stenosis in the long segment of the extrahepatic bile duct.

Four common manifestations of HIV/AIDS related biliary lesions by ERCP examination, which are described as the following. (1) General bile duct dilation, ampulla stenosis and contrast agent retention; (2) Sclerotic cholangitis; (3) Ampulla stenosis with accompanying intrahepatic and extrahepatic sclerotic cholangitis; (4) Stenosis of the long segment of extrahepatic bile ducts without intrahepatic biliary sclerosis.

Case Study 1

A female patient aged 20 years was confirmatively diagnosed as having AIDS by CDC. Her CD4 T cell count was 71/μl.

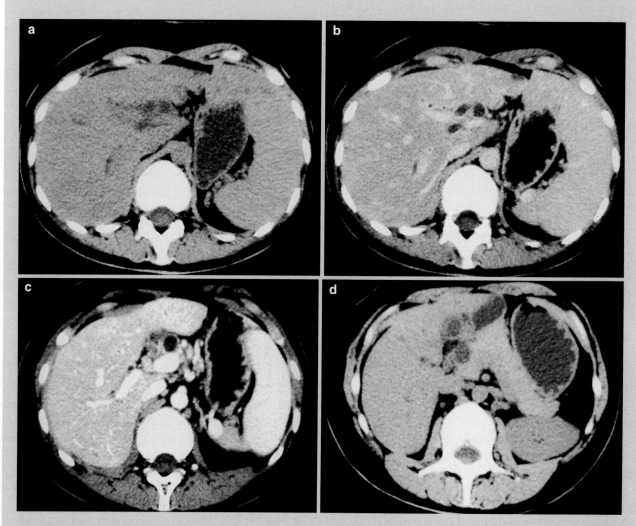

Fig. 20.14 (a–d) HIV/AIDS related low level biliary obstruction. **(a, b)** CT scanning demonstrates intrahepatic multiple biliary dilation with blurry borders. **(c, d)** Enhanced scanning demonstrates dilated bile duct with clear borders, spleen enlargement, slightly thickened gallbladder wall, slight enhancement and dilated gallbladder duct and general bile duct

Case Study 2

A female patient aged 43 years was confirmatively diagnosed as having AIDS by CDC. Her CD4 T cell count was 96/μl.

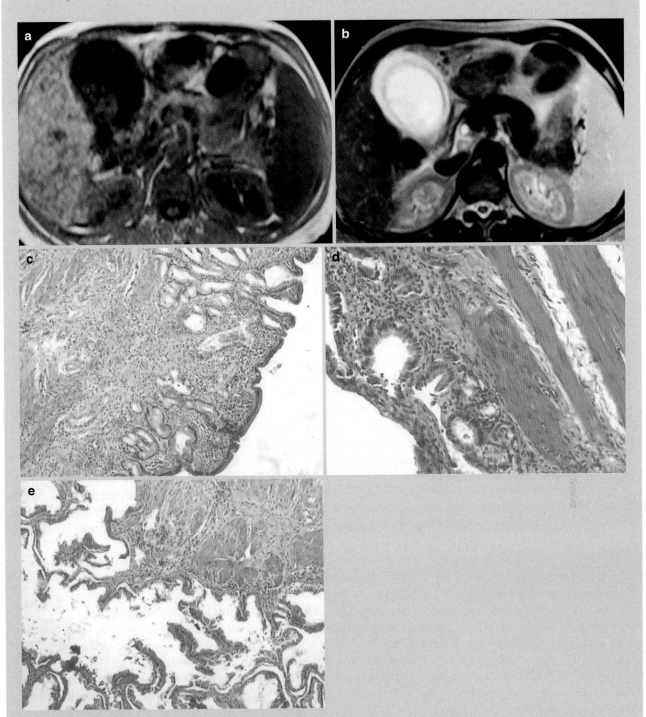

Fig. 20.15 (a–e) HIV/AIDS related cholecystitis and hepatolithiasis. (**a**, **b**) MR imaging demonstrates dilated gallbladder with thickened gallbladder wall, irregular slightly high T1WI signal and slightly low T2WI signal in the gallbladder lumen and enlarged spleen. (**c**) Medium magnification demonstrates dilated gallbladder, chronic cholecystitis and papillary hyperplasia of mucosa glands. (**d**) Low magnification demonstrates chronic cholecytitis. (**e**) Medium magnification demonstrates chronic cholecytitis and papillary hyperplasia of mucosa glands

20.5.6 Diagnostic Basis

The preliminary diagnosis of biliary diseases can be made based on clinical manifestations such as epigastric pain, fever and jaundice as well as laboratory findings of increased serum alkaline phosphatase. The definitive diagnosis can be made based on further diagnostic imaging.

20.5.7 Differential Diagnosis

Sclerotic cholangitis should be differentiated from infectious cholangitis based on clinical manifestations. By diagnostic imaging, the enhancement of the biliary wall is more obvious in the cases of infectious cholangitis.

20.6 HIV/AIDS Related Splenic Diseases

20.6.1 HIV/AIDS Caused Splenic Diseases

Its clinical manifestation mainly includes moderate splenomegaly, mostly in a weight of 300–600 g. In a few cases, megalosplenia occurs, with a spleen weight of over 800 g, and even more than 1,000 g. It is histologically characterized by: (1) a significant loss of lymphocytes in the splenic white pulp; (2) medullary cord filled up with macrophages that engulf massive hemosiderins; (3) disulfide bond linked virus protein p24 and hemoglobins to form into immunoreactive substances that diffusely distributed in the splenic macrophages.

Ultrasound and CT scanning demonstrate obviously enlarged or thickened spleen, in some cases megalosplenia, with clear boundaries and accompanying calcification spots in some cases. Splenomegaly usually is the early sign of HIV infection. The causes of splenomegaly are as the following: (1) HIV damages CD4 T lymphocytes in large quantity to impair their functions. Meanwhile the functions of mononuclear macrophages, B lymphocytes, CD8 T lymphocytes and NK cells are functionally impaired to infect the marrow stem cells. The increased blood flow in splenic red pulp causes normal or abnormal blood cells retain in the spleen or aggravate splenic damages, resulting in spleen congestion and enlargement. (2) AIDS can spread via the use of blood products. Most patients with AIDS have a past history of paid blood donation. They are probably infected by viral hepatitis. Therefore, the possibility of inflammatory cells infiltrations caused splenomegaly cannot be excluded.

20.6.2 HIV/AIDS Related Splenic Amyloid Diseases

Amyloid changes refer to pathological process with amyloid substances deposition in the reticular fiber, vascular wall or tissues of some organs. It usually involves multiple systems but in a few cases as local lesions. Amyloid lesions are found peripheral to the central artery of the spleen corpuscle in about 30–40 % AIDS patients by autopsy.

20.6.2.1 Pathogens and Pathogenesis

Its pathogen has not been fully understood. Some patients have a hereditary family history. It may be caused by protein metabolism disorder. It may also be caused by manufacturing of amyloid proteins under stimulation of antigens to cause plasmocytes dysfunction and then release of immunoglobulins. However, some scholars believe that its occurrence is related to long-term chronic inflammation.

20.6.2.2 Pathophysiological Basis

By gross cross sections observation, the lesions are semitransparent and nodular. Under a microscope, the lesions are nodular and cotton wool liked structureless substances in pink staining. Nakagawa Sadaaki categorized the lesions into four types, including Lymphoid follicles, red pulp, arterial wall and spleen trabecula as well as capsule, which can be concurrent.

20.6.2.3 Clinical Symptoms and Signs

The involvement of spleen usually is asymptomatic, or sometimes has symptoms of pain, infarction and spleen dysfunction. Spleen rupture is the initial clinical manifestation in patients with amyloid degeneration. Even in patients with normal sized spleen, spontaneous spleen rupture can occur; probably due to amyloid substances deposit induced an increase of brittleness of the blood vessels or spleen capsule.

20.6.2.4 Examinations and Their Selection

1. Ultrasound, CT scanning and MR imaging can define the location and range of the lesions as well as their relationship with the adjacent tissues. All of these are valuable data for clinical surgeries.
2. Pathological biopsy is an important examination for the definitive diagnosis.

20.6.2.5 Imaging Demonstrations

1. Ultrasound demonstrates splenomegaly, space occupying lesions with strong echo that can be clearly defined from their surrounding tissues.
2. CT scanning demonstrates splenomegaly and diffuse decrease of the spleen density and enhancement. The focal mass is demonstrated as poorly defined low density shadow or unobvious enhancement. In the case of primary amyloid degeneration, extensive calcification can be found in the spleen.
3. MR imaging demonstrates decreased T2WI signal.

20.6.2.6 Diagnostic Basis

The clinical and imaging manifestations of splenic amyloid lesions are non-specific. Its definitive diagnosis is dependent on pathological biopsy.

20.6.2.7 Differential Diagnosis

This disease should be differentiated from splenic tuberculosis, abscess, lymphoma and metastases. Patients with splenic tuberculosis experience long-term fever and tuberculin test positive as well as accelerated blood sedimentation. Round multiple foci are found in the spleen, with no enhancement or slight marginal enhancement and accompanied by splenic portal lymphadenectasis. Patients with splenic abscess experience high fever and chilliness. Enhanced CT scanning or MR imaging demonstrates obvious ring shaped enhancement of the abscess wall, with peripheral stripes of edema. Splenic lymphoma can be singular or multiple, with equal or low T1WI signal and slightly high T2WI signal. Enhanced imaging demonstrates slight enhancement of the foci, typical cases with map liked changes, and no ring shaped enhancement of the enlarged lymph nodes. Enhanced scanning of typical metastases demonstrates bull's eyes sign or target center sign.

20.6.3   HIV/AIDS Related Splenic Malignancies

The splenic malignancies are mostly malignant lymphoma and occasionally KS. According to literature reports, splenic involvement occurs in 60–80 % patients with AIDS complicated by malignant lymphoma.

20.6.3.1 Pathophysiological Basis

Due to red pulp filled up most of the spleen with blood, the section of the spleen is dark red. In the cases of malignant lymphoma, the tumor tissues are in nodular or flaky distribution with a dark red background. Pathologically, it can be divided into four types, including (1) homogeneous diffuse type; The spleen is evenly enlarged, with no obvious nodules. Microscopically, the tumor cells are diffusively distributed, with a diameter of less than 1 mm. (2) miliary nodules type; Grayish white nodules are diffusively distributed in the spleen, in a diameter of 1–5 mm. (3) multiple masses type; The focus is multiple in a diameter of 1–10 cm. (4) huge mass type; It is rarely found, with the focus diameter of above 5 cm. The spleen is occupied with singular mass, with normal splenic tissues in the residue small portion of spleen parenchyma. Microscopically, various types of B lymphocytes can be found in malignant lymphoma.

20.6.3.2 Clinical Symptoms and Signs

The principal symptoms of most patients are splenomegaly of various degrees, which is related to the severity of the impaired immunity and the pathological changes. The accompanying symptoms include fever, fatigue, poor appetite and weight loss.

20.6.3.3 Examinations and Their Selection

1. Laboratory tests demonstrate decreased platelets, hemoglobins and white blood cells, as well as accelerated blood sedimentation on hemogram, and lymphoma cells infiltration on myelogram.
2. Ultrasound, CT scanning and MR imaging are commonly used examinations for the diagnosis. They can be applied to detect intrasplenic lesions and enlarged lymph nodes in the abdominal cavity and retroperitoneum.

20.6.3.4 Imaging Demonstrations
Ultrasound

(1) The spleen is diffusively enlarged, with decreased or normal echo from the parenchyma and inner evenly distributed fine spots echo. (2) In some patients, singular or multiple round low-echo nodules or no-echo nodules scatter in the spleen parenchyma, without following obvious echo enhancement effect. Several nodules can fuse with lobular appearance. (3) Multiple nodular lymphomas are in honeycomb liked no echo, and the septa are in regular linear shaped strong echo stripes.

CT Scanning

The demonstrations can be divided into three patterns. (1) Enlarged spleen with increased density. (2) Singular or multiple low or equal density foci in the spleen with clear or blurry boundaries; slight enhancement of the foci by enhanced scanning; and sharper contrast to obviously enhanced normal spleen tissues. (3) Diffuse infiltration, with generally decreased spleen density and uneven enhancement by enhanced scanning. In addition, most cases have accompanying general lymphadenectasis of some other body parts.

MR Imaging

MR imaging demonstrations are related to the pathological changes of splenic malignant lymphoma. For the cases of evenly diffuse type and miliary nodules type, the foci are small, which cannot be demonstrated by MR imaging, with only demonstration of diffusively enlarged spleen. But for the cases of huge mass type, MR imaging demonstrates signal changes of the focus. The intrasplenic mass is demonstrated as equal or mixed equal and low T1WI signals; slightly higher or lower T2WI signal compared to the normal splenic tissues signal. Enhanced imaging with Gd-DTPA demonstrates blurry foci at first and obviously increased signal of the normal spleen tissue 1 min later due to its abundant blood supply but only slight enhancement of the focus, with more obvious contrast. Typical lymphomas present with map liked distribution. SPIO can increase the diagnostic accuracy of splenic malignant lymphoma. Since SPIO particles can be selectively absorbed by reticular endothelial cells but not by tumor cells, the signal intensity of the normal splenic tissues are decreased while lymphoma foci still maintain relatively high intensity signals, thus producing a more distinct contrast which can increase lesions detection rate. Furthermore, SPIO can be used to qualitatively identify splenomegaly. Non-neoplastic splenomegaly is usually caused by proliferative reaction or congestion with normal red pulp tissue structure; the reticular endothelial cells are not impaired which can still absorb massive SPIO particles, thus resulting in homogeneous signal decrease of enlarged spleen tissues. However, for neoplastic splenomegaly, damage and replication of red pulp by tumor cells decrease its interior reticular endothelial cells, therefore decreasing SPIO absorption. Therefore, the enlarged spleen presents consistent signals before and after enhanced scanning.

Case Study

A male patient aged 30 years was confirmatively diagnosed as having AIDS by CDC. Her CD4 T cell count was 98/μl.

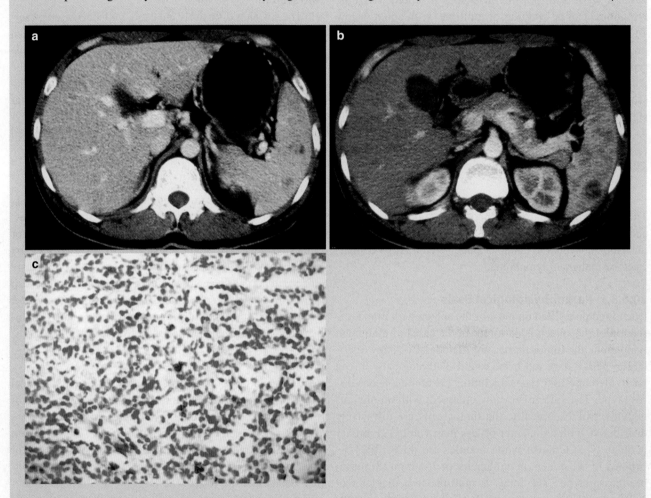

Fig. 20.16 (a–c) HIV/AIDS related splenic malignant lymphoma. (a, b) CT scanning demonstrates splenomegaly and multiple round liked low-density foci of various sizes and with clear boundaries in the spleen. The diameter of the largest foci is up to 18 mm. Enhanced scanning demonstrates slightly enhancement of the foci. (c) Immunohistochemistry demonstrates HIV-1P24 positive in the splenic lymphocytes, ×200

20.6.3.5 Diagnostic Basis

The key points for imaging diagnosis of splenic malignant lymphoma include splenomegaly, multiple nodules in the spleen and multiple lymphadenectasis in the abdominal cavity and retroperitoneum.

20.6.3.6 Differential Diagnosis

Splenic Metastases

Most cases of splenic metastases have a history of tumors. The intrasplenic tumor is in bull's eyes sign. The signal changes principally depend on the qualitative property of the primary tumors. In the combination with case history, its diagnosis can be defined.

Splenic Hemangiomas

Plain scanning demonstrates low density. Enhanced scanning demonstrates early marginal enhancement and delayed filling of the foci in high density.

20.6.4 HIV/AIDS Related Splenic Opportunistic Infections

Among AIDS patients, the spleen can develop various opportunistic infections. Klatt et al. [4] reported that the splenic opportunistic infections in 565 cases of AIDS are successively infection of MAC, Cryptococcus, tuberculosis mycobacterium bacilli, CMV, histoplasma capsulatum, Candida albicans and sporozoon Carinii according to its incidence. Splenic MAC infection not only tops all splenic opportunistic infections but also ranges second in all MAC infections, next to lymphoid MAC infection.

MAC infection can result in splenomegaly, with multiple nodules on the surfaces of the spleen and its sections with a diameter of up to 2 cm. Microscopy shows large quantity histocyte proliferation and its dense concentration can form spindle cell pseudotumors.

The clinically symptoms and signs of splenic abscess include fever, increased WBC count and pain. But immuno-suppressed patients with multiple splenic abscesses usually have no local symptoms.

20.6.4.1 Imaging Demonstrations

Ultrasound

(1) Slight to moderate splenomegaly; (2) No-echo area in the spleen with peripheral strong-echo stripes and mass liked, stripe liked and spots liked echoes in the no-echo area.

CT Scanning

In the early stage of the disease, the demonstrations include diffuse splenomegaly with slightly low but homogeneous density. In the cases with tissue liquefaction and necrosis, it presents low density area with no enhancement or slight enhancement. Generally, the abscess border is with relatively equal density, with enhancement by enhanced scanning. The cases of splenic fungal infections or mycobacterium bacilli infections are usually demonstrated to have miliary, multifocal or multilocular manifestations. About 64 % multilocular abscesses are fungal and 94 % unilocular abscesses are bacterial. Presence of gas or gas–liquid level in a few cases is characteristically splenic abscess. Calcification may be found in Candida microabscesses after treatment or in the focus of other fungal (commonly histoplasmosis capsulatum), mycobacterium bacilli and sporozoon Carinii infections.

MR Imaging

In contrast to normal spleen tissues, MR imaging demonstrates low T1WI signal and high T2WI signal. After intravenous injection of Gadolinium (Gd) the septa of bacteria abscesses and the abscess wall show enhancement, while fungal splenic abscesses show no enhancement.

Case Study

A male patient aged 48 years was confirmatively diagnosed as having AIDS by CDC. His CD4 T cell count was 45/μl.

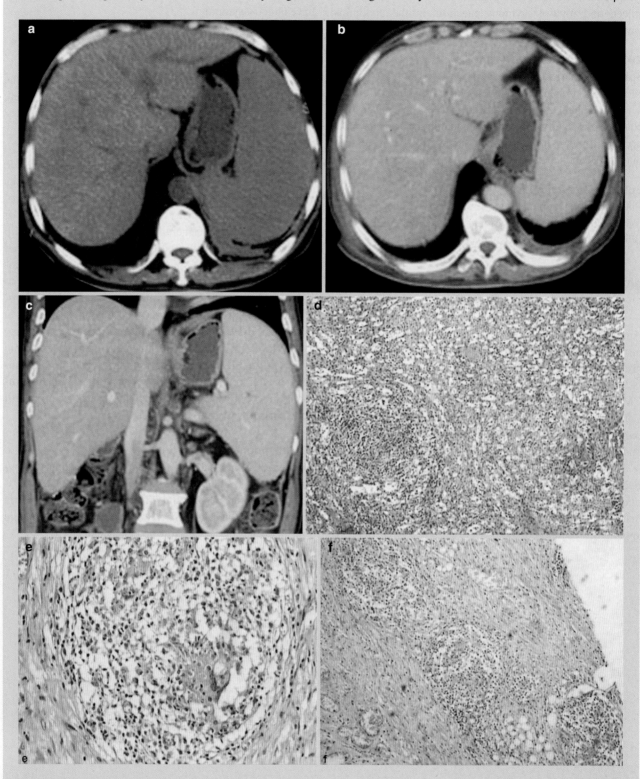

Fig. 20.17 (a–f) HIV/AIDS related splenic tuberculosis. (a) CT scanning demonstrates splenomegaly and multiple low density foci with various sizes and irregular shapes in the spleen. (b, c) Enhanced scanning demonstrates no obvious abnormal enhancement of the foci. (d) Low magnification demonstrates spleen congestion. (e) Medium magnification demonstrates chronic inflammation and formation of multinuclear cells. (f) Medium magnification demonstrates chronic inflammation and formation of multinuclear cells

20.6.4.2 Diagnostic Basis

Imaging demonstrations, in combination with clinical data can lead to the diagnosis. However, there is no demonstrations of local abnormalities by CT scanning cannot exclude the possibilities of early infection, especially blood-borne spreading fungal diseases.

20.6.4.3 Differential Diagnosis

Splenic abscess should be differentiated from splenic abscess and lymphangioma. Plain scanning of splenic abscess presents round or round liked low-density foci with clear boundaries, which have no wall and no enhancement by enhanced scanning. Plain scanning of lymphangioma indicates spleen enlargement, multiple round or irregular low-density foci of various sizes. Meanwhile, enhanced scanning presents no obvious enhancement of the foci at the arterial phase and still demonstrates low-density foci with clear boundaries at the portal and delayed phases. Ultrasound and CT guided puncture for biopsy can be performed for the definitive diagnosis.

20.7   HIV/AIDS Related Pancreatic Diseases

AIDS patients are predisposed to pancreatic lesions, clinically mainly manifested as abdominal pain. According to literature reports, AIDS patients are at 35–800 times higher risk than the general population in developing acute pancreatitis. Or in other words, 5–14 % HIV infected patients sustain acute pancreatitis. It has also been reported that 46 % AIDS patients in ICU are experiencing hyperamylasemia, but usually asymptomatic.

20.7.1   Pathogens and Pathogenesis

The occurrence of AIDS complicated by acute pancreatitis is related to the following factors. (1) Some drugs for the treatment of HIV infection and its related diseases have direct toxic effects on pancreatic acinar, such as Didanosine, Pentamidine, Lamivudine, Rifampicin and paromomycin, which have been reported to cause pancreatitis. (2) Some underlying basic diseases can make patients susceptible to pancreatitis, including immunodeficiency (with CD4 T cell count lower than 10.1×10^9/L), hyperamylasemia, and a past history of pancreatitis. (3) Opportunistic infections including CMV, Mycobacterium bacilli, toxoplasma, Cryptococcus, Candida, Aspergillus and herpes simplex virus infections can result in pancreatitis. (4) Alcohol abuse of some HIV-infected patients can lead to alcoholic pancreatitis.

20.7.2   Pathophysiological Basis

About 10 % AIDS patients present with pancreatic lesions like fatty necrosis, fibrosis, and acute/chronic inflammation. In addition to infiltration of inflammatory cells, serious cases may also have pancreatic necrosis. Toxoplasma and CMV infections can lead to pancreatic necrosis, manifested as destructed pancreatic acinar, presence of CMV inclusion bodies and cystic toxoplasmas at the necrotic borders. However, in the cases with pancreatic involvement of CMV and toxoplasma infections, manifestations of pancreatitis are not necessarily present. Many lesions are found by autopsy and it is also reported to have calcification spots in the pancreas.

20.7.3   Clinical Symptoms and Signs

Acute pancreatitis is mainly manifested as abdominal pain, abdominal distension, signs of peritonitis and shock. Chronic pancreatitis presents with dominantly persistent diarrhea or diarrhea without abdominal pain. Abdominal physical examination indicates evident tenderness, muscular tension as well as palpable masses in the cases with pseudoabscess.

20.7.4   Examinations and Their Selection

20.7.4.1 Laboratory Tests

It demonstrations increased serum or urine amylase, increased WBC count and neutrophil.

20.7.4.2 Ultrasound and CT Scanning

Both can be applied to define pancreatic enlargement, pancreatic abscesses, pancreatic cysts and biliary diseases.

20.7.4.3 MR Imaging and ERCP

Both can be applied to define biliary abnormalities and provide information about the conditions of the biliary ducts.

20.7.5   Imaging Demonstrations

20.7.5.1 Ultrasound

Acute edematous pancreatitis manifests diffuse enlargement of the pancreas, with homogeneous low echo in the enlarged pancreatic parenchyma and slight posterior enhanced echo. Acute necrotic pancreatitis presents significantly enlarged pancreas, irregular morphology, blurry boundary and enhanced heterogeneous echo from the pancreas parenchyma with small low echo areas or liquefied no-echo areas.

Chronic pancreatitis manifests slight enlargement or shrinkage of the pancreas generally with irregular contour.

There are unevenly enhanced echo from the parenchyma, and dilated common pancreatic duct. The cases with small stones inside show spots or patches of strong echoes and sound shadows. Sometimes pseudoabscess can be found.

20.7.5.2 CT Scanning

Acute edematous pancreatitis shows diffuse pancreatic enlargement of various degrees. The pancreas density is normal or slightly decreased which is homogeneous or heterogeneous, with clear or blurry pancreatic contours. In the cases with obvious effusions, pancreatic peripheral effusions can be found. Enhanced scanning demonstrates homogeneous enhancement of the pancreas with no necrotic area. Acute necrotic pancreatitis mainly presents with obvious pancreatic enlargement which is not diffuse. The pancreatic density is heterogeneous, increased or decreased, with no pancreatic peripheral fatty space. In addition, there are lesser peritoneal cystic effusion and pseudoabscess.

Chronic pancreatitis manifests normal, enlarged or shrunk pancreas, dilated pancreatic ducts, pancreatolithiasis, calcification of pancreatic parenchyma and pseudoabscess.

20.7.5.3 MR Imaging

Acute pancreatitis manifests pancreatic enlargement with irregular appearance. There is low T1WI signal and high T2WI signal. Pseudoabscess presents imaging demonstrations of round, clearly defined lesions with smooth sharp cystic wall. MR imaging demonstrates homogeneous signal, with low T1WI signal and high T2WI signal. The cases with complicated hemorrhage are demonstrated with high T1WI signal and low or high T2WI signal as well as irregular low signal ring in the chronic stage as a result of hemosiderin deposit.

Chronic pancreatitis manifests diffuse or local pancreatic enlargement or pancreatic shrinkage, with chaotic low T1WI signal and chaotic high T2WI signal. Calcified foci present with low signal or no signal.

Although imaging manifestations of pancreatic lesions in AIDS patients are similar with those in Non-AIDS patients, the clinicians should be aware of the following key points in the diagnostic imaging. (1) For the comparison of pancreas and liver parenchyma echoes, the liver usually presents low density due to adipose deposit or active hepatitis, and normal pancreas presents relatively higher density like pancreatitis. (2) The comparison with the kidney may be not reliable because the manifestation of renal high density in the cases of HIV/AIDS related nephropathy.

Case Study

A male patient aged 45 years was confirmatively diagnosed as having AIDS by CDC. His CD4 T cell count was 39/μl.

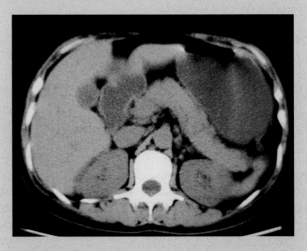

Fig. 20.18 HIV/AIDS related acute pancreatitis. CT scanning demonstrates slightly increased pancreas, with uneven density; and a few liquid density shadows near the pancreatic caudal

20.7.6   Diagnostic Basis

Pancreatitis generally has a definitive case history, signs and laboratory findings. In the combination with diagnostic imaging, its diagnosis can be defined.

20.7.7   Differential Diagnosis

Chronic pancreatitis, especially local enlargement of the pancreatic head induced by chronic pancreatitis, is sometimes difficult to be differentiated from pancreatic cancer, both present pancreatic head enlargement and caudate shrinkage. The key points for their differentiation are as the following. (1) Chronic inflammatory swelling of the pancreatic head is predominantly fibrosis in low T1WI and T2WI signal. (2) Dynamic enhanced scanning demonstrates enhancements similar to those of normal pancreas, while pancreatic head cancer shows low signal or low density at the arterial phase. (3) Detection of calcification and pseudocyst is highly suggestive of the inflammation. (4) Pancreatic cancer is more prone to cause invasion or embedding of the peripheral blood vessels. (5) Pancreatic cancer can show earlier metastasis to the liver and retroperitoneum.

20.8   HIV/AIDS Related Liver Cancer

Case Study 1

A male patient aged 46 years was confirmatively diagnosed as having AIDS by CDC. He had a past history of blood transfusion. In 2002, he was diagnosed as having hepatitis C, with progressive weight loss. His CD4 T cell count was 5/μl.

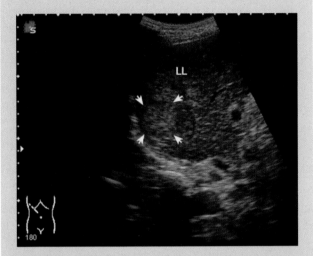

Fig. 20.19 AIDS complicated by space occupying lesions in the liver parenchyma (liver cancer). Ultrasound demonstrates diffuse echo changes in the liver, inflammatory changes of the gallbladder and enlarged spleen. There is a round liked parenchymal equal echo mass in size of 40×30 mm in the right hepatic lobe, with surrounding low echo and uneven interior echo (*arrows*). CDFI demonstrates abundant peripheral blood flow. *LL* left liver

Case Study 2

A male patient aged 53 years was confirmatively diagnosed as having AIDS by CDC. He had a past history of blood transfusion in 1996. In 2005, he was diagnosed as having hepatitis B and C, with abdominal upset. His CD4 T cell count was 58/μl.

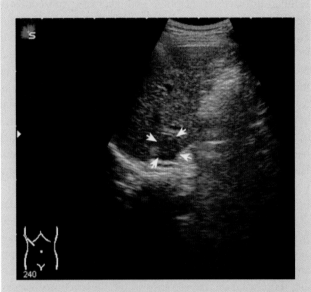

Fig. 20.20 AIDS complicated by space occupying lesions in the liver parenchyma (liver cancer). Color ultrasound demonstrates diffuse echo changes in the liver and widened portal vein, an irregular parenchymal low density mass in size of 23×25 mm with clear boundary in the right hepatic lobe near the envelope, with uneven interior echo (*arrows*). CDFI demonstrates poor blood flow signal in and peripheral to the mass

20.8.1   Discussion

AIDS patients, especially those infected via blood transfusion, are usually complicated by HBV and HCV infections. There chronic hepatic lesions usually progress into hepatocirrhosis and liver cancer. Hepatocirrhosis is a common chronic liver disease, with hepatic lesions caused by singular or multiple causes, presenting progressive, diffuse and fibrotic lesions in the liver. Its manifestations include hepatocellular diffuse degeneration and necrosis, subsequently fibrous tissues hyperplasia and hepatocellular nodular regeneration. The three changes alternatively and repeatedly occur to gradually reconstruct the hepatic lobular structure and blood circulation routes. The deformation and hardening of the liver finally result in hepatocirrhosis. Hepatocirrhosis is asymptomatic in its early stage. Later, a series of portal hypertension and liver dysfunction of diverse severities occurs, with further complications of upper digestive tract hemorrhage and hepatic encephalopathy to cause death. Hepatocirrhosis is not liver cancer because it is resulting from long-term repeated liver lesions due to singular or multiple causes, while liver cancer is due to hepatocellular degeneration; necrosis and even carcinogenesis resulted from interactions of multiple factors in multiple processes and multiple mutations of polygenes. The clinical symptoms and signs of hepatocirrhosis and liver cancer are quite different. For instance, hepatocirrhosis at the decompensatory stage mainly manifests weariness, fatigue, indigestion and liver function decrease and portal hypertension, with accompanying multiple systems symptoms as endocrine disorders and anemia. However, patients with liver cancer in their middle or advanced stages experience dominantly liver pain, as persistent distending pain or dull pain which can refer to the shoulders, and accompanying progressive emaciation, fatigue, low fever of unknown reasons, abdominal pain and diarrhea, although both hepatocirrhosis and liver cancer may be asymptomatic in the early stage.

Extended Reading

1. Apicella PL, Minrowitz SA, Weinreb JC. Extension of through hepatic neoplasms: MR and CT finding [J]. Radiology. 1994;1: 135–6.

2. Besson C, Goubar A, Chatelet FP, et al. Changes in AIDS-related lymphoma since the era of highly active antiretroviral therapy [J]. Blood. 2001;98(8):2339–44.

3. Kim SH, Han JK, Lee KH, et al. Abdominal amyloidosis: spectrum of radiological findings [J]. Clin Radiol. 2003;58(8): 610–20.

4. Klatt EC, Meyer PR. Pathology of the spleen in the acquired immunodeficiency syndrome [J]. Arch Pathol Lab Med. 1987;111(11): 1050–3.

5. Knowles DM. Etiology and pathogenesis of HIV/AIDS related non-Hodgkin's lymphoma [J]. Hematol Oncol Clin North Am. 2003;17(3):785–820.

6. Koh DM, Langroudi B, Padley SP. Abdominal CT in patients with HIV [J]. Imaging. 2002;14(1):24–34.

7. Li Hongjun. Clinical AIDS and imaging diagnosis. Beijing: China Medical Science and Technology Press; 2007.

8. Li xueqin, Li hongjun. A case report of liver related Kaposis sarcoma [J]. Beijing Med. 2010;32(9):773–4.

9. Li Hong-jun, Cheng Jing-liang. AIDS complicated with intestinal lymphoma: X-ray radiology, CT scan and pathological findings. Chin Med J. 2011;124(9):1427–30.

10. Lubat E, Megibow AJ, Balthazar EJ, et al. Extrapulmonary Pneumocystis carinii infection in HIV/AIDS: CT findings [J]. Radiology. 1990;174(1):157–60.

11. Monzawa S, Tsukamoto T, Omata K, et al. A case with primary amyloidosis of the liver and spleen: radiologic findings [J]. Eur J Radiol. 2002;41(3):237–41.

12. Moon Jr KL, Federle MP, Abrams DL, et al. Kaposi sarcoma and lymphadenopathy syndrome: limitations of abdominal CT in acquired immunodeficiency syndrome [J]. Radiology. 1984;150(2): 479–83.

13. Mortelé KJ, Segatto E, Ros PR. The infected liver: radiologic-pathologic correlation [J]. Radiographics. 2004;24(4):937–55.

14. Nyberg DA, Federle MP, Jeffrey RB. Abdominal CT findings of disseminated mycobacterium avium-intracellulare in HIV/AIDS[J]. Am J Roentgenol. 1985;145(2):297–9.

15. Semelka RC, Chung JJ, Hussain SM, Marcos HB, et al. Chronic hepatitis: correlation of early patchy and late linear enhancement patterns on gadolinium-enhanced MR images with histopathology initial experience [J]. J Magn Reson Imaging. 2001;13(3): 385–91.

16. Shirkhoda A. CT findings in hepatosplenic and renal candidiasis [J]. J Comput Assist Tomogr. 1987;11(5):795–8.

17. Trojan A, Kreuzer KA, Flury R, et al. Liver changes in AIDS. Retrospective analysis of 227 autopsies of HIV-positive patients [J]. Pathologe. 1998;19(3):194–200.

18. Valls C, Cañas C, Turell LG, et al. Hepatosplenic HIV/AIDS related Kaposi's sarcoma [J]. Gastrointest Radiol. 1991;16(4):324–42.

19. Yu RS, Zhang SZ, Wu JJ, et al. Imaging diagnosis of 12 patients with hepatic tuberculosis [J]. World J Gastroenterol. 2004;10(11): 1639–42.

20. Zhang XM, Mitchell DG, Shi H, et al. Chronic hepatitis C activity: correlation with lymphadenopathy on MR imaging [J]. Am J Roentgenol. 2002;179(2):417–22.

Contents

21.1 General Introduction to HIV/AIDS Related Peritoneal and Retroperitoneal Diseases

Abdomen is one of the most commonly involved body parts by AIDS, following the chest. It may involve the whole digestive tract and the liver, biliary tract, pancreas and some urinary and reproductive organs. It may also involve the tissues of mesentery, peritoneum and retroperitoneum. Currently, with the continuously increasing prevalence of AIDS, the manifestations and diagnosis of HIV/AIDS related abdominal diseases have gained increasing attention. In fact, many patients are definitively diagnosed as AIDS because they pay clinic visits due to gastrointestinal symptoms. Most of the abdominal symptoms in AIDS patients are non-specific, including abdominal pain, abdominal distension, diarrhea, fever, weight loss, abdominal mass, jaundice and gastrointestinal bleeding. These non-specific clinical manifestations, in addition to delayed specific laboratory tests, the diagnosis and treatment are usually delayed. HIV/AIDS related abdominal organs diseases will be described in detail in the relevant chapters and sections. In this chapter, we focus our attention on peritoneal and retroperitoneal diseases.

After HIV infection, it firstly involves the lymph nodes all over the body. Stimulated by the virus antigen, the immunocytes in the lymph nodes are activated to proliferate and differentiate to cause cellular and humoral immune responses in the lymph nodes. Clinically, it is manifested as lymphadenectasis, which is caused directly by HIV infection. Most diseases in AIDS patients are the complications after HIV infection progresses into the stage of AIDS. In the stage of AIDS, helper T lymphocytes significantly decrease due to long-term damage by HIV and its immune functions are also destroyed in different degrees. The patients are susceptible to opportunistic infections and malignancies, especially concurrence of multiple opportunistic infections when CD4 T cell count is extremely low. Occurrence of peritoneal and retroperitoneal diseases in AIDS patients are mostly peritoneal and retroperitoneal responses to the abdominal organs lesions.

H. Li (ed.), *Radiology of HIV/AIDS*,
DOI 10.1007/978-94-007-7823-8_21, © Springer Science+Business Media Dordrecht and People's Medical Publishing House 2014

That is to say, abdominal organs lesions commonly involve the peritoneum and retroperitoneum. Therefore, clinically, the imaging demonstrations and immunity of the patients should be in combination to be considered. In the imaging analysis, the abdominal organs lesions should be in combination with peritoneal and retroperitoneal lesions for a comprehensive understanding of their relationship for the diagnosis.

Opportunistic infections are the principal complications of HIV/AIDS, whose incidence is related to the virulence of the pathogenic bacteria or virus and the immunity of the patient. The chances of opportunistic infections significantly increase when CD4 T cell count is lower than 350–400×10^6/L. The common abdominal opportunistic infections in AIDS patients include tuberculosis, CMV infection, herpes virus infection, fungal infection, pneumocystis carinii infection and histoplasmosis. These infections not only involve abdominal organs, biliary system and intestinal mucosa, but also are disseminating to invade and involve the peritoneal cavity and retroperitoneal structures. HIV/AIDS complicated by mycobacterium non-tuberculosis infection are frequently reported and it occurs when the immunity is severely compromised.

Kaposi's sarcoma and lymphoma are more common in HIV/AIDS related malignancies. KS and malignant lymphoma of abdominal organs are discussed in the corresponding chapters and sections. In this chapter, HIV/AIDS related peritoneal and retroperitoneal lymphoma is the focus. Lymphoma is the second common in HIV/AIDS related malignancies, following KS. The risk of non-Hodgkin's lymphoma in AIDS patients is greatly higher than the general population and its pathogenesis is still unknown, which may be related to B lymphocytes proliferation caused by HIV or Epstein-Bar virus.

Due to compromised immunity of the AIDS patients, the incidence of various opportunistic infections and other related tumors obviously increases. Abdominal lesions in AIDS patients need various examinations, especially CT scanning, to define their diagnosis and differential diagnosis as well as to assess the therapeutic efficacy. Barium meal radiology is the most convenient method to detect the lesions of the gastrointestinal tract, which can demonstrate the lesions in the gastrointestinal lumen. Although endoscopy can visually display the lesions as well as collect tissues for biopsy, its manipulation is complex that can lead to obscure bleeding of the gastrointestinal mucosa to endanger the patients. CT scanning is advantageous in demonstrating the extragastrointestinal lesions, peritoneal lesions, abdominal lymph nodes lesions and abdominal organs lesions. Especially the enhancement of lesions range and lymph nodes can help to make a preliminary diagnosis before the results of bacteriological or histological examinations. However, MR imaging is rarely applied because CT scanning can well define the lesions and the further MR imaging

is thus unnecessary. The cost of MR imaging is also a reason. And the other reason is that AIDS patients are in a generally poor physical constitution and they show poor compliances in breath holding examinations for MR imaging. The importance of the diagnostic imaging is that they can assess the dynamic changes of the lesions and the therapeutic efficacy. The diagnostic imaging of peritoneum and retroperitoneum is a part of abdominal scanning/imaging. For patients with AIDS complicated by abdominal diseases, non-invasive diagnostic examination should be of choice to reduce their pain' and to reduce the risk of infection in medical staffs.

21.2 HIV/AIDS Related Peritoneal and Retroperitoneal Lymphadenectasis

21.2.1 HIV/AIDS Related Lymphadenectasis

21.2.1.1 Pathogens and Pathogenesis

Lymph node is a peripheral immune organ. The pathogenic microorganisms and toxins from tissues can gain their access into the lymph fluid via lymphatic capillaries. The immunocytes in the lymph nodes receive antigen stimulation to be activated for proliferation and differentiation. The following cellular and humoral immune responses occur in the lymph nodes to cause the clinical manifestation of lymphadenectasis.

Lymphadenectasis in non-AIDS patients can be divided into two types according to their distribution: (1) local lymphadenectasis, which is commonly seen in the cases of lymph nodes inflammation, lymph nodes tuberculosis and lymph node metastasis of malignancies; (2) general lymphadenectasis, which is common in the cases of infectious mononucleosis, lymphoma, various types of leukemia, and systemic lupus erythematosus. Clinically, according to the distribution of the enlarged lymph nodes, its differential diagnosis can be restricted into less possibility. Abdominal organs lesions, including infections and malignancies, can invade the lymph nodes via the lymphatic system. Therefore, occurrence of peritoneal and retroperitoneal lymphadenectasis cannot exclude the possibility of abdominal organs diseases, especially malignancies.

Pathologic changes of AIDS are predominantly found in lymphatic tissues and hematopoietic system. The lymph node is the key target organ. There are three common causes of HIV/AIDS related lymphadenectasis. By frequency, they are lymph nodes lesions caused by HIV itself, opportunistic infections and malignancies. In this section, we focus on the most common one, lymphadenectasis caused by HIV itself.

After HIV gains its access into the human body, Langerhans cells or dendritic cells pass it to CD4 T cells, whose homing causes in acute infection of the lymphatic tissue, with clinical manifestations of general lymphadenectasis, fever, rash and (or) symptoms of the central nervous system. After a varying durations of incubation period (clinically asymptomatic period), the virus replicates itself in a large quantity to successively involve the general lymphatic tissues. Meanwhile, specific immunity occurs and the viruses are confined in follicular dendritic cells of the lymphatic germinal centre. This is known as the chronic infection stage with clinical manifestations of AIDS associated syndrome and chronic lymphadenopathy. During the acute and chronic periods of lymphatic tissues infection, general lymphadenectasis may occur, with abdominal lymphadenectasis as its local manifestation.

In addition to HIV induced general lymphadenectasis, the indirect effects of HIV to induce destruction of CD4 T cells and cellular immunodeficiency are predominant. The results are occurrence of opportunistic infections and neoplasms.

In HIV infected patients, with the further damage to the immunity by the viruses, the CD4 T cell count is gradually decreasing to cause increasingly serious compromised immunity. When CD4 T cell count is below $200/\mu l$ in the stage of AIDS, opportunistic infections occurs successively. With the decrease of the CD4 T cell count, the incidence of opportunistic infections is increasing, with complications of various opportunistic infections as well as complex and diverse conditions. The gastrointestinal tract, communicating with the outside world, is a location that is most vulnerable to opportunistic infections. The causes of abdominal infectious lymphadenectasis are mainly tuberculosis infection, followed by intestinal infection. Fungal infections are relatively rare. Once the HIV infection progresses into the stage of AIDS, HIV exerts great destructive effects on the macrophages and CD4 T lymphocytes to cause a decrease or even loss of its suppression against mycobacterium tuberculosis, which further leads to recurrence and dissemination of the tuberculosis foci. Meanwhile, the obviously compromised immunity increases the possibility of reinfection by exogenous tuberculosis bacilli. All of these processes can result in tuberculous lymphadenectasis.

In AIDS patients, the lymphocyte count is decreasing, with deficiency of T cells and reverse ratio of TH/TS. There is also reduced activity of the natural killer cells. All these factors cause the decreases of immune surveillance and defensive function, which in turn impedes the body from effectively eliminating mutant cells to cause malignancies. In HIV/AIDS related tumors, the most common is Kaposi's sarcoma, followed by lymphoma that is commonly non-Hodgkin's B cell lymphoma. So far, it has been understood that the decrease of CD4 T cell count is the only reason for significantly increased risk of KS. It has been reported that impaired immunity, chronic antigen stimulation and overproduction of cytokines all contribute to the occurrence of lymphoma. EB virus may be the main reason for occurrence of lymphoma and non-Hodgkin's lymphoma. Apart from the

knowledge about KS and typical Non-Hodgkin's lymphoma, the pathogenesis of other tumors caused by compromised immunity remains elusive. But it has been known that their pathogenesis is related to the decrease of CD4 T cell count. HIV/AIDS related neoplasms cause general lymphadenectasis, with involvement of abdominal, retroperitoneal and mesenteric lymph nodes.

21.2.1.2 Pathophysiological Basis

During the early and chronic persistent periods, the pathological changes of lymph nodes are mainly reactive hyperplasia (follicular hyperplasia, I period). In this period, follicular hyperplasia is obvious, with irregular shapes like a map. The mantle zone is thinner or absent, with expansion of the germinal centre. Due to the destruction of dendritic cells in the follicular centre, lytic follicle occurs, which is not unique in AIDS. With the development of the lesions, follicles degenerate and the follicular central cells gradually reduce, with proliferation of interstitial cells, to form a characteristic concentric circle like an onion (follicular regression, II period). When it progresses into the period of follicles absence (III period), there is a disorderly lymphatic structure, with obviously decreased amount of follicles, proliferation of histocytes with scattered lymphocytes, plasmacytes and immunoblastic cells, and commonly post-capillary vein hyperplasia. In the period of lymph nodes exhaustion (IV period), total destruction of the lymph nodes structure occurs, with obviously decreased lymphocytes, diffuse or nodular proliferation of histocytes with or without accompanying fibrosis. Follicular regression and absence indicate the decline of the immune function. Therefore, opportunistic infections and/or neoplasms complicate HIV/AIDS in these two periods.

Lymphadenectasis caused by various HIV/AIDS related opportunistic infections and neoplasms will be discussed in the following sections.

21.2.1.3 Clinical Symptoms and Signs

As the fact that AIDS is a new type of infectious disease, with the immune system as the target organ of HIV, various diseases may occur when the immunity is compromised. Therefore, the clinical manifestations are diverse and complex. The clinical manifestations can be categorized into following five groups: (1) general manifestations including long-term fever, night sweat, weight loss of more than 10 %, abdominal pain, diarrhea and bloody stool; (2) persistent general lymphadenectasis, especially retroperitoneal and mesenteric lymphadenectasis with non-specific symptoms and signs; (3) multiple infections, especially opportunistic infections; (4) various neoplasms, especially KS and lymphoma; (5) multiple lesions of the nervous system. Therefore, AIDS patients commonly pay their clinic visits due to various common diseases, including all clinic sections. The physicians should comprehensively access the clinical symptoms and signs to consider the possibility of AIDS in the differential diagnosis.

21.2.1.4 Examinations and Their Selection

There are various causes for the abdominal lymphadenectasis in AIDS patients, with varying manifestations. The selection of appropriate diagnostic imaging facilitates the detection, comprehensive assessment, diagnosis and differential diagnosis. Ultrasound is widely applied for abdominal diseases. For the diagnosis of AIDS, a syndrome that can involve multiple organs with various manifestations, ultrasound is economical, practical and convenient, which is suitable for screening. Its application for reexamination is also convenient, which is applicable for following up observations of the therapeutic efficacy. However, due to the interference of gastrointestinal gas and coverage by the spinal column, ultrasound is less sensitive to early lesions of retroperitoneal lymphadenectasis and can favorably demonstrate the large or fused mass of lymphadenectasis. In addition, it can favorably show the indirect changes of the retroperitoneal blood vessels. Compared to ultrasound, CT scanning and MR imaging play increasingly more important roles in the diagnosis of HIV/AIDS related abdominal diseases. Both can comprehensively evaluate the abdominal lesions in AIDS patients, and even can provide information for accurate diagnosis. Although the imaging findings are not always specific, they play important role in formulating therapeutic plan and assessing therapeutic efficacy, such as accurate staging of the opportunistic infections. The nuclear medical examination, such as PET scanning, is rarely applied for the assessment of AIDS.

21.2.1.5 Imaging Demonstrations
CT Scanning

Abdominal lymphadenectasis is one of the manifestations of general extensive lymphadenectasis in AIDS patients. Superficial lymphadenectasis mainly distributes in the bilateral inguinal region, with manifestations of multiple nodules in a diameter of above 3 cm that may scatter or accumulate into a large mass. Deep lymphadenectasis such as retroperitoneal, mesenteric and pelvic lymphadenectasis is mostly multiple nodular in different sizes surrounding the major blood vessels with clear boundaries and rare fusion. The nodular density is even, with slight to moderate enhancement by enhanced scanning and no obvious necrotic area. Enlarged lymph nodes surrounding the abdominal aorta may cause anterior migration of the abdominal aorta and its enlarged distance from the spinal column and the inferior vena cava. The enlarged lymph nodes surrounding the abdominal trunk can straighten its running course. Enlarged lymph nodes surrounding the superior mesenteric artery and enlarged lymph nodes surrounding the renal vessels can also lead to similar migration.

MR Imaging

The distribution of retroperitoneal lymphadenectasis is the same as CT scanning demonstrations. Its MR imaging shows similar signals to general lymph nodes, with even and low T1WI signal against high signaling adipose background and slightly high and even T2WI signal in moderate and high signaling adipose tissues. By adipose suppression imaging, the enlarged lymph nodes are more clearly defined, in moderately high and even signal. The lymph nodes can accumulate into groups, but rarely fuse, with clear boundaries from each other. The surrounding blood vessels of the lymph nodes are in void low signals and are compressed by multiple enlarged lymph nodes to migrate, with rigid running course. But the vascular wall is smooth and intact with no invasion.

Ultrasound

Abdominal lymphadenectasis is obvious in HIV infected patients, with commonly accumulation of multiple enlarged lymph nodes and their fusion. The ultrasonogram demonstrates characteristic changes, including (1) Enlarged wide diameter of the lymph nodes, longitudinal to transverse ratio below 2, full morphology and huge mass formed by fusion of multiple enlarged lymph nodes. (2) Unclearly defined interface of the cortex and medulla in the enlarged lymph nodes, with low echo, enhanced echo of the envelope with unclear boundary that has peripheral infiltration in crab liked appearance. (3) Lymphadenectasis can be singular or multiple, principally multiple, with greater significance. (4) Changes of the adjacent blood vessels including straight running course of the abdominal trunk due to its surrounding lymphadenectasis, the left and right wings sign when enlarged lymph nodes encompassing the hepatic artery and splenic artery (hawk wing sign), forward migration of the abdominal aorta and its enlarged distance from the inferior vena cava due to its surrounding lymphadenectasis.

Case Study

A male patient aged 35 years was confirmatively diagnosed as having AIDS by the CDC. His CD4 T cell count was 85/ μl.

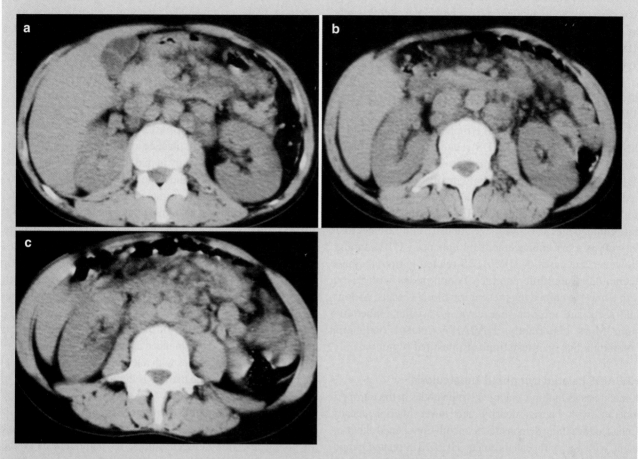

Fig. 21.1 (a–c) HIV/AIDS related retroperitoneal lymphadenecta- sis. (a–c) Epigastric plain CT scanning demonstrates multiple lymphadenectasis surrounding the abdominal artery, supramesen- teric artery and bilateral hepatic portal areas that accumulate into mass but with no fusion

21.2.1.6 Diagnostic Basis

As for HIV infected patients, general or local lymphadenectasis can be detected by physical examinations and diagnostic imaging. Their density and signal are even, with rare fusion. The causes of lymphadenectasis are multiple. According to the imaging demonstrations, the causes can be preliminarily distinguished. But the definitive diagnosis of HIV/AIDS related lymphadenectasis cannot be made. Most conclusions are the diagnosis of consistency.

21.2.1.7 Differential Diagnosis

HIV/AIDS Related Lymphoma

HIV/AIDS related abdominal lymphadenectasis should be differentiated from HIV/AIDS related lymphoma, which has its lesions confined within the retroperitoneum. HIV/AIDS related lymphoma can only involved the retroperitoneal lymph nodes. The distribution of the involved lymph nodes is in a similar range like HIV/AIDS related abdominal lymphadenectasis, with even density and rare necrosis as well as even enhancement by enhanced CT scanning. However, the cases of HIV/AIDS related lymphoma have accumulated multiple enlarged lymph nodes with fusion into a mass to embed the mesenteric blood vessels, abdominal aorta and inferior vena cava in vascular embedding sign. More importantly, HIV/AIDS related lymphoma commonly has manifestations of intestinal lymphoma.

HIV/AIDS Related Lymphoid Tuberculosis

It manifests as multiple enlarged lymph nodes in the retroperitoneum, with uneven density and lower interior density. Enhanced scanning demonstrates smooth ring shaped enhancement, with no central enhancement. HIV/AIDS related lymphadenectasis has even density foci, with rare interior necrosis. In addition, retroperitoneal lymphoid tuberculosis is commonly complicated by or secondary to intestinal tuberculosis, with corresponding clinical manifestations of intestinal tuberculosis, which facilitates the differential diagnosis.

Non-HIV/AIDS Related Lymphadenectasis

Before the clinical confirmative diagnosis of HIV infection, their differential diagnosis is difficult. HIV/AIDS related lymphadenectasis has evident features: (1) a wider range of involvement, rare local foci, common involvement of the abdomen, diffuse enlargement, large flaky fusion, sandwich sign in the mesentery and the major omentum in large pie liked appearance; (2) multiple organs involvement with commonly involved abdominal lymph nodes, liver and spleen, peritoneum and gastrointestinal tract. Compared to the cases of non-HIV/AIDS related lymphadenectasis, the involvement of the liver and spleen in the cases of HIV/AIDS related lymphadenectasis are more common, with diffuse nodular foci, which can be the basis for the gross differentiation of the two diseases.

Non-HIV/AIDS related lymphadenectasis occurs in many diseases, with distinctive features.

Typhoid Fever

In the cases of typhoid fever, there is peritoneal lymphadenectasis, with accompanying symptoms of high fever, ascites, hepatosplenomegaly, decreased peripheral WBC count and platelets, which are similar to malignant histiocytosis. After treatment, the heteromorphic lymphocytes are absent, with negative findings by blood culture and normal retroperitoneal lymph nodes.

Histiocytic Necrotic Lymphadenitis (HNL)

It is rarely seen in clinical practice and therefore can be misdiagnosed. It occurs commonly in middle aged and young adults, with 80 % patients being under the age of 30 years. The pathological examinations demonstrate characteristic necrosis of the lymph nodes, which is also known as extensive and coagulative necrosis of lymph nodes, with no infiltration of neutrophils. In the cortex area, there are extensive cellular necrosis, large quantity residue fragments which is known as necrotic fragments. The clinical symptoms include persistent high fever. Routine B mode ultrasound demonstrates retroperitoneal lymphadenectasis of different sizes, which can be pathologically confirmed. The cause of the disease may be related to virus infection or to virus induced autoimmune responses. It is believed to be lymph nodes with allergic reaction or slight collagen disease. Antibiotic therapy is ineffective.

Retroperitoneal Chronic Non-specific Lymphadenitis

The cause of the disease is complex, with more occurrences in young and middle-aged adults. Its pathogenesis is the chronic infection of the corresponding drainage tissues and organs and absorption of tissues destructive products, which can involve the lymph nodes of the drainage area to cause chronic inflammation. Chronic lymphadenitis has complex manifestations, including various responsive hyperplasias in the lymph nodes such as chronic diffuse lymphocytes proliferation, follicular hyperplasia, sinus histocytes proliferation. Its diagnosis needs to exclude specific lymphadenitis or lymphadenopathy such as lymphoid tuberculosis and systemic lupus erythematosus. Its diagnosis is difficult. Findings by once puncture and biopsy cannot define its diagnosis.

21.2.2 HIV/AIDS Related Mycobacterium Infectious Lymphadenectasis

21.2.2.1 Pathogens and Pathogenesis

Mycobacterium infection is one of the common abdominal opportunistic infections in AIDS patients and the most common pathogen is mycobacterium tuberculosis bacilli.

Generally decreased immunity is the pathogenic basis of TB. Factors including fatigue, coldness and dampness, malnutrition, vitamin deficiency, poor living environment and some virus infection contribute to decreased immunity. Tuberculosis induced by HIV infection has distinctive pathological changes and imaging demonstrations.

HIV infection targets to destroy CD4 T cells, leading to a progressive decrease of CD4 T cell count in the blood circulation. The impaired function of CD4 T cells destroys the defense mechanism of the human body to limit the responses from cells to the antigen of mycobacterium tuberculosis bacilli. Therefore, the stable incubated old TB foci are reactivated to cause secondary TB, namely endogenous reactivation. In addition, HIV infected patients are susceptible to exogenous reinfection due to the weak defense mechanism. The reinfected mycobacterium tuberculosis bacilli can rapidly cause the disease, with rapidly exacerbating conditions. The resistance of the mycobacterium bacilli to drugs can lead to outbreak and prevalence of TB.

Abdominal TB infection is often a result of blood-borne transmission, with complications of blood borne transmitted pulmonary TB and general lymph nodes TB. It has been reported that when the CD4 T cell count is below 350–400/μl, the infection rate of TB is obviously increasing, with concurrent increased infection rate of extrapulmonary TB, being up to 50 %. In patients with non-HIV/AIDS related TB, the incidence of extrapulmonary TB is only 10–15 %. Abdominal lymph nodes involvement is the most common manifestation of abdominal TB, found in 2/3 patients, commonly with multiple lymph nodes involvement. Abdominal TB in AIDS patients is more prone to disseminate, with involvement of mesenteric lymph nodes, peritoneum and abdominal organs including the liver, spleen, pancreas and gastrointestinal tract, especially ileum and colon.

In the patients with immune-deficiency, atypical mycobacteria infections rarely occur, but commonly occur in AIDS patients. The pathogen is commonly avium intracellular mycobacterium. Eight cases of AIDS complicated by Geneva mycobacteria infection have been reported and it is believed that its occurrence is at CD4 T cell count being lower than 100/μl. Puncture for biopsy can define the diagnosis.

21.2.2.2 Pathophysiological Basis

Early HIV infection can be complicated by TB, or TB may occur prior to HIV infection. The manifestation of TB is similar to those in immunocompetent patients. Microscopically, typical tuberculosis granuloma can be found, with slight caseous necrosis, less mycobacterium tuberculosis (MTB), more CD4 T cells, epithelioid giant cells and Langerhans cells around the foci to confine the foci. Because the destructive effects of HIV on the immune functions of CD4 T lymphocytes and macrophages, with the decrease of the CD4 T cells, the macrophages have decreased ability to inhibit the growth of mycobacterium tuberculosis to result in expanded caseous necrosis, decreased epithelioid giant cell and Langerhans cell and inhibited formation of tuberculous granuloma. In the advanced stage of HIV infection with complicated tuberculosis, the CD4 T cell count further decreases, with more serious immunodeficiency and even loss of immune responses. In the foci, there are insufficient epithelioid giant cells and Langerhans cells, extremely rare giant cells and lymphocytes, no granuloma formation but purulent coagulative necrosis and large quantity proliferation of mycobacterium tuberculosis bacilli. By biopsy or autopsy, it is found that TB is blood borne disseminating and non-responsive.

21.2.2.3 Clinic Symptoms and Signs

AIDS complicated by abdominal tuberculosis is manifested as active tuberculosis and systemic blood borne spreading. Clinically, patients show general symptoms of TB including fever, cough, expectoration and hemoptysis, night sweats, general soreness and pain, fatigue, anemia, emaciation, malnutrition and other toxic consumptive symptoms. Based on the involved organs by abdominal TB, there are corresponding symptoms and signs, commonly with abdominal pain, abdominal distention, diarrhea, abdominal tenderness and rebound pain in some patients, ascites sign positive and other gastrointestinal symptoms, lymphadenectasis and hepatosplenomegaly.

21.2.2.4 Examinations and Their Selection

AIDS complicated by abdominal mycobacterial bacilli infection can involve the gastrointestinal tract and parenchymal organs. Therefore, different diagnostic imaging examinations are necessary to comprehensively assess the abdominal lesions. Ultrasound examination is economical, practical and convenient, with wide application for assessment of abdominal parenchymal organs, following up examinations and assessment of curative effect. Ultrasound guided biopsy of parenchymal organs can shorten the time for definitive diagnosis. Barium meal radiology is simple and noninvasive that result in favorable compliance from the patients to assess the gastrointestinal involvement. Meanwhile, the comparatively not close contacts between the patients and medical staffs facilitate the occupational protection of the medical staffs. CT scanning and MR imaging are advantageous in assessing the abdominal parenchymal organs as well as abdominal and retroperitoneal lymph nodes. When the intestinal tract is well prepared, the gastrointestinal tract can be well assessed. Therefore, CT scanning and MR imaging, especially CT scanning, play important roles in assessing AIDS complicated by abdominal diseases. The above mentioned diagnostic imaging examinations can simultaneously assess retroperitoneal lymph nodes TB.

Nuclear medical examinations, including PET, have advantages of high sensitivity, but less significance for AIDS complicated by abdominal tuberculosis.

21.2.2.5 Imaging Demonstrations

HIV/AIDS related abdominal TB is commonly multiple organs infection with mesenteric, peritoneal and retroperitoneal lymph nodes TB. Abdominal organs TB are discussed in the corresponding chapter and sections.

CT Scanning Demonstrations

Abdominal lymph node TB is manifested as multiple soft tissue density nodules in the mesenteric, hepatic portal, hepatoduodenal ligament and surrounding abdominal aorta areas. The nodules are accumulated into mass with comparatively clear boundary. In the serious cases, there is sandwich liked changes in the mesentery, namely anterior and dorsal mesenteric lymphadenectasis with central mesenteric vascular vessels. Retroperitoneal enlarged lymph nodes are distributed around the major blood vessels, commonly leading to enlarged distance between the aorta and the spinal column as well as the inferior vena cava. Enhanced scanning demonstrates central necrosis of the nodules with no enhancement, marginal smooth ring shaped enhancement, and even the ring shaped enhancement of the small lymph nodes.

Abdominal organs tuberculosis can cause peritoneal tuberculosis, with manifestations of extensively thickened peritoneum and obviously thickened omentum in pie liked appearance and multiple nodules in the peritoneum to form abdominal effusion. Enhanced scanning demonstrates obvious enhancement of the nodules in the thickened omentum and peritoneum.

MR Imaging Demonstrations

MR imaging demonstrations for retroperitoneal lymph node TB are similar to those by enhanced CT scanning. The distribution of enlarged lymph nodes demonstrated by MR imaging is similar to that by CT scanning. Studies on MR imaging of abdominal lymph node TB have demonstrated that plain MR imaging displays low T1WI signal of the enlarged lymph nodes, with much lower central signal as well as high T2WI signal with higher signal of the central necrosis. By adipose suppression sequence, the signaling of retroperitoneal lymph nodes is more prominently characteristic. The mesenteric and retroperitoneal blood vessels are in vascular void low or no signal, passing through enlarged lymph nodes. Enhanced imaging demonstrates peripheral enhancement of the lymph nodes with no central enhancement. The characteristic demonstration is similar to that of CT scanning, which is determined by characteristic pathological changes of lymph node TB.

Ultrasound

The demonstrations are commonly round or oval shaped focus with a longitudinal and transverse diameters ratio of lower than 2. Some lymph nodes are in beads string distribution, with low and uneven echo. The medullar structure is absent. The lymph nodes with larger volume have cord liked slightly high echo structure at the lymph node hilum. Colored Doppler ultrasound demonstrates the blood flow in consistency of III type manifestations. In the cases with tuberculous lymph nodes abscess, the volume of lymph nodes is larger, being above 14 cm. The probe pressure demonstrates thick liquid flow. In the serious cases, rupture occurs to form fistula.

Case Study 1

A male patient aged 37 years was confirmatively diagnosed as having AIDS by the CDC. He was hospitalized due to anti-HIV positive for 5 years, fatigue and poor appetite for more than 1 month. About 5 years ago, he was detected to be HIV positive by physical examination, but receiving no therapies. And 1 month ago, he suffered from fatigue, poor appetite and intermittent fever with no known reasons. Two weeks ago, his CD4 T cell count was 7/μl. And he had a weight loss of 3 kg in the recent 1 month, with a peak body temperature of 40 °C, mild ane-

mia and left supraclavicular lymphadenectasis in a size of 4 mm×2 cm. The enlarged lymph node has no tenderness, but poor mobility. His cardiopulmonary is negative, with soft abdomen, no tenderness, no rebound pain, and impalpable liver and spleen. The mobile dull sound is negative. By laboratory tests, WBC $2.7–4.4 \times 10^9$/ml, N 89 %, Hb 72–89 g/L, PLT 127×10^9/ml, ALT 45–61 U/L, AST 71–94 U/L, ALB 22–26 g/L, ESR 140 mm/h, TB antibody(−), EBV(−), CMV(−), hepatitis B(−) and hepatitis C virus antibody(−).

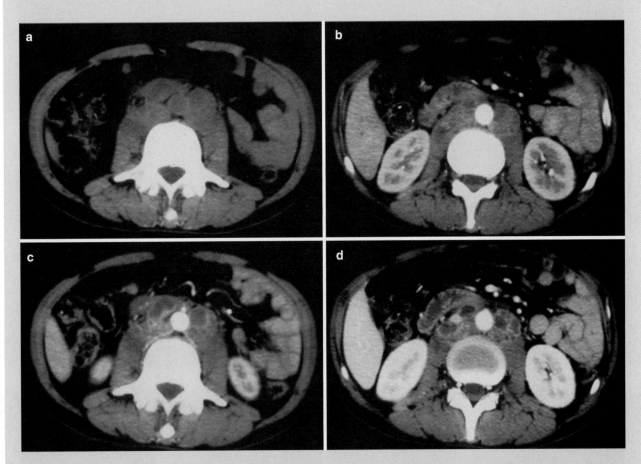

Fig. 21.2 (a–j) HIV/AIDS related retroperitoneal lymph node tuberculosis. (a) Abdominal plain CT scanning demonstrates equal density soft tissue mass around the abdominal aorta with unclearly defined boundary from the aorta, and anterior migration of the aorta. (b–f) Enhanced scanning demonstrates the early mass with slight or moderate uneven enhancement. (g, h) Delayed scanning demonstrates more intense enhancement of the mass, with interior multiple no enhancement areas and smooth inner wall. (i, j) Coronal reconstruction demonstrates the retroperitoneal lesion around the aorta, being accumulated multiple lymph nodes with central necrosis to fuse together, as well as enlarged liver and spleen

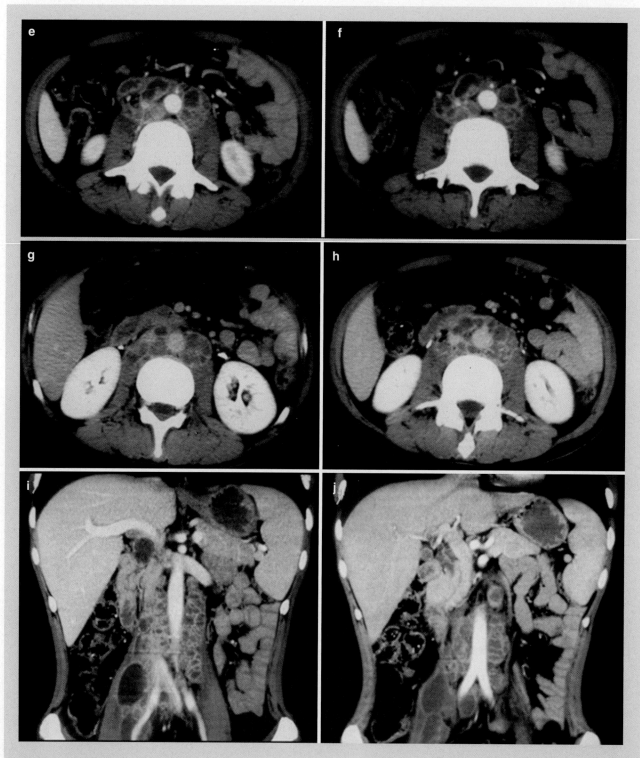

Fig. 21.2 (continued)

Case Study 2

A patient that was confirmatively diagnosed as having AIDS by the CDC. His/Her CD4 T cell count was 61/μl.

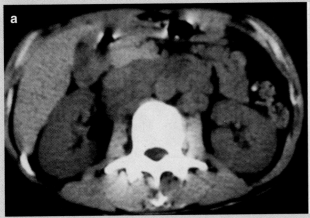

Fig. 21.3 (**a**, **b**) HIV/AIDS related retroperitoneal lymph node tuberculosis. (**a**) Epigastric plain CT scanning demonstrates multiple masses around the abdominal aorta, with irregular shape and unclear boundaries. (**b**) Enhanced scanning demonstrates slight to moderate even enhancement of the lesions, with no necrosis

Case Study 3

A patient that was confirmatively diagnosed as having AIDS by the CDC. He/She paid the clinic visit due to severe abdominal pain. By physical examination, there were severe abdominal tenderness and peritoneal irritation sign positive. His/Her CD4 T cell count was 11/μl.

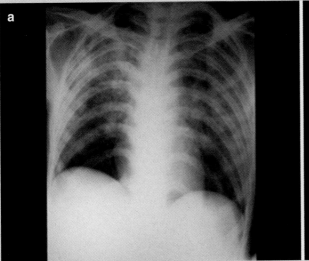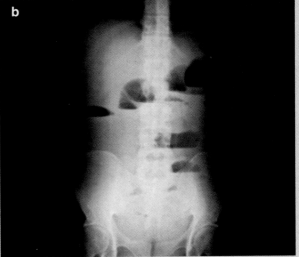

Fig. 21.4 (**a–e**) HIV/AIDS related intrapulmonary TB and extrapulmonary intestinal tract and intestinal lymph node TB. (**a**) Plain X-ray demonstrates flaky shadow in both lungs, especially the middle fields, with uneven density and multiple flakey fusion. There are also enlarge bilateral pulmonary hilar, which indicates hilar lymphadenectasis. (**b**) Abdominal plain X-ray at the standing posture demonstrates dilated jejunum with gas and fluid effusion in multiple ladder liked gas fluid level, indicating incomplete obstruction of the inferior jejunum. (**c**, **d**) Abdominal plain CT scanning demonstrates obviously dilated small intestines and large quantity effusion and small quantity gas. There are also local thickening of the small intestinal wall adjacent to the mesentery in the left abdomen, with lumen stenosis, which indicates the location of intestinal obstruction. (**e**) Pathohistology demonstrates tuberculosis nodules with central caseous necrosis and surrounding small quantity epithelial cells and lymphocytes

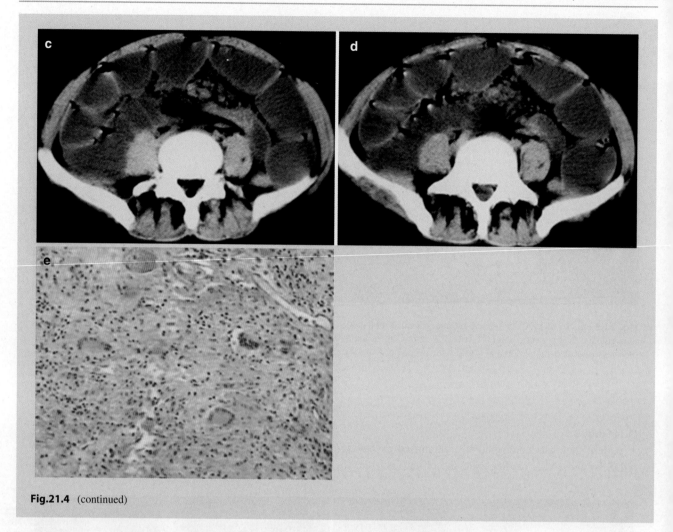

Fig.21.4 (continued)

21.2.2.6 Diagnostic Basis
Clinically Diagnosed HIV Infection
In the cases of clinically diagnosed HIV infection, there are general TB toxic manifestations and abdominal symptoms and signs. These symptoms and signs are mostly non-specific and the definitive diagnosis still needs direct evidence of TB.

Imaging Demonstrations
(1) Due to its principal blood borne transmission, the lesions have an extensive involvement to abdominal organs and retroperitoneal lymph nodes. (2) The lymph nodes are more likely to form tuberculosis abscess. Enhanced scanning demonstrates ring shaped enhancement, multiple marginal enhancement of lymph nodes fusion into multilocular sign.

21.2.2.7 Differential Diagnosis
Non-HIV/AIDS Related Abdominal Tuberculosis
Abdominal TB in immunocompetent patients is transmitted via gastrointestinal tract, mainly ileocecal TB and rare involvement of the abdominal organs. However, HIV/AIDS related abdominal tuberculosis is transmitted via blood borne route with an extensive involvement and common complications of pulmonary blood borne disseminating pulmonary TB or general lymph node TB foci. In terms of the abdomen, it commonly involves lymph nodes in the mesentery, hepatoduodenal ligament and surrounding superior abdominal aorta but rarely surrounding inferior abdominal aorta. CT scanning demonstrates non-HIV/AIDS related abdominal TB with enlarged abdominal lymph nodes in even soft tissue density. Enhanced scanning rarely demonstrates ring shaped enhancement. The incidence of abdominal lymphadenectasis is comparatively low, being about 42 %. Abdominal tuberculosis in AIDS patients tends to form tuberculosis abscess, with more complete central liquefaction and necrosis of the enlarged lymph nodes even in liquid density. Enhanced CT scanning demonstrates ring shaped enhancement and no central enhancement of the necrotic tissue, fusion of more than three adjacent lymph nodes with marginal enhancement into multilocular sign. It often involves multiple organs, more commonly the abdominal lymph nodes, liver and spleen, peritoneum and intestinal ileocecus. Compared to non-HIV/AIDS abdominal tuberculosis, the liver and spleen involvements are more common, with extensively distributed enlarged lymph nodes. These findings are of significance for the diagnosis and differential diagnosis of the disease.

Lymphoma
HIV/AIDS related lymph node tuberculosis can be misdiagnosed as lymphoma, which should be paid focused attention for their differential diagnosis. The distribution of HIV/AIDS related lymph node tuberculosis is relatively concentrated, with clearer tendency to fuse. Plain CT scanning demonstrates calcification of the lymph nodes. Enhanced scanning demonstrates ring shaped or multilocular enhancement of the lymph nodes. Clinically, the patients have toxic TB symptoms, with TB tuberculin test positive, TB signs by chest X-ray and complications of abdominal organs TB such as spleen TB. The lesions of lymphoma has an extensive distribution, commonly involving inferior area surrounding the abdominal aorta, the area below lumbar two to three vertebral level and retroperitoneal lymph nodes. Generally, the foci are in even density, with clear boundary and no calcification. Enhanced scanning demonstrates slight or moderate even enhancement, with no necrotic area. The typical manifestations of malignant lymphoma include multiple enlarged lymph nodes and their fusion to embed the mesenteric blood vessels, abdominal aorta and inferior vena cava, in vascular embedding sign, which is characteristic.

Metastatic Tumor
Patients with abdominal and retroperitoneal lymph node metastatic tumor usually have a past history of primary tumors. The enlarged lymph nodes are in a short distance from the primary tumor or in consistency of lymphadenectasis in the lymph drainage area. The foci are singular with a scattering distribution. The larger or fused lymph nodes have necrosis to be demonstrated as ring shaped enhancement by enhanced scanning. The ring shaped enhancement is thick with uneven thickness, with no interior liquefaction and necrosis area but in irregular patches with no calcification. Clinically, the patients have no toxic TB symptoms. When abdominal lymphadenectasis is found, its primary focus can be also found. In the short-term following up, the lymph nodes are obviously enlarged. However, patients with HIV/AIDS related abdominal lymph node TB have clinically toxic TB symptoms, tuberculosis tuberculin test positive, small foci in ring shaped enhancement by enhanced scanning, thin peripheral enhancement ring in even thickness like a ring stripe. There are also high enhancement, higher density of no enhancement area than water in the enhancement ring and calcification. Chest X-ray demonstrates signs of pulmonary TB. There are complications of abdominal organs TB, such as spleen TB.

Retroperitoneal Castleman's Disease (CD)
Plain CT scanning demonstrates even or uneven singular mass, with rare calcification. Enhanced scanning demonstrates multiple confined masses with obvious enhancement at the arterial phase, constant enhancement at the portal and equilibrium phases, which are characteristic demonstrations.

21.2.3 HIV/AIDS Related Penicillium Marneffei Infection

21.2.3.1 Pathogens and Pathogenesis
Penicillium marneffei (PM) is a deep pathogenic fungus initially isolated from the liver of Vietnam Rhizomys by Capponi in 1956. It can cause human confined or disseminated

deep fungal disease, Penicillium marneffei infection (PSM). PSM has an extremely low incidence in immunocompetent population, with confined foci. Its susceptible population is those with compromised immunity to cause disseminating infections. Therefore, PSM has a high incidence in AIDS patients as one of the most common opportunistic infections in AIDS patients of Southeast Asia. And its incidence is increasing. PM infection is an indicator for the definitive diagnosis of AIDS. Its transmission routes include contaminated soil by feces of Rhizomys. Human can infect the fungus via respiratory tract, gastrointestinal tract and skin defects and spread in the human body along with blood flow to invade the lungs, liver, spleen, kidney, bone marrow, skin and meninges, pericardium, peritoneum and mesentery, leading to symptoms of organs lesions.

21.2.3.2 Pathophysiological Basis

Penicillium marneffei is the only dual phase fungus, belonging to penicillium genus and Trichosporon order, which is also a special species of penicillium. The fungus is in dual phase morphological interchange at different culture temperatures, namely mould phase at the culture temperature of 25 °C and yeast phase at the culture temperature of 37 °C. Mould phase is multi-cellular mycelium, with certain biological morphology, such as broom liked conidiophores, chain liked conidium and spore chain; while yeast phase is single cell or double cells morphology. During the culture and growth of Penicillium marneffei, there is production of large quantity pigment in the color of bright rose or deep rose, which is characteristic. The pigment at the yeast phase is the secondary metabolites of the cells with strong hydrophobicity, which enables the conidium at the mould phase and cells at the yeast phase to adhere to the surface of alveolar macrophages and others cells. The pigment MAb can interrupt the pathological process of adhesion. In addition, the pigment can also prevent the permeation of the hydrophilic antifungal drugs, such as fluconazole, through Mdr expression, which improves its natural antifungal resistance of the Penicillium marneffei. The soluble substance of the mould phase pigment can trigger the production of anticonidium antibody (only IgG) to interrupt its spreading in the animal body. The phenomena indicate that the pathogenicity of the mould phase is weaker than the yeast phase. The conidium at the mould phase is the carrier of the pathogen while the cell at the yeast phase is the actual pathogen.

Penicillium marneffei often invades the mononuclear macrophage system to cause enlarged organs that have abundant mononuclear macrophages, such as the lymph nodes, liver and spleen. Macrophage granuloma can be formed, with multinuclear giant cells responses than are histologically divided three types. They are granuloma responses, purulent responses such as skin. Skin pustules and multiple pulmonary abscesses, weak responses and necrotic responses. Its pathogenesis is caused by the strong hydrophobicity of the

PM pigment at its yeast phase, which promotes the adhesion of conidium at the mould phase and cells at the yeast phase to the surface of alveolar macrophages and other parts macrophages. It has been reported that PM pneumonia is characterized by inflammatory granuloma with central necrosis, and accompanying infiltration of neutrophiles containing yeast liked PM cells. They proliferate by division rather than budding. Kudeken et al. studied PM infected immunocompetent rats and found that PM can induce a highly fatal inflammatory response [7], which is mediated by CD4 T lymphocytes after a complex process. In AIDS patients, due to the serious deficiency of CD4 T lymphocytes, the phagocytosis of macrophages is obviously weakened in the cases with complicated pulmonary PM infection to cause non-responsive necrotic inflammation and cavity formation. The effusion is relatively rare but proliferation is more common. In addition, PM can change the morphology of it and avoid the defense mechanism of the human body, which is the cause for its spreading in the human body. The pathogen can invade alveolus, pleura, interlobular septa, trachea wall, vascular bundles, mediastinum and pulmonary hilar lymph nodes in the lungs; and invade the liver, spleen, pancreas, retroperitoneal lymph nodes and other parenchymal organs to cause the enlargement of the organs and multiple abdominal abscesses.

21.2.3.3 Clinical Symptoms and Signs

Clinical manifestations include irregular fever, weight loss, anemia, cough, abdominal pain, diarrhea, and lymphadenectasis. Before the skin lesions occur, it tends to be misdiagnosed. In addition to skin mucosal involvement, other parts including lymph nodes, lungs, abdominal cavity and abdominal organs can also be involved. The clinical symptoms and signs of skin and lungs involvement is discussed in the corresponding chapters and sections. In this section, we focus on abdominal involvement. The lymph nodes involvements including lymphadenectasis of the neck, supraclavicular concave, axillary and inguen are hard and in different sizes with poor mobility and obvious tenderness. Deep lymphadenectasis occurs in retroperitoneum, mesentery and other deep organs. The pathological changes include macrophages granuloma, large quantity proliferation of yeast liked cells in a close and grape cluster liked arrangement. The manifestations of the digestive system include abdominal pain, diarrhea, varying frequency of bowel movements that is up to 20 times daily, watery or jelly liked stool; enlarged liver and spleen, abdominal tenderness, rebound pain and abdominal masses. Clinically, multiple infections of Penicillium marneffei occur; overlapping viral infections with hepatitis B virus and hepatitis C virus occur; other complications of fungal infection occurs including Candida albicans; some rare diseases can also occur, such as pulmonary TB, venous thrombosis and thrombocytopenia. Therefore, the clinical manifestations of Penicillium marneffei infection are diverse and complex.

21.2.3.4 Examinations and Their Selection

AIDS complicated by abdominal Penicillium marneffei infection has an extensive involvement, including organs, lymph nodes and abdominal cavity, with common symptoms of diarrhea, abdominal pain, abdominal distension, abdominal masses and jaundice. The simple diagnostic imaging should be firstly chosen for a comprehensive assessment. Ultrasound is the imaging examinations of choice for the abdominal organs assessment. However, it provides limited assessment for retroperitoneal or gastrointestinal lesions. CT scanning is more commonly applied for abdominal assessment in AIDS patients, especially some acute abdominal diseases. In addition, MR imaging can be performed, but its application is less common.

21.2.3.5 Imaging Demonstrations

CT Scanning

CT scanning demonstrates enlarged lymph nodes in the peritoneum and retroperitoneum. There are multiple soft tissue nodules in the mesentery, hepatic portal area, hepatoduodenal ligament and adjacent area of the abdominal aorta. The enlarged lymph nodes in the mesentery are in sandwich sign, which is actually anterior and dorsal mesenteric lymphadenectasis, with central mesenteric vascular vessels. Enhanced scanning demonstrates ring shaped enhancement of the lymph nodes, with no obvious central enhancement. The liver and spleen are diffusively enlarged, with focal or diffuse low density nodular foci in the liver and spleen parenchyma. Enhanced scanning also demonstrates diffuse and scattering small flaky areas with weak enhancement in the liver and spleen parenchyma, in fretwork change. There are low density foci with no enhancement surrounding the hepatic vascular vessels. The involvement of the intestinal wall is rare, with demonstrations of diffusively thickening of the intestinal wall. Multiple abscesses can be formed in the abdominal cavity, mesentery, retroperitoneum, with manifestations of cystic low density foci of different sizes in the abdominal cavity, mesentery, retroperitoneum, pancreas and both adrenal areas. Some abscesses may fuse. Enhanced scanning demonstrates marginal enhancement, with smooth wall in even thickness, and increased density of surrounding adipose that is turbid. The abdominal CT scanning demonstrations have been rarely reported, which may be related to insufficient knowledge about PM infection or less focus on the abdominal CT scanning demonstrations.

MR Imaging

There has been no study concerning MR imaging demonstrations of abdominal PM infection. It is speculated to be related to the more recent focus on the disease. Meanwhile, AIDS patients are rarely ordered MR imaging. However, MR imaging demonstrations may be similar to those by CT scanning.

Ultrasound

There are diffusively enlarged liver, thickened liver spot, but no confined echo abnormality. The spleen is diffusively enlarged. Multiple abscesses can be found in the abdominal cavity, commonly in peripheral hepatic space and paracolic sulci. The demonstrations include cystic liquid dark area and smooth inner wall of the cyst. Multiple lymphadenectasis in the mesentery and retroperitoneum, rarely have necrosis. The demonstrations include confluent pie liked or mass liked soft tissue lump, encompassing mesentery or retroperitoneal vascular vessels.

Case Study 1

A patient that was confirmatively diagnosed as having AIDS by the CDC. He/She complained of abdominal pain for 1 month. His/Her CD4 T cell count was 56/μl.

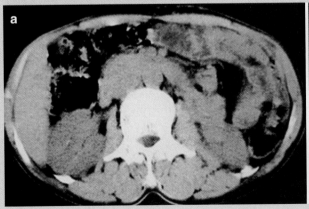 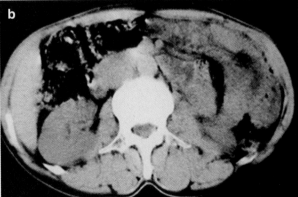

Fig. 21.5 (a–d) HIV/AIDS related abdominal Penicillium marneffei infection. (a, b) Epigastric plain CT scanning demonstrates obviously diffuse thickening of the small intestinal wall in the left upper abdomen. (c, d) Enhanced scanning demonstrates moderate enhancement of the thickened intestinal wall

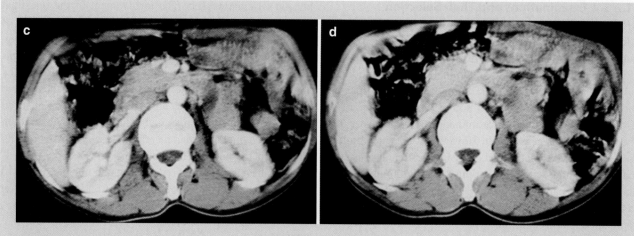

Fig.21.5 (continued)

Case Study 2

A patient that was confirmatively diagnosed as having AIDS by the CDC. He/She complained of abdominal pain. His/Her CD4 T cell count was 56/μl.

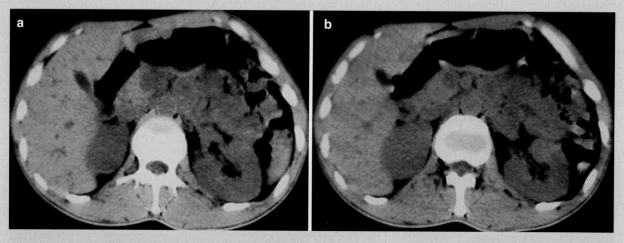

Fig. 21.6 (**a–e**) HIV/AIDS related Penicillium marneffei infection of abdominal lymph nodes. (**a–c**) Epigastric plain CT scanning demonstrates fused lymph nodes filling into the adipose space around the retroperitoneal major blood vessels with unclear boundary. (**d**) Enhanced scanning demonstrates obvious enhancement of the retroperitoneal blood vessels, slight enhancement of the fused lymph nodes, with sharp contrasts. (**e**) PSA staining demonstrates yeast phase of the Penicillium marneffei, in sausage liked appearance with both ends being dull round with obvious septa. Some are sphere shaped due to different perspective of the section. PAS ×1,000

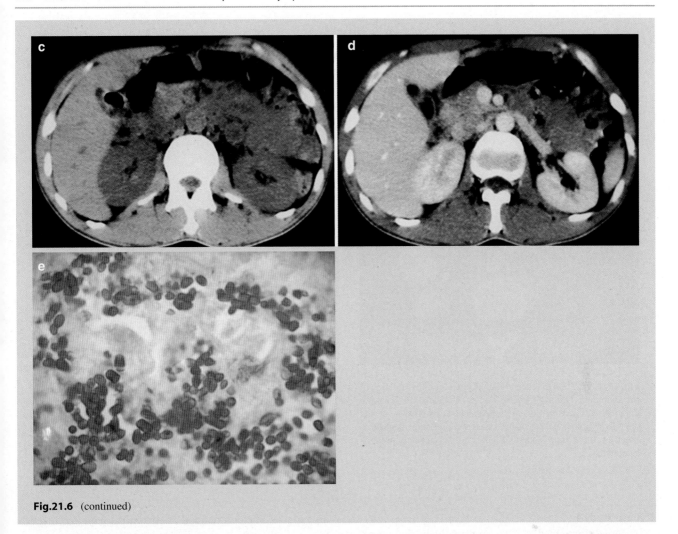

Fig. 21.6 (continued)

Case Study 3

A female patient that was confirmatively diagnosed as having AIDS by the CDC. Her husband had a history of drug abuse. She complained of abdominal pain and fever for more than 2 months, with accompanying face skin rash and diarrhea. Her CD4 T cell count was 5/μl.

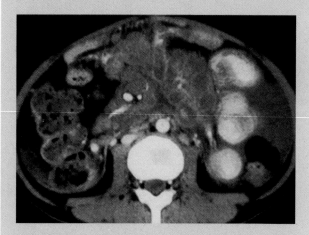

Fig. 21.7 HIV/AIDS related Penicillium marneffei infection of the abdominal lymph nodes. Abdominal enhanced CT scanning demonstrates retroperitoneal lymphadenectasis, fusion of the enlarged lymph nodes into a huge mass and ring shaped enhancement of the lymph nodes. It tends to be misdiagnosed as lymphoma

Case Study 4

A female patient that was confirmatively diagnosed as having AIDS by the CDC. Her husband had a history of drug abuse. She complained of abdominal pain and fever for more than 2 months, with accompanying face skin rash and diarrhea. Her CD4 T cell count was 5/μl.

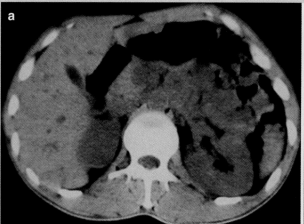
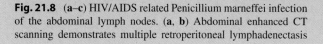
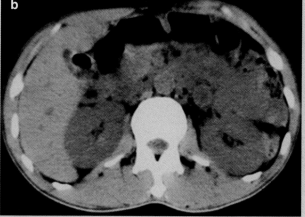

Fig. 21.8 (a–c) HIV/AIDS related Penicillium marneffei infection of the abdominal lymph nodes. (a, b) Abdominal enhanced CT scanning demonstrates multiple retroperitoneal lymphadenectasis with clear boundaries. (c) Enhanced scanning demonstrates slightly enhancement of the retroperitoneal lymph nodes

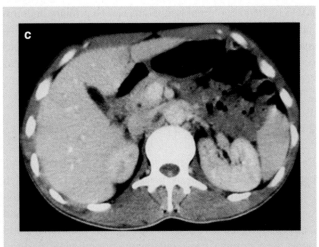

Fig.21.8 (continued)

21.2.3.6 Diagnostic Basis

AIDS complicated by Penicillium marneffei infection occurs only in patients with extremely compromised immunity. Therefore, its diagnosis should be based on the understanding of the patient's immunity. The diagnosis of HIV/AIDS related PSM should firstly understand its diagnostic basis. In addition, the patient's HIV infection, including its stage and CD4 T cell count should be fully understood.

HIV/AIDS related Penicillium marneffei infection is a general disease, involving multiple organs. In the diagnosis of abdominal PM infection, the imaging demonstrations of lymph nodes in the abdominal organs, abdominal cavity and retroperitoneum should be pain focused attention. In addition, the imaging demonstration of skin and chest should also be focused. During the treatment for HIV infected patients, patients with general infection such as skin necrotic papula should be paid focused attention on their clinical manifestations. For the cases with chills and fever (37.5–40.0 °C), shortness of breath, chest pain, nausea, vomiting, bloody stool, abdominal pain and diarrhea, the diagnostic imaging should be ordered. For the cases with abdominal lymphadenectasis, hepatomegaly and/or splenomegaly, as well as focal or diffuse parenchymal foci in the liver and spleen, especially cases with ring shaped enhancement in the liver and spleen parenchyma by enhanced CT scanning or perivascular low density foci and intestinal wall involvement, HIV/AIDS related PSM should be highly suspected. Especially, for the cases receiving common antibiotic therapy but ineffective, PSM should be considered. The related examinations and experimental treatment should be prescribed. The final definitive diagnosis should be based on blood culture or biopsy to find the double phase penicillium.

21.2.3.7 Differential Diagnosis

The imaging demonstrations of HIV/AIDS related PSM are non-specific. Similar demonstrations can also be found in cases of other opportunistic infections, such as disseminated histoplasmosis, cryptococcosis, tuberculosis and abscess. In addition, HIV/AIDS related PSM is commonly concurrent with other opportunistic infections, with diverse clinical manifestations, which presents difficulty for its diagnosis and differential diagnosis.

Blood-Borne Multiple Staphylococcus aureus Abscess

There are multiple cystic foci in the liver, spleen and retroperitoneum with clear boundaries which are in consistency with blood borne distribution. Accumulating and clustering rarely occur. Enhanced CT scanning demonstrates the bull's eyes sign, with smooth and even wall.

Abdominal and Retroperitoneal Lymphoma

It commonly involves the lymph nodes in the surrounding inferior area of the abdominal aorta below the lumbar second to third vertebrae level, in even density with rare necrosis. Enhanced CT scanning demonstrates even enhancement. Multiple enlarged lymph nodes can be fused to embedding the mesenteric vascular vessels, abdominal aorta and inferior vena cava, in a vascular embedding sign.

Abdominal Kaposi Sarcoma

The imaging demonstrations are characteristic, with typical demonstrations of distribution of the tumors along the vascular direction of the infiltrated organ. The involved lymph nodes have high density. In the cases with gastrointestinal tract involvement, the tumors are commonly fused to enlarge, with demonstrations of submucosal nodules and umbilicated as well as target sign or bull's eyes sign. In the cases with the lesions extending to the intestinal wall, the manifestations include polyps liked mass and irregular thickening of the folds. KS in the liver and spleen has manifestations of hepatomegaly, splenomegaly and enhancement of the small low density foci. The accompanying para-aorta lymphadenectasis may be only demonstrated as abdominal lymphadenectasis.

Abdominal Tuberculosis

The CT scanning demonstrations of both diseases are similar. Abdominal tuberculous lymphadenectasis tends to more commonly involve the hepatic hilum and retroperitoneal lymph nodes. The central necrosis is extensive. The lesions of the liver and spleen have manifestations of diffuse miliary small nodules. Abdominal lymphadenectasis in the cases of PSM tends to more commonly involve mesenteric lymph nodes, with slight necrosis or with no obvious necrosis. The degree of enhancement is more obvious. The hepatic lesions are comparatively extensive.

21.3 HIV/AIDS Related Retroperitoneal Lymphoma

The incidence of lymphoma in HIV infected patients is up to 4–10 %, second only to KS. The incidence of non-Hodgkin's lymphoma (NHL) is obviously higher than that of Hodgkin's lymphoma (HL). The pathogens and pathogenesis of lymphoma are still unknown, which may be related to the following factors.

1. Virus. HIV/AIDS related lymphoma is closely related to EBV and HHV-8, which belong to herpes virus family. The tissue culture of human Burkitt lymphoma has been found to contain EB virus. With its antigen to detect the patients' serum, it was found that 80 % patients are antibody positive. The HIV induced immunodeficiency may activate EB virus infection to cause lymphatic hyperplasia disease, lymphoma, which is commonly Burkitt lymphoma related to EB virus.
2. Radiation. Long-term exposure to radioactive substances may induce the occurrence of lymphoma.
3. Immunity. It has been internationally reported that the T lymphocytes in HIV infected and AIDS patients have persistent and abnormal activation and the degree of cellular activation is highly related to the progression of the disease. AIDS is induced by HIV infection, with large quantity HIV in the patients' serum. HIV can promote T lymphocytes to proliferate, while AIDS can exacerbate the compromised immunity of the human body to promote the development of T cell lymphoma. Reversely, lymphoma can promote the rapid progression of AIDS. With the same principle, chronic antigen stimulation by B cell can promote the occurrence of B cell lymphoma.
4. Impaired defense mechanisms to cause abnormalities of oncogenes and cancer suppressor genes. HIV infection destroys the body's defense mechanism, the oncogenes are activated and cancer suppressor genes impaired or even inactivated to cause the occurrence of tumors.
5. Mediation abnormalities of Cytokines/growth factors, whose mechanisms are still unknown.
6. Genetic factors. Congenital chromosome aberration causes immunodeficiency disorder. Or, congenital susceptibility due to DNA damage causes dysfunctional DNA repair. Both can be factors inducing oncogenesis.

The above six factors fully explain the etiology and pathogenesis of lymphoma, which are related to virus, radiation, immunosuppression, gene abnormalities and hereditary. Clinically, the occurrence and progression of the disease is mostly related to immunosuppression. Although HIV infects T cells, occurrence of NHL is mostly B lymphocytes lymphoma. HIV/AIDS related lymphoma has high malignancy, which can be originated from local lymph nodes or extranodal lymphoid tissues. In its advanced stage, the lesions extensively involve lymph nodes and lymphoid tissues. HIV/

AIDS related abdominal lymphoma can be primary abdominal lymphoma or primary retroperitoneal lymphoma or primary abdominal organs lymphoma. In this section, we focus on retroperitoneal lymphoma. Other abdominal lymphomas see corresponding chapter and section.

21.3.1 Pathogens and Pathogenesis

Retroperitoneal space refers to space in the loose tissue between retroperitoneum and posterior abdominal wall, which is a huge potential space for filling of organs and various tissues. It has a deep location, with large range, many tissues and many major blood vessels (including the abdominal aorta trunk, the abdominal trunk and the superior mesenteric artery) and their branches. Many lymphoid tissues accumulate around the blood vessels. In some retroperitoneal organs such as pancreas, duodenum, colonic mesentery and para-intestine, there are abundant lymphatic tissues. The occurrence of lymphoma in the space is due to the above mentioned six factors and its abundant content of lymphatic tissues.

21.3.2 Pathophysiological Basis

HIV/AIDS related lymphoma is commonly NHL, including the subtypes of diffuse large cell, small non-cleaved cell Burkitt and large cell immunoblast, accounting for 80–90 %. The rarely found HIV/AIDS related lymphomas are ki-1 anaplastic large cell, vascular large cell, mucosa related lymphoma, primary T cell lymphoma, Sezary syndrome, plasmocytoma or multiple myeloma. Although HIV infects T cells, the occurrence of NHL is mostly B cell lymphoma. The incidence of T cell lymphoma in AIDS patients is not higher than that of lymphoma in general population, which indicates that T cell lymphoma, is not prevalent in AIDS patients. The pathological type of HIV/AIDS related lymphoma has certain relationship with its clinical manifestations. Burkitt occurs in a younger age group, with an early occurrence than other subtypes, mostly in lymph nodes, bone marrow and muscles. Large cell immunoblast and diffuse large cell occur in an elder age group, with a late occurrence than other subtypes. It commonly occurs in the central nervous system, gastrointestinal tract, retroperitoneum, oral cavity, anus and other locations that are less involved by non-HIV/AIDS related lymphoma.

21.3.3 Clinical Symptoms and Signs

There are symptoms and signs of emaciation, fever and night sweating, diarrhea, thrush, intractable cough, pityriasis rosea, systemic lymphadenectasis, anemia and pneumocystis carinii pneumonia. Meanwhile, there is a cervical painless mass that is progressively enlarging, being hard with no mobility, no surface redness and swelling and no surface effusion. Multiple enlarged superficial lymph nodes are palpable in the neck, auxiliary and groin, with accompanying difficulty swallowing. Fever, night sweating and weight loss of more than 10 % are known as the B symptoms of AIDS. In the cases with HIV/AIDS related lymphoma, the incidence of B symptoms is up to 82 %. The occurrence of these symptoms indicates possibility of potential opportunistic infection, such as mycobacterial infection. After exclusion of such causes, it is most likely to be lymphoma related fever and weight loss. Generally speaking, manifestations of HIV/AIDS related lymphoma is mixed with manifestations of other complications. Symptoms and signs other than lymphadenectasis are non-specific.

21.3.4   Examinations and Their Selection

There are a variety of imaging examinations, showing different advantages in assessing retroperitoneal lymphoma. Ultrasound, as a basic and noninvasive examination, is simple and convenient for examinations and reexaminations to find the enlarged lymph nodes. In addition, it can be applied to observe structural changes and blood flow for dynamic observation and following up examinations. However, due to the deep location of retroperitoneum and the interference of gastrointestinal gas, it has a high rate of missed diagnosis. Abdominal CT scanning, especially enhanced scanning demonstrates foci more favorably than ultrasound, which is an important examination for the diagnosis. It can help to understand the relationship between retroperitoneal lymphoma and its surrounding tissues, its amount and its lesions range. CT scanning is also applied to guide lymph nodes puncture for biopsy. MR imaging is less commonly applied for abdominal examinations. It can also favorably demonstrate the distribution, size and involvement of retroperitoneal lymph nodes. Nuclear medicine examinations are less applied than MR imaging.

21.3.5   Imaging Demonstrations

21.3.5.1   CT Scanning

Generally lymphadenectasis is one of the common demonstrations of its diagnostic imaging. The superficial lymphadenectasis is commonly found in the neck, axillary, and inguen, with obviously enlarged lymph nodes in a diameter of above 3 cm. They can accumulate into mass. The larger lymphadenectasis may have central necrosis, with limited necrotic area. Abdominal lymphoma commonly involves surrounding inferior area of the abdominal aorta below the level of lumbar second to third vertebra, with even density and rare necrosis. Enhanced CT scanning demonstrates even enhancement, and fusion of multiple enlarged lymph nodes to embed mesenteric vascular vessels, abdominal aorta and the inferior vena cava, in a vascular embedding sign. It often involves the gastrointestinal tract, commonly the stomach and small intestine, with manifestations of irregular thickening of the mucosa, nodular changes and accompanying penetrating ulcer and lumen stenosis. There may be also enlargements of the liver, spleen and kidneys as well as focal changes. The intrahepatic lesions can be singular or multiple. Plain and enhanced CT scanning demonstrates low density nodular foci, with thin marginal enhancement.

21.3.5.2   MR Imaging

Multiple retroperitoneal lymphadenectasis can be found, with similar distribution and morphology to CT scanning demonstrations. The multiple enlarged lymph nodes fuse into mass to encompass the major vessels and the branches of abdominal aorta, such as the renal arteries, superior and inferior mesenteric arteries and abdominal trunk. By T1WI, it is a moderate even signal, with occasional liquid liked low density area of the central necrosis in the larger lymph nodes. By T2WI, it is a moderately high signal. By adipose suppression sequence, it is more clearly demonstrated. And the major vessels and their main branches are in extremely low signal due to void flow effect, penetrating the fused lymph nodes. The arterial branches run rigidly but with no obvious stenosis from invasion. The manifestations of intestinal lymphoma see the chapter and section of gastrointestinal lymphoma.

21.3.5.3   Ultrasound

Gastrointestinal lymphoma, due to the interference by the gas in the lumen, shows unfavorable ultrasound demonstrations. Intestinal filling of the intestine in a low tension state can improve its ultrasound demonstration. But due to the inconvenient procedures for preparation, it gains less clinical applications. Ultrasound can well define obvious retroperitoneal and mesenteric lymphadenectasis, with demonstrations of parenchymal nodules and fused mass as well as even interior echo and weak blood flow signal. In the cases with inner necrosis in the larger mass, it is demonstrated as low echo or liquid dark area, with rapid strong arterial blood flow signal penetrating through the nodules and masses.

Case Study 1

A patient that was confirmatively diagnosed as having AIDS by the CDC. He/She complained of abdominal pain. His/Her CD4 T cell count was 26/µl.

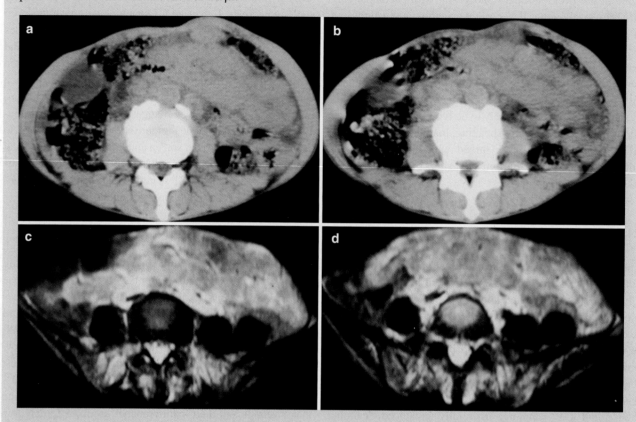

Fig. 21.9 (**a–d**) HIV/AIDS related retroperitoneal lymphoma. (**a**, **b**) Abdominal plain CT scanning demonstrates multiple lymph nodes surrounding retroperitoneal aorta with some enlarged. They are in moderate and even density, with unclear boundary and some fuse together. The distance between the aorta and the inferior vena cava is enlarged. (**c**, **d**) MR imaging demonstrates the middle and lower abdomen, with transverse sectional T2WI demonstrations of parenchymal moderately high signal of soft tissues surrounding the bilateral common iliac arteries. The void common iliac artery is thinner due to compression

Case Study 2

A patient that was confirmatively diagnosed as having AIDS by the CDC. He/She complained of abdominal pain. His/Her CD4 T cell count was 56/μl.

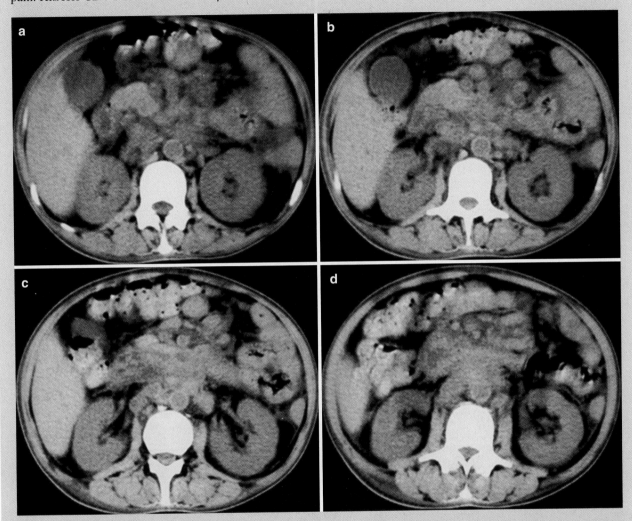

Fig. 21.10 (**a–d**) HIV/AIDS related retroperitoneal lymphoma. (**a–d**) Abdominal plain CT scanning demonstrates multiple lymph nodes with varying sizes and moderate density surrounding retroperitoneal major vessels, with unclear boundaries to each other. Some fuse into mass anterior to the aorta. There are forward migration of the duodenum due to compression and decreased density of the aorta lumen that is obviously lower than the arterial wall

Case Study 3

A patient that was confirmatively diagnosed as having AIDS by the CDC. He/She has a history of extramarital affair and a history of drug and food allergy. He/She had sustained AIDS for 8 years, with complaints of abdominal pain. His/Her CD4 T cell count was 44/μl.

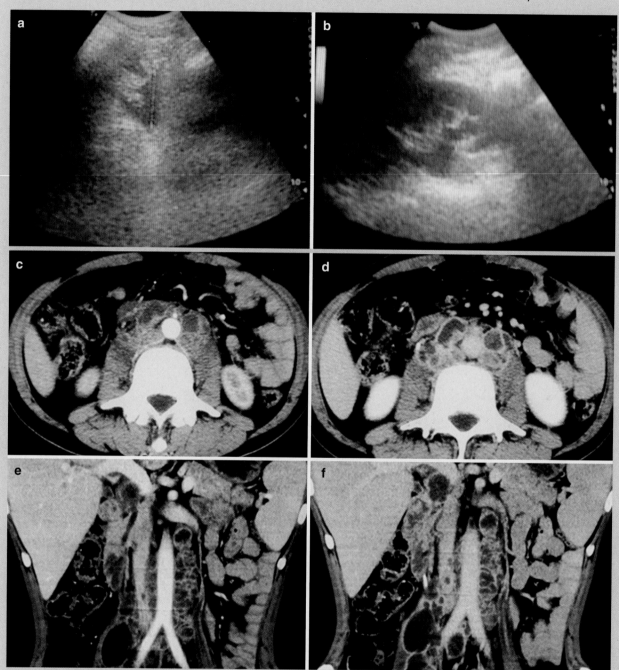

Fig. 21.11 (**a–f**) HIV/AIDS related retroperitoneal lymphoma. (**a, b**) Ultrasound demonstrates multiple round liked low echo. (**c, d**) Epigastric enhanced CT scanning demonstrates multiple enlarged lymph nodes accumulating around the aorta to form a mass and fuse together. Most interior tissues show liquefaction with no enhancement and moderate marginal enhancement. (**e, f**) Coronal 3-D reconstruction demonstrates multiple retroperitoneal enlarged lymph nodes accumulating around the aorta to fuse

Case Study 4

A patient that was confirmatively diagnosed as having AIDS by the CDC. He/She complained of low back pain for more than 1 month and finding of a cervical mass for half a month. One month ago, he/she suffered from lower back pain with no known causes that aggravated during activities but relieved during resting in posture of lying down. There was sometimes referred pain in the lower extremities with no definitive location and night sweating. Half a month ago, he/she found a mass at the left neck, with no redness, swelling and fever. His/Her CD4 T cell count was 86/μl.

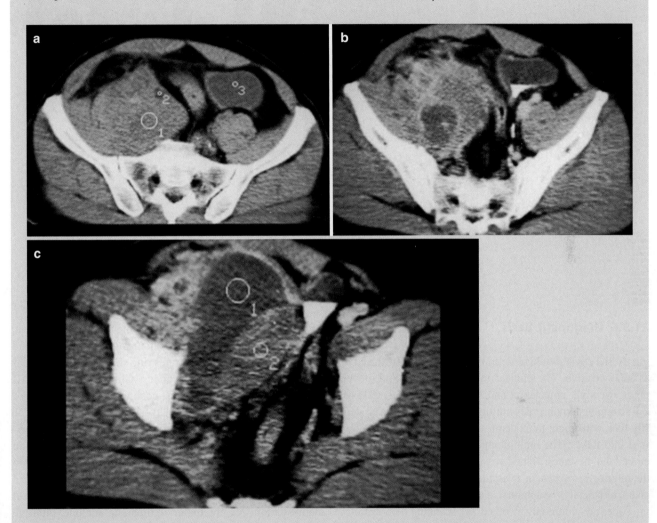

Fig. 21.12 (a–e) HIV/AIDS related pelvic lymphoma. (a–c) CT scanning demonstrates a huge solid and cystic soft tissue density mass in the right pelvis, with quite clear boundary. (d, e) MR imaging demonstrates the huge solid and cystic soft tissue density mass in the right pelvis in uneven abnormal signal. Enhanced imaging demonstrates uneven abnormal enhancement with clear boundary. By biopsy of cervical lymph nodes and right lower abdominal mass in a local hospital, the pathological analysis was diffuse B large cell lymphoma of lymph nodes (ABC immune subtype). The tumor cells have obvious heteromorphology, with differentiation towards plasmablast. The immune phenotype are CD20 (+/−), CD79a (+), CD38 (+) and CD30 (−), ALK (−), ki67 indicating a tumor cells proliferation index of above 90 %

Fig.21.12 (continued)

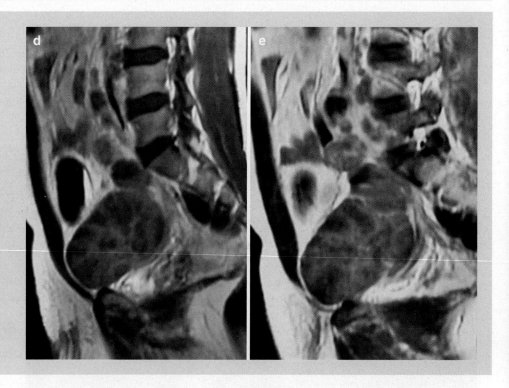

21.3.6 Diagnostic Basis

Firstly, the cases should be definitively diagnosed by the CDC as HIV positive. The clinical manifestations include fever, night sweating, emaciation and systemic lymphadenectasis. CT scanning demonstrates multiple retroperitoneal even density foci, with slight to moderate even enhancement. The foci fuse into flakes. The multiple enlarged lymph nodes fuse to embed the mesenteric blood vessels, the abdominal aorta and the inferior vena cava, in a vascular embedding sign, which is characteristically lymphoma. The stomach and the small intestines are commonly involved. CT scanning demonstrates irregular thickening of the mucosa in nodular changes, with accompanying penetrating ulceration and lumen stenosis. There are also enlargements of the liver, spleen and kidneys as well as multiple focal changes. In the clinically undiagnosed cases, if typical imaging demonstrations are found, HIV/AIDS related lymphoma should be high suspected. Further examinations should be ordered to define the diagnosis.

21.3.7 Differential Diagnosis

21.3.7.1 Retroperitoneal Lymph Node Tuberculosis

Both have imaging demonstrations of multiple enlarged lymph nodes in the retroperitoneum and the mesentery, but with different characteristics. In the cases of lymph nodes

TB, the enlarged lymph nodes distribute more concentrative. By CT scanning, lymph nodes calcification can be found and enhanced scanning demonstrates ring shaped or multilocular enhancement of the lymph nodes. Clinically, there is TB toxic symptoms, tuberculin test positive and complication of abdominal organs TB such as liver and spleen TB. The CT scanning demonstrations are similar to abscesses. The peritoneum is commonly involved, with extensive thickening in pie shape. In the cases of lymphoma, the foci are in even density with clear boundary but no calcification. Enhanced scanning demonstrates slight even enhancement. The typical manifestations of malignant lymphoma include multiple enlarged lymph nodes and their fusion can also embed the mesenteric vascular vessels, the abdominal aorta and the inferior vena cave, in a vascular embedding sign. The sign is characteristically lymphoma.

21.3.7.2 Retroperitoneal Lymph Node Reactive Hyperplasia

It has complex causes and is more common in young and middle aged adults. Its pathogenesis is chronic infection and absorption of the destroyed tissues of the corresponding tissues and organs drainage to involve the lymph nodes of the drainage area, leading to chronic lymphadenitis. Its manifestations are complex, including various reactive hyperplasia in lymph nodes, such as chronic diffuse lymphocyte proliferation, follicular hyperplasia and sinus histiocytosis. CT demonstrations are similar to those of lymphoma. There are retroperitoneal multiple enlarged lymph nodes and their fusion into flakes. Necrosis is rare and the vascular embedding sign is rare. The definitive diagnosis depends on the dynamic observation and puncture for biopsy after anti-inflammatory therapies.

21.4 HIV/AIDS Related Primary Coelom Lymphoma

HIV/AIDS related primary body cavity based lymphoma (BCBL) is also known as primary exudative lymphoma (PEL). It was firstly described in 1989 by Knowles et al. [6]. In blood and lymphatic system neoplasms classification by WHO in 2008, it is categorized as a subtype of diffuse large B cell lymphoma, commonly invading the serum including pleural, pericardium, peritoneum, articular membrane and rarely meninges. The manifestation is large quantity effusion in the serous cavity.

21.4.1 Pathogens and Pathogenesis

The malignant cell of PEL is a monoclonal B cell, expressing CD38 and HHV-8 gene and being EB virus positive. It is still unknown that the exact B cell subgroup that these malignant cells and the biological mechanism of their growth in only body cavity. Some scholars believe that they are undifferentiated B cells. However, it is also believed that the occurrence of PEL is not limited to one stage of B cell differentiation. They may represent the transformation of different differentiation stages of B cell.

The role that EB virus plays in the oncogenesis of PEL has not yet been clarified. It does not play an important role as it plays for the occurrence of primary central nervous system lymphoma (PCNSL). The role of HHV-8 infection in the oncogenesis is also unknown, during which a HHV-8 encoded latent nuclear antigen may play an important role. It causes HHV-8 DNA adhere to the chromosome of the host cells during mitosis to separate HHV-8 episome from the daughter cells. Studies have demonstrated that generally activated transcription factors (NF-κB), or other factors is related to survival of HHV-8 infected PEL cells. By competitive blockage of apoptosis signal, the suppressed NF-κB can result in induced apoptosis. HHV-8 genome encoded virus IL-6 is a cytokine that promotes plasma cells and angiogenesis. In vitro studies have demonstrated that PEL cells can secrete IL-6 and antisense oligonucleotide almost fully suppressed the growth of these cell lines. However, it fails to inhibit the growth of the non-HHV-8 infected two B cell lymphoma cell lines. The above in vitro experiments indicate that virus IL-6 is an autocrine growth factor that promotes the growth of PEL. In addition, PEL expressed human IL-10 is possibly another important autocrine growth factor.

21.4.2 Pathophysiological Basis

Lesions are commonly found in the serosa of the body cavity (pleura, pericardium and peritoneum). It destroys the integrity of the serosa to cause diffuse thickening of the serosa and large quantity malignant effusion. The typical manifestation is often only an involved body cavity, with no formation of visible lumps as well as no swelling of lymph nodes and organs. In very few cases, there are lesions out of the body cavities with/without effusions, with increased IL-6 and IL-10 in the effusion. Although PEL does not tend to spread throughout the body, it can lead to the destruction of local organs and tissues, with poor prognosis. The data show that the average survival time after its diagnosis is 75 days (6–240 days) and the effusion of malignant lymphoma is the direct cause of death.

21.4.3 Clinical Symptom and Signs

The common symptoms and signs include serous cavity effusions such as ascites, pleural effusion and pericardial effusion. Clinically, patients usually present a variety of serous cavity involvements, with large quantity effusion and related clinical manifestations. In the cases with large quantity pleural effusion, the clinical symptoms include chest distress, shortness of breath and difficulty breathing. The patients also suffer from abdominal distension, anorexia and indigestion, generally without abdominal pain, diarrhea and fever. The serous effusion contains highly malignant lymphocytes, but with no definitive mass foci. Therefore, pain is clinically rarely found and usually occurs late.

21.4.4 Examinations and Their Selection

Due to its only manifestation of serous cavity effusion with rare invasion to other organs, PEL can be defined by findings of serous cavity effusion through various imaging examinations. Chest X-ray demonstrates amount of pleural effusion and its dynamic changes, which is simple and economical. Plain abdominal X-ray can demonstrate large quantity abdominal effusion, but less sensitive to small quantity effusion. Therefore, it is of less value in assessing abdominal cavity. Ultrasound has unique values in assessing pleural, abdominal and pericardial effusions. Its advantages of noninvasiveness, simple manipulation and low cost render it to be applicable for dynamic observation and assessment of the body cavity based effusion. CT scanning and MR imaging can clearly and accurately assess the pleural, abdominal and pericardial effusions, especially MR imaging. However, due to the favorable information provided by simple and economical X-ray and ultrasound, MR imaging is less applied. In addition to assessing the body cavity based effusion by CT scanning and MR imaging, they can also assess the thickening of the serosa, mass and organ involvement. Therefore, they can apply for the differential diagnosis.

Imaging examinations only demonstrate the body cavity effusions, which is not sufficient for the diagnosis of PEL. The final definitive diagnosis should be based on the finding of malignant cells in the body fluids. Therefore, the serous effusion puncture for fluid examination is very important. By serous cavity puncture for fluid examination, malignant cells can generally be found. Morphologically, malignant cells are between diffuse large B cell lymphoma (immunoblast variant) and anaplastic large cell lymphoma, with a phenotype being CD45 and CD30 positive. It obviously lacks B cell and T cell related antigen expression. In addition, it has no c-MYC gene rearrangement, with detection of HHV-8 in the effusion.

21.4.5 Imaging Demonstrations

21.4.5.1 X-ray Examination

For the cases with pleural effusion, the orthostatic chest X-ray demonstrates unilateral or bilateral pleural effusion, in small or large quantity. Due to the coverage by pleural effusion, pleural thickening cannot be defined. The small quantity ascites cannot be defined by abdominal plain X-ray and the large quantity ascites can be defined by orthostatic abdominal plain X-ray for enlarged abdomen in frog belly liked state. The structures cannot be clearly defined. Supine lateral projection plain X-ray demonstrates anterior accumulation of intestines in floating appearance.

21.4.5.2 Ultrasound

It demonstrates even dark areas of the pleural, pericardial and abdominal effusions as well as its thickness. By abdominal ultrasound, parenchymal organs rarely show abnormal echo, with findings of small intestinal accumulation but no definite solid mass.

21.4.5.3 CT Scanning

Chest CT scanning demonstrates pleural effusion. With the increase of the effusion, the adjacent lung tissues show atelectasis due to compression. Enhanced scanning clearly demonstrates pleural thickening, with no definite solid mass. CT scanning demonstrates pericardial effusion as evenly thickened pericardium, with even and liquid density. Small quantity pericardial effusion and thickened pericardium is difficult to be distinguished and can be differentiated by enhanced scanning. Abdominal CT scanning demonstrates large quantity ascites in even density to fill the abdominal cavity. The ascites also is demonstrated to surround the liver and spleen as well as to push the small intestines forwards for accumulation. By hypotonic or enhanced scanning, the accumulated small intestines are demonstrated to have slight diffuse thickening of the wall, with adhesion and no obvious mass sign.

21.4.5.4 MR Imaging

The distribution of pleural, abdominal and pericardial effusions is the same as those by CT scanning. The effusions are in even liquid low signal on T1WI and even highest signal on T2WI, with no definitive solid mass signal and filling defect. FLAIR imaging demonstrates thickened pleura, pericardium and peritoneum, with accumulated intestinal tract. The thickened intestinal wall is adhered together with unnatural running course.

Case Study 1

A male patient aged 41 years was confirmatively diagnosed as having AIDS by the CDC. He complained of fever, cough, weak limbs, progressively weight loss, skin papula, abdominal prominence and ascites. By ascites examination, it was clear and yellow with no coagulation, Rivalta test negative, with a cell count 70×10 %, mononuclear 0.36, multinuclear 0.64. By blood biochemistry: TP 12.1 g/L, CL 97.4 mmol/L. His CD4 T cell count was 30/μl.

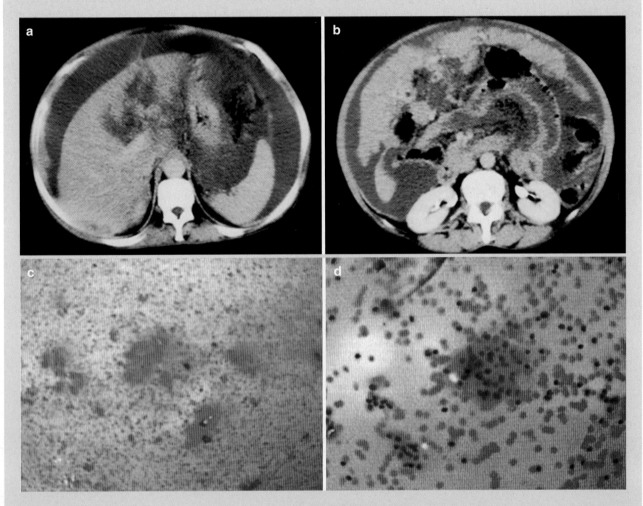

Fig. 21.13 (a–d) HIV/AIDS related primary abdominal effusive lymphoma. (a, b) Enhanced CT scanning demonstrates diffuse thickening of the peritoneum, no definite formation of lumps and no retroperitoneal lymphadenectasis. (c, d) Microscopic cytology of the ascites demonstrates large quantity protein contents, a few lymphocytes and mesothelial cells

21.4.6 Diagnostic Basis

The case should be clinically confirmed as having HIV infection. There are general serous pleural, abdominal and pericardial effusions and residues of joint capsule liquid. No accompanying lumps by diagnostic imaging. The definitive diagnosis depends on puncture for cytological and other related laboratory tests. The body fluid is serous, with detection of highly malignant lymphocytes, HHV-8 and EB virus positive.

21.4.7 Differential Diagnosis

HIV/AIDS related primary effusive lymphoma is mainly manifested as malignant effusion of the body cavity, thickened serosa but no definitive lumps. Therefore, diagnostic imaging demonstrations are less sufficient for the diagnosis. The body cavity based effusion can only indicate the diagnosis. The definitive diagnosis should be based on pathology to differentiate it from other lymphoma subtypes.

Appendix

Differentiation of HIV/AIDS related gastrointestinal lymphoma, PSM, abdominal TB and retroperitoneal lymphoma

	Clinical symptoms	Abdominal and retroperitoneal lymphadenectasis	Gastrointestinal involvement	Liver and spleen involvements
HIV/AIDS-related PSM	Irregular fever Cough with sputum Hemoptysis Abdominal pain Diarrhea Lymphadenectasis Skin rash Hepatosplenomegaly Abdominal mass	Mesentery, portal area, hepatoduodenal ligament, lymph nodes surrounding superior abdominal aorta, mesenteric lymphadenectasis in sandwich sign	With involvement of the stomach, duodenum and jejunum, thickened intestinal wall and accompanying upper gastrointestinal obstruction and acute pancreatitis	Hepatosplenomegaly with diffuse low density nodules, fretwork sign by enhanced CT scanning
HIV/AIDS related abdominal TB	B symptoms of AIDS TB toxic symptoms Abdominal pain Diarrhea Abdominal mass Hepatosplenomegaly	Involving the same areas as above, Sandwich sign Lymph nodes tend to form TB abscesses Ring shaped and multilocular enhancement by enhanced scanning that is characteristic Enlarged lymph nodes smaller than 4 cm	Mainly involving the terminal ileum, cecum, and ascending colon, irregular thickening of the intestinal wall or mass formation, peritoneal thickening like a pie	Miliary nodules in the liver and spleen, ring shaped enhancement
HIV/AIDS related retroperitoneal lymphoma	B symptoms of AIDS Systemic lymphadenectasis Hepatosplenomegaly Abdominal mass	Mainly involving the lymph nodes in surrounding inferior area of the abdominal aorta below the lumbar second to third vertebra, even density and necrosis Even enhancement by CT scanning Multiple lymphadenectasis with fusion to embed the mesenteric blood vessels, abdominal aorta and the inferior vena cava in a vascular embedding sign The vascular sign and even enhancement are characteristic manifestations	Mainly involving the stomach and small intestine, irregular thickening of the mucosa with nodular changes, with penetrating ulcerations and intestinal stenosis	Hepatosplenomegaly Singular or multiple focal lesions in low density foci by plain and enhanced CT scanning, with thin marginal enhancement Extrahepatic and intrahepatic bile ducts dilation
HIV/AIDS related gastrointestinal lymphoma	B symptoms of AIDS Abdominal pain Abdominal distension Diarrhea Abdominal tenderness and rebound pain Ascites sign positive General lymphadenectasis	Mostly involving mesenteric lymph nodes, with thickening of the mesentery in to pie appearance and central necrosis	Extensive diffuse thickening of the intestinal wall, and slightly lumen stenosis, which are its characteristic manifestations, infiltration and adhesion of intestinal lumen, irregular thickening of the mesentery	The liver and spleen can be involved, with no special changes

Notes: (1) B symptoms of AIDS including fever, night sweating and weight loss of above 10 %. (2) The sandwich sign is the anterior and dorsal enlargement of the lymph nodes in the mesentery, with central mesenteric vascular vessels

Extended Reading

1. Balthazar EJ, Noordhoorn M, Megibow AJ, Gordon RB. CT of small-bowel lymphoma in immunocompetent patients and patients with AIDS: comparison of findings. Am J Roentgenol. 1997;168: 675–80.
2. Herts BR, Megibow AJ, Birnbaum BA, Kanzer GK, Noz ME. High-attenuation lymphadenopathy in AIDS patients: significance of findings at CT. Radiology. 1992;185:777–81.
3. His ED, Foreman KE, Duggan J, et al. Molecular and pathologic characterization of an AIDS-related body cavity-based lymphoma, including ultrastructural demonstration of human herpesvirus-8: a case report. Am J Surg Pathol. 1998;22(4):493–9.
4. Jeffe WS. Primary body cavity-based AIDS-related lymphoma. Evaluation of a new disease entity. Am J Clin Pathol. 1996;105(2): 141–3.
5. Jimenez-Heffernan JA, Hardisson D, Palacios J, et al. Adrenal gland leiomyoma in a child with acquired immunodeficiency syndrome. Pediatr Pathol Lab Med. 1995;15(6):923–6.
6. Knowlwes DM, Inghirami G, Ubriaco A, et al. Molecular genetic analysis of three AIDS-associated neoplasms of uncertain lineage demonstrates their B-cell derivation and the possible pathogenetic role of the Epstein-Barr virus [J]. Blood. 1989;73(3):792–9.
7. Kudeken N, Kawakami K, Kusano N, et al. Cell-mediated immunity in host resistance against infection caused by Penicillium marneffei [J]. J Med Vet Mycol. 1996;34(6):371–8.
8. Mead JH, Mason TE. Lymphoma versus AIDS. Am J Clin Pathol. 1983;80(4):546–7.
9. Townsend RR, Laing FC, Jwffrey Jr R, Bottles K. Abdominal lymphoma in AIDS: evaluation with US. Radiology. 1989;171: 719–24.

HIV/AIDS Related Urogenital Disease

Contents

22.1 An Overview of HIV/AIDS Related Urogenital Diseases

HIV/AIDS may involve all of the systems and organs, including the urinary system. In HIV infected patients, about 30 % kidney dysfunctions. HIV infection can involve glomerulus, renal tubule, renal interstitium and blood vessels. HIV/AIDS related nephropathy (HIVAN) is the most common in the terminal stage of AIDS, which is the common reason for the end-stage renal failure (ESRF) and is related with the progression of AIDS and the occurrence of death. IgA nephropathy, heroin associated nephropathy and hypertensive nephropathy can also be found in AIDS patients. Opportunistic infections also involve kidneys. CMV infection is one of the most common opportunistic infections of kidney, accounting for about 12.8 %. It is believed to accelerate the development of HIVAN. Renal infection induced by fungal infections is likely to develop into intrarenal or perinephral abscesses, with possible concurrent involvements of the spleen and the liver. Usually, tuberculosis infection occurs prior to other opportunistic infections. Renal tuberculosis is a part of systemic TB. In cases of ARL, 6–12 % has the invaded kidney. KS is a commonly found renal neoplasm in AIDS patients. In the cases of HIV/AIDS related infections or cancer, 20–40 % has occurrence of acute kidney failure.

The invasion of HIV/AIDS to the reproductive system can cause diseases including HIV/AIDS related opportunistic infections and neoplasms. Of all the infective diseases, infections of Cryptococcus and CMV are more common. Of neoplastic diseases, KS is more common. In female patients, HIV infection has certain correlationship with the occurrence of cervical carcinoma.

H. Li (ed.), *Radiology of HIV/AIDS*,
DOI 10.1007/978-94-007-7823-8_22, © Springer Science+Business Media Dordrecht and People's Medical Publishing House 2014

22.2 HIV/AIDS Related Nephropathy

HIV/AIDS related nephropathy (HIVAN) is the leading cause for HIV/AIDS related renal diseases. HIVAN tends to occur in certain races and 90 % HIVAN patients are the black people. In the etiological factors for ESRF in the black people aged 20–64 years, HIVAN ranks the third. The prognosis of HIVAN is determined by the HIV infection instead of the kidneys. The diagnosis of HIVAN is the indicator of the advanced HIV infection.

22.2.1 Pathogen and Pathogenesis

Currently, the pathogenesis of HIVAN is still unknown, which is possibly related to the following factors: (1) direct infection of HIV to the kidney parenchymal cells, and then invasion of the renal epithelial cells including visceral epithelial cells and tubular epithelial cells; (2) indirect renal lesions after the coding products of HIV in the blood circulation being absorbed by renal cells; (3) indirect renal lesions caused by the cytokines released from HIV infected lymphocytes and mononuclear cells in the kidney. In addition, it may also be related to gene and environmental factors.

22.2.2 Pathophysiological Basis

The pathologic changes of HIVAN are characteristic, mainly including enlarged kidney volume, proliferation of epithelial cells, the whole or segmental contraction and collapse of the glomerular capillary wall with obvious podocyte proliferation, apoptosis in the glomerulus and renal interstitium. By light microscopy, the findings of whole collapse of any one glomerulus or segmental collapse in more than 20 % glomerulus should be suspected as the disease. Under an electron microscope, large quantity tubuloreticular inclusion bodies (in 80–90 % HIVAN patients) in endothelial cells and interstitial leukocytes of the glomerulus can facilitate to define the diagnosis.

22.2.3 Clinical Symptoms and Signs

Including serious albuminuria (above 3.5 g/day), azotemia, water electrolyte imbalance, hematuria by naked eyes, normal blood pressure, normal/enlarged kidney, acute progressive renal dysfunction. The normal blood pressure is characteristically HIVAN.

22.2.4 Examinations and Their Selection

22.2.4.1 Laboratory Tests
The urine precipitation examination demonstrates serious albuminuria (above 3.5 g/day), oval liposome and lipuria. A large quantity huge waxy casts is characteristically HIVAN.

22.2.4.2 CT Scanning and Ultrasound
The demonstrations are non-specific, with main manifestations of normal/enlarged kidney volume.

22.2.5 Imaging Demonstrations

22.2.5.1 CT Scanning
CT scanning demonstrates enlarged kidney volume. Plain CT scanning can occasionally demonstrate increased density of the kidney medulla, which may be caused by abnormalities of the renal tubule in the cases of HIVAN. Enhanced scanning demonstrates the kidney with stripes of enhancement.

22.2.5.2 Ultrasound
It demonstrates normal/enlarged kidney volume, with unclearly defined cortex and medulla. These demonstrations may be caused by focal/segmental sclerosis of glomerulus, and tubular dilation filled by protein casts. But echoes demonstrated by ultrasound fail to directly show the severity of renal lesions.

22.2.6 Diagnostic Basis

In the advanced stage of HIV infection, albuminuria occurs (being higher than 1 g/24 h), with increased creatinine. By the diagnostic imaging, the kidney is found enlarged and renal failure with other etiologic factors excluded. The cases with no typical clinical manifestations or ineffective treatment by antiretroviral therapy or other therapies should be performed kidney tissues biopsy to define the diagnosis.

22.2.7 Differential Diagnosis

22.2.7.1 IgA Nephropathy
It is commonly found in white people, with manifestations of hematuria by naked eyes or microscopy, slight/moderate renal dysfunction, albuminuria lower than 1 g/24 h, and a slow progression. Pathologically, it shows mesangium proliferation and IgA deposits. In some patients, interstitial inflammation occurs.

22.2.7.2 Heroin Associated Nephropathy

It has common manifestations of albuminuria and hypertension. By ultrasound, it is demonstrated to have decreased kidney volume. The process into end-stage renal disease is much slower than that of HIVAN (for 1–4 months). The renal tissues biopsy can facilitate the differential diagnosis.

22.3 HIV/AIDS Related Urogenital Tuberculosis

TB is the most common opportunistic infection of HIV/AIDS and extrapulmonary tuberculosis is more common. TB of urogenital system is one of the common extrapulmonary tuberculosis.

22.3.1 Pathogen and Pathogenesis

Almost all cases of renal tuberculosis occur secondary to pulmonary tuberculosis, and occasionally secondary to joint tuberculosis, lymphaden tuberculosis and intestinal tuberculosis. The invasion of tubercle bacilli to the kidneys is via 4 routes, blood, urinary tract, lymphatic vessel and direct extension. Blood borne spreading to the kidneys is recognized as the most common transmission route. Blood borne infection of renal TB is mostly simultaneous infections of both kidneys. However, in its progressive process, the severity of renal TB may be more serious in one kidney than the other. Due to the compromised immunity, the conditions may develop rapidly, with possible serious lesions in both kidneys. Pathological examinations have demonstrated that more than 80 % cases have simultaneous infection of both kidneys. But actually, the contralateral lesions are slight and can be self healed. Therefore, the clinical cases of renal TB is mostly unilateral, accounting for about 85 % and the cases of bilateral renal TB account for about 10 %.

Ureter tuberculosis is caused by downward spreading of the homolateral renal tuberculosis. And it can also be caused by the urinary reflux of mycobacterium tuberculosis in the bladder for the retrograde infection.

About 50–70 % of male patients with renal tuberculosis sustain the complication of reproductive system tuberculosis. Its occurrence in males originates from the prostate and the seminal vesicle. The condition with the most obvious clinical symptoms is epididymis TB. In the patients with renal TB complicated by reproductive TB, about 40 % have their epididymis tuberculosis occurring before or during the occurrence of renal tuberculosis.

22.3.2 Pathophysiological Basis

Along with the blood flow, mycobacterium tuberculosis invades the kidney to cause lesions, of which 90 % are located in the cortex and 10 % in the medulla. Cortex tuberculosis infection is self healing. However, in the cases with further progression, the medulla may be involved to form caseous necrosis and tuberculous abscesses. The abscess can penetrate into the kidney calices to cause cavities after the necrotic materials being discharged. The abscess rupture and access of mycobacterium tuberculosis into the urine via the tubules can cause mucosa lesions and ulceration in the kidney calices and pelvis. Subsequently, due to the formation of tuberculous granulation tissue, stenosis of the kidney calices and pelvis occurs with their wall thickened. Calyceal stenosis can cause the infection to involve the other kidney calices and further invade the adjacent renal parenchyma. The primary lesions in the renal parenchyma can also gradually enlarge to cause extensive lesions in the renal parenchyma to form multiple cavities. Therefore, tuberculous pyonephrosis occurs. This type is the most commonly found in the clinical practice. In some patients, if the compromised immunity improves, caseous materials thus are concentrated rather than liquefaction to cause extensive fibrous tissues hyperplasia and calcification, which is known as autonephrectomy or plaster kidney. Although the disease may clinically progress to calcified autonephrectomy, the actual pathological changes are caseous cavities, fibrous atrophy, and mixed hard nodules and calcification. Tubercle bacilli can still exist in the caseous substances.

Ureter tuberculosis often invades the ureteral mucosa, mucosal lamina propria and muscularis. In the early stage, ureteral mucosa is damaged, which leads to ulceration and lumen dilation. Subsequently, due to the formation of tuberculous granulation tissues, the ureteral wall is thickened and rigid, with stenosis and even occlusion. Urethral stenosis commonly occurs most commonly at the ureterovesical junction, followed by the ureteropelvic junction. Its occurrence at the middle segment is rare. The involved ureter can be partially or totally calcified.

Bladder tuberculosis is commonly caused by spreading of renal or ureteral tuberculosis. In the early stage, it is demonstrated to have bladder mucosal congestion, edema, irregular ulcers and (or) granuloma. The lesion begins adjacent to the ipsilateral ureteral opening, and then spreads to other parts to involve the delta or even the whole bladder. In the advanced stage, the lesions invade into the myometrium to cause serious fibroplastic proliferation and scar contraction, resulting in the shrinkage of the bladder capacity to less than 50 ml. It is known as bladder contracture. Bladder fibroplastic proliferation can cause ureteral stenosis or ureteral incompetence to form cave liked lesions. Both can lead to obstruction and urine reflux in the ureters, resulting in hydronephrosis. Ureteral incompetence also allows urine in the bladder flowing upwards to infect the contralateral kidney. In the cases of serious bladder lesions and deep ulceration, the bladder wall can be penetrated to involve the vagina or the rectum, resulting in vesico-vaginal fistula or vesico-rectal fistula.

The main pathological changes of urethral tuberculosis are ulcer and stenosis, which can cause dysuresia and urinary fistula and aggravate the kidney dysfunction.

22.3.3 Clinical Symptoms and Signs

The patients with renal tuberculosis commonly sustain the symptoms of urgent urination, frequent urination, painful urination and other bladder irritation symptoms, with accompanying hematuria, pyuria, backache, anemia, low grade fever, night sweating, poor appetite, weight loss, fatigue and other systemic symptoms.

22.3.4 Examinations and Their Selection

1. Routine urine test provides important clues for the early screening of renal tuberculosis.
2. Urinary tubercle bacilli culture is an important basis for the diagnosis of renal tuberculosis. It also monitors the drug resistance to tubercle bacilli.
3. Immunological assays of ELISA detects tubercle bacilli antibody for the diagnosis of renal tuberculosis, which has a coincidence rate of 82 % with the pathological examinations. It is the most important examination for the diagnosis of renal tuberculosis.
4. Intravenous urography (IVP) can demonstrate the calyx erosion and deformation and tuberculous abscesses of early renal tuberculosis. It can also demonstrate the general view of hydronephrosis caused by calyx and/or pelvic stenosis. Therefore, it is the examination of the choice for the early diagnosis of renal tuberculosis.
5. Percutaneous kidney puncture is an important method for the diagnosis. Especially for the nonfunctional kidney that fails to be demonstrated by IVP, it can be favorably applied for the understanding of the condition above obstructed urinary passage.
6. Ultrasound is of less significance for the early diagnosis of renal tuberculosis. However, for the cases with cavities or hydronephrosis, it is of great assistance.
7. CT scanning is less favorable than IVP in demonstrating the early lesions. However, it can well demonstrate the

calcification, thickened ureteral wall, renal functional assessment and severity of perinephral lesions, which is optimal for the examination of these lesions.
8. MR imaging is not the conventional imaging examination for the diagnosis of urinary tuberculosis. But for the cases with failed demonstration by pyelography or unfavorable conditions for enhanced CT scanning, MR imaging can define the diagnosis.
9. Cystoscopy is an important examination for the diagnosis of urinary tuberculosis.

22.3.5 Imaging Demonstrations

22.3.5.1 Renal Tuberculosis

Ultrasound demonstrates early renal TB as echo free areas from the kidney parenchyma, with fine small spots or patchy echoes. The advanced renal TB is demonstrated as hydronephrosis, with spots echoes in it. For the cases with calcification, the lesions are demonstrated with strong echo patches and posterior sound shadows. Tuberculous abscesses are demonstrated as low echo. CT scanning demonstrates focal low density lesions in the kidneys, liver and the spleen, with abdominal lymphadenectasis and decreased density areas in it. Tuberculous abscesses are demonstrated as low density. MR imaging is sensitive to early infiltrative foci of intrarenal tuberculosis, with focal or diffuse long T1 and long T2 signals. With the progression of the conditions, necrosis of the caseous lesion tissues occur to form cavities, with long T1 and long T2 signals of the cavities as well as equal T1, equal/short T2 signals of the cavity walls. When the lesions penetrate the kidney capsule, there are signal changes of perirenal adipose layer, with thickened perirenal fascia.

22.3.5.2 Ureteral Tuberculosis

CT scanning demonstrates no abnormalities or slight dilation of the ureter. In its advanced stage, the ureteral wall is thickened, with multiple irregular stenosis and dilation of the lumen, which can involve the whole ureter. MR imaging demonstrates unfavorably ureteral tuberculosis, sometimes with demonstrations of thickened ureteral wall and peripheral exudations.

22.3.5.3 Bladder Tuberculosis

Ultrasound demonstrates no early abnormalities. After the occurrence of diffuse fibrosis, the bladder wall can be found thickened. In the cases with their urine containing pus, blood and tissue fragments, fin spots echoes can be found. CT scanning demonstrates irregular inner layer of the bladder wall, thickened bladder wall and shrinkage of bladder lumen. MR imaging has similar demonstrations to CT scanning.

Case Study 1

A female patient aged 47 years was confirmatively diagnosed as having AIDS by the CDC. She had a history of paid blood donation in the year of 1994 and sustained symptoms in 2008 of low grade fever, night sweating and weight loss. The urine test demonstrated tubercle baccili positive and his CD4 T cell count was 88/μl.

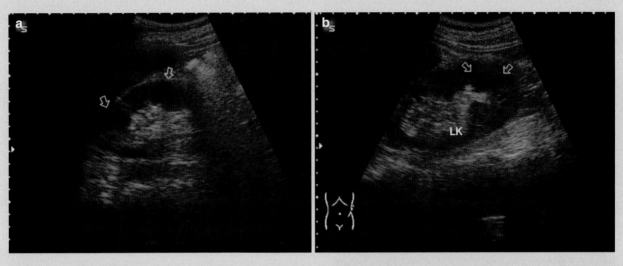

Fig. 22.1 (**a**, **b**) HIV/AIDS related renal tuberculosis. (**a**, **b**) Color Doppler demonstrates normal kidney size, unsmooth capsule, uneven echo from the renal parenchyma with multiple irregular low echo areas (*arrows*), unclear boundary and uneven internal echo. CDFI demonstrates unobvious internal blood flow signal. *LK* left kidney

Case Study 2

A male patient aged 41 years was confirmatively diagnosed as having AIDS by the CDC. He sustained symptoms in 2008 of frequent urination, and bloody urine found by naked eyes. The urine test found tubercle baccili positive. His CD4 T cell count was 67/μl.

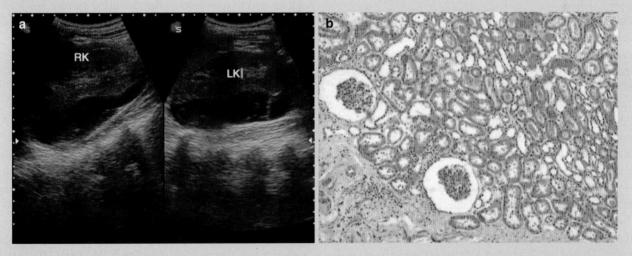

Fig. 22.2 HIV/AIDS related renal tuberculosis. (**a**) Color Doppler demonstrates normal kidney size, smooth capsule, uneven echo from the renal parenchyma with multiple irregular low echo, unclear boundary and uneven internal echoes. CDFI demonstrates unobvious internal blood flow signal. (**b**) Microscopy at a low magnification demonstrates chronic inflammatory cell infiltration in the renal cortex. *LK* left kidney, *RK* right kidney

Case Study 3

A male patient aged 36 years was confirmatively diagnosed as having AIDS by the CDC. He complained in 2008 of frequent urination, left lower back pain for 6 months. The urine test demonstrated tubercle baccili positive and his CD4 T cell count was 71/μl.

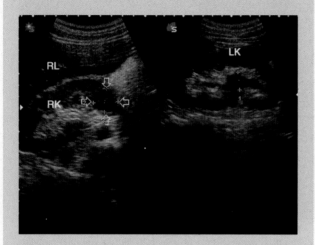

Fig. 22.3 HIV/AIDS related renal tuberculosis. Color Doppler demonstrates normal kidney, tough capsule, uneven echo from the renal parenchyma. An irregular shaped low echo area in size of 22 × 23 mm can be found in the right lower kidney (*arrows*), with unclear boundary and mixed internal echoes. CDFI demonstrates unobvious internal blood flow signal. The left renal collecting system is separated a width of 18 mm. *LK* left kidney, *RK* right kidney, *RL* right liver

22.3.6 Discussion

Due to their compromised immunity, AIDS patients are susceptible to renal tuberculosis, which is the most common and earliest urinary TB. It can spread from the kidney to involve the whole urinary system. Therefore, renal tuberculosis actually represents urinary tuberculosis.

Renal tuberculosis occurs commonly in age group of 20–40 years old-old, accounting for 70 %. The male patients are more than female patients, with a ratio of 2:1. About 80 % cases of renal tuberculosis are unilateral, with similar lesions in the left and right kidney.

Renal tuberculosis commonly originates from pulmonary tuberculosis, and rarely from bone and joint tuberculosis. Tubercle bacilli disseminate from the primary lesions to the renal cortex along with the blood flow to form multiple micro-TB lesions. When the defense system is weakened, it progresses into renal medullary tuberculosis, which is the clinical renal TB.

Early renal tuberculosis is commonly asymptomatic, with abnormal findings in the urine test including acidic urine, small quantity protein in the urine, erythrocytes in the urine and the finding of tubercle bacilli. (1) Urgent urination and painful urination: The symptom of frequent

urination occurs the earliest in the cases of renal TB. It is progressively serious and is the last symptom that resides. In some rare cases, ureteral lesions can cause early occlusion and the TB lesions cannot extend to the bladder, with no resulted symptoms of frequent, urgent and painful urination. (2) Hematuria and pyuria: Hematuria is more common and can be found by naked eyes or microscopic observations. It concurs with frequent urination and is commonly terminal hematuria caused by bladder tuberculosis. In some rare cases, intrarenal lesions can cause the whole course hematuria that can be observed by the naked eyes. (3) Renal pain and masses: Patients with renal tuberculosis generally do not have symptoms of lower back pain, but it can occurs in the advanced stage when the patient suffers from tuberculous pyonephrosis or occurs when lesions spread to perinephral area. In the cases with complication of contralateral hydronephrosis, contralateral lower back pain shows up. (4) Systemic symptoms: The systemic symptoms are commonly unobvious. Some symptoms including low grade fever, night sweating, weight loss and anemia occurs in the advanced stage of renal tuberculosis or in the cases with complication of other organs active TB. Ultrasound demonstrates no early abnormalities. In the cases with obvious renal tissue lesions, abnormal echoes are demonstrated, with enlarged kidney volume. In the cases with tuberculous renal abscesses, the fluid dark areas can be demonstrated in the kidney area.

22.3.7 Diagnostic Basis

Urinary TB can be clinically diagnosed based on urine culture and tissues biopsy. But the urine culture has a low positive rate. In the clinical practice, the definitive diagnosis is mainly based on IVP, CT scanning and cystoscopy.

22.3.8 Differential Diagnosis

22.3.8.1 Intracellular Mycobacterium Avium Infection

The cases of intracellular mycobacterium avium infection usually have obviously enlarged liver and spleen, low density abscesses in the kidney, liver and spleen, diffuse thickening of the jejunum wall and enlarged lymph nodes in soft tissue density. About 82 % cases intracellular mycobacterium avium infection firstly have HIV/AIDS related diseases, among which tuberculosis infection is the initial HIV/AIDS related diseases.

22.3.8.2 ARL

In the cases with renal involvement by ARL, CT scanning demonstrates low density lesions in both kidneys, while ultrasound demonstrates typical low echoes. Meanwhile, there is direct invasion of the kidney by enlarged lymph nodes or blockage of ureters to cause hydronephrosis. CT or US guided puncture for biopsy can facilitate to define the diagnosis.

22.4 HIV/AIDS Related Renal Failure

22.4.1 Acute Renal Failure

Acute renal failure (ARF), a clinical syndrome, has a variety of causes. Its clinical manifestations include acute degeneration of the renal function, in vivo retention of metabolites retention, as well as water, electrolytes and acid–base balance disorders. Clinical studies have shown that acute renal dysfunction is one of the most common clinical manifestations in the kidneys of HIV infected patients.

22.4.1.1 Pathogen and Pathogenesis

HIV/AIDS complicated by ARF can be etiologically divided into prerenal, renal, post-renal ARF. Prerenal ARF is caused by decreased blood volume due to gastrointestinal bleeding, vomiting, diarrhea, high fever and anorexia. In the cases with large quantity proteinuria, hypoproteinemia, cachexia, the liquid may remain in the third lacuna and sometimes causes ARF. Renal ARF is commonly caused by acute tubular necrosis induced by antiviral drugs or non-antiviral drugs, HIV/AIDS related nephropathy, immune complex nephritis after infection, and other types of nephritis. Drug induced tubular obstruction, and internal/external obstruction of the ureter lead to post-renal ARF. Acute tubular necrosis has a higher mortality rate and poorer prognosis.

22.4.1.2 Pathophysiological Basis

About 20–40 % AIDS patients sustain ARF, which the main pathological changes of enlarged and pale kidney with increased weight, pale cortex and dark red medulla on the cross section. Light microscopy demonstrates degeneration, shedding and necrosis of the tubular epithelial cells, filling of the shed tubular epithelial cells, casts and exudates in the tubular lumen. Electron microscopy demonstrates broken and shed microvilli on the cavity surface of tubular epithelial cells, swollen TEC mitochondria, absent mitochondria crest and ruptured mitochondrial membrane, increased primary and secondary lysosomes and increased phagocytic vacuoles. In the cases with seriously damaged TEC, disintegration, dissolution and complete necrosis of mitochondria, golgi complex and other organelles can be found (Fig. 22.4).

22.4.1.3 Clinical Symptoms and Signs

The clinical symptoms can be divided into oliguria and non-oliguria. The oliguria type has a typical progress, with primary lesions, ARF metabolic disorder and complications. (1) The oliguria period generally lasts for 5–7 days, with mainly manifestations of less urine, and even no urine, accompanying gastrointestinal, nervous and circulatory

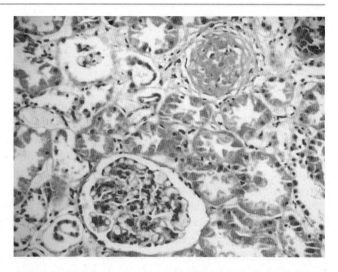

Fig. 22.4 HE staining demonstrates renal interstitium fibrosis and tubular dilation, with accompanying focal glomerular sclerosis. HE ×200

symptoms. Patients in serious conditions tend to have bleeding with diffuse intravascular coagulation. By laboratory tests, biochemical and the electrolytes are abnormal, with increased creatinine and blood urea nitrogen, acidosis, hyperpotassaemia and hyponatremia. (2) The diuretic period lasts for 1–3 weeks, with a urine volume up to 3,000–5,000 ml and relatively low specific gravity of urine. A few patients may have dehydration and low blood pressure. Most systemic symptoms gradually alleviated and the patients are susceptible to various infections and complications. (3) The renal functions gradually recover to normal in the recovery period, with normal or slightly increased urine volume. There are also different degrees of malnutrition, increased specific gravity of the urine and low endogenous creatinine clearance rate. Glomerular filtration function returns to normal within 3–12 months.

22.4.1.4 Examinations and Their Selection

Urine Test

It can facilitate to differentiate prerenal ARF from renal parenchymal ARF.

Blood Biochemical Examinations

They are important examinations to understand the renal function.

Ultrasound, CT Scanning and MR Imaging

They can demonstrate the size and shape of the kidneys as well vascular, ureteral and bladder obstructions, which is main basis for the exclusion of postrenal ARF. Moreover, they provide important information for the differential diagnosis of ARF and CRF.

Kidney Tissues Biopsy

For ARF of unknown causes, kidney tissues biopsy is a reliable tool for the diagnosis. It can help to understand the pathological changes and their severity of the renal lesions.

In addition, it is facilitative for the therapeutic planning and prognosis assessment.

22.4.1.5 Imaging Demonstrations

All of the ultrasound, CT scanning and MR imaging can demonstrate the size of the kidneys, but clinically, ultrasound is more commonly used. Ultrasound can accurately demonstrate the volume of the kidneys. In addition, echoes from the renal parenchyma are facilitative for the differential diagnosis. In the cases with AFR, the kidneys have symptoms of obvious congestion, edema and therefore enlarged kidney volume. The pyramids in the renal parenchyma are in low echoes, with has clear demonstrations. CT scanning and MR imaging can demonstrate enlarged kidney volume. For the cases of postrenal ARF, there are ureteral and bladder obstruction caused by calculus and masses, which is important for the diagnosis and classification of AFR.

22.4.1.6 Diagnostic Basis

The diagnosis of AFR requires detailed reports of the case history, treatment history, medication history. In combination with clinical manifestations, laboratory findings and imaging findings, the diagnosis can be defined. Kidney tissues biopsy can be performed if necessary.

22.4.1.7 Differential Diagnosis

Chronic Renal Failure (CRF)

The cases of chronic renal failure commonly have a past history of chronic renal disease, with accompanying severe anemia, calcium and phosphorus metabolism disorders as well as renal osteopathy. By laboratory tests, BUN (mg/dl)/Scr (mg/dl) is no higher than 10. By diagnostic imaging, there is reduced renal volume. But in the cases of CRF and early period of ARF, no increase and decrease of the kidney volumes can be found. Therefore, their differential diagnosis should be based on other laboratory tests including nails examination or hair creatinine test. Pathological biopsy can be performed for their differentiation.

HIVAN

Sometimes AFR is difficult to be differentiated from HIVAN in its rapid progression. The cases of HIVAN commonly have a past history of proteinuria as well as some special risk factors.

22.4.2 Chronic Renal Failure

Chronic renal failure (CRF) is an irreversible disease of chronic progressive renal parenchyma with a variety of causes. It is a syndrome with a group of manifestations including urotoxin retention, water and electrolytes disorder, renal anemia as well as calcium and phosphorus metabolism disorder. CRF is the serious period of renal dysfunction.

22.4.2.1 Pathogens and Pathogenesis

HIVAN is a common cause of AIDS complicated by chronic progressive renal insufficiency. It commonly progresses into end-stage renal disease within 6–12 months. In the black people aged 20–64 years, it is the third common cause of end-stage renal disease, following diabetes and hypertension.

22.4.2.2 Pathophysiological Basis

The pathophysiological process is mainly related to the following factors: (1) increased blood pressure in glomerular capillary; (2) systemic hypertension; (3) glomerular blood coagulation; (4) increased serum lipid level; (5) activity changes of local renal cytokines and angiotensin system; (6) high tubular metabolism.

22.4.2.3 Clinical Symptoms and Signs

The clinical symptoms and signs of CRF are caused by a variety of toxins and metabolites retention to involve the whole body systems. The early symptoms are weakness, low spirit; later poor appetite, nausea, vomiting and other gastrointestinal symptoms. Its further progress can show symptoms and signs of anemia, palpitations, itchy skin, limbs sensory abnormalities and numbness.

22.4.2.4 Examinations and Their Selection

Urine Test

It is a routine test which facilitates the diagnosis.

Blood Test

It plays an important implicative role for the diagnosis of CRF.

Renal Function Examinations

It is an important diagnostic examination, which helps understanding the renal functions.

Diagnostic Imaging

It is of great value in the etiological diagnosis of CRF.

22.4.2.5 Imaging Demonstrations

The cases of early CRF may have normal renal volume. But in the cases of advanced CRF, the demonstrations include reduced renal volume, thinner renal cortex (thickness being less than 1.5 cm). The size of two kidneys and the thickness of renal parenchyma demonstrated by CT scanning can help to predict the renal function. The diagnostic imaging can also demonstrate urinary calculus, obstruction, neoplasms and other pathological changes. CT scanning and MR imaging findings are complementary to each other, which is important for the diagnosis.

22.4.2.6 Diagnostic Basis

The diagnosis is mainly based on the case history of chronic primary or secondary renal disease, clinical manifestations, and urine test and blood biochemical examinations. The diagnostic imaging facilitates the etiological diagnosis of CRF.

22.4.2.7 Differential Diagnosis

The early CRF should be differentiated from ARF and the detailed knowledge see the section about ARF.

22.5   HIV/AIDS Related Cervical Carcinoma

Cervical carcinoma is a common gynecological malignancy. Currently, it is well known that the high risk type of human papillomavirus (HPV) infection is the major cause of cervical carcinoma. HIV infection can induce T lymphocytic lesions to cause persistent immunodeficiency, complications of opportunistic infections and malignancies. It has been reported by Caceres et al. that HIV/AIDS is related to the occurrence of cervical carcinoma [1].

22.5.1 Pathogens and Pathogenesis

HPV is a class of heterotype viruses but with the same structures. It is a small double-stranded circular DNA virus, mainly invading the skin and mucosal squamous epithelium. The HIV infection induced immunosuppression increases the incidence of HPV associated genital neoplasms. And its incidence is increasing along with the increase of immuno-suppression. HIV positive female are more susceptible to cervical carcinoma than HIV negative females. The incidences are 39.3 and 13.9 % respectively.

22.5.2 Pathophysiological Basis

Cervical carcinoma is mainly derived from squamous cells, accounting for about 90–95 %; and adenocarcinoma accounts for only 5–10 %. By the naked eyes observation, it can be divided into four categories: erosive, exogenous, endogenous and ulcerative. By microscopy, it can also be divided into four types: atypical dysplasia, in situ carcinoma, microscopic early invasive carcinoma and squamous cells infiltrative carcinoma.

22.5.3 Clinical Symptoms and Signs

The commonly manifestations include irregular vaginal bleeding and increased vaginal secretions. In its advanced stage, there are symptoms of pain, frequent urination, painful urination, tenesmus, bloody stool or bowel movement difficulties. In the advanced stage of carcinoma, there may be cachexia due to long-term consumptive progression of the carcinoma.

22.5.4 Examinations and Their Selection

22.5.4.1 Cervical Smear for Cytological Examination

It is the commonly used examination for the screening of cervical carcinoma.

22.5.4.2 Cervix and Cervical Canal Biopsy

The findings are the basis for the diagnosis of cervical carcinoma and its precancerous lesions.

22.5.4.3 Ultrasound

It is the conventional examination for the diagnosis and following up assessments.

22.5.4.4 CT Scanning

It is commonly applied in the diagnosis and treatment of advanced cervical carcinoma. In addition, it is also applied to monitor its recurrence and the efficacy of radiotherapy.

22.5.4.5 MR Imaging

It is the examination of choice in the diagnosis of cervical carcinoma, its staging and therapeutic planning.

22.5.4.6 PET/CT Scanning

It is sensitive to the neoplastic tissues, lymph nodes metastasis and recurrent lesions. However, it cannot be the conventional examination for the diagnosis of cervical carcinoma due to its high cost.

22.5.5 Imaging Demonstrations

22.5.5.1 Ultrasound

Ultrasound demonstrates cervical hypertrophy, irregular shape, heterogeneous echo and heterogeneous echo of cervical parenchymal mass. There are also uterine effusion, vaginal and parametrial tissues infiltration as well as abdominal and pelvic lymphadenectasis.

22.5.5.2 CT Scanning

Tumor Being Confined Within the Cervix

There is enlarged cervix with smooth edge. By enhanced scanning, the density of the tumor is lower than normal cervical tissues. In the tumor, there is an even lower density area which may be necrosis or ulceration. Cervical canal obstruction can cause uterine effusion.

Paracervical Tumor Infiltration

There is irregular or blurry cervical lateral edge, and obvious s irregularly thickened cords liked shadows or soft tissue masses in the paracervical soft tissues. The peripheral adipose spaces at the urethral end are unclear.

Tumor Invasion into the Rectum or Bladder

There is serrate liked thickening of the rectum or bladder wall or tumor nodules protruding into the rectum or bladder.

Pelvic Involvement

Lymph Nodes Metastasis

The pelvic lymph node has a diameter of above 1.5 cm or the lymph node adjacent to the abdominal aorta has a diameter of above 1.0 cm indicates lymph nodes metastasis.

22.5.5.3 MR Imaging

(1) T1WI is in medium to low signal and T2WI is in a medium to high or high signal. (2) DWI of tumors are in obvious high signals, demonstrating significantly restricted diffusion; and obviously decreased ADC values than normal cervical tissues. (3) Enhance imaging demonstrates early enhancement of the tumors. The late enhancement degree is lower than the normal cervical matrix. The enhancement curve is in an outflow type. (4) Parametrial invasion has manifestations of tumor tissues in irregular high signal protruding into the parametrium, with interrupted cervical matrix. (5) Vaginal invasion is demonstrated to have interrupted irregular signal of the normal vaginal wall. (6) The pelvic lymph node metastases is demonstrated to have medium to low signal by T1WI and increased T2WI signal of the involved lymph nodes by metastasis. The application of adipose suppression demonstrates can clearly demonstrate the lesions. Enhanced imaging demonstrates enhancement of the lymph nodes.

Cases Study 1

A female patient aged 41 years was confirmatively diagnosed as having AIDS by the CDC. She had a history of extramarital sexual behaviors, with irregular vaginal bleeding. Her CD4 T cell count was 127/μl.

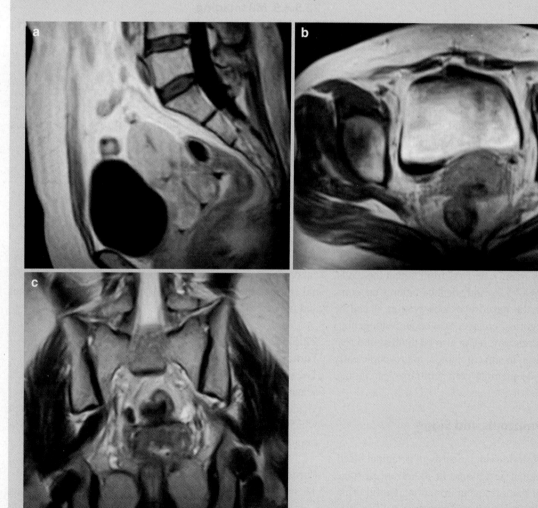

Fig. 22.5 (**a–c**) HIV/AIDS related cervical in situ carcinoma. (**a**) Sagittal T1WI demonstrates slightly lower signal nodules in the cervix, invasion of the cervical matrix, and no invasion the parametrium and vagina. (**b**) Axial T2WI demonstrates the nodules in slightly higher signal. (**c**) Coronal imaging demonstrates nodular thickening of the uterine wall

22.5.6 Diagnostic Basis

According to the case history and clinical manifestations, especially the cases with contact vaginal bleeding, should be suspected to be cervical carcinoma. The general examinations and gynecological examinations should be performed. Based on the actual conditions of the patients, cytological examinations or biopsy should be ordered to facilitate the diagnosis. The diagnostic imaging is of great value in the preoperative staging of carcinoma and postoperative following up observations.

22.5.7 Differential Diagnosis

When cervical carcinoma invades upwards into the uterus, it should be differentiated from endometrial carcinoma invasion of the cervix. Cervical smear and enhanced CT/MRI for enhancement of the tumor can help the differential diagnosis. Cervical carcinoma should be also differentiated from benign cervical tumors and cervical polyps. The latter two diseases do not invade the surrounding tissues, and their diffusion weighted imaging demonstrates the lesions with slight restricted diffusion than the carcinoma tissue.

22.6 HIV/AIDS Related Kidney Tumors

22.6.1 HIV/AIDS Related Renal Carcinoma

22.6.1.1 Discussion

No matter how large the renal carcinoma is, about 80 % patients are asymptomatic in the early stage. Only by physical examinations or B mode ultrasound examination, the space occupying lesions or palpable abdominal masses can be found. The symptoms of renal carcinoma include:

Case Study

A male patient aged 40 years was confirmatively diagnosed as having AIDS by the CDC. He complained of weight loss and gross hematuria. He received surgical removal of the right kidney for the pathological examination as clear cell renal carcinoma and his CD4 T cell count was 90/μl.

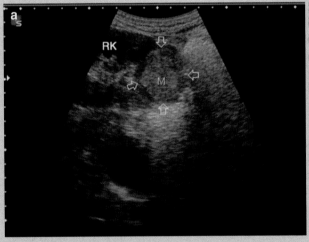
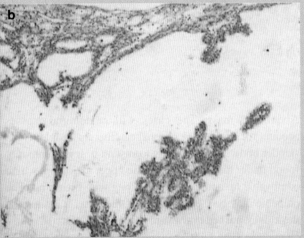

Fig. 22.6 (a–e) HIV/AIDS related space occupying lesions in the right kidney (renal carcinoma). (**a**) Color Doppler demonstrates normal size of the kidneys, smooth capsule, heterogeneous echo of the renal parenchyma, irregular parenchymal high echo mass in the inferior parenchyma with clear boundary and uneven internal echoes (*arrows*). CDFI demonstrates abundant internal blood flow signal. (**b**) Microscopy at a low magnification demonstrates cystic wall with papilla in the inner wall. (**c**) Microscopy at a medium magnification demonstrates he papillary structures. (**d**, **e**) Microscopy at a high magnification demonstrates transparent cytoplasm of the cancer cells. *M* carcinoma, *RK* right kidney

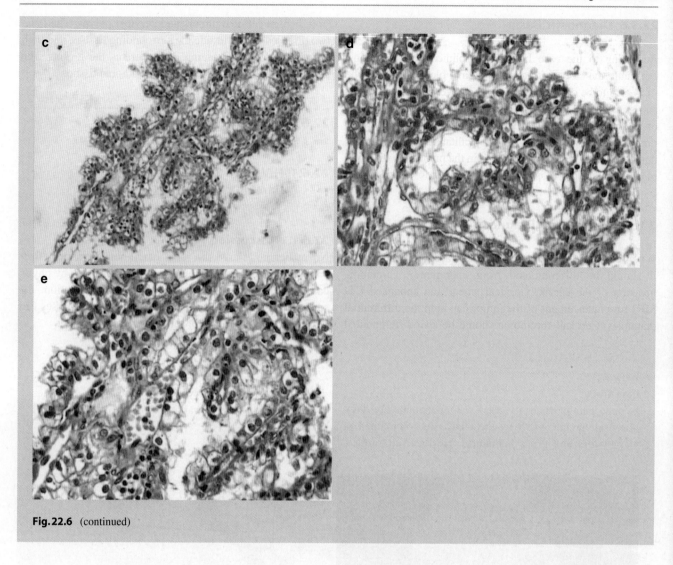

Fig. 22.6 (continued)

1. Abdominal mass: The cases with abdominal masses account for about 20 % of renal carcinoma. People with a slender body are more likely to sustain it. It is commonly found under the costal arch in the upper abdomen, which is movable up and downwards along with breathing. The palpable may be the mass itself. Otherwise, it is the base the kidney pushed downwards by the carcinoma.

2. Hematuria: The kidneys communicate to the outside via urine. Therefore, hematuria is one of the most common clinical symptoms of renal carcinoma; which is caused by the invasion of the carcinoma to the mucosa of the renal pelvis or calices. About 40–60 % patients sustain varying degrees of hematuria, which is usually intermittent, painless and visible by the naked eyes. Sometimes the blood is strip liked clots, which are ureteral casts. In the cases with obstruction of the ureters by blood clots, renal colic occurs.

3. Pain: The pain caused by renal carcinoma is located at the lower back, which is usually dull with an incidence of 20 %. In addition to the tumor growth stretching the renal capsule, the causes also include the invasion of the carcinoma to the surrounding organs or psoas muscles, which is more serious and longer lasting.

Serious hematuria may cause blood clots formation, which further lead to ureteral obstruction. As a result, renal colic occurs, which can be pathologically classified:

1. Conventional or clear cell renal carcinoma is the most common type, accounting for 70–80 % of renal carcinoma. Microscopically, the carcinoma cells are large in a shape of round or polygon. They have abundant cytoplasm, which is transparent or granular. Its stroma is rich in capillaries and blood sinuses. The cases of this type are commonly sporadic, and rarely hereditary with accompanying VHL syndrome. The occurrence of this type of renal carcinoma is related to the genetic changes in VHL.

2. Papillary carcinoma accounts for 10–15 % of renal carcinoma, including basophilic cell subtype and eosinophilic cell subtype. The carcinoma cells are cubic or short columnar in a papillary arrangement. The papillary axial stroma often has psammoma bodies and foam cells, with possible occurrence of edema. This type also includes two subtypes, hereditary and sporadic. The occurrence of papillary renal carcinoma is not obviously related to VHL syndrome. Sporadic papillary renal carcinoma is genetically caused by trisomy of the 7, 16 and 17 chromosomes and loss of y chromosome in male patients [t (X, 1)]. However, hereditary papillary renal carcinoma is genetically caused by trisomy of the 7 chromosome. The occurrence of hereditary clear cell renal carcinoma is related to the mutation of protooncogene in the 7 chromosome, MET gene.

3. Chromophobe renal carcinoma accounts for about 5 % of renal carcinoma. Microscopically, the cells are in different sizes, lightly stained or slightly eosinophilic cytoplasm, thick concentration of the cytoplasm adjacent to the cellular membrane and halo surrounding the nucleus. This type is possibly derived from the epithelial cells of the collecting tubules, with favorable prognosis. Cytogenetic examinations demonstrate multiple chromosomes deletions and serious hypodiploid. Chromosome deletion occurs in 1, 2, 6, 10, 13, 17 or 21 chromosomes. Renal carcinoma also includes collecting duct carcinoma and renal cell carcinoma (unclassified). Collecting duct carcinoma rarely occurs, accounting for less than 1 % renal carcinoma. Renal cell carcinoma (unclassified) includes those cannot fit into the above types, which accounts for 3–5 % renal carcinoma.

It has been reported that HIV infection induced compromised immunity is possibly related to genitourinary parenchymal carcinoma. The relationship has been proved in AIDS complicated by renal cell carcinoma, vascular0 sarcoma, testicular seminoma and germinoma. So far, the relationship has not been fully confirmed, which still has possibility of accidental occurrence. The occurrence of renal cell carcinoma in young AIDS patient indicates compromised immunity induced by HIV infection promotes or advances its occurrence.

22.6.2 HIV/AIDS Related Renal Hodgkin's Lymphoma

Hodgkin's lymphoma (HL), which was known as Hodgkin's disease (HD5), is a special kind of lymphoma with characteristic microscopic demonstrations of diverse cellular components and findings of R-S cells. It is not listed as the diagnostic indicator of AIDS. However, according to literature reports, its occurrence in AIDS patients is not uncommon. In the cases with HIV-1 infection and HL, the diagnosis of AIDS should be considered. HIV/AIDS related lymphoma is composed of aggressive undifferentiated non-Hodgkin's lymphoma, including small nucleus with no division type, large nucleus with division and central follicle type, immunoblast type and undifferentiated cell type. However, it is still controversial to list HL as the diagnostic indicator of AIDS. AIDS patients with undifferentiated non-Hodgkin's lymphoma or Hodgkin's disease have lower degree of tumor differentiation, compared to non-HIV/AIDS patients with lymphoma. HIV/AIDS related lymphoma is commonly accompanied by invasive growth, with involvement of extranodal tissues. Diagnostic imaging studies indicated that in patients with HIV/AIDS related lymphoma; 6–12 % has their kidneys involved. HIV/AIDS related Hodgkin's lymphoma with renal involvement commonly has manifestations of low density lesions of bilateral kidneys. In contrast, non-HIV/AIDS related renal lymphoma has the manifestation of diffusely enlarged kidney. Ultrasound demonstrates typical low echo areas. Reactive hyperplasic lymphadenectasis is one of the common signs of HIV/AIDS related lymphoma, intracellular mycobacterium avium infection and Kaposi's sarcoma. In the cases with extensive lymphadenectasis, HIV/AIDS related lymphoma, intracellular mycobacterium avium infection and Kaposi's sarcoma should be suspected. Puncture for biopsy is necessary to define the diagnosis and the puncture can be performed under the guidance of CT scanning or ultrasound.

Case Study

A male patient aged 38 years was confirmatively diagnosed as having AIDS by the CDC. He had a history of blood transfusion after car accident, with no obvious upset in daily life activities. His CD4 T cell count was 67/μl.

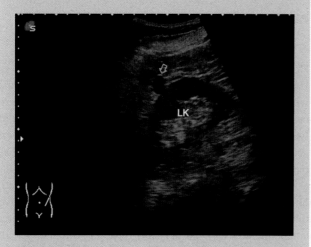

Fig. 22.7 HIV/AIDS related space occupying lesions in the left kidney (renal Hodgkin's lymphoma). Color Doppler demonstrates normal size of the kidneys, quite smooth capsule, quite even parenchymal echoes, and an irregular low echo area protruding outwards from the capsule with clear boundary and uneven internal echoes (*arrow*). CDFI demonstrates abundant blood flow signal. *LK* left kidney

22.6.3 HIV/AIDS Related Kaposi's Sarcoma

KS is one of the common complications of AIDS. It occurs commonly in sexually transmitted AIDS patients, but rarely in AIDS patients infected via intravenous drug abuse and blood or blood products. Although KS was discovered a long time ago, its origin and innate character have not been fully understood. Concerning its origin, there are generally two theories: (1) Its origination from endothelial cells, which is supported by the evidence that CD34 is the most sensitive marker with specificity for HIV/AIDS related KS. (2) Its origination from the mesenchyma, which is supported by the evidence that KS cells express marks of both endothelial cells and macrophages. The markers of endothelial cells are VIII factor related antigen and vascular endothelial cells specific adhering. The markers of macrophages include macrophages antigen PAM-1, CD68 and CD14, which is similar to the expressions of endothelial macrophages in the splenic lymph nodes. Therefore, it is believed that these cells are intermediate cells with features of both macrophages and endothelial cells and KS is caused by proliferation and accumulation of intermediate cells. Therefore, the occurrence of KS is believed to be caused by proliferation and differentiation of vascular endothelial cells or differentiation of primary immature mesenchymal cells to vascular endothelial cells. Due to different degrees of differentiation, vascular liked structures or spindle shaped cellular bundles of different degrees of maturity can be formed, in different histological types. It is likely that angioma type has favorable differentiation, with ability or tendency to form vascular vessels, while singular or dedifferentiated spindle cells have unfavorable differentiation that fails to form vascular vessels. However, these cells have potential ability for multiple directional differentiations to express multiple cellular markers, with endothelial cells differentiation is the predominant direction. More evidence has been found to support the speculations that KS is actually a multi-focal reactive vascular hyperplasia or multi-central hyperplasia. The manifestations include (1) KS has an extensive disseminated distribution or has multi-central growth, with no definitive evidence of metastasis, which is similar to viremia induced multi-focal reactive vascular hyperplasia. (2) KS can be extensively reversed, resolved or degraded. However, they are progressive lesions in AIDS patients, which is possibly due to their serious immunodeficiency and susceptibility to opportunistic infections. (3) Reactive hyperplasia with accompanying inflammatory cells infiltration is in line with inflammatory hyperplasic diseases. (4) Extensive lesions are more commonly found in male patients, which are related to the endocrine conditions of the human body. The lymph node is the third commonly involved body part, which can be found in 95 % cases, following skin and oral mucosa. Extensive retroperitoneal KS has the manifestation of retroperitoneal lymphadenectasis. Enhanced imaging demonstrates obvious enhancement of the enlarged lymph nodes in the retroperitoneal cavity and pelvis.

22.7 HIV/AIDS Related Urete and Bladder Diseases

Case Study 1

A male patient aged 51 years was confirmatively diagnosed as having AIDS by the CDC. He had a history of paid blood donation in 1995, with complaint of right lower back pain for 3 days and hematuria. His CD4 T cell count was 47/μl.

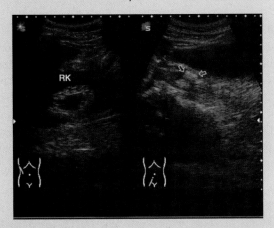

Fig. 22.8 HIV/AIDS related right ureteral stones and hydronephrosis. Color Doppler demonstrates separated right renal collecting system, a strong echo at the inferior segment of the right ureter with accompanying posterior sound shadow (*arrows*), from which above the ureter has different degrees of dilation. *RK* right kidney

Case Study 2

A male patient aged 35 years was confirmatively diagnosed as having AIDS by the CDC. He had a history of paid blood donation in 1992, with complaints of lower abdominal pain for 10 days and urinary retention. His CD4 T cell count was 54/μl.

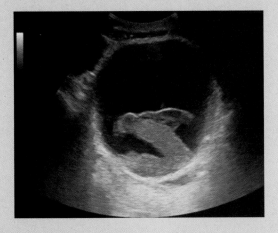

Fig. 22.9 HIV/AIDS related space occupying lesions in the bladder. Color Doppler demonstrates a strip liked abnormal echo in the bladder, which is not obviously movable. CDFI demonstrates unobvious internal blood flow signal

22.8 HIV/AIDS Related Other Renal Diseases

Case Study

A male patient aged 42 years was confirmatively diagnosed as having AIDS by the CDC. He had a history of paid blood donation in 1995, with complaint of progressive weight loss in 2005. His CD4 T cell count was 35/μl.

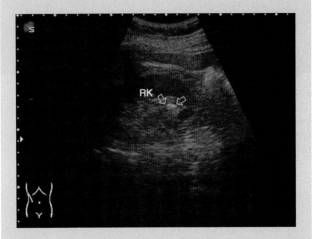

Fig. 22.10 HIV/AIDS related right renal calculus. Color Doppler demonstrates a strong echo area in size of 8×4 mm in the middle and inferior renal calices of the right kidney (*arrows*), with accompanying posterior sound shadow. *RK* right kidney

22.8.1 HIV/AIDS Related Renal Calculus

22.8.1.1 Discussion

Renal calculus is mostly located in the renal pelvis and renal calices, and rarely in renal parenchyma. The clinical manifestations have great individual difference, which are dependent on the causes, components, size, amount, location, mobility, obstructive infection and severity of renal parenchymal lesions. The slight cases can be asymptomatic, while the serious cases may have anuria, renal failure, toxic shock and even death. The incarcerated stones at the ureteropelvic junction or descending along the ureter can cause renal colic, which is sudden paroxysmal intolerable sharp pain radiating from the lower back or lateral abdomen downwards to the bladder area, genital area and medial thigh. Sometimes, the patients have profuse sweating, nausea and vomiting. Due to the serious damages of the stones to the mucosa, bloody urine is visible by the naked eyes. Pain and uremia are commonly induced by more physical activities. In the cases with renal calculus complicated by infections, pyocytes can be found in the urine, with symptoms of frequent and painful urination. In the cases with secondary acute pyelonephritis

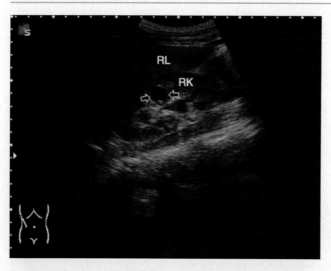

Fig. 22.11 HIV/AIDS related right kidney cyst. Color Doppler demonstrates a cystic area with no echo in the middle of the right kidney (*arrows*), with clear boundary and favorable sound transparency. CDFI demonstrates unobvious internal blood flow signal. *RK* right kidney, *RL* right liver

or renal pyonephrosis, there are fever, chills, shivers and other systemic symptom.

22.8.2 HIV/AIDS Related Renal Cyst

A female patient aged 50 years was confirmatively diagnosed as having AIDS by the CDC. She had a history of paid blood donation in 1993, with symptoms in 2006. Her CD4 T cell count was 39/μl.

22.8.2.1 Discussion

Most cases of renal cyst are asymptomatic, with normal findings by physical examinations. Occasionally, a palpable mass can be found in the kidney areas. In the cases with renal cyst complicated by infection, tenderness can be found in the flank area. In the cases of huge cyst, a mass can be found in the Lumbar abdomen area. In some patients, the following symptoms may occur due to the cyst itself and increased intracystic pressure or cystic infection.

Case Study 1
A female patient aged 40 years was confirmatively diagnosed as having AIDS by the CDC. She sustained

symptoms in 2006, with complaints of left lower back upset for half a year. Her CD4 T cell count was 55/μl.

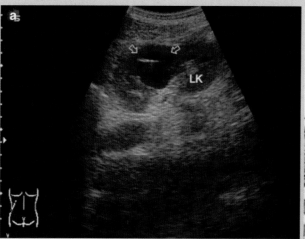

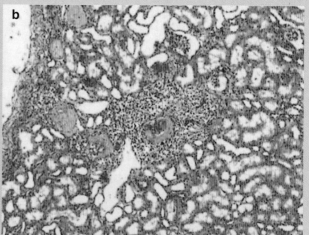

Figs. 22.12 (**a–e**) HIV/AIDS related left kidney cyst. (**a**) Color Doppler demonstrates a cystic area with no echo in the middle of the left kidney (*arrows*), with clear boundary and favorable sound transparency; and a strip shaped septum with slightly higher echo. CDFI demonstrates unobvious internal blood flow signal in the cystic area. (**b, c**) Microscopy at a low magnification demonstrates infiltration of chronic inflammation cell in the renal cortex. (**d, e**) Microscopy at a low magnification demonstrates cystic wall of the renal cyst and atrophic renal parenchyma due to compression. *LK* left kidney

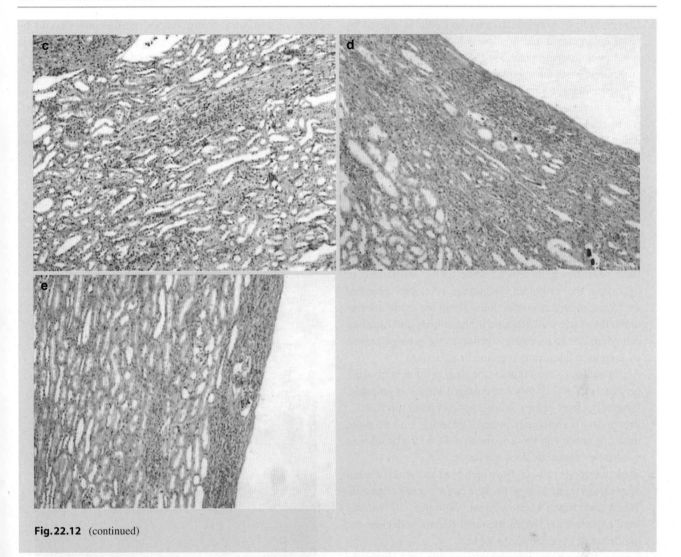

Fig. 22.12 (continued)

Case Study 2

A female patient aged 38 years was confirmatively diagnosed as having AIDS by the CDC. She had symptoms in 2004, with complaint of waist upset for 1 year. Her CD4 T cell count was 61/μl.

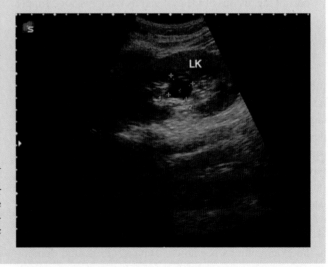

Fig. 22.13 HIV/AIDS related left renal pelvic cyst. Color Doppler demonstrates a cystic area with no echo in the left renal pelvis of the middle kidney, with clear boundary and favorable sound transparency. CDFI demonstrates unobvious blood flow signal in this cystic area. *LK* left kidney

1. Lower back or abdominal upset and pain is caused by renal enlargement and dilation, which results in tractive renal pedicle due to increased tension of the renal capsule. Otherwise, the symptom can be caused by the compressed adjacent organs. In addition, renal polycystic causes increased water content in the kidneys. Therefore, the heavy kidneys droop and tract to cause the lower back pain. The pain is dull and blunt, fixed unilaterally or bilaterally and radiating downwards and towards the lower back and the back. In the cases with intracystic bleeding or infection, the pain can be suddenly aggravated. In the cases with calculus or urinary obstruction by blood clots after bleeding, renal colic occurs.

2. Hematuria is visible microscopically or by the naked eyes. Its occurrence is periodical, with more serious lower back pain during its attack. Some factor can induce or aggravate the symptom, including strenuous physical exercises, trauma and infections. There are many arteries under the cystic wall. Rupture of the arteries and bleeding can occur due to excessive traction to the arteries caused by increased intracystic pressure or infections.

3. Abdominal mass sometimes is the chief complaint from the patient. In 60–80 % patients, enlarged kidney is palpable. Generally, larger kidney indicates poorer renal function.

4. Proteinuria is commonly in small quantity, with no more than 2 g protein in the urination of 24 h. Renal disease syndrome commonly does not occur.

5. Hypertension is resulted from increased secretion of renin after compressed kidney by cyst causes renal ischemia. When renal functions are normal, more than 50 % cases have hypertension. When the renal functions decline the incidence of hypertension is higher.

6. Renal dysfunction is progressive due to obviously decreased renal tissues, which is caused by the space occupying lesions of the cyst and its compression. Simple renal cyst has been not fully understood in terms of hereditary or acquired. Its origination is possibly similar to that of multicystic kidney, with the only difference in severity.

From other perspective, by artificially induced renal tubular obstruction and local ischemia, some animals sustain simple renal cyst. The results indicated that the lesions can be acquired. The enlarged cyst compresses and destructs the renal parenchyma, which fails to impair the renal functions. An isolated cyst can occur at the location to compress the ureter, which causes progressive hydronephrosis, followed by complications of infection. Ultrasound can define the amount and size of the cysts as well as the cystic wall. In addition, it facilitates the differential diagnosis from renal parenchymal masses. Therefore, ultrasound is the examinations of choice. Typical ultrasound demonstrations include no echo from the lesions area, smooth cystic wall with clear boundaries. In the cases with irregular echoes or confined strong echoes, malignancy should be alert of. In the cases with secondary infections, the cystic wall can be thickened, with fine echoes from the lesions area. In the cases with intracystic bleeding, the echo is strong. When ultrasound demonstrates multiple cysts, it should be differentiated from multilocular cyst and multicystic kidney.

22.8.3 HIV/AIDS Related Kidney Transplantation

Case Study

A male patient aged 46 years was confirmatively diagnosed as having AIDS by the CDC. He received kidney transplantation in 1995 and his CD4 T cell count was 89/µl.

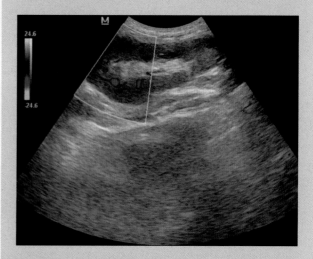

Fig. 22.14 HIV/AIDS related renal transplantation. Color Doppler demonstrates a kidney image in the right lower abdomen, with normal size but irregular morphology. It has slightly low uneven echo in the parenchyma. CDFI demonstrates abundant blood flow signal

22.8.4 HIV/AIDS Related Renal Purulent Infection

Due to the compromised immunity, AIDS patients have greatly increased risk of serious bacterial urinary infection including pyelonephritis and renal abscess. The imaging demonstrations of HIV/AIDS related bacterial pyelonephritis and renal abscess are the same as those in non-HIV/AIDS related bacterial pyelonephritis and renal abscess. Puncture to suction fluid for biopsy can define renal abscess.

22.8.5 HIV/AIDS Related Renal Pneumocystis Carinii Infection

Due to the prolonged survival period of AIDS patients, pathogenic factors changes of pneumocystis carinii and effective drug therapies, extrapulmonary pneumocystis carinii infections is more common in AIDS patients. Extrapulmonary pneumocystis carinii commonly invades the lymph nodes, spleen, liver, bone marrow, gastrointestinal tract, eyes, thyroid, adrenal gland and kidney. CT scanning of renal pneumocystis carinii infection demonstrates low density lesions, which are nonspecific. Low density lesions can also be found in the cases of lymphoma, small abscesses infected by bacteria and candida, and Kaposi's sarcoma.

22.8.6 HIV/AIDS Related Renal Candida Infection

Genital candidiasis (GC) is mainly caused by Candida albicans, which spreads via sexual contacts and contacts to the contaminated bath tubes, bath towels and underwear. In HIV positive patients, candidiasis is the most common mucosal opportunistic infection. Oral candidiasis is the early sign of immunosuppression, occurring prior to other symptoms. In patients with immunodeficiency, disseminated candidiasis occurs, with triad of fever, papular skin defects and diffuses muscular tenderness, which can be the indicator for its diagnosis. Disseminated candidiasis can cause focal abscesses in the kidney, commonly with accompanying splenic and hepatic involvements. Ultrasound demonstrates small candidal abscesses in typical low echoes. CT scanning demonstrates multiple small low density nodules and enhanced scanning demonstrates obvious ring shaped enhancement.

Extended Reading

1. Caceres W, Cruz-Amy M, Diaz-Melendez V. AIDS-related malignancies: revisited [J]. P R Heath Sci J. 2010;29(1):70–5.
2. D'Agati V, Appel GB. Renal pathology of human immunodeficiency virus infection. Semin Nephrol. 1998;18(4):406–21.
3. Dikov DI, RoLand J, Chatelet FP. An autopsy study of the prostate in acquired immunodeficiency syndrome. Arch Pathol Lab Med. 1998;122(10):875–9.
4. Heyns CF, Fisher M. The urological management of the patient with acquired immunodeficiency syndrome [J]. BJU Int. 2005; 95(5):709–16.
5. Klatt EC, Nichols L, Noguchi TT. Evolving trends revealed by autopsies of patients with the acquired immunodeficiency syndrome. Arch Pathol Lab Med. 1994;118(9):884–90.
6. Kuhlman JE, Browne D, Shermak M, et al. Retroperitoneal and pelvic CT of patients with AIDS: primary and secondary involvement of the genitourinary tract [J]. Radiographics. 1991;11(3):473–83.
7. Li Hong-jun. Clinical and imaging diagnosis of AIDS [M]. Beijing: China Medical Science Press; 2007.
8. Liu De-chun. Clinical pathology of AIDS [M]. Hefei: Anhui Science & Technology Publishing House; 2002.
9. Palefsky JM, Holly EA. Chapter 6: Immunosuppression and co-infection with HIV [J]. J Natl Cancer Inst Monogr. 2003;31:41–6.
10. Schoenfeld P, Humphreys MH. Renal aspects of HIV disease. In: Cohen PT, Sande MA, Volberd-ing PA, editors. The AIDS knowledge base. 2nd ed. Boston: Little Brown Company; 1997. 5.17-1-5. 17–14.
11. Schwartz EJ, Klotrnan PE. Pathogenesis of human immunodeficiency virus (HIV)-associated nephropathy. Semin Nephrol. 1998; 18(4):436–45.
12. Soriano-Rosas J, Avila-Casado MC, Carrera-Gonzalez E, et al. AIDS-associated nephropathy: 5 year retrospective morphologic analysis of 87 cases. Pathol Res Pract. 1998;194(8):567–70.
13. Symeonidou C, Standish R, Sahdev A, et al. Imaging and histopathologic features of HIV-related renal disease [J]. Radiographics. 2008;28(5):1339–54.

HIV/AIDS Related Musculoskeletal Diseases

23

Contents

23.1   An Overview of HIV/AIDS Related Musculoskeletal Diseases

In recent years, the widespread use of immunosuppressive therapy and supportive therapy prolong the survival period of AIDS patients. Therefore, chronic immunosuppression occurs, including various inflammatory diseases and arthritis, which is possibly related to HIV infection

Soft tissue diseases and skeletal diseases in AIDS patients are rarely reported, which is related to the less common occurrence of skeletal complications than central nervous complications and respiratory complications. However, musculoskeletal diseases are possibly the initial disease of AIDS, which should be paid focused attention. Due to its less

H. Li (ed.), *Radiology of HIV/AIDS*,
DOI 10.1007/978-94-007-7823-8_23, © Springer Science+Business Media Dordrecht and People's Medical Publishing House 2014

common occurrence, less attention is paid on musculoskeletal complications and delayed treatment. Therefore, its progression is accelerated. The diagnostic imaging is important for the early diagnosis of musculoskeletal infectious diseases. In this chapter, we focus on the diagnostic imaging of HIV/AIDS related musculoskeletal diseases.

23.1.1 Muscular and Soft Tissue Infections

Myositis may occur secondary to various bacterial infections. In the cases with no trauma and osteomyelitis, the volume, morphology, CT value and MRI signal can be varying, with normal subcutaneous adipose tissue or with lymphedema and cellulitis. Muscular necrosis occurs at sterile conditions or secondary to/complicated by bacterial infections. MR imaging is more sensitive to CT scanning in demonstrating muscular and facial changes, which facilitate the differentiation from superficial non-necrotic soft tissue inflammation.

23.1.2 Abscesses

Soft tissue abscess is usually liquid accumulation with clear boundary and thick wall. The surrounding soft tissue has inflammatory responses. The diagnostic imaging plays an important role in defining the location and range of soft tissue abscesses, which can also guide the puncture of abscesses for biopsy and drainage. Especially CT scanning and MR imaging, both have definitive demonstrations for the diagnosis. One of the main causes of abscesses in HIV positive patients is their sharing of needles for intravenous drug use. Other causes include blood borne spreading and direct spreading from adjacent osteomyelitis or purulent arthritis. The pathogenic bacteria of abscesses include Staphylococcus aureus, purulent streptococcus, Salmonella, tubercle bacilli and atypical mycobacteria. The range and progression of abscesses are dependent on the immunity status of the patients.

23.1.3 Osteomyelitis

Osteomyelitis is one of the common complications of skeletal infection, which commonly occurs in the progressive period of HIV infection. It has a rapid progression but hideous symptoms. And its pathogenic bacteria are commonly Staphylococcus aureus and Salmonella.

23.1.4 Ischemic Necrosis

Due to the immunological factors after HIV infection, vasculitis and vascular involvement can cause ischemia and necrosis of bones.

23.1.5 Rheumatic Diseases

It is still controversial concerning the correlation between rheumatic arthritis, non-purulent inflammations and HIV infection, mainly because of the etiological controversies of arthritis. Therefore, the diagnosis by radiologists is important for the therapeutic options by orthopaedic surgeons and rheumatologists. In patients with Reiter's disease, skin and skeletal psoriasis, spinal arthritis with serological negative findings or spinal osteoarthrosis, and inexplicable facet lesions, HIV infection should be suspected.

23.1.6 Neoplasms

Along with the compromised immunity in HIV positive patients, the incidence of neoplasm is increasing. Kaposi's sarcoma, a more common neoplasm, invades multiple organs but rarely involves the bone and bone marrow.

The prevalence of HIV infection adds new lesions for the diagnostic imaging of musculoskeletal system. The knowledge about HIV/AIDS related musculoskeletal diseases facilitates the diagnosis and differential diagnosis.

23.2 HIV/AIDS Related Osteomyelitis

23.2.1 Pathogens and Pathogenesis

After any part of human body is infected, the pathogen can involve the bone marrow, bone and periosteum along with blood flow and spread to the surrounding soft tissue. In the osteoblasts, the bacteria can directly invade the bone marrow to cause osteomyelitis. Its spreading is mainly via the following three transmission routes: (1) Blood borne infection has an inappropriately treated purulent infective lesion before its onset. The transmission route is that the bacteria gain their access to the bone tissue along with blood flow to cause osteomyelitis. (2) Traumatic infection is caused by the direct invasion of the pathogenic bacteria to the bone tissue, leading to osteomyelitis. (3) Spreading infection is caused by direct spreading of the adjacent purulent lesions to the bone tissues to cause osteomyelitis.

23.2.2 Pathophysiological Basis

When the immunity is compromised, local inflammation shows an acute onset to form large quantity pus fluid and invade the periosteum and bone marrow, resulting in osteomyelitis. Chronic purulent osteomyelitis repeatedly occurs, with newly formed dead space and necrotic bone during each period of attack to complicate the dead cavities and sinuses. Meanwhile, due to the long term local deficiency in blood supply and repeated inflammatory stimulations, local bone hyperplasia and sclerosis occur.

23.2.3 Clinical Symptoms and Signs

The symptoms of acute osteomyelitis are local redness and swelling, fever, pain, hard lump with limited mobility. The symptoms of chronic osteomyelitis include trauma surface erosion, white and foul secretion at the opening of the fistula. In the serious cases, the bone is destructed and cannot heal in a long period of time. Necrotic bones, sinuses or dead spaces are formed, with discharge of necrotic osteocomma from the sinus tract.

23.2.4 Examinations and Their Selection

23.2.4.1 Laboratory Tests
The blood WBC count can be normal, but ESR and C reactive protein increase.

23.2.4.2 X-ray
It has demonstrations of irregular thickening and sclerosis of the bone, with cavities of different sizes and necrotic bones.

23.2.4.3 CT Scanning
In the cases with unclearly defined demonstrations by X-ray, CT scanning can be ordered to define the diseased bone and paravertebral abscesses.

23.2.4.4 Biopsy
For neoplasms, biopsy can be performed for bacterial culture and drug sensitivity test.

23.2.4.5 Lipiodolography
To confirm the relation between dead bone, dead space and sinus tract.

23.2.5 Imaging Demonstrations

1. Conventional X-ray is not sensitive to early osteomyelitis. Abnormal demonstrations can be found when peritoneum is reactive and bone is destructed to cause obvious osteolysis.
2. CT scanning demonstrates soft tissue swelling, reactive peritoneum, intramedullary density changes, localized cortical bone erosion and rough bone trabecula.
3. MR imaging has a sensitivity and specificity of 82–100 % and 53–94 %, respectively, in the diagnosis of osteomyelitis. There are low T1WI signal and high T2WI signal. Enhanced imaging can increase the assessment range of bone and soft tissue infections.

Case Study 1

A female patient aged 29 years was confirmatively diagnosed as having AIDS by the CDC. Her CD4 T cell count was 110/μl.

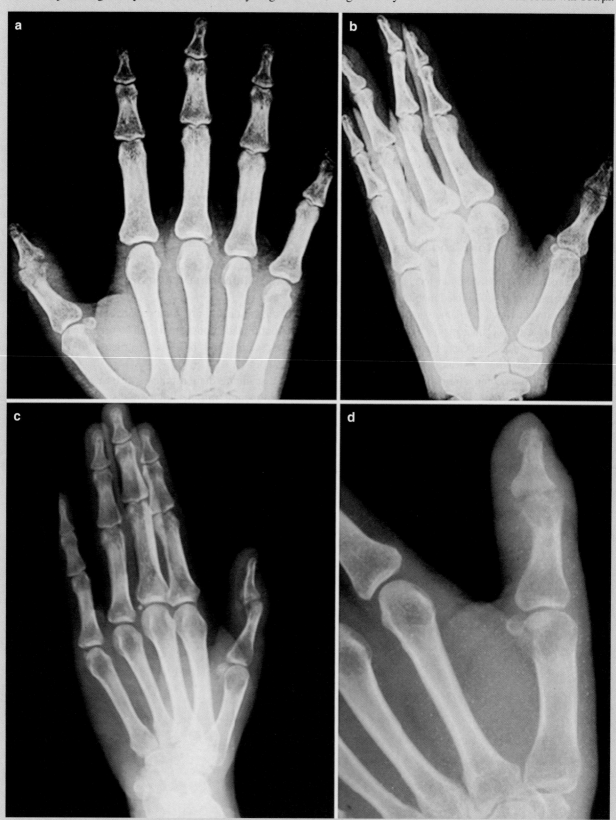

Fig. 23.1 (a–d) HIV/AIDS related tuberculous osteomyelitis. (a–d) DR demonstrates surrounding soft tissue swelling of the thumb interphalangeal joint, osteoporosis surrounding the joint, blurry joint space, worm bitten liked changes of articular facet and multiple small cystic low density areas

Case Study 2

A male patient aged 45 years was confirmatively diagnosed as having AIDS by the CDC. He had been found to be HIV antibody positive for 5 years, with complaint of joint pain for more than 20 days. He was in a chronic episode, with a history of unhealthy sexual behaviors. His CD4 T cell count was153/μl.

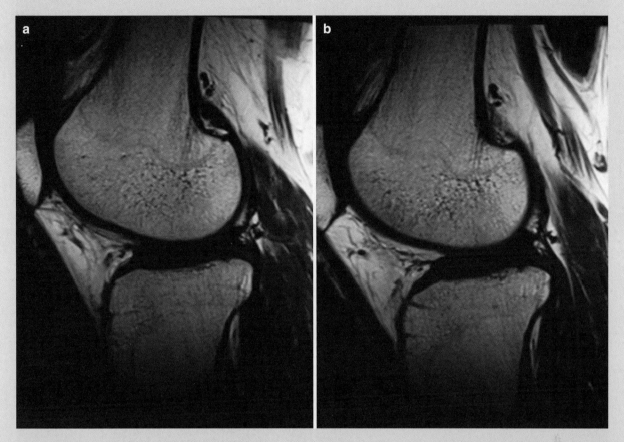

Fig. 23.2 (**a–n**) HIV/AIDS related gonarthromeningitis, wrist osteomyelitis and pelvic osteomyelitis. (**a–d**) MRI demonstrates strip liked long T1 and long T2 signal in the articular cavity of both knees. (**e–h**) It is demonstrated to have decreased T1WI signal in the lunate bone marrow and triangular bone marrow of the right wrist, high T2 signal after adipose suppression, intact cortical bone, strip liked long T1 and long T2 signal in the trapezoid bone, capital bone and scapholunate joint. (**i–j**) It is demonstrated to have strip liked long T1 and long T2 signals in the radioscaphoid joint space and extensive worm bitten liked bone destruction in the bilateral pelvic bones. (**k**) Microscopy at a low magnification demonstrates caseous necrosis, epithelioid cells and lymphocytes. (**l**) Microscopy at a low magnification demonstrates caseous necrosis and inflammatory granulation tissue. (**m**) Microscopy at a medium magnification demonstrates epithelioid cells and multinucleated giant cells. (**n**) Microscopy at a medium magnification demonstrates necrotic tissues and necrotic bones

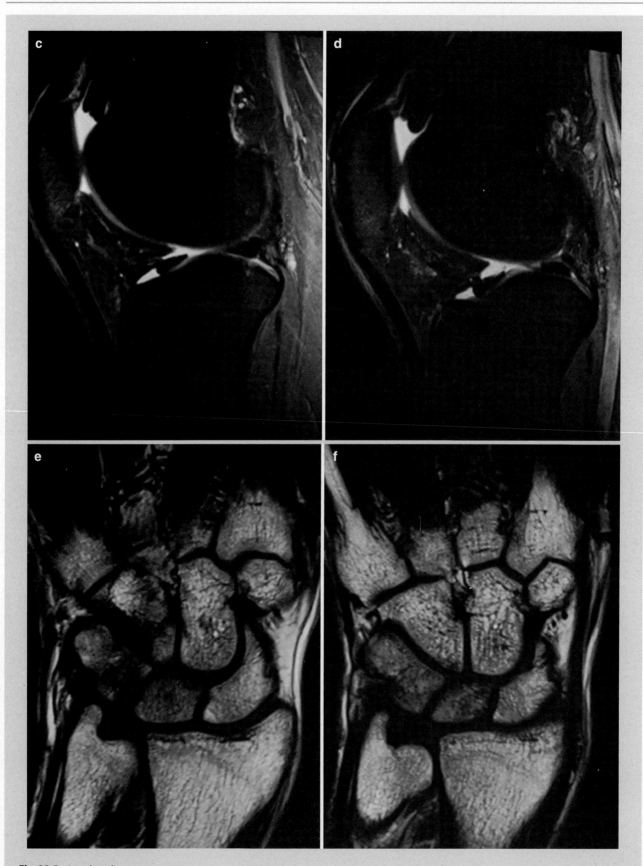

Fig. 23.2 (continued)

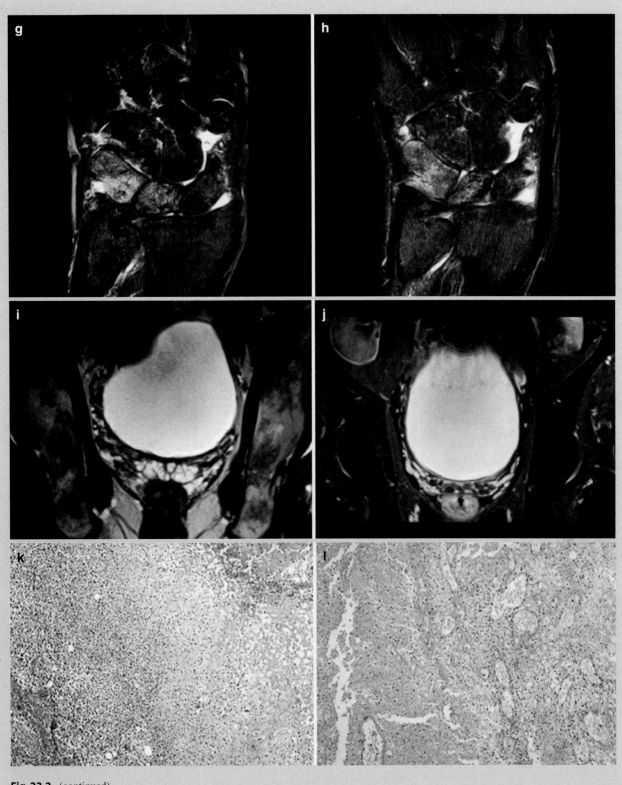

Fig. 23.2 (continued)

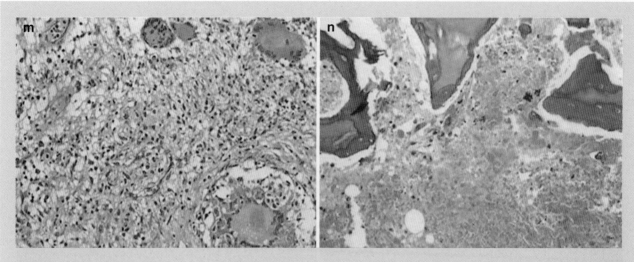

Fig. 23.2   (continued)

Case Study 3

A male patient aged 38 years was confirmatively diagnosed as having AIDS by the CDC. He had a history of paid blood donation, with complaint of fever, posterior curvature of the back for 3 months and both lower limbs fatigue for 1 month. His CD4 T cell count was 26/µl.

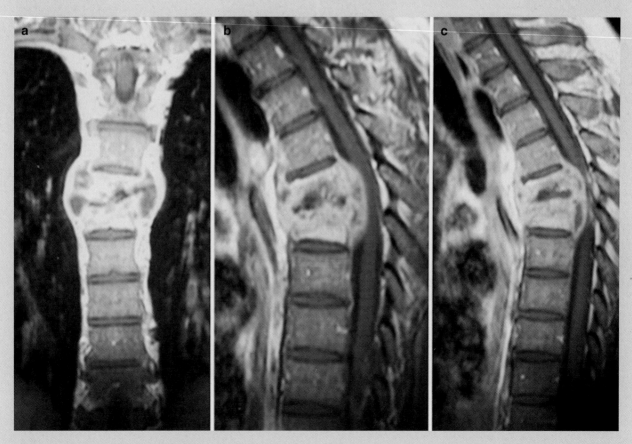

Fig. 23.3   (**a–c**) HIV/AIDS related extrapulmonary thoracic spinal tuberculosis. (**a–b**) It is demonstrated to have T7-8 vertebral compressed fracture in a wedge shape with fusion, narrowed joint space with surrounding cold abscesses to protrude into the spinal canal, and obviously compressed spinal cord. (**c**) Enhanced scanning of the thoracic vertebrae demonstrates patchy abnormal enhancement of the thoracic vertebrae, linear and even abnormal enhancement of the abscess wall

Case Study 4

A male patient aged 35 years was confirmatively diagnosed as having AIDS by the CDC. He had a history of paid blood donation, with complaint of fever, heel pain for 2 months. His CD4 T cell count was 406/μl.

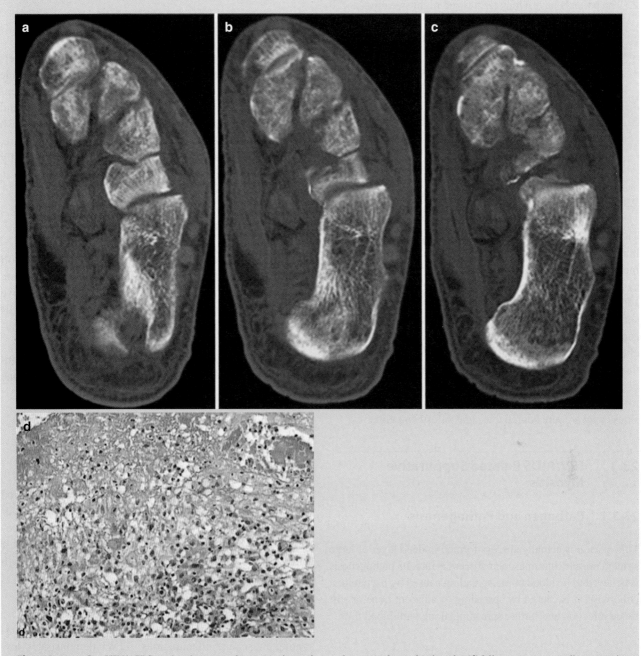

Fig. 23.4 (**a–d**) HIV/AIDS related extrapulmonarycalcaneal tuberculous osteomyelitis. (**a–c**) It is demonstrated to have round liked bone defects in the posterior calcaneus with clear boundary and sparse calcaneal trabecula. (**d**) Microscopy at a medium magnification demonstrates epitheloid cells and caseous necrosis

23.2.6   Diagnostic Basis

1. The patients mostly have a source lesion of TB or a past history of TB.
2. The patients have a long term fever, night sweating, accelerated ESR and other symptoms of TB.
3. Conventional X-ray demonstrates destructed bone, blurry facet and soft tissue swelling.
4. CT scanning demonstrates more favorably fine bone destruction, facet involvement, peritoneal reaction and surrounding soft tissues of the joints.
5. MR imaging demonstrates intramedullary edema in long T2 signal, which is more sensitive to the pathological changes of the soft tissues.

23.2.7   Differential Diagnosis

The disease should be mainly differentiated from malignant bone tumor and aseptic bone necrosis. The following findings including swelling degrees of the soft tissue, abscess liked cysts, soft tissue masses, residual bone shell at the margin of soft tissue masses or shell liked calcification, neoplasm in the soft tissue mass or tumor chondral calcification have significance for the differential diagnosis. In the cases with osteomyelitis, the range of soft tissue swelling is more extensive than those in bone malignancy. Increased surrounding bone density of destructed bone areas is an important feature of acute osteomyelitis. Gas and adipose liquid signs as well as formation of sinus canal are rare but reliable signs of osteomyelitis.

23.3   HIV/AIDS Related Suppurative Myositis

23.3.1   Pathogen and Pathogenesis

This disease is actually abscess formed in deep layer of large striated muscle. Intramuscular abscess is rare. Its pathogenesis is believed to be blood borne spreading caused by bacteremia. Otherwise, it is caused by spreading of adjacent bone or soft tissue infection and further spreading along with blood flow.

23.3.2   Pathophysiological Basis

Purulent myositis occurs commonly in immunocompromised patients, especially AIDS patients. The lesions are most commonly found in quadriceps femoris, gluteus, arm and shoulder muscles. According to statistics, about 40 % of the cases have multiple abscesses.

23.3.3   Clinical Symptoms and Signs

The early symptoms include spasm pain, and then upsets caused by progressively serious edema and low grade fever, muscle rigidity, tissue edema and aggravating tenderness. In early period of muscle rigidity, puncture and aspiration may have negative findings, and then yellowish thick purulent fluid can be obtained. By bacterial culture, staphylococcus aureus can always be found, occasionally Pyogenic streptococcus or Escherichia coli.

23.3.4   Examinations and Their Selection

MR imaging has a higher resolution in demonstrating soft issue lesions than CT scanning. MR imaging provides more direct images from multiple perspectives, which is sensitive to the early lesions in the muscles and bones. Therefore, MR imaging is the examination of choice and the optimal examination for suppurative myositis.

For the cases with further progressive lesions, CT scanning can provide supplementary information on bone destruction.

23.3.5   Imaging Demonstrations

23.3.5.1   CT Scanning
CT scanning demonstrates swollen muscles with decreased CT values due to edema, clearly defined intramuscular abscesses. Enhanced scanning demonstrates intramuscular necrosis and no enhancement of the necrotic areas, ring shaped enhancement of muscular abscesses with clear boundary.

23.3.5.2   MR Imaging
MR imaging is more sensitive than CT scanning in demonstrating muscular inflammations. T1WI demonstrates low signal in the muscles. T2WI demonstrate high signal from the intramuscular pus fluid. Enhanced imaging demonstrates low signal and high signal ring shaped enhancement surrounding the necrotic tissue.

Case Study

A female patient aged 34 years was confirmatively diagnosed as having AIDS by the CDC. Her CD4 T cell count was 40/μl.

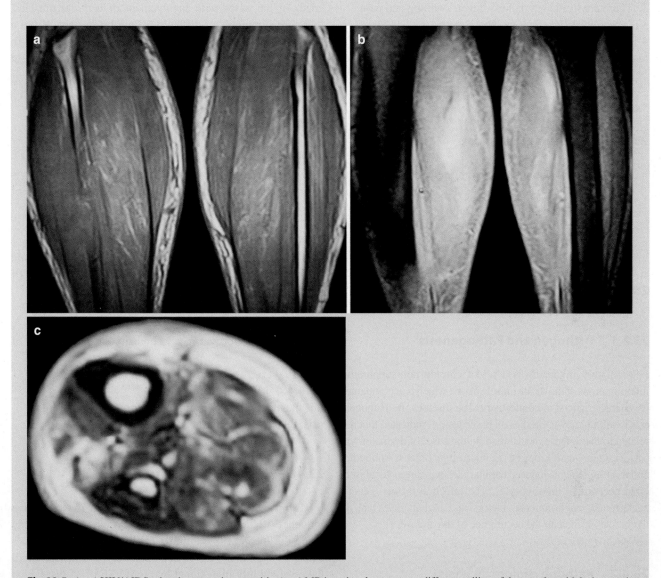

Fig. 23.5 (**a–c**) HIV/AIDS related suppurative myositis. (**a–c**) MR imaging demonstrates diffuse swelling of the muscles with lesions, strip liked T1WI low signal in the muscles and high T2WI signal

23.3.6 Diagnostic Basis

1. The patient had a history of infection.
2. There are local skin redness, fever, swelling and pain.
3. Increased WBC count by laboratory tests.
4. CT scanning and MR imaging demonstrations of soft tissue abscess with central liquefaction in low density shadows. Otherwise, MR imaging demonstrates long T1WI and long T2WI signals.

23.3.7 Differential Diagnosis

1. Benign lesions mainly include muscular hematoma, diabetic muscular infarction, nodular neurofibroma and infections secondary to bone fracture.
2. Malignant lesions mainly include synovial sarcoma, liposarcoma, neurofibroma.

23.4 HIV/AIDS Related Inflammatory Myopathy

23.4.1 Pathogen and Pathogenesis

Inflammatory myopathy is a set of chronic non-suppurative inflammations of the striate muscle tissue, which is accompanied by characteristic skin connective tissue diseases. Its pathogenesis is still unknown. Studies on tissue lesions indicated that it is related to the defense mechanism. In the cases of dermatomyositis, vascular vessels may be the main target organs. Antibodies and its complements induced capillary lesions causes focal ischemic necrosis of the myocytes. The infection factors, genetic background, environmental factors and malignancies are all likely to contribute to the occurrence of the disease.

23.4.2 Pathophysiological Basis

Polymyositis (PM) and dermatomyositis (DM) occur in any age group. The main pathological changes include infiltration of affected muscle tissue by inflammatory cells as well as degenerative or necrotic muscle fibers.

23.4.3 Clinical Symptoms and Signs

The disease has a hideous onset, with muscle weakness as its initial symptom. The clinical manifestations include symmetrically gradual exacerbation of proximal muscle weakness of the upper and lower extremities. In the cases with involvement of pelvic muscles, there are symptoms of unsteady walking, disability to standing up from sitting by him/her, difficulty standing after waking up and down stairs, running and squatting. In the cases with involvement of shoulder muscles, arm elevating and hand gripping are weakened. In the cases with involvement of cervical muscles, there are symptoms of difficulty lifting his/her head from a pillow by him/her, or sitting up from the supine posture. In the serious cases, turning over and sitting with head upright are difficult.

23.4.4 Examinations and Their Selection

23.4.4.1 Laboratory Tests
The determination of serum muscular enzyme spectrum is the most commonly used examination for the diagnosis of the disease, which is simple and reliable.

23.4.4.2 Electromyography
About 90 % PM (DM) are demonstrated to have myogenic lesions by EMG, which can be used for the diagnosis of myositis and following up examination for the mobility.

23.4.4.3 Muscle Biopsy
It should be performed in all clinically suspected cases of myositis.

23.4.4.4 MR Imaging
It is the most sensitive examination for the diagnosis of myositis, which is also noninvasive.

23.4.5 Imaging Demonstrations

MRI spin echo sequence (FSE) of T2WI is the most sensitive sequence to detect myositis and the demonstrations can guide the location of sampling for biopsy. The lesions are equal T1 signal by T2WI but bilaterally symmetric small flakes of slightly high signal by rapid FSE of T2WI, which also demonstrates normal morphology of muscular bundles with clear boundaries.

23.4.6 Diagnostic Basis

1. In spring and winter, after acute upper respiratory tract infection, obvious muscular pain and mild weakness occur in the proximal limbs. By physical examination, muscular tenderness can be found.
2. Increased serum muscular enzyme and EMG demonstrates myogenic lesions.
3. Flu virus liked particles in myoctye by serum influenza virus antibody titer monitoring, or electronic microscopy for muscle biopsy.

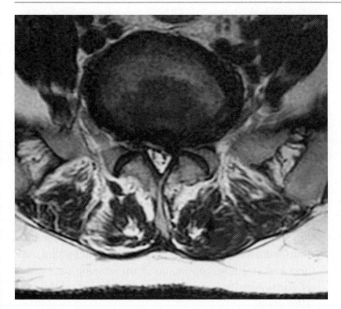

Fig. 23.6 HIV/AIDS related polymyositis. MR imaging demonstrates flaky long T2 signal in the L5 segmental erector muscle of spine, which is more obvious in the right side

4. MRI FSE T2WI demonstrates equal T1 signal. MRI rapid FSE T2WI demonstrates bilaterally symmetric small flakes of slightly high signal, no abnormal morphology of the muscular bundles with clear boundaries.

23.4.7 Differential Diagnosis

23.4.7.1 Periodic Paralysis
Periodic paralysis is more common in the young and middle aged adults, which has periodic attacks. The symptom is mainly muscular weakness of proximal limbs, muscular soreness and distention and no muscular tenderness. During its attack, the blood potassium level decreases, with low potassium manifestations by ECG, which can be relieved by potassium supplementation therapy.

23.4.7.2 Polymyositis
The conditions are serious.

23.5 HIV/AIDS Related Pine Moth Arthritis

23.5.1 Pathogen and Pathogenesis

Pine moth osteoarthritis, a seasonal endemic disease, has been successively found in the southern provinces of China. It mainly invades the skin, bone and joint. The epidemiological studies and animal experiments have demonstrated that it is related to the contact of pine moth, therefore nominated as pine moth osteoarthritis. All the patients have a history of touching the insect or touching the insect contacted objects. In China, the found pine moths are up to 40 kinds, with D. punctatus as the most common. Its pathogenesis is still unknown, with the following three speculations: (1) In the poisoning theory, it is proposed that toxin gains its access into the blood circulation to cause toxemia. Due to the strong affinity between the toxin and the connective tissue, tissues surrounding the joint respond to cause lesions. (2) The allergic reaction theory is supported by the facts that the early symptoms can be rapidly controlled by anti-allergic drugs. In addition, X-ray demonstrations and pathologic changes of the tissues around the joint are also similar to those of rheumatoid arthritis. Therefore, it is speculated as allergic reactions. (3) The theory of infection is supported by the research findings of suppurative fluid from the diseased joint or skin callosity as well as staphylococcus aureus, Staphylococcus albus and Pseudomonas aeruginosa. In addition, the X-ray demonstrations and the pathologic changes are in line with low toxic infections.

23.5.2 Pathophysiological Basis

The pathologic manifestation is aseptic inflammation. The involved joints have initial symptoms of reactive edema, congestion, small quantity bloody thick exudates from the synovium, which has a tough surface and no filtration of inflammatory cells. When the lesions progress, the joint synovium is obviously thickened, being up to several centimeters, and infiltration of inflammatory cells. The thickened synovium adheres to the surrounding thickened connective tissues. The continuous thickening of the synovium and its surrounding soft tissue may push local skin to disturb the blood supply and cause necrosis and sinus canal. Otherwise, due to the tough surface of the articular cartilage and its insufficient blood supply, the subchondral bone may be destructed to be filled by granulation tissue. There are also narrowed joint space, thickened periosteum, and formation of fibrous joint stiffness or bony stiffness.

23.5.3 Clinical Symptoms and Signs

23.5.3.1 Systemic Symptoms
The systemic symptoms are commonly slight or the patients are asymptomatic. Fever is commonly with a body temperature of 37.5–38.5 °C and rarely up to 39 °C. Other systemic symptoms include chills, headache, dizziness, general weakness and anorexia.

23.5.3.2 Local Symptoms
The lesions are commonly found in the hands, feet, wrists and ankles. According to different range and manifestations

of invasion, it can be divided into four types: (1) Osteoarticular type accounts for above 55 % and is commonly found in the exposed small joints bone ends of four extremities. The clinical symptoms include local redness, swelling, fever, pain and functional disturbance. The pain is more serious at nights and sometimes is paroxysmally serious. In its advanced stage, joint deformity and stiffness occur with proximal muscular atrophy of the joint. (2) Dermatitis type is less common that the previous type, accounting for only 25 %. The local manifestations include burning pain, unbearable itch, and pain, which tend to occur in the exposed parts of four extremities. (3) Mass type accounts for about 5 %, commonly with formation of local induration in the four extremities, both sides of lumbar and sacral spine, and perineum. The induration is painful and gradually enlarges, leading to liquefaction. (4) The mixed type accounts for 5–15 %.

23.5.4   Imaging Demonstrations

The X-ray demonstrations can be pathologically divided into acute phase and chronic phase. (1) During the acute phase, within 6 months of onset, X-ray demonstrations include surrounding tissues swelling of the affected joints, osteoporosis, bone destruction and joint lesions. There are unilateral or bilateral singular or multiple small round worn bitten lesions at the bone ends, with clear boundaries, commonly in the bone protuberance area with attachment of tendons. Singular layer thin strip or irregular periosteal proliferation occurs. (2) In the chronic phase, after 6 months, there are bone hyperplasia and sclerosis as well as joint stiffness. Local tissue edema is manifested as increased density of soft tissues surrounding joints, decreased transparency of subcutaneous adipose and swollen joint capsule. In the advanced stage, the demonstrations

include bone hyperplasia and sclerosis surrounding the destructed bone, with clear boundary and thickened diaphysis. The articular space has early asymmetric stenosis, being blurry and with unsmooth joint facets. The joint may have subluxation, and even self fusion and stiffness.

23.5.5   Diagnostic Basis

1. The patient had a history of touching pine moth or pine moth contaminated objects.
2. The exposed body parts are vulnerable to its attacks, such as hands, feet, wrist and ankles.
3. Pine moth osteoarthritis is different from other inflammations, with a rapid onset and symptoms of itchy skin, redness and swelling, continuous sharp jumping pain which is paroxysmally exacerbated and severe at nights and after noon.
4. Swelling of soft tissues in purplish red surrounding the joint, joint serious pain and articular dysfunctions.
5. Laboratory examinations demonstrate increased eosinophils and accelerated ESR.
6. Electrocardiography demonstrates myocardial lesions.
7. X-ray demonstrates soft tissue swelling surround the joint in the acute phase, with osteoporosis, bone destruction and joint lesions. In the chronic phase, bone hyperplasia and sclerosis as well as joint stiffness can be demonstrated.

23.5.6   Differential Diagnosis

In the cases with suspected history of touching pine moth or pin moth contaminated objects, the possibilities of rheumatoid arthritis, suppurative arthritis and joint tuberculosis should be excluded by the differential diagnosis.

Case Study

A male patient aged 29 years was confirmatively diagnosed as having AIDS by the CDC. His CD4 T cell count was 51/ μl.

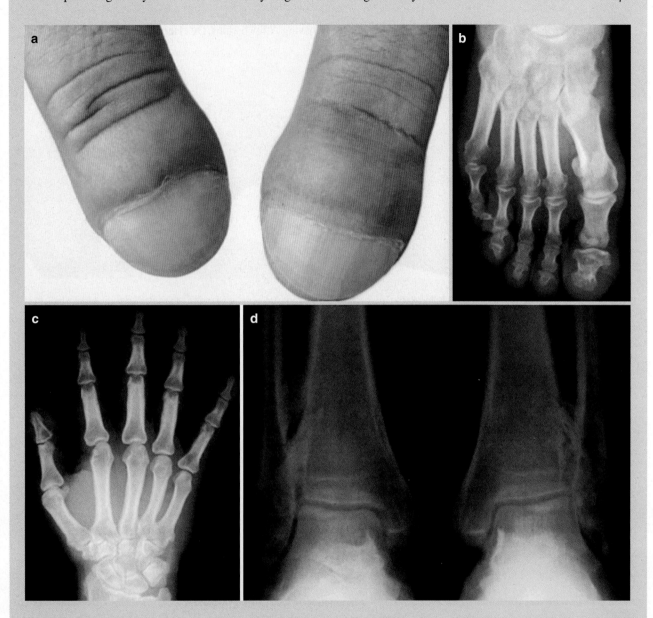

Fig. 23.7 (**a–d**) HIV/AIDS related Pine moth osteoarthritis. (**a**) The gross observations demonstrates an appearance of bone end enlargement and joint swelling. (**b**) DR demonstrates swollen articular facets and swollen surrounding soft tissues. (**c**) DR demonstrates swollen articular facets of the distal metacarpal bone, narrowed articular space of metacarpophalangeal joint, and swollen surrounding soft tissues. (**d**) DR demonstrates ankle joint osteoporosis and tough external cortex

23.6   HIV/AIDS Related Hemophilia

Case Study 1
A female patient aged 39 years was confirmatively diagnosed as having AIDS by the CDC. Her CD4 T cell count was 10/μl.

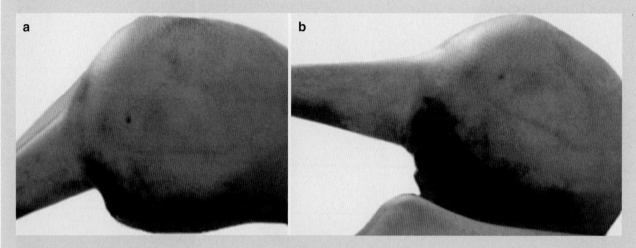

Fig. 23.8 (**a–b**) HIV/AIDS related hemophilia. (**a–b**) Gross observation demonstrates an appearance of swollen knee joint like a ball, skin ulceration in purplish black at the joint skin folds

Case Study 2
A male patient aged 49 years was confirmatively diagnosed as having AIDS by the CDC. His CD4 T cell count was 30/ μl.

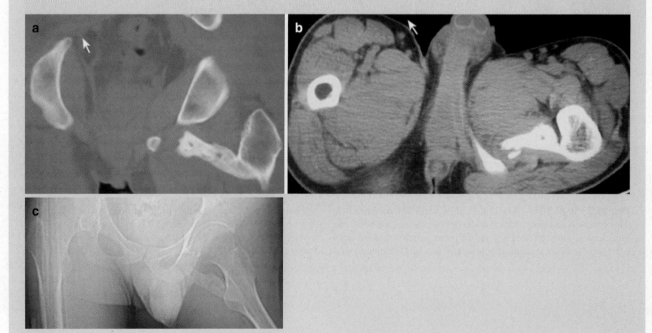

Fig. 23.9 (**a–c**) HIV/AIDS related hemophilia. (**a–b**) CT scanning demonstrates strip liked ossification plaque as a bony bridge between the left femoral trochanter space to the pubic symphysis (*arrow*). (**c**) DR demonstrates ossification plaque as a bony bridge between the left femoral trochanter space to the pubic symphysis

23.7 HIV/AIDS Related Rheumatoid Diseases

23.7.1 Pathogen and Pathogenesis

Rheumatoid arthritis is a disease that is closely related to environmental factors, cells, viruses, genetic factors, sex hormones as well as psychiatric and mental conditions. It is believed to be a autoimmune disorder. In people with HLA-DR4 and DW4 antigens, their HLA gene can generate antigen receptor as the carrier of T cell and immunity related antigens. Therefore, in the cases of exterior stimulating factors recognized by macrophages, T cell is triggered and a series of immune mediators are released to show immunological responses.

23.7.2 Pathophysiological Basis

Rheumatoid arthritis is pathologically characterized by:
1. Diffuse or localized infiltration of lymphocytes or plasma cells in the tissue, and even formation of lymphatic follicles.
2. Vasculitis accompanied by endothelial hyperplasia as well as lumen stenosis and obstruction or fibrinoid necrosis of the vascular wall.
3. Rheumatoid granuloma formation has different manifestations at different locations: (1) Synovial lesion is the beginning of articular diseases, with congestion and edema of the synovium. There are infiltration of lymphocytes, plasma cells and small quantity multinucleated cells on the surface of the synovium, with coverage by fibrin exudates. (2) There is obvious proliferation of fibroblasts at the cellular infiltration around the capillaries. The synovial cells are in column liked or fence liked arrangement, with obviously thickened synovium in villosity appearance, namely granuloma formation. (3) Due to granuloma tissue on the synovium, the vascular vessels direct to intrachondral coverage and invasion, which spreads to the center of the cartilage to interrupt its nutrients supply from the synovia. The cartilage is gradually absorbed. Meanwhile, due to the release of protein degrading enzyme and collagenase in the lysosomes, the cartilage matrix is resolved and destructed to cause narrowed articular space, rough articular facets, vascularization as well as fibrous stiffness or bony stiffness to affect its functional mobility. (4) Subcutaneous rheumatoid nodules is formed by gathering of fibrocytes, lymphocytes and mononuclear cells, which progress into dense connective tissue to form granuloma, which is the reliable evidence for the diagnosis of rheumatoid diseases. In the cases of tendinitis, tenosynovitis and bursal synovitis, there is infiltration of lymphocytes, monocytes and plasma cells. In the serious cases, rupture of tendon occurs, with adhesion and joint deformation.

23.7.3 Clinical Symptoms and Signs

Rheumatoid diseases occur commonly in small joints of the hands, wrists and feet. The lesions are symmetric and the disease is recurrent. In its early phase, there are articular redness, swelling, fever, pain and functional disturbance. In the advanced phase, the joints have different degrees of stiffness and deformation, with accompanying bone and skeletal muscular atrophy. There may be symptoms of fever, fatigue, pericarditis, subcutaneous nodules, pleuritis, arteritis and peripheral neuropathy.

23.7.4 Examinations and Their Selection

23.7.4.1 Laboratory Tests
Laboratory tests demonstrate typical antistreptolysin O test positive, most rheumatoid factors positive, abnormal IgM in about 70 % patients with rheumatoid diseases and IgG positive.

23.7.4.2 Plain X-ray
Plain X-ray is the examination of choice for screening diagnosis.

23.7.4.3 MR Imaging
It is the examination of choice for early diagnosis of rheumatoid arthritis.

23.7.5 Imaging Demonstrations

23.7.5.1 X-ray
(1) Osteoporosis is one of the common early manifestations in the cases of rheumatoid arthritis. The obvious changes include bone end and local bone lesions of the adjacent joint. (2) Narrowed articular space as well as destructed articular facet and subchondral bone; hyperplasia and sclerosis of chondral bone or partial bony fusion in the advanced stage. (3) Periosteal elevation due to the stimulation by tendinitis and arthroedema; feather liked periosteal hyperplasia and layered subperiosteal new bone that is parallel to the short bone shaft in the middle segment of tendon of phalanx and ligament attachment point; (4) Ligament ossification caused by rheumatoid arthritis has extensive distribution, with irregular ossified margin and extremely uneven density. The demonstrations can be cauliflower liked, feather liked, bone spike liked or lips liked to protrude towards the soft tissue, with accompanying local bone sclerosis. (5) In the advanced stage, subluxation of joint may occur. Especially, radial migration of the finger at the metacarpophalangeal joint is characteristically rheumatoid arthritis hand. There are also narrowed articular space and even its absence, which may progress into joint fibrous or bony stiffness.

23.7.5.2 CT Scanning

CT scanning can clearly demonstrate soft tissue swelling around the joint and its density changes. It can also demonstrate small erosive defects of the marginal bone in the articular facets of bone ends and bone destruction in the bones. The scanning of hip joints and atlanto-axial joint can provide more information for the diagnosis than conventional X-ray. In the cases with negative findings of hands and wrists, CT scanning can be ordered for early diagnosis of bone erosive lesions.

23.7.5.3 MR Imaging

MR imaging can also demonstrate the erosion of intra-articular transparent cartilage, thickening or rupture of the tendon and ligament as well as spinal cord involvement. Vascularization is demonstrated as low-medium signal on both T1WI and T2WI. Rheumatoid subcutaneous nodules are cystic, with accompanying surrounding enhancement and parenchymal even enhancement.

23.7.6 Diagnostic Basis

23.7.6.1 Clinical Evidence

(1) Morning articular stiffness persists for at least an hour. (2) Swelling of at least three joints. (3) Swelling of hand joints, palm joint or proximal interphalangeal joint. (4) Joint swelling is symmetric. (5) X-ray demonstrates osteoporosis of hand joints or their adjacencies or obvious decalcification. (6) Subcutaneous nodules. (7) Rheumatoid factors positive. The manifestations in items of (1), (2) and (3) should persist for at least 6 weeks.

23.7.6.2 Evidence from Diagnostic Imaging

(1) X-ray demonstrates osteoporosis, narrowed articular space as well as articular facet and sub articular facet bone destruction. In the advanced stage, there may be bone hyperplasia and sclerosis of articular facet as well as partial bony fusion. (2) CT scanning demonstrates soft tissue swelling around the joint and its density changes, worm bitten liked defects and bone destruction in the marginal bone of the bone end articular facet. (3) MR imaging demonstrates erosion of intra-articular transparent cartilage, thickened or rupture of the tendon and ligament, and spinacord involvement.

23.7.6.3 Evidence from Laboratory Tests

(1) Antistreptolysin O test positive and most rheumatoid factors positive. (2) More than 70 % patients with rheumatoid diseases are IgM abnormal and IgG mostly positive.

23.7.7 Differential Diagnosis

23.7.7.1 Ankylosing Spondylitis

It is characterized by (1) common occurrence in males; (2) its occurrence commonly in the age group from 15 to 30 years old; (3) its occurrence being related to the genetic factors, with high familial incidence and HILA-B27 gene positive rate being up to 90–95 %; (4) Serum rheumatoid factors negative and rheumatoid nodules rare; (5) common violations of the sacroiliac joint and the spinal cord, and sometimes large joints of the four limbs to cause joint ankylosis, intervertebral

ligament calcification and bamboo liked spine; (6) Rare involvement of the hands and feet joints; (7) Limb joint disease, mostly asymmetric.

23.7.7.2 Reiter's Syndrome

It commonly occurs in male aged 20–40 years, with repeated attacks of arthritis. It commonly invades the lower limbs, the sacroiliac joint and the spine. Arthritis commonly involves the knees, ankles, phalangeal and interphalangeal joints.

23.7.7.3 Psoriatic Arthritis

It commonly occurs in finger ends interphalangeal joints, thumb interphalangeal joints and foot interphalangeal joints. The sacroiliac joint and the spine are also commonly invaded. Early joint pathological changes can be stiffness, with later involvement of the sacroiliac joint and the spine.

23.7.7.4 Enteropathic Arthritis
Peripheral Arthritis

Initial occurrence of chronic enteritis is followed by arthritis.

Enteritis Complicated by Ankylosing Spondylitis

The lesions are mainly found in the sacroiliac joint and the spine.

23.7.7.5 Infectious Arthritis

Infectious arthritis is mainly manifested as migrating pain of large limb joints, osteoporosis, erosion and narrowed articular space.

23.7.7.6 Rheumatic Arthritis

It is common in children and young adults, with initial symptoms of acute fever as well as joint swelling and pain. It commonly invades the large joints and is migrating. There are also serum rheumatoid factors negative, antistreptolysin O test positive, antistreptokinase positive and antihyaluronidase positive.

23.7.7.7 Tuberculous Arthritis

It commonly occurs in young adults with pulmonary or lymphaden TB. It commonly invades the fingers, wrists, shoulders, ankles and knee joints. Tuberculin test is positive.

23.7.7.8 Systemic Lupus Erythematosus

It is commonly found in female young adults, with butterfly liked erythema on the face and multiple organs lesions in the heart, kidney, lung and brain. Raynaud disease is common in such cases. Serum anti-ribosomal is positive. The finding of lupus cells is an important basis for its diagnosis.

23.7.7.9 Arthrolithiasis

It commonly occurs in males, and is found in the first metatarsophalangeal joint, with involvement of the joints in ankles, knees, elbows, wrists and fingers.

23.8 HIV/AIDS Related Skeletal Syphilis

23.8.1 Pathogen and Pathogenesis

Congenital syphilis is also known as prenatal syphilis, which is transmitted to the fetus via the placenta during pregnancy. Currently, its pathogenic mechanism remains unknown. After the access of treponema pallidum into the fetus via the placenta, it multiplies in large quantity in the fetal liver, spleen, adrenal gland and other organs and tissues to cause stillbirth and premature birth. Pregnancy syphilis has an increased harmful risk, being 2.5 times higher than normal pregnancy. The perinatal mortality rate of the fetus/baby reaches as high as 50 % in the cases of pregnancy complicated by syphilis. The survivors show clinical symptoms at different ages. The occurrence at the age under 2 years is known as early syphilis and above 2 years is known as late syphilis.

23.8.2 Pathophysiological Basis

The main pathological changes include vascular endothelial cells swelling and proliferation as well as luminal occlusion. There is also caseous change or fibrous tissue proliferation of the distal local tissue to form scars. Therefore, the organs are structurally destructed and functionally impaired.

23.8.3 Clinical Symptoms and Signs

The clinical manifestations of early congenital syphilis include macula and papula in the head, hip and limbs; skin sclerosis, skin redness and luster in the palms and pelma; systemic or local edema; shedding of the hair, eyebrows and eyelashes. There may be also spindle shaped swelling of the fingers and toes as well as limbs pseudoparalysis induced by syphilitic osteomyelitis and periostitis. Other symptoms include low grade fever, unfavorable breast feeding, no weight gain, weakness, vomiting and abdominal distension, often with accompanying bleeding and anemia. Late congenital syphilis has clinical manifestations of stromal keratitis, saber leg, horse saddle nose, syphilis tooth, knee joint swelling and pain, retarded intelligence development, deafness and optic nerve atrophy at the age above 5–6 years.

23.8.4 Examinations and Their Selection

1. Treponema pallidum examination is to collect secretions from the skin or mucosa defects for direct smear. The observation under a dark-field microscope can find the Treponema pallidum.
2. Rapid plasma reagin (RPR) of annular slide test demonstrates black agglutination after reaction between the test reagents and the positive serum, which is the basis for the diagnosis.
3. Serum Treponema pallidum test findings can define the diagnosis with Treponema pallidum as the antigen to detect the specific antibodies in the serum.
4. Determination of Treponema pallidum IgM antibody can be an indicator for assessing the therapeutic efficacy and defining the diagnosis.
5. X-ray is the examination of choice for the diagnosis of congenital bone syphilis.

23.8.5 Imaging Demonstrations

The X-ray demonstrations include: (1) Syphilitic bone disease has the pathological changes commonly in the diaphysis of limbs long bone. Its bilaterally symmetric occurrence causes pathological separation of the diaphysis and epiphysis to avoid destruction of the bone epiphysis. (2) Some thickened periosteum fuses with cortex to thicken the diaphysis. (3) The early ossification strip of the diaphysis and epiphysis end is thickened and blurry, with transparent strip and dense line, which form sandwich liked changes. (4) The diaphysis and epiphyseal end has bone destructions and defects, which are unilateral with clear boundary and is known as cat bitten sign. (5) The periosteum is obviously thickened to wrap the diaphysis in onion liked changes.

Case Study

A baby boy aged 3 months was confirmatively diagnosed as having AIDS by the CDC. He had skin rashes for 10 days, with acute onset. By examinations, his serum syphilis antibody (TPPA) was positive; and RPR titer was 1:256. The diagnosis was congenital syphilis. His mother was an HIV positive patient and was found to have syphilis after delivery.

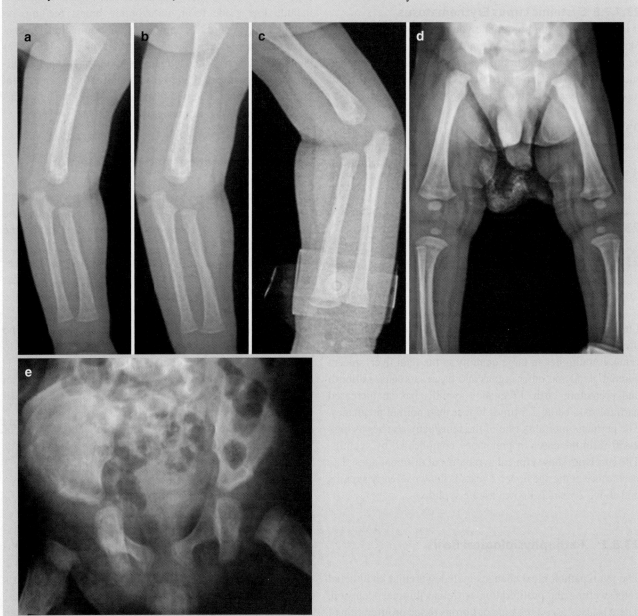

Fig. 23.10 (a–e) HIV/AIDS related bone syphilis. (a-b) It is demonstrated to have bilateral femur and tibia as well as bilateral fibula diaphysis in layered and onion liked hyperplasia and subcortical transparent strip line, blurry early calcified strip of the epiphysis end with increased density. (c) It is demonstrated to have bilateral diaphysis layered and onion liked hyperplasia of the humerus, ulna and radius; subcortical transparent bright strip line; blurry early calcified strip with increased density and being rough and irregular; and spots transparent areas in the medullary cavity of the bilateral humerus, radius and ulna. (d, e) It is demonstrated to have patchy low density shadows in the inferior margin of the right ilium, which is likely to be bone defects of cat bitten sign with blurry boundary; and transparent bright line at the left medial inferior margin

23.8.6   Diagnostic Basis

1. Neonatal congenital syphilis has prodromes of low grade fever, unfavorable breast feeding, no weight gain, weakness and vomiting. The parents usually have a history of syphilis, and the neonatal usually have jaundice, edema, hepatosplenomegaly and lymphadenectasis. In 3–12 weeks after birth, there are symptoms of skin rash, rhinitis and bloody secretions, or childhood horse saddle nose and syphilis tooth.
2. The blood syphilis antibody (TPPA) is positive.
3. X-ray demonstrates onion liked periosteum hyperplasia of the limbs long bones to form bone shell, worm bitten liked bone destructions in cat bitten sign, as well as thickened and blurry early calcified strip at the epiphyseal end.

23.8.7   Differential Diagnosis

23.8.7.1 Cortical Bone Hyperplasia
HIV/AIDS related bone syphilis should be differentiated from cortical bone hyperplasia. Both have multiple and symmetric layers of periosteum in long tube appearance. However, in the cases of cortical bone hyperplasia, epiphyseal end is not involved, with self healing after several months.

23.8.7.2 Scurvy and Rickets
Syphilitic osteochondritis should be differentiated from scurvy and rickets. The cases of syphilitic osteochondritis have serum syphilis enzyme positive and sandwich liked sign. However, scurvy and rickets rarely occur in babies aged less than 6 months.

23.8.7.3 Suppurative Osteomyelitis
Syphilitic osteomyelitis should be differentiated from suppurative osteomyelitis. The cases of syphilitic osteomyelitis are commonly RPR positive, with accompanying multiple symmetrical periostitis and epiphyseal inflammation. There is fine or no bony necrosis. The cases of suppurative osteomyelitis have an acute onset, with bone destructions spreading rapidly from the epiphyseal end to the diaphysis. There are large areas bone destruction and large bony necrosis, with obvious bone hyperplasia to form bone shell.

23.9   HIV/AIDS Related Vertebral Metastases

23.9.1   Pathogen and Pathogenesis

The body institution is an important factor for the occurrence of bone neoplasm. In some cases, the occurrence of bone neoplasm is related to lesions. In some other cases, its occurrence is related to infections and long-term exposure to large quantity of radioactive substances. Primary bone neoplasm is derived from bones, cartilages, hemopoietic tissues or bone marrow, fibrous tissues, vascular vessels, adipose, nerves, dorsal cord, epithelium and other unknown origins. Secondary bone neoplasm, namely metastatic neoplasm, can be from any neoplasm because almost all neoplasm can spread to the bone. The metastatic neoplasms are rarely sarcoma and neuroblastoma.

23.9.2   Pathophysiological Basis

The internal and external blood supplies and lymph flow of the vertebral bodies and canals are abundant, with slow blood flow. The venous system in the vertebral canal has no venous valve, which enables tumor embolus to remain there. Therefore, the vertebral canal is susceptible to metastatic neoplasms.

23.9.3   Clinical Symptoms and Signs

The common symptoms are as the following: (1) The pain is commonly gradually exacerbating lower back pain which is often persistent and dull with paroxysmally severe. At nights, it is worse. In the cases of tumor compression or nerve root stimulation, radiating pain occurs. (2) The cases with benign tumor usually have a normal body temperature, while the cases of malignancies usually have low grade fever. (3) Masses. (4) Cachexia manifestations. (5) Local swelling is manifested as superficial venous filling and high skin, which is the sign of penetrating of the bone malignancies through cortical bone into the soft tissue and rapidly growing. (6) Spinal dysfunctions. (7) Spinal cord and nerve lesions. (8) Vertebral bone neoplasm may compress or invade the sympathetic nerves to cause sweating dysfunction, which results in dry skin with no sweating in the lower limbs.

23.9.4   Examinations and Their Selection

23.9.4.1 X-ray
It is the most basic examination, which is of the choice. However, the demonstrations cannot define the qualitative diagnosis in most cases of spinal neoplasms.

23.9.4.2 CT Scanning
Compared to X-ray, CT scanning has obviously improved diagnostic rate for spinal neoplasms. By CT scanning, spinal neoplasm is divided into osteolytic lesions, mixed lesions and osteogenic lesions. It can demonstrate those fine lesions that are failed to be demonstrated by the X-ray. It demonstrates more clearly invasion of neoplasm to both interior and exterior tissues. Especially, the enhanced scanning and 3-dimensional reconstruction greatly improve the diagnosis and differential diagnosis of spinal neoplasm.

23.9.4.3 MR Imaging

It has a high resolution to the soft tissue, with multiple perspective demonstrations of spinal destruction by the neoplasm with no false shadow. Especially by adipose suppression techniques and Gd-DTPA enhanced imaging for venous enhancement, the diagnosis can be greatly improved.

23.9.4.4 Radioactive Nuclide Examination

It can be applied for the early diagnosis of neoplasms, which has great significance in defining the lesion range and metastasis as well as assessing the therapeutic efficacy.

23.9.4.5 Biopsy

CT guided puncture for biopsy can define the pathological type of spinal neoplasms and its qualitative diagnosis.

23.9.5   Imaging Demonstrations

23.9.5.1 X-ray

The lesions are originated from the appendices and spread toward the vertebral body, being cystic and dilated, with unilocular and multilocular changes. It has a clearly defined borderline from the normal bone, with no surrounding sclerosis. The lesions penetrate into the soft tissue to form soft tissue masses.

23.9.5.2 CT Scanning

The vertebral bodies are in round spots liked or decorative pattern liked changes. The lesions are in osteolytic low density, with clear boundary. The thickened bone trabecula is in round spots liked high density, with intact cortical bone and surrounding soft tissue swelling.

23.9.5.3 MR Imaging

Most neoplasms are in low to moderate signal by T1WI and high signal by T2WI. Non-calcified neoplasms are in high signal by spin echo and gradient echo of T2WI. Lesions of calcification and sclerosis are in low signals by T1WI and T2WI. The invasion of the cortical bone is in high signal by T1WI and T2WI. Edema and neoplasm are in similar signal by T1WI and T2WI, which is difficult to differentiate. Enhanced imaging can differentiate the enhanced neoplasm from edema.

Case Study

A female patient aged 59 years was confirmatively diagnosed as having AIDS by the CDC. She had a surgical history for breast carcinoma 8 months ago and her CD4 T cell count was 5/μl.

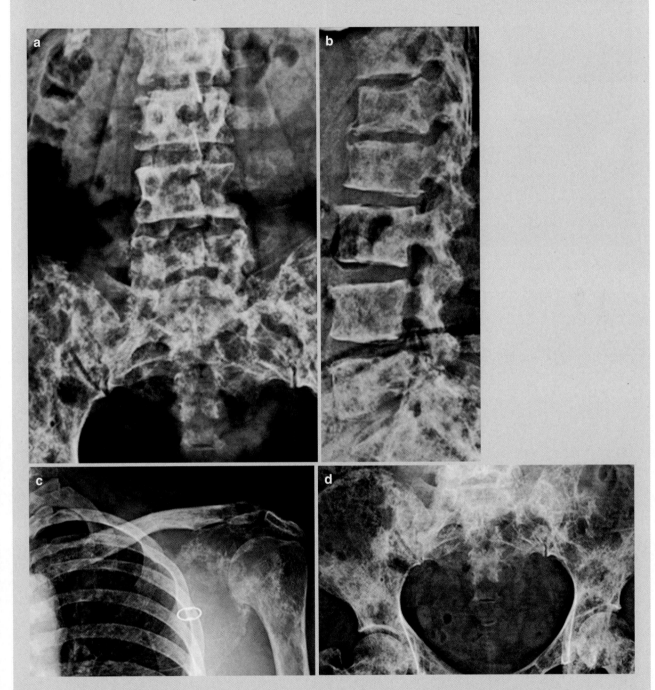

Fig. 23.11 (**a–h**) HIV/AIDS related bone metastasis of breast cancer. (**a–b**) Lumbar anteroposterior and lateral radiology demonstrates multiple low density areas in the bone of lumbar vertebrae and cacroiliac joint. (**c**) DR demonstrates multiple low density areas in the bones of should joint. (**d**) DR demonstrates multiple low density areas in the bones of pelvis. (**e–f**) CT scanning demonstrates multiple low density areas in the bones of vertebral body and interrupted bone trabecula. (**g**) Microscopy at a low magnification demonstrates breast invasive micropapillary carcinoma. (**h**) Microscopy at a medium magnification demonstrates breast invasive micropapillary carcinoma

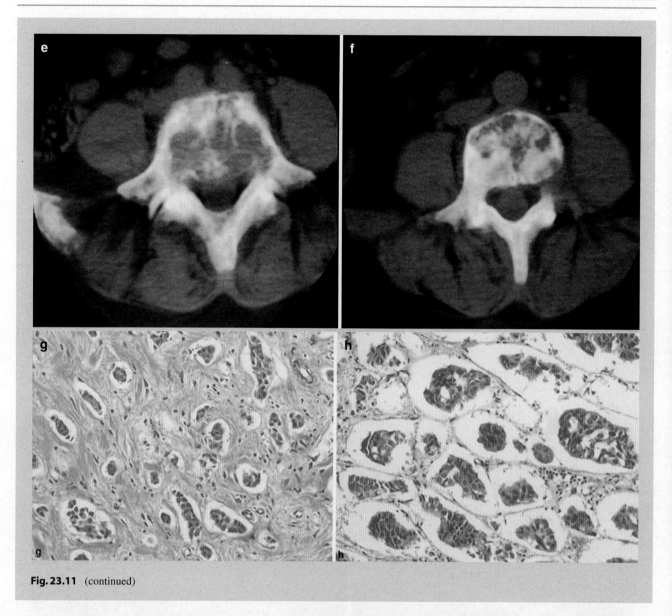

Fig. 23.11 (continued)

23.9.6 Diagnostic Basis

23.9.6.1 Clinical Manifestations
The clinical symptoms include pain, neurological functional impairment, masses and pathological fracture.

23.9.6.2 Diagnostic Imaging
(1) X-ray has a low sensitivity to vertebral destructions. The lesions can be found with at least 30–50 % component destruction. (2) CT scanning demonstrates cortical bone destruction and trabecular destruction, as well as tumors invasion into the epidural space or paravertebral soft tissues. (3) MR imaging demonstrates the whole spine, epidural space and paravertebral tumors as well as the compressed segments of the spinal cord and the nerve roots, the severity of the compression. (4) PET-CT scanning demonstrates thick stained areas of lesion metabolites. (5) Laboratory tests demonstrate indices within normal limits. In some patients, there are accelerated ESR, anemia and increased alkaline phosphatase, as well as abnormal level of biomarkers in the metastatic tumors.

23.9.6.3 Pathological Biopsy

23.9.7 Differential Diagnosis

23.9.7.1 Bone Tuberculosis
HIV/AIDS related bone metastasis should be differentiated from bone tuberculosis. The cases of bone TB have low grade fever, night sweating and other toxic symptoms. The lesions erode the intervertebral discs and corresponding margins of the vertebral body, with paravertebral cold abscesses, which facilitate the differential diagnosis.

23.9.7.2 Degenerative Spinal Cord Diseases
HIV/AIDS related bone metastasis should be differentiated from degenerative spinal cord diseases. The cases of degenerative spinal cord diseases have manifestations of vertebral bone hyperplasia, intervertebral discs degeneration, vertebral canal stenosis and ligament calcification.

23.9.7.3 Spinal Suppurative Inflammation
HIV/AIDS related bone metastasis should be differentiated from spinal suppurative inflammation. The cases with spinal suppurative inflammation have manifestations of bone destruction, narrowed vertebral space, commonly formation of necrotic bone and mostly no formation of abscesses.

Extended Readings

1. Fleckenstein JL, Burns DK, Mrphy FK, et al. Differential diagnosis of bacterial myositis in AIDS:evaluation with MR imaging. Radiology. 1991;179:653–8.
2. Steinbach LS, Tehranzedah J, Fleckenstein JL, et al. Human immunodeficiency virus infection: musculoskeletal manifestations. Radiology. 1993;186:833–8. WB Saunders, 1996. 210–222.
3. Hughes RA, Row IF, Shanson D, et al. Septic bone, joint and muscle lesions associated with human immunodeficiency virus infection. Br J Rheumatol. 1992;31:381–8.
4. Jarzem P, Tsoukas C, Burke D, et al. Hemophilia, septic arthritis and human immunodeficiency virus (abstract no.TH.B.P.7). Int Conf AIDS. 1989;5:416.
5. Johnson SC, Stamm CP, Hicks CB. Tuberculous psoas muscle abscess following chemoprophylaxis with isoniazid in a patient with human immunodeficiency virus infection. Rev Infect Dis. 1990; 12:754–6.
6. Go BM, Ziring DL, Kountz DS. Spinal epidural abscess due to Aspergillus sp in a patient with acquired immunodeficiency syndrome. South Med J. 1993;86:957–60.

Contents

H. Li (ed.), *Radiology of HIV/AIDS*,
DOI 10.1007/978-94-007-7823-8_24, © Springer Science+Business Media Dordrecht and People's Medical Publishing House 2014

24.1   An Overview of HIV/AIDS Related Pediatric Diseases

Since the prevalence of HIV/AIDS, there had been 3.2 million children patients with HIV/AIDS worldwide till the year of 2002. The diagnostic criteria for pediatric AIDS formulated by the CDC of the United States are: children under the age of 13 years, with characteristic opportunistic infection or neoplasm caused by cellular immunodeficiency that excludes primary immunodeficient diseases, other congenital diseases and the cases with a history of immunodepressant used. Pediatric HIV/AIDS is the most commonly infected via vertical transmission from mother to children, and blood transfusion and the use of blood products are the second commonly transmission route. The vertical transmission occurs in the late period of pregnancy and before/after delivery. The HIV gains its access to the fetus via the placenta (intrauterine infection) or via contacting secretions containing HIV during delivery. It is believed that the transmission rate is related to the viral load of the mother. In the cases with HIV RNA above 50,000 copies/ml, vertical transmission occurs.

Compared to AIDS in adults, pediatric HIV/AIDS is characterized by: (1) The latent period after HIV infection is short, with acute onset of the disease and rapid progression. (2) The growth retardation deviated from common growth curve is a typical manifestation of pediatric HIV infection. (3) Bacteria infections recur, commonly lymphatic interstitial pneumonia. (4) Encephalopathy syndrome is common in infants and young children, which has an early onset, rapid progression and poor prognosis. (5) About 50 % infected children have accompanying diffuse lymphadenectasis and repeated diarrhea. About one third infected children have accompanying thrombocytopenia. Some infected children have eczema liked skin rashes and repeated otitis media.

24.2   HIV/AIDS Related Lymphoid Interstitial Pneumonia

Lymphoid interstitial pneumonia (LIP) is a lung disease with respiratory distress caused by HIV infection of children. Its pathological changes are characterized by specific pulmonary infiltration of lymphocytes. It was firstly reported by Carrhigton and Liebow in 1966 [1]. Since then, its occurrence in children with HIV/AIDS is continually reported. LIP in children under 13 years of age is defined as the diagnostic indicator of HIV/AIDS by the CDC of the United States.

24.2.1 Pathogen and Pathogenesis

LIP has an incidence of 16–50 % in children with HIV, commonly at the age of 2–3 years. Currently, it is believed that LIP in children with HIV infection is caused by the immunological responses. Most studies indicate that the proliferating lymphocytes in HIV infected patients are CD8 or cytotoxic/inhibited T lymphocytes. These cells cause immunological impairments via different ways, including T cells activation caused by immunological identification of antigens, production of lymphokines by CD4 lymphocytes such as interleukin-2 and proliferation of effector cells responsible for tissue lesions caused by lymphokines that is mainly CD8 cells in HIV/AIDS. Currently, the following three factors are believed to be related to the pathogenesis of HIV/AIDS. (1) HIV infection causes proliferation of lymphocytes in the body. The lung lesions can be relieved by using the Zidovudine therapy. HIV antigens and antibodies can be found in the bronchoalveolar lavage fluid of LIP patients. (2) HIV and EB virus synergetic infection: Most children with LIP have concurrent EBV infection. Otherwise, EB virus genome can be found that causes lymphatic tissue hyperplasia in lungs of HIV positive children. EB virus infection is transmitted via contacts, with LIP patients as its susceptible population. (3) The immunogenetics basis: It has been demonstrated that more HLA-DR6 can be found in HIV positive patients, with occurrence of CD8 lymphocytosis syndrome and LIP. Generally, the factors of immunological nonspecific stimulation, HIV specific stimulation or EB virus infection and HIV infection contribute to the onset of LIP in HIV positive patients.

24.2.2 Pathophysiological Basis

Gross lung specimen demonstrates diffuse thickening of the pulmonary interstitium. Microscopy demonstrates mass liked mixed cells infiltration in the septa of pulmonary lobes, alveolar wall, bronchus, bronchioles and perivascular tissues, which is mainly mature lymphocytes and occasionally generative center with no nucleus cleavage. Lymphatic follicle with generative center is common. There are hyperplasia of type II alveolar epithelium, and increased macrophages in the alveolar cavity.

24.2.3 Clinical Symptoms and Signs

The onset is chronic, with symptoms of cough, dyspnea and hypoxia. Lung auscultation may be negative or may find weakened respiration sound, wheezing and end-inspiratory dry rales. Most of the children patients have bronchospasm, with no cough before demonstration of lesions by chest X-ray. The patients with long term illness course have clubbing fingers/toes and parotid/lymphaden enlargement. The pulmonary functions impaired children have serious hypoxia which causes oxygen dependency. Due to the decrease of lymphocytes and CD4 T cell count, the critical cases with lift threatening conditions are rare, but the patients are more susceptible to opportunistic infections.

24.2.4 Examinations and Their Selection

24.2.4.1 Laboratory Tests
Laboratory tests may demonstrate slight anemia, immuno-globulin manufacturing abnormalities and about 80 % patients with LIP have serum protein abnormality.

24.2.4.2 Pulmonary Function Examinations
Pulmonary function examinations commonly demonstrate restricted pulmonary ventilation disturbance, decreased functional diffusion and hypoxemia.

24.2.4.3 Alveolar Lavage
Alveolar lavage fluid has certain diagnostic value for LIP. The increases of lymphocytes, CD3 T cells, and polyclone CD20 B cells in bronchoalveolar lavage fluid indicate the diagnosis of LIP.

24.2.4.4 Chest X-ray and CT Scanning
Both are commonly used examinations, but with non-specific findings.

24.2.4.5 Lung Biopsy
The diagnosis of LIP depends on histological examination.

24.2.5 Imaging Demonstrations

24.2.5.1 Chest X-ray
Chest X-ray demonstrates non-specific findings for the diagnosis of LIP. Both lungs have diffuse interstitial infiltration that is mostly symmetric network or find network and nodular shadows. Otherwise, they are thick network and nodular shadows or thick nodular shadows. The network liked shadows are linear or leather liked, with a distribution in the basement of the lungs. The lesions can also be located in the upper lungs or middle lobes, with air bronchogram sign. Hilar/Mediastinal lymphadenectasis is rare, and pleural effusion is rare.

24.2.5.2 CT Scanning
High-resolution computed tomography (HRCT) has main demonstrations of diffuse ground glass liked changes, blurry centrilobular nodules and subpleural small nodules (1–4 mm), thickened interlobular septa, thickened broncho-vascular bundles and scattering thin-walled cysts. The demonstrations of turbid interlobular grids, honeycomb liked deformation and bronchiectasis are rare. By HRCT, thin walled cysts can be found in 68–82 % children with LIP, which have diameters of 1–3 mm in a small quantity. Pulmonary involvement can be found in less than 10 % cases, with demonstrations overlapping with ground glass liked changes. The pulmonary ground glass liked changes pathologically demonstrate diffuse infiltration of alveolar septum lymphocytes and plasmocytes. Generally, demonstrations by CT scanning of thin sections of ground glass liked changes predict that the lesions can be absorbed or are healing. Due to the infiltration of lymphocytes in the surrounding tissues of bronchioles, the airway is obstructed and dilated to finally cause cysts. The primary lesions of parenchymal changes can also progress into cysts and the formation of cysts is irreversible. The pulmonary parenchymal changes can be partially absorbed and partially progress into honeycomb liked lung. Generally, the newly emerging cysts mostly occur at the site of primary centrilobular nodules. And the honeycomb liked changes commonly occur in the areas with original pulmonary parenchymal changes.

Case Study

A boy patient aged 2 years was confirmatively diagnosed as having AIDS by the CDC. His CD4 T cell count was 25/μl.

Fig. 24.1 HIV/AIDS related lymphoid interstitial pneumonia. It is demonstrated to have infiltration of large quantity lymphocytes around alveoli

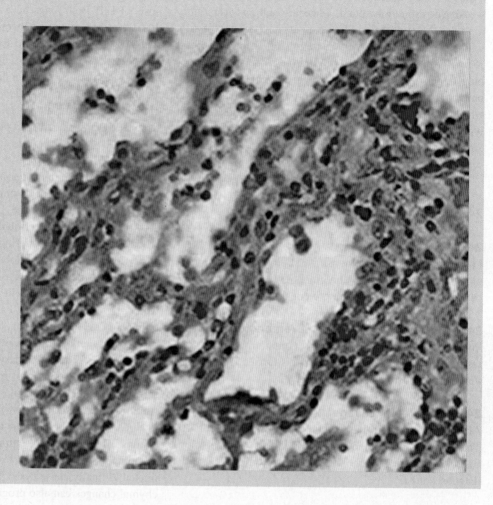

24.2.6 Diagnostic Basis

Clinical manifestations in pediatric AIDS patients include cough, dyspnea and hypoxia, which have a slowly progressive course. The occurrence of lymphocytosis and hyperglobulinemia with no other isolated pathogens in combination with chest diagnostic imaging findings can define the clinical diagnosis. Based on the findings of bronchoalveolar lavage fluid examination and lung biopsy, the definitive diagnosis can be made.

24.2.7 Differential Diagnosis

24.2.7.1 Pneumocystis Carinii Pneumonia

The characteristic CT scanning demonstrations of PCP are bilaterally symmetric extensive ground glass liked shadows in both lungs. Otherwise, the shadows are in patchy or map liked distribution. However, early PCP is difficult to be differentiated from LIP by the diagnostic imaging. Bronchoalveolar lavage contributes to the differential diagnosis.

24.2.7.2 Miliary Pulmonary Tuberculosis

Most cases of military pulmonary tuberculosis have symptoms of acute infections. The pulmonary lesions are mostly located in the upper and middle lungs, with even size and in bilaterally symmetric distribution. Pathological examinations contribute to the differential diagnosis.

24.2.7.3 Cytomegalovirus Pneumonia

The clinical manifestations are non-specific. Chest X-ray demonstrates diffuse network nodular shadows or flaky thin shadows. The definitive diagnosis depends on the histological diagnosis.

24.3 HIV/AIDS Related Pulmonary Bacterial Infection

Respiratory system is the most commonly involved body part by opportunistic infections of AIDS. Bacterial pneumonia is one of the major causes of death in AIDS patients. It has been reported that in every 10 cases of death in AIDS patients each year, 1 case is from bacterial pneumonia, and the cases of HIV positive bacterial pneumonia are 78 times as many as those of HIV negative bacterial pneumonia.

24.3.1 Pathogen and Pathogenesis

AIDS children are susceptible to bacterial pneumonia, which is related to their immune deficiency. B cell dysfunction leads to decreased production of antigen specific antibody, T cell functional impairment and neutrocytopenia, which, in combination with intravenous drug use and other factors, result in their susceptibility to various bacteria. Currently, the reported pathogenic bacteria include streptococcus pneumonia, hemophilus influenza, pseudomonas, staphylococcus aureus and legionella.

24.3.2 Pathophysiologic Basis

By microscopic observation, pneumonia caused by streptococcus pneumonia has lesions in different sizes with small spots and flakes of focal inflammation. The lesions are more serious in the inferior lobes and dorsal segment of both lungs. The lesions are in dark red and slightly protrude in the section that is smooth with no particle. In the young children, fusion of multiple small lesions is common, and sometimes even involves the whole lung lobe. Under a microscope, at the center and peripheral areas of the lesions, there are inflammatory bronchi and the lesions are filled with neutrophilic granulocyte as well as lytic and shed epithelial cells. The surrounding alveoli are initially filled with exudates containing abundant proteins, followed by occurrence of neutrophilic granulocyte, erythrocytes as well as shed and enlarged alveolar epithelial cells. The cellulose is rarely found. In the advanced stage of pneumonia, the exudates are commonly transformed into purulent fluid.

By the naked eyes observation, staphylococcus aureus pneumonia has coverage of the pleural surface by a thick layer of fibrinous purulent secretions, protruding grayish yellow or yellowish parenchymal changes under the pleura, extensive hemorrhagic necrosis and multiple small abscesses in the lungs. Once the subpleural small abscesses rupture, pyothorax or pneumopyothorax occurs, sometimes with involved bronchi to form bronchopleural fistula. Microscopic observation demonstrates alveoli filled with bloody edema, occasionally macrophages and small quantity neutrophils. There are also large quantities of Staphylococcus aureus and necrotic tissue debris in the abscess, bronchial lumen filled with pyocyte, seriously damaged mucosa, collapsed parenchymal changes on the cross section to form most abscesses.

24.3.3 Clinical Symptoms and Signs

The involvement of lungs in HIV positive patients has non-specific symptoms and signs. The clinical manifestations include cough, fever and shortness of breath. The symptoms are obvious, being more acute and serious than those in adult patients. Fever and shortness of breath are especially common in HIV/AIDS children. Its further progression may cause bacteremia and sepsis. By physical examinations, there are tachypnea, tachycardia, pulmonary dry and moist rales and pulmonary parenchymal changes.

24.3.4 Examinations and Their Selection

24.3.4.1 Laboratory Tests
Laboratory tests demonstrate increased C-reactive protein concentration, which is important for the diagnosis and differential diagnosis of bacterial pneumonia. Pathogenic examinations are the basis for the definitive diagnosis.

24.3.4.2 Diagnostic Imaging
Chest X-chest and CT scanning are commonly used imaging examinations, which contribute greatly to the diagnosis and prognosis prediction.

24.3.5 Imaging Demonstrations

Chest X-ray demonstrates pneumococcus pneumonia as high density blurry shadows in the lungs fields, commonly with concurrent pleural effusion or pyothorax. Sometimes nodular lesions and clubbed lesions can also be found at the base of lungs. CT scanning demonstrates thickened bronchial wall and bronchiectasis.

Chest X-ray and CT scanning demonstrate legionella pneumonia as involvement of singular or multiple lung lobes, with a rapid progression. Cavities and empyema are common. Interstitial infiltration may also occur.

Chest X-ray and CT scanning demonstrate bronchogenic staphylococcus aureus pneumonia as multiple small patches of high density shadows in the middle zone of both lungs, with blurry boundary and accompanying transparent areas, which are lesions of focal obstructive emphysema. Dynamic observation of the intrapulmonary lesions demonstrates that the lesions can progress from patches of parenchymal changes into extensive large flakes or segments of lesions within several hours or 1 day. Round or oval shaped low density air sacs occur within 1–2 days after the onset. The rapid progression demonstrated by the diagnostic imaging is characteristic. Sometimes, pulmonary cavities containing gas–liquid level can be found. Pleural effusion, empyema, and pyopneumothorax are also common. By chest X-ray, the secondary blood-borne staphylococcus aureus pneumonia is demonstrated to have patches or spherical high density shadows in middle and lower fields of both lungs.

Case Study 1

A boy patient aged 4 years was confirmatively diagnosed as having AIDS by the CDC. His CD4 T cell count was 25/μl.

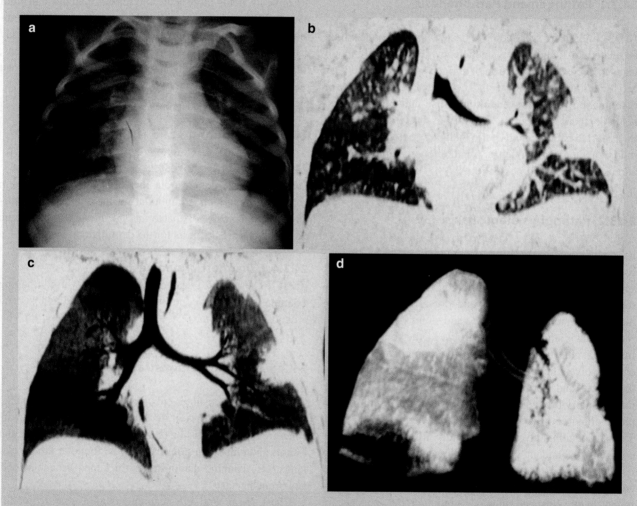

Fig. 24.2 (a–g) HIV/AIDS related bacterial infection. (a) Chest X-ray demonstrates multiple shadows with increased density in both lungs, which is more obvious in the right upper lung. (b–d) Coronal plain CT scanning demonstrates high density parenchymal changes shadows in both lungs, which is more obvious in the left lung. (e, f) Sagittal plain CT scanning demonstrates parenchyma lesions. (g) CT scanning of the mediastinal window demonstrates parenchyma lesions in the left lung, left pleural effusion and pleural hypertrophy

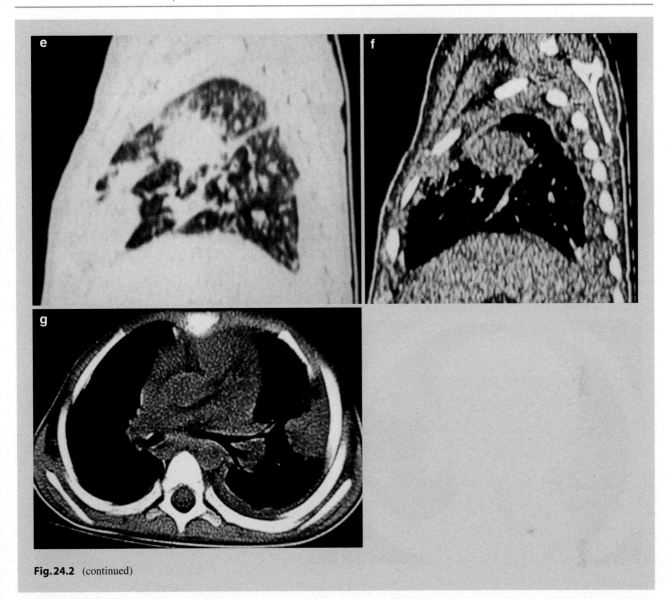

Fig. 24.2 (continued)

Case Study 2

A boy patient aged 3 years was confirmatively diagnosed as having AIDS by the CDC. He had symptoms of cough and fever and his CD4 T cell count was 45/μl.

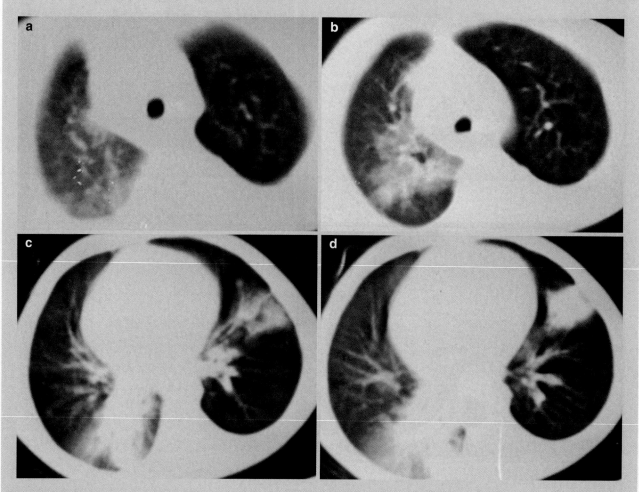

Fig. 24.3 (**a**) CT scanning demonstrates increased density shadows in the upper lobe of the right lung, and small flakes of ground glass liked shadows. (**b**) CT scanning demonstrates large flakes of high density parenchymal shadows in the upper lobe of the right lung, with blurry boundary. (**c**, **d**) CT scanning demonstrates high density parenchyma shadows in both lungs, with air bronchogram sign in them

Case Study 3

A boy patient aged 11 years was confirmatively diagnosed as having AIDS by the CDC. His CD4 T cell count was 29/μl.

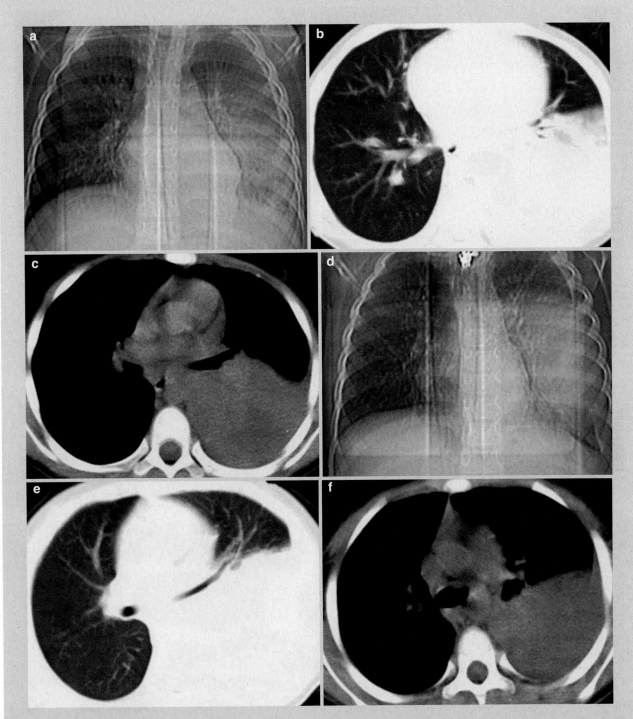

Fig. 24.4 (**a–f**) HIV/AIDS related bacterial infection. (**a–c**) It is demonstrated the lesions pre-treatment. (**d–f**) It is demonstrated the lesions post-treatment. (**a**) DR demonstrates large flakes of shadows with increased density in left lung. (**b**) Pulmonary window demonstrates high-density parenchymal shadows in the left lung, with smooth anterior margin; and cords liked shadows in the medial segment of the middle lobe of the right lung. (**c**) Mediastinal window demonstrates parenchymal changes of soft tissue density in the left lung, with irregular low density areas in them. (**d**) DR demonstrates progressed lesions in the left lung, lesions with increased density, and extended range with lesions. (**e**) Pulmonary window demonstrates high density parenchymal shadows in the left lung, compressed and narrowed bronchi in the upper lobe of the left lung, with forward migration. (**f**) Mediastinal window demonstrates even density of lung tissues with parenchymal changes, straight and smooth anterior margins of the lesions

Case Study 4

A girl patient aged 9 years was confirmatively diagnosed as having AIDS by the CDC. She was infected via vertical transmission of HIV, with manifestations of fungal stomatitis, drug induced hepatitis, moderate anemia and hepatitis C. Her CD4 T cell count was 6/μl.

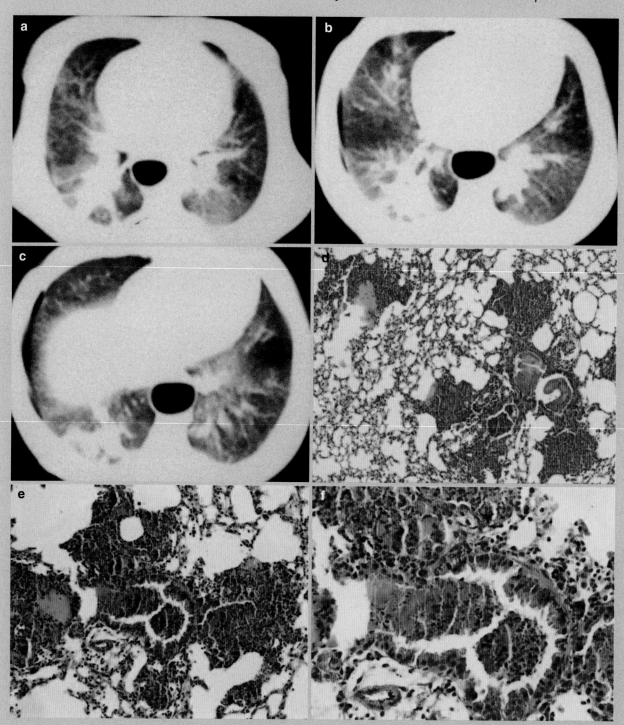

Fig. 24.5 (**a–f**) HIV/AIDS related bacterial infection and pneumothorax. (**a–c**) Pulmonary window demonstrates multiple patches and large flakes of shadows with increased density in both lungs, abnormal transparent area without lung markings in the lateral zone of the right lung. (**d–f**) HE staining demonstrates many inflammatory cells infiltration in the lung tissues around the bronchioles, and inflammatory exudates in the bronchiole lumen (HE×10, ×20, ×40)

Case Study 5

A boy patient aged 8 years was confirmatively diagnosed as having AIDS by the CDC. His CD4 T cell count was 13/μl.

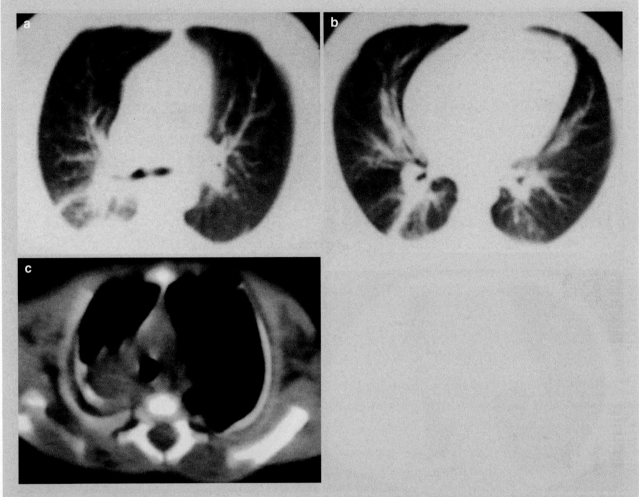

Figs. 24.6 (a–c) HIV/AIDS related bacterial infection. (a, b) CT scanning demonstrates high density parenchyma shadows and multiple cords liked shadows in the right lung, and ground glass liked shadows in the left lung. (c) CT scanning of the mediastinal window demonstrates decreased volume of the right lung, and soft tissue density of the lung tissues with parenchymal changes

Case Study 6

A boy patient aged 6 years was confirmatively diagnosed as having AIDS by the CDC. His CD4 T cell count was 63/μl.

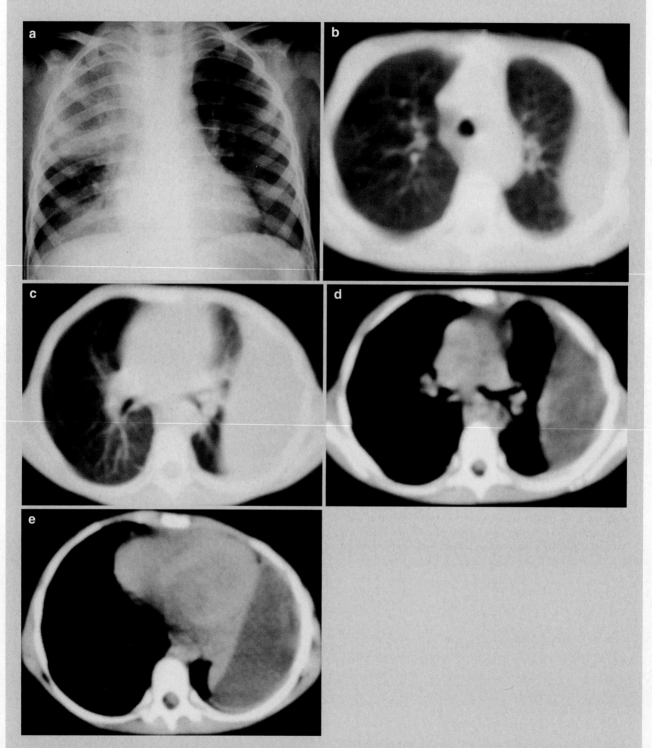

Fig. 24.7 (a–e) HIV/AIDS related bacterial infection and encapsulated pleural effusion. (**a**) Chest X-ray demonstrates parenchymal changes in the right lung, which is more obvious in the upper right lung; and blurry flakes of shadows in the left lower lung. (**b**, **c**) CT scanning of the pulmonary window demonstrates increased density of both lungs, left encapsulated pleural effusion, compressed left lung with shrinkage of lung volume. (**d**, **e**) Mediastinal window demonstrates left encapsulated pleural effusion and left pleural hypertrophy

24.3.6 Diagnostic Basis

1. The most common clinical manifestations are cough, fever and shortness of breath. There is also moist rale of lungs.
2. Laboratory tests demonstrate obviously increased total WBC count.
3. The imaging demonstrations include lobar or segmental high density shadows of parenchymal changes, air bronchogram sign with blurry boundary.

24.3.7 Differential Diagnosis

Pulmonary infection in AIDS children should be firstly differentiated from PCP, which is the most common pulmonary opportunistic infection in AIDS children. Therefore the sputum specimen should be conventionally stained. In combination with the clinical manifestations and imaging findings, differential diagnosis can be made. However, complications of various bacterial infections occur in AIDS children with PCP, which should be paid focused attention. Meanwhile, it should also be differentiated from pulmonary tuberculosis. The clinical manifestations, results of PPD test and the findings of pathogenic examinations should be integrated for the differential diagnosis.

24.4 HIV/AIDS Related Pneumocystis Carinii Pneumonia

Pneumocystis carinii pneumonia is an opportunistic infections of the respiratory system caused by the Pneumocystis carinii. In the past, it was only found in severely malnourished infants and children with leukemia undergoing immunosuppressive therapy. With the increasing incidence of AIDS, the incidence of PCP is obviously increasing, which is one of the common opportunistic infections in AIDS children and the common cause of death. PCP occurs commonly in infants aged 3–12 months, and rarely in young children aged above 1 year.

24.4.1 Pathogen and Pathogenesis

Pneumocystis carinii belongs to the fungus, with lungs as its most common target of invasion. In immunocompetent people, it can be clear out of the body by concurrent actions of cellular immunity and activated macrophages. In AIDS patients, due to their decreased CD4 T cell count and compromised immunity, its clearance ability against Pneumocystis carinii is also decreasing, which enables them to multiply in a large quantity in the alveoli to obstruct the capillaries. Thereafter, large quantity of foamy substances exudates from the alveolar cavity, together with inflammatory cells infiltration and pulmonary interstitial fibrous tissue proliferation, causes a serious of clinical manifestations and X-ray demonstrations.

24.4.2 Pathophysiologic Basis

By the naked eyes observation, the lung tissue has parenchymal changes. In some serious cases, the lungs are swelling and enlarged, with increased weight. The lungs are solid like the liver, in brown, with increased resistance during dissections. The float and sink test demonstrates positive findings. Microscopy demonstrates interstitial pneumonia and alveolar pneumonia, which are characterized by filling of pink foamy or honeycomb liked material in the dilated terminal bronchioles and in the alveolar cavities. The pink foamy or honeycomb liked material contains piles of worms and their disintegrated components; shed alveolar epithelial cells, lymphocytes, plasmocytes, eosinophils, histocytes or alveolar macrophages. There are also congestion and thickening of the pulmonary interstitium with accompanying infiltration of macrophages, lymphocytes and plasma cells. In the serious cases, the lung tissue has parenchymal changes, which are caused by large quantity proliferation of pneumocystis carinii in the alveoli. The infiltration is predominated by plasma cells in infants, and lymphocytes in children, with findings of macrophages and eosinophils.

24.4.3 Clinical Symptoms and Signs

Due to the immaturely developed organs and compromised immunity in AIDS children, the disease has an acute onset and rapid progression. The clinical manifestations include shortness of breath, cyanosis, serious hypoxia, as well as unobvious cough and fever. By auscultation, rales can be rarely heard, but obvious three depressions sign.

24.4.4 Examinations and Their Selection

24.4.4.1 Laboratory Tests
The findings include decreased WBC count and decreased lymphocytes, which are non-specific. The increased CD4 T cell count (commonly lower than 0.1×10^9/L) has prognostic significance. Increased serum lactate dehydrogenase and decreased protein can serve as the basis for the diagnosis. Pathogenic and serological examinations are necessary for the definitive diagnosis.

24.4.4.2 Imaging Examinations
Chest X-ray demonstrations are the basis for diagnosis and assessment of PCP. HRCT scanning can demonstrate characteristic PCP lesions earlier and more clearly than chest X-ray.

24.4.5 Imaging Demonstrations

24.4.5.1 Chest X-ray

Early plain chest X-ray may have normal demonstrations. With the progress of the disease, it rapidly develops into ground glass liked infiltration around the bilateral hilum and diffuse symmetric network or network nodular shadows. Pneumatocele, pneumothorax and subcutaneous/mediastinal emphysema are common. The rarely found chest X-ray

demonstrations include lobar parenchyma, restrictive shadows or nodules, miliary lesions, endobronchial lesions and pleural effusion.

24.4.5.2 CT Scanning

HRCT scanning clearly demonstrates ground glass liked lesions in the lungs, pneumatocele, intrapulmonary network liked and military shadows, which are characteristic demonstrations.

Case Study

A girl patient aged 12 years was confirmatively diagnosed as having AIDS by the CDC. Her father was an intravenous drug abuser, her mother was infected by HIV via sexual transmission and she was infected by vertical transmission from her mother. Her CD4 T cell count was 263/μl and CD4 percentage was 6 %.

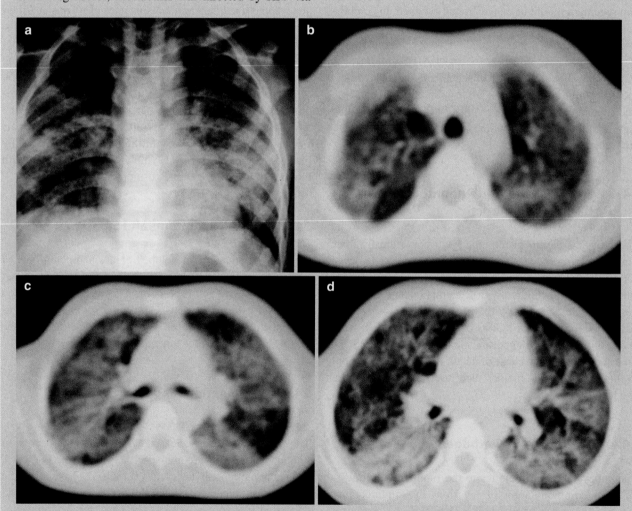

Fig. 24.8 (a–f) HIV/AIDS related pneumocystis carinii pneumonia. (a) Chest X-ray demonstrates multiple flakes of blurry shadows in both lungs. (b–f) Plain CT scanning demonstrates ground glass liked shadows in both lungs, and multiple round liked transparent areas in the outer zone of the lungs

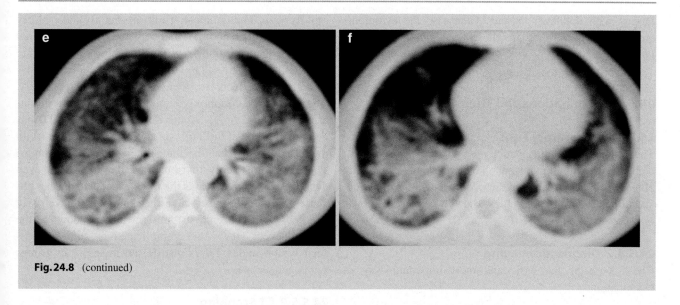

Fig. 24.8 (continued)

24.4.6 Diagnostic Basis

1. Clinical manifestations are shortness of breath, cyanosis, and severe hypoxia, but three depression signs obvious.
2. The increased lactate dehydrogenase and decreased protein also can be used as the evidence for the diagnosis.
3. Comparing to imaging demonstrations of adults pulmonary PCP, the imaging demonstrations of children patients change rapidly, with a short duration. Within a short period of time, multiple pathogens infections may occur, with complex and diverse imaging demonstrations.

24.4.7 Differential Diagnosis

HIV/AIDS related pneumocystis carinii pneumonia should be differentiated from pulmonary edema, bacterial pneumonia and mixed infections. Based on imaging demonstrations, the differential diagnosis is difficult, and the differential diagnosis can be made in combination to clinical manifestations and laboratory tests.

24.5 HIV/AIDS Related Miliary Tuberculosis

HIV/AIDS related miliary tuberculosis is one of the earliest opportunistic infections in children with HIV/AIDS.

24.5.1 Pathogen and Pathogenesis

Due to the dramatic drop of CD4 T cell count and compromised immunity in children with HIV/AIDS, the invasion of tubercle bacilli into the human body may cause its replication in a large quantity and spreading to involve multiple systems and organs.

24.5.2 Pathophysiologic Basis

The type of tuberculosis infection in children with HIV/AIDS is related to the immunity of human body. However, almost all cases are primary tuberculosis, which is related to non-HIV/AIDS related TB in children. Non-HIV/AIDS related TB in children is manifested as primary syndrome or intrathoracic lymphaden TB, while HIV/AIDS related TB in children has primary lesions with no demonstrations of primary syndrome, with rare occurrence of lymphatic cords draining towards the pulmonary hilum and hilar lymphadenectasis. In addition, cavities, calcification, pleural effusion as well as patchy and nodular lesions in the upper lung fields also occur rarely in children with HIV/AIDS complicated by pulmonary TB. Due to the seriously compromised immunity, tubercular nodules and caseous necrosis are rarely formed.

24.5.3 Clinical Symptoms and Signs

The clinical manifestations are commonly long-term irregular fever, night sweating, cough, shortness of breath and fatigue with unknown reasons. Otherwise the symptoms are intermittent diarrhea, weight loss, anemia and systemic lymphadenectasis.

24.5.4 Examinations and Their Selection

24.5.4.1 Laboratory Tests

The erythrocyte sedimentation rate changes can help to define the activity of pulmonary TB as well as its therapeutic efficacy and prognosis. Due the inhibited cellular immunity and allergic responses, PPD test shows weakened response or even no response.

24.5.4.2 Diagnostic Imaging

Chest X-ray is the basic and most important way of examination.

24.5.5 Imaging Demonstrations

24.5.5.1 X-ray

Chest X-ray demonstrates HIV/AIDS related pulmonary TB in children with complex and diverse findings, which rapidly vary. The demonstrations are mainly flaky blurry shadows, miliary nodular shadows and hilar/mediastinal lymphadenectasis, among which flaky blurry shadows are more common. The shadows have a higher central density and gradually decreased density towards the periphery. The lesions are commonly singular or multiple in unilateral or bilateral lungs. Acute miliary pulmonary TB has demonstrations of miliary sized nodular shadows with increased density that distribute extensively in both lungs. The lesions are evenly distributed, with even size and even density, which is known as the three evens. However, subacute and chronic cases have the lesions of uneven size and density in uneven distribution, which is known as the three uneven. HIV/AIDS complicated by hilar/mediastinal lymph nodes TB is manifested as multiple groups lymphadenectasis.

24.5.5.2 CT Scanning

CT scanning demonstrations are similar to those by chest X-ray, but with more clear and accurate demonstrations in terms of the size, shape, range, contour and density of the lesions as well as their relationship with the surrounding tissues. Therefore, the diagnosis can be defined and the outcomes of the lesions can be understood.

Case Study

A girl patient aged 8 years was confirmatively diagnosed as having AIDS by the CDC. Her CD4 T cell count was 78/μl.

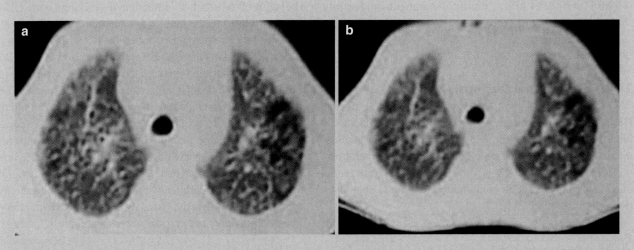

Fig. 24.9 (**a–c**) HIV/AIDS related miliary pulmonary TB. (**a–c**) Plain CT scanning demonstrates increased density of both lungs and multiple nodular shadows with different sizes

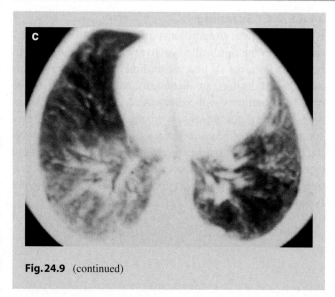

Fig. 24.9 (continued)

24.5.6 Diagnostic Basis

The cases of children have long term irregular fever, with chest X-ray demonstrations of flaky blurry shadows, miliary nodular shadows and hilar/mediastinal lymphadenectasis that vary in a short period of time. Such cases should be firstly suspected as HIV/AIDS complicated by pulmonary TB. PPD test and acid-fast bacilli test are positive.

24.5.7 Differential Diagnosis

24.5.7.1 Bacterial Pneumonia
In general, their differential diagnosis can be made by case history, symptoms and examinations. However, the diagnosis of some cases with complex demonstrations should be defined by diagnostic therapies.

24.5.7.2 Lymphocytic Interstitial Pneumonia
There are network liked and nodular infiltrative shadows of different sizes in both lungs, with enlarge hilum and thickened hilar shadow. The etiological examinations facilitate the differential diagnosis.

24.6 HIV/AIDS Related Aspergillus Infection

Aspergillus is one of the most widely distributed fungi in the nature, and it is also the main pathogen to cause human opportunistic fungal infection. Currently, is an important cause of opportunistic infections and death in immunocompromised patients.

24.6.1 Pathogen and Pathogenesis

Pediatric HIV/AIDS related aspergillus infection is induced by dysbacteriosis or inhibited immune responses in the body.

24.6.2 Pathophysiological Basis

In immunocompromised or immunodeficient children, due to the decreased lymphocytes and/or neutrophilic granulocyte, the defense ability of the respiratory tract is decreased. The inhalation of aspergillus invades the bronchial wall, the lung tissue and even the vascular vessels to cause exudative and necrotic lesions, with secondary suppurative pneumonia and pulmonary abscesses. After the discharge of the pus fluid and necrotic materials, cavities can be formed, sometimes with occurrence of aspergilloma. After the invasion of hyphae into the vascular vessels, local vascular embolism occurs or thrombus is induced to occur, which can cause regional infarction/necrosis. The hyphae can also be disseminated to the heart, brain, pituitary, eyes and esophagus along with the blood flow to cause disseminated or septic aspergillosis. This serious of pathological changes are caused by the invasive aspergillus, with typical manifestations in AIDS children.

24.6.3 Clinical Symptoms and Signs

The clinical symptoms are diverse, which is related to the amount of inhaled aspergillus and the allergic responses from the human body to fight against the invasion of aspergillus. Some patients are asymptomatic and some others have an acute onset, with symptoms of fever, cough and expectoration, which may be misdiagnosed as acute pneumonia. There are also some other patients with low grade fever, night sweating and cough, which are similar to pulmonary tuberculosis.

24.6.4 Examinations and Their Selections

24.6.4.1 Etiological Examinations
Sputum or bronchial lavage fluid culture or smear can detect the pathogen.

24.6.4.2 Diagnostic Imaging
CT scanning is the diagnostic examination of the choice.

24.6.5 Imaging Demonstrations

24.6.5.1 Chest X-ray

Pulmonary aspergillosis is characterized by aspergilloma, which is demonstrated as round or round liked dense shadows in the lung cavities that have an even density and smooth boundary, with air crescent sign. Bronchial mucus impaction is common in the upper lobes of both lungs, which is demonstrated as column shaped dense shadows and distributes along with pulmonary segment or subsegment of the bronchi. Due to bronchial obstruction by mucus, distal pulmonary parenchymal changes and atelectasis occur.

24.6.5.2 CT Scanning

By CT scanning, aspergilloma is usually isolated spherical lesion in the thin walled cavity, which has sharp smooth boundary in sizes of several millimeters to several centimeters. The lesions are demonstrated to have soft tissue density, sometimes with calcification. But enhanced scanning demonstrates no enhancement. Air crescent sign is common and the location of aspergilloma varies along with the body postures, but being always proximal. In addition, there are nodules and masses with blurry boundaries, cavities, parenchymal changes, reticular nodules and mediastinal lymphadenectasis.

Case Study

A girl patient aged 5 years was confirmatively diagnosed as having AIDS by the CDC. She had symptoms of intermittent fever for more than 2 years that has aggravated for 1 month. Her CD4 T cell count was 43/µl and the HIV viral load was 5.34×10^6 copies/ml.

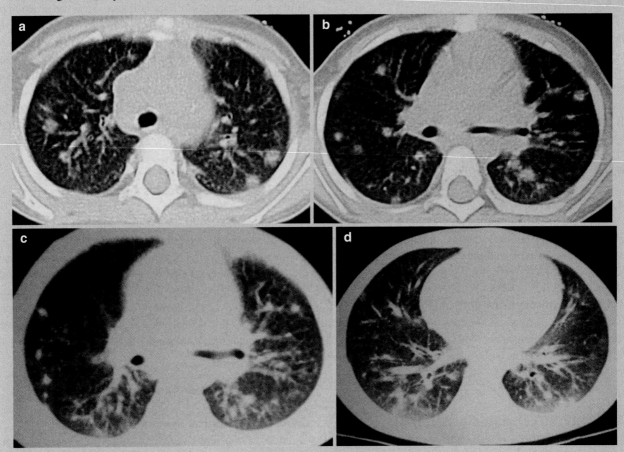

Fig. 24.10 (**a–d**) HIV/AIDS related aspergillus infection. (**a–d**) Pulmonary window demonstrates multiple small flakes of dense shadows in both lungs, with diverse morphology, different sizes, blurry boundary and uneven density

24.6.6 Diagnostic Basis

1. Fever, cough, expectoration and other symptoms.
2. There is regular morphology of aspergilloma in the pulmonary cavities, which also has even density, smooth boundary and is isolated and movable. Air crescent sign can be found between the aspergilloma and the cavity wall, which is characteristically pulmonary aspergilloma.
3. Pathological findings of aspergillus hyphae are the evidence for the definitive diagnosis.

24.6.7 Differential Diagnosis

24.6.7.1 Cavity Pulmonary Tuberculosis

Cavity pulmonary tuberculosis occurs after exacerbation of pulmonary TB, which is commonly singular. Chest X-ray demonstrates large flakes of blurry shadows, with irregular blurry semi-transparent areas of decreased density in them. The cavity is commonly thick walled. The tuberculin test is positive. The cases of aspergillosis have symptoms of paroxysmal cough and hemoptysis. The aspergilloma is commonly found in the upper lungs, being in singular or multiple with different sizes. The larger one may compress the bronchus to cause pulmonary atelectasis, with the X-ray demonstration of parenchymal shadow in the cavity with surrounding ring shaped transparency. The spherical parenchymal shadow is movable along with the posture changes. By aspergillin test, the result is positive.

24.6.7.2 Bacterial Pulmonary Abscesses

In the slight cases of aspergillosis, the fungi parasitize on the mucosal surface of the bronchus, with no invasion to the bronchial wall. The clinical symptoms are similar to those of bronchitis. Disseminated aspergillus pulmonary abscess has similar manifestations to staphylococcus aureus sepsis induced pulmonary abscess. However, staphylococcus aureus induced pulmonary abscess can be complicated by pulmonary bullae, which rarely occurs in the cases of aspergillus induced pulmonary abscess. The cavities induced by bacterial pulmonary abscess are different from those induced by aspergillus pulmonary abscess. The lesions of pulmonary aspergillus abscess are not surrounded by parenchymal inflammation.

24.7   HIV/AIDS Related Cerebral Atrophy and Infarction

24.7.1 Cerebral Atrophy

24.7.1.1 Pathogen and Pathogenesis

Currently, studies have demonstrated that HIV can pass through the blood–brain barrier to directly cause AIDS encephalitis. Simple brain atrophy is commonly early manifestation of HIV encephalitis.

24.7.1.2 Pathophysiologic Basis

Cortical atrophy in patients with AIDS is actually secondary to decreased deep cerebral tissues rather than primary reduction of cortical cells. The pathological changes include cerebral arteritis, vascular intimal fibrosis with thrombotic occlusion and vascular intimal hyperplasia with stenosis.

24.7.1.3 Imaging Demonstrations

Cerebral atrophy has complex clinical manifestations, which are non-specific. The common clinical manifestations are central nerves related motor disorder, epilepsy episodes and intelligence disorders of varying degrees.

24.7.1.4 Examinations and Their Selection
CT Scanning

CT scanning is the most reliable examination for the diagnosis of cerebral atrophy.

MR Imaging

MR imaging can clearly demonstrate the abnormal changes of the brain tissues, which facilities the qualitative and quantitative diagnosis.

24.7.1.5 Imaging Demonstrations
CT Scanning

The common demonstrations include widened sulcus, possibly widened fissure and symmetric dilation of the brain ventricles.

MR Imaging

The demonstrations of cerebral atrophy are similar to those by CT scanning.

Case Study

A girl patient aged 9 years was confirmatively diagnosed as having AIDS by the CDC. She had memory loss, generally developed intelligence and unstable walking for more than 3 months. Her CD4 T cell count was 28/μl.

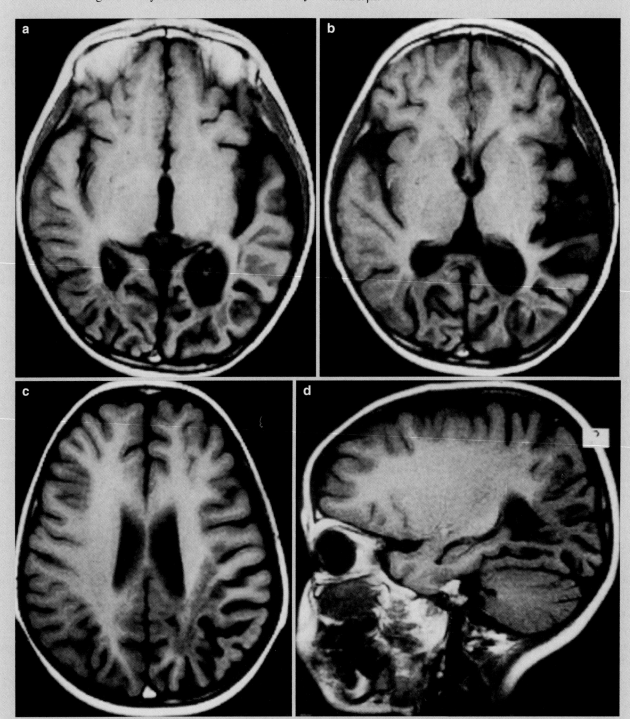

Fig. 24.11 (**a–d**) HIV/AIDS related cerebral atrophy. (**a–d**) MR imaging demonstrates widened and deepened sulci in bilateral brain, widened bilateral lateral fissures as well as dilated third ventricle and bilateral lateral ventricles

24.7.1.6 Diagnostic Basis

1. The clinical manifestations are memory loss and cognitive functional decline.
2. Imaging demonstrations include widened cerebral sulcus, possibly widened cerebral fissure, symmetric dilation of the brain ventricles and decreased total brain volume.

24.7.1.7 Differential Diagnosis

HIV/AIDS related cerebral atrophy should be differentiated from opportunistic virus infection induced brain atrophy. Opportunistic virus infection induced brain atrophy occurs due to seriously compromised immunity after HIV infection in children. The imaging demonstrations are concurrent cerebral atrophy and intracerebral abnormal density/signal. In such cases, HIV/AIDS complicated by cerebral atrophy should be firstly suspected.

24.7.2 Cerebral Infarction

Pediatric cerebral infarction can occur at any age groups. It is common in children aged 6 months to 8 years, with a low incidence and favorable prognosis.

24.7.2.1 Pathogen and Pathogenesis

Infection is the most common cause of pediatric cerebral infarction, accounting for 40–60 %. In various infections, virus infection is the most common. HIV can also cause pediatric cerebral infarction.

24.7.2.2 Pathophysiologic Basis

Pediatric cerebral infarction is commonly found in the cerebral cortex. Due to its rapid development of the cerebral cortex and abundant blood supply, the infection commonly involves cerebral arteries to cause cerebral arteritis.

24.7.2.3 Clinical Symptoms and Signs

Acute hemiplegia is its first symptom, which is followed by the symptoms of drowsiness, hemiplegia, and aphasia, which are progressively serious.

24.7.2.4 Examinations and Their Selection
CT Scanning

CT scanning is the diagnostic examination of choice for the diagnosis of cerebral infarction.

MR Imaging

MRA is the diagnostic examinations of choice for the diagnosis of super-acute cerebral embolism.

24.7.2.5 Imaging Demonstrations
CT Scanning

The lesions are spots and patches of low density shadows, mostly located in the cerebral cortex.

MR Imaging

The lesions are in spots and small flakes of long T1 and long T2 signals. MRA demonstrates beads string liked stenosis of the cerebral arteries and sparse cerebral arteries.

24.7.2.6 Diagnostic Basis

The diagnosis can be defined in combination with case history, clinical manifestations and imaging demonstrations.

24.7.2.7 Differential Diagnosis

It should be differentiated from traumatic cerebral infarction. The case history facilitates their differentiation.

24.8   HIV/AIDS Related Hepatic Lymphoma

Primary hepatic lymphoma (PHL) refers to lymphoma confined to the liver, with no evidence of lymphatic involvements in the spleen, lymph nodes, bone marrow and other lymphatic tissues. PHL is extremely rare in clinical practice, accounting for 0.1 % of hepatic malignancies and 0.4 % of extranodal lymphoma. It is common in patients after receiving organ transplantations and in patients with AIDS.

24.8.1 Pathogen and Pathogenesis

The cause and pathogenesis of PHL remains unclear until recently. Studies have demonstrated that the occurrence of PHL is possibly related to HCV and HBV infections. In addition, the occurrence of PHL may be related to EB virus infection. In the cases immunosuppression, such as HIV infection and the use of immunosuppressants, due to the functional defects of T lymphocytes, EB virus can persistently stimulate the proliferation of B lymphocytes, which may eventually progress into lymphoma.

24.8.2 Pathophysiologic Basis

Pathologically, hepatic lymphoma can be classified into two types: nodule type and diffuse infiltration type.

24.8.2.1 Nodule Type

This type is common in cases of primary lymphoma. The singular mass may be accompanied by central fibrosis or necrosis. Sometimes, multiple nodules can be found.

24.8.2.2 Diffuse Infiltration Type

This type is common in cases of secondary lymphoma.

24.8.3 Clinical Symptoms and Signs

The children mostly pay their clinic visit due to space occupying lesions in the liver. Other symptoms and signs are rarely found. The systemic symptoms of lymphoma are greatly varied according to its types and different stages. Some patients may be even asymptomatic. The symptomatic cases may commonly have symptoms of fever, weight loss (for more than 10 %) and night sweating. And the other less common symptoms include poor appetite, fatigue and skin itching. The systemic symptoms are related to the age of onset, involved range and immunity. The involved hepatic parenchyma can cause hepatic area pain. In the cases with intrahepatic diffuse infiltration or compression of the common bile duct by enlarged lymph nodes, jaundice may occur. Approximately 15 % of Hodgkin's disease with involved liver sustains jaundice.

24.8.4 Examinations and Their Selection

24.8.4.1 Laboratory Tests

The findings of laboratory tests are non-specific.

24.8.4.2 Diagnostic Imaging

The diagnostic imaging can define the location, shape and size of the lesions as well as their relationship with the surrounding tissues. Enhanced CT scanning and MR imaging facilitate the qualitative and quantitative diagnosis.

24.8.4.3 Pathological Examinations

The qualitative diagnosis can be made based on the pathological examinations.

24.8.5 Imaging Demonstrations

24.8.5.1 CT Scanning

Plain CT scanning demonstrates round liked or irregular low density lesions in the liver, with quite clear boundaries and no calcification. By enhanced scanning, uneven or even enhancement can be found in the arterial phases, but the enhancement degree is lower than that of the normal liver tissue; ring shaped enhancement in the portal phase and equilibrium phase; uneven central density of the lesions; and no enhancement of central necrosis in some larger lesions. The portal vein can be demonstrated to penetrate through the lesions or migrated due to compression. Delayed scanning demonstrates no shrinkage of the round liked lesions, which is different from that in the cases of hepatic angioma and hepatic abscess.

24.8.5.2 MR Imaging

Singular lesion is in long T1 and slightly long T2 nodular signal. Dynamic enhanced imaging by GD-DTPA demonstrates no enhancement. The diffuse type has demonstrations of intrahepatic diffuse long T1 and slightly long T2 uneven signal as well as splenomegaly or similar signaling, which indicate the diagnosis.

24.8.5.3 Ultrasound

The common demonstrations are low echo with space occupying effect. In some cases, there are equal echoes with space occupying effects, with surrounding low echo ring to form target shaped space occupying effect. In some rare cases, there are also no echo space occupying lesions. In the cases with PHL lesions around the portal vein with more adipose tissues, the ultrasound demonstrates strong echo of space occupying effects.

Case Study 1

A boy patient was confirmatively diagnosed as having AIDS by the CDC. He had abdominal pain, weight loss and night sweating for 3 months.

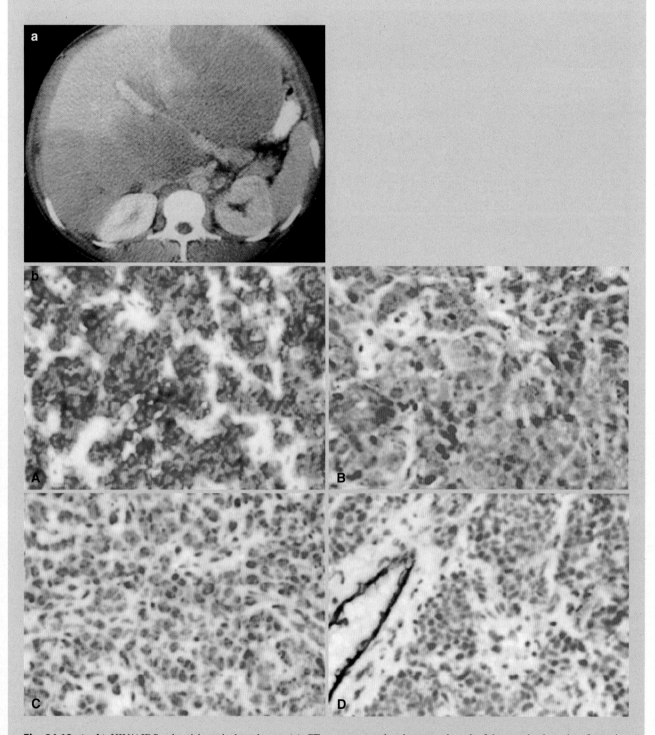

Fig. 24.12 (**a**, **b**) HIV/AIDS related hepatic lymphoma. (**a**) CT scanning demonstrates multiple low density mass shadows in the liver, the degree of enhancement being significantly lower than the surrounding liver parenchyma, and homogeneous enhancement; compressed and narrowed trunk of the portal vein and no formation of thrombosis. (**b**) Immunohistochemistry demonstrates CD20 positive (*A*), CD10 positive (*B*), high expression of Ki-67 (*C*), endothelial cells stained positive (*D*) and CD34 negative

Case Study 2

A girl patient aged 4 years was confirmatively diagnosed as having AIDS by the CDC. She had abdominal upset, poor appetite and fatigue. Her CD4 T cell count was 36/μl.

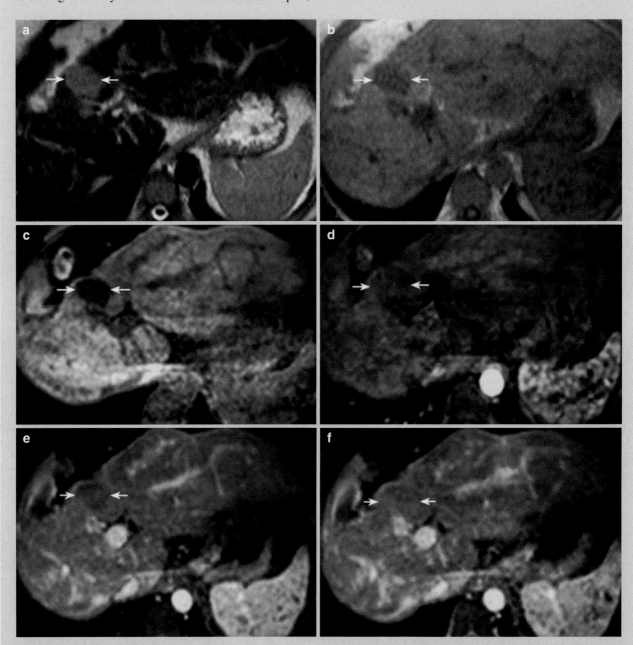

Fig. 24.13 (**a–f**) HIV/AIDS related hepatic lymphoma. (**a, b**) MR imaging demonstrates long T1 and long T2 nodular signal in hepatic segment IV, with clear boundary and even signal (pointed by *arrows*). (**c**) Adipose suppression T1WI sequence demonstrates decreased signal from the lesion in hepatic IV segment (pointed by *arrows*). (**d–f**) Enhanced imaging demonstrates slight enhancement of the lesions in the arterial phase, comparatively low signal in the portal phase and equal signal in the delayed phase (pointed by *arrows*)

24.8.6 Diagnostic Basis

1. The clinical symptoms are commonly caused by hepatic infiltration. There are no palpable superficial lymph nodes.
2. Intrahepatic space occupying effect (detailed information in the part of imaging demonstrations).
3. Pathological demonstrations of lymphoma cells.
4. Immunohistochemical findings of CD20 positive, CD10 positive and high expression of Ki-67.

24.8.7 Differential Diagnosis

The clinical manifestations, laboratory findings and imaging demonstrations of PHL are non-specific. Clinically, it is commonly misdiagnosed as primary liver cancer, liver metastasis and liver abscess.

24.8.7.1 Primary Hepatocellular Carcinoma (HCC)

Dynamic enhanced scanning facilitates their differentiation. The lesions of primary HCC commonly have abundant blood supply, with early lesions enhancement by enhanced scanning and low density lesions by delayed scanning. The demonstration of lesions capsules can define the diagnosis. PHL is an ischemic disease, with no obvious enhancement or slight even enhancement by enhanced scanning and no capsules. HCC is commonly accompanied by involved portal veins, while PHL has no such lesions.

24.8.7.2 Hepatic Metastasis

The cases of hepatic metastasis commonly have a case history of primary neoplasm. The metastasis usually has multiple lesions of different sizes, with scattering distribution. Sometimes, the lesions are in target sign or bull eyes sign. Enhanced scanning may demonstrate hepatic metastasis as marginal enhancement, which has overlapping demonstrations with hepatic lymphoma. Therefore, their differentiation is difficult and the combination with the case history is very important for the diagnosis.

24.8.7.3 Hepatic Abscess

Plain CT scanning demonstrates typical liver abscess as low density lesions with obvious surrounding edema. Enhanced scanning demonstrates obvious enhancement of the abscess wall. In combination with the case history, clinical manifestations and laboratory tests, its differentiation from PHL can be clarified.

24.9 HIV/AIDS Related Hepatoblastoma

Hepatoblastoma (HB) is hepatic malignancy composed of embryonic epithelial tissue or embryonic mesenchymal tissue. It is the most common malignancy in the liver of children, accounting for 45 % of pediatric hepatic malignancies. It is commonly found in children aged within 5 years.

24.9.1 Pathogen and Pathogenesis

The detailed pathogenesis of hepatoblastoma has not yet fully understood, but it is generally believed that it is an embryonic tumor, which is possibly due to abnormal proliferation and differentiation of hepatocytes during the embryonic development. There may be still immature hepatic embryonic tissue in the infancy and postneonatal periods. Such histologically abnormal persistent proliferation causes immaturely developed tissue mass, which may be transformed into malignant blastoma. The pathological process may be triggered in the late fetus period or in the adulthood. Clinically, the occurrence in infancy and early childhood is more common.

24.9.2 Pathophysiologic Basis

HB is more commonly found in the right hepatic lobe, accounting for 60–70 %. It size varies from 5 to 15 cm, with bleeding and necrosis in the tumors. The tumor is composed of undifferentiated embryonic stem cells, and sometimes with other mesenchymal tissue components, such as osteoid tissue, cartilage or fibrous tissue.

The cross section of the tumor demonstrates diverse colors, which are dependent on the contents of bile and adipose. The well differentiated tumors are light yellowish green, with homogeneous quality; while the poorly differentiated tumors are white, with fish liked quality, bleeding and necrosis. Its difference from adult hepatic carcinoma, also a characteristic demonstration, is that the pediatric cases rarely have complication of hepatocirrhosis. HB has two types of growth, endogenous and exogenous. Its pathological morphology includes giant mass type, nodular type, diffuse type and cystic type, among which the giant mass type is the most common.

24.9.3 Clinical Symptoms and Signs

About 50 % cases of HB are asymptomatic. The patients commonly pay their clinic visits due to abdominal protrusion and epigastric mass. Some children patients have poor appetite and weight loss. About 1/3 children patients have accompanying cleft lip, adrenal missing and other deformities. The boy patients have sexual precocity as the first symptom, with increased serum chorionic gonadotrophin level. By physical examination, there is epigastric palpable hard lump with clear boundary and surface nodules. Some tumors grow across the midline or the navel.

24.9.4 Examinations and Their Selection

24.9.4.1 Laboratory Tests
About 80 % children cases are serum AFP positive. AFP test is one of the important evidence for the assessment of total HB removal or its recurrence.

24.9.4.2 Ultrasound
Ultrasound is simple and convenient for demonstrating the lesions, which is the diagnostic examinations of choice for the diagnosis of HB. Repeated examination is applicable.

24.9.4.3 CT Scanning
CT scanning is superior to MR imaging in demonstrating hemorrhage, calcification and pseudocapsule.

24.9.4.4 MR Imaging
MR imaging can demonstrate the vascular vessels with no use of contrast agent, which facilitates to demonstrate the relationship between the lesions and the vascular vessels. It also accurately demonstrates the involved range of the tumor, with no radiation damage, which is especially appropriate for pediatric examination.

24.9.4.5 Biopsy
It is the main basis for the diagnosis of HB, which also provides information for the cytological diagnosis and histological categorization.

24.9.5 Imaging Demonstrations

24.9.5.1 CT Scanning
The singular lesion is commonly found in the right hepatic lobe, and rarely in the left lobe and caudate lobe, which is commonly an intrahepatic huge lump. Otherwise, multiple nodules in a diffuse distribution are found. The lump can be clearly or unclearly defined from the surrounding normal hepatic parenchyma, with uneven density and possibly fissure liked or irregular necrotic areas. The calcification of the tumor is cords liked or large particle liked. By enhanced scanning, the enhancement of the lump is uneven in the arterial phase, together with no enhancement of the fibrous tissues and necrosis; the enhancement of the lump in equal and low density in the portal phase; low density lump in the equilibrium phase or delayed phase; and delayed slight enhancement of some areas in the lump with abundant fibrous stroma.

24.9.5.2 MR Imaging
MR imaging demonstrates the lumps in long T1 and long T2 signal or mixed signal. T2WI demonstrates pomegranate liked changes, which are multiple small cystic shadows with high signal, and fibrous septa in low or equal signal. In the cases with bleeding or adipose component, local T1W1 high signal can be found. MR imaging is inferior to CT scanning in demonstrating the calcification. Dynamic enhanced imaging demonstrates early enhancement of the lump, and surrounding halo ring liked enhancement of the lump in about 40 % cases.

Case Study 1
A boy patient aged 14 years was confirmatively diagnosed as having AIDS by the CDC. He had been found HIV positive for 5 years and paid his clinic visit due to the initial symptom of diarrhea. His CD4 T cell count was 7/μl.

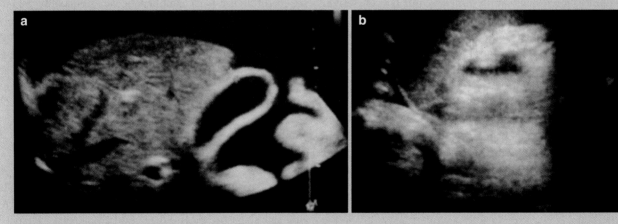

Fig. 24.14 (**a**, **b**) HIV/AIDS related hepatoblatoma. Ultrasound demonstrates uneven strong echo of an isolated lump, with cystic areas or spots irregular calcification in the lump

Case Study 2

A boy patient aged 13 years was confirmatively diagnosed as having AIDS by the CDC. He complained of right hypochondrium pain for 8 days. By laboratory tests, AFP above 1,000 µg/L; CEA 5.96ug/ml; and CD4 T cell count 36/µl.

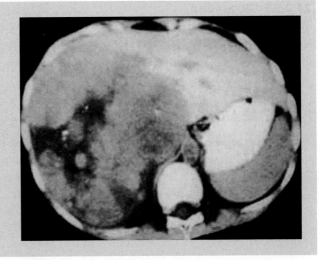

Fig. 24.15 HIV/AIDS related hepatoblatoma. Plain CT scanning demonstrates a lump in the right hepatic lobe with a size of 13 × 14 cm with unclear boundary and uneven density, irregular lower density area and necrotic area in the lump, and scattering small spots liked calcification in the lump

Case Study 3

A pediatric patient was confirmatively diagnosed as having AIDS by the CDC. The diagnosis was hepatoblastoma.

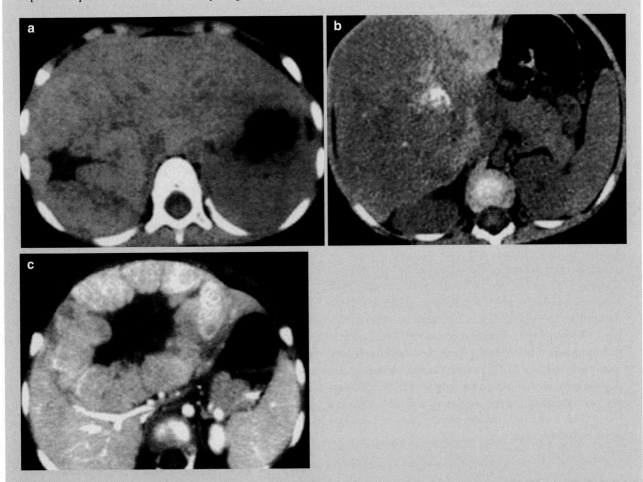

Fig. 24.16 (a–c) HIV/AIDS related hepatoblatoma. (a) CT scanning demonstrates slightly higher density lump in the right hepatic lobe, and irregular shaped necrosis in the lump. (b) CT scanning demonstrates multiple patchy calcifications in the lower density lump, and posterior migration of the right kidney due to the compression. (c) Enhanced scanning demonstrates obvious enhancement of the lump, and no enhancement of the necrosis in the lump

24.9.5.3 Ultrasound

The ultrasound demonstrates isolated lump with uneven strong echo, with cystic areas and spots liked irregular calcification in the lump.

24.9.6 Diagnostic Basis

1. There are hepatic space occupying lesions in infants and young children (aged within 5 years), with increased serum AFP level. In addition, the serum AFP level is parallel to the growth of the lump. That is to say, the lump recedes, with decreased serum AFP level, while the lump recurs or metastasizes, with increased serum AFP level. By liver functional examination, the levels of lactate dehydrogenase, transaminase or alkaline phosphatase may be normal or slightly to moderately elevated. The cases with these findings should be firstly suspected as having hepatoblastoma.
2. By pathological biopsy, the lump is composed of undifferentiated embryonic hepatocytes, sometimes with other mesenchymal tissue components, such as osteoid tissue, cartilage or fibrous tissue.
3. The diagnostic imaging has important value in diagnosing hepatoblastoma. CT scanning is the most commonly used examination. Its characteristic demonstrations include singular or multiple lumps in round or round liked shape. By plain scanning, the lump is in low or equal density, with central lower density area and clear boundary. Calcification is common, in spots and fine strips liked appearance. Otherwise, there are large flakes calcifications, being concentrated in one area. By enhanced scanning, the lesions have slight to obvious enhancement, with their density possibly being lower than the surrounding normal hepatic tissues and higher than the surrounding normal hepatic tissues. The morphology of enhanced lesions is ring shaped arch shaped, grid shaped or unevenly high density of the whole lesion. By delayed scanning, the lesions are in equal or low density. MR imaging demonstrations of hepatoblastoma are similar to those of hepatocellular carcinoma, with no special findings. MR imaging is slightly superior to CT scanning in demonstrating the lump itself, local invasion, lymph node metastasis and surrounding major vascular structures. By angiography, the lump has obviously abundant blood supply, with thickened supplying arteries, large volume of blood flow, more intratumoral branch lines and obvious lump embedding sign.

24.9.7 Differential Diagnosis

24.9.7.1 Primary Hepatocellular Carcinoma

By CT scanning and MR imaging, the demonstrations of HB are similar to those of hepatic cancer. However, the lump of hepatic cancer has irregular shape, with blurry boundary, no capsule and paratumor lesions in different sizes. The liver tissues may have hepatocirrhosis manifestations apart from the lump, which is more common in children above 3 years old. This is the key point for the differentiation.

24.9.7.2 Liver Rhabdomyosarcoma

The lesion has clear boundary, which may be found in the portal area or in the right or left hepatic lobe with uneven low density space occupying effect. Bleeding, necrosis and calcification are rarely found. Liver rhabdomyosarcoma occurs in children aged 5–11 years. Serum AFP negative can facilitate the differential diagnosis.

24.9.7.3 Liver Metastases

Pediatric liver metastasis should be differentiated from HB. The cases of HB have manifestations of invasion of large fusion of nodular lesions to the hepatic parenchyma, with various morphology of calcification, which is similar to those of HB. The key points for differential diagnosis are the finding of primary lesions. In addition, the cases of HB have increased AFP level, while the cases of liver metastasis have no increased AFP level.

24.10 HIV/AIDS Related Osteoporosis and Epiphyseal Sclerosis

24.10.1 Osteoporosis

24.10.1.1 Pathogen and Pathogenesis

The causes of pediatric osteoporosis remain unclear. It has been speculated that during the critical period of development in the childhood, there is imbalanced skeletal growth and muscular growth. Therefore, the bone and bone volume are increased but with no corresponding increase of the bone density. Comparing to the normal bone, osteoporosis occurs.

24.10.1.2 Pathophysiological Basis

The histological changes of osteoporosis include thinner cortical bone, dilated Haversian canal and Volkmann canal as well as decreased, thinner or even absent bone trabecula.

24.10.1.3 Clinical Symptoms and Signs

The main symptoms include back pain and scoliosis. The incidence rate of fracture is relatively low. Osteoporosis of disuse and fractures may occur in long-term bedridden patients.

24.10.1.4 Examinations and Their Selection

Plain X-ray

It is the examination of the choice.

MR Imaging and Ultrasound

Both can be used for bone mineral measurement.

24.10.1.5 Imaging Demonstrations
X-ray

The main manifestation is decreased bone density. In the long bone, there is thinner and decreased trabecula in the cancellous bone, widened spaces as well as stratified and thinner cortical bone. In the spine, the intravertebral structure shows longitudinal stripes, and thinner surrounding cortical bone. In the serious cases, the intravertebral structure is absent. The vertebral body is flattened, with inwards depressions of the superior and inferior margins. The intervertebral space is widened in spindle shape, which causes the vertebral body in a fish spine shape.

CT Scanning

CT scanning demonstrations are almost the same as those by X-ray.

24.10.1.6 Diagnostic Basis

The fundamental basis for the diagnosis of osteoporosis is the decrease of bone density. The definitive diagnosis should also integrate the case history and X-ray demonstrations.

24.10.1.7 Differential Diagnosis

Osteoporosis should be differentiated from osteomalacia. Osteomalacia refers to insufficient bone calcification in one unit volume, with normal organic components of bone but decreased inorganic components and calcium salt. However, the cases of osteoporosis are manifested as proportional decrease of the organic and inorganic components. Reduced bone density, thinner cortical bone and thinner trabecula are the common demonstrations of osteoporosis and osteomalacia by X-ray and CT scanning. The difference is that the lesions of osteomalacia have blurry boundaries due to their large quantity contents of uncalcified osteoid tissue. As a result of softened bone, the weight-bearing bones often have various deformations, with possible occurrence of fake fracture line, which is known as looser band.

24.10.2 Epiphyseal Sclerosis

Osteoepiphysis is the secondary ossification center in children, which is formed in different period after birth. Due to epiphyseal cartilage inflammation caused by various reasons, ischemic necrosis occurs, with complete closure of the epiphyseal line and stasis of bone growth.

Plain X-ray is the examination of the choice. X-ray and CT scanning demonstrate fine strips liked dense lines transversing throughout the diaphysis at both ends of the diaphysis and epiphyseal cartilage. MR imaging demonstrates fine stripes signals at both ends of the diaphysis and epiphyseal cartilage. By T1WI and T2WI, the demonstrations are low signals. The disease can be definitively diagnosed based on demonstrations by X-ray and CT scanning.

Case Study

A patient boy aged 5 years was confirmatively diagnosed as having AIDS by the CDC. He had been found to be HIV positive for 2 years. His CD4 T cell count was 110/μl.

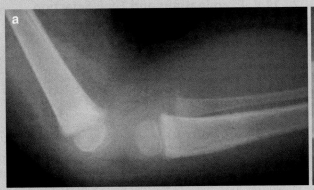 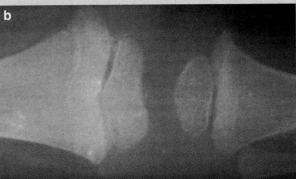

Fig. 24.17 (a, b) HIV/AIDS related epiphyseal sclerosis. (a, b) Plain X-ray demonstrates fine stripes of dense lines in the lower humerus and in the upper ulna

24.11 HIV/AIDS Related Congenital Syphilis Infection

Congenital syphilis caused by spreading of Treponema pallidum to the fetus through placenta. Approximately 90 % of children with congenital syphilis have their bones violated. According to times of onset, congenital bone syphilis can be divided into two types: early and late. Early congenital bone syphilis occurs in children aged within 2 years, which is more common in the neonatal period. Late congenital bone syphilis occurs in children aged above 2 years, which is more common in children aged 5–15 years. Treponema pallidum infection and HIV infection are interactive to be synergic and promotive.

24.11.1 Pathogen and Pathogenesis

The co-infection of syphilis and HIV-1 has obvious impact on the immunity of the patients with HIV infection. When complicated by syphilis, the AIDS patients have obviously decreased CD4 T cell count. Syphilis negatively affects the immunity of HIV positive patients (decreased CD4 T cell count) and increases the viral load of HIV-1. CC-chemokine receptor 5 (CCR5) is a kind of G protein-coupled receptor, which is a main auxiliary receptor for HIV to infect the lymphocytes and collaborates with CD4 receptor to promote HIV infection. The expression level of CCR5 is an important factor influencing the transmission and progression of HIV infection. CD4 T cell count is obviously decreased in the HIV positive patients, with obviously increased surface CCR5 expression, which indicates that CCR5, as an auxiliary receptor for HIV to infect the lymphocytes, obviously increases in the cases with HIV infection, which indicates that CD8 T lymphocytes obviously proliferate and are activated to play their role in killing the virus. CD8 T cells can secrete RANTES, MIP21α, and MIP21β to activate the anti-HIV responses, which could inhibit RT, env, gag, vid, Nef in HIV and meanwhile can inhibit the replication of HIV in the CD4 T cells. Once CTL is suppressed, the immune activity of anti-HIV T lymphocytes declines.

24.11.2 Pathophysiologic Basis

Early congenital bone syphilis has main pathological changes of osteochondritis, periostitis and osteomyelitis. Osteochondritis is a common disease, with lesions commonly found in the long bones of the four limbs that are especially common in the femur and tibial metaphysis with rapid growth. Because the metaphysis has abundant bloody supply and rapid growth, Treponema pallidum in the blood flow stagnates here to seriously damage the cartilage ossification. Formation of granulation tissue destroys the metaphysis, with dissolved and destructed trabecula, to finally separate the epiphysis from the metaphysis. The separation part is zigzag liked, with absent normal straight interface between the metaphysis and epiphysis. Instead, there is a broad zigzag liked grayish white band. The nose and the hard palate often have saddle nose and palate perforation due to destruction of gumma. Periostitis and osteomyelitis can occur in isolation, but mostly occurs following osteochondritis.

24.11.3 Clinical Symptoms and Signs

The bone lesions of early congenital syphilis simultaneously involve multiple systems. The children commonly have manifestations of joint swelling, affected limbs pain, dependent limbs motions (namely Parrot pseudo paralysis), irritative responses to the stimulations of touch, crying and fighting against embrace. The bone lesions and its clinical symptoms are not necessarily corresponding. According to data reports, the bone lesions in most children patients occur within 6 months old. The bone lesions are extensive, but the symptoms are not obvious.

Late congenital bone syphilis has the typical change of sliced shin, with manifestations of tibial periosteal hypertrophy, extended and swelling tibia, the tibia in arch shape and forward curve like a saber, and tenderness.

24.11.4 Examinations and Their Selection

24.11.4.1 Laboratory Tests
Treponema pallidum hemagglutination assay (TPHA) and rapid plasma reagin (RPR) is more sensitive and more specific test for Treponema pallidum, which can be applied to detect Treponema pallidum.

24.11.4.2 X-ray
It is a necessary examination for the diagnosis of congenital bone syphilis. The locations for X-ray examination should include the long bones of the four limbs, short bones, scapula and ilium. In such way, the invaded bone locations, lesions range and severity can be comprehensively and accurately assessed to guide the therapy administration.

24.11.5 Imaging Demonstrations (X-ray)

Early congenital bone syphilis is characterized by multiple bones involvement and occasionally singular bone involvement. The tibia, femur and humeral metaphysis are susceptible to the disease, with no involvement of the bone center. In addition to the long bones of the limbs, the lesions can also be found in the ribs, clavicles, facial bones and spine. The following demonstrations by X-ray are common: (1) Osteochondritis (metaphyseal inflammation) is the earliest and most characteristic demonstration. The lesions are mainly in the long bones of the limbs, which are bilaterally symmetric. The early demonstrations include widened and thickened calcification area, and a following transverse irregular transparent area due to bone destruction caused by syphilis granuloma, namely the sandwich sign. With the progression of the disease, the metaphyseal bone can be seriously destructed and defected, which is commonly unilateral with clear boundary, namely the cat bitten sign. The bilateral metaphysis of the long bones, especially bilateral proximal medial tibia may have symmetric destruction, which is known as Wimberger sign. In the serious cases, there is pathological fracture of the long bone metaphysis, with accompanying distal migration of the fracture or incarceration. (2) Periostitis has manifestations of unilayer or multi-layer onion liked hyperplasia

of the peritoneum. There is linear transparent incarceration between most hyperplasic peritoneum and cortical bone. (3) Osteomyelitis (diaphysitis) is commonly caused by extension of osteochondritis to involve the diaphysis, with manifestations of worm bitten liked bone destruction. (4) Irregular bones and short bones changes have main manifestations of transparent lines along the margins of the irregular bones and sharp angle liked change. The transparent lines are common in the ilium, while the sharp angles are common in the calcaneus and the astragalus. The short bone changes in the cases of syphilis are similar to the long bones. The bone changes occur in the metacarpal bones and phalanges, but are rare. (5) Soft tissue swelling may occur in the involved joints.

The X-ray demonstrations of late congenital bone syphilis are similar to those of acquired bone syphilis, with periostitis as the most common bone manifestation. The second common manifestation is ostitis or osteomyelitis. The lesions are commonly found in the long bones, commonly tibia. The lesions are commonly confined to the anterior tibia in knife sliced liked change which is known as knife sliced sign of tibia. Ostitis and osteomyelitis have main manifestation of bone sclerosis, with thickened cortical bone, irregular bone trabecula and increased density in the marrow cavity. The bone destruction area can be demonstrated, but the necrotic bone is rarely found.

Case Study

A boy aged 1 year was definitively diagnosed as having AIDS by the CDC. He was hospitalized due to skin rashes and bucking while drinking milk for 10 days. By laboratory tests, TPHA positive, RPR titer 1:256, and CD4 T cell count 159/μl.

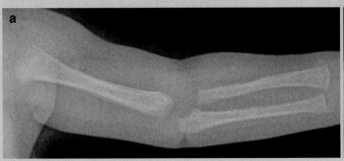
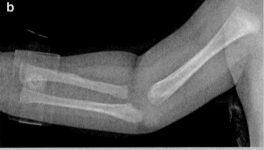

Fig. 24.18 (a–f) HIV/AIDS related early congenital bone syphilis. (**a, b**) DR demonstrates layer and union liked hyperplasia of the bilateral humerus, ulna, radius diaphysis, subcortical cords liked transparent lines; blurry early calcification of the metaphysis with increased density and being rough and irregular; spots transparent areas in the bone marrow cavities of the bilateral humerus, ulna and radius. (**c–e**) It is demonstrated to have layer and union liked hyperplasia of the bilateral femur, tibia and fibula diaphysis, subcortical transparent lines, and blurry early calcification in the metaphysis with increased density and being rough and irregular. (**f**) CT demonstrates patches of low density shadows at the inferior margin of the right ilium, with blurry boundary; and subcortical transparent lines at the inferior margin of the left ilium

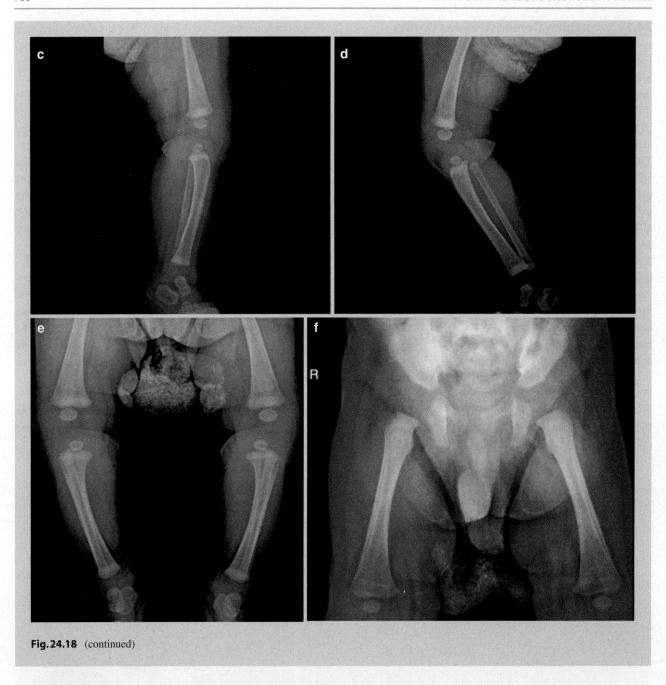

Fig. 24.18 (continued)

24.11.6 Diagnostic Basis

The parents of the patient have case history of syphilis, and the serological test of the patient is positive. The newborns, especially premature birth, have fade skin, scaling, maculopapule and pustular eruption in the limbs, face and trunk, as well as hepatosplenomegaly, jaundice and other symptoms. By X-ray examination, the children have extensive multiple symmetric osteochondritis, periostitis and osteomyelitis of the limb long bones, with some accompanying specific X-ray demonstrations such as the cat bitten sign. Such cases should highly suspect as congenital syphilis. The following serological test can define the diagnosis of early congenital bone syphilis.

The diagnosis of late congenital bone syphilis is based on the case history in combination to the X-ray demonstrations and laboratory tests findings.

24.11.7 Differential Diagnosis

24.11.7.1 Infants Cortical Hyperplasia
Syphilic peritonitis should be differentiated from infant's cortical hyperplasia. Both have multiple symmetric stratified periosteums in the long bones. However, infant's cortical hyperplasia commonly has no metaphyseal involvement and occurs commonly at the age of 2.5 months. In infants

aged above 5 months, its occurrence is rare. The disease can be self healing within several months, with no effects on the growth and development of the infant.

24.11.7.2 Rickets

Syphilic osteochondritis should be differentiated from rickets. Syphilic osteochondritis has serum syphilis ELISA positive, possibly with the sandwich sign. The cases of rickets have thickened early calcification, but have no zigzag liked changes, no transparent transverse strip and soft tissue swelling. In its active period, the cup opening liked change can be found, which, in combination with the clinical manifestations, facilitates to define the diagnosis.

24.11.7.3 Suppurative Osteomyelitis

Syphilic osteomyelitis should be differentiated from suppurative osteomyelitis. Both have bone destruction and thickened peritoneum. Syphilic osteomyelitis has RPR positive, with accompanying multiple symmetric periostitis and metaphysitis, with fine or absent necrotic bone. Suppurative osteomyelitis has an acute onset, with the bone destruction spreading rapidly from the metaphysis to the diaphysis to cause large area bone destruction and large necrotic bone. There are also obvious hyperosteogeny to form bone shell.

24.11.7.4 Scurvy

In the cases of scurvy, there are thickened early calcification and its inferior transparent transverse stripe. However, the thickened early calcification has no zigzag liked changes, but protrudes right wards to form a characteristic spike liked change. In addition, there is ring shaped dense stripe in the metaphysis of scurvy children. But in the cases of bone syphilis, the metaphysis is commonly not involved. Scurvy has commonly a latent period of 4–6 months. The infants aged within 3 months are asymptomatic, with normal X-ray demonstrations.

Extended Reading

1. Carrington CB, Liebow A. Limited forms of angiitis and granulomatosis of Wegener's type. Am J Med. 1966;41(4):497–527.
2. Donnelly L, Bisset G. Hepatic imaging: pediatric hepatic imaging. Radiol Clin North Am. 1998;36:413–27.
3. Elsayes KM, Menias CO, Willatt JM, et al. Primary hepatic lymphoma: imaging findings. J Med Imaging Radiat Oncol. 2009; 53(4):373–9.
4. Johkoh T. Imaging of idiopathic interstitial pneumonias. Clin Chest Med. 2008;29(1):133–47.
5. Pearl R, Irsh M, Caty M, et al. The approach to common abdominal diagnoses in infants and children :part II. Pediatr Clin North Am. 1998;45:1287–326.
6. Rampalo AM, Joesoef MR, O'Nonnell JA. Clinical manifestations of early syphilis by HIV status and gender: results of the syphilis and HIV study. Sex Transm Dis. 2001;28(3):158–65.
7. Rizzi EB, Schinina V, Cristofaro M, et al. Non-Hodgkin's lymphoma of the liver in patients with HIV/AIDS: sonographic, CT, and MRI findings. J Clin Ultrasound. 2001;29(3):125–9.
8. Siskin GP, Haller JO, Miller S, Sundaram R. AIDS related lymphoma :radiologic features in pediatric patients. Radiology. 1995;196:63–6.
9. Soave R, Sepkowitz KA. The immunocompromised host. In: Reese RE, Betts RF, editors. A practical approach to infectious diseases. 3rd ed. Boston: Little, Brown and Company; 1991. p. 566–618.
10. Stark D, Bradley Jr W. Magnetic resonance imaging, vol. 1. 3rd ed. St. Louis: Mosby; 1999.
11. Stoane JM, Haller JO, Orentlicher RJ. The gastrointestinal manifestations of AIDS in children. Radiol Clin North Am. 1996;34:779–90.
12. Tardieu M. Stroke and cerebral infarcts in children infracted with human immunodeficiency virus. Arch Pediatr Adolesc Med. 1994;48:965–70.
13. Wood BP. Children with AIDS; radiographic features. Invest Radiol. 1992;27:964–70.
14. Wrzolek MA, Brudlowska J, Kozlowski PB, et al. Opportunistic infections of the central nervous system in children with HIV infection: report of 9 autopsy cases and review of literature. Clin Neuropathol. 1995;14:187–96.

Contents

25.1 An Overview of HIV/AIDS Related Skin Diseases

In AIDS patients, skin diseases are common including infectious and exogenous infectious skin diseases. The infectious skin diseases are commonly fungal and viral infection of the skin, and bacterial infection of the skin rarely occurs.

The common skin diseases include seborrheic dermatitis, psoriasis, skin and nail fungal infection, herpes virus infection, insect skin infection and bacterial infection.

25.1.1 Bacillary Angioma or Bacillary Peliosis

Bacillary epithelioid angiomatosis (BA) is also known as bacillary angiomatosis (BP) or epithelioid angiomatosis. It was first reported by Stoler in 1983 to be a multiple cutaneous vascular proliferative disease in AIDS patients that is different from Kaposi sarcoma [15]. The findings of small bacilli in the skin lesions were also reported. The disease was then believed to be a newly found infectious disease in AIDS patients which causes cutaneous and organ minor vascular proliferation. Bacillary angioma can cause vascular proliferation in multiple organs, including lymph nodes, skin, gastrointestinal tract and lungs. The manifestations of skin lesions are various, including reddish vascular lesions that are smooth and tend to rupture; spot lesions of cellulitis, KS liked lesions, dry squamous lesions with lupus base and subcutaneous nodules. Bacillary vascular diseases may be chronic and last for 1 year. There is commonly collar desquamation around the lesions, which is the key point for the

H. Li (ed.), *Radiology of HIV/AIDS*,
DOI 10.1007/978-94-007-7823-8_25, © Springer Science+Business Media Dordrecht and People's Medical Publishing House 2014

differential diagnosis from Kaposi's sarcoma. In addition, it also should be differentiated from vascular sarcoma, pyogenic granuloma and other pathogenic sepsis.

25.1.2 Herpes Simplex Virus Caused Primary or Recurrent Oral and Genital Diseases

The lesions are commonly found in the oral cavity, perioral area, vulva, mucosa and perianal skin; occasionally in the groin and buttocks, being small blisters or erosions, and even shallow ulceration.

25.1.3 Zoster

Varicella-zoster virus causes skin and mucosa infections that are distributed along the skin area. In HIV positive patients, the manifestations are pain, necrosis and hemorrhage. The patients have painful skin blisters, which is different from HIV negative patients with zoster. Zoster in HIV negative population recurs.

25.1.4 Molluscum Contagiosum

It is a benign skin infection caused by pox virus, which transmits via direct contacts. It usually occurs in the head and neck as well as pudendum. They are semicircular papules in the colors of flesh, white and yellow. It should be differentiated from disseminated cryptococcosis infection or other fungal infections with similar clinical manifestations.

25.1.5 Oral Candidiasis

It is a fungal disease in the oral mucosa or tongue which is caused by Candida, which commonly indicates the occurrence of HIV infection. Thrush is the most common manifestation. Other manifestations include erythema, hyperplasia or plaques. HIV patients usually have three symptoms: pseudomembrane, erythema and angular cheilitis.

25.1.6 Seborrheic Dermatitis

About 25–83 % of HIV positive patients have seborrheic dermatitis which has always a local occurrence near the midline of the body. Sometimes, it occurs in ears, chest, upper back, axilla and groin.

25.1.7 Genital Candidiasis

Genital yeast infection is caused by a variety of pathogens belonging to the Candida species. It is common in females and is more common and serious in HIV positive females. Refractory vaginal Candida infection may be the primary clinical manifestation in HIV positive women, which can also have manifestations of genital inflammation, white thick secretion on the vaginal folds and ulcers on the viginal wall.

25.1.8 Scabies

It is one of the reasons of pruritus in HIV positive patients. And it is common underdeveloped areas.

Studies have demonstrated that the incidence of neoplasms closely related to virus infections. Therefore, the neoplasms are known as opportunistic neoplasms.

25.1.9 Kaposi's Sarcoma

It is a neoplasm originated from blood vessels in the skin, mucosal surface or organs, which is the most common neoplasm in HIV positive patients. Currently, it is believed to be induced by HHV-8. Epidemic or HIV/AIDS related KS is a neoplasm with short duration that can be disseminated. It prevalence is commonly regional in homosexual HIV positive patients. The condition progresses slowly or rapidly, with poor prognosis. Epidemic KS commonly spreads to the skin, lymphatic system, lungs, gastrointestinal tract, liver or heart. The clinical manifestations are characterized by asymptomatic skin defects with pigment sedimentation or skin defects in the head, neck and the oral cavity. Extensive oral involvement has manifestations of fallen tooth, pain and ulcer. In the advanced stage, edema and pain occur in the lower limbs ends, penis, scrotum or face. CD4 T cell count may increase by about 200–500/μl.

25.2 HIV/AIDS Related Fungal Infections

25.2.1 HIV/AIDS Related Mucocutaneous Candidiasis

25.2.1.1 Pathogen and Pathogenesis
Candida is a yeast liked fungus of gemmation, which has a wide distribution in the nature world. It can also be parasitize in normal human skin and the oral, gastrointestinal, anal and vaginal mucosa, with no occurrence of diseases. It is a typical conditional pathogen. Candida albicans is a common

pathogen. Only when the immunity of the human body is compromised, Candida albicans can cause diseases. The pathogenesis of Candida includes three aspects: (1) The compromised cellular immunity of the human body. Its manifestations include candida antigen skin test negative. When stimulated in vitro by Candida antigen, the lymphocyte transformation rate is low and reduced/absent macrophage migration inhibitory factor synthesis. The amount of phagocytes is reduced, with loss of the chemotaxis and declining ability to swallow and kill the pathogens. (2) The pathogen. The spore wall of Candida albicans is mainly composed of glycogen and mannan which could strengthen the adhesion of Candida albicans to cause infection. (3) Iatrogenic factor. Iatrogenic factor includes the administrations of broad spectrum antibiotics, adrenal cortical hormone, and immunosuppressants, which provide chances for the invasion of the pathogens.

25.2.1.2 Pathological Basis

The histopathological changes include inflammatory (such as the skin, lungs), purulent (such as kidney, lung and brain) or granulomatous (such as skin). Special organs and tissues can also have special manifestations. For instances, ulceration occurs in the esophagus and small intestine; proliferative changes occur in the cardiac valves; micro-abscesses occur in the cases of acute disseminated diseases with spores and hyphae in the abscesses and external infiltration of the neutrophils and histocytes. Surrounding the spore, there occasionally are eosinophilic materials, like astral body. Sometimes, the hyphae invade into the vascular wall. The histopathological findings of hyphae have diagnostic value.

25.2.1.3 Clinical Symptoms and Signs

Candida erythema commonly occurs in the skin folds, such as the gluteal fold, groin, under the breast, axillary, umbilical fossa, as well as the labia. The manifestations include erythema erosion and dipping whitish membranous scales, with clear boundary, surrounding red macula, blisters or pustules, and sense of itches. It is common in patients with diabetes, overweight and hidrosis. Due to the immunodeficiency of

AIDS patients, systemic skin candidiasis may occur, with manifestations of widespread erythema and scales lesions with clear boundary, scattered surrounding papules or vesicles. It is often accompanied by thrush or gastroenteritis.

25.2.1.4 Examinations and Their Selection

Direct Microscopy

It is the most commonly used examination.

Staining

Microscopy after staining has a higher detection rate, comparing to the direct microscopy.

Isolation and Culture

The patients with smears negative findings should receive Candida culture.

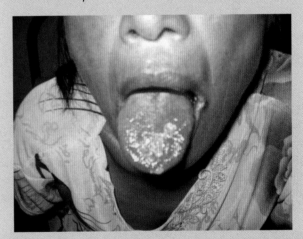

Case Study 1

A female patient aged 43 years was confirmatively diagnosed as having AIDS by the CDC. Her CD4 T cell count was 78/μl.

Fig. 25.1 HIV/AIDS related oral mucosa candidiasis. The gross observation demonstrates diffuse scattering whitish mucous plaques on the surface of the tongue

Case Study 2
A female patient aged 55 years was confirmatively diagnosed as having AIDS by the CDC. Her CD4 T cell count was 98/μl.

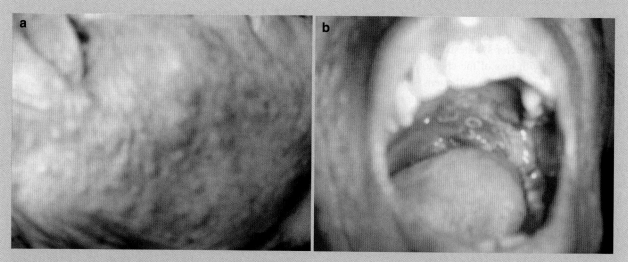

Fig. 25.2 (**a, b**) HIV/AIDS related skin and oral mucosa candidiasis. (**a**) The gross observation demonstrates diffuse scattering grayish white papules on the face. (**b**) The gross observation demonstrates white plaques and ulcers in the oral upper palate.

25.2.2 HIV/AIDS Related Cryptococcal Infection

25.2.2.1 Pathogen and Pathogenesis
Compromised immunity is an important factor inducing cryptococcal infection. Cryptococcal infection is rarely infected via skin contacts to Cryptococcus contaminated objects. Systemic cryptococcal disease with local manifestations is more common, which may be caused by spreading from meningeal, pulmonary or other lesions.

25.2.2.2 Pathophysiological Basis
The basic pathological changes have two kinds: early diffuse infiltrative exudative changes, and later granuloma formation. In the early lesions, there are large quantity Cryptococcus neoformans gathering, encapsulated thallus by colloid capsule that avoids direct contacts between the thallus and the surrounding tissues. Therefore, the inflammatory responses of the tissue are not obvious. Granuloma formation occurs sever months after the infection, with proliferated giant cells, macrophages and fibroblasts, infiltration of lymphocytes and plasma cells, and occasional occurrence of necrosis and small cavities.

25.2.2.3 Clinical Symptoms and Signs
Skin Cryptococcus infection has manifestations of acne liked skin rash, papules, hard nodules, and granuloma. The lesions have central necrosis, ulceration and fistula. The mucosal lesions are commonly found in the oral cavity and nasopharynx, with manifestations of nodules, ulceration and granuloma, with coverage of the surfaces with adhesive exudative thin membrane.

25.2.2.4 Examinations and Their Selection
Pathogenic Examinations
India ink staining is a rapid, simple and reliable method. Its repeated application has a high detection rate.

Serological Tests
The examination of the antibody has low positive rate, with low specificity. It is applied as a facilitative examination for the diagnosis.

Case Study 1

A female patient aged 34 years was confirmatively diagnosed as having AIDS by the CDC. Her CD4 T cell count was 118/μl.

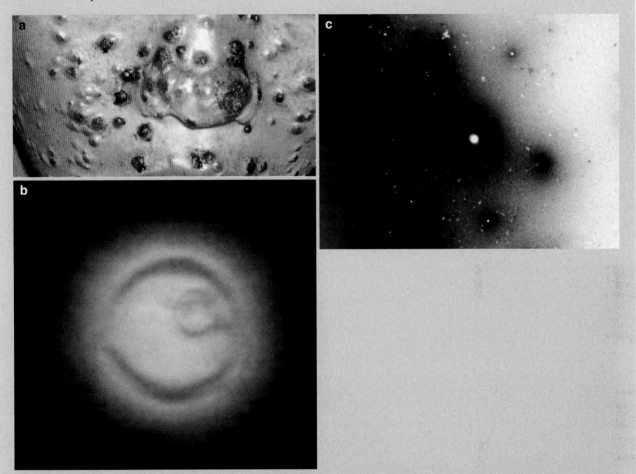

Fig. 25.3 (a–c) HIV/AIDS related skin cryptococcal infection. (a) The gross observation demonstrates diffuse scattering purplish black papules on the face. (b, c) Ink staining and light microscopy demonstrate cryptococcal cystozooid

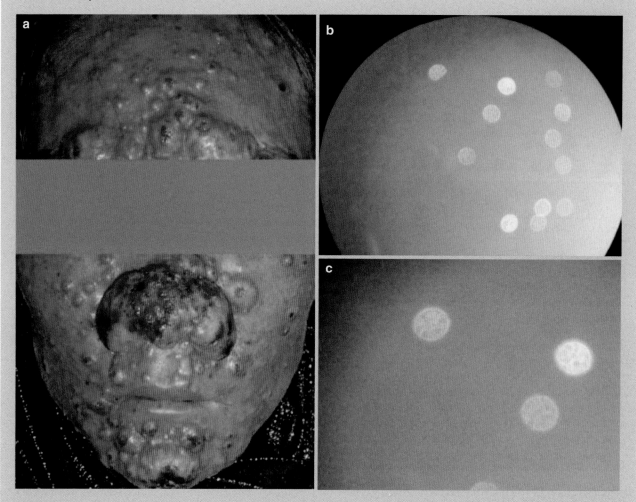

Fig. 25.4 (**a–c**) HIV/AIDS related skin cryptococcal infection. (**a**) The gross observation demonstrates diffuse scattering purplish red papules on the face. (**b, c**) Ink staining and light microscopy demonstrate cryptococcal cystozooid

25.2.3   HIV/AIDS Related Histoplasmosis Infection

25.2.3.1 Pathogen and Pathogenesis

Histoplasma is a biphasic fungus. It is in the yeast phase in the tissues and grows in the cells. By HE staining, round or oval globules can be found, with surrounding transparent halo like a capsule and a diameter of merely 2–4 um. PAS bacteria are slightly larger, with surround red stained cell wall to take the place of the capsule liked halo (actually the

fungus has no capsule). It is highly contagious and can cause laboratory infection. The disease is caused by capsular histoplasmosis, which invades the human body via the skin. Its access into the human body causes primary or disseminated infections in people with compromised immunity.

25.2.3.2 Pathophysiological Basis

The pathological basis is the non-specific inflammatory infiltration of primary histoplasmosis. Occasionally, the macrophages and necrotic area can be found. In the macrophages, there are large quantity pathogenic fungi; and histocytes with swallowed spores can also be found in the regional lymph nodes. In the early period, there is central proliferation, with more or less fungi in the macrophages. After that, tissue necrosis occurs, with surrounding granuloma changes and final fibrosis to heal.

25.2.3.3 Clinical Symptoms and Signs

Skin histoplasmosis has hard plaques, nodules and subcutaneous nodules of erythema liked changes.

25.2.3.4 Examinations and Their Selection
Pathogenic Examinations

The finding of Histoplasma capsulatum in specimens has decisive significance for the diagnosis of the disease. Culture is still the only basis for the definitive diagnosis.

Serological Tests

In the early period, the latex agglutination test is positive. Immunodiffusion facilitates to differentiate the active lesions from non-active lesions. It is commonly positive in 2–5 weeks after the onset of symptoms.

Fluorescent Antibody Assay

It can facilitate the diagnosis. Complement fixation test can also be used for the screening test.

25.2.4 HIV/AIDS Related Superficial Fungal Infections

Case Study 1

A male patient aged 46 years was confirmatively diagnosed as having AIDS by the CDC. His CD4 T cell count was 153/ μl.

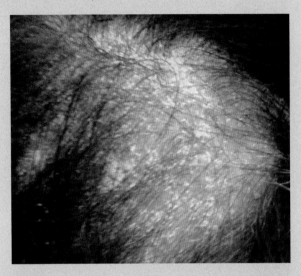

Fig. 25.5 HIV/AIDS related superficial fungal infection. The gross observation demonstrates vertex sparse hairs, and white scalp decrustation

Case Study 2

A female patient aged 36 years was confirmatively diagnosed as having AIDS by the CDC. Her CD4 T cell count was 73/μl and she sustained skin aspergillus infection.

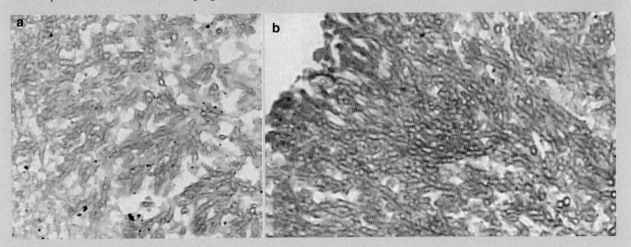

Fig. 25.6 (**a, b**) HIV/AIDS related fungal infection. Pathological biopsy demonstrates diffuse Aspergillus hyphae under a microscope

Case Study 3
A male patient aged 46 years was confirmatively diagnosed as having AIDS by the CDC. His CD4 T cell count was 13/ μl.

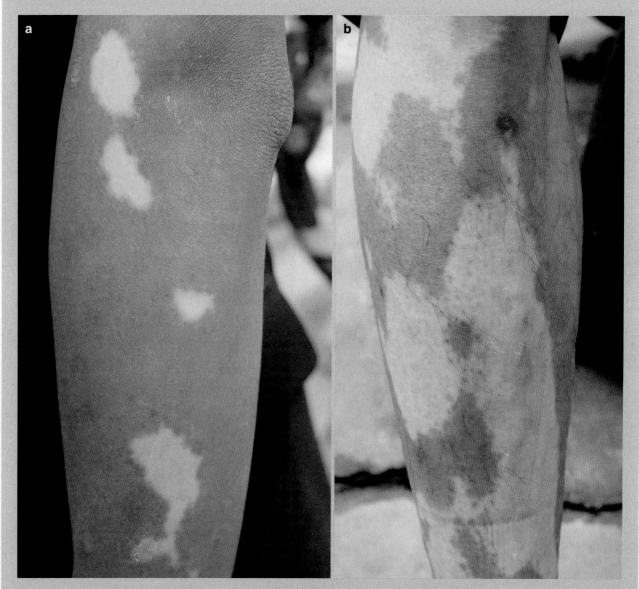

Fig. 25.7 HIV/AIDS related superficial fungal infection. (**a, b**) The gross observation demonstrates pink and white plaques on the skin surface

25.3   HIV/AIDS Related Parasitic Infections

25.3.1   HIV/AIDS Related Cutaneous Leishmaniasis

25.3.1.1 Pathogen and Pathogenesis

Since the mid 1980s, leishmaniasis in HIV patients has been increasing dramatically. Leishmaniasis is a zoonotic disease caused by Leishmania and it transmits between arthropods and mammals, with occurrence in more than 80 countries. It has been estimated that the total number of infected patients is up to more than 15 million and the newly emerging cases are more than 0.4 million per year. For the HIV positive patients, leishmania may be a opportunistic pathogenic parasite.

25.3.1.2 Pathophysiological Basis

The amastigote of leishmania can parasitize in macrophages and other phagocytic cells, such as monocytes and neutrophil. It causes chronic diffuse cells (including macrophages, lymphocytes and plasma cells) infiltration and the formation of micro granuloma with intact structure in patients with immunodeficiency.

25.3.1.3 Clinical Symptoms and Signs

Cutaneous leishmaniasis has two types: confined and diffuse. The manifestations include singular papula and nodule, with no occurrence of ulceration.

25.3.1.4 Examinations and Their Selection
Pathogenic Diagnosis

The finding of amastigote in cytological or histological examinations can define the diagnosis.

Immunological Diagnosis

The immunological assays include leishmania antibodies examination and cytoimmunological assay, both with high sensitivity.

25.3.2   HIV/AIDS Related Toxoplasma Infection of Skin

25.3.2.1 Pathogen and Pathogenesis
Skin toxoplasmosis is caused by toxoplasma gondii.

25.3.2.2 Pathophysiological Basis

It is pathologically manifested as (1) inflammatory cell infiltration, and sometimes formation of granulomas to involve the blood vessels and skin appendages; (2) vascular changes of capillary dilation, endothelial cells proliferation, venules necrosis and perivasculitis; (3) squamous epithelial cells pro-liferation, with the demonstration of epitheliomatous symptom in some serious cases.

25.3.2.3 Clinical Symptoms and Signs
The manifestations include skin rashes, commonly in the face, trunk and limbs; and secondary scarlet fever liked desquamation. There are also high fever and general upset.

25.3.2.4 Examinations and Their Selection
Pathogenic Examinations

The finding of the pathogen by histopathological examinations is a reliable basis for the diagnosis.

Immunological Assays

It is the main basis to define the diagnosis.

25.4   HIV/AIDS Related Viral Infections

25.4.1   HIV/AIDS Related Skin Herpes Simplex Virus Infection

25.4.1.1 Pathogen and Pathogenesis
This disease caused by herpes simplex virus of DNA virus. Herpes simplex virus (HSV) can be divided into two types: HSV-1 and HSV-2. HSV-1 often causes the lips and corneal herpes while HSV-2 causes genital herpes which mainly spreads by direct contacts to the lesions (sexual contacts) to result in skin lesions. They can be primary and recurrent herpes.

25.4.1.2 Pathophysiological Basis
Approximately 22 % cases of AIDS are complicated by herpes simplex. According to the diagnostic criteria by the CDC, chronic mucous herpes simplex or disseminated herpes simplex indicate the HIV infection has progressed in to AIDS.

25.4.1.3 Clinical Symptoms and Signs
Clinically, the lesions are erosions and ulcers with irregular margins, which is formed by rupture of intensive small blisters. Herpes simplex has atypical manifestations, with palm blisters or bullous lesions.

25.4.1.4 Examinations and Their Selection
Pathological Examinations

The finding of macrophages or intranuclear inclusions by biopsy has diagnostic significance.

Serological Tests

The finding has diagnostic significance, but it has false negative findings.

Case Study 1

A female patient aged 36 years was confirmatively diagnosed as having AIDS by the CDC. Her CD4 T cell count was 18/μl.

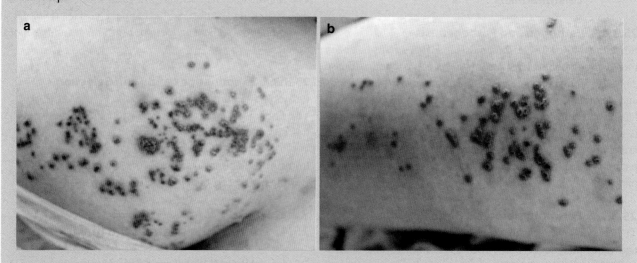

Fig. 25.8 (a, b) HIV/AIDS related skin herpes simplex virus infection. The gross observation demonstrates herpes simplex ulceration and scab on the buttocks and thighs, and newly emerging herpes

Case Study 2

A male patient aged 35 years was confirmatively diagnosed as having AIDS by the CDC. His CD4 T cell count was 88/ μl.

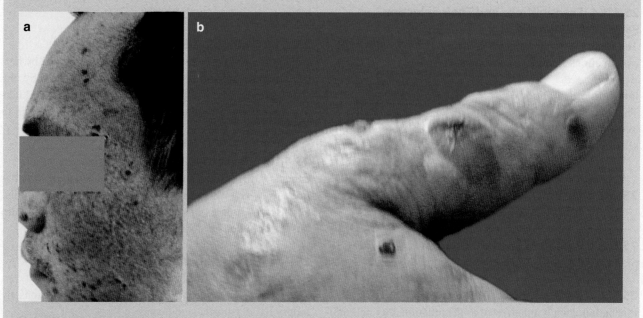

Fig. 25.9 (a, b) HIV/AIDS related skin herpes simplex virus infection. The gross observation demonstrates old scars and newly emerging large blisters on the face and finger

Case Study 3

A boy aged 5 years was confirmatively diagnosed as having AIDS by the CDC. His CD4 T cell count was 102/μl.

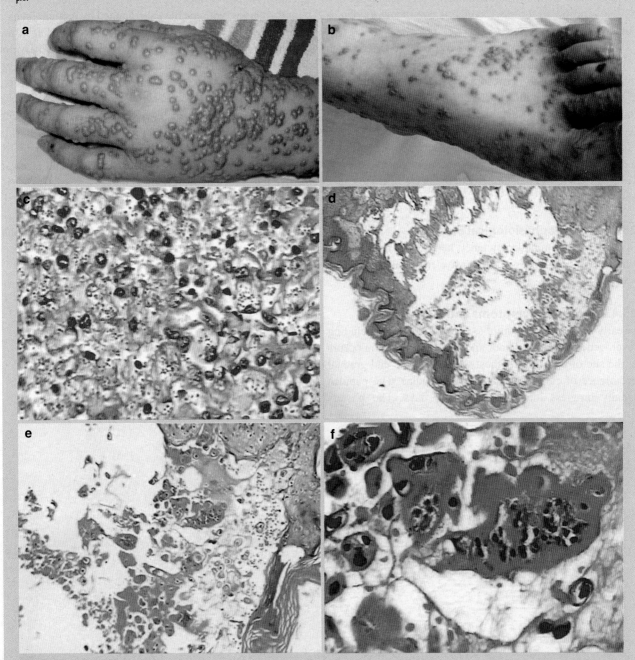

Fig. 25.10 (a–f) HIV/AIDS related skin herpes simplex virus infection. (**a, b**) The gross observation demonstrates diffuse scattering newly emerging blisters on the hand back and the foot back, and rupture and fusion of some blisters. (**c**) Biopsy of cervical lymph nodes by PAS staining and high magnification demonstrates lymphocytes, mononuclear cells and viral particles. (**d**) Skin rash biopsy with PAS staining and 40×-1 demonstrates lymphocytes, mononuclear cells and viral particles. (**e**) Skin rash biopsy with PAS staining and 100×-1 demonstrates. (**f**) Skin rash biopsy with PAS staining and 400×-1 demonstrates lymphocytes, mononuclear cells and macrophages inclusions

25.4.2   HIV/AIDS Related Skin Varicella-Zoster Virus Infection

25.4.2.1 Pathogen and Pathogenesis

Herpes zoster is an acute inflammatory skin disease caused by the varicella-zoster virus, which is commonly known as spider sore.

The pathogen of the disease is herpes zoster virus, which is philic to the nerves and the skin. The virus invades into the human body through the respiratory tract mucosa to cause chickenpox or latent infection. The virus can be incubated in the dorsal root of the spinal nerve or ganglia neurons. With the immunity is compromised, the latent virus grows and replicates to cause inflammation or necrosis of the invaded ganglion. As the result, neuralgia occurs. Meanwhile, the virus spreads to the skin along with the nerve fibers to cause clustering blisters.

25.4.2.2 Pathophysiological Basis

In patients with immunodeficiency, herpes zoster is disseminating, with accompanying extensive mucosal and organs necrosis

25.4.2.3 Clinical Symptoms and Signs

In early stage, there are mild systemic symptoms including fever, general upset and poor appetite. Skin irritation occurs at the site of upcoming rashes, with local pain and gradual occurrence of clustering mung sized papulae. The papulae rapidly progress into blisters in 1–2 days. The blisters develop into strip liked arrangement along the proximal nerve. Several days later, the blister wall is relaxed with cloudy blister fluid, which is gradually absorbed to form dry scar. After healing, erythema or pigmentation temporarily remains. The skin rashes are in strip liked arrangement along with the nerves, with the base surrounded by red halo, which commonly does not exceed the midline. The skin defects are common in the areas innervated by the intercostal nerve or the first branch of trigeminal nerve. The skin defects can also be found in the waist and abdomen, limbs and ears. Local lymph nodes are commonly swollen and painful. Neuralgia is characteristically varicella-zoster virus infection, with occurrence before the skin rashes or together with skin rashes. After skin rashes recede, the blisters may persist for months or longer. The skin rashes on the head and face can involve the cornea to cause viral keratitis.

25.4.2.4   Examinations and Their Selection

The diagnosis is mainly based on the clinical examinations, with no use of other diagnostic examinations.

Pathological Examination
Biopsy has important diagnostic significance.

Virus Culture
It facilitates accurate diagnosis.

HSV Antibody Test
It facilitates the definitive diagnosis of the disease.

Case Study
A female patient aged 38 years was confirmatively diagnosed as having AIDS by the CDC. Her CD4 T cell count was 62/μl.

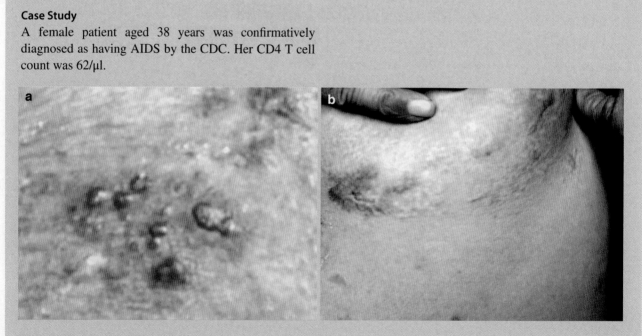

Fig. 25.11 (**a**, **b**) HIV/AIDS related skin herpes zoster virus infection. (**a**) The gross observation demonstrates purplish red herpes in sternocostal area, with fusion of some herpes. (**b**) The gross observation demonstrates healing scar after treatment

25.4.3 HIV/AIDS Related Skin Poxviridae Infection

25.4.3.1 Pathogen and Pathogenesis

Self-inoculation viral skin disease caused by pox viruses is known as molluscum contagiosum. Molluscum contagiosum cannot repeatedly grow in cell culture and its pathogenesis remains unknown.

25.4.3.2 Pathophysiological Basis

It is pathologically characterized by cytoplasmic inclusions in the epidermic cells, which are known as molluscumbody. The molluscumbody compress the nucleus of the infected cell to cause it in meniscus shape and located at the edge of the cells. The molluscumbody changes from eosinophilic to basophilic. Multiple basophilic molluscumbody in a diameter of 35 um can be found in the corneum. In the cases with ruptured corneum, the inner molluscumbody are discharged to form a volcanic crater liked lesion. In the cases with follicular molluscum contagiosum, multiple dilated follicles can be found in the dermis, filled by molluscumbody. Under an electron microscope, viral particles can be observed in the cytoplasm.

25.4.3.3 Clinical Symptoms and Signs

The pox viruses have a latency period ranging from 1 week to 6 months. The typical lesions are infected local epidermal cells proliferation to form macula in a diameter of 2–8 mm. The lesion may be singular or multiple, in round or semispherical shape, with waxy luster. It has central hilar depression, containing caseous embolus and the macula is in the color of flesh or pink. In the early period, the lesions are hard. With their maturity, it becomes soft, which can be compressed to squeeze the caseous material. Clinically, the disease can be divided into two types: (1) Pediatric type is infected via direct skin contacts or along with infectious vector. The molluscum can be found on the face, trunk and the limbs. (2) Adult type is transmitted via sexual behaviors. The molluscum can be found in the genital organs, buttocks, lower abdomen, suprapubic area and medial thighs. In patients with anal sexual behaviors, the molluscum can be found in the anus.

25.4.3.4 Examinations and Their Selection

The diagnosis mainly depends on the clinical diagnosis. For some individual atypical cases, pathological diagnosis should be performed to define the diagnosis.

Direct Examination of the Virus Particle Smear and Staining

The squeezed caseous material can be found molluscumbody positive by Wright staining.

Electron Microscopy

The specimen for biopsy demonstrates molluscum virus positive.

Histopathological Examination

The findings are characteristic for the diagnosis.

25.4.4 HIV/AIDS Related Skin Cytomegalovirus Infection

25.4.4.1 Pathogen and Pathogenesis

Cytomegalovirus belongs to herpes virus group and has typical structure of the herpes virus. It is a kind of large DNA virus with a diameter of about 80–110 nm, and its shell is a symmetric icosahedron containing 162 shell grains. Around the shell there is a single or double layer of lipoid protein envelope. It grows slowly in vitro, with a replication cycle of 36–48 h. It has one serum type, which can be further divided into more than three subtypes. It can only grow in the living cells, which can be cultured with human fibroblasts.

25.4.4.2 Pathophysiological Basis

Under a light microscope, the infected cells by cytomegalovirus have enlarged nucleus, with formation of inclusion bodies. Between the surrounding inclusions and the nucleus membrane, there is a circular halo, which is known as the eagle eyes cells, which have significance for the morphological diagnosis.

25.4.4.3 Clinical Symptoms and Signs

The skin lesions are manifested as purplish plaques.

25.4.4.4 Examinations and Their Selection

Polymerase chain reaction (PCR) can be applied to quantitatively detect the viral load of the specimen. Currently, it is believed to be the optimal method for the diagnosis of invasive CMV infection.

25.4.5 HIV/AIDS Related Skin Human Papillomavirus Infection

25.4.5.1 Pathogen and Pathogenesis

Human papilloma virus invades the human body to cause epidermal neoplasm liked proliferation with close relationship to sexual transmission, which is known as genital warts (CA). Its pathogen is human papilloma virus (HPV), with a diameter of 50–55 nm and 72 virus shell particles. The virus has an icosahedral shell containing a double-stranded circular DNA with 7,900 base pairs.

25.4.5.2 Pathophysiological Basis

The incubation period of the pathogen ranges from 5 weeks to 9 months, and an average of 1–3 months. CA is more common in sexually active young and middle-aged adults and its peak age of occurrence is 20–25 years old. In HIV positive patients, its incidence is 3–6 %.

Histologically, genital CA has manifestations of epidermal hyperkeratosis, parakeratosis, and acanthosis. In the epidermal layer, koilocytes with empty halo of perinuclear cytoplasm can be found, with enlarged foamy prickie cells that have chromatin, obviously hyperplasic basal cells and occurrence of dual-nuclear or multi-nuclear cells. In addition, chronic inflammatory cells infiltration occurs in the dermis.

25.4.5.3 Clinical Symptoms and Signs

The latency period of HIV/AIDS related skin human papilloma virus infection ranges from 1 to 8 months, with an average latency period of 3 months. It commonly occurs in the cutaneous mucosal infiltration areas adjacent to the external genitals and the anus. The lesions are commonly found in the balanus, coronary sulcus, frenulum of prepuce, urethra opening and penis of the male patients. And the lesions are commonly found in the anus and the rectum in the homosexual patients. In female patients, the lesions are commonly found in the major and minor labia, vagina orifice, vagina, urethra, cervix, perineum, mons pubis and groin. Apart from the genitals, the lesions can also be found in the axillaries, umbilical fossa and breasts. In the cases with oral sex history, the lesions can also be found in the oral cavity. The lesion have an early morphology of small soft pink excrescence with a pointed top, which gradually enlarges and increases with fusion into various morphologies. At this time, the lesion has an uneven surface, which is moist and soft in papillary liked, cauliflower liked and crest liked appearance. Its root is commonly accompanied by a pedicle that is prone to erosion with stench. The wart has a whitish, dark grayish and reddish surface, which is prone to bleeding. The lesions located in the dry body parts are small and flat. Cervical condyloma has smooth surface or is in granular and groove shapes, with no typical papillary morphology.

25.4.5.4 Examinations and Their Selection

The diagnosis can be defined mainly based on the clinical manifestations.

Acetic Test

It has a high sensitive to HPV than routine observation of histological changes.

Pathological Examination

Histochemical Examination

Peroxidase anti-peroxidase (PAP) method has a high specificity and provides the diagnostic information more rapidly, which facilitates the diagnosis.

Genetic Diagnosis

The recently developed PCR has high sensitivity and specificity. It is also simple and rapid. Therefore, it provides a new way for the detection of HPV.

Case Study 1

A male patient aged 35 years was confirmatively diagnosed as having AIDS by the CDC. His CD4 T cell count was 42/ μl.

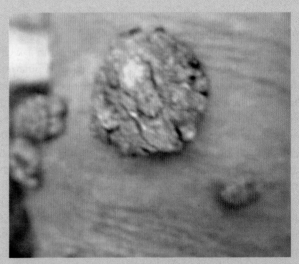

Fig. 25.12 HIV/AIDS related skin human papilloma virus infection. The gross observation demonstrates multiple condylomas in the penis, with different sizes and in cauliflower or mushroom shape

Case Study 2

A male patient aged 48 years was confirmatively diagnosed as having AIDS by the CDC. His CD4 T cell count was 62/ μl.

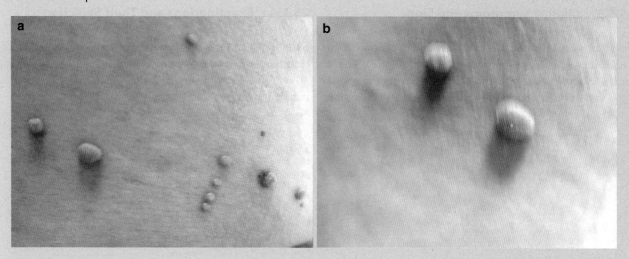

Fig. 25.13 (**a, b**) HIV/AIDS related skin human papilloma virus infection. The gross observation demonstrates multiple condylomas in the abdominal skin, with different sizes and in nodular or mushroom liked shape

25.4.6 HIV/AIDS Related Skin Epstein-Barr (EB) Virus Infection

25.4.6.1 Pathogen and Pathogenesis

Epstein-Barr virus belongs to human herpes virus, which has a worldwide distribution. It spreads along with saliva droplets and its infection mostly occurs in young children, with no obvious symptoms. Oral hairy leukoplakia caused by EB infection is characteristically HIV infection, which is believed to be an indicator of HIV infection progressing into AIDS.

25.4.6.2 Pathophysiological Basis

Oral hairy leukoplakia is more common in male patients, with lesions in any part of the oral cavity. It is most commonly found in the buccal mucosa and the ventral tongue mucosa. The histopathological change is the abnormal proliferation of mucosal epithelium, with manifestations of parakeratosis of many epithelial cells and accompanying vacuolated cells.

25.4.6.3 Clinical Symptoms and Signs

Most oral mucosal lesions are whitish plaques in different sizes, with no protrusion out of the mucosal surface but a rough sensation. Some lesions may have erosion or ulceration, which is locally painful. The plaques cannot be abraded. In AIDS patients, hairy whitish plaques are commonly found in the lateral border of the tongue.

25.4.6.4 Examinations and Their Selection
Pathologic Examination
It is the basis for the definitive diagnosis.

Blood Tests
The total WBC count increases and lymphocytes are up to 60–90 %. In the lymphocytes, 10–25 % is the heterophilic lymphocytes, which has diagnostic value.

25.5 HIV/AIDS Related Bacterial Infections

25.5.1 Pathogen and Pathogenesis

Although there are large quantity bacteria on the normal skin, they fail to cause diseases. The skin is a favorable defense against bacterial infections. However, AIDS patients, due to their compromised immunity and decreased skin resistance to the bacterial invasion, are susceptible to skin infections.

25.5.2 Pathophysiological Basis

The impact of bacterial skin infection is limited, with small pustules. They may spread within several hours to involve a large area of skin. The severities of skin infection range from a small acne to life threatening lesions. For instances, staphylococcal scalded skin syndrome usually occurs in patients with immunodeficiency.

25.5.3   Clinical Symptoms and Signs

Bacterial skin infection has early confined scab infection, which seems to be pustule. Usually within 1 day, scarlet flush area appears around the scab, with pain. Otherwise, large skin flush area appears with blisters that are susceptible

to rupture. Subsequently, the epidermis begins to desquamate, and even large area epidermal desquamation by a gentle touch or oppression.

25.5.4   Examinations and Their Selection

Skin biopsy or laboratory culture of skin specimens can differentiate it from staphylococcal scalded skin syndrome and other diseases with similar manifestations, such as drug induced toxic epidermal necrolysis.

Case Study

A female patient aged 39 years was confirmatively diagnosed as having AIDS by the CDC. Her CD4 T cell count was 123/μl.

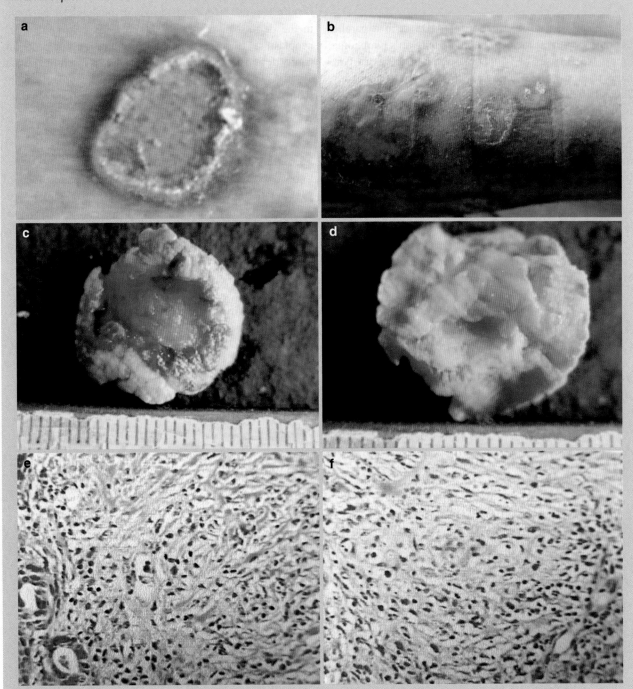

Fig. 25.14 (a–f) HIV/AIDS related bacterial infections. (a, b) The gross observation demonstrates multiple depressive ulcers in the shank skin. (c, d) The naked eyes observation after removal demonstrates a tissue mass in size of a button (anterior and dorsal views). (e, f) Microscopy demonstrates skin mucosal erosion and ulceration, with surface inflammatory exudates, necrosis, submucosal granuloma proliferation, scar formation, quite favorable conditions of the sebaceous gland and the sweat gland, and mesenchymal infiltration of neutrophils, eosinophils and lymphocytes

25.6 HIV/AIDS Related Malignancies of Skin

25.6.1 HIV/AIDS Related Skin Malignant Lymphoma

The epidemiological distribution of AIDS is in a parallel relationship with the incidence of non-Hodgkin's lymphoma. Almost 95 % cases of lymphoma occur in the extra lymphatic tissues, with occurrence in any part of the body. Clinically, AIDS complicated by lymphoma tends to be the histological type and invasiveness of high malignancy, with poor prognosis. Death commonly occurs within 6 months. The common non-specific skin lesions include pruritus and prurigo. Pruritus is a common manifestation of Hodgkin's diseases, accounting for 85 % and it could occur prior to other skin rashes. Zoster also commonly occurs in the cases of Hodgkin's diseases, accounting for 5–16 %. Skin lymphoma often indicates advanced lymphoma in other body parts and its blood borne dissemination. The cases of rarely occurring primary skin Hodgkin's diseases and mycosis fungoides have long survival period.

25.6.2 HIV/AIDS Related Cutaneous Kaposi's Sarcoma

25.6.2.1 Pathogen and Pathogenesis

Kaposi's sarcoma is multi-focal angioma caused by herpes virus type 8. The skin lesions originate from middle dermis and extend to the epidermis.

25.6.2.2 Pathophysiological Basis

It occurs commonly in young and middle-aged adults aged 20–50 years with AIDS. The skin lesions are widely distributed, commonly in the head, neck, trunk and pelma. Histopathological, all types of skin KS has basically same manifestations. Neoplasm tissues in masses can be found in the dermis, and irregular fissures can be found in the neoplasms. Endothelial cells proliferation is predominantly found in the cavities and obvious erythrocytes out of the cavities. There are also different quantities spindle shaped cells, which have deep stained large nuclei and are heteromorphous.

25.6.2.3 Clinical Symptoms and Signs

Kaposi's sarcoma is probably the initial manifestation of AIDS, with only lesions of protruding purplish, pink or reddish papula. Otherwise, the lesions are round or oval shaped brown/purple plaques. The lesions are initially found in the skin or mucosa of the upper trunk, and they can be extensively disseminated in the skin.

25.6.2.4 Examinations and Their Selection
Differential Leukocyte Count

In the cases with lymphatic involvement, the mononuclear cells increase, with following increased eosinophilic granulocytes.

Histopathological Examination

Case Study 1

A male patient aged 39 years was confirmatively diagnosed as having AIDS by the CDC. His CD4 T cell count was 23/ μl.

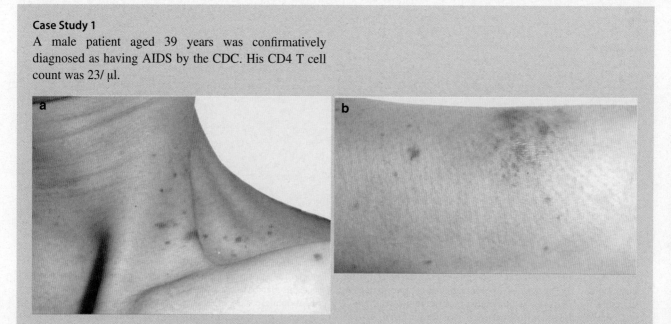

Fig. 25.15 (a, b) HIV/AIDS related skin Kaposi's sarcoma. The gross observation demonstrates multiple spots and flakes of purplish red ecchymosis in the left clavicular fossa and the neck

Case Study 2

A male patient aged 25 years was confirmatively diagnosed as having AIDS by the CDC. His CD4 T cell count was 76/ μl.

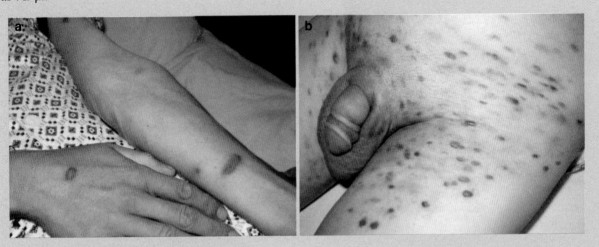

Fig. 25.16 (**a, b**) HIV/AIDS related skin Kaposi's sarcoma. The gross observation demonstrates multiple scattering purplish red protrusions in the hand back, forearms and abdomen and perineal region

Case Study 3

A female patient aged 53 years was confirmatively diagnosed as having AIDS by the CDC. Her CD4 T cell count was 51/μl.

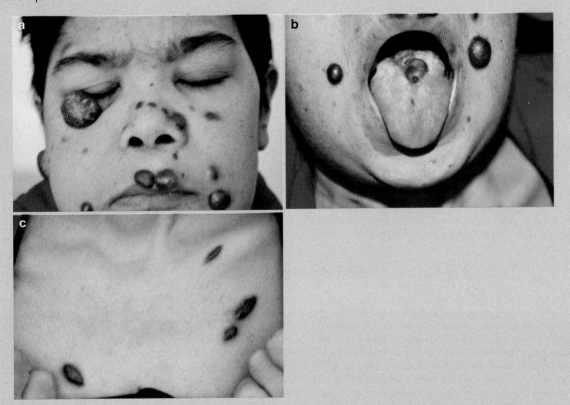

Fig. 25.17 (**a–c**) HIV/AIDS related skin Kaposi's sarcoma. The gross observation demonstrates multiple nodular purplish brown nodules or protrusions in the face, oral cavity and the chest

Case Study 4

A male patient aged 36 years was confirmatively diagnosed as having AIDS by the CDC. He had a homosexual history and was hospitalized due to fever and cough for 2 months as well as chest distress for more than 20 days. Since July 2010, he began to have a

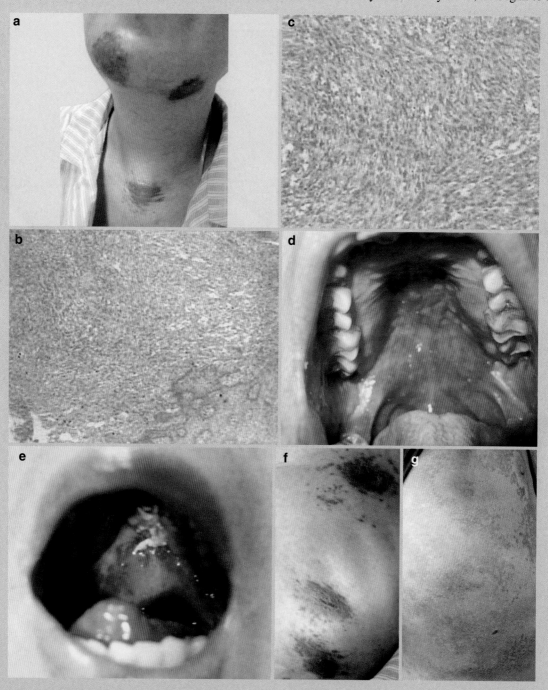

Fig. 25.18 (**a–g**) HIV/AIDS related skin kaposi's sarcoma. (**a**) The gross observation demonstrates multiple large flakes of purplish red protrusions in the jaw and the chest. (**b**, **c**) HE staining demonstrates skin tissue surface hyperkeratosis, perivascular cells proliferation and infiltration in the dermis, minor vascular hyperplasia, small vascular lumen and thin endothelium; thick squamous epithelium, spindle cells proliferation under it in parenchymal flaky and bundle liked distribution and some in luminal distribution; large cellular volume; obvious local vascular hyperplasia and filling of erythrocytes in the lumen. By specialized examinations, HHV8 positive, Ki-67 positive and lower than 10 %; immunohistochemical: Vim positive and CD34 positive. (**d**, **e**) The gross observation demonstrates nodular purplish red neoplasmic protrusions in the throat and the hard palate. (**f**) The gross observation after the treatment demonstrates purplish gray patches of protrusions in the chest. (**g**) The gross observation demonstrates purplish gray patches of protrusions in the skin surface, with scabs and ecdysis

body temperature of 37.5–37.8 °C, cough with yellowish bloody sputum and dark purplish patches of skin rashes. By examinations, anti-treponema pallidum antibody positive, CD4 T cell count 5/μl and a body temperature on admission of 39.1 °C, with low spirits as well as dark purplish patches of skin rashes in the face, eyelid, lower mandible, hairline, chest and abdomen. The large rash is in a size of 2 × 3 cm, protruding from the skin with surface desquamation. By palpation, bilateral neck has multiple enlarged lymph nodes, the largest in size of 19 × 10 mm. By laboratory tests, WBC $5.98 × 10^9$/L, N 78.74 %, RBC $2.22 × 10^{12}$/L, HGB 71 g/L, PLT $204 × 10^9$/L, CD4 T cell count 12/μl. By sputum smear, fungal spores and hyphae are detected. The clinical diagnosis was Kaposi's sarcoma.

Before the treatment:

25.7   HIV/AIDS Related Vascular Lesions of Skin

25.7.1   HIV/AIDS Related Skin Bacillary Epithelioid Angiomatosis (BEA)

25.7.1.1 Pathogen and Pathogenesis

Bacillary epithelioid angiomatosis is an important HIV/AIDS related angiomatosis. In 1983, Stoler et al. firstly reported the cases with HIV/AIDS complicated by multiple subcutaneous vascular nodules [15], within which there are small bacilli. By Warthin-Starry staining, the bacteria were clearly demonstrated, which was then nominated as bacillary epithelioid angiomatosis.

By electron microscopic observation of the skin defects tissue section, small bacilli similar to cat scratch diseases can be found, in size of about $0.5 × 1.5$ μm and in a distribution of cluster or bundle. Currently, successful bacilli culture has been reported. However, its categorization has not been finally defined. Some scholars believe that it is related to the newly found bacilli in the cases of cat scratch diseases. And some scholars believe that they are actually bacilli in the cases of cat scratch diseases and cause granuloma lesions in the cases with competent immunity but vascular hyperplasia lesions in the cases with compromised immunity. Its pathogenesis is still unknown.

25.7.1.2 Pathophysiological Basis

This disease commonly occurs in the process of the HIV infection. In 1992, it was defined as one of HIV/AIDS related bacterial infectious diseases, with male patients accounting for 90 % [4]. By Warthin-Starry staining, the masses composed of gathering bacilli can be clearly demonstrated. Generally, the pathological changes include: (1) Common epidermal ulceration; (2) The skin lesions with no surrounding adnexal epithelium; (3) Obvious mixed inflammatory cells infiltration in the dermis that is predominantly neutrophils, leukocytoclastic and nuclear dusts; (4) Three layered cellular wall of bacillus under an electron microscope. The important pathological manifestations include: (1) The blood vessels with lobular hyperplasia in the dermis have large prominent cuboidal endothelial cells; (2) Purplish granular clots composed of clustering bacteria; (3) By Warthin-Starry silver staining, the bacillary clots are dark brown, which are located in the interstitium adjacent to the blood vessels.

25.7.1.3 Clinical Symptoms and Signs

This disease commonly occurs in the process of HIV infection, with more male patients. The skin defects can be divided into dermal type and subcutaneous type. The dermal lesions are red or dark red in size of a needle point. The papulae then enlarge and progress into semispheric, pointed doom liked or pedicled nodules in hardness of elephantoid. In the advanced stage, the lesions may be manifested as ulcer and serous effusion in amounts ranging from singular to hundreds, which can be found in any part of the human body. The singular skin defect in the face or hand may be similar to pyogenic granuloma, with residue mild pigmentation after its absence. By Warthin-Starry staining and electron microscopy, the granular substance is demonstrated to be bacteria, being the same as the bacteria in the lesions. Webster categorized its clinical manifestations into three types: (1) Pyogenic granuloma is dark red, with the lesions in sizes of 1 to several centimeters, surface scales and basal pedicles. (2) The subcutaneous nodules are fixed and soft, with involvement of the lower bone tissues in the serious cases. (3) Pigmented hard nodules are black in oval shape, with rough surface and central epidermal keratinization.

25.7.1.4 Examinations and Their Selection

1. Gross observation of the appearance.
2. Pathological examinations.

The diagnosis mainly depends on the histopathological changes.

25.7.1.5 Differential Diagnosis

It is important to differentiate the disease from Kaposi sarcoma and Kaposi's Sarcoma with pyogenic granuloma.

25.8 HIV/AIDS Related Skin Dermatitis and Other Dermatologic Diseases

25.8.1 HIV/AIDS Related Eosinophilic Folliculitis

HIV/AIDS related eosinophilic folliculitis (HIV-EF) is a HIV/AIDS related folliculitis characterized by persistent increase of blood eosinophils and large quantity eosinophils infiltration in the skin hair follicles. In the 1970s, HIV-EF was confused with Ofuji disease (eosinophilic pustular folliculitis). Until 1986, Soeprono firstly reported three cases of HIV/AIDS complicated by eosinophilic folliculitis [14]. And until 1991, Rosenthal D formally proposed the nomination of HIV-EF, which clearly defined the disease from Ofuji disease [12]. Such cases are rarely reported and most cases are male homosexuals aged between 30 and 70 years. So far, only six cases of female patients have been reported, including 1 case of heterosexual female patient reported in Hong Kong. The pathogenesis of HIV-EF has been unknown. In the literature reports, the patients have a CT4 T cell count

being lower $200/\mu l$. Therefore, compromised immunity caused by HIV infection plays an important role in the pathogenesis of HIV-EF. In addition to HIV infection, there are also other theoretical explanations for its occurrence. For instances, Blauvelt A et al. found the conditions of patients with HIV-EF improved after receiving Permethrin therapy [3], which indicated that HIV-EF is related to demodex infection. Smith KJ et al. successfully treated one case of HIV-EF simply with metronidazole therapy [13], which indicated the incidence of HIV-EF is related to opportunistic bacterial infections, especially Gram-negative bacteria infection. Fearfield LA et al. believe that HIV-EF is an autoimmune disease [5], with infiltration of eosinophils and CD8 T cells due to exposure of sebaceous gland concealed antigen. It has been recognized that the incidence of HIV-EF is related to fungal infections, but the skin pathological examination failed to find the definitive pathogens, which was speculated to be caused by the extremely small quantity of the fungi in the follicular infection. In the theory, the extremely small quantity fungi can induce the exposure of the concealed antigens, thus trigger serious hypersensitivity.

Case Study

A male patient aged 34 years was confirmatively diagnosed as having AIDS by the CDC. He had a history of unhealthy sexual behaviors and a history of gonorrhea that was cured. In addition, he had no histories of intravenous drug use, blood products use, drugs and food allergies. He was hospitalized due to recurrent itchy skin rashes for 6 years that was exacerbating for 10 days. About 6 years ago, the patient had sustained systemic erythema, papula and accompanying pruritus in the face, neck and limbs, with no known reasons. By laboratory tests, blood WBC $3.55 \times 10^9/L$, NEUT% 43.1 %, absolute lymphocytes $0.65 \times 10^9/L$, eosinophil ratio 29.3 %, eosinophils absolute value $6.04 \times 10^9/L$, liver function and myocardiac enzymes normal, Anti-O, C-reactive protein normal, RF normal, humoral immune IgA, IgG and IgM normal, complement C_3 0.807 g/L, C_4 0.115 g/L, sputum, stool and blood cultures normal, normal sinus rhythm by EKG, chest CT scanning normal, B mode ultrasound demonstrations of normal liver, gallbladder, spleen, pancreas, both kidneys and ureter. He was defined to be HIV-1 antigen positive by the city CDC on 26th, June, with CD4 T cell count of $9/\mu l$ and HIV-RNA of $5.12 \times 10^7/ml$.

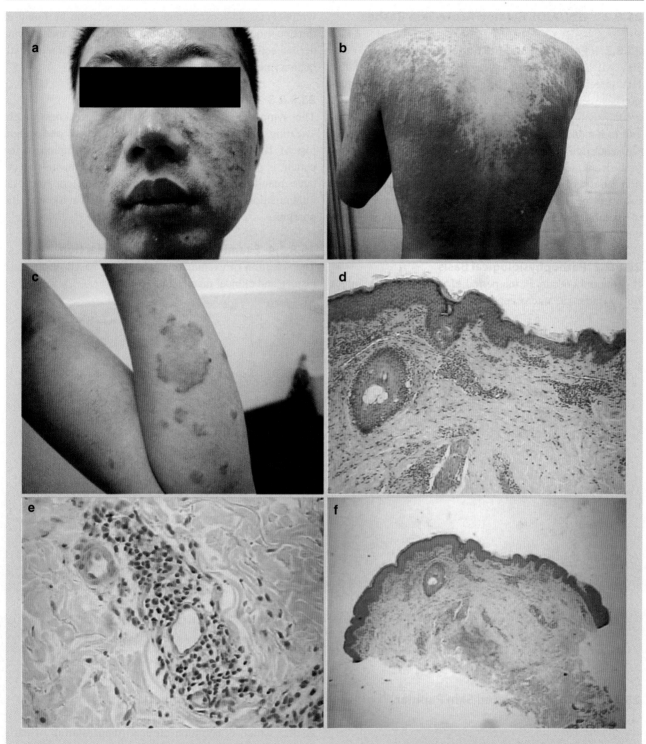

Fig. 25.19 (a–f) HIV/AIDS related eosinophilic folliculitis. (a–c) The gross observation demonstrates extensive erythema and papula in the face, back and forearms. (d–f) Pathological examinations demonstrate normal epidermis, scattering flakes of inflammatory cells infiltration in the hair follicles and sebaceous gland that is predominantly histocytes and lymphocytes, large quantity eosinophils, vascular dilation in the superficial dermis and no growth of pathogenic microorganisms. The diagnosis is HIV/AIDS related eosinophilic folliculitis (HIV-EF)

25.8.2   HIV/AIDS Related Acute Skin Rashes

25.8.2.1 Pathogen and Pathogenesis
HIV/AIDS related acute skin rashes occurs 1–3 weeks after HIV infection. About 30–50 % cases of primary HIV infection have accompanies skin rashes and mucosal rashes, which are mostly macula and papula in amounts ranging from several to hundreds and in sizes of 2–5 mm. They do not fuse with each other but with pruritus. They are commonly found in the trunk, face and upper limbs, possibly with desquamation and roseola, occasionally with hemorrhage, necrosis and palm and toes involvements that are similar to manifestations of syphilis. The skin rashes may be caused by responses of the human body to the HIV infection.

25.8.2.2 Pathophysiological Basis
It commonly occurs in the period of viremia of HIV infection. Under a microscope, perivascular infiltration of lymphocytes, histocytes, and plasma cells can be found in the upper dermis. Sometimes, the findings also include epidermal cells necrosis in the herpes, with infiltration of small quantity neutrophils.

25.8.2.3 Clinical Symptoms and Signs
The symptoms include persistent fever, weakness, night sweating, general superficial lymphadenectasis and weight loss of 10–40 % within 3 months. The emaciation of the patient is particularly obvious. The skin and mucus defects have manifestations of diffuse papula, zosters, mucosal inflammation and ulceration of the oral cavity and the pharynx.

25.8.2.4 Examinations and Their Selection
The selection of examinations should be based on the case history and clinical manifestations

Case Study
A male patient aged 43 years was confirmatively diagnosed as having AIDS by the CDC. His CD4 T cell count was 61/ μl.

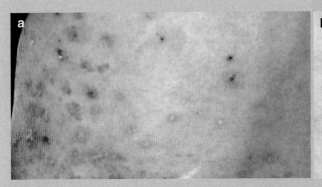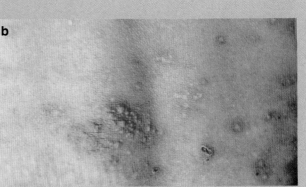

Fig. 25.20 (**a, b**) HIV/AIDS related dermatitis. The gross observation demonstrates multiple spots of papula in the skin of the back, with some papula gathering together

25.8.3   HIV/AIDS Related Skin Papular Prurigo

25.8.3.1 Pathogen and Pathogenesis
The pathogen of the disease remains unknown. It has been generally recognized that it is related to allergy. Some patients have a family history of allergies, in such cases the pediatric prurigo is related to atopic dermatitis. Some patients have prior papular urticaria and in such cases the prurigo is related to insect bites.

25.8.3.2 Pathophysiological Basis
In HIV positive patients, 20–72 % cases have skin papular rashes, which is common clinical manifestation of early HIV infection. The pathological changes of the disease are non-specific chronic inflammation, epidermal hyperkeratosis and parakeratosis, acanthosis, intraepidermal edema, superficial epidermal blisters, mild edema in the dermis, and perivascular infiltration of lymphocytes. The pathological changes of nodular prurigo include obvious epidermal hyperkeratosis and acanthosis in papillomatosis, as

well as superficial infiltration of histocytes and lymphocytes in the dermis.

25.8.3.3 Clinical Symptoms and Signs

The lesions are mainly distributed in the head, neck and upper trunk, which can also have a systemic distribution. They are in sizes of 2–5 mm and some fuse into flakes.

Extremely itch is its characteristic manifestation. The manifestations also include isolated and scattering solid papula, which are intensely itchy.

25.8.3.4 Examinations and Their Selection

The selection of examinations is mainly based on the case history and the clinical manifestations.

Case Study

A female patient aged 29 years was definitively diagnosed as having AIDS by the CDC.

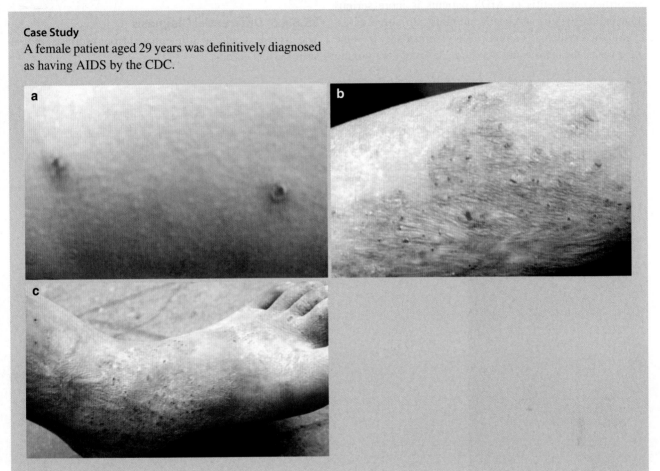

Fig. 25.21 (a–c) HIV/AIDS related skin papula prurigo. The gross observation demonstrates multiple spots of papula on the skin of the back, forearms and ankles, with scabs gathering into flakes

25.8.4 HIV/AIDS Related Skin Seborrheic Dermatitis

25.8.4.1 Pathogen and Pathogenesis

The etiology of HIV/AIDS related seborrheic dermatitis is still unknown. Generally, it is believed to be related to gonadal secretion disorders, specifically hypersecretion of male hormones. In addition, it is possibly related to the immunity (immunodeficiency in AIDS patients), hereditary factors, hormones, neurological and environmental factors. Based on excessive seborrhea, fungal and bacterial infections with symptoms of acnes may be secondary to seborrheic dermatitis.

Allergic responses to fungi and bacteria can also be secondary to seborrheic dermatitis. In the cases with autoimmune responses, eczema liked lesions and disseminated soborrheic dermatitis may be secondary to soborrheic dermatitis.

25.8.4.2 Pathophysiological Basis

About 80 % AIDS patients have seborrheic dermatitis. There is infiltration of lymphocytes, histocytes and eosinophils in the superficial dermis, deep perivascular area, and among the collagen fibers. And there are also confined epidermal prickle cells edema and dermal papillary edema. In some serious cases, intraepidermal blisters occur.

25.8.4.3 Clinical Symptoms and Signs

Seborrheic dermatitis may occur in the prodromal period of AIDS. The skin lesions are commonly found in the cheeks, zygomatic areas, scalp, posterior ears and chest. The rashes are slightly yellowish erythema or pink spots in different sizes with irregular clear boundary. The erythema is covered by large flakes of oily scaly scab. Seborrheic dermatitis in AIDS patients is more serious than patients with competent immunity. In some cases, zygomatic erythema is similar to erythematosus. In some other cases, the manifestation is large flakes of keratinizing

desquamation, like psoriasis, which can develop into erythroderma.

25.8.4.4 Examinations and Their Selection

1. Specialized dermatological examinations.
2. The examinations and their selection should be based the clinical manifestations.

25.8.4.5 Differential Diagnosis

The disease should be differentiated from psoriasis, pityriasis rosea and eczema.

Case Study

A female patient aged 29 years was definitively diagnosed as having AIDS by the CDC. Her CD4 T cell count was 120/μl.

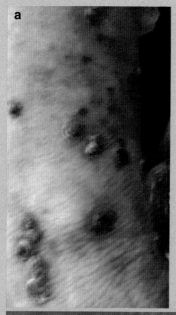

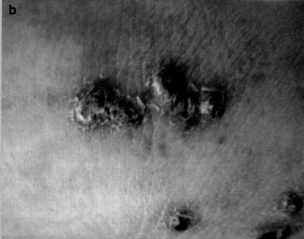

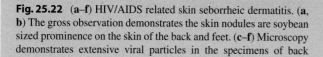

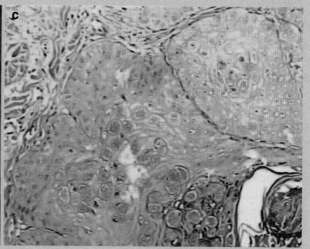

Fig. 25.22 (a–f) HIV/AIDS related skin seborrheic dermatitis. (**a**, **b**) The gross observation demonstrates the skin nodules are soybean sized prominence on the skin of the back and feet. (**c–f**) Microscopy demonstrates extensive viral particles in the specimens of back lesions, which are in line with manifestations of molluscum contagiosum. The skin lesions in the feet are in line with pathological manifestations of seborrheic dermatitis and slight to moderate atypical proliferation of some regional squamous epithelial cells

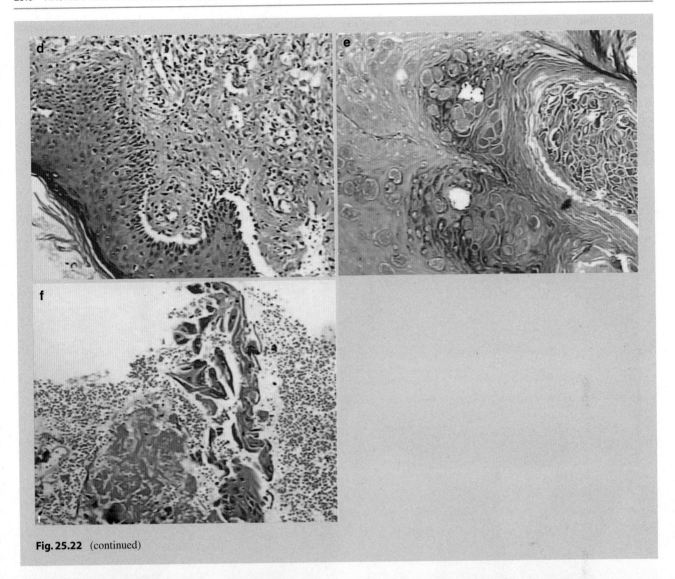

Fig. 25.22   (continued)

25.8.5   HIV/AIDS Related Skin Contact Dermatitis

25.8.5.1 Pathogen and Pathogenesis

Contact dermatitis is an acute inflammatory response caused by skin contacts of external allergens or irritants, with lesions on the contact site. The most common drug induced skin rashes in AIDS patients are caused by the combined use of sulfonamides and trimethylbenzyl amine pyrimidine for Pneumocystis carinii diseases. Reports indicated that 50–70 % cases have such responses, with manifestation of erythema papula that may involve the whole body and be accompanied by fever. About two thirds patients have to discontinue the therapy.

25.8.5.2 Pathophysiological Basis

According to different pathogenesis, the disease can be generally divided into two types: primary irritation and allergic response. The allergic response type is more common in clinical practice.

Primary Irritation Type of Contact Dermatitis

It is a direct response of the skin or mucosa to external stimuli. The occurrence is dependent on the intensity of the irritants and is unlikely to be related to the organism of the human body. Generally, the dermatitis inducing substances have intense irritability and people with contacts to it can sustain the disease. Otherwise, long term repeated contacts can cause the disease.

Allergic Response Type of Contact Dermatitis

The pathogen of this type of contact dermatitis is less irritable. Only allergic people can sustain the disease after contacts to the irritants. T cells and B cells play important roles in the occurrence of allergic response type of contact dermatitis.

25.8.5.3 Clinical Symptoms and Signs

Contact dermatitis have incubation period. The period from contact to irritants to the occurrence of dermatitis ranges from several minutes to several days. More intense irritability of the contacted materials can cause shorter incubation period. In the cases of allergens as the irritants, the disease occurs within 4–20 days after initial contact and 24 h after the repeated contact. The lesions are commonly confined on the contact site, with clear boundary. Clinically, there are changes of acute dermatitis, with skin lesions of erythema, swelling, blisters, papula erosion and exudation. In some serious cases, necrosis, ulceration and edema can be found. After long term repeated contacts to the irritants, the changes are chronic dermatitis, with locally dry lesions, desquamation or rhagadia, subjective intense itch with occasional sensations of burning and severe pain, as well as slight systemic symptoms.

25.8.5.4 Examinations and Their Selection

1. The patch test can be applied to facilitate the diagnosis.
2. After removal of the irritants, no contact causes no recurrence, which can define the diagnosis.

Case Study

A male patient aged 39 years was definitively diagnosed as having AIDS by the CDC. His CD4 T cell count was 18/µl.

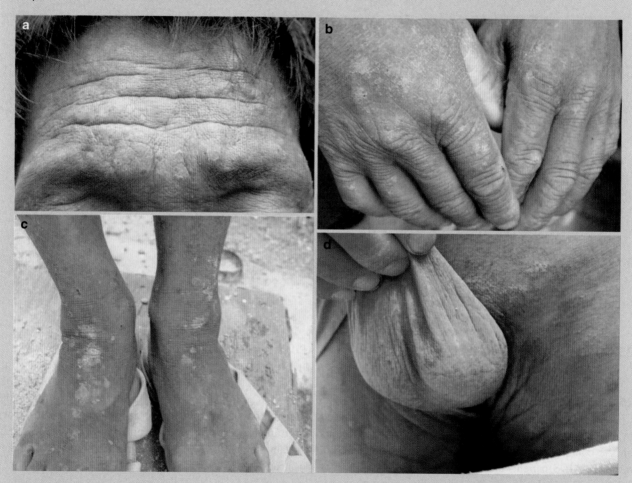

Fig. 25.23 (a–d) HIV/AIDS related skin contact dermatitis. The gross observation demonstrates multiple local skin swelling in the face, dorsal hands, dorsal feet and perineal region

25.8.6   HIV/AIDS Related Medicament Tetter

AIDS patient may have contact dermatitis, but its occurrence is rare. Clinically, the contact irritant is difficult to be differentiated from drug. The histological changes include vacuolation of basal cells and necrosis of keratinocytes necrosis. But in the cases with contact dermatitis, there is no infiltration of eosinophils and neutrophils, which can be the basis for the differential diagnosis.

Case Study 1
A male patient aged 29 years was definitively diagnosed as having AIDS by the CDC. His CD4 T cell count was 80/μl.

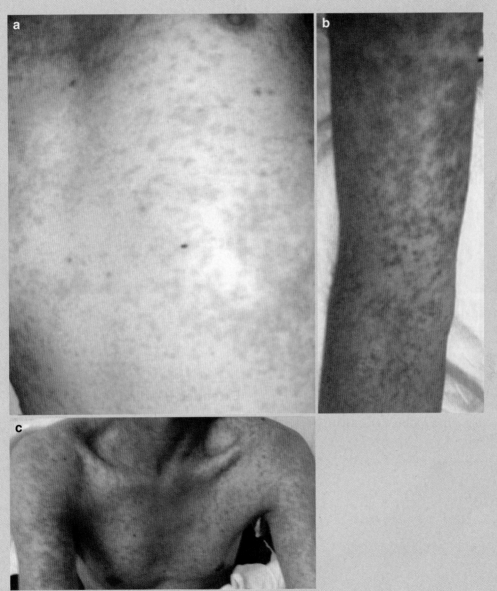

Fig. 25.24   (**a–c**) HIV/AIDS related skin drug rash. The gross observation demonstrates diffuse scattering multiple spots of red rashes on the skin of the chest and forearms

Case Study 2

A female patient aged 37 years was definitively diagnosed as having AIDS by the CDC. Her CD4 T cell count was 90/μl.

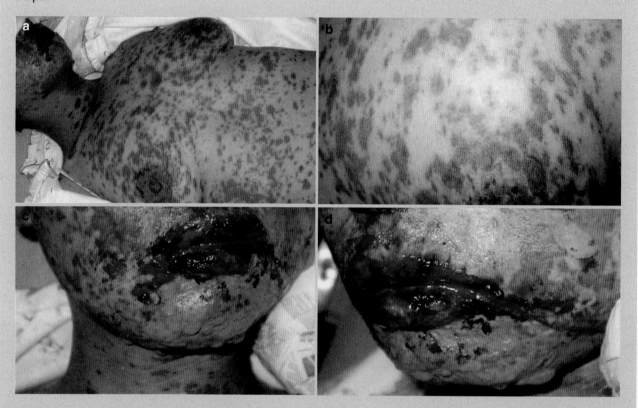

Fig. 25.25 (a–d) HIV/AIDS related skin drug rash. The gross observation demonstrates diffuse scattering multiple spots of purplish red rashes on the skin of the chest and face, swollen face, oral mucosal swelling and ulceration

Case Study 3

A female patient aged 49 years was definitively diagnosed as having AIDS by the CDC. Her CD4 T cell count was 70/μl.

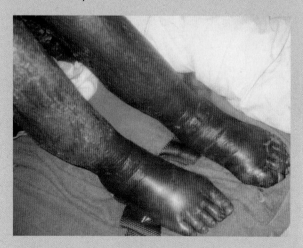

Fig. 25.26 HIV/AIDS related serious erythematous exfoliative dermatitis. The gross observation demonstrates purplish red and swollen skin of the both lower limbs

Extended Reading

1. Basurab T, Russell-Jones R. HIV-associated eosinophilic folliculitis: case report and review of the literature. Br J Dermatol. 1996;134(3):499–503.
2. Berger TG, Heon V, et al. Itraconazole therapy for human immunodeficiency-virus-associated eosinophilic folliculitis. Arch Dermatol. 1995;131(3):358–60.
3. Blauvelt A, Plott RT. Eosinophilic folliculitis: associated with the acquired immunodeficiency syndrome responds well to permethrin. Arch Dermatol. 1995;131(3):360–1.
4. Cockerell CJ, Bergstressor PR, Myrie Williams C, et al. Bacillary epithelioid angiomatosis occurring in an immunocompetent individual. Arch Dermatol. 1992;126:787–90.
5. Fearfield LA, Rowe A, et al. Itchy folliculitis and human immunodeficiency virus infection: clinicopathological and immunological features, pathogenesis and treatment. Br J Dermatol. 1999;141(1):3–11.
6. Ferrandiz C, Riberia M, et al. Eosinophilic pustular folliculitis in a patients with acquired immunodeficiency syndrome. Int J Dermatol. 1992;31:193–5.
7. Harris DWS, Ostlere L, et al. Eosinophilic pustular folliculitis: in an HIV-positive man response to cetirizine. Int J Dermatol. 1992;126:392–4.
8. Hayes BB, Hille RC, et al. Eosinophilic folliculitis in 2 HIV-positive women. Arch Dermatol. 2004;140(4):463–5.

9. Ho MH, Chong LY, Ho TT. HIV-associated eosinophilic folliculitis in a Chinese woman: a case report and a survey in Hong Kong. Int J STD AIDS. 1998;9:489–93.

10. Misago N, Norisawa Y, et al. HIV-associated eosinophilic pustular folliculitis: successful treatment of a Japanese patient with UVB phototherapy. J Dermatol. 1998;25(3):178–84.

11. Otley CC, Avram MR, et al. Isotretinoin treatment of human immunodeficiency virus-associated eosinophilic folliculitis: results of an open pilot trial. Arch Dermatol. 1995;131(9):1047–50.

12. Rosenthal D, Leboit PF, et al. Human immunodeficiency virus-associated eosinophilic folliculitis. Arch Dermatol. 1991;127:206–9.

13. Smith KJ, Skelton HG. Metronidazole for eosinophilic pustular folliculitis in human immuno-deficiency virus type 1-positive patients. Arch Dermatol. 1995;131(9):1089–91.

14. Soeprono FF, Schinella RA. Eosinophilic pustular folliculitis in patients with acquired immunodeficiency syndrome. J Am Acad Dermatol. 1986;14:1020–2.

15. Stoler MH, Bonfiglio TA, Steigbigel RT, et al. An atypical subcutaneous infection associated with acquired immunodeficiency syndrome [J]. Am J Clin Pathol. 1983;80(5):714–8.

Contents

26.1   MR Functional Imaging in Neurological Diseases

Functional magnetic resonance (MR) imaging is a valuable technique for the analysis and assessment of metabolism and water diffusion from the perspectives of histology, cytology and even molecular biology based on conventional MR technology. It has exhibited a promising application in the diagnosis and differential diagnosis of HIV/AIDS.

Functional magnetic resonance imaging (fMRI) is applied for the research and assessment of human or animals functions by using MRI. Generally, it includes diffusion weighted imaging (DWI), diffusion tensor imaging (DTI), perfusion weighted imaging (PWI), blood oxygenation level dependent (BOLD) fMRI, and magnetic resonance spectroscopy (MRS).

26.1.1   Diffusion Weighted Imaging (DWI)

DWI is a valuable tool for diffusion assessment and imaging by using the characteristic diffusive movements of water molecules. Being different from conventional T1WI and T2WI, DWI enables more microcosmic studies by MRI, which provides information about spatial structure of the human tissues and the functional water molecules exchange between tissue components at different physiological and pathological conditions.

Diffusion is one of the important physical processes in physiological functional activities of the human body, which is also a random motion of molecules, namely the self-diffusion of water molecules (known as Brownian motion). Molecular diffusion of pure water is the same in all directions, namely isotropy. In biological tissues, however, the water diffusion is restricted by various local factors, with manifestation of different diffusion in different directions, namely anisotropy. Anisotropic discrepancy is related to the physical properties of the medium and the obstacles restricting molecular motion. Therefore, anisotropic information

H. Li (ed.), *Radiology of HIV/AIDS*,
DOI 10.1007/978-94-007-7823-8_26, © Springer Science+Business Media Dordrecht and People's Medical Publishing House 2014

about the water molecules diffusion per unit volume can be obtained to demonstrate the subtle anatomical structure and functional changes of organisms.

The principle of DWI is the addition of two equally intense but directionally opposite gradient pulses before and after the 180° pulse of spin-echo T2-weighted sequence. For static water molecules (with low diffusion), the dephasing of the proton spin induced by the first gradient pulse is re-focused by the second gradient pulse, with no attenuation of the signaling. For water molecules in motion, the dephasing of the proton spin induced by the first gradient pulse leaves its original position, which fails to be re-focused by the second gradient pulse, with attenuation of the signaling. The degree of signaling attenuation is dependent on the water molecules diffusing capacity and diffusing sensitivity coefficient at specific temperature and pressure, while the diffusing sensitivity coefficient is determined by the duration and strength of diffusing gradient field. Their relationship can be expressed by the following formula: $SI = exp - bD$, in which D is the diffusing coefficient, a larger D value representing the faster diffusion; and b is the diffusing sensitivity coefficient. The b value can be calculated by $b = \gamma 2G2\delta 2 (\Delta - \delta/3)$, in which γ represents magnetogyric ratio, G strength of the diffusion pulse, δ duration of the diffusion pulse, and Δ the time interval between two pulses. The b value is positively related to the degree of diffusion weight. Concerning DWI, there are many factors influencing the molecular diffusion (such as blood flow/CSF flow and cytomembrane). Therefore, D value is replaced by the diffusion coefficient (ADC) which integrates these factors. ADC chart can be figured out according to different b values, with the following formula: $ADC = (lnS1/lnS2)/(b1 - b2)$. In the formula, S1 and S2 represent two different signal strength of DWI. The signal strength in ADC chart has a positive correlation with the capacity of molecular diffusion. Rapid signal attenuation and high value of ADC indicate rapid molecular diffusion in the tissues, which is demonstrated as low DWI signal but high signal in ADC chart; and vise versa. DWI signal is affected by both T2 value and the diffusion, while ACD chart avoids the effect of T2. Therefore, ADC chart more authentically demonstrates the changes of the diffusion, but is affected by the diffusion sensitive gradient direction.

26.1.2 Diffusion Tensor Imaging (DTI)

DTI is the most recently developed technology of magnetic resonance imaging based on the DWI. It is the only effective and noninvasive examination to observe and track cerebral white matter fiber tracts.

The principle of DTI is that the dispersion of water molecules is isotropic in infinitely homogeneous liquid in vitro. At the physiological conditions of the human body, the three-dimensional diffusion of the water molecules is affected by multiple local factors, including cytomembrane and high molecular substances. Especially in the myelinated nerve fibers, the diffusion rate of the water molecules along the axons is much faster than that in the vertical direction. Such direction highly dependent diffusion is known as anisotropic diffusion. In the brain tissues, the diffusion of the CSF is isotropic and the diffusion of cerebral gray matter is generally anisotropic. However, due to the components of axons with similar directions in the cerebral white matter fiber tracts, the diffusion is therefore highly anisotropic.

Fractional anisotropy (FA) is the most commonly used quantitative anisotropic index, whose magnitude is related to the integrity of myelin sheath, compactness and parallelism of fibers, which varies from 0 (direction independent diffusion) to 1 (unidirectional diffusion). The FA value of the brain white matter association fibers (corpus callosum) is the highest. That is to say, it has the highest degree of anisotropy, which is followed by the brain white matter projecting fibers (internal capsule) and the association fibers (semioval center). When the axons and myelin of white matter fiber bundles are involved by various lesions, the FA value of the involved region decreases in different degrees. The FA value can be represented by vectogram and color coding FA image, and its brightness is positively related to the magnitude of FA value.

Diffusion tensor tractography (DTT) is also known as fiber tractography, which is a noninvasive imaging examination based on the diffusion tensor data for three-dimensional demonstration of cerebral white matter fiber bundles in the living bodies. Due to its capacity in demonstrating the coursing direction and the three-dimensional morphology of the fibers and functional tracts, it facilitates in understanding the normal brain functions and the pathogenesis of the diseases influencing brain functions.

DTI is a most recently developed imaging examination based on the DWI, which is superior to the unidimensional imaging by routine DWI. It quantitatively analyzes the molecular motion by using tensor at the voxel level, with the advantage of three-dimensional quantitative analysis of the water molecules diffusion in the tissues to describe the diffusion directions and the average degree. In addition, it can provide imaging based on the anisotropy of water molecules diffusion in the tissues to demonstrate the minor functional and structural changes of the living tissues. Therefore, the integrity of the white matter as well as the lesions (which interrupt the continuity of the tissues) can be assessed.

26.1.2.1 The Basic Principle of DTI
Definition of DTI

Diffusion is random movement of the liquid molecules, which is known as Brownian motion. At an unconstrained condition, the motion is isotropic. However, in tissues of organisms such as the cerebral white matter, the three-dimensional diffusion of water molecules is affected by multiple extracellular and intracellular factors, such as neuron membrane and wall as well as high molecular materials.

Therefore the motion range of water molecules is direction dependent, namely anisotropy. Tensor is a mathematical structure used to three-dimensionally describe the ellipsoidal features, usually with three spatial coordinates of X, Y and Z. The Z coordinate is the axis across the main magnetic field, whose direction is the main direction of diffusion.

Tensor is generally represented by diffusion coefficient D. But in human body, the D value fails to inclusively represent the diffusion features of the water molecules. Therefore, apparent diffusion coefficient (ADC) is used to indicate the degree of water molecules diffusion. In the cerebral white matter, the factors influencing ADC value include the density of fibers, the degree of myelinization, the average diameter of fibers and the voxel direction similarity. The basic quantitative measurement of the DTI is the three eigenvector values of $\mu1$, $\mu2$ and $\mu3$ as well as eigenvalues of $\lambda1$, $\lambda2$ and $\lambda3$ of the MRI (magnetic resonance imaging) voxel. In each voxel, the main diffusion directions and the diffusion degree in each direction are obtained along the three main coordinate of ellipsoid. Due to the relative strength of the eigenvalue, the anisotropically diffusing voxels form ellipsoid.

DTI is a technology with quantitative anisotropy of water molecules to observe the microstructure of the tissues and to measure the degree and direction of water molecules diffusion. DTI can be applied for quantitative research and fiber tractography (FT). The following indices of measurement serve the quantitative research:

Trace Apparent Diffusion Coefficient (Trace ADC)

ADC value indicates the speed of water molecules diffusion but fails to indicate their anisotropy. The value is the mean of water molecules diffusion in all directions of the tissue. With the ADC value as the imaging signal intensity, the ADC map can be fitted out to directly demonstrate the speed of water molecules diffusion. The faster diffusion speed is demonstrated by the greater ADC value, the stronger ADC imaging signal and the brighter ADC imaging. For instance, the signal of cerebrospinal fluid is high while that of the cerebral white matter is low. The mean ADC value of three mutually perpendicular directions is known as the mean diffusivity (MD), which is direction independent and does not demonstrate the anisotropy of the tissue. Rather, it demonstrates the magnitude of water molecules diffusion in the tissue. The increased MD indicates unrestrained water molecules diffusion in all directions due to myelin defects or loss. The more free water in the tissue indicates the higher diffusion degree. The transverse diffusion coefficient ($\lambda\perp$) is the water molecules activity in the direction perpendicular to axon axis, which provides information specific to myelination changes. The longitudinal diffusion coefficient ($\lambda\parallel$) is water molecules activity in the direction along the axon axis, which is more correlated with the essential characteristics of axons, or indicates extra-axonal or extracellular changes.

Anisotropy

It includes fractional anisotropy (FA) and relative anisotropy (RA). FA is the ratio of fractional anisotropy of the diffusion tensor to the total diffusion tensor, which indicates a small fraction of anisotropic diffusion coefficient. RA is the ratio of diffusion anisotropy to diffusion isotropy. The value of FA represents intensity of water molecules motion in the main vector axis of diffusion. Both FA and RA are non-vectored (values, non-directional), which are zero for the totally isotropic tissue. With the increase of anisotropy, the RA value can be up to $\sqrt{2}$ and the FA can be up to 1. With the FA values as the imaging signalling intensity, the FA image can be fitted out, which directly demonstrates the proportion of anisotropy and indirectly demonstrates the speed of water diffusion in the tissue. In the direction of fiber tract coursing, the diffusion motion is minimally restricted, with the fastest speed, largest FA value, the most intense signalling in the FA image and the brightest image. However, in the direction vertical to the fiber tract coursing (the second and third vectors), the diffusion motions are maximally restricted, with the slowest motion. In FA image, the cerebral white matter is the most highly anisotropic in high signal; while the cerebrospinal fluid is the least anisotropic in low signal. The FA value is an index for assessing the anisotropy and integrity of the cerebral white matter, which decreases in the cases of changed environmental of the microstructure (such as tissue density), defective or lost myelin, and decreased fibers. In the normal brain tissue, the factor with largest impact on the diffusion anisotropy is the arrangement and density of white matter fibers. That is to say, the more regularly dense arrangement of the fibers (the thicker myelin sheath) has the higher degree of anisotropy, with the higher FA value and the brighter FA image. In the normal brain tissues, the FA values are different in different brain tissues. For instance, the FA value of association fibers is the highest, followed by projection fibers and subcortical association fibers.

Volume Ratio (VR)

VR is the ratio of the diffusing ellipsoid volume to the spherical volume with a diameter of 2e, varying from 1 to 0. The VR value of 1 indicates isotropic diffusion. The closer its value is to 0, the higher degree of anisotropy the tissue has. The exponential ADC (EADC) excludes the effect of tissue T2, which, compared to ADC, can more conveniently and more accurately localize and measure the restriction degree of diffusion. Anisotropy index (AI) is equal to $1 - VR$, which increases along with the increase of anisotropy.

Three Eigenvalues of $\lambda1$, $\lambda2$ and $\lambda3$

The three eigenvalues is usually represented with the help of the three diameters of the ellipsoid. The three values demonstrate the diffusion degrees along the longest diameter of the ellipsoid (the longest axis), anteroposterior diameter (the middle axis) and the mediolateral dimension (minimal axis), respectively.

Fiber tractography (FT) refers to a new visualization fiber imaging technology by applying DTI data and specialized software (such as fiber tracking software), which is also known as diffusion tensor tractography (DTT). It can clearly demonstrate the coursing, direction and integrity of fiber bundles, especially the cerebral white matter fiber tracts. Clinically, the combination of FT image with the corresponding trace ADC and FA images is commonly applied to demonstrate and illustrate the fiber images.

Data Collecting

DTI demands high-quality MRI images, namely more complicated magnetic resonance scanner with stable and uniform magnetic field as well as faster and stronger magnetic field gradient to reduce motion artifact, eddy current and heterogeneity of magnetic field. In addition, a mathematical framework is also necessary to convert discrete and rough diffusion tensor data into smooth and macroscopic coursing of the cerebral white matter tracts. Before DTI imaging, the gradient field strength and slew rate should be set. Meanwhile, the imaging planes should be selected according to the region of interest (ROI), in addition to the index settings of section thickness and intervals.

Image Processing

There are mainly four methods to study the cerebral white matter changes by applying DTI technology.

1. The region of interest (ROI) is selected to manually measure the values of anisotropy for comparison with those of the control group. The recent research data of ROI can be applied to demonstrate the cerebral white matter and its functions related structures.

2. Based on the similarities of adjacent voxels in shape and size in the ellipsoid, 2D color tensor images and 3D tracts tensor images can be established for direct visual observation.
   2D color tensor images

   The DTI is sensitive to anisotropic water molecules diffusion, which can construct visualized anatomic structures images based on colored directional encoding of various white matter tracts. According to its definition, the three main vector components of each voxel eigenvector are assigned with three colors, namely red in X coordinate, green in Y coordinate and blue in Z coordinate. That is to say, the rightward and leftward coursing tracts are red, the anterior and posterior coursing tracts are green and the cephalic and caudal coursing tracts are blue. The thickness of the color represents the magnitude of FA value.

   3D tracts tensor images

   3D white matter fiber tracts tensor images can be reconstructed by using computer software. The specific methods mainly include two types: (1) Linear extension algorithm directly utilizes the tensor information within each pixel for extension step by step. (2) Total energy minimization algorithm can explore a passage between

two predetermined pixels with minimal energy loss, including fast marching method and SA (simulate annealing). Fiber assignment using continuous tracking (FACT) technology is to trace local vector information of each pixel and bidirectional (forwards and backwards) linear extension from the seed pixel for reconstruction of the nerve fiber pathway. The extending direction is determined by the main direction of seed pixel eigenvector. The extension is terminated till the FA value of voxel being less than 0.2 or the angle between two connected pixels being above 45°. The algorithm can well demonstrate the complex fiber pathways for more favorable reconstruction of the white matter fiber tracts.

3. Voxel-based morphometry (VBM) is applied to analyze the whole brain. The standard VBM examination is based on the pixel analysis, which requires spatial standardization firstly. That is to say, the brain structure images of an individual should be standardized into a standard three-dimensional space. Subsequently, the standardized brain structure images are effectively segmented to obtain three types images of gray matter, white matter and cerebrospinal fluid. After that, the images to be studied should be smoothed. Finally, 3D pixels statistics can be applied to measure the anisotropy and diffusion changes of the whole brain.

4. Concerning the method of fMRI and DTI images fusion, the fMR imaging provides the fiber tracer seeds to register both fMRI and DTI images into statistical parametric mapping (SPM) system. In the FA image, the white matter ROI directly adjacent to the corresponding activated cortex can be chosen as the seed points for 3D white matter fiber tracts tracer imaging. According to the voxel with most obvious change based on BOLD fMRI signal, three adjacent seed points are selected in both cerebral hemispheres. Such a way of selection is due to the obviously different connectivity patterns resulted from the white matter fibers images originated from adjacent voxels. To harvest different cortical connectivity patterns is in line with the intracerebral cortical complex connectivity. Therefore, the selection of three adjacent seed points can reduce the probability of important connecting path loss resulted from the minor errors in placing the seed points. Meanwhile, after SPM software processing, the three seed points produced connecting fibers can be merged. It also has the advantage that the functional area information provided by fMRI can prevent the large artificial error caused by random selection of the seed points. Especially in cases with intracerebral space occupying lesions, the normal anatomical markers are migrated.

26.1.2.2 Application of DTI in HIV/AIDS Related Dementia

HIV can pass through the blood brain barrier to replicate itself in brain tissue, which evolves into nerve tropic HIV strain to invade the nerve cells. In the cases with direct invasion of HIV-1 to the brain, the neuropathological changes occur to cause continuously progressive loss of intelligence and motion function, namely cognitive and behavioral problems, which is known as AIDS dementia complex (ADC), HIV-1 related dementia complex, HIV encephalopathy or HIV-1 related cognitive/motion syndrome. The manifestation is white matter and subcortical HIV encephalopathy and about 20–90 % HIV infected patients have such lesions, including extensively responsive astrocytosis, blood borne macrophages infiltration, inherent microglia activation and the formation of multinucleated giant cells. Some patients with HAD only have slight pathological changes, such as atrophic lesions in frontal and temporal region. HAD is commonly diagnosed in the advanced stage of AIDS. However, the early diagnosis and accurate diagnosis of HAD is the key to improve the therapeutic efficacy and quality of life of the patients.

Before the application of HAART therapy, the average survival period of HAD patients is 6 months. After the application of HAART therapy, the average survival period of such patients is prolonged seven times as long as those with no HAART therapy. Meanwhile, the newly emerging incidence and mortality of HAD both decrease. Therefore, early detection is critically important for the therapeutic efficacy of HAD. In the developed countries with application of HAART therapy, the incidence of HAD has decreased by about 50 %, compared to that in 1990s. Some studies in China indicated that the period from the diagnosis of HAD to the occurrence of death is averagely 4.17 months, which is shorter than that reported internationally. Moreover, the number of newly emerging cases of HAD increases in some regions. For instance, about 1,300 cases paid their clinic visit to the HIV section, neurology department in Johns Hopkins University during 1994–2000, with a slight increase. In Australia, the incidence of HAD increased from 5.2 % in 1993–1995 to 6.8 % in 1996–2000. HAD remains to be an important public health problem, especially in the developing countries with insufficient supply of antiviral drugs. Therefore, HIV is another main cause of dementia in addition to Alzheimer's disease and vascular dementia worldwide.

Currently, the diagnosis of HAD is based on typical clinical manifestations and exclusion of other causes. Otherwise, its diagnosis can also be made based on neuropsychological behavior test. But it only defines the damage severity of cognitive execution function but fails to detect the pathological state of HAD. It has been documented that 22.4–47.5 % patients with AID sustain clinical symptoms of neurological lesions. However, autopsy revealed that about 87–90 % patients with AIDS have pathological changes of central nervous system. In asymptomatic patients, 5.5–43 % has neuropsychological disturbance. The discrepancy of the incidences is due to the insufficient sensitivity of the diagnostic examination. Recently, neuroimaging technology has gained a rapid development, with advantages in its directness compared to speculations proposed based on neuropsychological behavior test and other assistant examinations, which effectively decreases the testing errors.

The mechanism of nerve cells damage and apoptosis caused by HIV infection remains unknown. Therefore, the studies for its pathogenesis and early diagnosis are necessary but challenging. DTI facilitates our understanding to the pathology and physiology of HAD, which also provides basis for the diagnosis of HAD. In addition, it has special significance in assessing cerebral functions of HIV positive patients. In recent years, some scholars have attempted to assess HAD related white matter lesions by using DTI technology.

A preliminary study using DTI has demonstrated that DTI is particularly sensitive to microstructure of white matter and the microstructural abnormality is related to the severity of the disease. Filippi et al. studied the diffusion and anisotropy in HAD patients by using DTI and the patients have a viral load ranging from undetected to 400,000 [39]. It has been found that with the increase of viral load, the anisotropy of the corpus callosum genu and splenium decreases. In addition, along with the increase of viral load, the patients have increased diffusion of subcortical white matter. However, the viral load cannot be detected in patients receiving HAART therapy and their anisotropy and diffusion are normal. Pomara [86] & Ragin [88], et al. found that the fractional anisotropy is a more sensitive index. In their study, the FA values of the frontal and whole brain significantly decreased compared to the control group.

Y. Wu et al. [117] performed a study by using DTI technology, which has demonstrated that the corpus callosum and frontal white matter have diffusion abnormalities. Their further study for the relationship between the diffusion abnormalities and the severity of cognitive deterioration demonstrated that the FA value of the corpus callosum splenium in patient with HAD significantly decreases compared to the normal control. In addition, the diffusion abnormalities are related to the severity of dementia and the rate of motion functional loss. The MD value also significantly increases, which is related to the rate of motion functional loss. The FA value is also related to the visual and oral memory. The quantitative neuroimaging assessment of the integrity of the corpus callosum is a potentially effective marker for brain lesions in HAD patients. David F. Tate et al.. proposed that most scholars pay their focused attention to the quantitative changes of the DTI indices but ignore the diffusion direction [25]. Their study by fiber tractography found that the tractography indices can provide information about the clinical cognitive ability of patients, suggesting the importance of microstructural changes of the white matter in assessing the cognitive ability.

Adolf Pfefferbaum et al. studied 42 cases of AIDS patients without dementia and 88 age-matched healthy volunteers

[84]. In the study, the researchers measured 11 association fiber tracts and projecting fiber tracts as well as 6 association fiber tracts, with the indices of FA value, apparent diffusion coefficient, horizontal diffusion coefficient and longitudinal diffusion coefficient. The study of frontal striatum fiber tracts in AIDS patients without dementia found higher diffusions (mainly longitudinal) of the posterior corpus callosum, internal and external capsules, and the superior cingulate bundle. Neuroimaging evidence indicates that HIV positive patients without dementia have association fibers and association fiber tracts lesions, which accelerate the progression of HIV infection into AIDS. Otherwise, HAART therapy can alleviate the conditions.

Edith V. Sullivan et al. studied 40 cases of HIV positive patients without dementia and 83 healthy volunteers [100]. All the subjects received quantitative balance experiments, digital symbol test and finger movement speed and flexibility test. The DTI quantitative examination was performed to assess the infratentorial brain area, supratentorial ventricular system, callosum, pontocerebellar tract as well as internal and external capsular motion fiber system. The correlationship between the DTI indices and the results of behavioral tests was analyzed. It has been found that the ratio of infratentorial to the whole brain in HIV positive patients is 3 % less than that of the healthy control. The HIV positive patients have behavioral problems in single foot balance test, digital symbol replacement task. The proportion of their whole infratentorial brain tissues is significantly related to the balance. However, the size of cerebral ventricles and the callosum, as well as the integrity of the internal and external capsular fiber bundle and pontocerebellar tract are not related to the balance ability.

Yasheng Chen et al. studied 8 cases of HAD [24], 21 cases of HIV positive patients without dementia (HND) and 18 healthy volunteers. The region of interest was the white matter of the whole brain, including the frontal, parietal, temporal and occipital white matters, the corpus callosum, and the internal capsule, with measurement indices of FA, MD, transverse diffusion coefficient and longitudinal diffusion coefficient. Compared to the healthy control, all the indices have significant differences from the patients with HND and HAD. The MD and longitudinal coefficient of parietal white matter have significant difference between patients with HAD and HND. Patients with HND and HAD had extensive abnormalities in the brain and the abnormalities of the four DTI indices in HAD patients were more serious. The longitudinal diffusion coefficient based on the voxel analysis is more sensitive to HIV infection than the transverse diffusion coefficient, indicating the demyelination is the primary lesion the white matter.

DTI is a valuable imaging technology in studying the microstructures of living HAD patients, which can provide anatomic details that routine MR imaging fails to demonstrate. With the advantages of histopathological visualization of microstructures and the functional brain imaging, DTI is an effective tool for the brain comprehensibility, noninvasiveness and functions. However, in the related studies, the anatomic ROI and the research methodology are different. Therefore, the results greatly vary. Moreover, due to the heterogeneous magnetic field and the sensitivity to motion artifact of the planar echo sequence, the images are geometrically deformed to a certain degree. Therefore, in neuromorphological studies, the imaging is not so favorable for low noise small white matter fiber tracts and fiber overlapping areas. Currently, the brain diffusion in patients with HAD is still a hot research area internationally. And the current problems can be resolved with the development of MRI device and imaging processing techniques. With the development of DTI research, its application in functional brain diseases is promisingly wider.

26.1.3 Perfusion Weighted Imaging (PWI)

Perfusion refers to the process of delivery of oxygen and nutrients to the tissues and cells when blood flows through the capillary bed. To some extent, it defines the hemodynamic state and functions of tissues or organs. Because the physiological and pathological changes of tissues and organs are closely related to the changes of blood flow perfusion, the changes monitoring can therefore reveal the pathological process of tissues and organs for early diagnosis or early functional assessment.

PWI is a functional imaging, which demonstrates vascular changes and blood flow perfusion, and provides hemodynamic information of the tissues and organs by using rapid magnetic resonance imaging sequence and image processing techniques. Currently, the procedures include intravenous injection of the contrast reagent for rapid imaging sequence. Specifically, intravenous bolus injection of contrast reagent gadolinium is performed for a high concentration of gadolinium to flow through the examined area in a short period of time. During this period, the rapid imaging technology such as EPI is used to scan the examined area to harvest the images when the contrast reagent initially passes through the vascular bed of the ROI. Because gadolinium has impact on the magnetic susceptibility of local tissue, it therefore increases the heterogeneity of local magnetic field and obviously shortens the T1 and T2 relaxation times. It has greater impact on the T2 relaxation time, which is demonstrated by more obviously shortened T2 relaxation time and decreased signaling. The degree of signaling decrease is positively related to the local reagent concentration. Therefore, it demonstrates the blood perfusion capacity of local tissue. The indices demonstrating blood flow distribution in the capillary bed include: (1) capacity indices, such as regional cerebral blood volume (rCBV); (2) speed indices, such as mean transition time (MTT) and local perfusion time to peak (TTP); (3) flow volume indices, such as regional cerebral blood flow (rCBF). Based on the signaling decrease of local tissue along with time, a signal intensity-time curve can be obtained, as well as a concentration of the contrast reagent-time curve. The area under the curve demonstrates the blood capacity of the cerebral tissue, namely rCBV. The processing of regional rCBV through the working station can show its corresponding greyness or color, namely rCBV image. In the same ways, rCBF image of the contrast reagent, MTT image and TTP imaging can also be obtained.

26.1.4   Blood Oxygenation Level Dependent fMR Imaging (fMRI-BOLD)

Functional magnetic resonance imaging (fMRI) has been widely applied in scientific research of the brain and clinical practice due to its noninvasive and radiation-free as well as effective demonstration of anatomic structures and their functions since it was proposed in 1990s. It plays an important role in neuroscience research, which has been proved to be a powerful tool in demonstrating motions, visual sense, auditory sense and the rest state as well as functional brain network.

BLOD-fMRI is a noninvasive examination of the brain function, which is based on the difference of oxyhemoglobin and deoxygenated hemoglobin. It demonstrates the functional activities of certain brain area in real time with high time and spatial resolutions, which facilitates the understanding of brain activities more objectively, accurately and directly. Due to its advantages, BLOD-fMRI has been widely applied in modern scientific research, such as neuroscience, cognitive and psychological sciences. And some breakthroughs have been achieved. The principle is that neurons in some brain areas are activated when the area is executing certain tasks or is stimulated. The results are increased blood flow volume and blood flow capacity of the adjacent venous blood and capillary bed, which further leads to increased content of local oxyhemoglobin and no marked increase of oxygen consumption. Therefore, the balance between oxygen supply and oxygen consumption is interrupted, with subsequent decrease of deoxygenated hemoglobin in this area. Deoxygenated hemoglobin is a paramagnetic substance. MRI is sensitive to changes of the magnetic field, which can detect the brain activated functional area by specific rapid imaging sequence and data processing method and has obvious T2 shortening effects. Therefore, in the activated state, the decreased deoxygenated hemoglobin in the brain area causes relatively prolonged relaxation time and increased intensity of MR signal, which is demonstrated as high signal by brain functional MR imaging. Generally, deoxygenated hemoglobin plays a role of endogenous contrast agent in BLOD-fMRI.

When HIV invades the central nervous system, the virus can be firstly found in the microgliacytes and phagocytes. Its infection of the neurons fails to directly induce the death of HIV related neurons. However, the mechanism of HIV related brain lesions is not fully elucidated. Multiple HIV related diseases can affect the brain functions. The knowledge of these abnormal manifestations and the imaging features of the brain lesions is important for the early diagnosis and therapeutic planning. The diagnostic imaging examinations including CT and PET are performed for patients in resting state. However, fMRI can demonstrate the functional activated brain area during tasks or after stimulations. In addition, it can detect early changes caused by HIV infection, such as minor cognitive motor disorder (MCMD) and HIV associated dementia (HAD).

HIV positive patients with common neurological functional impairments usually have cognitive, behavioral and motion difficulties, whose severity varies with the progression of the conditions. MCMD is believed to participate the functional degeneration of certain nerve cells while cell death occurs in the HAD stage. HAD has difficulties in attention, memory, learning, problem solving and social activities, with manifestations of emotional apathy and fatigue.

Currently, functional imaging studies in HIV positive patients are rarely conducted by using fMRI. The researchers selected different experimental tasks to assess the early central nervous system lesions in HIV positive patients. The experimental tasks include working memory test such as zero-back, one-back and two-back, attention and mathematic calculation assessment as well as respond speed test. When the subjects executed simple reaction task and work memory test, bilateral lateral prefrontal cortex (LPFC), posterior parietal cortex (PPC) and caudate nuclei were all activated. Compared to the controls, complex tasks usually induce activated supplementary motor cortex (SMA) such as in the two-back test. In addition, compared to the controls, greater activation was found in the left and middle parietal lobe when HIV positive patients executed simple reaction task and one-back task. However, the activation significantly increased in frontal area including LPEC and SMA when they executed complex tasks such as mathematic calculation and two-back tasks. The brain activated areas are characterized by: (1) adjacent to the activation areas of healthy control; different activation range between HIV positive patients and healthy controls. During the process of BOLD-fMRI, with the increased difficulty of the task, HIV positive patients showed prolonged reaction time and decreased reaction accuracy, which also occurred in the healthy controls.

The activation in HIV positive patients demonstrates that the neural activities are saturated in the normal activation area and the execution of the tasks needs functional assistance by peripheral nerve materials, indicating the existence of reserve system in the nerve network. In different tasks, the nerve pathways play their role for such assistance. HIV infection plays a destructive role to the brain nerve materials, which may have impact on the brain nerve pathways. Therefore, when HIV positive patients execute simple tasks, large amount of energy reserve is consumed, with a small proportion of residual energy for executing more complex tasks.

BLOD-fMR imaging is a new research tool for early brain lesions of HIV positive patients. In the future studies, its use in combination with magnetic resonance spectroscopy (MRS), diffusion weighted imaging (DWI) and MR perfusion imaging (PWI) for the diagnosis provides new insights for the assessment of brain functions in patients with HIV/AIDS.

26.1.5 Magnetic Resonance Spectroscopy (MRS)

MR spectroscopy (MRS) is the only noninvasive examination for histochemical features of living body. In many diseases, metabolic changes occur prior to pathomorphological changes. MRS has a highly potential sensitivity to the metabolic changes for early diagnosis of these diseases. MRS demonstrates physiopathological changes of cell metabolism in human body, while routine MRI demonstrates physiopathological changes of the organs and tissues gross morphology. However, both are physically based on the magnetic resonance. MRS is an examination for quantitative analysis of specific atomic nucleus and their compounds, which utilizes the magnetic resonance and chemical migration and is the only non-invasive examination to quantitatively analyze metabolism and biochemical changes of the living tissues and organs. It is virtually molecular imaging. Based on chemical migration, it explores the frequency discrepancies of different substances, with the results represented with ppm. Currently, the atom nucleus applied in medical spectrum studies includes 1H, 31P, 13C and 19F. Especially, 1H and 31P are the most widely used in medical sciences. Currently, as the only non-invasive examination for metabolic and biochemical changes of the living tissues and organs, it quantitatively analyzes specific atomic nucleus and their compounds and has been widely used in clinical and basic studies of neoplasms, ischemic cerebral stroke, cerebral hemorrhage, senile dementia, neonatal intensive care, prognosis of brain trauma, white matter lesions, infectious diseases and AIDS. The commonly applied procedures now is single voxel PRESS 1HMRS, which has convenient and simple manipulation. However, its disadvantage firstly is compulsory appropriate area setting of single voxel and one-dimensional data that fails to provide spatial distribution of the metabolic abnormalities. Moreover, the correct voxel localization has to be based on the understanding of the lesions position in advance, which restricts its application. The recently developed two-dimensional or M-dimensional MRS technologies are targeting on these disadvantages. Chemical migration imaging for one time can be applied for multiple voxel MRS for two-dimensional or three-dimensional data. After computer processing of these data, metabolic images can be obtained. These images can be registered with routine MR T1 or T2 images for favorable background contrast, therefore a more direct view for the examination and diagnosis.

26.1.5.1 The Basic Principal of MRS

Two factors determine the resonance frequency of magnetic resonance signal. The first factor is the gyromagnetic ratio that indicates the inherent property of the atoms. And the other factor is magnetic intensity at the place of the nucleus. The magnetic field of nucleus is determined by the external main magnetic field B_0 while the magnetic intensity of the nucleus is related to the extranuclear electron cloud and adjacent atomic cloud. The electron cloud can shield the effect of the main magnetic field to cause weaker magnetic intensity of the nucleus than external main magnetic field. This magnetic field discrepancy caused by electron cloud is known as the chemical migration. Therefore, in certain external magnetic field, different nucleus is in different chemical environment to cause minor difference in resonance frequency and different peak of magnetic resonance spectrum. As a result, different metabolites and their concentrations can be recognized. By MRS, the concentrations of many important compounds can be detected, based on which the changes of tissue metabolism can be analyzed. By 1H-MRS, the resonance peak of 12 brain metabolites and neurotransmitters can be determined, including NAA, Cr, PCr, Cho, Mi, Gln, Glu and Lac. Many biomolecules contain 31P, which participates in cellular energy metabolism of cells and biomembrane related phospholipids metabolism. 31-PMRS has been widely used in analysis of brain tissues energy metabolism and acid–base balance to measure the contents of PCr, PI α-ATP, β-ATP and γ-ATP, as well as the intracellular pH value.

26.1.5.2 Clinical Application of MRS
MRS Changes of Normal Human Brain
The MR spectrum changes of normal human brain can demonstrate the growth and differentiation of the neurons, brain energy metabolism and the myelin sheath disintegration. NAA is commonly found in mammalian nervous system, almost all of which can be found in the nerve pairs. Currently, NAA is believed to be an internal marker of the neuron functions. In healthy people, the ratio of NAA/Cr is high and the decrease of NAA indicates absence or destruction of the neurons. Both Cho and Cr can be found in neurons and gliocytes. However, cell studies have demonstrated that the contents of Cho and Cr in oligodendrocytes and astrocytes are obviously higher than those in neurons. Therefore, the increases of Cho and Cr suggest the occurrence of gliosis. The decrease of NAA or increases of Cho and Cr results in the decrease of NAA/(Cho + Cr) which is often used as the indicator of the neuron function. In addition, 1H-MAS has demonstrated that NAA increases twice as high as that at birth within one year, with corresponding increase of the creatine signal. Along with the age, NAA/Cr and Glu-n/Cr increase and MI/Cr decreases. 31P-MRS has demonstrated that along with the age, the PME signal weakens compared to other metabolites and the creatine phosphate increases. These findings indicate that by quantitative analysis of the brain tissue metabolites by MRS, the development and maturity of the brain tissue can be understood. In addition, these findings also indicate that age related changes should be aware of during observation of pathological spectrum.

MRS of Epilepsy

1H-MRS has demonstrated that lateral to the epilepsy lesion and adjacent to the middle temporal lobe, the NAA peak value decreases by 22 %, with increases of Cho and Cr values by 25 and 15 % respectively. The decrease of NAA indicates the absence, defect or dysfunction of neurons in the lesion. The increases of Cho and Cr suggest gliocyte proliferation. The previous studies tend to use NAA/(Cho+Cr) as the marker of lateralization and abnormality. In healthy people, the bottom value of NAA/(Cho+Cr) is 0.72. The two-side discrepancy being above 0.05 or significant two-sided decreases than those in healthy people can be defined as abnormality. The decreased ratio indicates hippocampal sclerosis. The lateralization sensitivity of NAA/(Cho+Cr) is 87 % and the accuracy, 96 %. In addition, 1H-MAS can be also applied to determine epilepsy activity related neurotransmitters, including r-aminobutyric acid (GABA), glutamic acid (Gln), and hydrochloric acid of glutamic (Glu).

MRS of Brain Neoplasms

1H-MAS is an effective way to study brain neoplasm materials and energy metabolism, which contributes to the diagnosis and differential diagnosis of brain neoplasms. It can provide information about the histological grading as well as assessment for recurrence and therapeutic efficacy. The 1H-MAS demonstrates differences between tumor tissues and the normal brain tissues. The increase of Cho value indicates increased membrane metabolism and the decrease of NAA peak value indicates the migration of neurons due to compression. 1H-MAS demonstrates meningiomas and brain metastatic tumors as deficient NAA signal and decreased creatine peak value. In addition, 1H-MAS demonstrates meningioma as abnormal alanine signal. In the cases of brain metastatic tumor, the characteristic finding is the paired resonance peak, which is the occurrence of lipid fluidity. In the cases of low-grade malignant glioma, the creatine signal peak is almost the same as the normal brain tissue. However, the Cho signal peak doubles, with small NAA signal in the tumor, which is in consistency with the invasive growth of glioma. These findings demonstrate that a small amount neurons remains in the tumor. In about 50 % cases of glioma, lactate signal can be found. The highly malignant part is demonstrated to have significantly decreased or even absent NAA and Cr peak values. Some other demonstrations are similar to those of low grade malignant glioma. The difference is due to the heterogeneity of glioma structure, namely the proportional difference of parenchymal and necrotic components. The necrotic lesions are demonstrated as decreased Cho peak value and increased lactate peak value. The increased lactate peak value indicates poor prognosis, which plays an important role in radiotherapeutic planning.

MRS of Cerebral Ischemia and Infarction

The demonstrations include decreased NAA signal peak value and decreased Cho peak value. The decrease of the Cho peak value is different from the demonstration of encephaloma. In the cases of cerebral ischemia and infarction, the decrease of NAA is obviously larger than the decrease of total Cr and Cho values. The brain ischemia lesions caused by neonatal hypoxia have demonstrations of obviously decreased NAA peak value of the basal ganglia, and different strength of lactate signal. The higher signalling indicates more serious hypoxia.

MRS of Alzheimer's Disease

The decrease of NAA can sensitively and accurately demonstrate demyelination of neurons in the cases of Alzheimer's disease. Previous studies have shown that patients with AD have obviously decreased NAA level but increased MI level. Their levels in the white matter are closely related to the severity and duration of dementia. The ratio of NAA/MI can be used to differentiate AD from normal brain.

MRS of Other Conditions

In addition to the above mentioned clinical applications, MRS plays important roles in the diagnosis of brain metabolic diseases and white matter demyelinating disease, as well as in assessing the prognosis of multiple sclerosis, traumatic brain injury. For instances, children with non-ketone glycine hyperlipidemia have excessive glycine signal by 1H-MAS. Patients with Canavan's disease have specific increase of NAA signal. In the acute plaque period of demyelinating diseases, the concentration of choline chemical compound is t by 1H-MAS, but decreased NAA concentration when the conditions are stable. These findings indicate that 1H-MRA can be used to monitor the clinical changes of the acute phase, chronic phase and advanced plaque phase. In recent years, many scientific studies have paid focused attention on the specific peak values of demyelinating diseases. From the perspectives of monitoring and therapeutic efficacy, the data is valuable.

26.1.5.3 1H-MRS Resonance Peak of Human Brain Metabolites and its Clinical Significance

NAA

The main peak is located at 2.02 ppm and is the highest in normal MRS. NAA are mainly located in the neuron and its axon, which is believed to be the internal marker of the neuron. Many brain diseases including inflammations, infections, neoplasms, dementia and gliosis can cause neuron dysfunction and therefore decreased NAA. By MRS, decreased NAA is rarely found which can only be found in cases of Canavan's disease.

Choline

The resonance peak is located at 3.22 ppm. Cho includes choline phosphate, phosphatidylcholine and glycerophosphate choline, which is the marker of membrane flip. Its content in the white matter is higher than that in the gray matter.

The increased Cho indicates increased cellular membrane synthesis or increased cell count, which is the demonstration of wound repair, neoplasms, gliosis and demyelination. The decreased Cho indicates cell density decline,, which is the demonstration of dementia, cerebral stroke and AIDS.

Creatine/Creatine Phosphate (Cr)

The resonance peak is located at 3.0 and 3.94 ppm. In the normal brain MRS, it is the second or third highest peak. Cr is an important compound for energy use and storage, which is a marker of cellular energy state. In infants, its level is low, which increased with age. It pathological increase can be found in the cases of trauma, hyperosmolar state, while its pathological decrease can be found in the cases of hypoxia, stroke and neoplasms.

Lactate (Lac)

The resonance peak is located at 1.33–1.35 ppm, which is double peaks and is absent in normal brain tissue. Lac is a glycolytic terminal product, whose occurrence indicates terminated effective aerobic respiration. In the cases with occurrence of long TE from short TE, the Lac peak can be reverse. The Lac peak occurs in the cases of brain neoplasms, abscesses, cysts and infarction.

Muscular Inositol (mI)

The resonance peak is located at 3.56 and 4.06 ppm. mI plays roles in adjusting osmotic pressure, nourishing cells, anti-oxidation and generating surfactants. It is the marker of neuroglia, and its increase is believed to be a sign of gliosis.

Glutamine and Glutamic Acid Complex (Glx)

The resonance peak is located at 2.2–2.4 ppm ($\beta+\gamma$ peak), 3.6–3.8 ppm (α peak). Glx has effects of activating toxicity and increases in the cases of brain tissue ischemia and hypoxia as well as hepatic encephalopathy.

Lipids (Lip)

The resonance peak is located at 1.33–1.35 ppm, which is absent in normal brain tissue. Its increase can be found in the cases of high-grade tumor, abscess, acute inflammation and acute stroke.

26.1.6 Clinical Application of Functional MR Imaging

Functional MR integrates the nerve activities with high resolution magnetic resonance imaging, which is a only non-invasive examination to accurately position the human brain functions. It not only provides basis for the diagnosis of the diseases, but also facilitates our understanding to the pathophysiology of some diseases, such as HIV associate dementia.

1. HIV encephalitis (HIV associated dementia)

HIV virus is neurotropic and the central nervous system and peripheral nervous system are susceptible to its invasion. About 37–75 % of HIV infected patients develop HIV encephalitis. In some serious cases, dementia occurs. MRS demonstrates decreased NAA peak and increased Cho peak in the lesions. DWI demonstrates significantly decreased FA value and significantly increased ADC value of the cerebral white matter.

2. Opportunistic infections

CMV encephalitis is the most common opportunistic infection in HIV positive patients. Its infection rate at the terminal stage of AIDS is up to 40 %.

Toxoplasma encephalitis is the most common opportunistic infection of the central nervous system of AIDS patients, commonly leading to abscess and granuloma. The typical demonstrations by DWI include even high signal and low ADC value. The MRS demonstrates decreased NAA, Cr, Cho and mI peak values in the lesions, and decreased ratios of NAA/Cr, NAA/Cho.

Cryptococcus neoformans meningoencephalitis is caused by invasion of Cryptococcus neoformans via the respiratory tract and along with blood flow to meninges and brain parenchyma. It the most common fungal infection of the central nervous system in AIDS patients, which commonly occurs in the advanced stage of AIDS.

Herpes simplex encephalitis is relatively rare. It is commonly caused by reactivated Herpes simplex virus spreading to the brain due to compromised immunity.

3. Glioma

It is the most common primary intracranial tumor. AIDS complicated by glioma is rarely found. MRS, DWI and DTI can facilitate its diagnosis and differential diagnosis, which provide information about the histological grading, postoperative recurrence and therapeutic efficacy.

26.1.6.1 HIV Encephalitis

HIV encephalitis is also known as AIDS encephalopathy, HIV associated dementia (HAD) and AIDS dementia complex (ADC). It is the most common and serious neurological complication in AIDS patients. HIV fails to directly infect the neurons, but can infect macrophages and microglia in the brain tissues. These cells produce the inflammatory responses and release post-inflammatory cytokines and free radicals to impair the cerebral neurons, namely HIV encephalitis. And in some serious cases, dementia occurs. Gliocytes in the human brain is 10 times as many as the neurons and thus the impairment has a cascade effect.

In the early stage of HIV encephalitis, no obvious morphological changes of the brain can be found. With its development, varying degrees of brain atrophy occurs, with manifestations of local brain atrophy that is more obvious in the frontal and temporal lobes. In the advanced stage, the cerebral ventricles expand, with obvious brain tissues atrophy and brain weight loss. HIV encephalitis commonly involves the white matter or/and deep nuclei. The pathological changes include brain parenchymal and perivascular infiltration of lymphocytes and macrophage. There is also reactive proliferation of the astrocytes, as well as the formation of glial nodules by microglia, astrocytes and macrophages. The lesions of HIV encephalitis are generally in size of 0.2–2.0 cm, which distribute under the white matter and cerebral cortex and mainly symmetrical periventricular and semi-oval central white matter. The white matter lesions often extend to the subcortical area and the extensive lesions may involve the basal ganglia, cerebellum and brainstem.

HIV encephalitis is clinically characterized by cognitive impairment, decreased motion ability and behavioral changes. The diagnosis is based on the clinical symptoms as well as exclusion of other diseases that are not related to HIV infection.

The typical CT scanning demonstrations include bilaterally symmetric/asymmetric cerebral white matter lesions. In some rare cases, the lesions are unilaterally found. By plain CT scanning, the lesions are in low density. In the advanced stage, the lesions fuse together to form large flakes of low density lesions, with no space occupying effect. By enhanced scanning, no enhancement can be found. The lesions are commonly found in the periventricular white matter, semioval center, frontal and parietal lobes, and even subcortical area. Meanwhile, accompanying cerebral atrophy occurs. By MR imaging, diffuse cerebral white matter lesions can be demonstrated, with slightly low T1WI signal, high T2WI signal and no space occupying lesions. By enhanced imaging, no enhancement can be found.

In the period of no neurological symptoms of HIV infection and negative findings by conventional MRI, MRS can detect early abnormalities of brain metabolism. It can also be used to assess the involvement of the central nervous system. For HIV infected patients with no neurological symptoms, there are significantly decreased ratios of NAA/Cr and NAA/Cho in bilateral semioval center and thalamus, no significant change of Cho/Cr and mI/Cr ratios, more obvious change of NAA/Cr ratio in the white matter than in the gray matter and more obvious decrease of mI/Cr ratio in the gray matter. In addition, Cho/Cr ratio decreases less in the white matter than in the gray matter. The ratios of mI/Cr and Cho/Cr increase in bilateral basal ganglia. The NAA/Cr ratio decreases in the white matter of the frontal lobe, but Cho/Cr ratio increases. The mI/Cr ratio significantly changes in the basal ganglia, while NAA/Cr ratio decreases more in the white matter. For HIV infected patients with neurological symptoms, the NAA peak value and NAA/Cr ratio decrease, but the Cho and mI peak values increase. Lip and Lac peak values commonly increase. In the following ups after the treatment, some patients showed gradual decreased of the NAA/Cr ratio, but in some other patients, the ratio increases. In HDC patients, NAA/Cr and NAA/Cho ratios decrease in the frontal cortex, with increased mI/Cr and Cho/Cr ratios. mI/Cr ratio in the white matter increases. NAA/Cr ratio decreases in parietal cortex, with increased Cho/Cr and mI/Cr ratios. NAA/Cr ratio decreases in bilateral basal ganglia, with significantly increased NAA/Cr, Cho/Cr and mI/Cr ratios. mI/Cr and Cho/Cr ratios increase in the semioval center and the NAA value

drops in hypothalamus. For children, the Cho/Cr ratio increases in the frontal gray matter, frontal white matter and the left parietal white matter.

For HIV positive patients without dementia, quantitative fiber tracer demonstrates increased diffusion coefficient in the posterior corpus callosum, internal capsule, external capsule and the superior cingulum and increased longitudinal diffusion coefficient (an index for axonal defect) in the posterior corpus callosum, fornix and superior cingulum. In untreated patients, the transverse diffusion coefficient (an index for myelin lesions) increases in the major forceps, inferior cingulum and superior longitudinal fasciculus. In patients with cognitive impairments, the FA values of multiple areas white matter significantly decrease, with significantly increased ADC values. Meanwhile, the MD values of the corona radiata, optic radiation, posterior limb of the internal capsule as well as the genu and splenium of the corpus callosum increase. Studies have shown that the FA value of the whole brain of HIV positive patients decreases, which is related to the severity of dementia. It has also been demonstrated that the ADC value of the whole brain is related to psychomotor dysfunctions.

PWI demonstrates that the rCBV of deep gray matter and cortical gray matter increases in HIV positive patients, indicating subcortical inflammatory responses. The rCBF values in bilateral frontal inferior lateral cortex and unilateral parietal inferior medial area decrease in early HAD patients. The white matter perfusion increases in the bilateral parietal inferior posterior area. The increased parietal white matter perfusion may be related to the reactive inflammatory responses or proliferative responses of the neuroglia, which may cause the increase of blood flow velocity. The abnormity of rCBF is related to the CD4 T cell count, the viral load and the severity of HIV dementia. Specifically, the lower rCBF value indicates more serious HIV encephalopathy.

Chang et al. studied the working memory performance of the patients [5]. The finding indicates indicate that the lateral frontal cortex, posterior parietal cortex and the accessional motion area are activated. In patients with serum negative findings, the total activated volume and the brain activated areas in BOLD images increased when they performed more difficult tasks. The brain activation and the difficulty of the tasks or attentional load may demonstrate the regulatory effect of the attention by the neural circuits. However, HIV positive patients showed increased total activation area when performing simple tasks, with locally increased activation. But these increases were absent whey they performed difficult tasks, which indicated that HIV positive patients require stronger stimulation (such as increase of attentional regulation) to the neural circuits to perform the simple tasks, which plays an role in compensating decreased neural processing efficacy due to brain lesions. In contrast, in healthy people or HIV positive patients, the activation volume is saturated when they perform more difficult tasks, indicating exhausted neural network resources. Therefore, the increased activation volume in HIV positive patients is most likely to be directly related to the attention.

Case Study

A female patient aged 48 years was confirmatively diagnosed as having AIDS by the CDC. She had diarrhea, vomiting and occasional epilepsy seizures since May 2011. Her CD4 T cell count was 95/μl.

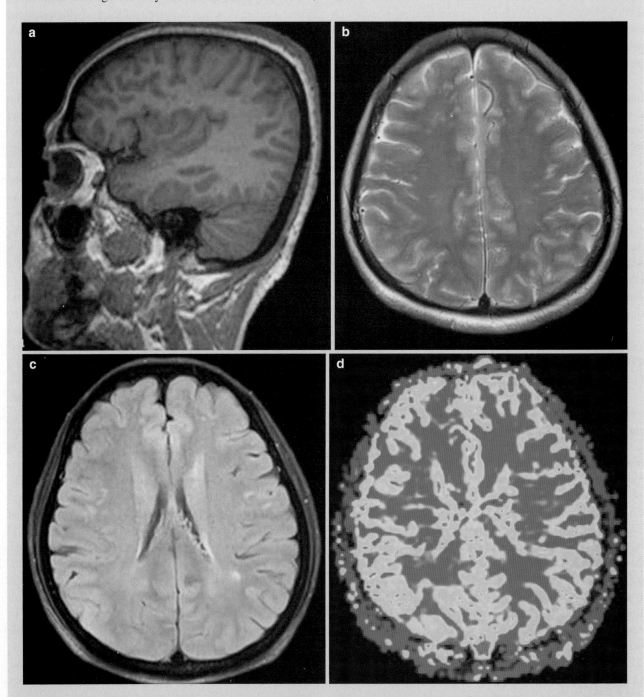

Fig. 26.1 (**a-i**) HIV/AIDS related HIV encephalitis. (**a-b**) MR imaging demonstrates multiple spots long T1 and long T2 signal in the subcortical white matters in bilateral frontal and parietal lobes, with unclear boundaries, that is more obvious in the bilateral frontal lobes. (**c**) Fat and water suppression T2WI demonstrates high signal. (**d**) Perfusion imaging demonstrates bilaterally symmetric CBF. (**e**) DTI demonstrates strips of decreased signal areas in the bilateral frontal and parietal lobes and decreased FA values. (**f-g**) 3D white matter fiber tracts tracer imaging demonstrates sparse fiber tracts in the left frontal and parietal lobes than the contralateral. (**h-i**) MRS demonstrates obviously decreased NAA/Cr in the white matter of the left frontal and parietal lobes

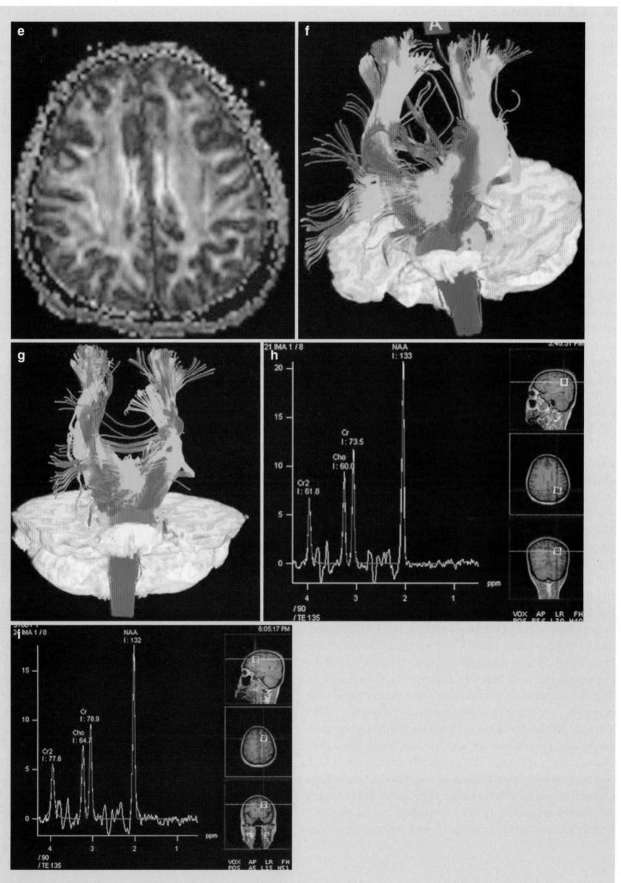

Fig. 26.1 (continued)

26.1.6.2 Toxoplasmosis Encephalitis

Toxoplasmosis encephalitis is a common complication of the central nervous system of AIDS patients, with an incidence of about 10–30 %. It is also a common cause of death in AIDS patients. Toxoplasma widely infests parasites in the healthy population, with no specific selectivity to the parasitized tissues. All nucleated cells except erythrocytes in the human body can be parasitized by toxoplasmas. Toxoplasmosis encephalitis in AIDS patients is commonly a result of activated latent infection. The toxoplasmas incubating in the cysts escape or cysts rupture to cause acute necrosis of the brain tissue. In combination with the participation of delayed hypersensitivity, glial nodules are formed in local brain tissue. The pathological manifestations include different degrees of coagulation necrosis and granulomatous inflammation, yellowish necrotic malacia, later calcification as well as edema and space occupying lesions. Clinically, the manifestations include low grade fever, headache and nervous system positioning symptoms in over 90 % cases. In some serious cases, death occurs. The findings of free or intracellular trophozoites in tissues, body fluids or nucleated cells can define the diagnosis.

Toxoplasmosis encephalitis commonly occurs in the basal ganglia (70–75 %), with multiple lesions and possible involvement of the cerebellum, brainstem and the interface of cortex and medulla. The diameters of the lesions are about 4.0–5.0 cm. The imaging demonstrations are characterized by bilateral multiple lesions but rare unilateral lesions. CT scanning demonstrates low density lesions with accompanying perifocal edema and space occupying effect. MR imaging demonstrations are different in different stages of the disease. In the stage of necrotic abscesses, high T2WI signal is found. In the stage of organic abscesses, equal T2WI signal is found. Generally, T1WI is in equal or slightly low signals. Enhanced CT scanning or MR imaging demonstrates obvious enhancement of the lesions, with even enhancement of the small nodules and spiral shaped, ring shaped or mass shaped uneven enhancement of the large lesions. The asymmetric and uneven target sign of the lesions enhancement indicates collapse of the abscess wall. The enhancement of lesions adjacent to the ependyma has diagnostic significance. After treatment, the high T2WI signal of the lesions is transformed into equal signal, indicating the progression of necrotic abscesses stage into organic abscesses stage. DWI typically demonstrates high signal, with pathological basis of coagulation hemorrhage and necrosis of local brain tissue. In the necrosis area, there are mainly inflammatory cells, toxoplasmas and proteins. Protein has a strong absorption to water molecules and thus to cause restricted water molecules diffusion. As a result, DWI demonstrates even high signal, with a low ADC value. MRS demonstrates decreased NAA, Cr, Cho and mI peak values, significantly decreased NAA/Cr and NAA/Cr ratios, lower NAA/Cr ratio in the acute stage than in the remission stage, increased Cho/Cr ratio, and obvious occurrence of Lip peak or its concurrence with Lac peak. After anti-toxoplasm treatment, NAA/Cr ratio returns to normal, but in some patients Cho/Cr ratio may decrease or continuously increase. PWI demonstrates decreased rCBV of toxoplasmosis encephalitis lesions, which may be caused by insufficient blood vessels in the lesions.

HIV/AIDS complicated by toxoplasmosis encephalitis should be differentiated from primary CNS lymphoma. Primary CNS lymphoma is commonly singular, with slighter peritumor edema than toxoplasmosis encephalitis but more obvious space occupying effect. It commonly invades the ependyma and corpus callosum. Enhanced scanning demonstrates map liked or sawteeth liked enhancement of the lesions. It shows no responses to anti-toxoplasmosis therapy but is sensitive to radiation therapy. DWI facilitates their differential diagnosis. For the cases with an ADC ratio (ADC value of lesion ROI to ADC value of contralateral ROI of normal brain tissue) being above 1.6, the diagnosis of toxoplasma infection should be considered. For the cases with the ADC ratio being lower than 1.0, the diagnosis of lymphoma should be considered. For the cases with the ADC ratio between 1.0 and 1.6, large overlapping of both diseases occurs. Therefore, for the cases of difficulty diagnosing, directed biopsy should be performed for the differential diagnosis. In addition, HIV/AIDS complicated by toxoplasmosis encephalitis should also be differentiated from tuberculosis meningitis. The localization of the lesions facilitates the differential diagnosis. The lesions of toxoplasmosis encephalitis are commonly found in the basal ganglia, while the lesions of tuberculosis meningitis are commonly found adjacent to the brain surface. The difference of the lesions location is possibly related to the infection route of the pathogens. Both toxoplasmas and TB can spread along with blood flow to seriously damage the blood brain barrier via multiple routes, especially the supplying area by the medullary branches of the middle cerebral artery. Deep brain is firstly infected by toxoplasmas, while meninges are firstly infected by tubercle bacilli, which may be related to the distribution of the lesions. The lesions of toxoplasma encephalitis are distributed in the nerve nuclei of the deep brain and the periventricular white matter, while the lesions of TB encephalitis are distributed in the brain surface, the cerebral cortex and the transitional area of the cortex and medulla.

Case Study

A male patient aged 34 years was confirmatively diagnosed as having AIDS by the CDC. He had no obvious symptoms, decreased coordination function and memory loss. His CD4 T cell count was 186/μl.

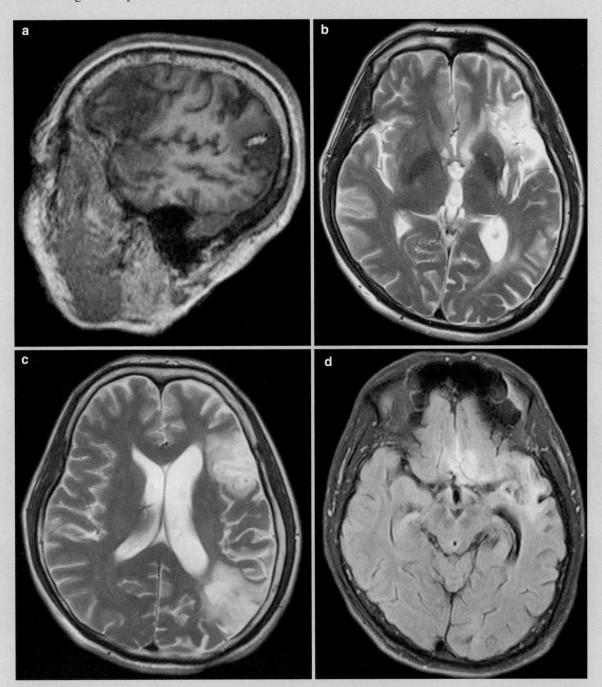

Fig. 26.2 (**a–m**) HIV/AIDS related toxoplasma encephalopathy, cytomegalovirus infection, TB meningitis, herpes meningitis sequela. (**a–c**) MRI demonstrates mass liked and cloudy long T1 and long T2 signals in the gray matter of the left frontal lobe, temporal lobe, frontal-temporal interface and parietal-occipital interface, with involvement of the white matter. The signals are uneven, and some signals are cerebrospinal fluid signal shadows. There are also widened cerebral fissure. (**d, e**) Tirm demonstrates high signals. (**f**) DWI demonstrates high signals. (**g**) Enhanced imaging with Gd-BOPTA demonstrates small mass liked enhancement of the lesion area in the left frontal lobe and occipital lobe. (**h**) Perfusion imaging demonstrates lower CBF of the lesion area than the contralateral part in the left frontal lobe and occipital lobe. (**i**) DTI demonstrates weakened signal of the white matter in the left frontal lobe, temporal lobe, frontal-temporal interface and parietal-occipital interface, with obviously decreased FA value. (**j, k**) 3D white matter fiber tracts tracer imaging demonstrates sparser transverse fiber tracts in the left frontal, temporal and occipital lobes than the contralateral areas. (**l**) MRS demonstrates decreased NAA/Cr ratio being 1.23 in the lesion area. (**m**) Simple movement test of the right hand demonstrates smaller range and amplitude of the motion activated areas of the left pre- and post-central gyri than those in healthy people

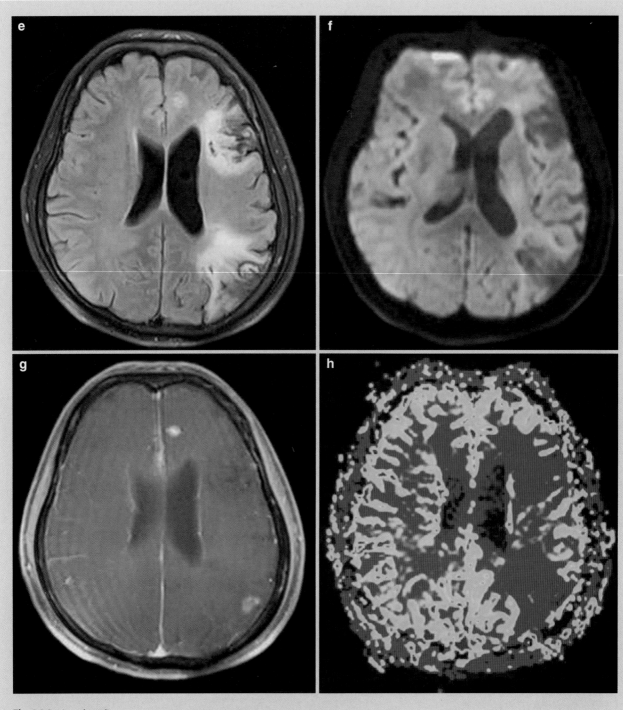

Fig. 26.2 (continued)

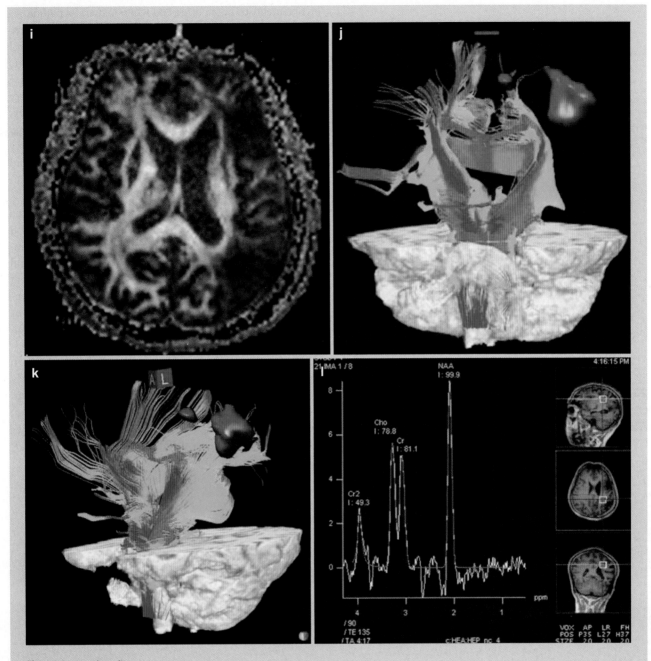

Fig. 26.2 (continued)

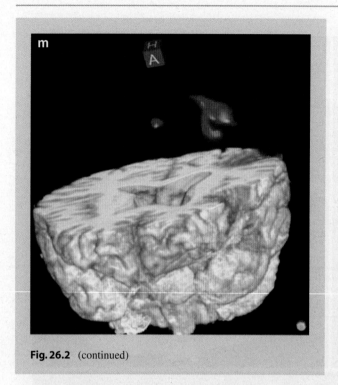

Fig. 26.2 (continued)

26.1.6.3 Cytomegalovirus Encephalitis

CMV infection has an incidence of 40 % in end-stage of AIDS, with common involvements of the cerebrum, cerebellum, spinal cord and spinal nerve roots. CMV encephalitis is more common in the temporal lobe, with possible involvements of both cortex and white matter. Its pathological manifestations greatly vary. The slight cases may have no inflammatory changes but only small quantity viral inclusions. The serious cases may have serious necrotic ependymitis and meningoencephalitis. The disease has a subacute process, with clinical manifestations of memory loss, apathy, consciousness disturbance and delirium. Approximately 30 % patients complain of headache and 50 % patients complain of focal neurological defects. By laboratory tests, the CMV titer in cerebrospinal fluid increases. By brain tissue biopsy, eosinophilic CMV inclusions can be found in the cells.

The imaging demonstrations of cytomegalovirus encephalitis are non-specific. The incidence of cerebral atrophy and ventricular dilation is about 40 %. CT scanning demonstrations can be normal, or can be cerebral atrophy with dilated ventricles. In some cases, scattering or diffuse low density lesions can be found in the paraventricular white matter. Enhanced scanning demonstrates ring shaped or nodular enhancement. MR imaging demonstrates periventricular diffuse white matter lesions or irregular strip liked lesions, with low T1WI signal and high T2WI signal. In the large lesions, there are commonly weakened signal areas. Enhanced imaging demonstrates diffuse irregular enhancement under the ependyma. However, there is no enhancement of the white matter lesions, which is the key difference from progressive multifocal leukoencephalopathy.

Case Study 1

A male patient aged 18 years was confirmatively diagnosed as having AIDS by the CDC. He had fever, head- ache and functional disturbance of the left limbs. His CD4 T cell count was 60/μl.

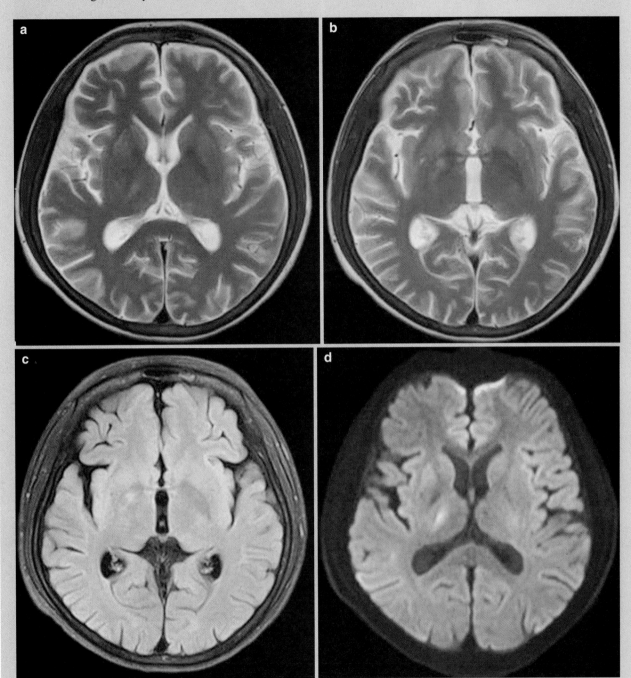

Fig. 26.3 (a–k) HIV/AIDS related CMV encephalitis. (**a**, **b**) MRI demonstrates flakes of slightly higher T2WI signal in the right basal ganglia, with blurry boundary. (**c**) Tirm demonstrates high signals. (**d**, **e**) Diffusion imaging demonstrates high signal. (**f**) Enhanced imaging demonstrates obvious abnormal enhancement of the tentorium and occipital meninges. (**g**) Perfusion imaging demonstrates higher CBF in the right basal ganglia than the contralateral part. (**h**) DTI demonstrates symmetric signals in the white matter of bilateral basal ganglia. (**i**, **j**) 3D white matter fiber tracts tracer imaging demonstrates almost bilaterally symmetric fiber bundles. (**k**) MRS demonstrates increased NAA peak value

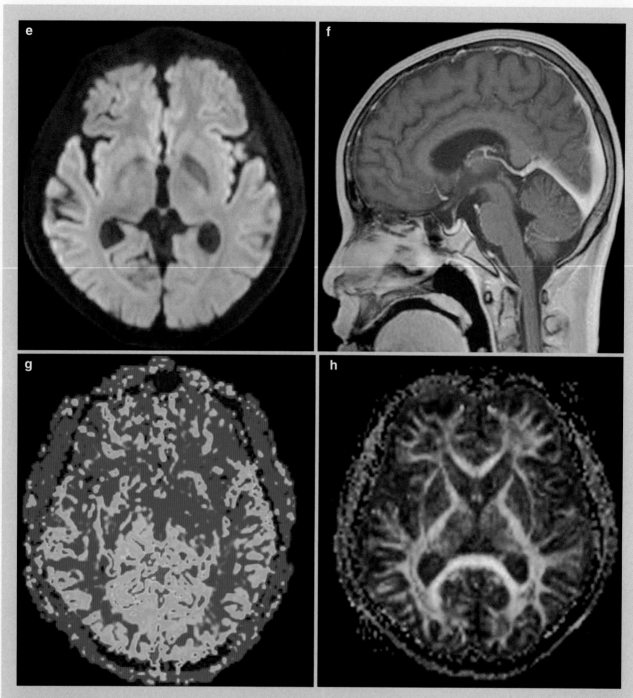

Fig. 26.3 (continued)

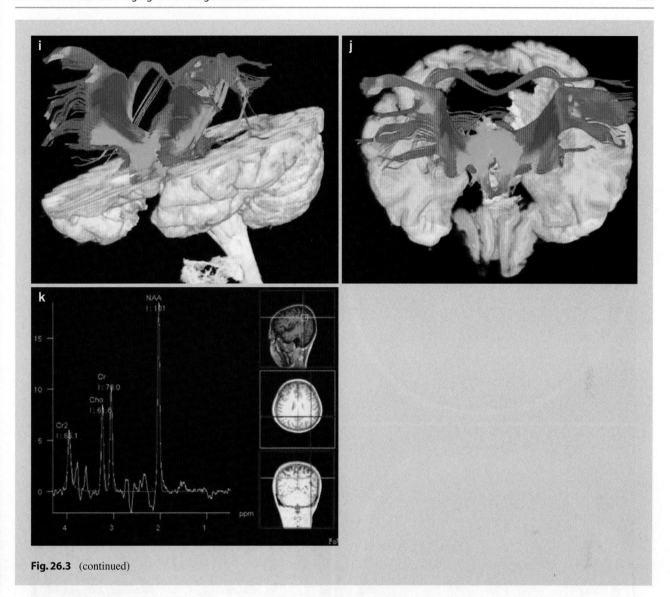

Fig. 26.3   (continued)

Case Study 2

A female patient aged 38 years was confirmatively diagnosed as having AIDS by the CDC. She had no obvious neurological symptoms and signs. Her CD4 T cell count was 566/μl.

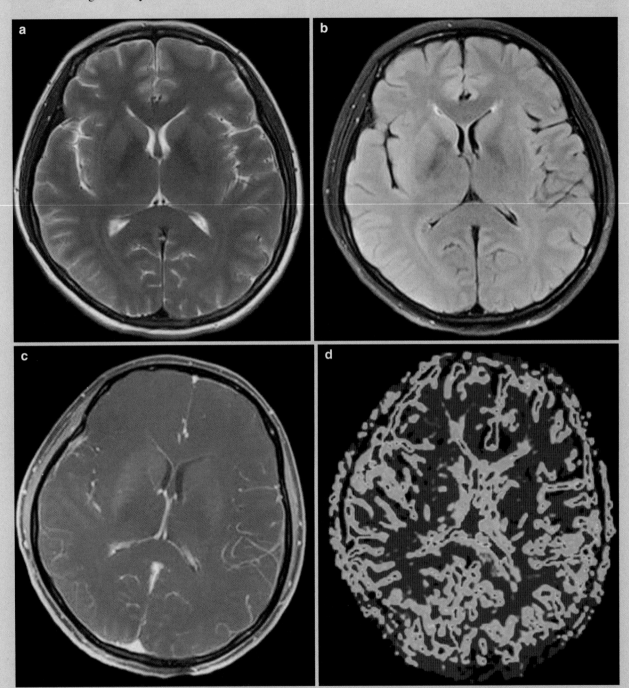

Fig. 26.4 (**a–i**) HIV/AIDS related CMV infection and TB lymphadenitis. (**a**, **b**) MRI demonstrates no abnormal signal in the brain parenchyma, and clear borderline between the cortex and the medulla. (**c**) Enhanced imaging demonstrates no abnormal enhancement. (**d**) Perfusion imaging demonstrates bilaterally symmetric CBF in both cerebral hemispheres. (**e**) DTI demonstrates no obvious abnormalities, and bilaterally symmetric FA values of bilateral brain white matter and nuclei. (**f**, **g**) 3D white matter fiber tracts tracer imaging demonstrates bilaterally symmetric fiber tracts. (**h**) Frontal MRS (single voxel) demonstrates normal NAA/Cr peak and Cho/Cr peak. (**i**) Simple motions test of the right hand demonstrates higher amplitude of the motion activated areas in the left pre- and post-central gyri than healthy people

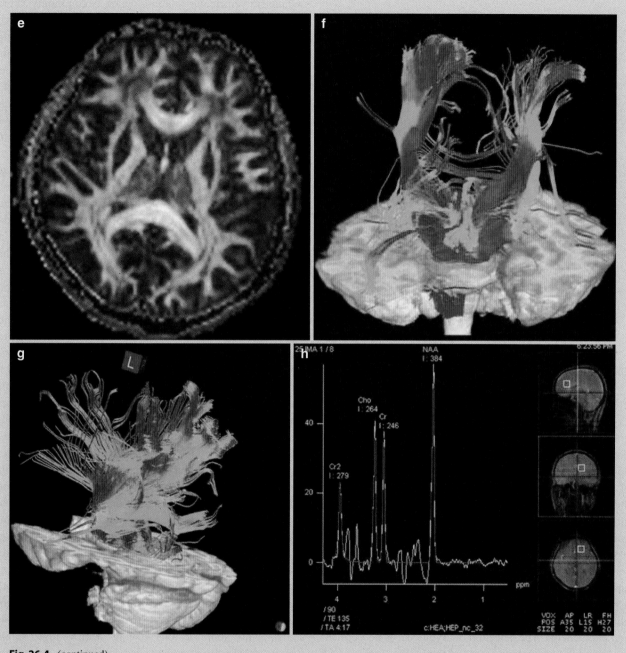

Fig. 26.4   (continued)

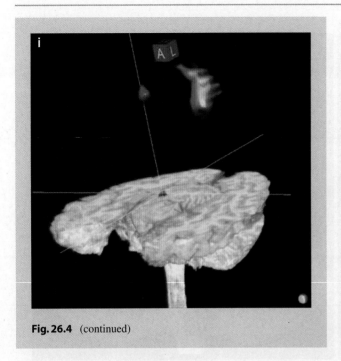

Fig. 26.4 (continued)

26.1.6.4 Cryptococcus Neoformans Meningoencephalitis

Intracranial Cryptococcus neoformans infection is Cryptococcus neoformans infection of the meninges and brain parenchyma, which is the most common fungal infection of CNS in AIDS patients. And it is the second common opportunistic infection in AIDS patients, with an incidence of approximately 5–7 %. The pathogen gains its access into the human body via the respiratory tract and reaches the brain along with blood flow. Due to the lack of antibodies and the complement system in the cerebrospinal fluid and its content of dopamine is favorable to the growth of Cryptococcus neoformans; the intracranial cryptococcus neoformans and the central nervous system have a high affinity. The disease has a subacute or chronic onset, with no specific symptoms. The clinical manifestations include headache, fever, vomiting and papilledema. The detection of cryptococcus neoformans by India ink staining and smear of the CSF as well as CSF culture can define the diagnosis.

Early invasion of the pathogens to the brain parenchyma causes diffuse encephalitis. CT scanning and MR imaging demonstrate brain edema, spots low density lesions in the brain parenchyma, long T1 and long T2 signal area. Enhanced scanning or imaging demonstrates no obvious abnormal enhancement. The involvement of the meninges causes thickened and enhanced meninges in the brain surface, the brain sulci, and basal cistern of the brain. The secondary occurrence of cerebrospinal fluid circulation disturbance has manifestation of slight hydrocephalus. CT scanning and MR imaging demonstrate slight to moderate symmetric ventricular dilation, which is commonly lateral ventricles. With the progression of the conditions, the cryptococcus reproduces and accumulates along the perivascular Virchow-Robin space (V-R space) to invade the deep brain. Multi-focal colloidal pseudo-capsule occurs in the deep white matter of bilateral semispheres, basal ganglia, thalamus and midbrain tegmentum supplied by the deep perforating branches. The colloidal pseudo-capsules in the V-R space cause the expansion of V-R space. CT scanning demonstrates spots of slight lower density areas with blurry boundaries. MR imaging demonstrates multiple spots long T1 and long T2 signals, being similar to lacunar infarction. No surrounding edema and mild enhancement are characteristic neuroimaging findings of the disease. The pseudo-capsules in the brain parenchyma are demonstrated as multiple oval cysts with clear boundaries by MR imaging. Multiple small cysts can fuse with each other to form large cystic lesions, which are demonstrated as multilocular or unilocular cystic space occupying lesions in long T1 and long T2 signals. The space occupying effect and surrounding edema are obvious. Enhanced imaging demonstrates ring shaped obvious enhancement of the cystic wall. In the cases with the lesions penetrating the blood–brain barrier to form granulomas in the brain parenchyma or along the ependyma or choroid plexus, cryptococcal occurs. Pathologically, it is composed of histocytes, giant cells, lymphoid cells and fibroblasts. Cryptococcosis is rarely found, commonly in the giant cells and histocytes. Cryptococcal granuloma is generally more common in the chronic phase, which is more obvious in the cases with more than 3 months course and is the demonstration of strong body responses. The CT scanning and MR imaging demonstrations are non-specific. Plain scanning/imaging demonstrates cortical singular or multiple round and oval liked lesions in the cerebral hemispheres and cerebellar hemispheres. Plain CT scanning demonstrates equal or slightly higher or low density lesions, while plain MR imaging demonstrates slightly lower T1WI signal and low or equal T2WI signal, with some lesions having central high signal. Enhanced scanning/imaging demonstrates nodular, ring shaped or even enhancement. In the cases of large granuloma, flower ring liked and nodular enhancement can be found. In the large lesions, there are internal low T2WI signal septa, which show no enhancement by enhanced imaging. Accompanying space occupying effect of compressed ventricles or cisterns can be found. In the cases with invasion of Cryptococcosis along the ependyma, intraventricular granuloma may occur. MR imaging demonstrates obstructive hydrocephalus and ring shaped enhancement lesions. The lesions may fuse, with perifocal edema. MRS demonstrates decreased NAA, Cr, Cho and mI peak but increased Lip peak in it.

Case Study 1

A male patient aged 33 years was confirmatively diagnosed as having AIDS by the CDC. He had low grade fever, headache, apathy and logagnosia. His pathological sign of neural reflex was positive and his CD4 T cell count was 11/μl.

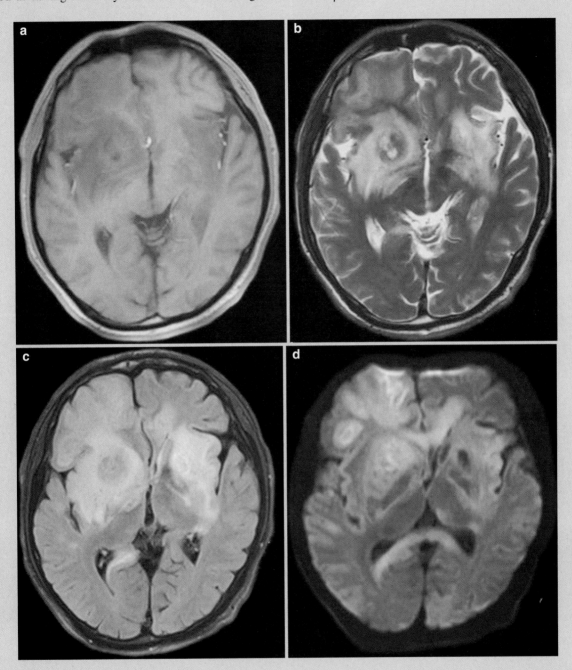

Fig. 26.5 (**a–j**) HIV/AIDS related disseminated fungal infection, progressive multifocal leukoencephalopathy, CMV encephalitis and cryptococcal abscess. (**a, b**) MRI demonstrates multiple focal mass liked and large flakes of equal long T1 and equal long T2 signal in the bilateral basal ganglia, bilateral corona radiata, bilateral frontal and parietal cortex and subcortical white matter, bilateral temporal cortex, genu and splenium of the corpus callosum, and the right thalamus; short T1 and short T2 signal in some lesions with clear boundaries, and the largest lesion being in a diameter of 20 mm. (**c**) FLAIR sequence demonstrates high signal of most lesions. (**d**) DWI demonstrates restricted high signal; some lesions being in ring shape which is more commonly in the right frontal lobe and basal ganglia with central low signal shadows and peripheral high signal; perifocal swelling of the gyrus in the right frontal lobe with narrowed sulcus; obvious space occupying lesions in the right basal ganglia; obviously deformed right lateral ventricle due to compression; and compressed third ventricle, suprasellar cistern, interpeduncular cistern and optic chiasm. (**e**) Enhanced imaging demonstrates multiple ring shaped enhancement lesions in the right frontal lobe, temporal lobe, left cerebellar hemisphere, bilateral basal ganglia, genu and splenium of the corpus callosum, and abnormal enhancement shadows in the bilateral lateral ventricular ependyma, left temporal gyrus and the tentorium. (**f**) Perfusion imaging demonstrates increased CBF in the right lesions area compared to the contralateral part. (**g**) DTI demonstrates decreased FA values of most lesions, which are more obvious in the right temporal lobe and the right basal ganglia. (**h, i**) 3D white matter fiber tracts tracer imaging demonstrates sparse fiber tracts in bilateral frontal lobes. (**j**) MRS demonstrates NAA/Cr is 0.76 which is decreased; and Cho/Cr is 0.69, which is also decreased

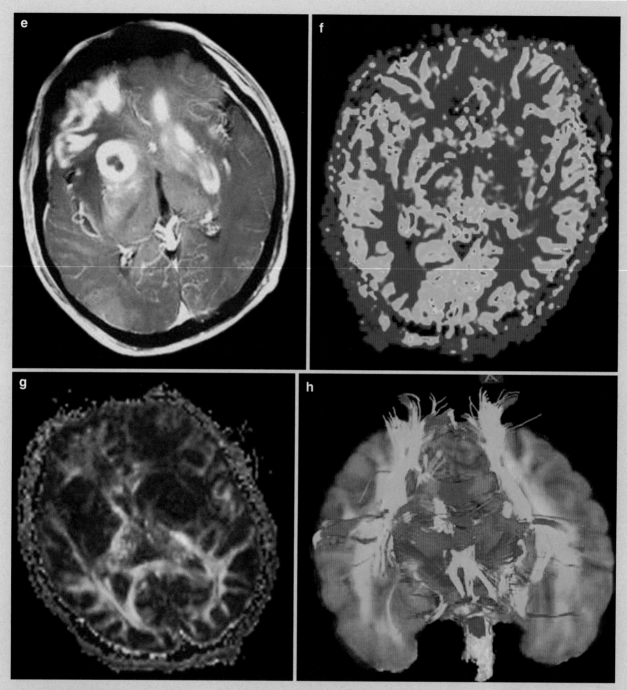

Fig. 26.5 (continued)

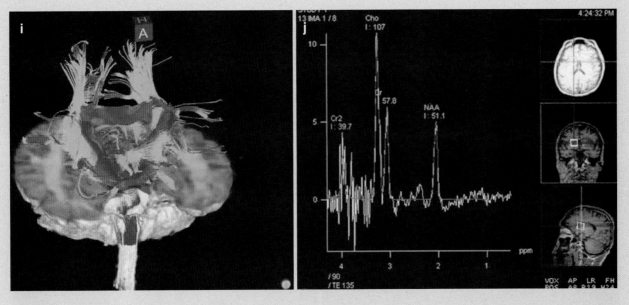

Fig. 26.5 (continued)

Case Study 2

A male patient aged 32 years was confirmatively diagnosed as having AIDS by the CDC. He had fever, headache, nausea, vomiting and chills for half a month. His CD4 T cell count was 32/μl.

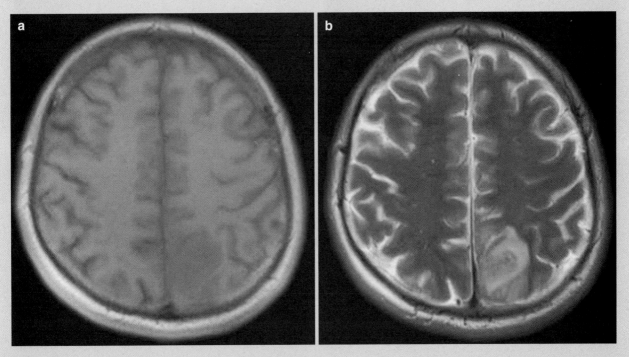

Fig. 26.6 (**a**–**o**) HIV/AIDS related cryptococcal meningitis. (**a**–**c**) MRI demonstrates multiple patchy abnormal long T1 and long T2 signal along the gyri in the bilateral frontal lobes and left local parietal lobe, with clear boundaries; shallow local cerebral sulci, and narrowed gyri. (**d**, **e**) FLAIR sequence demonstrates high signal of the lesions. (**f**, **g**) DWI demonstrates slightly higher signal shadows of the lesions. (**h**–**j**) Enhanced imaging demonstrates abnormal enhancement shadows in the sulci of bilateral frontal lobes and bilateral parietal lobes. (**k**) Perfusion imaging demonstrates symmetric CBF in the bilateral cerebral hemispheres. (**l**) DTI demonstrates decreased FA values of the bilateral frontal lobes and the left parietal lobe, compared to the contralateral parts. (**m**, **n**) 3D white matter fiber tracts tracer imaging demonstrates decreased longitudinal fiber bundles in the bilateral frontal lobes and the left parietal lobe. (**o**) MRS demonstrates that NAA/(Cr + Cr2) is 0.58, which is decreased; and Cho/Cr is 0.33, which is decreased

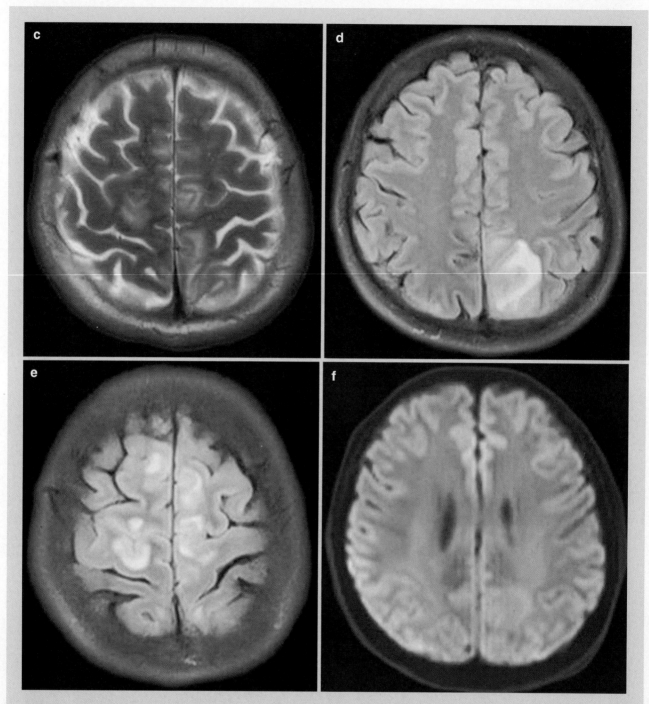

Fig. 26.6 (continued)

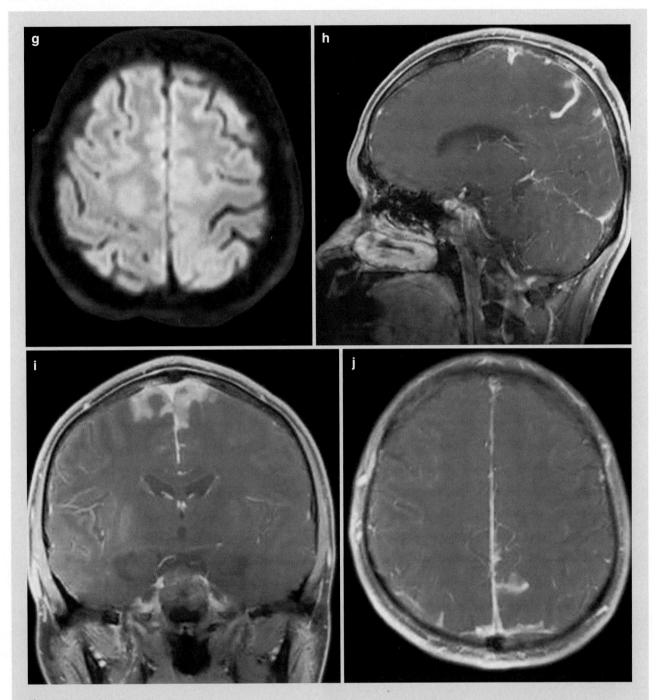

Fig. 26.6 (continued)

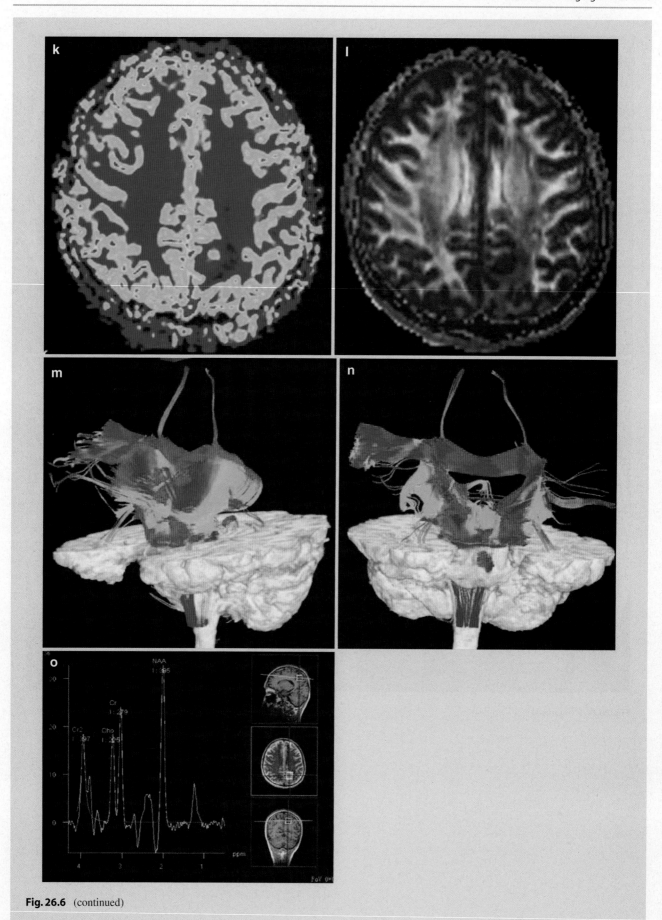

Fig. 26.6 (continued)

26.1.6.5 Herpes Simplex Encephalitis

HIV/AIDS related herpes simplex encephalitis is a rare complication of AIDS and most occurrences are due to the compromised immunity. The activated virus spreads to the brain to cause the disease. The lesions are commonly asymmetrically distributed, which are more common in the temporal lobe, hippocampus, frontal orbital surface, parietal lobe and the cingulatus, with involvements of the hypothalamus, medulla oblongata and pons. By the naked eyes observation, necrosis can be found in the bilateral temporal lobes, which are asymmetric with accompanying hemorrhage. Under a microscope, the brain parenchyma has hemorrhage, necrosis and liquifaction, with occurrence of acute hemorrhagic necrotizing encephalitis. The clinical manifestations are not typical, with symptoms of headache and fever as well as seizures, drowsiness, ataxia, aphasia and other neuropsychiatric symptoms.

CT scanning demonstrates flakes of low density lesions in the temporal lobe, limbic system and the frontal lobe, with accompanying central small focal high density hemorrhagic foci. In the cases with involved bilateral hemispheres, extensive cerebral edema can be found, with narrowed ventricles and cisterns which even can be absent. MR imaging demonstrates flakes of long T1 and long T2 signal in the temporal lobe, frontal lobe and parietal lobe, with clear boundaries and space occupying effect. Brain tissues edema is obvious, but generally with no involvement of the putamen, which are characteristic MR findings. MRS demonstrates significantly decreased NAA, significantly increased Lac peak, increased Cho and Lip peaks, and slightly decreased Cr peak.

Case Study 1

A male patient aged 31 years was confirmatively diagnosed as having AIDS by the CDC. He had fever, with a body temperature lower than 38°C, weakness of the right limbs, and aphasia for 1 week. His CD4 T cell count was 266/μl.

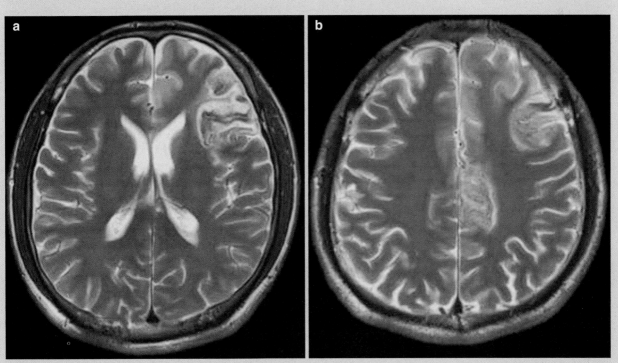

Fig. 26.7 (a–n) HIV/AIDS related herpes encephalitis. (**a**, **b**) MRI demonstrates multiple patchy long T2 signals in the left frontal lobe, hippocampus, parietal lobe, cingulate gyrus and insular lobe, unclear borderline between the cortex and medulla, and blurry boundaries of the lesions. (**c**, **d**) Tirm demonstrates high signals of the lesions. (**e**, **f**) DWI demonstrates high signals. (**g**, **h**) Enhanced imaging demonstrates obvious enhancement of the lesions, with uneven enhancement and adjacent meningeal enhancement. (**i**) Perfusion imaging demonstrates higher CBF of the left frontal and parietal lobes than that of the contralateral part. (**j**, **k**) DTI demonstrates lower FA values of the left frontal and parietal lobes than those of the contralateral parts. (**l**, **m**) 3D white matter fiber tracts tracer imaging demonstrates sparser fiber tracts in the left frontal and parietal lobes than those in the contralateral parts. (**n**) MRS demonstrates NAA/(Cr+Cr2) is 0.62, which is decreased; and Cho/(Cr+Cr2) is 0.58, which is decreased

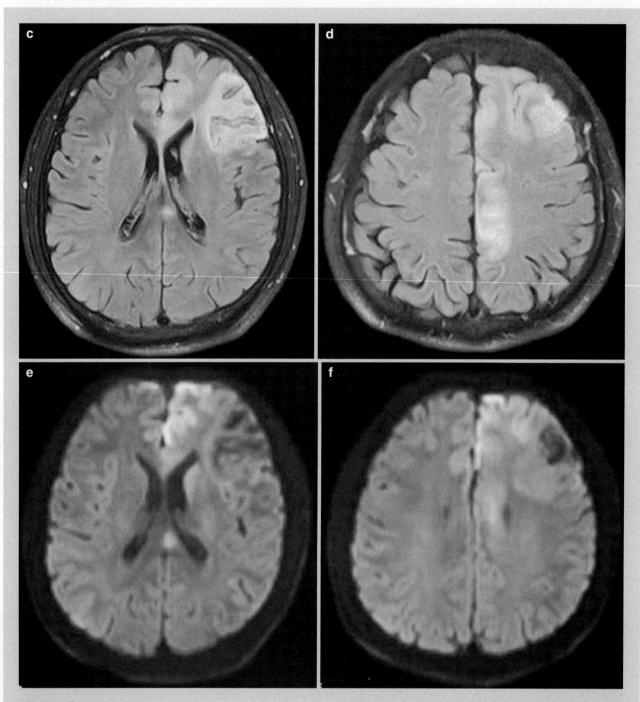

Fig. 26.7 (continued)

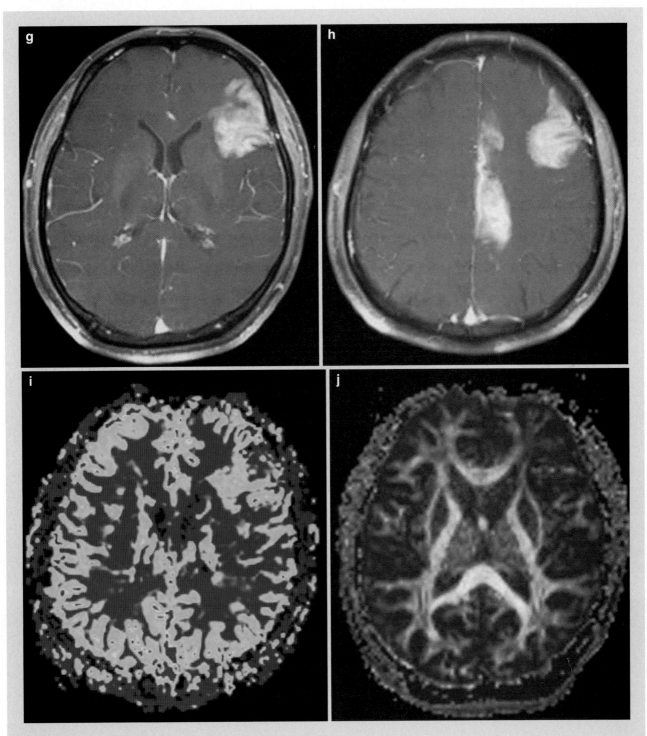

Fig. 26.7 (continued)

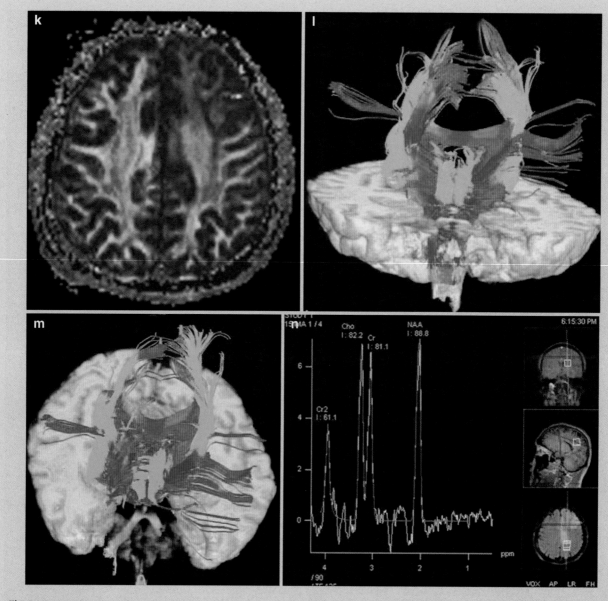

Fig. 26.7 (continued)

Case Study 2
A girl aged 8 years was confirmatively diagnosed as having AIDS by the CDC. She had weakness of the right limbs for more than 2 months, with a CD4 T cell count of 21/μl.

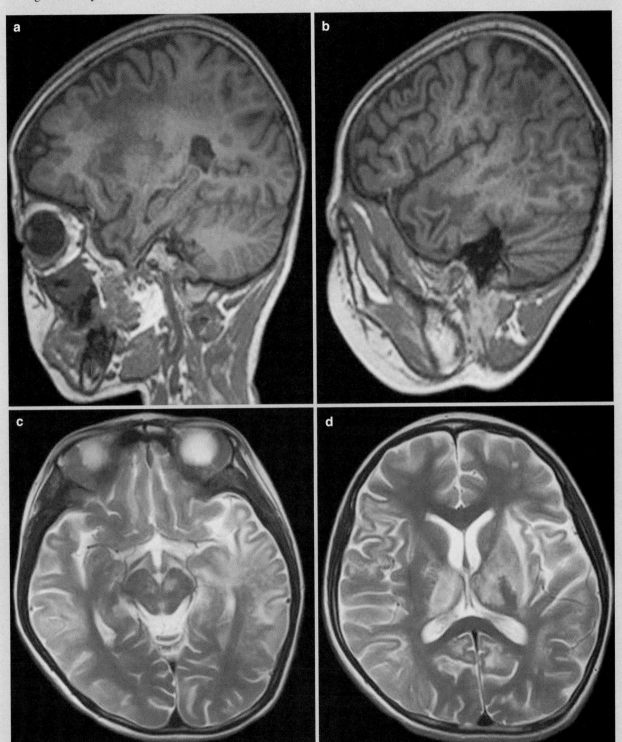

Fig. 26.8 (**a–m**) HIV/AIDS related herpes virus encephalitis sequela. (**a–e**) MR imaging demonstrates flakes and spots of long T1 and long T2 signals in bilateral brain white matter, thalamus, basal ganglia and brain stem. (**f**) T2 adipose and water depression imaging demonstrates scattering high signals and fusion of some lesions. (**g**) DWI demonstrates perifocal high signals. (**h**) Enhanced imaging demonstrates no obvious enhancement of the lesions. (**i**) Perfusion imaging demonstrates decreased CBF of the lesion area. (**j**) DTI demonstrates lower FA value of the lesions than those of contralateral part. (**k, l**) 3D white matter fiber tracts tracer imaging demonstrates sparser left fiber tracts than the contralateral part. (**m**) MRS demonstrates obviously decreased NAA peak, widened sulci and fissures and dilated ventricular system

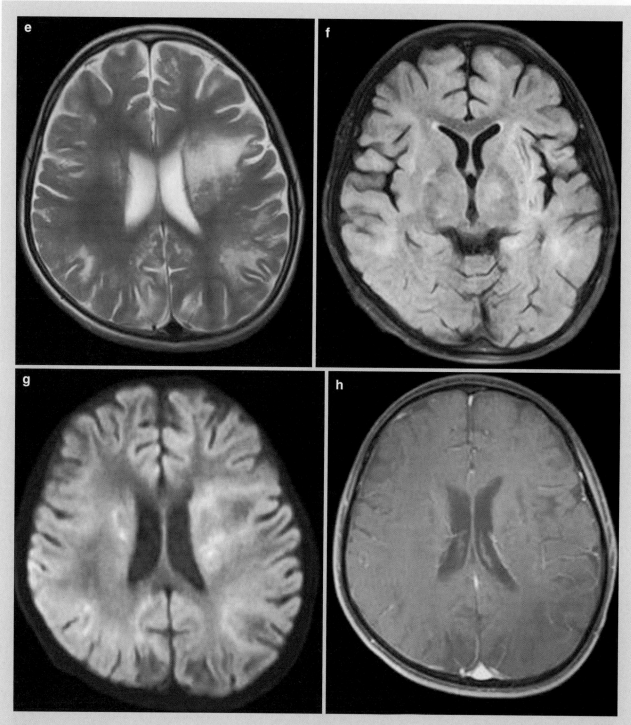

Fig. 26.8 (continued)

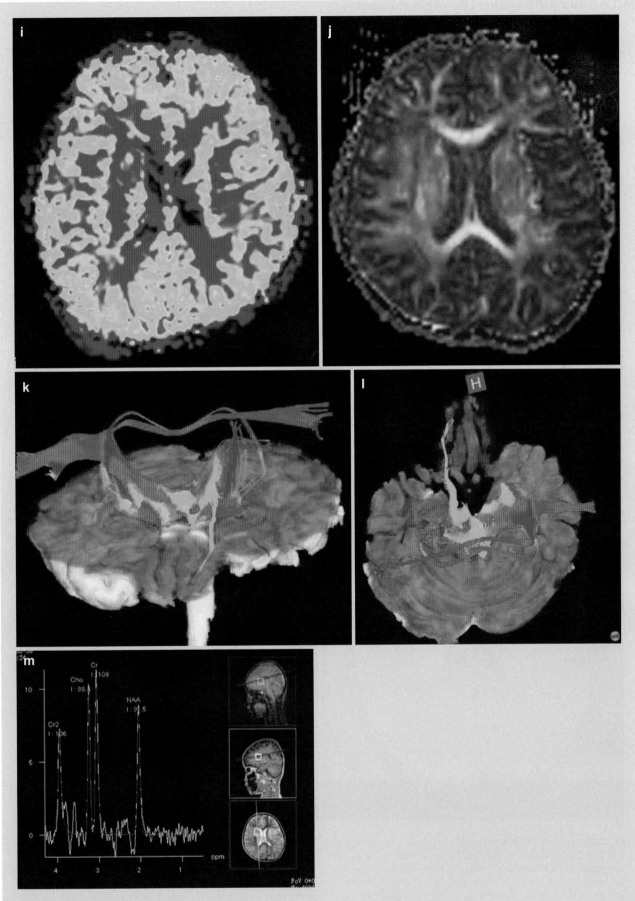

Fig. 26.8 (continued)

26.1.6.6 HIV/AIDS Related Leukoencephalopathy

Case Study 1
A male patient aged 45 years was confirmatively diagnosed as having AIDS by the CDC. He had no obvious neurological symptoms and signs. And his CD4 T cell count was 140/ μl.

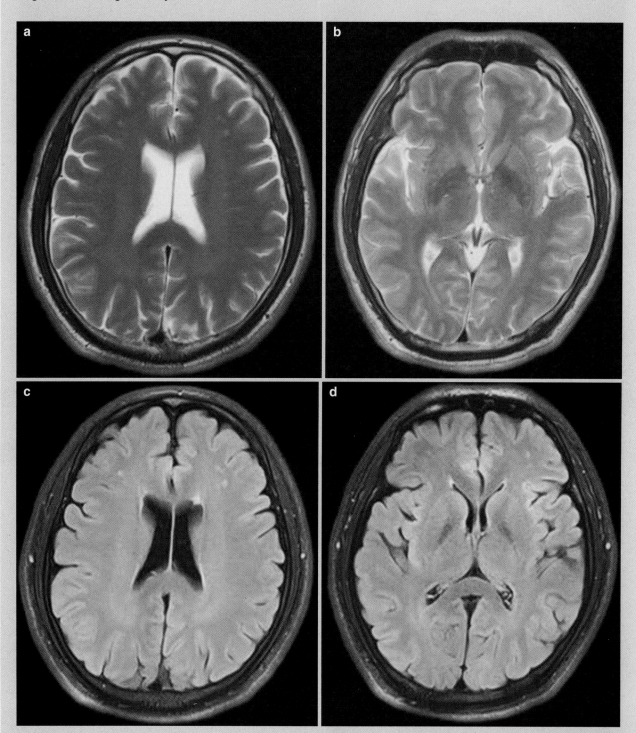

Fig. 26.9 (**a–h**) HIV/AIDS related bilateral basal ganglia malacia and white matter degeneration of the semioval centrum. (**a, b**) MR imaging demonstrates multiple spots and flakes of long T2 signal in the bilateral basal ganglia, multiple small patchy long T2 signal in the white matter of the frontal lobe. (**c, d**) T2 adipose and water depression imaging demonstrates high signal, and clear borderline between the cortex and medulla. (**e**) Perfusion imaging demonstrates symmetric CBF of bilateral cerebral hemispheres. (**f**) DTI demonstrates weakened signal of the white matter in the bilateral frontal lobes, and decreased FA values. (**g, h**) 3D white matter fiber tracts tracer imaging demonstrates have bilaterally symmetric fiber bundles

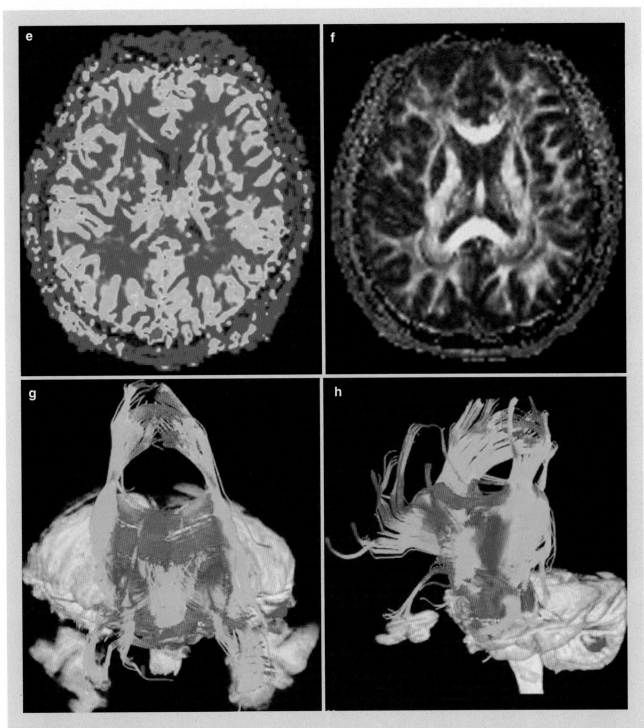

Fig. 26.9 (continued)

Case Study 2

A male patient aged 63 years was confirmatively diagnosed as having AIDS by the CDC. He had intermittent fever, cough and headache. And his CD4 T cell count was 70/μl.

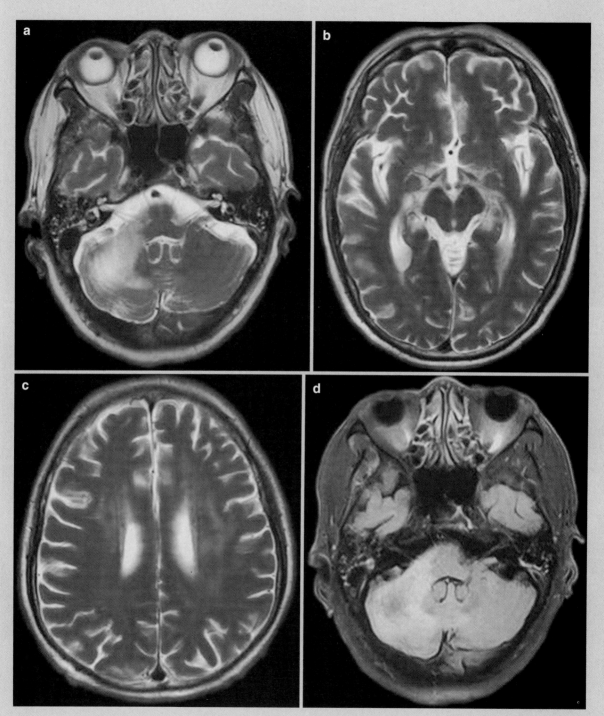

Fig. 26.10 (**a–n**) HIV/AIDS related progressive focal leukoencephalopathy, cerebellar stem encephalitis and cerebral atrophy. (**a–c**) MR imaging demonstrates have multiple patchy long T2 signal in the bilateral semioval centrum, with blurry boundaries and bilaterally symmetric distribution; large flakes of long T1 long T2 signal in the right cerebellum and brain stem, with blurry boundaries. (**d–f**) Water and adipose depression T2WI imaging demonstrate high signal of the lesions. (**g**) DWI demonstrates high signal. (**h, i**) Enhanced imaging by intravenous injection of Gd-BOPTA demonstrates no obvious enhancement of the lesions in the bilateral semioval centrum, and slight enhancement of the right cerebellar lesions adjacent to the meninges. (**j**) Perfusion imaging demonstrates bilaterally symmetric CBF of the bilateral cerebral hemispheres. (**k**) DTI demonstrates decreased FA values in bilateral temporal, frontal and parietal lobes. (**l, m**) 3D white matter fiber tracts tracer imaging demonstrates sparse fiber tracts in the bilateral temporal lobes. (**n**) MRS demonstrates obviously decreased NAA/Cr peak

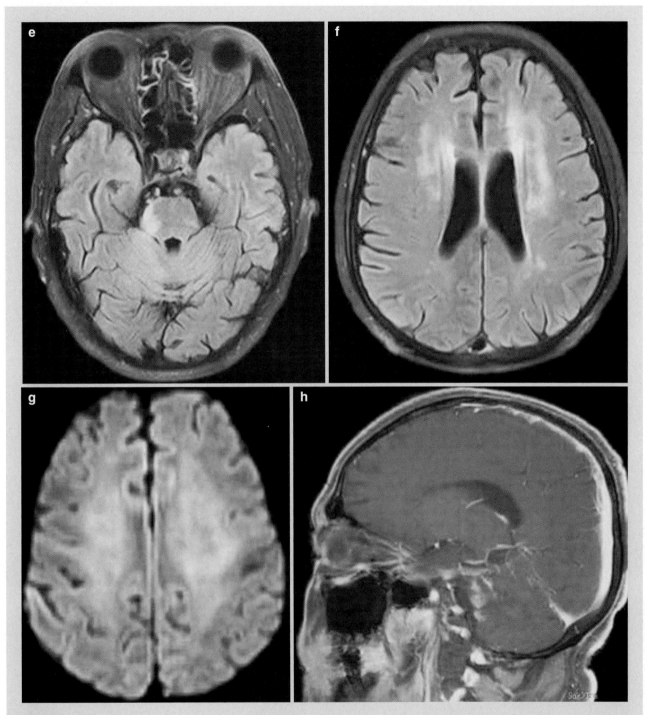

Fig. 26.10 (continued)

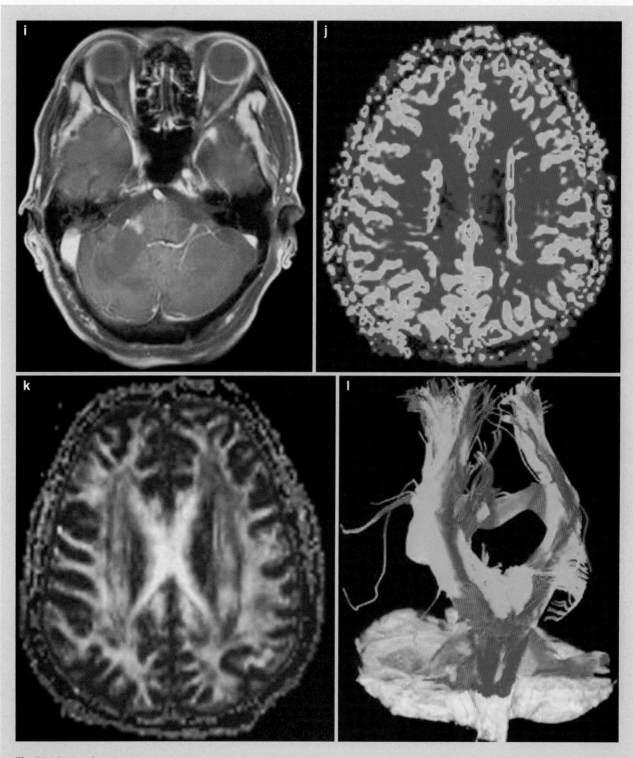

Fig. 26.10 (continued)

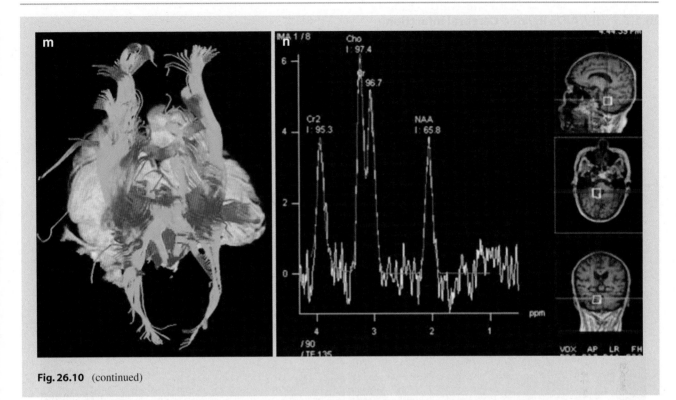

Fig. 26.10 (continued)

26.1.6.7 HIV/AIDS Related Cerebral Infarction

Case Study 1

A female patient aged 47 years was confirmatively diagnosed as having AIDS by the CDC. She had no obvious neurological symptoms and signs. Her CD4 T cell count was 52/ μl.

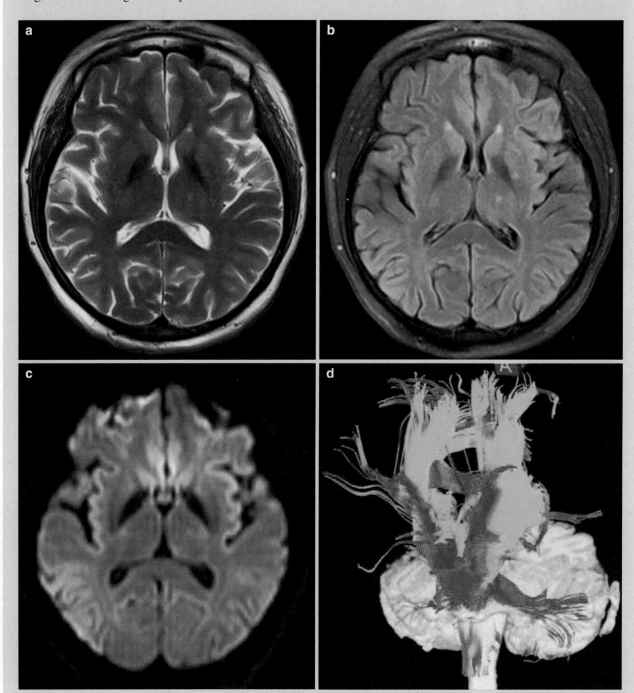

Fig. 26.11 (a–f) HIV/AIDS related lacunar infarction. (a) T2WI demonstrates small patchy high signal in the left basal ganglia. (b) Trim demonstrates high signal. (c) DWI demonstrates high signal. (d–e) 3D white matter fiber tracts tracer imaging demonstrates more transverse fiber tracts in the left side than in the right side. (f) Simple motion test of the right hand demonstrates larger range and magnitude motion activated areas in the left pre- and post-central gyri

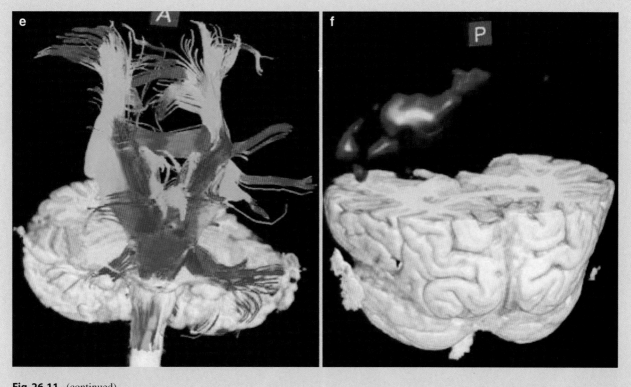

Fig. 26.11 (continued)

Case Study 2

A male patient aged 33 years was confirmatively diagnosed as having AIDS by the CDC. He had low grade fever and his CD4 T cell count was 14/μl.

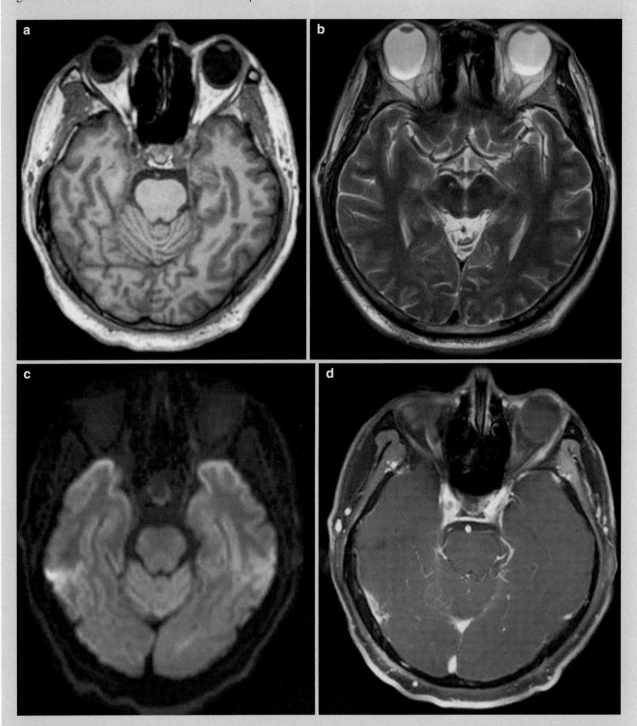

Fig. 26.12 (**a–h**) HIV/AIDS related lacunar infarction. (**a–c**) MR imaging demonstrates small spots long T1 and long T2 signal in the right pons, and high DWI signal, with clear boundary. (**d**) Enhanced imaging demonstrates no abnormal enhancement. (**e**) DTI demonstrates weakened signal of the white matter in the bilateral temporal lobes and decreased FA values. (**f, g**) 3D white matter fiber tracts tracer imaging demonstrates sparse fiber tracts in the bilateral temporal lobes. (**h**) Simple motion test of the right hand demonstrates larger range and magnitude of motion activated areas in the left pre- and post-central gyri, posterior parietal cortex, and the cerebellum than healthy people

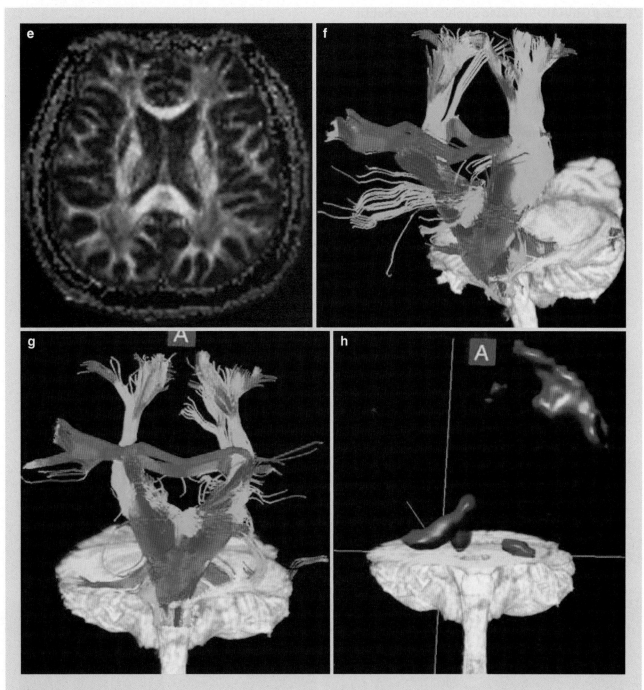

Fig. 26.12 (continued)

26.1.6.8 HIV/AIDS Related Syphilis Encephalitis

Case Study

A male patient aged 35 years was confirmatively diagnosed as having AIDS by the CDC. He had cognitive impairment and behavioral problems. His CD4 T cell count was 74/μl.

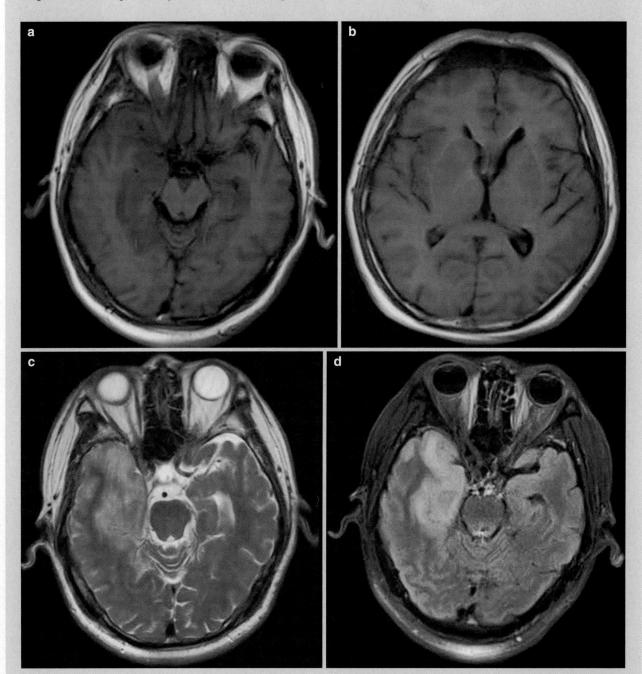

Fig. 26.13 (**a–j**) HIV/AIDS related syphilis encephalitis. (**a–c**) MR imaging demonstrates multiple large flakes of long T1 long T2 signals in the right temporal lobe, frontal lobe and occipital lobe, with unclear boundaries; flatter right lateral ventricle due to compression. (**d, e**) Water and adipose depression T2WI demonstrates high signal and high DWI signal. (**f–h**) Enhanced imaging by intra- venous injection of Gd-BOPTA demonstrates gyri liked enhance- ment in the right temporal lobe, and obviously thickening and enhancement of the longitudinal sinus and tentorium. (**i**) DTI dem- onstrates lower FA value in the right temporal lobe than the contra- lateral part. (**j**) MRS demonstrates obviously decreased NAA/Cr peak

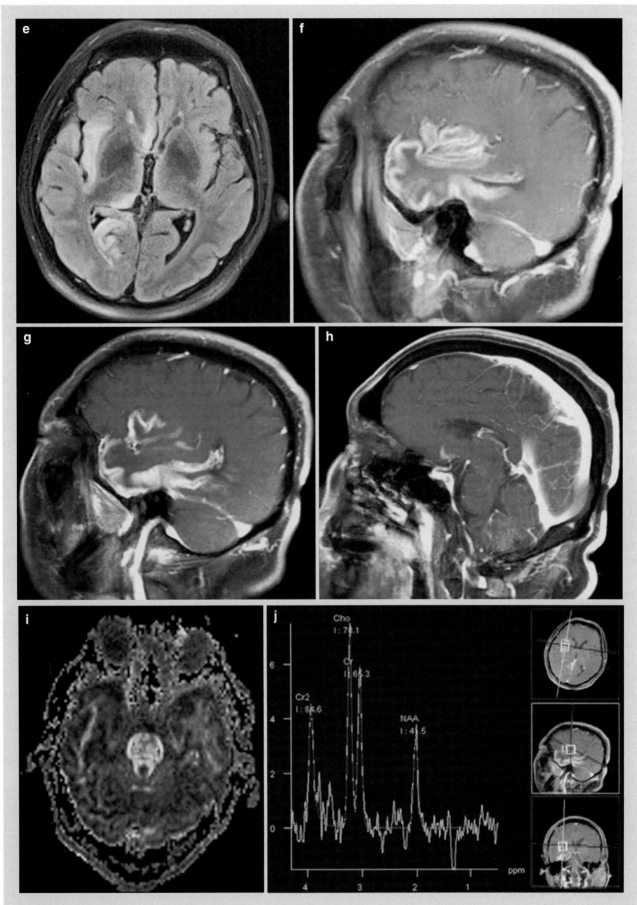

Fig. 26.13 (continued)

26.1.6.9 Glioma

Glioma originates from the nerve stromal cell components, including astrocytoma, oligodendroglioma, ependymoma, pleomorphic glioblastoma and others, which is one of the most commonly CNS neoplasms. Glioma accounts for 40–50 % of brain parenchymal tumors. Based on their pathohistological features, it can be divided into low grade and high grade gliomas.

By CT scanning, low density or low and equal mixed density masses can be found, with peritumor edema and obvious space occupying effect. Enhanced scanning demonstrates irregular ring shaped enhancement and accompanying wall nodules. By MR imaging, lower or equal T1WI signals and high T2WI signals can be found, commonly with slight to moderate peritumor edema and space occupying effect. Enhanced imaging demonstrates uneven or flower ring liked enhancement of the lesions.

MRS demonstrates Gliomas as decreased NAA and Cr as well as increased Cho. However, in the cases of glioblastoma, the Cho value decreases due to the diluted Cho content caused by micronecrosis in the tumors. The increases of Lip and Lac are due to the micro-necrosis and anaerobic metabolism in the tumors. Meanwhile, each metabolite peak is different in the different areas of the tumor. For the cases of high grade gliomas, Cho and NAA decrease in the central necrotic area and increase in tumor entities and the peripheral area. For the cases of low grade gliomas, Cho and NAA at the central necrotic area increase, while decrease at the peripheral area, with no Lac and Lip. This is the key point for its differentiation from the high grade gliomas. Therefore, the increase of Lip may indicate early malignant conversion of the gliomas. Gliomas are highly invasive neoplasms, with tumor cells infiltration in its surrounding area and edema area. The increase of Cho/NAA concurs with normal manifestation of the simple edema area. Therefore, MRS can further define the boundary and range of the gliomas, which greatly facilitates the pathological biopsy and radiotherapeutic planning. In addition, studies have demonstrated that the change of Cho and increases of Cho/Cr and Cho/NAA are markers indicating the progression of gliomas. When the increase of Cho is 45 % higher than its normal level, progression of glioma is indicated. When the increase of Cho is within 35 % of the normal level, the gliomas are commonly in a stable condition. Cho/NAA, Cho/Cr and NAA/Cr ratios have significance in the differential diagnosis for its recurrence after radiation therapy. The increases of the Cho/NAA and Cho/Cr, as well as the decrease of NAA/Cr indicate recurrence of gliomas after radiation therapy.

PWI indices are closely related to the vascular density in glioma tissues, which indicate the hemodynamic changes and the number of neovascularization of the tumors rather than the severity blood–brain barrier damages. Related immunohistochemical studies also have demonstrated that the microvessel density (MVD) of the tumors and the expression of vascular endothelial growth factor (VECF) are obviously related to the pathological grading of the gliomas

and the rCBV value of the tumors. The glioma MVD and the expression of VEGF of high grade glioma is obviously higher than those of low grade glioma. The high grade glioma also has higher rCBV value.

DWI demonstrates glioma as high signal, slightly high signal, equal signal or low signal. It is generally believed that the high signal indicates edema or fresh necrosis of the tumor cells, while the low signal suggests hemorrhage or calcification. DWI demonstrates edema as equal low or slightly high signal. ADC images show slightly high or high signal, with clearly defined boundaries from the lesions. DWI demonstrates necrotic as obviously low signal and its ADC is high signal. Studies have shown that the ACD value of the same grade gliomas gradually decreases from peritumoral edema, tumor core area to the contralateral normal white matter. The ADC values of the tumor area and peritumoral area are negatively correlated with tumor grade. Namely, the higher grade tumor has a lower ADC value. The reason may be the large quantity of cells in the high grade gliomas and these cells have a close arrangement and smaller intercellular space, less extracellular water molecules and more intracellular compound protein molecules to restrict the free diffusion of the water molecules. In addition, increased cellular atypia and increased ratio of cellular nucleus to cytoplasm ratio more seriously restrict the water molecules diffusion, which causes lower ADC value, obvious low signal in ADC images and equal or high signal in DWI images. Therefore, the ACD value can be used to assess the therapeutic efficacy of tumors. Specifically, the increase of the ACD value indicates effective treatment, while the decreased or constant ACD value suggests poor therapeutic efficacy.

DTI technology and FT technology contribute to the grading, differential diagnosis and surgical planning of glioma. In the cases with tumor invasion, the spacial arrangement of the fiber tracts can be damaged in certain extent, with decreased FA value. Therefore, the changes of FA value can be an indicator of intactness of the fiber tracts. Low grade glioma can cause migration and edema of the white matter fiber tracts rather than destroying and infiltration. The clear demonstrations of the intratumor or surrounding fiber tracts can facilitate its differentiation from the high grade glioma.

Bold-fMRI can clearly define the tumor tissue from the normal tissues, which greatly help to define the range of the tumors to avoid surgical damages to the functional cortex. Meanwhile, it has potential for the differential diagnosis and for the assessment of the brain nerves functions before and after operation.

Recent studies have demonstrated that ^{18}F-FDG PET/CT can directly and comprehensively demonstrate metabolic status of the glioma cells. Their uptake of the imaging agent is not related to the severity of the blood–brain barrier damage, but to the expression of VECF. The SUV ratio of the tumor tissue to the brain white matter is believed to be the best semi-quantitative indicator for differentiation of the low grade glioma from high grade glioma.

Case Study 1

A male patient aged 42 years was confirmatively diagnosed as having AIDS by the CDC. He had headache and weakened muscular strength of the left limbs. His CD4 T cell count was 134/μl.

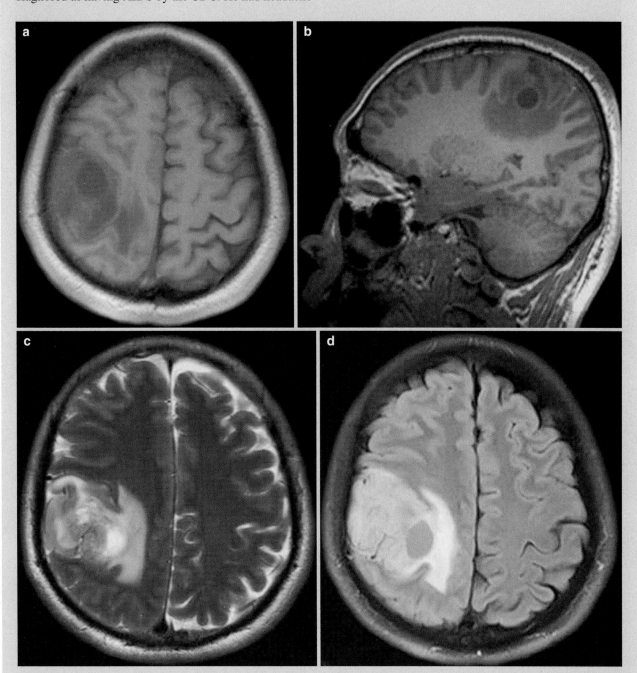

Fig. 26.14 (**a–k**) HIV/AIDS related astrocytoma. (**a–c**) MR imaging demonstrates irregular mixed signals at the interface of the gray matter and the white matter in the right parietal lobe; slightly short T1 or slightly long/equal T2 signal of the lesions; multiple long T1 and long T2 signal in the lesions with obvious space occupying effect; and surrounding flakes of long T1 and long T2 edema signal. (**d**) Water and adipose depression T2WI imaging demonstrates high signal. (**e**) DWI demonstrates high signal, and low DWI signals of the liquifaction and necrosis. (**f**) Enhanced imaging by intravenous injection of Gd-BOPTA demonstrates uneven peripheral flowers ring liked enhancement, obvious enhancement of the parenchymal part and no enhancement of the liquifaction and necrosis. (**g, h**) DTI demonstrates obviously decreased FA values in the right parietal lobe compared to the contralateral part. (**i, j**) 3D white matter fiber tracts tracer imaging demonstrates absent fiber tracts of the white matter in the right lesions area, some interrupted bridging fiber tracts. (**k**) MRS demonstrates that NAA/Cr is 0.7, which is decreased; and Cho/(Cr + Cr2) is 0.67, which is also decreased

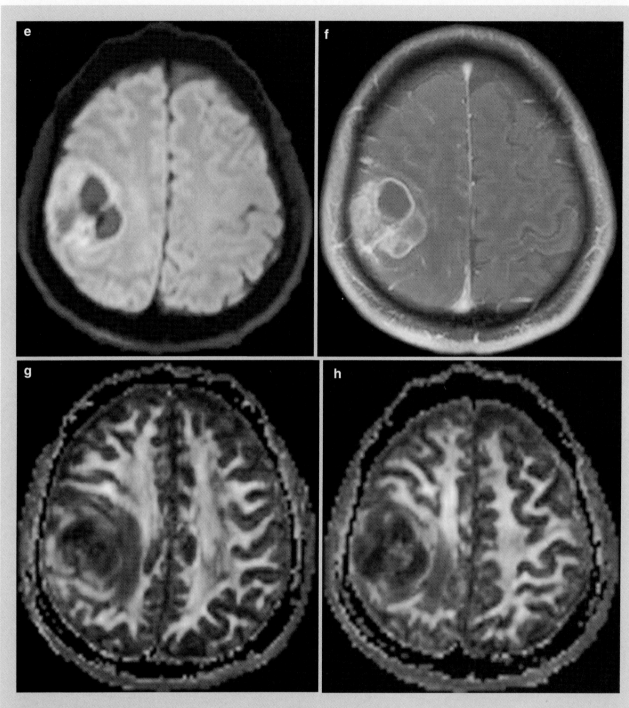

Fig. 26.14 (continued)

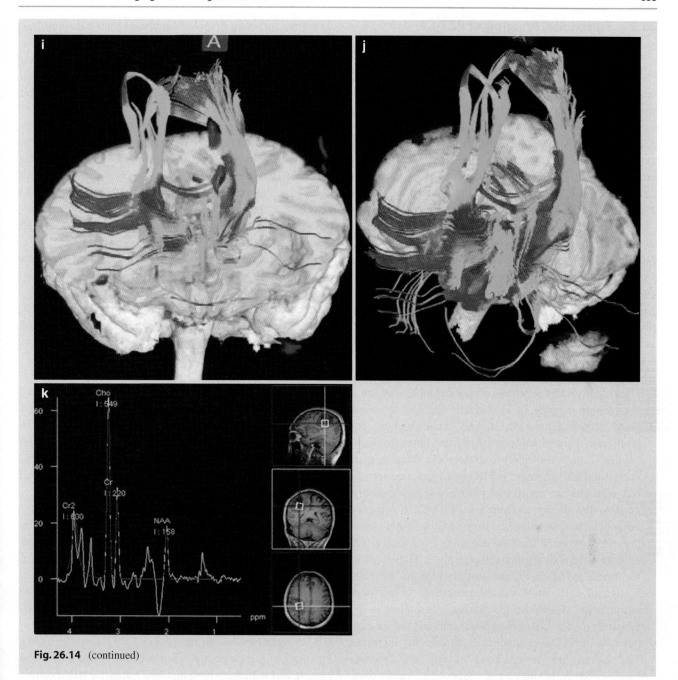

Fig. 26.14 (continued)

26.2 Functional Imaging of PET-CT for HIV/ AIDS

Functional imaging is a science of cellular and molecular imaging for quantitative and qualitative analysis of the biological processes of living humans or animals. The commonly used molecular imaging examinations include radionuclide imaging, MR imaging, optical imaging and ultrasound molecular imaging. Among these technologies, radionuclide imaging is the firstly applied imaging technology in molecular imaging. PET molecular imaging has gained most attentions, which is the frontier of the nuclear medicine.

PET imaging is a series of pairs of probes in 180° arrangement with following wiring. In vitro tracers including ^{11}C, ^{18}F, ^{15}O and ^{13}N produce γ-photon with annihilation radiation. The collected information is processed by a computer to demonstrate sectional images of the target organ and to provide quantitative physiological parameters. But it has disadvantages of low spatial resolution, high false positive rate, and no accurate anatomical localization of abnormal signals at the molecular level.

The applications of molecular PET imaging include:

1. The recent studies of protein functional molecular imaging include imaging of hexokinase and glucose transporter protein expression, choline kinase imaging, cell proliferation and endogenous thymidine kinase imaging. ^{18}F-FDG is the most widely used metabolic imaging agent in clinical PET imaging. ^{18}F-FDG gains its access into the cell with glucose transporter protein and is phosphorylated by hexokinase to form 6-P-^{18}F-FDG. However, it cannot be phosphorylated by isomerase into 6-phosphate fluorodeoxyglucose fructose due to the structural difference from the natural glucose 6-phosphate. Thus it cannot be further metabolized and just remains in the cells. Malignant cells proliferation accelerates to consume more energy. Therefore, the glucose metabolism is significantly higher than normal tissue cells and the accumulation of ^{18}F-FFDG in tumor cells significantly increases. The lesions are demonstrated as radioactive uptake images. SUV is the most commonly used semiquantitative index in diagnostic PET examination, demonstrating local tissue metabolism. SUVmax being no less than 2.5 is recognized to be a relatively objective index to differentiate malignancies from benign tumors. However, as non-specific tumor tracers, ^{18}F-FDG can be uptake in different degrees in some benign diseases, such as benign tumors, active inflammation and tuberculosis. In some cases, the uptake of ^{18}F-FDG can reach a high level, resulting in false positive findings.

2. Gene expression in molecular imaging includes antisense imaging and reporter gene expression imaging.

3. Receptor molecular imaging includes dopaminergic system and 5-hydroxytryptamine nervous system as well as acetylcholine receptor, among which the dopaminergic system is the common focus in scientific studies.

PET/CT is the integration of PET technology and multislice spiral CT technology into one framework of machine for simultaneous images collection of the nuclear medicine and CT scanning. The two kinds of images can be merged. The merged images demonstrate functional information and complicated anatomic information. Therefore, the advantages of the two technologies are combined, with a high clinical value.

PET/CT molecular imaging is applied for the diagnosis of following HIV/AIDS related diseases:

1. CNS diseases

   It can be used for the diagnosis of HIV encephalitis, opportunistic infections, cerebral cysticercosis and cerebral white matter demyelination.

2. Chest diseases

   PET/CT can be applied for the diagnosis and differential diagnosis of pulmonary benign tumors, pulmonary malignancies, pulmonary TB and pulmonary fungal infections. In addition, it can also be used to assess the activity of pulmonary TB. Meanwhile, it has a high detection rate for lesions at the structurally complex location or small lymph nodes with a diameter of less than 1.0 cm.

3. Abdominal diseases

   It can be used for the diagnosis of AIDS complicated by liver cancer, abdominal organs tuberculosis and other abdominal diseases.

26.2.1 Brain PET-CT for HIV/AIDS

HIV encephalopathy: Brain ^{18}F-FDG PET imaging shows low cortical metabolic areas and subcortical (such as basal ganglia and thalamus) high metabolic areas in HIV positive with or without neurological symptoms. It is recognized that the subcortical high metabolism is characteristically early HIV dementia, while cortical and subcortical low metabolism is a sign of advanced HIV infection. AIDS children without neurological symptoms show cortical low metabolic lesions in the temporal and occipital lobes, predominantly right side. AIDS children with neurological symptoms show cortical diffuse low metabolic lesions and subcortical high metabolic lesions.

Case Study 1

A patient who was confirmatively diagnosed as having AIDS by the CDC. He/She had fever, and following numbness and weakness of the left limbs in early 2010, and was diagnosed as having encephalitis. He/She received anti-viral therapy and physiotherapy. His/Her CD4 T cell count was 33/μl.

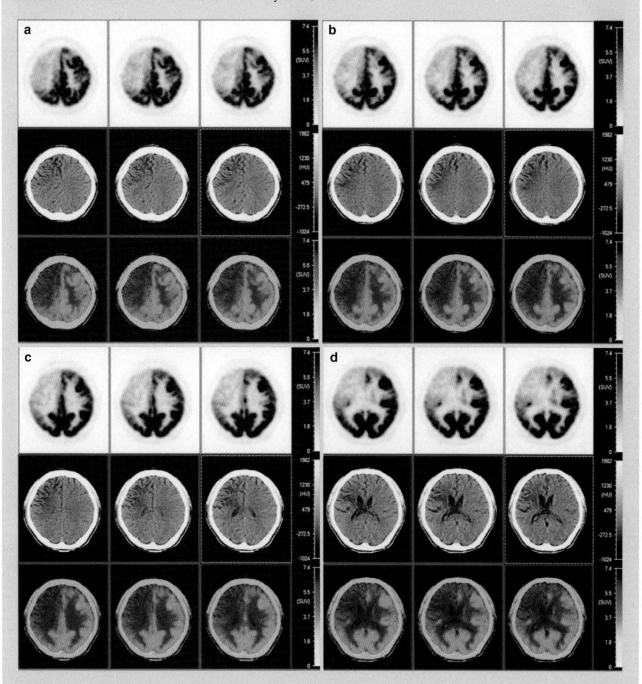

Fig. 26.15 (**a–g**) HIV/AIDS related HIV encephalopathy. (**a–d**) The imaging reexamination after treatment demonstrates decreased density of the brain white matter in bilateral frontal lobes, right temporal lobe, right basal ganglia and the left cerebellar hemisphere. PET demonstrates the decrease of the radioactive uptake in the corresponding locations, and no abnormal increase or decrease of the radioactive uptake in other parts of brain parenchyma. (**e–g**) PET/CT demonstrates lowest metabolic activity in the right basal ganglia

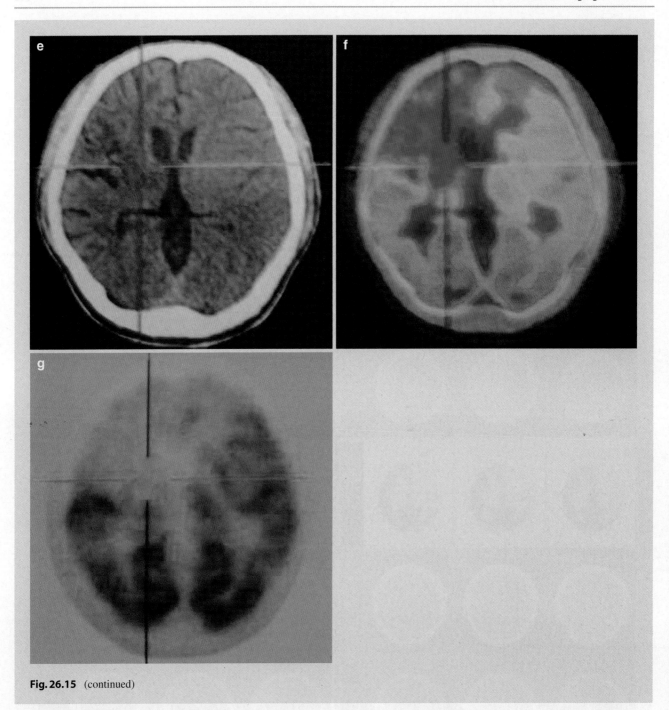

Fig. 26.15 (continued)

Case Study 2

A female patient aged 31 years was confirmatively diagnosed as having AIDS by the CDC. She had intermittent fever for half a year, cough for 4 months, dizziness and accompanying paroxysmal distensile headache, nausea and vomiting for 1 month. Her CD4 T cell count was 149/μl.

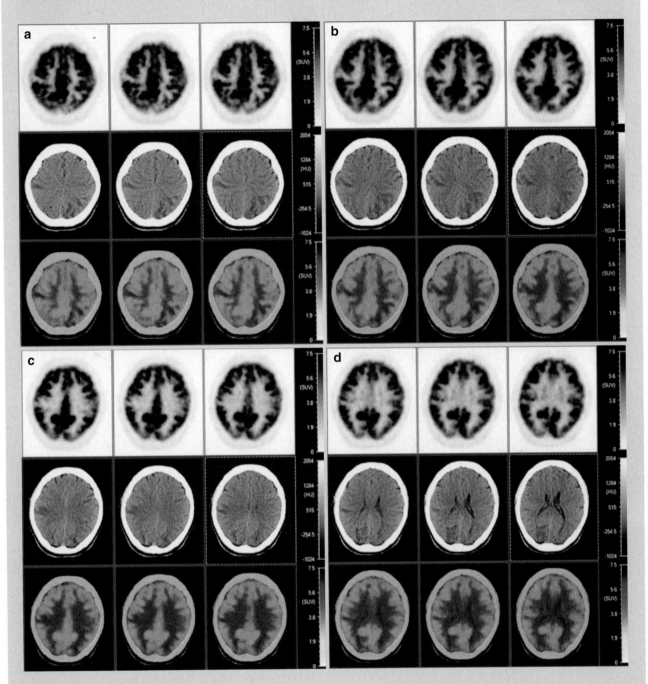

Fig. 26.16 (a–g) HIV/AIDS related cerebral tuberculoma. (a–d) Plain CT scanning demonstrates multiple strips and flakes of low density shadows in the frontal, parietal and occipital lobes. PET imaging demonstrates slightly increased radioactive uptake of the lesions in the right frontal lobe, with SUVmax is about 8.42; and slightly decreased radioactive uptake of the other brain parts. (e–g) PET-CT demonstrates the lowest metabolic activity of the lesions in the right side

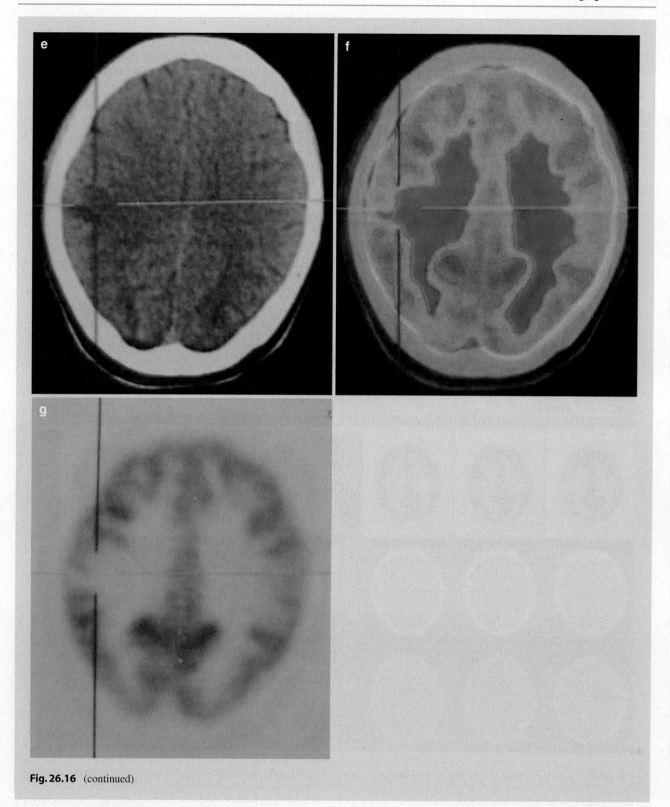

Fig. 26.16 (continued)

Case Study 3

A male patient aged 35 years was confirmatively diagnosed as having AIDS by the CDC. He had intermittent fever and cough for more than 4 months. His CD4 T cell count was 287/μl and his VL was less than 50.

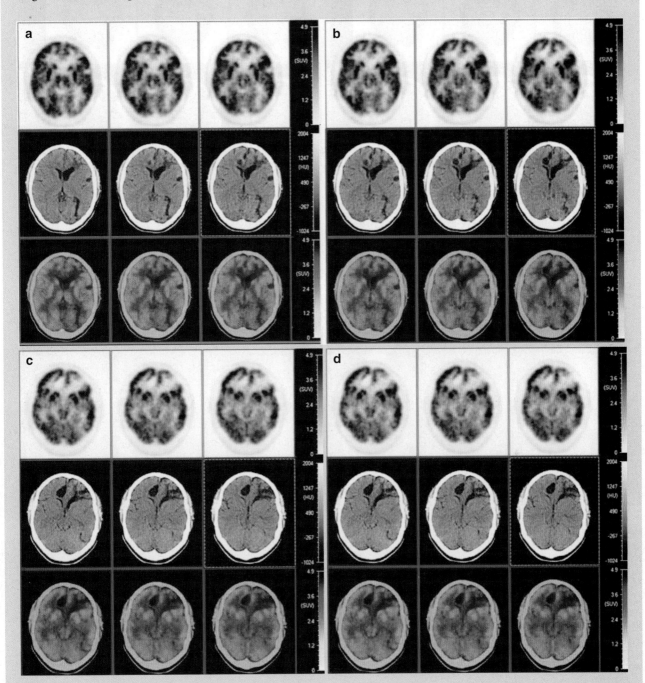

Fig. 26.17 (a–k) HIV/AIDS related cerebral cysticercosis. (a–f) MR imaging demonstrates decreased radioactive uptake in bilateral frontal lobes, left temporal lobe and right parietal lobe. CT scanning with the same scanner demonstrates cystic density shadows in bilateral frontal lobes, left temporal lobe and right parietal lobe (g–i), another flaky low density shadow in the left parietal lobe (k), Bilateral lateral ventricles are asymmetry, the left ventricle is widened. (j) CT scanning demonstrates scattered spots and nodular high density, no abnormal increase or decrease of radioactive uptake by PET imaging of the corresponding areas. There are multiple intracranial stripes, flakes and nodular low density shadows, with decreased metabolic activities in the corresponding areas. In addition, multiple spots and nodular high density lesions can be found in the brain, with no increased metabolic activity

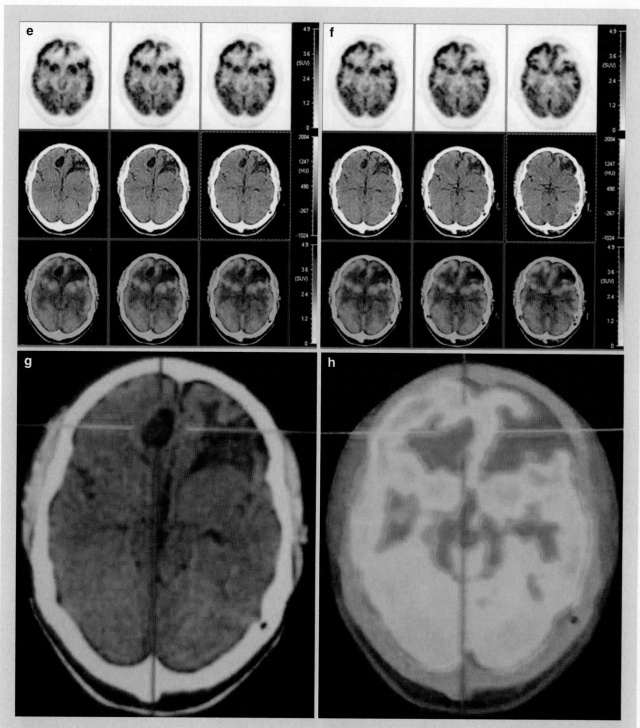

Fig. 26.17 (continued)

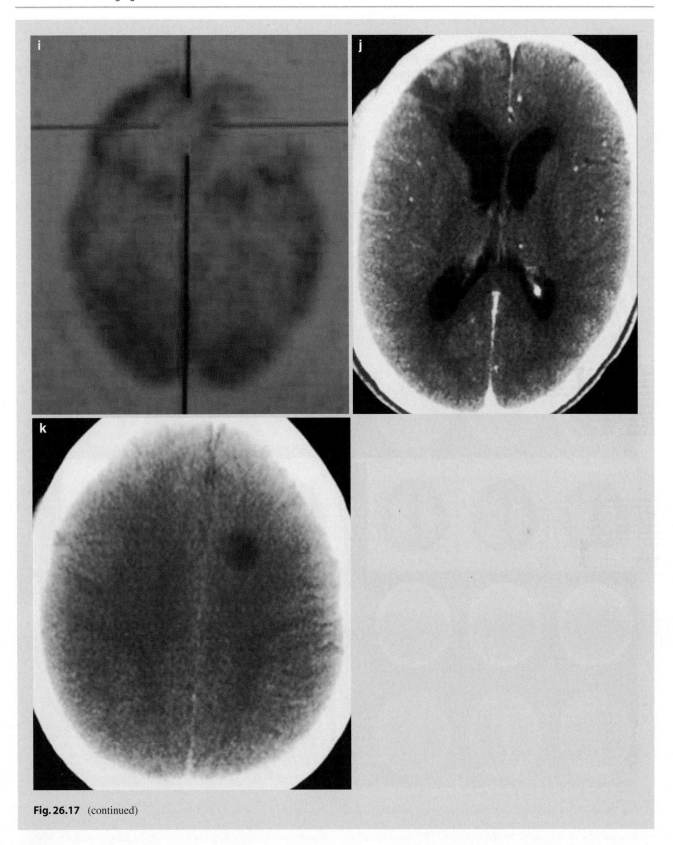

Fig. 26.17 (continued)

Case Study 4

A male patient aged 37 years was confirmatively diagnosed as having AIDS by the CDC. He had intermittent headache for 3 months, consciousness disturbance for 10 days, fever for 7 days, weakened pain of the right lower limb and IV grade muscular strength. One week ago, he received brain MR imaging, with findings of multiple intracranial space occupying lesions. Intracranial puncture for biopsy was then performed.

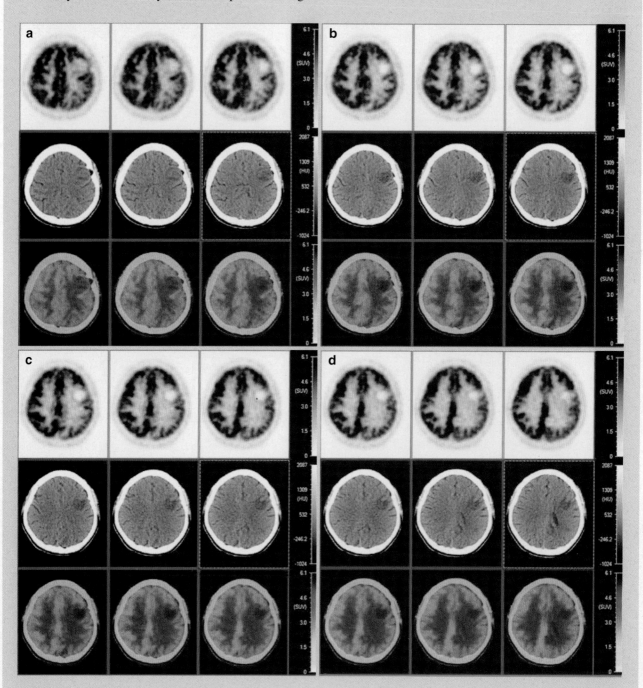

Fig. 26.18 (**a–o**) HIV/AIDS related brain fungal infection. (**a–i**) After brain tissue biopsy, there are partial left cranial defect and irregular low-density areas on the left skull. PET imaging of the corresponding areas shows radioactive defect. Slightly low density shadows with unclear boundaries can be found in the right occipital lobe, left parietal lobe adjacent to the brain falx, left temporal lobe and the left frontal lobe. PET imaging of the corresponding areas demonstrates radioactive decrease or defect. (**j–o**) MR imaging demonstrates multiple large flakes of long T1 long T2 edema lesions in the brain, ring shaped long and short T1, long and short T2 mixed signals in the left temporal lobe. Enhanced imaging demonstrates intracranial multiple ring shaped enhancement of the lesions

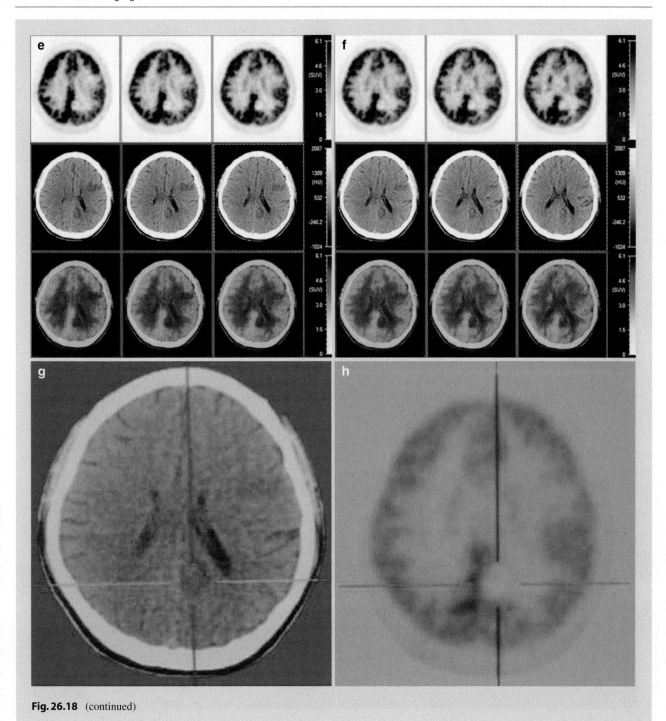

Fig. 26.18   (continued)

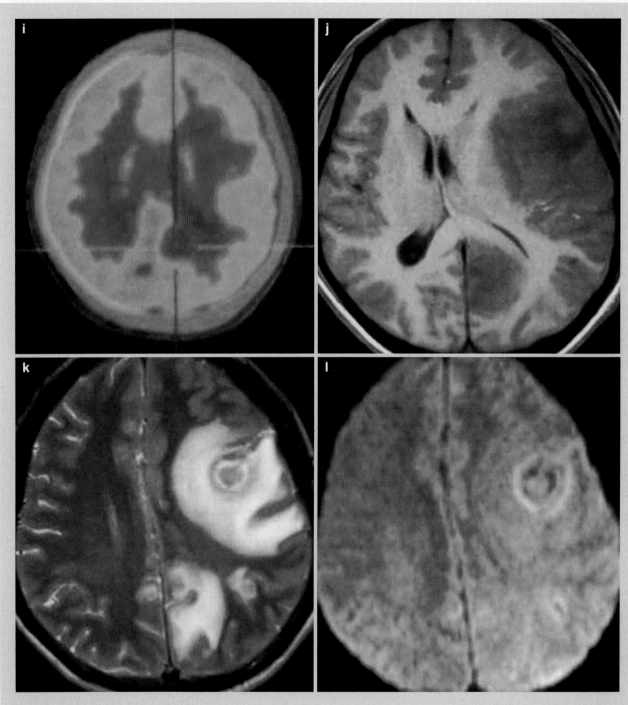

Fig. 26.18 (continued)

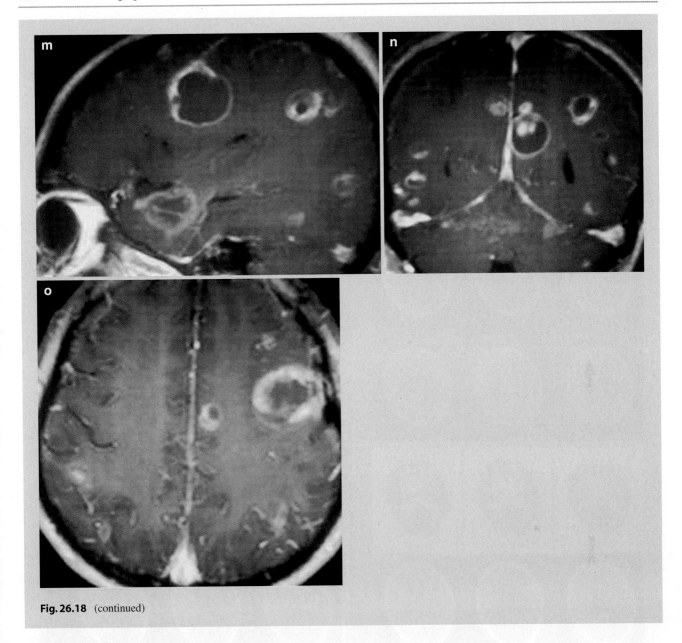

Fig. 26.18 (continued)

Case Study 5

A female patient aged 46 years was confirmatively diagnosed as having AIDS by the CDC. She had intermittent fever for 3 months, and consciousness disturbance for 1 month. Her CD4 T cell count was 266/μl. Lumbar puncture demonstrated that cerebral pressure normal, no abnormalities of CSF biochemical examination and CSF culture.

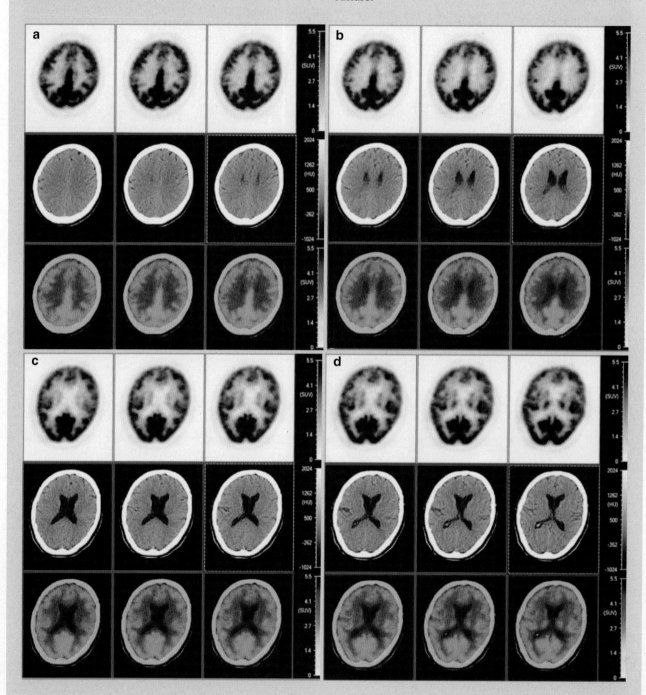

Fig. 26.19 (a–l) HIV/AIDS related cerebral infarction and tuberculoma. (a–e) PET-CT demonstrates normal morphology of the cerebral cortex, even and bilaterally symmetric radioactive distribution in bilateral cerebral hemisphere cortex, thalamus, basal ganglia, cerebellum and brain stem, with no abnormal increase or decrease of radioactivity distribution. CT scanning demonstrates all sections with no obvious abnormal density changes of the brain parenchyma. There are bilaterally symmetric ventricles, no dilation of ventricles, no widened of the cisterns and sulci, no migration of the midline structures, and no obvious abnormalities in the brain stem and the cerebellum. Cerebral glucose metabolic imaging demonstrates no foci of abnormally increased metabolic activity. (f–l) Cranial MR imaging demonstrates spots long T1 and long T2 signal in the white matter of bilateral basal ganglia and bilateral frontal and parietal lobes. Enhanced imaging demonstrates multiple round liked enhancement of lesions in the brain

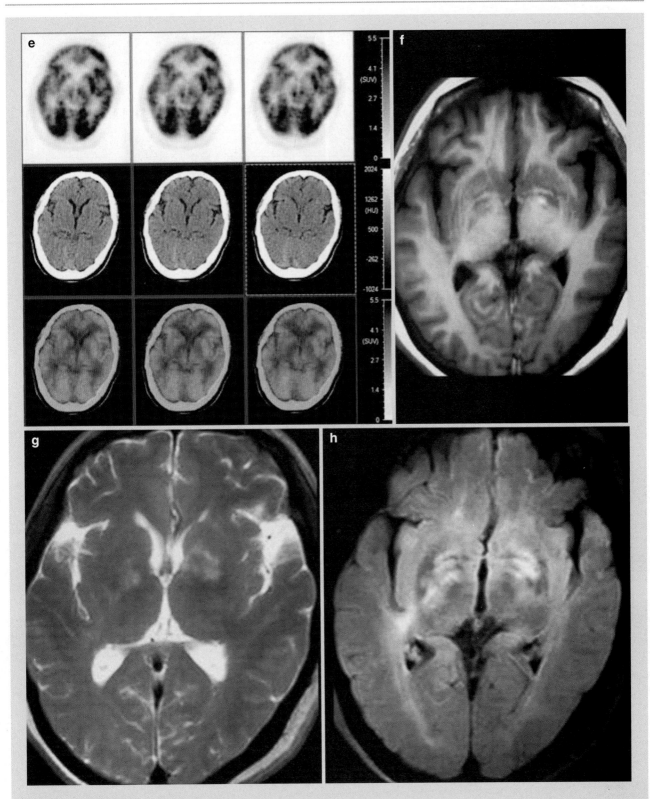

Fig. 26.19 (continued)

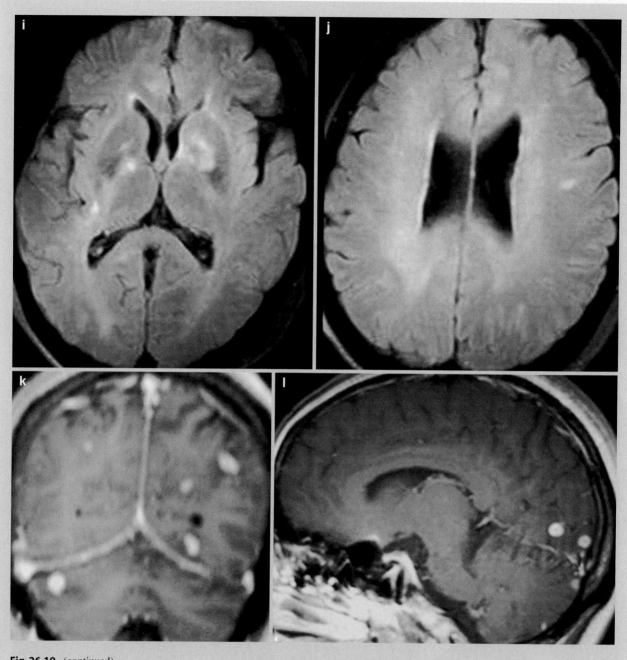

Fig. 26.19 (continued)

26.2.2 Pulmonary PET-CT for HIV/AIDS

26.2.2.1 Pulmonary Tuberculosis

Tuberculosis is one of the common complications of AIDS, which is also one of the early opportunistic infections. Its incidence is 30 times as high as that in immunocompetent population. Due to the seriously compromised immunity in AIDS patients, the imaging demonstrations of TB are diverse and complex, which are non-specific.

The imaging demonstrations of AIDS complicated by tuberculosis are related to the immune status of the patients. In the cases of early HIV infection, the CD4 T cell count shows no decrease. At this time, the imaging demonstrations are similar to the immunocompetent patients of TB. In the cases of middle and advanced HIV infection, the CD4 T cell count obviously decreases or extremely decreases. At this time, the immunity is moderately or seriously inhibited, with manifestations of primary pulmonary TB. Compared to HIV negative patients, the HIV positive patients have enlarged mediastinal lymph nodes, atypical infiltration and more miliary tuberculosis lesions. However, cavity formation, thickened bronchial wall, nodules, micronodules and thickened lobular septa rarely occur. These findings indicate that HIV positive patients with TB have less focal parenchymal lesions of the lungs, but more diffuse lesions.

^{18}F-FDG PET imaging demonstrates old tuberculosis as negative, but active tuberculosis is demonstrated as increased ^{18}F-FDG uptake. Most of the lesions are proliferative lesions or tuberculous nodules of proliferative lesions containing large quantity epithelioid cells, the Langhans giant cells and lymphocytes. The metabolisms of these inflammatory cells are active, with increased uptake of ^{18}F- FDG and even SUVmax being above 10. Pulmonary TB, by ^{18}F-FDG PET imaging, can be divided into four basic types: (1) Focal concentrated ^{18}F-FDG of TB lesions; (2) Pulmonary lesions complicated by concentrated ^{18}F-FDG of hilar or mediastinal lymph nodes; (3) Pulmonary lesions complicated by concentrated ^{18}F-FDG of supraclavicular, mediastinal and abdominal lymph nodes; (4) Extensive concentrated ^{18}F-FDG in the pleura. By dual-phase ^{18}F-FDG PET imaging, SUVmax of pulmonary tuberculosis delays, with its significantly increase compared to normal SUVmax. Its amplitude of increase is similar to malignant lesions. Therefore, for the diagnosis of atypical lesions, CT or HRCT demonstrations by the same scanner should be combined, including the assessment of satellite lesions and ground glass liked changes. Combined imaging with ^{11}C-Choline or ^{18}F-FLT can be performed if necessary.

Immunity is seriously compromised in patients with AIDS complicated by pulmonary tuberculosis, which fails to confine the tubercle bacilli. Therefore, the infection can further involve the lymph nodes, hilum and mediastinum to cause hilar and mediastinal scrofula. Based on occurrence of ^{18}F-FDG uptake by lymph nodes, the detection rate of lymph nodes by PET is higher than that by CT. One of the reasons is that PET facilitates detecting lymph nodes in the complicated structures, such as double supraclavicular fossa, hilum, posterior mediastinum and peri-diaphragm lymph nodes. Another reason is that PET can detect small lymph nodes with a diameter of less than 1.0 cm. Due to the high sensitivity of ^{18}F-FDG and poor specificity of tumor, the high $^{18F\text{-}FDG}$ uptake of hilar and mediastinal lymph node tuberculosis can hardly be differentiated from lymph node metastases or lymphoma metastasis. CT density analysis of the intake positive lymph nodes by the same scanner can exclude the false positives findings by PET. The cases of PET positive but CT scanning by the same scanner demonstrates calcification or higher density than in the mediastinal lymph nodes of the major blood vessels mostly have benign lesions.

Case Study 1

A male patient aged 59 years was confirmatively diagnosed as having AIDS by the CDC. He had intermittent headache, cough and expectoration for half a year. By physical examination, a palpable swollen lymph node in size of 1 cm×2 cm in the left neck, which is flexible and movable, with tenderness. Auscultation demonstrated decreased breathing sound of the left lung. Bronchoscopy demonstrated narrowed right trunk and segments of the right upper lobe due to external compression, large quantity white sticky secretions in the apical segment. The lavage fluid examination demonstrated tuberculosis, mycelium and spores as well as commonly found bacteria, with negative findings. His CD4 T cell count was 38/μl.

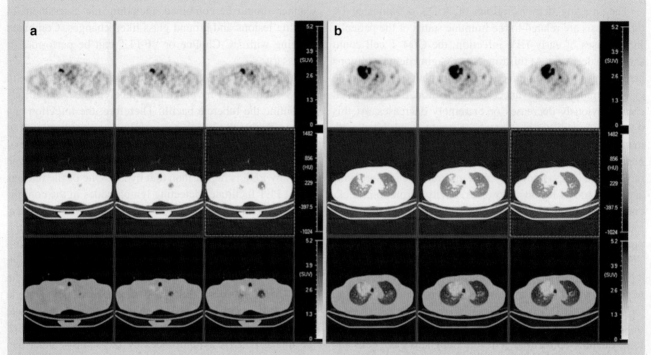

Fig. 26.20 (a–e) HIV/AIDS related hilar lymph node tuberculosis. (a–e) PET-CT demonstrates nodules in different sizes and flakes of increased radioactive uptake areas in the right hilum and right upper lung lobe adjacent to the mediastinum, with SUVmax is about 10.37. Plain CT scanning of the corresponding areas by the same scanner demonstrates flaky and nodular shadows. There is nodular lesions with increased radioactive uptake in the right supraclavicular fossa, mediastinum, and 1 L/2R/4R areas; larger lesion in the 4R area with higher radioactive uptake in a size of about 1.4×2.6 cm. The SUVmax is about 10.66. Plain CT scanning of the corresponding areas with the same scanner demonstrates soft tissue nodules shadows in different sizes. Plain CT scanning with the same scanner demonstrates a small nodule shadow in the left upper lung lobe, with a diameter of about 0.4 cm and large area of surrounding ground glass liked shadows. PET imaging of the corresponding areas demonstrates slightly higher radioactive uptake, with SUVmax is 8 about 1.22. Plain CT scanning with the same scanner demonstrates patch shadow near the left hilum of the lung; PET imaging of the corresponding areas demonstrates slightly higher radioactive uptake, with SUVmax is about 2.88. Plain CT scanning with the same scanner demonstrates multiple small nodular shadows in both lungs, high density of some lesions. PET imaging of the corresponding areas demonstrates no obvious increase of the radioactive uptake

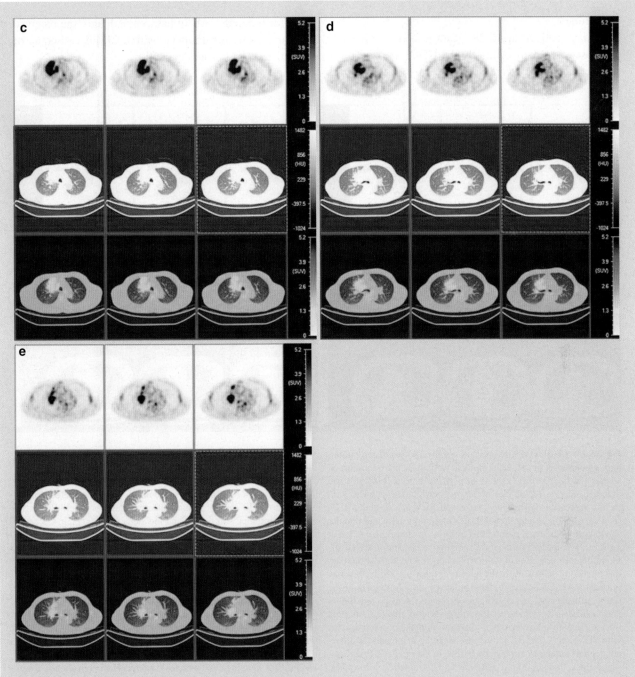

Fig. 26.20 (continued)

Case Study 2

A female patient aged 28 years was confirmatively diagnosed as having AIDS by the CDC. She had fever, cough, fatigue and weight loss for 7 months, lower back pain for 6 months. About half a month ago, she received abdominal abscess drainage, with a CD4 T cell count of 357/μl and VL was less than 50.

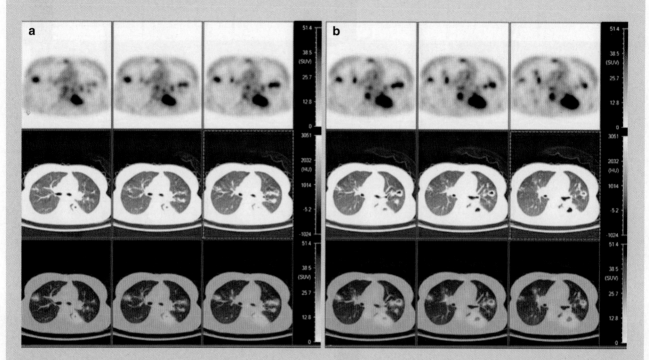

Fig. 26.21 (**a–q**) HIV/AIDS related systemic disseminated pulmonary tuberculosis (lungs, right thoracic wall, systemic bones, brain, spleen and both kidneys). (**g, i, o, p**) After abscess puncture and drainage, there are puncture points in the right lower back, with locally increased radioactive uptake and SUVmax is about 4.75. (**a–e, h, q**) CT scanning demonstrates multiple patchy and nodular shadows in both lungs, round liked transparent areas in some larger lesions. PET imaging of the corresponding areas demonstrates different degrees increases of radioactive uptake, the highest radioactive uptake by the lesions in the left lower lung lobe, with SUVmax is about 9.42. CT scanning demonstrates multiple nodules in the retroperitoneal and pelvis, with lower central density but higher peripheral density. The larger lesion is in size of 1.8×2.8 cm. PET imaging demonstrates increased radioactive uptake of some lesions, with SUVmax is 6.65. (**f, j, l–n**) PET imaging demonstrates different degrees radioactive uptake by lesions in the right 5–6 costal cartilage areas, thoracic 11–12 vertebrae and surrounding soft tissues, lumbar 3 to sacral vertebrae and surrounding tissues, left iliac and ischium surrounding soft tissues and right psoas major muscle; the highest radioactive uptake of the lesions in the surrounding areas of left iliac, with SUVmax is about 13.43. Plain CT scanning with the same scanner demonstrates thoracic subcutaneous soft tissue nodules in the right 5–6 costal cartilage areas, focal bone defects of the thoracic 11–12 vertebrae and different degrees swelling of the above mentioned soft tissues and low density areas. Plain CT scanning with the same scanner demonstrates multiple slightly higher density nodules in the spleen and both kidneys. PET imaging of the corresponding areas demonstrates no abnormal radioactive uptake lesions and no abnormal increase of radioactive uptake by the lesions of the neck and axillary lymph nodes, no increase of radioactive uptake by bilateral groin lymph nodes. (**k**) MRI imaging demonstrates scattering multiple nodular lesions with slightly higher density in the bilateral brain hemispheres and right cerebellar hemisphere. The largest lesion is in the left head of the caudate nucleus, in a size of about 1.0×0.8 cm and surrounding low density areas. PET imaging demonstrates the largest lesion in slightly lower radioactive distribution and no abnormal increase or decrease of radioactive uptake by other lesions

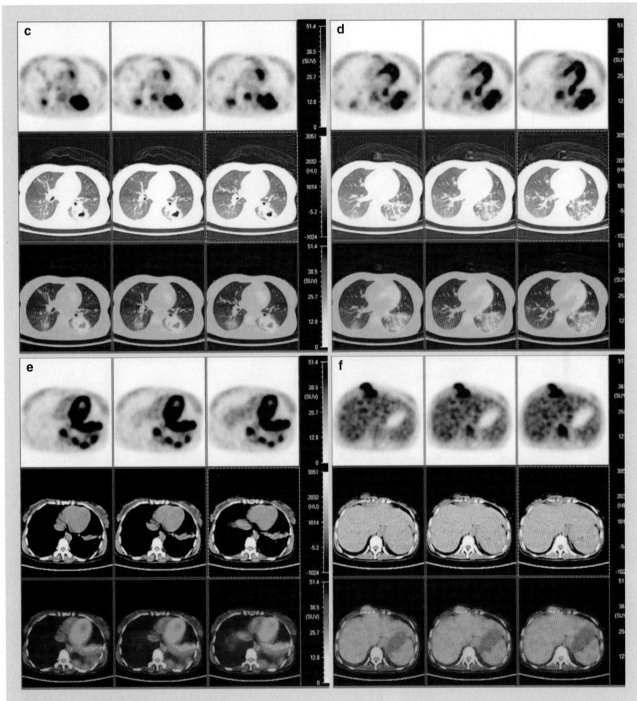

Fig. 26.21 (continued)

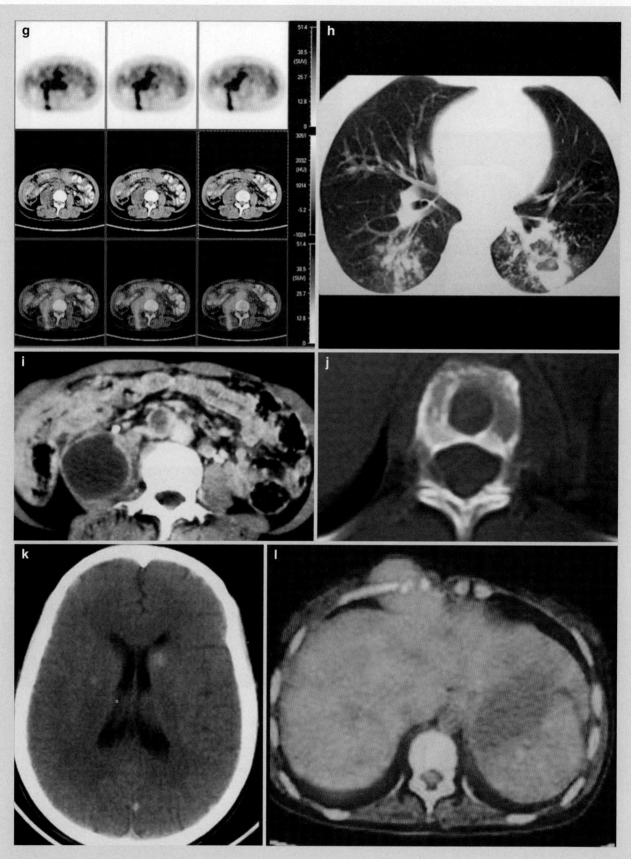

Fig. 26.21 (continued)

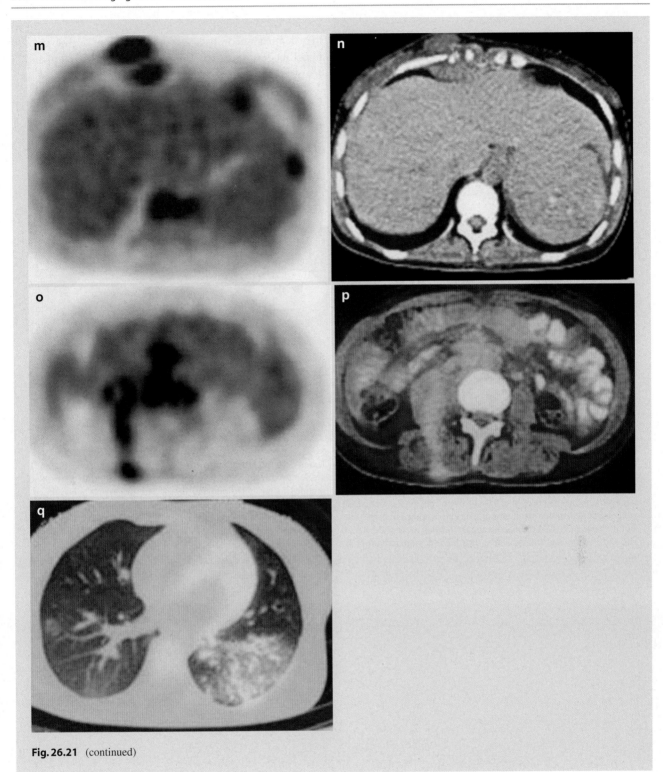

Fig. 26.21 (continued)

Case Study 3

A male patient aged 68 years was confirmatively diagnosed as having AIDS by the CDC. He had fever, cough, expectoration and fatigue. CT scanning 2 years ago demonstrated space occupying lesions in the right upper mediastinum. His CD4 T cell count was 229/μl and VL was less than 50.

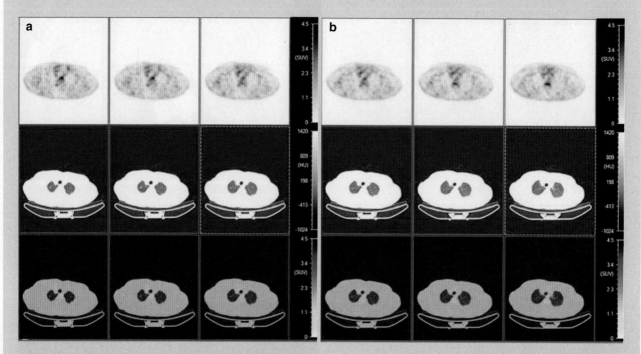

Fig. 26.22 (a–f) HIV/AIDS related mediastinal lymph node tuberculosis. (a–d) Demonstrations of multiple nodules in different sizes in the right upper lung lobe and the both lower lung lobes; the largest lesion in the left lower lung lobe in size of 0.9 cm × 1.1 cm. PET imaging demonstrates no abnormal radioactive uptake in both lungs but multiple increased radioactive uptake lesions in the mediastinal 4R and 7 areas and bilateral hila. The highest radioactive uptake lesion is in the left hilum, with a SUVmax is about 5.49. Plain CT scanning with the same scanner demonstrates multiple soft tissue nodules in the corresponding areas. The largest nodule is in the mediastinal 4R area, in size of about 2.1 × 1.0 cm. (e, f) Scanning demonstrates solid mass in the right upper lung apex, with coarse edge

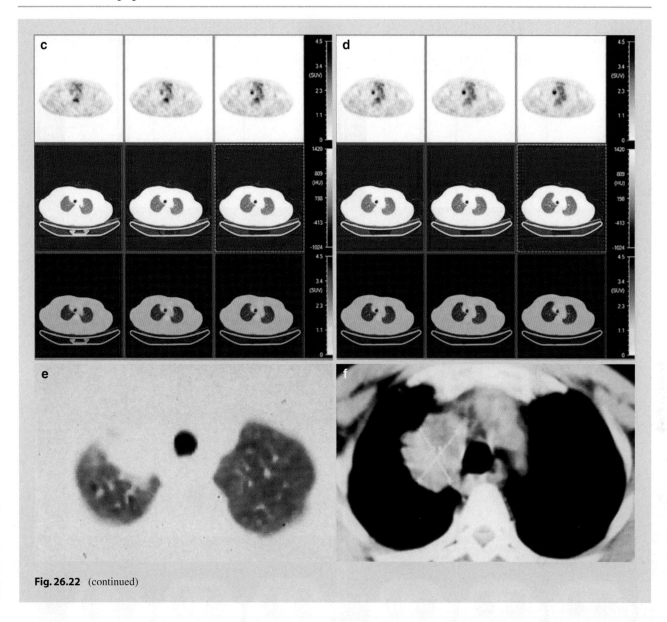

Fig. 26.22   (continued)

A male patient aged 36 years was confirmatively diagnosed as having AIDS by the CDC. He had lower back pain and his CD4 T cell count was less than 100/μl.

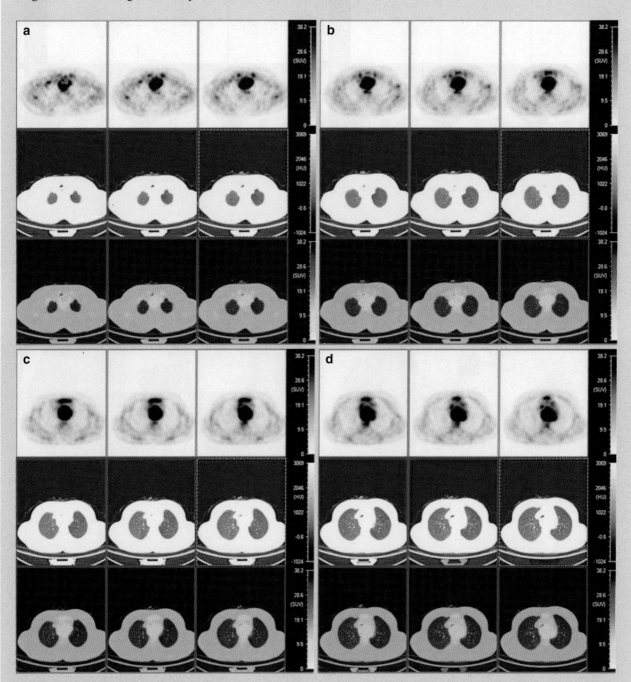

Fig. 26.23 (a–d) HIV/AIDS related pulmonary tuberculosis, mediastinal lymph node tuberculosis and sternum tuberculosis. (a–d) Plain CT scanning with the same scanner demonstrates multiple spots, flakes and strips of high density shadows in the both lungs. PET imaging of the corresponding areas demonstrates different degrees increase of radioactive uptake, with SUVmax is about 2.07. There are multiple strips of increased radioactive uptake areas in the bilateral pleura, which is higher in the right pleura. The SUVmax is about 4.16. Plain CT scanning with the same scanner demonstrates thickened pleura. CT scanning demonstrates water liked density shadows in the bilateral basal thoracic cavity. There are also multiple nodular lesions with higher metabolic activities in the mediastinum and bilateral hilus, which is higher in the mediastinum 7 area.

The SUVmax is about 4.44. Plain CT scanning with the same scanner demonstrates soft tissue shadows in different sizes and larger lesions in the mediastinum in size of about 2.5 cm × 1.2 cm. nodular lesions with increased radioactive uptake can be found in the left bronchus, with SUVmax is about 4.44. Plain CT scanning with the same scanner demonstrates irregular morphology of the left bronchus, with narrowed lumen and local soft tissue shadows. Focal lesions with increased radioactive uptake can be found in the bilateral extremitas sternalis claviculae and the mucronate cartilage, with SUVmax is about 6.71. Plain CT scanning with the same scanner demonstrates unevenly decreased bone density of the extremitas sternalis claviculae, with surrounding swollen soft tissue shadows, which can be also found around the mucronate cartilage

Case Study 5

A female patient aged 46 years was confirmatively diagnosed as having AIDS by the CDC. She had intermittent fever, cough and expectoration. About 1 year ago, she received stent implantation for esophageal carcinoma. Her CD4 T cell count was 97/μl.

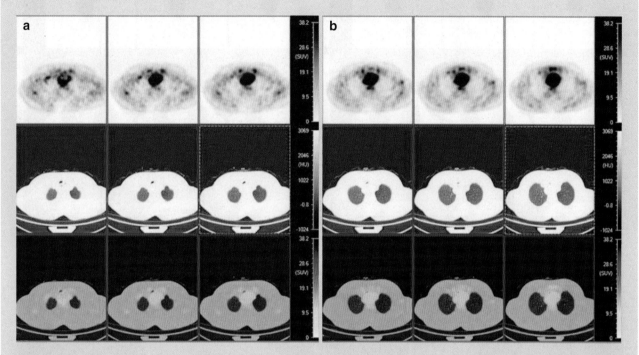

Fig. 26.24 (a–g) HIV/AIDS related esophageal carcinoma and accompanying pulmonary TB. (**a–d**) After stent implantation for esophageal carcinoma, there is mental stent shadow in the esophagus; PET demonstrations of irregular increased radioactive uptake lesions from the sternal angle downwards to the thoracic seventh vertebra, with a range of 8.4×9.6×12.3 cm and SUVmax is about 8.81; plain CT scanning demonstrations by the same scanner of irregular thickening of the esophageal wall, multiple nodular lesions with increased radioactive uptake in the abdominal cavity adjacent to the preventriculus and posterior peritoneum, with larger lesions and higher radioactive uptake in the posterior peritoneum, with a range of 2.5×2.9×2.8 cm and SUVmax is about 5.22; plain CT scanning demonstrations by the same scanner of enlarged spleen and the spleen thickness at the spleen hilus being about 5.6 cm; PET imaging demonstrates higher radioactive uptake by the spleen than that by the liver, with SUVmax is about 3.23. Plain CT scanning with the same scanner demonstrates cords liked shadows in both lungs. PET imaging of the corresponding areas demonstrates no obvious increase of the radioactive uptake. (**e**) Esophageal barium meal demonstrates mental stent in the middle esophagus, irregular stenosis and stiffness of the esophagus at both ends of the stent. (**f, g**) Chest CT scanning demonstrates soft tissue mass shadows in the mediastinum and internal mental stent shadow

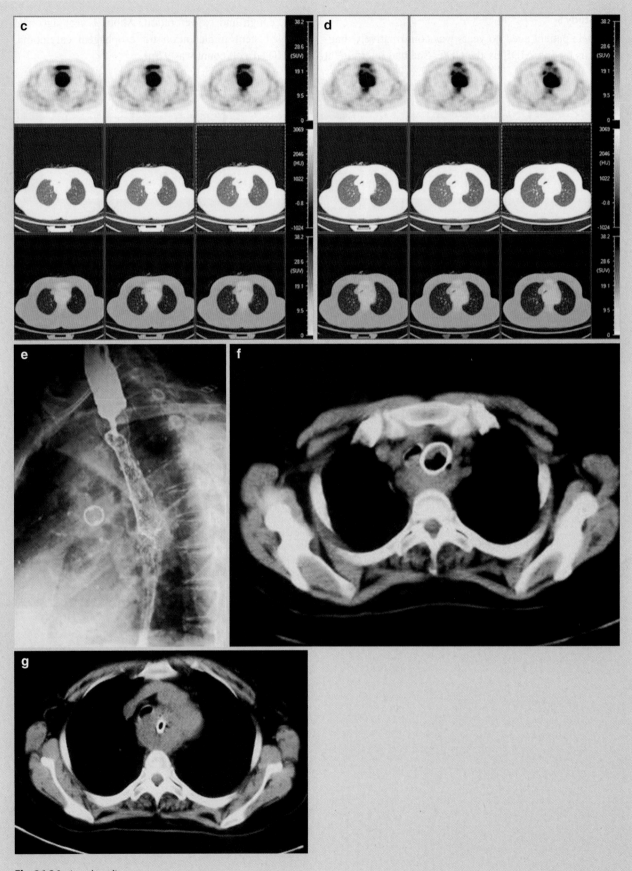

Fig. 26.24 (continued)

26.2.2.2 Hepatocellular Carcinoma (HCC)

The occurrence of HCC is closely related to hepatitis B and hepatocirrhosis. About 50–90 % cases of HCC is complicated by hepatocirrhosis. And about 30–50 % cases of hepatocirrhosis is complicated by hepatocellular carcinoma. The clinical symptoms occur commonly in the middle and advanced stages, with manifestations of liver pain, weight loss, fatigue, abdominal mass and jaundice in the advanced stage. About 60–90 % cases of HCC have AFP positive. Pathologically, hepatocellular carcinoma can be categorized into giant mass, nodular type and diffuse type. The carcinoma is supplied by the hepatic artery and about 90 % cases have abundant blood supply to the tumor.

The CT scanning classification of hepatocellular carcinoma is the same as the pathological classification. The giant mass and nodular types have singular/multiple round or round liked low density masses, and rare cases have equal or high density masses. The mass is in expansive growth, with marginal pseudocapsule as well as clear and smooth margin, which is the sign for the diagnosis by CT scanning. Diffuse nodular type has an extensive distribution, with unclear boundary. Enhanced scanning demonstrates typical "rapid in and rapid out" sign. MR imaging demonstrates similar findings as CT scanning. On T1WI imaging, the tumor is demonstrated as slightly low or equal signal. On T2WI imaging, the tumor is demonstrated as slightly high or equal signal.

Enhanced imaging by SPIO contrast, T2WI still demonstrates slightly high signal due to the lack of Kupffer cells in the tumor.

^{18}F-FDG is a glucose analog substance, which is transported into the cells by glucose transporter protein on the surface of the cell membrane. After the transportation, it is phosphorylated with contributions from hexokinase to form ^{18}F-FDG-6-phosphate, which has no free access to the cell membrane and remains in the cells. But there are abundant glucose-6-phosphatase in the liver tissue. The enzyme can dephosphorylate the ^{18}F-FDG-6-phosphate to produce free ^{18}F-FDG, which finally is transported from the intracellular to the extracellular. Therefore, the concentrated ^{18}F-FDG uptake of HCC cancer cells depends mainly on the level of phosphorylation and dephosphorylation. The more active biological behaviors of cancer cells can cause the higher the malignancy degree, the greater heterogeneity of the tumors and the poorer synthesis of glucose-6-phosphatase, which lead to lower level of dephosphorylation and high uptake of ^{18}F-FDG by the lesions. However, the liver tumor cells show special glucose uptake. The high concentration of glucose-6-phosphatase in well differentiated tumor cells can accelerate the metabolic process of ^{18}F-FDG. Therefore, the low content of ^{18}F-FDG in highly differentiated HCC tumor cells does not necessarily indicate high metabolism. PET/CT imaging commonly demonstrates negative findings, with false negative.

Case Study

A female patient aged 59 years was confirmatively diagnosed as having AIDS by the CDC. She had abdominal distension for half a year and changed bowel movement for more than 10 days.

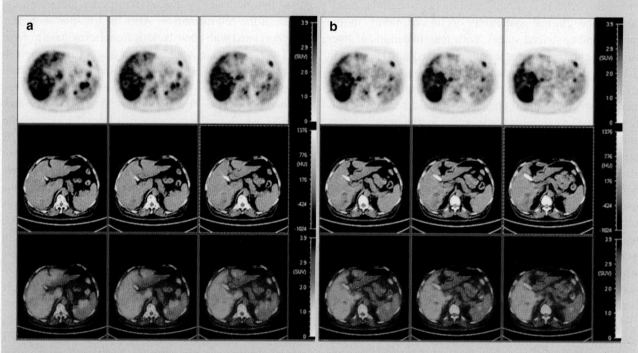

Fig. 26.25 (a–h) HIV/AIDS related hepatocellular carcinoma with peritoneal metastasis. (a–e) PET-CT scanning demonstrates irregular lesions with increased radioactive uptake in the right hepatic lobe, with SUVmax is about 6.86. Plain CT scanning of the corresponding areas with the same scanner demonstrates low density with unclear boundaries. There are also focal lesions with increased radioactive uptake in the left hepatic lobe with SUVmax is about 4.16. Plain CT scanning of the corresponding areas with the same scanner demonstrates low density shadows with unclear boundaries. CT scanning demonstrates small quantity arch shaped water density under the hepatocapsule. Mass liked lesions with increased radioactive uptake can be found at the splenic hilum, with an active range of 2.7×2.8×2.3 cm and SUVmax is about 6.19. Plain CT scanning of the corresponding areas with the same scanner demonstrates soft tissue nodular shadows in different sizes. Multiple nodular lesions with increased radioactive uptake can be found in the anterior hepatocapsule, posterior peritoneum and abdominal cavity and higher radioactive uptake by the lesions in the posterior peritoneum, with SUVmax is about 5.85. Plain CT scanning of the corresponding areas with the same scanner demonstrates soft tissue nodular shadows in different sizes. Mass liked lesions with increased radioactive uptake in the right lower abdomen (at the level of lumbar fourth vertebra), with an active range of 4.6×3.9×3.6 cm and SUVmax is 4.81. Plain CT scanning of the corresponding areas with the same scanner demonstrates soft tissue uneven density, and unclearly defined lesions from the surrounding intestinal tracts. (f–h) MR imaging demonstrates round uneven equal to long T2 signal in the right hepatic lobe. Enhanced imaging demonstrates uneven enhancement and internal irregular enhancement of the lesions

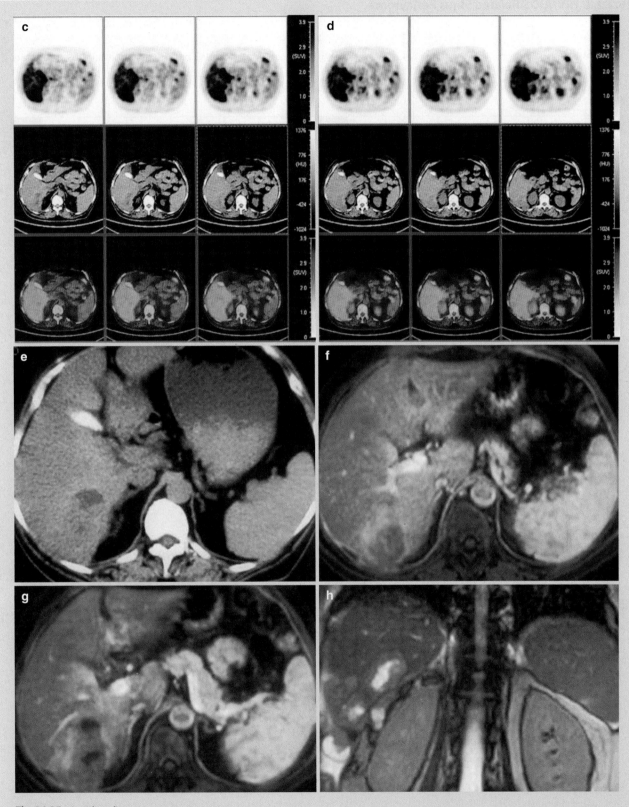

Fig. 26.25 (continued)

26.2.2.3 HIV/AIDS Related Sinus Pericytoma

Case Study
A male patient aged 57 years was confirmatively diagnosed as having AIDS by the CDC. He had left headache, eye orbital pain, left exophthalmos with tears and gradually exacerbated numbness for more than 8 months.

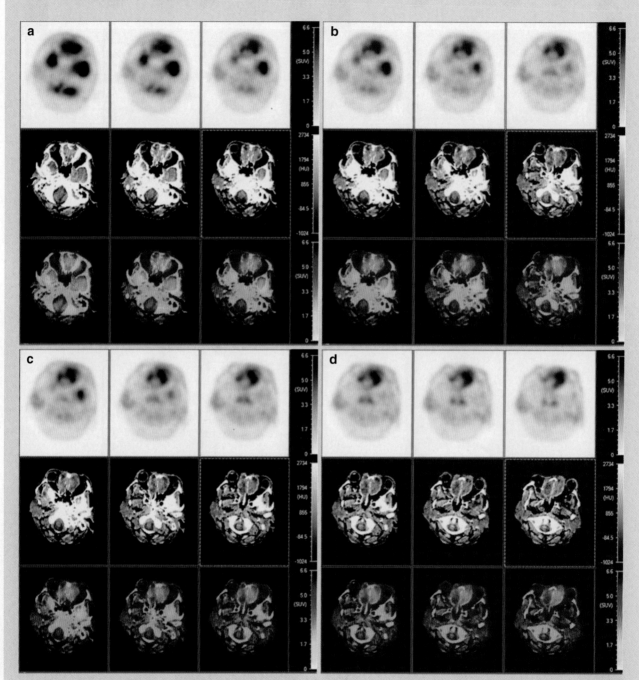

Fig. 26.26 (**a–h**) HIV/AIDS related sinus pericytoma. (**a–d**) PET imaging demonstrates lesions with increased radioactive uptake in the ethmoid sinus and the frontal sinus, with SUVmax is about 5.27 and an active range of 3.0×4.8×3.2 cm; and focal areas with decreased radioactive uptake in the right sinus cavity. (**e, f**) Plain CT scanning with the same scanner demonstrates soft tissue shadows filling the ethmoid sinus cavity with uneven density, focal low density shadow in the right ethomoid sinus cavity, unclearly defined ethomoid sinus, frontal sinus, internal orbital wall and basal cranial bone wall that protrudes outwards, migrated internal rectus muscle of both eyes due to compression, unclearly defined lesions from the frontal lobe. CT scanning demonstrates liquid density in the right maxillary sinus cavity, widened bilateral cisterns and sulcus. (**g, h**) Enhanced MR imaging demonstrates uneven enhancement of the soft tissues of the ethmoid sinus, with internal no enhancement area

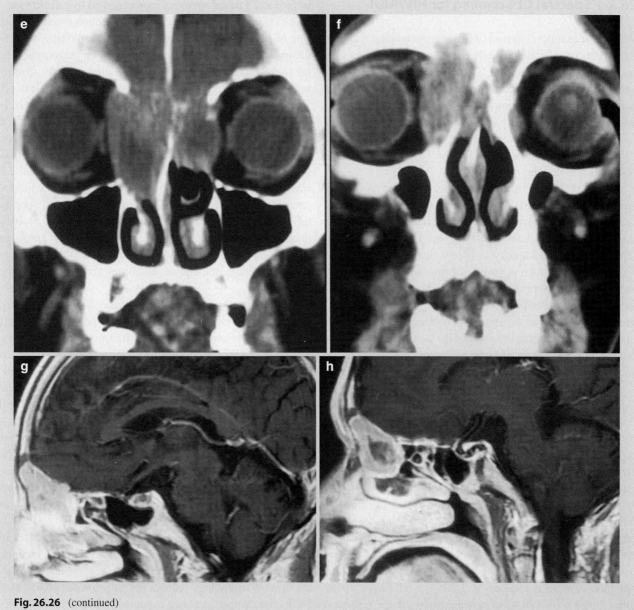

Fig. 26.26 (continued)

26.3   Spectral CT Scanning for HIV/AIDS

With the recent development of CT energy imaging technology, spectral CT scanning has been a research field attracting focused attention. Energy CT imaging has evolved from energy subtraction to monoenergetic spectrum and now it has developed into a new field. Currently, the clinically applied devices for energy CT scanning is gemstone spectral CT scanner with the core technology of instantaneous dual kVp. Another is dual-source CT (DSCT) whose core technology is double tubes.

As one of the functional imaging technologies, gemstone spectral imaging (GSI) has the functions that previous CT scanning failed to perform. Its basis of imaging is by using instant high and low voltage (80 kVp and 140 kVp) and their rapid switching technology to obtain two sets of absorbed projection data, which is then translated into density data of the substances. X-ray attenuation coefficient can be measured through high-speed switch of high and low voltages. This attenuation can be further converted to produce the same attenuation of the densities of the two substances. This process is known as the substance composition analysis and substance separation.

New material (gemstone) detector can be traced back to Garnet with special optical properties. After addition of lanthanon, its molecular structure is similar to gemstone. The detector has cubic structural unit, with favorable X-ray flash properties, specifically rapid conversion speed, high efficiency, high resolution, low noise and extremely low afterglow effect. It has the fastest initial speed, which is 100 times as fast as the conventional CT detector, which ensures the relatively independent data processing of high and low energy high-speed sampling. The sampling rate of the detector increases by 2.5 times, with great increase of the spatial resolution. Compared to the materials of other detectors, the radiation damage is reduced by 1/20. The automatic zoom tubes driven by instant energy change high-voltage generator enables the high-speed switching from 80 kVp to 140 kVp within 0.5 ms. It allows instantaneous data collection of the high and low energy. Two sets of data are independently and instantaneously collected, which completely freezes the movement of the patient. The two energy samplings are at almost the same time from the same perspective, which enables spectral analysis in the projection data space. 101 mono-spectral images of 40–140 KeV from 40–140 KeV can be generated. Their observations and working procedures can be optimized by GSI browser. Reconstruction of the spectral images and the post-processing engine, together with GSI browser, enable a multi-parameter imaging, including conventional hybrid energy image (kVp), material density images and single energy images (KeV).

Spectral CT imaging is a brand new field, which analyzes and amplifies the traditional CT scanning principles and details to improve CT scanning from the previous single-parameter imaging to multi-parameter imaging. It is a diagnostic examination of multi-parameter imaging, which improves CT scanning to an unprecedented five-dimensional space (x, y, z, time and energy) for separation and identification of substances. Therefore, different histological classification of tumors and tumor grading can be performed. The previous mixed energy imaging is improved to spectral multi-energy imaging. An important tool of spectral CT scanning is the signal energy imaging, which effectively avoids artifacts caused by hardened contrast reagent and the volume effect and thus reduces the missed diagnosis and misdiagnosis of small lesions. The detection rate of small lesions and multiple lesions can be improved. Spectral CT imaging generates images based on the X-ray attenuation coefficient, which facilitates the differentiation of specific tissues. Through comparison of various spectral CT analysis diagram (scatter plots, histograms) and energy spectrum curve, some regularities can be found, which contributes to the localization, qualitative diagnosis and grading of the tumors.

Generally speaking, spectral CT imaging is an advanced analysis for the physical and chemical properties of materials and also a more complicated multi-parameter imaging examination based on the conventional CT imaging principles. It demonstrates X-ray specific attenuations of different materials and tissues in the human body. Therefore, it has great potential contributions to the scientific research and clinical practice.

From the perspective of reconstruction, the gemstone spectral CT scanning for energy images is based on GSI mode scanning. In addition to the conventional MSCT scanning parameters, the gemstone spectral CT also supplements a new technique for reconstruction, which is known as Adaptive Statistics Iterative Reconstruction (ASIR). It advances the conventional filtered back projection (FBP) to suppress the statistical noise by using an iterative method, resulting in clearer images. Along with the same images quality, the new technology reduces the radiation dose by 50 %.

In clinical practice, once examination can achieve single-energy images including water based images, iodine based images, and the optimized quality images as well as the mixed energy images. The application of gemstone spectral CT imaging in the diagnosis of HIV/AIDS is believed to include the following aspects:

26.3.1 Pulmonary Spectral CT Scanning for HIV/AIDS

Along with the decrease of CD4 T cell count, the probability of complications of opportunistic infections greatly increases in AIDS patients. As a result, their survival rate and quality of life significantly decrease. HIV/AIDS complicated by pulmonary opportunistic infections is the major cause of death in AIDS patients. The imaging examinations play an irreplaceable role in the diagnosis and differential diagnosis of HIV/AIDS complicated by pulmonary infections. Currently, studies about CT demonstrations of pulmonary opportunistic infections in AIDS patients have been focused on the morphological analysis of the lesions by MSCT. However, with the introduction of gemstone spectral CT imaging and the application of its powerful image processing software, the detection rate, sensitivity and specificity of the diagnosis have been greatly improved. It also provides more advanced technology to functionally study the lesions of pulmonary infections.

It can be clinically applied to differentiate bacterial pneumonia from tuberculosis pneumonia and fungal pneumonia. Pathologically, the three diseases have their charac-teristic pathological typology and morphology, therefore, with different demonstrations in terms of internal compo-nents of the lesions, their water contents, X-ray attenuation. The lesions of pulmonary infections have pathological mani-festations of exudation, with its most content of water rather than cellulose. The water based images obtained by spectral CT imaging can define the water increase in the lesions for quantitative analysis of different lesions. In addition, scatter diagram, histogram and spectrum curve of the water contents can assess the discrepancies of the lesions as well as the lesions from the normal lung tissues.

Case Study 1

A male patient aged 44 years was confirmatively diagnosed as having AIDS by the CDC. The transmission route is not clear. He had cough with whitish thick sputum and fever with a highest body temperature of 40°C in Sep. 2010. By laboratory tests, HIV positive, CD4 T cell count 90/μl. By sputum culture, pseudomonas aeruginosa was found.

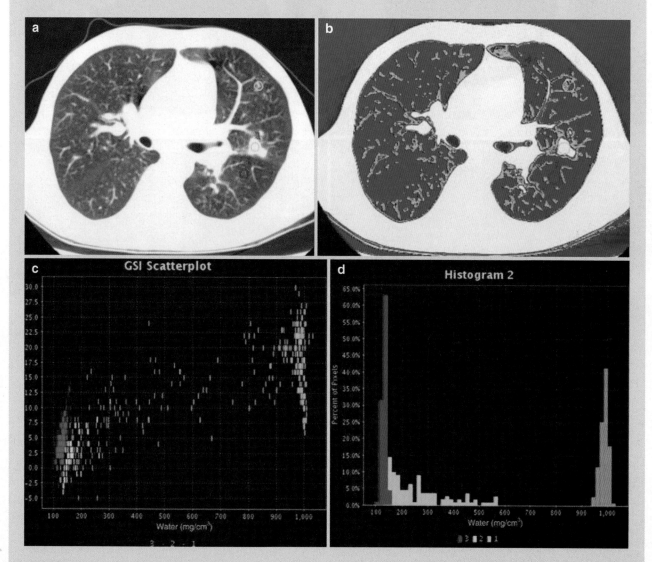

Fig. 26.27 (**a–d**) The pathological typological differences are demonstrated in this figure. The three ROIs are demonstrated (**a**) to have different properties: (1) Parenchymal lesions; (2) Exudative lesions; (3) Normal lung tissue. (**b**) is an colored artifacts image showing density changes of the three regions. (**c**) Is the ROI scatter diagram of lesions with different pathological types. (**d**) Is the ROI histogram of lesions with different pathological types

Case Study 2

A male patient aged 58 years was confirmatively diagnosed as having AIDS by the CDC. He had been found HIV positive for 3 years. In recent 2 months, he had intermittent fever, with body temperatures ranging from 38.5 to 39.3°C, and accompanying cough. By laboratory tests, HIV positive, CD4 T cell count 20/μl. After anti-inflammatory treatment, the lesions obviously decreased and he had no symptoms.

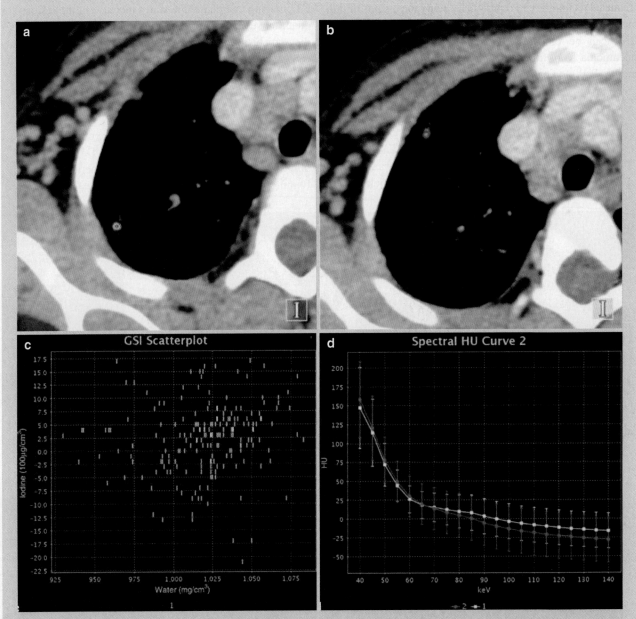

Fig. 26.28 (**a–d**) Bacterial pneumonia. (**a–b**) CT scanning demonstrates multiple small nodules and thin flakes of shadows in both lung fields, with quite clear boundaries and more commonly found in the external zone of both lungs. (**c**) Is the energy spectrum curve of ROIs of **a** and **b**. (**d**) Is the scatter diagrams of ROI of **a** and **b**

Case Study 3

A girl aged 5 years was confirmatively diagnosed as having AIDS by the CDC. Her transmission route was unknown. In recent 2 years, she had intermittent fever with body temperature ranging from 37.5 to 40°C and received symptomatic anti-infective therapy after the diagnosis of bacterial pneumonia and upper respiratory tract infection, with poor therapeutic efficacy. Her HIV antibody test was positive in Jun. 2011. T lymphocytes were CD3 79 %, CD3 and CD8 69 %, CD3 and CD4 9 %, CD16 and CD56 9 % and CD19 9 %. Fungal spores and mycelium were found in sputum smear. After receiving intravenous antifungal drugs, her body temperature returned to normal and the lesions obviously decreased.

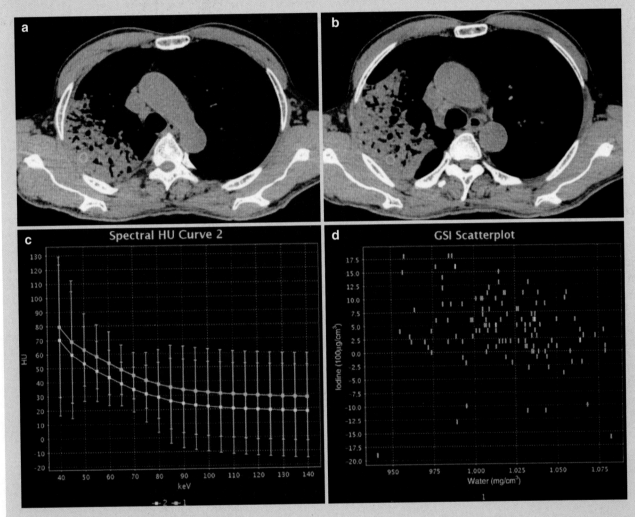

Fig. 26.29 (a–d) Fungal pneumonia. (a, b) CT scanning demonstrates flakes of soft tissue density parenchymal shadows in the right lung, with blurry boundaries, their internal bronchial gas sign, involved and thickened lateral pleura. (c) Is the ROI energy spectrum curve of a and b. (d) Is the ROI scatter diagrams of a and b

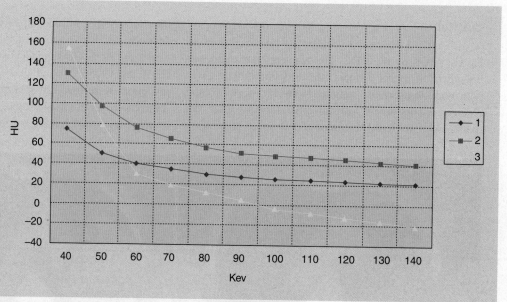

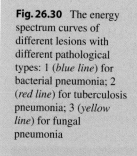

Fig. 26.30 The energy spectrum curves of different lesions with different pathological types: 1 (*blue line*) for bacterial pneumonia; 2 (*red line*) for tuberculosis pneumonia; 3 (*yellow line*) for fungal pneumonia

26.3.2 Spectral CT Scanning for HIV/AIDS Related Lymphadenopathy

Spectral CT scanning can be applied for the differentiation of lymph node tuberculosis and lymphoma. Although they are two different diseases, their differentiation has great difficulty in clinical practice, especially for AIDS patients. The basic reason is the obviously increased incidence of the both disease in AIDS patients. However, therapies targeting on the diseases can seriously damage the body systems. Therefore, their diagnosis and differential diagnosis are of great importance in clinical practice. The gemstone spectral CT scanning can amplify the different pathological types of lesions by different energy X-ray to demonstrate their differences and to obtain different energy values of lesions, including their water content, scatter diagram, histogram and spectrum curve. All these functions play important role in their diagnosis and differential diagnosis.

Case Study 1

A male patient aged 49 years was confirmatively diagnosed as having AIDS by the CDC. He was found HIV positive for 1 year due to the diagnosis of HIV/AIDS of his wife. In recent 6 months, he had fever, with a highest body temperatures of 38°C and no known reasons, with accompanying dizziness, headache, but without cough, expectoration and chills. By laboratory test in a local hospital, the CD4 T cell count was 37/μl. Earlier in 1993, he had paid blood donations for several times, with no histories of operation and trauma. By CSF smear as well as bacterial and fungal cultures, Cryptococcus negative. The laboratory blood test, tuberculin test and blood sedimentation test indicate TB-DOT and TB-Ab weakly positive. The findings support the diagnosis of pulmonary tuberculosis.

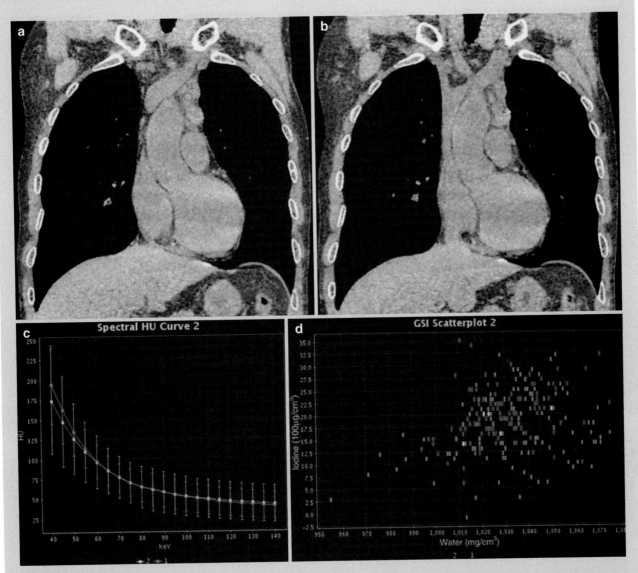

Fig. 26.31 (a–d) Lymph node tuberculosis. (a–b) Water based images demonstrate multiple enlarged lymph nodes shadows in the mediastinum. (c) Is the ROI energy spectrum curve of a and b. (d) Is the ROI scatter diagram of a and b

Case Study 2

A male patient aged 32 years was confirmatively diagnosed as having AIDS by the CDC. His girl friend was found HIV positive but did not receive HAART therapy. He had symptoms of fever, with a highest body temperature of 39.4°C about 5 days ago, with accompanying night sweating, chills and fatigue. By physical examinations, large quantity whitish plaques in the oral mucosa, and tenderness of the middle lower abdomen. By laboratory tests, erythrocyte sedimentation rate (ESR) 90 mm/L; T cells subsets, CD4 T cell count 35/µl, CD3 T cell count 455/µl and CD8 T cell count 404/µl. HBsAb, HBeAb and HBcAb were positive. Tumor markers series, CA12-5 70.41 U/mL which was increased. He was misdiagnosed as lymph node tuberculosis. Puncture for pathological biopsy defined the diagnosis of non-Hodgkin's lymphoma.

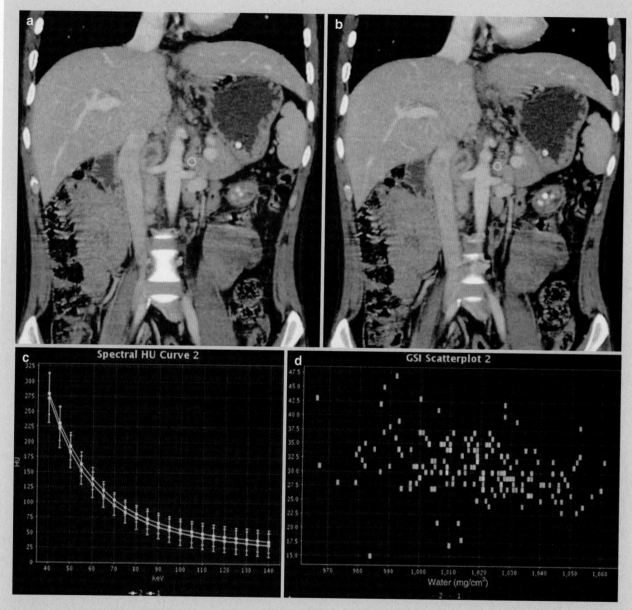

Fig. 26.32 (a–d) Non-Hodgkin's lymphoma. (a, b) CT scanning demonstrates multiple enlarged lymph nodes shadows in the retroperitoneum adjacent to the abdominal aorta. (c) Is the ROI energy spectrum curve of a and b. (d) Is the ROI scatter diagram of a and b

26.3.3 Spectral CT Scanning for HIV/AIDS Related Neoplasms

Due to the different originations and pathological types, the lesions of neoplasms have different components, water contents and iodine contents in enhanced imaging.

Therefore, the energy spectrum imaging can detect different energy attenuation curves of different lesions, with findings of different water contents and iodine contents. In addition, the composition materials in the masses are also different to cause differences in histogram and scatter plot.

Case Study

A male patient aged 51 years was confirmatively diagnosed as having AIDS by the CDC. He was firstly detected as HIV positive and has begun anti-viral therapy by combined use of AZT, 3TC and NVP. His wife died of AIDS. He had symptoms of intermittent cough for 20 years with small quantity whitish thick sputum and left chest pain. The laboratory blood test, tuberculin test and sedimentation test are negative. Sputum smear shows no acid fast bacilli. The tumor marker CA19-9 41.93 U/mL. Bronchoscopy diagnosis is red neoplasm in a bronchus of left upper lung lobe that completely obstructs the bronchus and protrudes towards the left major bronchus, obvious stenosis of a bronchus in the left lower lung lobe in line shape that the examination lens fail to pass through. The preliminary diagnosis is squamous cell carcinoma.

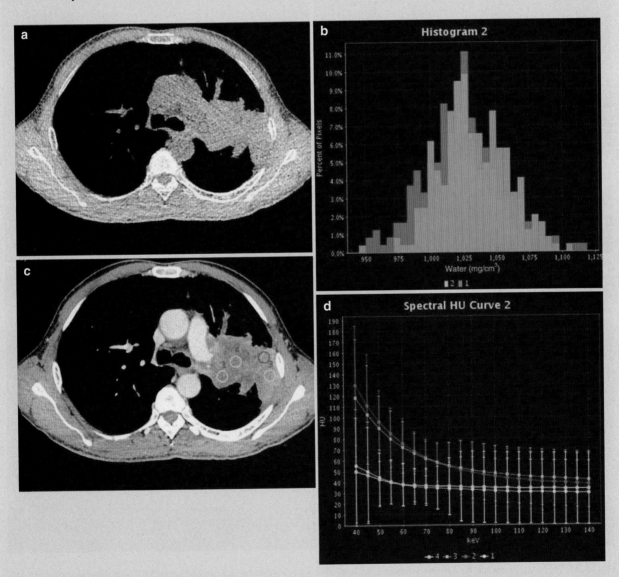

Fig. 26.33 (**a–d**) Squamous cell carcinoma of the left lung. (**a**) Water based image demonstrates mass liked soft tissue density shadows in the left lung. (**b**) Is the histogram of water contents at the points 1 and 2 in **a**, which demonstrates differences in the ROI water content peak and interval of the two points. (**c**) Enhanced imaging demonstrates uneven enhancement in the mass, with slightly high density of the peripheral area, which is demonstrated as pulmonary atelectasis region. (**d**) Is the four ROI energy spectrum curves, demonstrating differences of the different pathological types

26.3.4 Spectral CT Scanning for Angiography of HIV/AIDS

Mono-energetic imaging demonstrates vascular lesions. With the best contrast noise ratio curve in mono-energetic imaging technology, the specific best KeV values in different phases of the target blood vessel can be obtained to show the best contrast noise ratio image of the vascular vessel. A best balance between the image noise and the image contrast can be achieved to technologically enlarge the time window of angiography. Therefore, the image quality is significantly improved, which greatly facilitates the clear demonstration of the lesions and their accurate diagnosis.

Case Study

A female patient aged 35 years was confirmatively diagnosed as having AIDS by the CDC. Her transmission route may be during abortion in a small clinic 8 years ago, with unknown details. She had symptoms in Sep. 2006, with signs of intermittent fever and a highest body temperature of 37.8 °C, chest pain, fatigue and dysphagia. By laboratory test: HIV positive.

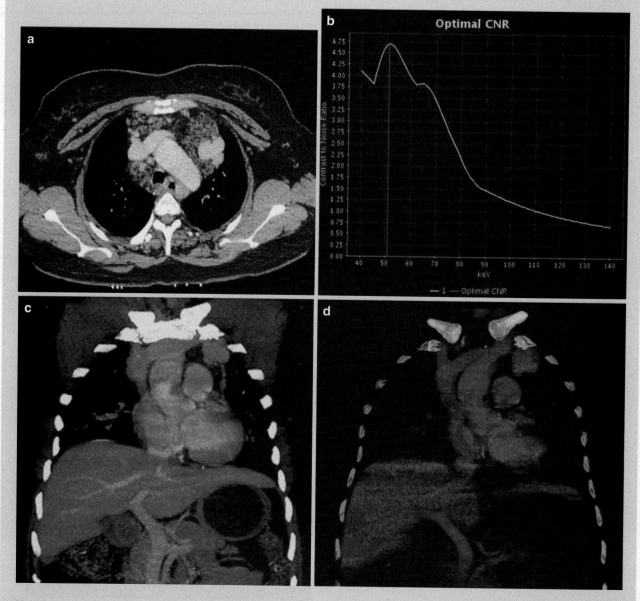

Fig. 26.34 (a–f) Angeioma. (a, b) Are three-dimensionally reconstructed images with the best KeV values of the superior vena cava and its surrounding area based on the best contrast noise ratio curve. (c, d) Are original mixed-energy MIP and VR images before processing. (e, f) Are processed MIP and VR images after reconstruction with 51 KeV values

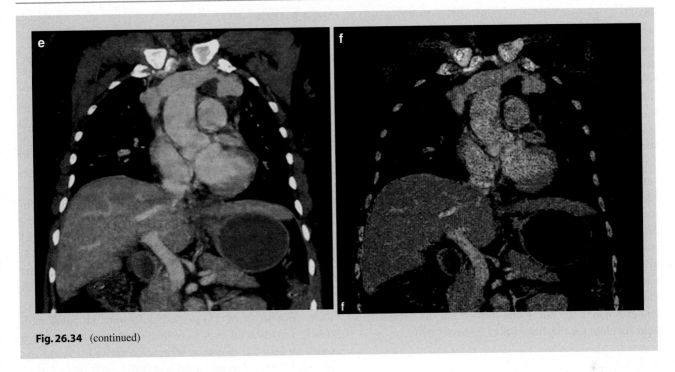

Fig. 26.34 (continued)

26.4 Clinic Application of Body Composition Assessment Methods in HIV/AIDS

Acquired Immune Deficiency Syndrome (AIDS) is caused by Human Immunodeficiency Virus (HIV). Subjects who are infected with HIV may develop AIDS over a period of years. Although the treatment with highly active antiretroviral regimens (HAART) has led to reductions in the development of HIV-related illness and increases patient's survival time remarkably, it has also led to the development of short- and long- term adverse effects of enormous concern. One of the most prominent side effects is the HIV lipodystrophy syndrome (HIV-LD), whose incidence is up to about 30–50 %. Its exact pathologic mechanism has been unknown. The morphological signs of lipodystrophy were first described approximately 2 years after the introduction of protease inhibitors (PIs) by Carr. HIV-infected patients being treated with these of drugs presented with progressive and selective thinning of the subcutaneous fat tissue in the cheeks, arms and legs, associated with/without intra-abdominal and dorso-cervical fat accumulation. However, there has been no clear definition of lipodystrophy. Clinical examination of a change in body fat or self-report of a change in body fat from a particular site was often used to describe the patients with lipodystrophy. Its limitation is no unified quantitative diagnostic criteria as well as normal reference data. How to evaluate the changes of body composition in patients with HIV-LD becomes one of important clinical problems. To evaluate changes in body composition for clinical study and researches, several methods have been developed, which are reviewed briefly as following:

26.4.1 Skinfold Thickness Measurement

Skinfold thickness measurement can be used in clinical and epidemiological investigation. Sites for anthropometric measurements included triceps, biceps, subscapular, upper iliac, and upper abdominal skin folds, plus waist and hip circumference. Total body fat content was estimated from anthropometric measurements using the equations of Durnin and Womersley. The index of waist-to-hip ratio is widely accepted to determine the parameters of abnormal fat abnormal distribution, with a criteria of >0.9 for male, >0.8 for female, respectively. It is inexpensive and is easily applied. However, there are some limitations which include lower accuracy, and multiple factors related anthropometric measurement, such as age, gender, race, as well as sizes of abdominal organs and muscles.

26.4.2 Sonographic Assessment

Sonography has been considered as an additional tool to quantify regional fat distribution in HIV-infected patients. Fatty atrophy can be diagnosed by ultrasound to measure the fat thickness at the sites of malar and extremities, which sensitivity is ranged to 67–71 %, specificity to 65–71 %, as well as positive and genitive predictive values to 11–20 % and

96–97 %, respectively. Although method of ultrasound is better than that of skinfold measurement in evaluation of abdominal fat, waist-hip ratio and lower extremity, there are no significant differences for accuracy and reproducibility between the both methods. It is quite easy to measure abdominal visceral fat by ultrasound. There is significant correlation between ultrasound and CT measurement for abdominal visceral fat content, with correlation coefficient $r=0.74$, $P<0.01$. In summarize, comparing with DXA, CT and MRI, ultrasound has some potential advantages, which include simplicity, rapidity, availability, harmlessness, good acceptance by the patient, and lower cost. The result for measurements of abdominal visceral fat and lower extremity fat is highly correlated between ultrasound with a acceptant differences with intra- or inter- operators. However, ultrasound is prone to be influenced by operator experience, abdominal intraluminal gas and obesity. In addition to lack of the normal reference value and no quantitative standard for fat content evaluation, the ultrasound method has not been used as gold standard for the diagnosis of lipodystrophy.

26.4.3 Bioelectrical Impedance Analysis

Bioelectrical impedance analysis (BIA) has some advantage with simpler, harmlessness, and repeatable characteristics. BIA can just evaluate total body fat content, but cannot distinguish regional adipose tissue separately. Also, it has low accuracy to assess the abnormal fat distribution of patients with HIV-LD. Measurement of accuracy and longitudinal and cross-sectional study should be considered for the further evaluation.

26.4.4 CT and MRI

Since the ninety of the twentieth century, CT and MRI have been developed in the field of abdominal fat evaluation. We could compute the ratio of visceral fat and subcutaneous fat, or the ratio of visceral fat and total body fat. Abnormal fat distribution should be considered if the ratio of visceral fat and total body fat is >0.45. The results of fat measurement with CT between single-slice and multi-slice is significantly correlated. Singe-slice CT scan has the advantages with low radiation dose and less examination time. Both single-slice CT and MRI have reproducibility and high accuracy rate and have similar ability comparing with other methods for evaluating the of subcutaneous fat atrophy. High cost, radiation, special operator and software dependent are the limitations for CT application. MR measurement can avoid the radiation, but long scan times, high costs for examination and equipment, as well as other disadvantages, however, limit its wide-spread use in clinical study and research.

26.4.5 DXA

It is meaningful of the DXA measurement to apply in clinical working, especially in assessment changes of body composition. DXA can measurement total and regional body composition including fat mass, lean mass and bone mass. The DXA reproducibility research for body fat measurement in patients with HIV lipodystrophy showed that RMS-CV% of total and arms fat were 1.6 and 4.0 %, respectively. Duo to high sensitivity in assessment changes of body composition for HIV-infected patients with lipodystrophy, DXA has been considered as the preferred methods of evaluation fat mass in clinical. Many researches had reported for fat measurement application by DXA in patients with HIV-LD. Tungsiripat M et al. [110] reported that there were correlations evaluation limbs fat content changes in HIV-LD patients between results of DXA measurement with those of patient-self-assessment and clinicians questionnaire, $r=-0.27$, -0.48; $P<0.01$ respectively. Bonnet et al. [11] first put forward fat mass ratio (FMR, i.e. trunk fat mass% to lower limbs fat mass%) as a index for HIV-LD diagnosis. The ration derived from theory, of which 80 % of trunk fat mass is perivisceral fat and 98 % of limbs fat mass is subcutaneous fat. The lipodystrophy in HIV-patient might be the result of loss of subcutaneous fat mass, and accumulation in perivisceral fat mass, or both. Threshold value FMR by DXA to defines lipodystrophy is set up to ≥ 1.5. Further, Paula Freitas [40] researched gender related FMR threshold value to diagnose lipodystrophy, which were FMR >1.961 for male and FMR >1.329 for female, respectively. For male-FMR, the 95 % confidence interval was 0.66–0.82, the sensitivity was 58.3 %, specificity of 83.7 %, positive predictive value of 89.6 %, and negative predictive value of 45.5 %. For female-FMR, the 95 % confidence interval was 0.63–0.86, the sensitivity was 51.4 %, specificity of 94.6 %, positive predictive value of 90.5 %, and negative predictive value of 66.0 %. Since the body fat distribution was vary with race, research for Chinese HIV-LD patients has rarely reported. It is necessary to establish our own diagnostic criteria based on large samples research for Chinese HIV-LD patients. In China, HAART long-term side effects gradually emerged until recent years since the generic antiretroviral drugs made in China has been used from 2003 to date. With the application of DXA, some studies have been reported on the changes of body composition of HIV-infected patients with or without HIV-LD. Jin-Peng Yao et al. [53] studied DXA fat measurement results retrospectively in 66 HIV-infected patients (the Han nationality), who received HAART therapy from January 2002 to December 2009. The results showed that the longer time of HIV infection and HAART regimen are, the lower fat mass in HIV-infected patients has (Fig. 26.1). Significant fat loss in HIV-LD patients was found at both limb and trunk (Figs. 26.2 and 26.3), which was different from the results of trunk fat accumulation with limb fat reduction in previous foreign reports.

Fig. 26.35 Relationship between the loss of total-body fat mass with the time of HAART therapy. Total-body fat mass of HIV-infected patients in male was negatively related to the time of therapy on HAART (regression coefficient was −0.563, P <0.01). However, there is no significant relationship between the loss in female with the time of HAART therapy

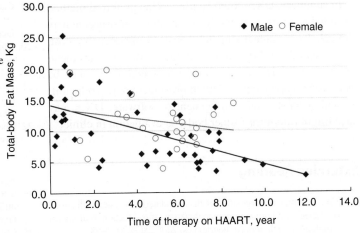

Fig. 26.36 Total and regional fat mass measured by DXA for male. P values represent differences between the LD patients, non-LD patients with controls by ANOVA analysis

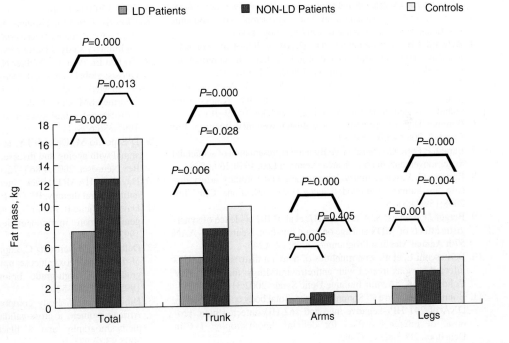

Fig. 26.37 Total and regional fat mass measured by DXA for females. P values represent differences between the LD patients, non-LD patients with controls by ANOVA analysis

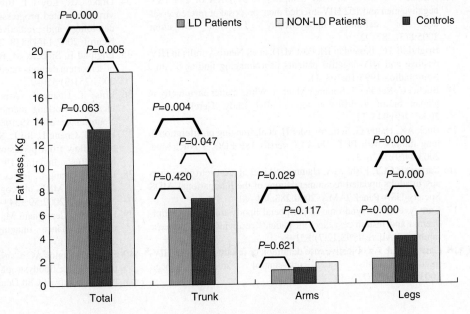

In summary, DXA could be used as the preferred method for reliable analysis of body composition measurement in clinical. Its advantages include: easy to operate, low cost, high reproducibility and accuracy for measurement. Limitation for DXA evaluation is visceral fat cannot be measured independently. With improvement of reproducibility and accuracy and development of software, DXA may have bright future for further body fat evaluation in clinic.

Extended Reading

1. Alice B, James G, Elisabeth J, et al. Central nervous system infections associated with human immunodeficiency virus infection: radiologic-pathologic correlation. Radiographics. 2008;28(7):2033–58.
2. Anders KH, Guerra WF, Tomiyasu U, et al. The neuropathology of AIDS UCLA experience and review. Am J Pathol. 1986;24:537–58.
3. Anno I, Itai Y. Evaluation of brain perfusion using dynamic functional MRI. Nihon Rinsho. 1997;55 Suppl 1:348–53.
4. Aylward EH, Brettschneider PD, McArthur JC, et al. Magnetic resonance imaging measurement of gray matter volume reductions in HIV dementia. Am J Psychiatry. 1995;152(7):987–94.
5. Aylward EH, Henderer JD, McArthur JC, et al. Reduced basal ganglia volume in HIV-1-associated dementia: results from quantitative neuroimaging. Neurology. 1993;43(10):99–104.
6. Bammer R. Basic principles of diffusion-weighted imaging. Eur J Radiol. 2003;45(3):169–84.
7. Baraldi P, Porro CA, Serafini M. Bilateral representation of sequential finger movements in cortical area. Neurosci Lett. 1999;269:95–8.
8. Barbaro G. Vascular injury, hypertension and coronary artery disease in human immunodeficiency virus infection. Clin Ter. 2008;159(1):51–5.
9. Berger JT, Juengst S, Aizenstein HJ, et al. fMRI evidence of synergistic effects of AIDS and age on brain function. Neurology – AAN 57th Annual Meeting Programme. 2005; 64:A245.
10. Bernasconi E, et al. Abnormalities of body fat distribution in HIV-infected persons treated with antiretroviral drugs: the Swiss HIV Cohort Study. J Acquir Immune Defic Syndr. 2002;31(1):50–5.
11. Bonnet E, Delpierre C, Sommet A, et al. Total body composition by DXA of 241 HIV-negative men and 162 HIV-infected men: proposal of reference values for defining lipodystrophy. J Clin Densitom. 2005;8(3):287–92.
12. Bonnet E, et al. Total body composition by DXA of 241 HIV-negative men and 162 HIV-infected men: proposal of reference values for defining lipodystrophy. J Clin Densitom. 2005;8(3):287–92.
13. Brightbill TC, Ihmeidan IH, Post MJD, et al. Neurosyphilis in HIV-positive and HIV-negative patients neuroimaging findings. Am J Neuroradiol. 1995;16:703–11.
14. Buchel C, Raedler T, Sommer M, et al. White matter asymmetry in human brain: a diffusion tensor MRI study. Cereb Cortex. 2004;14(9):945–51.
15. Buck AK, Halter G, Schirrmeisler H, et al. Imaging proliferation in lung tumors with PET; 18F-FLT versus 18F-FDG. J Nucl Med. 2003;44(9):1426–31.
16. Carpenter CCJ, Fishl MA, Hammer SM, et al. Antiretroviral therapy in adults updated recommendations of the International AIDS Society-USA Panel. JAMA. 2000;283:381–90.
17. Carr A, et al. A syndrome of peripheral lipodystrophy, hyperlipidaemia and insulin resistance in patients receiving HIV protease inhibitors. AIDS. 1998;12(7):F51–8.
18. Carr A, et al. An objective case definition of lipodystrophy in HIV-infected adults: a case–control study. Lancet. 2003;361(9359):726–35.
19. Cavalcanti RB, et al. Reproducibility of DXA estimations of body fat in HIV lipodystrophy: implications for clinical research. J Clin Densitom. 2005;8(3):293–7.
20. Chanc KH, Kim JM, Song YG, et al. Dose race protect an oriental population from developing lipodystrophy in HIV-infected individuals on HAART? J Infect. 2002;44:33–8.
21. Chang L, Ernst T, Leonido-Yee M, Speck O. Perfusion MRI detects rCBF abnormalities in early stages of HIV-cognitive motor complex. Neurology. 2000;54(2):389–96.
22. Chang L, Speck O, Miller E, et al. Neural correlates of attention and working memory deficits in HIV patients. Neurology. 2001;57:1001–7.
23. Chang L, Tomasi D, Yakupov R, et al. Adaptation of the attention network in human immunodeficiency virus brain injury. Ann Neurol. 2004;56:259–72.
24. Chen Y, An H, Zhu H, et al. White matter abnormalities revealed by diffusion tensor imaging in non-demented and demented HIV+patients. Neuroimage. 2009;47(4):1154–62.
25. Chen W, Ding Z, Tate DF, et al. A novel interface for interactive exploration of DTI fibers. IEEE Trans Vis Comput Graph. 2009;15(6):1433–40.
26. Choi SJ, Lim KO, Monteiro I, et al. Diffusion tensor imaging of frontal white matter microstructure in early Alzheimer's disease: a preliminary study. J Geriatr Psychiatry Neurol. 2005;18(1):12–9.
27. Corbett EL, Watt CJ, Walker N, et al. The growing burden of tuberculosis: global trends and interactions with the HIV epidemic. Arch Intern Med. 2003;163:1009–21.
28. Courtney SM, Ungerleider LG. Transient and sustained activity in a distributed neural system for human working memory. Nature. 1997;386:608–11.
29. D'Esposito M, Deouell LY, et al. Alterations in the BOLD fMRI signal with ageing and disease: a challenge for neuroimaging. Nat Rev Neurosci. 2003;4:863–72.
30. David E. HAART attack: metabolic disorders during long-term antiretroviral therapy. BETA. 1999;12(2):10–4.
31. Davis L, Hjelle B, Miller V, et al. Early viral brain invasion in iatrogenic human immunodeficiency virus infection. Neurology. 1992;42:1736–9.
32. Delbeke D, Meyerowitz C, Lapidus RL, et al. Optimal cutoff levels of 18F-fluorodeoxyglucose uptake in the differentiation of low-grade from high-grade brain tumors with PET. Radiology. 1995;195(1):47–52.
33. Dioum A, et al. Body composition predicted from skinfolds in African women: a cross-validation study using air-displacement plethysmography and a black-specific equation. Br J Nutr. 2005;93(6):973–9.
34. Drake AK, Loy CT, Brew BJ, et al. Human immunodeficiency virus-associated progressive multifocal leucoencephalopathy: epidemiology and predictive factors for prolonged survival. Eur J Neurol. 2007;14(4):418–23.
35. Englund E, Sjöbeck M, Brockstedt S, et al. Diffusion tensor MRI post mortem demonstrated cerebral white matter pathology. Neurol. 2004;251(3):350–2.
36. Ernst T, Chang L, Arnold S. Increased glial markers predict increased working memory network activation in HIV patients. Neuroimage. 2003;19:1686–93.
37. Ernst T, Chang L, Itti L, Speck O. Correlation of regional cerebral blood flow from perfusion MRI and SPECT in normal subjects. Magn Reson Imaging. 1999;17(3):349–54.
38. Ernst T, Chang L, Jovicich J, et al. Abnormal brain activation on functional MRI in cognitively asymptomatic HIV patients. Neurology. 2002;59:1343–9.
39. Filippi M, Cercignani M, Inglese M, et al. Diffusion tensor magnetic resonance imaging in multiple sclerosis. Neurology. 2001;56(3):304–11.
40. Freitas P, Santos AC, Carvalho D, et al. Fat mass ratio: an objective tool to define lipodystrophy in HIV-infected patients under antiretroviral therapy. J Clin Densitom. 2010;13(2):197–203.

41. Freitas P, et al. Fat mass ratio: an objective tool to define lipodystrophy in HIV-infected patients under antiretroviral therapy. J Clin Densitom. 2010;13(2):197–203.

42. Fuster-Garcia E, Navarro C, Vicente J, et al. Compatibility between 3T 1H sv-MRS data and automatic brain tumour diagnosis support systems based on databases of 1.5T 1H SV-MRS spectra. Magn Reson Mater Phys. 2011;24:35–42.

43. Gendelman HE, Lipton SA, Tardieu M, et al. The neuropathogenesis of HIV-1 infection. J Leukoc Biol. 1994;56:389–98.

44. Gillams AR, Allen E, Hrieb K, et al. Cerebral infarction in patients with AIDS. Am J Neuroradiol. 1997;18:1581–5.

45. Goletti D, Weissman D, Jackson RW, et al. Effect of Mycobacterium tuberculosis on HIV replication: role of immune activation. J Immunol. 1996;157(3):1271–8.

46. Goo JM, Im JG, Do KH, et al. Pulmonary tuberculoma evaluated by means of FDG PET: findings in 10 cases. Radiology. 2000;216(1):117–21.

47. Goodkin K, Shapshak P, Verma A. The spectrum of neuro-AIDS disorders: pathophysiology diagnosis and treatment. Washington, DC: American Society for Microbiology; 2009. p. 281–9; 247–267.

48. Hara T, Kosaka N, Suzuki T, et al. Uptake rates of 18F-fluorodeoxyglucose and 11C-choline in lung cancer and pulmonary tuberculosis: a positron emission tomography study. Chest. 2003;124(3):893–901.

49. Harris GJ, Pearlson GD, McArthur JC, Zeger S, LaFrance ND. Altered cortical blood flow in HIV-seropositive individuals with and without dementia: a single photon emission computed tomography study. AIDS. 1994;8(4):495–9.

50. Hartmann M, Heiland S, Sartor K. Functional MRI procedures in the diagnosis of brain tumors: perfusion- and diffusion-weighted imaging. Rofo. 2002;174(8):955–64.

51. Hatano H, et al. Metabolic and anthropometric consequences of interruption of highly active antiretroviral therapy. AIDS. 2000;14(13):1935–42.

52. Jinpeng Yao WY, Li T, et al. The pilot study of DXA assessment in Chinese HIV-infected men with clinical lipodystrophy. J Clin Densitom. 2011;14(1):58–62.

53. Jinpeng Y, Wei Y, Ping TJ, et al. Bone mineral content analysis of male patients with HIV-associated lipodystrophy syndrome. Chin J Osteoporos Bone Min Res. 2010;3(3):164–7.

54. Jovicich J, Peters RJ, Koch C, et al. Brain areas specific for attentional load in a motion tracking task. J Cogn Neurosci. 2001;13:1048–58.

55. Kaufmann SH, Ladel CH. Role of T cell subsets in immunity against intracellular bacteria: experimental infections of knockout mice with Listeria monocytogenes and Mycobacterium bovis BCG. Immunobiology. 1994;191:509–19.

56. Kaul M, Garden GA, Lipton SA. Pathways to neuronal injury and apoptosis in HIV-associated dementia. Nature. 2001;410(6831):988–94.

57. Kim IJ, Lee JS, Kim SJ, et al. Double-phase 18F-FDG PET-CT for determination of pulmonary tuberculoma activity. Eur J Nucl Med Mol Imaging. 2008;35(4):808–14.

58. Kotler DP, et al. Studies of body composition and fat distribution in HIV-infected and control subjects. J Acquir Immune Defic Syndr Hum Retrovirol. 1999;20(3):228–37.

59. Lentz MR, Kim WK, Lee V, et al. Changes in MRS neuronal markers and T cell phenotypes observed during early HIV infection. Neurology. 2009;72:1465–72.

60. Letendre SL, Ellis RJ, Everall I, et al. Neurologic complications of HIV disease and their treatment. Top HIV Med. 2009;17:47–56.

61. Li HJ, Gao YQ, Cheng JL, et al. Diagnostic imaging, preautopsy imaging and autopsy findings of 8 AIDS cases. Chin Med J. 2009;122(18):2142–21482.

62. Lichtenstein KA, et al. Clinical assessment of HIV-associated lipodystrophy in an ambulatory population. AIDS. 2001;15(11):1389–98.

63. Lichtenstein KA, et al. Incidence of and risk factors for lipoatrophy (abnormal fat loss) in ambulatory HIV-1-infected patients. J Acquir Immune Defic Syndr. 2003;32(1):48–56.

64. Liow JS, Rehm K, Stgother SC, et al. Comparison of voxel-and volume-of-interest-based analyses in FDG PET scans of HIV positive and healthy individuals. J Nucl Med. 2000;41(4):612–21.

65. Lohman T, Martorelli R, Roche AF. Anthropometric standardization reference manual: the Airlie consensus report. Chicago: Human Kinetics; 1988.

66. Major EO, Rausch D, Marra C, Clifford D. HIV-associated dementia. Science. 2000;288:440–2.

67. Martinez E, et al. Risk of lipodystrophy in HIV-1-infected patients treated with protease inhibitors: a prospective cohort study. Lancet. 2001;357(9256):592–8.

68. Martinez E, et al. Sonographic assessment of regional fat in HIV-1-infected people. Lancet. 2000;356(9239):1412–3. Padilla S, et al. Ultrasonography and anthropometry for measuring regional body fat in HIV-infected patients. Curr HIV Res. 2007;5(5):459–66.

69. McArthur JC, Haughey N, Gartner S, et al. Human immunodeficiency virus- associated-dementia: an evolving disease. J Neurovirol. 2003;9(2):205–21.

70. Miller J, et al. HIV lipodystrophy: prevalence, severity and correlates of risk in Australia. HIV Med. 2003;4(3):293–301.

71. Mohamed MA, Berker PB, Skolasky RL, et al. Brain metabolism and cognitive impairment in HIV infection: a 3-T magnetic resonance spectroscopy study. Magn Reson Imaging. 2010;28:1251–7.

72. Mukhergee P. Diffusion tensor imaging and fiber tractography in acute stroke. Neuroimaging Clin N Am. 2005;15(3):655–65.

73. Navia BA, Jordan BD, Price RW. The AIDS dementia complex: I. Clinical features. Ann Neurol. 1986;19:517–24.

74. O'Dcherty MJ, Barrington SF, Campbell M, et al. PET scanning and the human immunodeficiency virus-positive patient. J Nucl Med. 1997;38(10):1575–83.

75. O'Doherty MJ, et al. PET and HIV-positive patients. J Nucl Med. 1997;38(10):1575–83.

76. Offiah CE, Turnbull IW. The imaging appearances of intracranial CNS infections in adult HIV and AIDS patients. Clin Radiol. 2006;61:393–401.

77. Offiah CE, Turnbull IW. The imaging appearances of intracranial CNS infections in adult HIV and AIDS patients. Clin Radiol. 2006;61:393–401.

78. Ogawa S, Menon RS, et al. Functional brain mapping by blood oxygenation level-dependent contrast magnetic resonance imaging. Biophys J. 1993;64:803–12.

79. Orme IM, Collins FM. Protection against mycobacterium tuberculosis infection by adoptive immunotherapy. Requirement for T cell deficient recipients. J Exp Med. 1983;158:74–83.

80. Padma MV, Said S, Jacobs M, et al. Prediction of pathology and survival by FDG PET in gliomas. J Neurooncol. 2003;64(3):227–37.

81. Palella Jr FJ, et al. Anthropometrics and examiner-reported body habitus abnormalities in the multicenter AIDS cohort study. Clin Infect Dis. 2004;38(6):903–7.

82. Paul RH, Sacktor WC, Valcour V. HIV and the brain: new challenges in the modern era. New York: Humana Press; 2009. p. 49–108.

83. Paul RH, Yiannoutsos CT, Miller EN, et al. Proton MRS and neuropsychological correlates in AIDS dementia complex: evidence of subcortical specificity. J Neuropsychiatry Clin Neurosci. 2007;19:283–92.

84. Pfefferbaum A, Rosenbloom MJ, Rohifing T, et al. Frontostriatal fiber bundle compromise in HIV infection without dementia. AIDS. 2009;23(15):1977–85.

85. Pierce MA, Johnson MD, Maciunas RJ, et al. Evaluating contrast-enhancing brain lesions in patients with AIDS by using positron emission tomography. Ann Intern Med. 1995;123(8):594–8.

86. Pomara N, Crandall DT, Choi SJ, et al. White matter abnormalities in HIV-1 infection: a diffusion tensor imaging study. Psychiatry Res. 2001;106(1):15–24.

87. Post MJD, Tate LG, Quencer RM, et al. CT, MR, and pathology in HIV encephalitis and meningitis. AJR Am J Roentgenol. 1988;151:373–80.

88. Ragin AB, Storey P, Cohen BA, et al. Whole brain diffusion tensor imaging in HIV-associated cognitive impairment. Am J Neuroradiol. 2004;25(2):195–200.

89. Rosca EC, Rosca O, Chirileanu RD, et al. Neurocognitive disorders due to HIV infection. HIV AIDS Rev. 2011;10:33–7.

90. Rosen BR, Belliveau JW, Chien D. Perfusion imaging by nuclear magnetic resonance. Magn Reson Q. 1989;5(4):263–81.

91. Rottenberg DA, Moeller JR, Strother SC, et al. The metabolic pathology of the AIDS dementia complex. Ann Neurol. 1987;22(6):700–6.

92. Rottenberg DA, Sidtis JJ, Strother SC, et al. Abnormal cerebral glucose metabolism in HIV-1 seropositive subjects with and without dementia. J Nucl Med. 1996;37(7):1133–41.

93. Sacktor N. The epidemiology of human immunodeficiency virus-associated neurological disease in the era of highly active antiretroviral therapy. J Neurovirol. 2002;8 Suppl 2:115–21.

94. Safrin S, Grunfeld C. Fat distribution and metabolic changes in patients with HIV infection. AIDS. 1999;13(18):2493–505.

95. Saves M, et al. Factors related to lipodystrophy and metabolic alterations in patients with human immunodeficiency virus infection receiving highly active antiretroviral therapy. Clin Infect Dis. 2002;34(10):1396–405.

96. Schielke E, Tatsch K, Pfister HW, et al. Reduced cerebral blood flow in early stages of human immunodeficiency virus infection. Arch Neurol. 1990;47(12):1342–5.

97. Schwartz RB, Komaroff AL, Garada BM, et al. SPECT imaging of the brain: comparison of findings in patients with chronic fatigue syndrome, AIDS dementia complex, and major unipolar depression. AJR Am J Roentgenol. 1994;162(4):943–51.

98. Sepkowitz KA. AIDS – the first 20 years. N Engl J Med. 2001;344(23):1764–72.

99. Sharma SK, Mohan A. Extrapulmonary tuberculosis. Indian J Med Res. 2004;120:316.

100. Sulllivan EV, Rosenbloom MJ, Rohlfing T, et al. Pontocerebellar contribution to postural instability and psychomotor slowing in HIV infection without dementia. Brain Imaging Behav. 2011;5(1):12–24.

101. Suwanwela N, Phanuphak P, Phanthumchinda K, et al. Magnetic resonance spectroscopy of the brain in neurologically asymptomatic HIV-infected patients. Magn Reson Imaging. 2000;18:859–65.

102. Tarasów E, Wiercińska-Drapało A, Jaroszewicz J, et al. Antiretroviral therapy and its influence on the stage of brain damage in patients with HIV - 1H MRS evaluation. Med Sci Monit. 2004;3:101–6.

103. Tipping B, de Villiers L, Wainwright H, et al. Stroke in patients with human immunodeficiency virus infection. J Neurol Neurosurg Psychiatry. 2007;78:1320–4.

104. Toaff JS, Metser U, Goqfried M, et al. Differentiation between malignant and benign pleural effusion in patients with extra pleural primary malignancies- assessment with positron emission tomography- computed tomography. Invest Radiol. 2005;40(4):204–9.

105. Toosi Z, Sierra-MaderoJ G, Blinkhorn RA, et al. Enhanced susceptibility of blood monocytes from patients with pulmonary tuberculosis to productive infection with human immunodeficiency virus type 1. J Exp Med. 1993;177:1511–6.

106. Toshihiko H, Noboru K, Tsuneo S, et al. Uptake rates of 18F-FDG and 11C-choline in lung cancer and pulmonary tuberculosis. Chest. 2003;124(3):893–901.

107. Tracey I, Hamberg LM, Guimaraes AR, et al. Increased cerebral blood volume in HIV-positive patients detected by functional MRI. Neurology. 1998;50(6):1821–6.

108. Tucker KA, Robertson KR, Lin W, et al. Neuroimaging in human immunodeficiency virus infection. J Neuroimmunol. 2004;157:153–62.

109. Tungsiripat M, O'Riordan MA, Storer M, et al. Subjective clinical lipoatrophy assessment correlates with DEXA-measured limb fat. HIV Clin Trial. 2009;10(5):314–31.

110. Tungsiripat M, O'Riordan MA, Storer N, et al. Subjective clinical lipoatrophy assessment correlates with DEXA-measured limb fat. HIV Clin Trials. 2009;10(5):314–9.

111. Valcour V, Sithinamsuwan P, Letendre S, et al. Pathogenesis of HIV in the central nervous system. Curr HIV/AIDS Rep. 2011;8:54–61.

112. Van Horn JD, Ellmore TM, Esposito G, Berman KF. Mapping voxel-based statistical power on parametric images. Neuroimage. 1998;7(2):97–107.

113. Vanham G, Edmonds K, Qing L, et al. Generalized immune activation in pulmonary tuberculosis: coactivation with HIV infection. Clin Exp Immunol. 1996;103(1):30–4.

114. Viskovic K, et al. Assessment of ultrasound for use in detecting lipoatrophy in HIV-infected patients taking combination antiretroviral therapy. AIDS Patient Care STDS. 2009;23(2):79–84.

115. Wanke C, Polsky B, Kotler D. Guidelines for using body composition measurement in patients with human immunodeficiency virus infection. AIDS Patient Care STDS. 2002;16(8):375–88.

116. Wilkinson ID, Lunn S, Miszkiel KA, et al. Proton MRS and quantitative MRI assessment of the short term neurological response to antiretroviral therapy in AIDS. J Neurol Neurosurg Psychiatry. 1997;63:477–82.

117. Wu Y, Storey P, Cohen BA, et al. Diffusion alterations in corpus callosum of patients with HIV. AJNR Am J Neuroradiol. 2006;27(3):656–60.

118. Yao JP, Yu W, LI TS, et al. Change in body composition in female patients with human immunodeficiency virus-related lipodystrophy syndrome. Zhongguo Yi Xue Ke Xue Yuan Xue Bao. 2011;33(4):421–6.

119. Yiannoutsos CT, Nakas CT, Navia BA, et al. Assessing multiple-group diagnostic problems with multi dimensional receiver operating characteristic surfaces application to proton MR spectroscopy (MRS) in HIV-related neurological injury. Neuroimage. 2008;40:248–55.

120. Yousry TA, Schmid UD, Alkhadhi H, et al. Localization of the motor hand area to a knob on the precentral gyrus. A new landmark. Brain. 1997;120(1):141–1571.

121. Zhang YZ, Li HJ, Cheng JL, Bao DY. CT image demonstrations of HIV-seropositive tuberculosis and their relationship with CD4+ T-lymphocyte count. Chin Med J. 2010;124(5):693–703.

122. Zumla A, Malon P, Henderson J, et al. Impact of HIV infection on tuberculosis. Postgrad Med J. 2000;76(3):259–68.

Index

H. Li (ed.), *Radiology of HIV/AIDS*,
DOI 10.1007/978-94-007-7823-8, © Springer Science+Business Media Dordrecht and People's Medical Publishing House 2014

图书在版编目（CIP）数据

实用艾滋病影像学 = Radiology of HIV-AIDS：A practical approach：英文 / 李宏军主编. —北京：人民卫生出版社，2013
ISBN 978-7-117-18058-0

Ⅰ. ①实… Ⅱ. ①李… Ⅲ. ①获得性免疫缺陷综合征－影象诊断－英文 Ⅳ. ①R512.910.4

中国版本图书馆 CIP 数据核字（2013）第 226395 号

| 人卫社官网 www.pmph.com | 出版物查询，在线购书 |
| 人卫医学网 www.ipmph.com | 医学考试辅导，医学数据库服务，医学教育资源，大众健康资讯 |

实用艾滋病影像学
（英文）

主　　编：李宏军
出版发行：人民卫生出版社（中继线 010-59780011）
地　　址：中国北京市朝阳区潘家园南里 19 号
　　　　　世界医药图书大厦 B 座
邮　　编：100021
网　　址：http://www.pmph.com
E - mail：pmph @ pmph.com
购书热线：010-59787592　010-59787584　010-65264830
开　　本：889×1194　1/16
版　　次：2014 年 4 月第 1 版　2014 年 4 月第 1 版第 1 次印刷
标准书号：ISBN 978-7-117-18058-0/R·18059
打击盗版举报电话：010-59787491　E-mail：WQ @ pmph.com
（凡属印装质量问题请与本社市场营销中心联系退换）

32检